AF344465

PHARMACEUTICALS
IN MEDICAL IMAGING
▼▼▼

Dennis P. Swanson, R.Ph. M.S.
Associate Professor and Assistant Dean
School of Pharmacy
University of Pittsburgh
Pittsburgh, PA

Henry M. Chilton, Pharm. D.
Associate Professor
(Radiopharmacy—Nuclear Medicine)
Bowman Gray School of Medicine
Wake Forest University
Winston-Salem, N.C.

James H. Thrall, M.D.
Juan M. Taveras Professor of Radiology
Harvard Medical School
Radiologist-in-Chief
Massachusetts General Hospital
Boston, MA

PHARMACEUTICALS IN MEDICAL IMAGING

▼▼▼

Radiopaque Contrast Media
Radiopharmaceuticals
Enhancement Agents
for Magnetic Resonance Imaging
and Ultrasound

Dennis P. Swanson, R.Ph., M.S.
Henry M. Chilton, Pharm. D.
James H. Thrall, M.D.

MACMILLAN PUBLISHING CO., INC.
New York

COLLIER MACMILLAN CANADA, INC.
Toronto

COLLIER MACMILLAN PUBLISHERS
London

Copyright © 1990, Macmillan Publishing Company, a division of Macmillan, Inc.
Printed in the United States of America

Macmillan Publishing Company
866 Third Avenue, New York, New York 10022

Collier Macmillan Canada, Inc.

Collier Macmillan Publishers · London

Library of Congress Cataloging-in-Publication Data
Swanson, Dennis P.
    Pharmaceuticals in medical imaging: radiopaque contrast media, radiopharmaceuticals, enhancement agents for magnetic resonance imaging and ultrasound/Dennis P. Swanson, Henry M. Chilton, James H. Thrall.
        p. cm.
    Includes index.
    ISBN 0-02-420780-2
    1. Contrast media. 2. Radiopharmaceuticals—Diagnostic use.
3. Paramagnetic contrast media. 4. Diagnostic imaging.
I. Chilton, Henry M. II. Thrall, James H. III. Title.
    [DNLM: 1. Contrast Media. 2. Diagnosis, Radioisotope.
3. Magnetic Resonance Imaging. 4. Ultrasonic Diagnosis. WN 445
S972p]
RC78.7.C65S93 1989
616.07′572—dc 19
DNLM/DLC
for Library of Congress   89-2299
                                                                        CIP

Printing: 1 2 3 4 5 6 7 8   Year: 9 0 1 2 3 4 5 6 7

Foreword

During the past 15 years, advances in radiology have been no less than astounding—there has been an explosion of new imaging technologies in nuclear medicine, including ultrasound, computed tomography, and magnetic resonance imaging. In addition to gains in instrument technologies, each imaging advance has also been accompanied by new developments in pharmaceuticals that are employed in these diagnostic methodologies. In some cases, these new pharmaceuticals represent the vital character of the examination, as in nuclear medicine, for example, which relies on radiopharmaceutical localization for image determination. In others, the pharmaceuticals complement the imaging technique by enhancing the diagnostic examination that may be obtained. For example, paramagnetics may be used with magnetic resonance imaging, or iodinated contrast media with computed tomography to provide significant diagnostic information that might not otherwise be obtainable. In still other cases, pharmaceuticals are employed as interventional aids to evoke some change in a diagnostic parameter within an examination. Examples include the use of diuretics in renal nuclear medicine studies and vasodilators in studies of myocardial perfusion.

The net impact of these developments is that never before have radiologists and staff faced a greater need for understanding the properties of the large number of pharmaceuticals employed in medical imaging. A thorough knowledge of these agents is vitally important for selecting the appropriate pharmaceutical, preparing the patient properly, and optimizing conditions to ensure that the highest degree of clinical information will be obtained from each study. The vast number of pharmaceuticals employed in radiology necessitates an ability to recognize and treat adverse reactions. In this regard, radiologists also should be aware of the medicolegal implications of using certain pharmaceuticals. Finally, we must be able to make cost-effective selections to accommodate the patient's budget and that of the hospital.

The authors of this text recognized the need for a single source of up-to-date information about major pharmaceuticals available for use in a radiology department. To the practicing radiologist, radiologic technologist, pharmacist, and radiological research scientist, this book will serve as a much-needed reference source. It is of particular value for radiology and nuclear medicine residents and radiologic technology and pharmacy students as they are exposed to the pharmaceuticals that are as vital a part of the field of radiology as the imaging devices themselves.

The authors are ideally qualified to present this material. Dennis P. Swanson, R.Ph., on the faculty of a well respected school of pharmacy, is particularly interested in and knowledgeable about routine contrast media employed in diagnostic radiology. Henry M. Chilton, Pharm.D., specializes in radiopharmaceuticals and is involved daily in clinical practice and research in a busy nuclear medicine section in a major medical center. James H. Thrall, M.D., a radiologist who has been professionally involved in many aspects of medical imaging, currently is chairman of one of the major teaching and research radiology departments in the country.

Undoubtedly, this is the first of many editions to come. Growth of pharmaceuticals for medical imaging can be expected to continue as rapidly in the future as in the past; frequent updates, therefore, will be necessary. This comprehensive text provides all persons interested in radiological procedures an excellent source of much-needed information in a single reference. It will be a welcome addition to our department library and to countless others, I am certain.

C. Douglas Maynard, M.D.
Professor and Chairman
Department of Radiology
Bowman Gray School of Medicine
Wake Forest University

Preface

The objective of this work is to present a practical text discussing the clinical role and use of pharmaceuticals in medical imaging. Utilization of drugs has become increasingly important in the practice of radiology for both diagnosis and therapy. Radiographic indications for iodinated contrast media continue to increase. The problems in appropriately selecting and applying these agents have been further accentuated by the recent introduction of the better tolerated but extremely expensive low osmolality media. The number and diversity of radiopharmaceuticals also continues to expand with exciting horizons in the areas of radiolabeled antibodies, new single photon agents for the study of the cerebral and myocardial perfusion, and myriad agents for positron emission tomography. Early experience suggests that enhancement agents will assume an important role in magnetic resonance imaging. Although not yet clinically important, agents are also under investigation to enhance diagnostic ultrasound.

The use of pharmaceuticals for direct image enhancement and as adjuncts in diagnostic imaging procedures has become a pervasive and important element of radiology practice. Information has not been available in one text or reference, and instruction on the pharmaceuticals used in medical imaging has been fragmentary for radiologists, residents in radiology, radiologic technologists, and other applied health personnel, including pharmacists. It is the authors' hope and intention to provide, in this initial edition, a unified work that will serve as both a text and a reference for those involved in medical imaging and with the pharmaceuticals used in medical imaging.

This book is divided into three major sections, covering radiopaque contrast media, radiopharmaceuticals, and enhancement agents for magnetic resonance imaging and ultrasound, respectively. Within each chapter the discussion of each specific drug or drug group incorporates a standard format that is maintained throughout the book. Each chapter begins with a presentation of the chemistry and "pharmacology" (i.e., pharmacokinetics, mechanisms of location, physiological effects) of the drug/drug group, followed by a discussion of factors influencing pharmaceutical selection and correct use of the drug in the clinical setting. Included in the latter category are considerations related to patient preparation, diagnosis, drug–drug interactions, adjunctive techniques to improve diagnosis, and appropriate pharmaceutical dosages. Figures have been selected to illustrate drug behavior including altered patterns resulting from faulty technique or pharmaceutical failure. Although the book is not aimed at providing interpretative criteria to the reader, recognition of drug biodistribution is emphasized as it influences image interpretation.

Most of the material discusses diagnostic agents currently available and approved for use in the United States. However, in such a rapidly evolving area we have felt it appropriate to include a discussion of certain investigational agents and agents that represent paradigms for future development. Given the richness of the literature and the number of agents under current development, we recognize that subsequent editions of this text will be necessary to keep it current.

The "laboratory" for the radiopaque contrast media section of this book was

Henry Ford Hospital, where two of us (DPS and JHT) served on staff for several years. We are indebted to our colleagues at Henry Ford Hospital and Bowman Gray School of Medicine for their help as contributors to this work and, more important, for their assistance in evolving the concept of pharmacy practice in a Department of Radiology. We are also indebted to numerous other colleagues who have served as contributors to this publication, and to the various scientists and clinicians who served, through their research and publications efforts, as our mentors. We hope that each of these individuals will join us in the thought that what we now present to you, the reader, is really an initial step in recognizing the importance of pharmaceuticals in radiology and medical imaging and in ensuring inclusion of this subject matter in the basic science and clinical curriculum of physicians, pharmacists, and technologists.

Contributors

Joe P. Windham, Ph.D.
Adjunct Associate Professor
Medical College of Ohio
Toledo, Ohio;
Division of Diagnostic Radiology and
    Medical Imaging
Henry Ford Hospital
Detroit, MI

P.C. Shetty, M.D.
Clinical Assistant Professor of Radiology
University of Michigan Medical School
Ann Arbor, MI;
Director, Division of Angiography and
    Interventional Radiology
Department of Diagnostic Radiology
    and Medical Imaging
Henry Ford Hospital
Detroit, MI

David J. Kaston, M.D.
Fellow in Angiography
Department of Diagnostic Radiology
    and Medical Imaging
Henry Ford Hospital
Detroit, MI

Christopher K. Shier, M.D.
Resident in Radiology
Department of Diagnostic Radiology
    and Medical Imaging
Henry Ford Hospital
Detroit, MI

Ned Gregorio, R.Ph.
Graduate Student in Radiopharmacy
College of Pharmacy
University of New Mexico
Albuquerque, New Mexico

Mark Weingarden, M.D.
Director of Uroradiology
Department of Diagnostic Radiology
    and Medical Imaging
Henry Ford Hospital
Detroit, MI

Michael B. Alpern, M.D.
Clinical Assistant Professor of Radiology
University of Michigan Medical School
Ann Arbor, MI;
Director of Computed Tomography
Department of Diagnostic Radiology
    and Medical Imaging
Henry Ford Hospital
Detroit, MI

Roushdy S. Boulos, M.D.
Clinical Assistant Professor of Radiology
University of Michigan Medical School
Ann Arbor, MI;
Division of Neuroradiology
Department of Diagnostic Radiology
    and Medical Imaging
Henry Ford Hospital
Detroit, MI

Robert D. Halpert, M.D.
Associate Professor
Chief, Division of Gastrointestinal
    Radiology and Director,
    Ambulatory Care Radiology;
Department of Radiology
University of Texas Medical Branch
Galveston, TX

Stuart M. Simms, M.D.
Clinical Associate Professor
University of Michigan Medical School;
Ann Arbor, MI;
Director, Division of Gastrointestinal
    Radiology
Henry Ford Hospital
Detroit, MI

Burton I. Ellis, M.D.
Clinical Assistant Professor of Radiology
University of Michigan Medical School
Ann Arbor, MI;
Director, Division of Skeletal Radiology
Department of Radiological Sciences
    and Medical Imaging
Henry Ford Hospital
Detroit, MI

Carol J. Maywood, M.D.
Clinical Instructor of Radiology
University of Michigan Medical School
Ann Arbor, MI;
Director, Division of Ambulatory
    Radiology
Department of Radiological Sciences
    and Medical Imaging
Henry Ford Hospital
Detroit, MI

Rajinder P. Sharma, M.D.
Division of Angiography and
    Interventional Radiology
Department of Diagnostic Radiology
    and Medical Imaging
Henry Ford Hospital
Detroit, MI

Neil A. Petry, R.Ph., M.S.
Assistant Professor of Pharmacy and
    Internal Medicine;
Director of Nuclear Pharmacy Division
    of Nuclear Medicine
University of Michigan Medical School
Ann Arbor, MI

Brahm Shapiro, M.D., Ch.B., Ph.D.
Professor of Internal Medicine
Division of Nuclear Medicine
University of Michigan Medical School
Ann Arbor, MI

Terry J. Dick, Pharm.D.
Staff Pharmacist
Nuclear Pharmacist
Division of Nuclear Medicine
University of Michigan Medical School
Ann Arbor, MI

James A. Ponto, R.Ph., M.S.
Clinical Associate Professor
College of Pharmacy;
Nuclear Pharmacist,
Department of Radiology
University of Iowa Hospital and Clinics,
Iowa City, IA

Susan C. Jackels, Ph.D
Associate Professor of Chemistry
    and Radiology
Department of Chemistry
Wake Forest University
Winston-Salem, NC

Richard L. Witcofski, Ph.D.
Professor of Radiology
Department of Radiology
Bowman Gray School of Medicine
Wake Forest University
Winston-Salem, NC

Robert J. Cowan, M.D.
Professor of Radiology
Director, Division of Nuclear Medicine
Department of Radiology
Bowman Gray School of Medicine
Wake Forest University
Winston-Salem, NC

Nat E. Watson, Jr., M.D.
Associate Professor of Radiology
Department of Radiology
Bowman Gray School of Medicine
Wake Forest University
Winston-Salem, NC

James D. Ball, M.D.
Associate Professor of Radiology
Department of Radiology
Bowman Gray School of Medicine
Wake Forest University
Winston-Salem, NC

William C. Eckelman, Ph.D.
Vice-President
Diagnostics Research and Development
The Squibb Institute for Medical
  Research
New Brunswick, NJ

Ronald J. Callahan, Ph.D.
Director of Nuclear Pharmacy
Massachusetts General Hospital;
Assistant Professor of Radiology
Harvard Medical School
Boston, MA

Manuel L. Brown, M.D.
Professor
Department of Radiology
Mayo Clinic
Rochester, MN

Marion D. Francis
Staff Scientist,
Woods Corners Laboratories,
  Bone Metabolism
Norwich Eaton Pharmaceuticals,
Proctor and Gamble,
Norwich, NY

Scott W. Burchiel, Ph.D.
Professor (Pharmacology and
  Immunology)
The University of New Mexico
College of Pharmacy
Albuquerque, NM

Sanjay Saini, M.D.
Instructor of Radiology
Harvard Medical School
Division of Gastrointestinal Imaging
Massachusetts General Hospital
Boston, MA

Joseph T. Ferrucci, M.D.
Professor of Radiology
Harvard Medical School
Division Head, Division of
  Gastrointestinal Imaging
Massachusetts General Hospital
Boston, MA

Nancy Rollins, M.D.
Department of Radiology
Children's Hospital
Houston, TX

Contents

Section I: Radiopaque Contrast Media   1

CHAPTER 1:   **Angiographic Contrast Media   1**
Dennis P. Swanson, R.Ph., M.S.
P.C. Shetty, M.D.
David J. Kastan, M.D.
S. Ned Gregorio, R.Ph.
Nancy Rollins, M.D.

Pharmacoangiography   48
Christopher K. Shier, M.D.

CHAPTER 2:   **Urographic Contrast Media: Excretory and Retrograde   78**
Dennis P. Swanson, R.Ph., M.S.
Mark Weingarden, M.D.

CHAPTER 3:   **Contrast Media for Computed Tomography: Intravascular, Intracavitary, Xenon, Reticuloendothelial   99**
Dennis P. Swanson, R.Ph. M.S.
Michael B. Alpern, M.D.

CHAPTER 4:   **Myelographic Contrast Media   125**
Dennis P. Swanson, R.Ph., M.S.
Roushdy S. Boulos, M.D.

CHAPTER 5:   **Gastrointestinal Contrast Media: Barium Sulfate and Water-Soluble Iodinated Agents   155**
Dennis P. Swanson, R.Ph., M.S.
Robert D. Halpert, M.D.

CHAPTER 6:   **Cholecystographic and Cholangiographic Contrast Media   184**
Dennis P. Swanson, R.Ph., M.S.
Stuart M. Simms, M.D.

CHAPTER 7:   **Miscellaneous Radiopaque Contrast Media   221**

I.   Arthrographic Contrast Media
Dennis P. Swanson, R.Ph., M.S.
Burton I. Ellis, M.D.

II. Hysterosalpingographic Contrast Media
Dennis P. Swanson, R.Ph., M.S.
Carol J. Maywood, M.D.

III. Lymphographic Contrast Media
Dennis P. Swanson, R.Ph., M.S.
P.C. Shetty, M.D.

IV. Bronchographic Contrast Media
Dennis P. Swanson, R.Ph., M.S.
Rajinder P. Sharma, M.D.

CHAPTER 8: **Adverse Reactions to Contrast Media: Etiology, Incidence, Treatment, and Prevention** **253**
James H. Thrall, M.D.

Section II: Radiopharmaceuticals **279**

CHAPTER 9: **Fundamentals of Radiopharmaceuticals** **279**
Henry M. Chilton, Pharm. D.
Richard L. Witcofski, Ph.D.

CHAPTER 10: **Radiopharmaceuticals for Central Nervous System Imaging: Blood-Brain Barrier, Function, Receptor-Binding, Cerebral Spinal Fluid Dynamics** **305**

I. Radiopharmaceuticals for Conventional Brain Imaging
Henry M. Chilton, Pharm. D.
James H. Thrall, M.D.

II. Receptor-Specific Radiopharmaceutical
William C. Eckelman, Ph.D.

III. Imaging of Cerebral Spinal Fluid Dynamics
Robert J. Cowan, M.D.

CHAPTER 11: **Radiopharmaceuticals for Endocrine Imaging** **343**

I. Thyroid Imaging
James H. Thrall, M.D.

II. Parathyroid Scintigraphy
James H. Thrall, M.D.

III. Adrenocortical Imaging
Dennis P. Swanson, R.Ph., M.S.

IV. Adrenomedullary Imaging
Neil A. Petry, R.Ph., M.S.
Brahm Shapiro, M.D., Ch.D., Ph.D.

CHAPTER 12: **Radiopharmaceuticals for Lung Imaging   394**
Henry M. Chilton, Pharm.D.
James D. Ball, M.D.

I. Regional Pulmonary Perfusion Imaging

II. Ventilation Imaging

CHAPTER 13: **Radiopharmaceuticals for Cardiac Imaging: Myocardial Infarction, Perfusion, Metabolism and Ventricular Function (Blood Pool)   419**
Henry M. Chilton, Pharm.D.
Ronald J. Callahan, Ph.D.
James H. Thrall, M.D.

CHAPTER 14: **Radiopharmaceuticals for Abdominal and Gastrointestinal Imaging: Reticuloendothelial, Hepatobiliary and Intestinal   462**
Henry M. Chilton, Pharm. D.
Manuel L. Brown, M.D.

CHAPTER 15: **Radiopharmaceuticals for Genitourinary Imaging: Glomerular and Tubular Function, Anatomy, Urodynamics, and Testicular   501**
Henry M. Chilton, Pharm. D.
James A. Ponto, R.Ph., M.S.
Nat E. Watson, Jr., M.D.
James H. Thrall, M.D.

CHAPTER 16: **Radiopharmaceuticals for Bone and Bone Marrow Imaging   537**
Henry M. Chilton, Pharm. D.
Marion D. Francis,
James H. Thrall, M.D.

CHAPTER 17: **Radiopharmaceuticals for Imaging Tumors and Inflammatory Processes: Gallium, Antibodies, and Leukocytes   564**
Henry M. Chilton, Pharm. D.
Scott W. Burchiel, Ph.D.
Nat E. Watson, Jr., M.D.

CHAPTER 18: **Therapeutic Applications of Radiopharmaceuticals: Thyroid Disease, Polycythermia Vera, and Malignant Effusion   599**
James A. Ponto, R.Ph., M.S.
Henry M. Chilton, Pharm. D.

CHAPTER 19: **Radiopharmaceuticals for Hematological Applications   616**

I. Blood Volume Measurements
Dennis P. Swanson, R.Ph., M.S.

II. Schilling Test
    James A. Ponto, R.Ph., M.S.

III. Radioferrokinetic Studies
    Dennis P. Swanson, R.Ph., M.S.

IV. Venous Thromobosis Detection
    Dennis P. Swanson, R.Ph., M.S.

Section III: Enhancement Agents for Magnetic Resonance Imaging and Ultrasound   645

CHAPTER 20: **Enhancement Agents for Magnetic Resonance Imaging: Fundamentals   645**
    Susan C. Jackels, Ph.D.

CHAPTER 21: **Enhancement Agents for Magnetic Resonance Imaging: Clinical Applications   662**
    Sanjay Saini, M.D.
    Joseph T. Ferrucci, M.D.

CHAPTER 22: **Enhancement Agents for Ultrasound: Fundamentals   682**
    Dennis P. Swanson, R.Ph., M.S.

Appendices

A: Units of Radioactivity   688

B: Method for Prevention of Thyroid Uptake of Radioiodine   689
    Henry M. Chilton, Pharm. D.

C: Drugs for the Mitigation of Internal Radiocontamination   690
    Dennis P. Swanson, R.Ph., M.S.
    Terry J. Dick, Pharm. D.

RADIOPAQUE CONTRAST MEDIA

CHAPTER

1

▼▼▼

Angiographic Contrast Media

Dennis P. Swanson
P.C. Shetty
David J. Kastan
and Nancy Rollins

Angiography is the specific demonstration and study of blood vessels using roentgen (x-ray) techniques. Angiographic procedures are typically classified according to the organ or general anatomic location of the circulatory system under investigation (e. g., cerebral angiography, peripheral angiography), with subclassification according to the specific branch (e. g., artery, vein) of the vascular tree being studied or injected with the contrast medium (Table 1.1). These procedures are valuable in the diagnosis and evaluation of a variety of diseases that involve or cause alterations in normal vascular anatomy or physiology.

Since blood vessels and circulating blood have densities similar to surrounding soft tissues, angiography requires the intravascular administration of a radiopaque contrast medium. The concentrations and volumes of contrast media utilized in angiographic procedures are determined by the specific clinical application and the characteristics of the radiological equipment used to obtain the images (see Dosage).

Digital subtraction angiography (DSA) is a hybrid angiographic procedure that utilizes a phosphor-image intensifier system as the x-ray sensitive recording medium in place of the photographic film-screen combination utilized for conventional angiography. The DSA image intensifier system is directly coupled to a video camera to produce a digital (i. e., numerical) display of the image as opposed to the analog format of conventional film-based techniques. The digital format of DSA results in a mechanism whereby background anatomical densities ("mask image") can be directly subtracted from subsequent contrast-enhanced angiographic images to provide an increased sensitivity for detection of the administered contrast (Figure 1.1). This factor

Table 1.1 COMMON ANGIOGRAPHY PROCEDURES

ORGAN/ANATOMIC REGION UNDER INVESTIGATION	ANGIOGRAPHY PROCEDURE(S)
Abdominal viscera (selective)	Celiac arteriography
	Mesenteric arteriography (inferior, superior)
Adrenal	Adrenal arteriography
Aorta	Aortic arch
	Aortography (abdominal, lumbar, thoracic)
Cerebral	Carotid arteriography (common, exterior, interior)
	Vertebral arteriography
Heart	Coronary arteriography (selective)
	Ventriculography (right, left)
Kidney	Renal arteriography
Liver	Hepatic arteriography
	Splenoportography
Lung	Pulmonary arteriography
	Bronchial arteriography
Pancreas	Pancreatic arteriography
Peripheral	Femoral arteriography
	Venography
	Venacavography
Spleen	Splenoportography

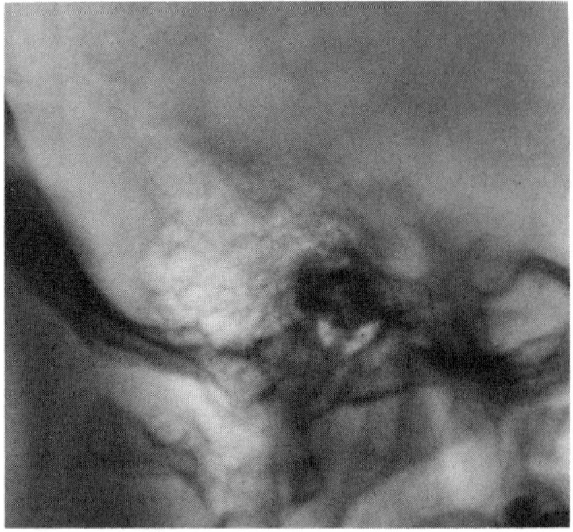

A

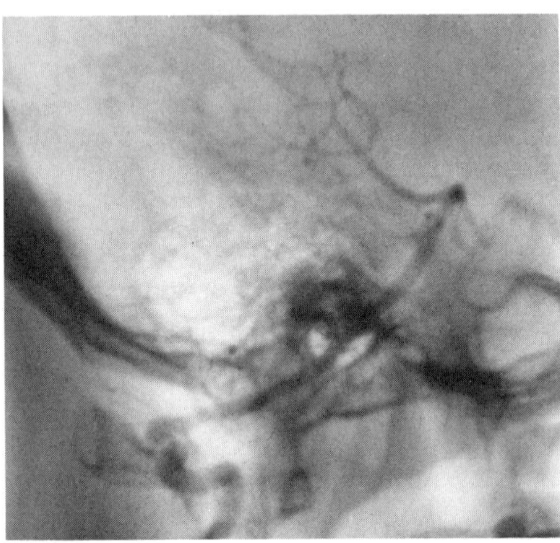

B

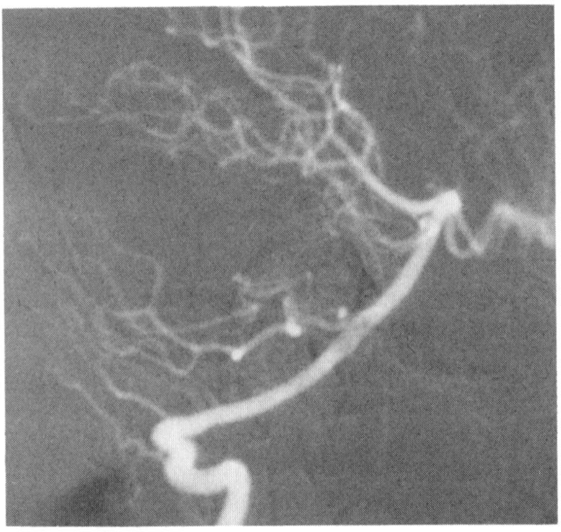

C

permits the intravenous administration of a contrast medium for various angiographic studies that would normally require the increased vascular iodine concentration of a direct arterial injection if the conventional film-based techniques were utilized. Similarly, if an arterial route of administration is employed, the percent weight/volume or iodine concentration of the contrast medium required for DSA is substantially lower than the corresponding requirement for conventional angiography, because of the increased contrast sensitivity of DSA. Currently, the major disadvantages of DSA compared to conventional angiography are its poorer spatial resolution and its greater susceptibility to image degradation as a result of patient motion.

The contrast media used for conventional film-based and digital subtraction angiography are the same and are discussed below. Significant differences that may exist between these techniques in regard to concentration requirements or routes of administration will be presented within the Dosage section of this chapter.

I. Chemistry

HISTORY

Angiographic studies on living human subjects were first reported in the early 1920s incorporating the intravascular administration of water-insoluble iodized poppy-seed oil (Lipiodol). Although this iodized oil was tolerated in low doses (5–20 ml), its high viscosity led to the formation of radiopaque globules and fragmentation of the opaque column, thus rendering this agent unsatisfactory for routine angiographic use. During this

---

Figure 1.1 *Example of Digital Subtraction Angiography Sequence.*

A. Mask image: Lateral view of the posterior fossa of the skull. B. Angiographic image: Contrast can be seen in left vertebral artery, basilar artery, and their distributions to the posterior fossa. Overlying bony structures obscure much of vascular detail. C. Subtracted image (image A subtracted from image B): Vascular detail is much improved following image subtraction.

same period, a 20% w/v solution of the water-soluble inorganic salt, strontium bromide, was utilized to produce arteriograms and venograms of acceptable quality. Subsequent reports emphasized the clinical use of inorganic sodium iodide for angiographic and urographic studies due to the higher atomic number and, hence, increased x-ray absorption of iodine versus bromine. However, the large doses of sodium iodide required for adequate angiography opacification resulted in adverse reactions associated with iodism, hypersensitivity to iodine, and the effects of free iodide on thyroid metabolism (see Abrams HL, 1983a).

In an attempt to eliminate the adverse effects of free iodide, attention was directed to the use of organic iodides for angiographic procedures. This interest was stimulated by the observation that the monoiodinated drug, Selection (Figure 1.2), could produce adequate radiographic opacification of the kidneys following renal excretion of an intravenous dose that was moderately well tolerated. Subsequent chemical modifications of Selec-

tan were aimed at improving its radiographic efficacy by increasing its rate and degree of renal excretion through the addition of hydrophilic carboxylic acid groups (e. g., Uroselectan, Figure 1.2), and by increasing the number of iodine atoms attached to the organic moiety (e. g., iodopyracet, iodomethamate derivatives, Figure 1.2). The latter diiodinated agents were used extensively for angiographic and urographic procedures during the 1930s and 40s (Abrams HL, 1983a; Grainger RG, 1982).

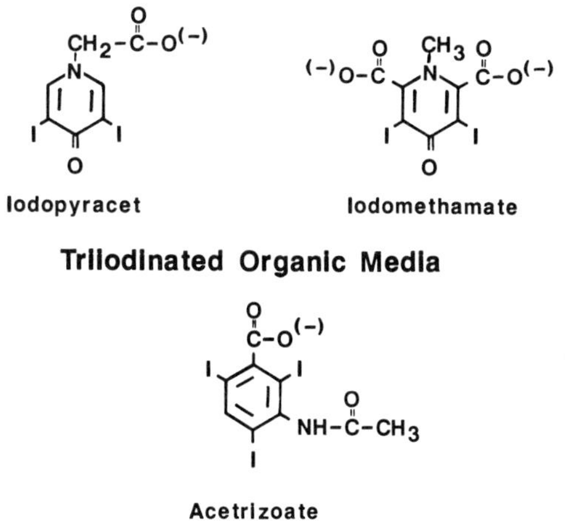

In the early 1950s, it was observed that acetylation of amino*triiodo*benzoic acid significantly reduced the toxicity of this agent and increased the water solubility of its sodium salt. The resulting acetrizoate (Figure 1.2) derivatives were subsequently used for angiography and urographic procedures based on their increased iodine concentration compared to equimolar solutions of the previously used diiodinated agents. It was soon recognized, however, that substitution of an additional aliphatic side chain at the vacant position of the acetrizoate derivative would greatly decrease its degree of protein binding. Decreased protein binding resulted in a corresponding increase in the rate and degree of renal excretion and a decrease in hepatobiliary excretion (Hoppe JO, 1959). Furthermore, later studies suggested that the degree of protein binding exhibited by a contrast medium may directly correlate with its overall systemic toxicity (Lasser EC, et al, 1962).

RATIO-1.5 IONIC CONTRAST MEDIA

The ionic contrast media currently utilized extensively in the United States for angiographic and urographic procedures are the meglumine, sodium, or combination meglumine-sodium salts of the fully substituted triiodobenzoic acid derivatives, diatrizoic acid and iothalamic acid (Figure 1.3). In Europe and Canada, a similar triiodobenzoic acid derivative, metrizoic acid (Figure 1.3), is available in various combination formulations of its

MonoIodinated Organic Media

DiIodinated Organic Media

TriIodinated Organic Media

Figure 1.2 Chemical structures of early angiographic contrast media.

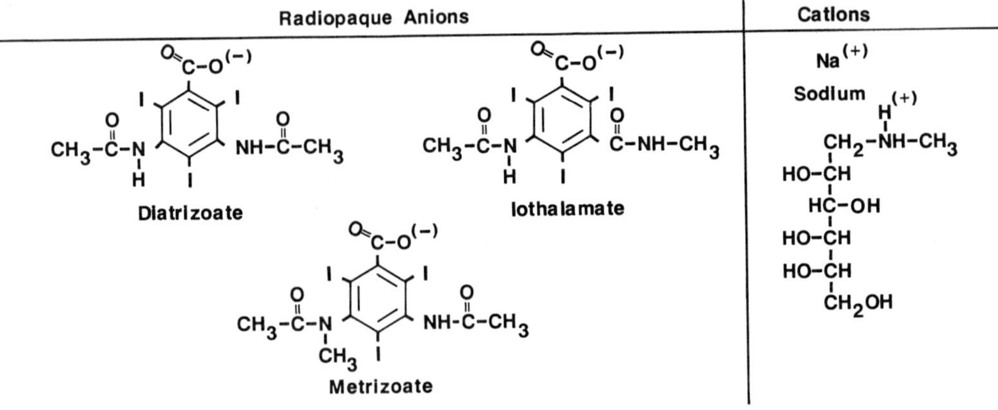

Figure 1.3 Chemical structures of ratio-1.5 ionic contrast media commonly utilized for angiography procedures.

meglumine, sodium, calcium, and magnesium salts. The cationic salts of these moderately strong organic acids are freely soluble in water; the resulting solutions being clear, colorless to pale yellow, and sterile and pyrogen-free if intended for intravascular administration. Preparations of these agents are stable to heat and cold, but are sensitive to light. Crystal formation, which may be occasionally observed in concentrated formulations, can usually be remedied by heating the contrast medium to 37°C with gentle shaking.

As might be expected based on the similarities in their chemistry, the pharmaceutical properties (i. e., iodine concentration, osmolality, viscosity) of equivalent cationic formulations of diatrizoate, iothalamate, and metrizoate are similar (Tables 1.2–1.4), as are their pharmacokinetic properties and relative chemical toxicities (Table 1.5). Commercially available preparations of these ionic media vary extensively in regard to their percent weight/volume and iodine concentrations and their relative ratios of sodium versus meglumine salts (Tables 1.2–1.4). As will be discussed under Physiological Effects, the cationic nature of these agents is an important factor in regard to their relative effects on vascular and organ physiology.

Table 1.2   RATIO-1.5 ANGIOGRAPHIC CONTRAST MEDIA[a]: ≤250 mg IODINE/mL

GENERIC NAME	CONCENTRATION (%w/v)	BRAND NAME®[b]	MG IODINE / ML	OSMOLALITY[c] (mOsm/kg)	VISCOSITY (cps)[c] 25°C/37°C	SEQUESTRANT(S)[d]
Diatrizoate meglumine	30	Urovist-Meglumine DIU/CT (B)	141	640	1.9/1.4	0.005% CaEDTA
Diatrizoate meglumine	30	Reno-M-Dip (S)	141	566	1.9/1.4	0.04% EDTA
Diatrizoate meglumine	30	Hypaque Meglumine DIU 30% (W)	141	633	1.9/1.4	0.01% CaEDTA
Diatrizoate sodium	25	Hypaque Sodium 25% (W)	150	696	1.6/1.2	0.01% CaEDTA
Iothalamate meglumine	30	Conray-30 (M)	141	600	2.0/1.5	0.01% CaEDTA
Iothalamate meglumine	43	Conray-43 (M)	202	1000	3.0/2.0	0.01% CaEDTA

[a] U.S. market, only
[b] (B) Berlex Imaging
(M) Mallinckrodt
(S) Squibb Diagnostics
(W) Winthrop-Brcon Laboratories
[c] From: Fischer HW. Catalog of intravascular contrast media. *Radiology* 1986, 159:561–563.
[d] CaEDTA = Calcium edetate disodium
EDTA = Edetate disodium

Iodine Concentration. The concentrations of ionic contrast media are typically expressed as percent weight-in-volume (% w/v), or the total grams of salt dissolved in 100 mL of the final formulation. However, the most important factor is their iodine concentration since it is this component of the medium that is responsible for x-ray absorption and opacification. Equal % w/v salt concentrations of equivalent cationic formulations of iothalamate and diatrizoate possess equal iodine concentrations, whereas an equivalent salt concentration of a metrizoate medium contains a slightly lower iodine concentration due to the increased molecular weight associated with the additional methyl group of metrizoic acid (Table 1.6).

At equal salt concentrations, a pure sodium salt of iothalamate or diatrizoate has a greater iodine concentration (59.9% of w/v concentration) than a pure meglumine salt (47.1% of w/v concentration). This occurs because the molecular weight of the meglumine cation (195.2) is approximately 8.5 times the molecular weight of the sodium cation (22.9). The iodine concentrations of combination meglumine-sodium formulations of the ionic media are dependent on their cationic ratios and are intermediate to the iodine concentrations of equal % w/v concentrations of pure meglumine or sodium salts (Table 1.7).

Viscosity. As the molecular weight of a substance in solution or the concentration

Table 1.3   RATIO-1.5 ANGIOGRAPHIC CONTRAST MEDIA[a]: 250 mg IODINE/mL-349 mg IODINE/mL

GENERIC NAME	CONCENTRATION (%w/v)	BRAND NAME®[b]	MG IODINE ML	OSMOLALITY[c] (mOsm/kg)	VISCOSITY (cps)[c] 25°C/37°C	SEQUESTRANT(s)[d]
Diatrizoate meglumine	60	Angiovist-282 (B)	282	1400	6.1/4.1	0.01% CaEDTA
Diatrizoate meglumine	60	Reno-M-60 (S)	282	1500	4.6/4.0	0.4% EDTA, 0.32% NaCit.
Diatrizoate meglumine	60	Hypaque-M 60 (W)	282	1415	6.2/4.1	0.01% CaEDTA
Diatrizoate meglumine (52%)–sodium (8%)	60	Angiovist-292 (B)	292	1500	5.9/4.0	0.01% CaEDTA
Diatrizoate meglumine (52%)–sodium (8%)	60	MD-60 (M)	292	1539	6.2/5.0	0.04% EDTA, 0.32% NaCit.
Diatrizoate meglumine (52%)–sodium (8%)	60	Renografin-60 (S)	292	1420	5.9/4.0	0.04% EDTA, 0.32% NaCit.
Diatrizoate meglumine (28.5%)–sodium (29.1%)	57.6	Renovist II (S)	309	1517	5.6/3.8	0.04% EDTA, 0.32% NaCit.
Diatrizoate sodium	50	Urovist Sodium 300 (B)	300	1550	3.3/2.4	0.01% CaEDTA
Diatrizoate sodium	50	MD-50 (M)	300	1522	3.2/2.4	0.01% CaEDTA
Diatrizoate sodium	50	Hypaque Sodium 50% (W)	300	1550	3.4/2.4	0.01% CaEDTA
Iothalamate meglumine	60	Conray-60 (M)	282	1400	6.0/4.0	0.009% CaEDTA
Iothalamate sodium	54.3	Conray-325 (M)	325	1700	4.0/3.0	0.01% CaEDTA

[a] U.S. market only
[b] (B) Berlex Imaging
(M) Mallinckrodt
(S) Squibb Diagnostics
(W) Winthrop-Breon Laboratories
[c] From: Fischer HW, Catalog of intravascular contrast media, *Radiology* 1986, 159:561–563
[d] CaEDTA = Calcium edetate disodium
EDTA = Edetate disodium
NaCit = Sodium citrate

Table 1.4   RATIO-1.5 ANGIOGRAPHIC CONTRAST MEDIA[a]: 350 mg IODINE/mL-500 mg IODINE/mL

GENERIC NAME	CONCENTRATION ($\%$w/v)	BRAND NAME®[b]	MG IODINE / ML	MG SODIUM / ML	OSMOLALITY[c] (mOsm/kg)	VISCOSITY (cps)[c] 25°C/37°C	SEQUESTRANT(s)[d]
Diatrizoate meglumine	76	Diatrizoate meglumine U.S.P. 76% (S)	358	0.91	1980	15.0/9.2	0.04% EDTA, 0.32% NaCit.
Diatrizoate meglumine (66%)–sodium (10%)	76	Angiovist-370 (B)	370	3.61	2100	13.8/8.4	0.01% CaEDTA
Diatrizoate meglumine (66%)–sodium (10%)	76	MD-76 (M)	370	4.48	2140	14.7/9.1	0.04% EDTA, 0.32% NaCit.
Diatrizoate meglumine (66%)–sodium (10%)	76	Renografin-76 (S)	370	4.48	1940	13.8/8.4	0.04% EDTA, 0.32% NaCit.
Diatrizoate meglumine (66%)–sodium (10%)	76	RenoCal-76 (S)	370	3.61	1870	15.0/9.1	0.01% CaEDTA
Diatrizoate meglumine (66%)–sodium (10%)	76	Hypaque-76 (W)	370	3.68	2016	13.3/8.3	0.01% CaEDTA
Diatrizoate meglumine (34.3%)–sodium (35%)	69.3	Renovist (S)	370.5	13.5	1900	9.1/5.7	0.04% EDTA, 0.32% NaCit.
Diatrizoate meglumine (50%)–sodium (25%)	75	Hypaque-M 75% (W)	385	9.0	2108	12.7/8.0	0.01% CaEDTA
Diatrizoate meglumine (60%)–sodium (30%)	90	Hypaque-M 90% (W)	462	10.9	2938	34.7/19.5	0.01% CaEDTA
Iothalamate meglumine (52%)–sodium (26%)	78	Vascoray (M)	400	9.4	2400	17.0/9.0	0.01% CaEDTA
Iothalamate sodium	66.8	Conray-400 (M)	400	24.2	2300	7.0/4.5	0.01% CaEDTA
Iothalamate sodium	80	Angio-Conray (M)	480	28.3	2400	14.0/9.0	0.01% CaEDTA

[a] U.S. market only

[b] (B) Berlex Imaging
(M) Mallinckrodt
(S) Squibb Diagnostics
(W) Winthrop-Breon Laboratories

[c] From: Fischer HW. Catalog of intravascular contrast media. *Radiology* 1986 159:561–563.

[d] CaEDTA = Calcium edetate disodium
EDTA = Edetate disodium
NaCit. = Sodium citrate

Table 1.5 INTRAVENOUS TOXICITY OF SELECTED ANGIOGRAPHIC CONTRAST MEDIA[a]

CONTRAST MEDIUM	MG IODINE / ML	$LD_{50}\left(\dfrac{MG\ IODINE}{KG}\right)$	
		Mouse (male)	Rat (female)
Iothalamate sodium (66.8%)	400	7,000	8,000
Diatrizoate meglumine (66%)–sodium (10%)	370	7,500	9,000
Metrizoate meglumine (66%)–sodium (10%)–calcium (1%)	370	8,000	10,100
Ioxaglate meglumine (39.3%)–sodium (19.6%)	320	13,400	—
Metrizamide (76.7%)	370	18,600	12,100
Iohexol (79.7%)	370	22,100	11,300
Iopamidol (75.5%)	370	24,200	15,000

[a] Adapted from: Shaw DD, et al, 1985

Table 1.6 COMPARATIVE IODINE CONCENTRATIONS OF SELECTED RATIO-1.5 ANGIOGRAPHIC CONTRAST MEDIA: EQUIVALENT CATIONIC FORMULATIONS

CONTRAST MEDIUM	CONCENTRATION (%w/v)	MG IODINE / ML
Diatrizoate meglumine	60	282
Iothalamate meglumine	60	282
Metrizoate meglumine	60	278

Table 1.7 COMPARATIVE IODINE CONCENTRATIONS OF SELECTED RATIO-1.5 ANGIOGRAPHIC CONTRAST MEDIA: MEGLUMINE VERSUS SODIUM SALTS

CONTRAST MEDIUM	CONCENTRATION (%w/v)	MG IODINE / ML
Diatrizoate meglumine (60%)	60	282
Diatrizoate meglumine (52%)–sodium (8%)	60	292
Diatrizoate sodium (60%)[a]	60	359

[a] Theoretical agent: Diatrizoate sodium is not commercially available at a 60% w/v concentration.

Table 1.8 COMPARATIVE VISCOSITIES OF SELECTED RATIO-1.5 ANGIOGRAPHIC CONTRAST MEDIA: (A.) MEGLUMINE VERSUS SODIUM SALTS AT EQUIVALENT %W/V CONCENTRATIONS; (B.) MEGLUMINE VERSUS SODIUM SALTS AT EQUIVALENT IODINE CONCENTRATIONS

	CONTRAST MEDIUM	CONCENTRATION (%w/v)	MG IODINE / ML	VISCOSITY (CPS)[a] 25° C	VISCOSITY (CPS)[a] 37° C
A.	Diatrizoate meglumine	76	358	15.0	9.2
	Diatrizoate meglumine (66%)–sodium (10%)	76	370	13.9[b]	8.6[b]
	Diatrizoate meglumine (50%)–sodium (25%)	75	385	12.7	8.0
B.	Diatrizoate meglumine (52%)–sodium (8%)	60	292	6.0[b]	4.3[b]
	Diatrizoate sodium	50	300	3.3[b]	2.4[b]

[a] From: Fischer HW Catalog of introvascular contrast media. *Radiology* 1986 159: 561–563
[b] Average of available products

of a given contrast medium increases, so does its viscosity. Hence, at equal % w/v salt concentrations, the viscosity of a meglumine contrast medium is significantly greater than a corresponding pure sodium or combination meglumine-sodium derivative (Table 1.8A). This increased viscosity of meglumine versus sodium media is even more apparent when equiiodine concentrations are compared (Table 1.8B).

Osmolality. The ionic contrast media currently used for angiographic and urographic procedures can dissociate in solution to form two osmotically active particles, the radiopaque anion and a cation, per every three atoms of iodine. Hence, these agents are frequently described as ratio-1.5 media because the ratio between the "number of iodine atoms" and "number of osmotic particles" in an ideal

Table 1.9 COMPARATIVE OSMOLALITIES OF SELECTED RATIO-1.5 ANGIOGRAPHIC CONTRAST MEDIA: MEGLUMINE VERSUS SODIUM SALTS AT EQUIVALENT IODINE CONCENTRATIONS

CONTRAST MEDIUM	CONCENTRATION (%w/v)	MG IODINE / ML	OSMOLALITY[a] (mOsm/kg)
Diatrizoate sodium	50	300	1541[b]
Diatrizoate meglumine (28.5%)–sodium (29.1%)	57.6	309	1517
Diatrizoate meglumine (52%)–sodium (8%)	60	292	1486[b]
Diatrizoate meglumine	60	282	1438[b]

[a] From: Fischer HW, Catalog of intravascular contrast media, *Radiology* 1986 159: 561–563
[b] Average of available products

solution is 3:2. At equal iodine concentrations, sodium salts of ionic media tend to have greater osmolalities than corresponding pure meglumine or combination meglumine-sodium salts (Table 1.9) due to their greater degree of disassociation in solution (i.e., increased number of distinct osmotically active particles in solution) or the greater molecular weight of the meglumine cation. Depending on the iodine concentration and cationic ratio required for a specific angiographic procedure, the osmolalities of these media may typically exceed the osmolality of blood (300 mOsm/kg) by factors of 5 to 7 (Tables 1.2–1.4). The hypertonicity of these ratio-1.5 media is a major causative factor for many of their undesirable effects on vascular and organ physiology (see Physiological Effects).

RATIO-3 LOW OSMOLALITY CONTRAST MEDIA

In an attempt to reduce the osmolality-related adverse effects of ionic contrast media, several approaches were proposed (Almén T, 1985) for the development of water-soluble contrast agents with an increased iodine-to-osmotic particle ratio (Figure 1.4). These approaches included the synthesis of an ionic medium wherein both the anion and cation would contain three iodine atoms (i.e., 6 iodine atoms/2 osmotic particles, ratio-3 medium); the polymerization of two triiodobenzoic acid derivatives to form a single dimeric anion, which when formulated with a sodium or meglumine cation would result in a ratio-3 medium (i.e., 6 iodine atoms/2 osmotic particles); or the preparation of a ratio-3 nonionic agent (i.e., 3 iodine atoms/1 osmotic particle) by replacing the carboxyl group and non-iodine side chains of a ratio-1.5 ionic medium with polyhydroxyalkyl groups in order to confer water solubility without ionization. An additional advantage of the latter approach would be the complete elimination of sodium and meglumine cations, which, as previously mentioned, contribute to the undesirable physiological effects of angiographic or urographic contrast media.

Research efforts on these approaches have subsequently led to the development

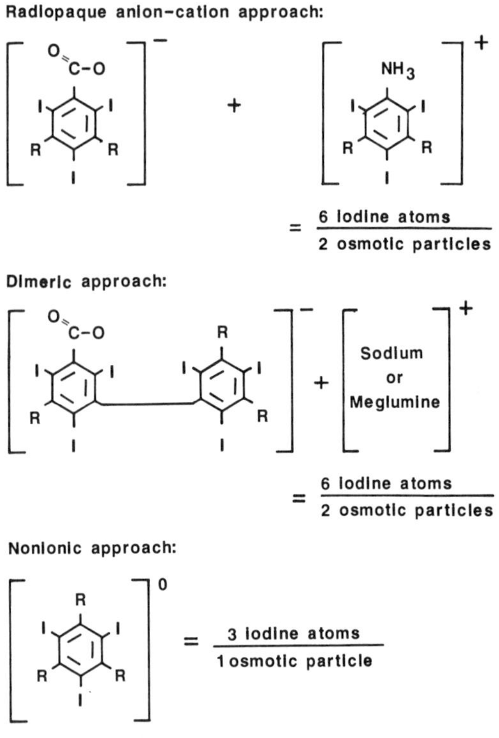

Figure 1.4 Chemical approaches to the development of ratio-3 angiographic contrast media.

and availability of two distinct categories of low-osmolality contrast agents, the nonionic and the ionic-dimeric media.

NONIONIC CONTRAST MEDIA

The first commercially available nonionic contrast medium, metrizamide (Figure 1.5), is a derivative of the ionic agent, metrizoate (Figure 1.3), wherein the carboxyl group of metrizoate is covalently attached to meglumine to confer water solubility without ionic dissociation. Hence, ideal solutions of metrizamide consist of three iodine atoms per one osmotically active particle, or a ratio-3 medium. Although experimental and clinical studies demonstrated reduced intravascular (Table 1.5) and subarachnoid toxicity (see Chapter 4, Myelographic Contrast Media) with metrizamide compared to the ratio-1.5 ionic media, its use has been primarily limited to myelography procedures due to problems associated with its high cost of production and price, its instability to heat and sterilization by autoclaving, and its instability in solution, which requires on-site reconstitution of the lyophilized metrizamide powder prior to administration.

Subsequent research on nonionic contrast media, aimed primarily at the development of agents with improved stability and reduced cost, resulted in the second generation nonionic media, iohexol and iopamidol (Figure 1.5). These ratio-3 media can be heat sterilized and are stable in solution, thereby decreasing their cost and increasing their convenience of use in comparison to metrizamide. Based on these considerations, the use of metrizamide for angiographic procedures is no longer warranted.

Iodine Concentration. On a per mole basis, iopamidol contains slightly more iodine (49%) than iohexol (46.4%). Based on the quantity of administered iodine, the intravascular toxicity of iohexol and iopamidol are similar and less than metrizamide (Table 1.5). The three nonionic media are approximately one-half to one-third as toxic as the ratio-1.5 ionic media (Table 1.5).

Viscosity. At equal, high-iodine concentrations and room temperature (25°C),

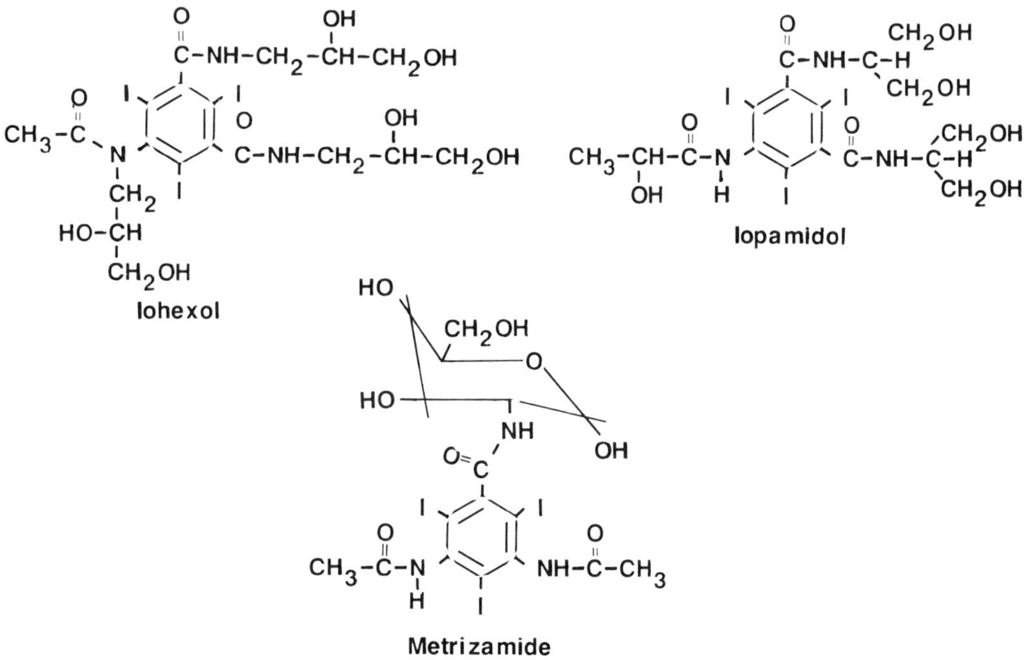

Figure 1.5 Chemical structures of ratio-3 nonionic contrast media currently indicated for angiography procedures.

Table 1.10   COMPARATIVE OSMOLALITIES AND VISCOSITIES OF SELECTED RATIO-1.5 AND RATIO-3 ANGIOGRAPHIC CONTRAST MEDIA: EQUIVALENT IODINE CONCENTRATIONS

CONTRAST MEDIUM	CONCENTRATION (%w/v)	MG IODINE / ML	OSMOLALITY[a] (mOsm/kg)	VISCOSITY (cps)[a] 25° C/37° C
Diatrizoate meglumine (52%)–sodium (8%)	60	292	1486[b]	6.0/4.3[b]
Diatrizoate sodium	50	300	1541[b]	3.3/2.4[b]
Iohexol	64.7	300	709	10.4/6.8
Iopamidol	61	300	616	8.8[c]/4.7
Ioxaglate meglumine (39.3%)–sodium (19.6%)	58.9	320	600	15.7/7.5

[a] From: Fischer HW, Catalog of intravascular contrast media, *Radiology* 1986 159: 561–563
[b] Average of available products
[c] Determined at 20°C

Table 1.11   RATIO-3 ANGIOGRAPHIC CONTRAST MEDIA

GENERIC NAME	CONCENTRATION (% w/v)	BRAND NAME®[a]	MG IODINE / ML	OSMOLALITY[b] (mOsm/kg)	VISCOSITY (cps)[b] 25°C/37°C	SEQUESTRANT[c]
Iopamidol	26	Isovue-128 (S)	128	290	2.1[d]/1.4	0.017% CaEDTA
Iohexol	51.8	Omnipaque 240 (W)	240	504	4.4/3.1	0.01% CaEDTA
Iohexol	64.7	Omnipaque 300 (W)	300	709	10.4/6.8	0.01% CaEDTA
Iopamidol	61.2	Isovue-300 (S)	300	616	8.8[d]/4.7	0.039% CaEDTA
Ioxaglate meglumine (39.3%)–sodium (19.6%)	58.9	Hexabrix (M)	320	600	15.7/7.5	0.01% CaEDTA
Iohexol	75.5	Omnipaque 350 (W)	350	862	18.5/11.2	0.01% CaEDTA
Iopamidol	75.5	Isovue-370 (S)	370	796	20.9[d]/9.4	0.048% CaEDTA

[a] (M) Mallinckrodt
(S) Squibb Diagnostics
(W) Winthrop-Breon Laboratories
[b] From: Fisher HW, Catalog of intravascular contrast media, *Radiology* 1986 159: 561–563
[c] CaEDTA = Calcium edetate disodium
[d] Determined at 20°C

the viscosity of iopamidol is less than iohexol, but greater than that of equal iodine concentrations of the ratio-1.5 ionic media (Table 1.10). Reducing the % w/v concentration or increasing the temperature of the nonionic media to 37°C significantly reduces their respective viscosities and decreases the relatively differences between agents; however, the same order is retained (Table 1.11).

Osmolality. The ratio-3 nonionic contrast media should theoretically demonstrate a 50% reduction in the osmolality exhibited by equiiodine concentrations of the ratio-1.5 ionic media. However, the actual reduction in osmolality achieved by these ratio-3 media is greater than 50% (Table 1.10) due to aggregation of the nonionic molecules in solution. Molecular aggregation further reduces osmolality by both decreasing the total number of osmotically active particles in solution and increasing their molecular weight (Dawson P, 1984a).

Within the nonionic media group, the osmolality of iopamidol is less than an equiiodine concentration of iohexol (Table 1.10). This phenomenon probably reflects their respective degrees of molecular aggregation in solution.

IONIC-DIMERIC CONTRAST MEDIA

Research on the polymeric approach to the development of low-osmolality contrast media subsequently led to the availability of ioxaglic acid (Figure 1.6). This

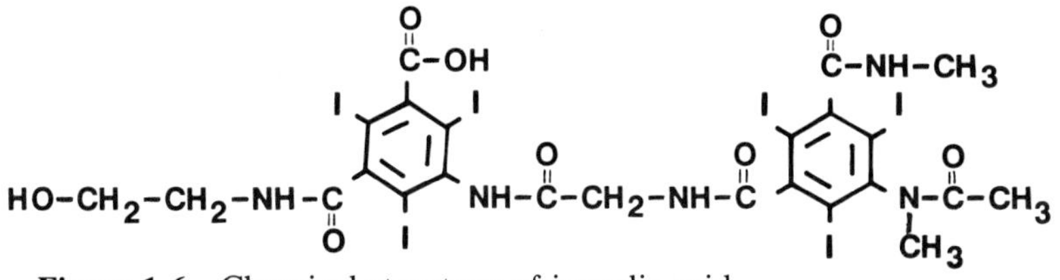

Figure 1.6   Chemical structure of ioxaglic acid.

agent consists of two triiodobenzoic acid molecules linked together to form a single dimeric anion containing six iodine atoms. Formulated as a combination meglumine-sodium (2:1 ratio) salt, this contrast medium dissociates in solution to form two osmotically active particles, and is therefore a ratio-3 medium. Hence, a different approach has been used to produce a low-osmolality contrast agent that is theoretically equivalent to the ratio-3 nonionic media in regard to osmolality per given degree of opacification.

Iodine Concentration.   Ioxaglate meglumine-sodium has a molar iodine concentration (54.3%) that is greater than the ratio-3 nonionic media or pure meglumine salts of ratio-1.5 ionic media, but less than sodium salts of ratio-1.5 ionic media. Its intravascular toxicity, based on the administered iodine dose, is intermediate to the ratio-1.5 ionic and ratio-3 nonionic agents (Table 1.5).

Viscosity.   At equivalent iodine concentrations, the viscosity of ioxaglate meglumine-sodium is similar to the ratio-3 nonionic media, iohexol and iopamidol, and is greater than the ratio-1.5 ionic agents (Table 1.10). As with each of the previously described media, heating ioxaglate meglumine-sodium significantly decreases its viscosity.

Osmolality   The ratio-3 ionic-dimer, ioxaglate meglumine-sodium, should also theoretically demonstrate a 50% reduction in the osmolality exhibited by equi-iodine concentrations of ratio-1.5 ionic media. However, as with the ratio-3 nonionic agents, the actual decrease in osmolality achieved with the ioxaglate salt is greater than 50% (Table 1.10). In fact, this agent demonstrates a lower osmolality per given iodine concentration than any of the previously described ratio-3 nonionic media (Table 1.10), probably due to its increased molecular size.

It is interesting to note that the factor of 2-3 decrease in osmolality exhibited by the ratio-3 nonionic or ionic-dimeric agents appears to correlate with their respective decrease in intravascular toxicity when compared to the ratio-1.5 ionic media (Table 1.5). Although osmolality is a major factor associated with the undesirable physiological effects of intravascular contrast media, these ratio-3 agents do exert toxicity related directly to their chemical properties. The disassociation between hyperosmolar and direct chemotoxic effects is illustrated by the intravascular toxicity of ioxaglate meglumine-sodium. This agent demonstrates the lowest osmolality per given iodine concentration of any media discussed; however, its intravascular toxicity (LD_{50}) is intermediate to the ratio-1.5 ionic and the ratio-3 nonionic media. Other examples of chemotoxic differences between the ratio-3 low-osmolality agents will be presented under the discussion of specific physiological effects.

SEQUESTERING AGENTS

Each of the commercially available ratio-1.5 ionic and ratio-3 low-osmolality contrast media contains low concentrations of either calcium edetate disodium or a combination of edetate disodium and sodium citrate (Tables 1.2–1.4, 1.11). These "sequestering" agents are incorporated into contrast media formulations to chelate various divalent and polyvalent cationic impurities that may be present in small quantities in the Water for Injection, U.S.P., used for reconstitution of these agents. Such heavy metal, ionic impurities adversely influence the rate of deiodination of the contrast moiety or may lead to its precipitation (Wang YJ, 1980).

The commonly utilized combination of additives, edetate disodium (0.04% w/v) and sodium citrate (0.32% w/v), can directly chelate 13 mMols of calcium per liter, whereas the calcium-binding effect of the calcium edetate disodium sequestrant has been preneutralized (Thomson KR, et al, 1978). As a result of respective differences in their degree of in vivo calcium binding, contrast media containing the combination edetate disodium/sodium citrate additives exhibit greater effects on electrical and mechanical physiology of the heart (see Physiological Effects) compared to formulations containing calcium edetate disodium.

BUFFERING AGENTS

Commercially available formulations of range of 6.5–7.5. Acidic pH values below contrast media contain phosphate, bicarbonate or TRIS-buffers to maintain their pH in the U.S.P. designated physiologic range of 6.5–7.5. Acidic pH values below this range may lead to precipitation of the radiopaque anion, whereas pH values on the alkaline side of, or higher than, this range lead to instability of the contrast moiety with release of free iodide and the formation of cytotoxic aromatic amines (Felder E, 1984). Furthermore, solutions with pH values significantly above or below this physiologic range have direct vasodilatory properties (Nyman U, et al, 1980a).

The nature of the buffer, (e. g., phosphate, bicarbonate, TRIS, etc.) used to maintain the pH of the contrast medium appears to be of minimal importance in regard to the production of undesirable physiological effects.

II. Pharmacokinetics

The use of a radiopaque contrast medium for angiography is based upon its ability to directly opacify the vessels in its path of flow. Maximum vascular iodine concentrations and opacification occur immediately after a direct, bolus injection of

the angiography medium into the arterial or venous system of interest.

Following bolus injection of an angiographic contrast medium, the vascular iodine concentration decreases rapidly as a result of flow-induced dilution within the vascular compartment. Due to the presence of a concentration gradient, the angiographic medium passively diffuses into and mixes with the extravascular, extracellular fluid of the interstitial spaces, thus resulting in a further, but slower decrease in its plasma concentration. In normal tissues, there is negligible membrane-binding or cellular uptake of any of the angiographic media; their distribution being confined to the plasma and extracellular fluid. Based solely on diffusion kinetics, approximately two hours would be required for equilibrium to be established between the intravascular and interstitial concentrations of the medium. This process is, however, effectively completed within 10 minutes as a result of concomitant renal elimination of the intravascular contrast agent. As urinary excretion continues, the plasma concentration becomes less than the interstitial concentration and reverse diffusion of the medium occurs. With normal renal function, 50% of the administered dose of an angiographic medium is eliminated from the body within 2 hours, nearly 100% within 24 hours. The normal plasma half-life is approximately 30–60 minutes (Cattell WR, et al, 1967; Talner LB, 1972; Dawson P, et al, 1984).

Although the various contrast media do demonstrate minor differences in their rates of equilibration and differential organ clearance, these factors are of no importance in angiographic procedures, wherein the critical pharmacokinetic parameter is simply the vessel-of-interest iodine concentration immediately after injection. This latter factor is determined by the volume and iodine concentration of the administered contrast medium and its rate of injection. For good angiographic evaluations of a given vessel, the rate and volume of the contrast medium injection must be sufficient to opacify the entire lumen of the vessel during the early phase of imaging (see Dosage).

III. Physiological Effects

The ideal contrast medium for angiographic procedures should produce opacification of the region(s)-of-interest without exerting biochemical or physiological effects. Hence, any physiological effect produced by an intravascular contrast medium is undesirable whether or not it is manifested as an observable adverse reaction. Unfortunately, angiographic contrast media produce myriad physiological effects as a result of their pseudo-allergic manifestations, hyperosmolarity, or direct molecular toxicity. In certain individuals, the undesirable physiological effects of angiographic contrast media can manifest as observable adverse reactions.

PSEUDO-ALLERGIC REACTIONS

Many of the observable reactions to intravascular contrast media are unpredictable and occur independent of the dose or concentration of the injected agent above a certain threshold level. Their presentation, ranging from mild urticaria and flushing to severe anaphylaxis, resembles an allergic hypersensitivity reaction although a casual relationship based on the classical antigen-antibody interaction has not been firmly established. Hence, these reactions are appropriately classified as being pseudo-allergic in origin. Several additional theories have been proposed to explain the etiology of these reactions, including direct contrast-induced release of histamine and serotonin from cellular (basophil, mast cells, platelets) storage sites, activation of the acute complement-coagulation system, and neurogenic factors associated with fear or the discomfort of the radiological procedure. Since many of the observable adverse reactions to intravascular contrast media are associated with or attributed to a pseudo-allergic origin, a separate chapter (Chapter 8) of this section has been devoted to a more complete discussion of their incidence and nature, causative mechanisms, preventative measures, and appropriate treatment.

CHEMOTOXIC EFFECTS

An angiographic contrast medium can exert direct physiological effects on the vasculature and organs being perfused by the medium. Unlike pseudo-allergic reactions, the incidence and severity of these chemotoxic effects are directly dependent on the dose and concentration of the injected agent. Several factors contribute to the chemotoxic effects of an angiographic contrast medium including the direct molecular toxicity of its organic iodine moiety or cation (if applicable), the nature of its sequestering agent(s), and its hyperosmolality. The relative chemotoxic potential of each of these factors as it relates to the specific physiological effects of angiographic contrast media is presented below.

The chemotoxic effects of angiographic contrast media are also dependent on their site and rate of administration. Certain organs, such as the lung, heart, brain, and kidney, are extremely sensitive to the chemotoxic effects of contrast media. Since the chemotoxic potential of an angiographic medium is dose and concentration dependent, direct injection of the medium into the arterial blood supply of one of these organs would be expected to increase the incidence and intensity of respective physiologic effects on that organ as compared to the diluted effects of a more peripheral injection. Similarly, rapid angiographic injections expose the vasculature and sensitive organs to a high dose and concentration of the medium, whereas slower infusions of an equivalent total dose reduce the acute chemotoxic potential but prolong the overall time of exposure. In consideration of these statements, the specific physiological effects of angiographic contrast media on each of the sensitive organs are discussed in association with the specific angiographic procedures that expose these organs to the highest dose and concentration of the media (Table 1.1). However, it must be recognized that the effects of a contrast medium on a specific organ relate not only to selective angiography of that organ, but also to any procedure that exposes that organ to a high dose and concentration of the medium. For example, with left ventriculography and aortography, the effects of the injected contrast medium on the brain must be considered. Similarly, all

Table 1.12   VASCULAR EFFECTS OF ANGIOGRAPHIC CONTRAST MEDIA

PHYSIOLOGICAL EFFECT(S)	RESPONSE(S)	RESPONSIBLE CHEMOTOXIC FACTOR(S)
Hypervolemia (systemic)	↓ Hematocrit ↑ L. ventricular end-diastolic/atrial pressures ↑ Cardiac output	Hyperosmolality
Echinocyte formation	↓ Erythrocyte aggregation	Molecular toxicity
Desicocyte formation	↓ Erythrocyte aggregation ↑ Blood viscosity · ↑ Capillary resistance	Hyperosmolality
↓ Platelet aggregation ↑ p. Thromboplastin, Thrombin times	↑ Clotting time	Molecular toxicity
Vessel dilation · ↓ Vascular resistance	↑ Blood flow ↓ Blood pressure (systemic) · Reflex tachycardia Pain	Hyperosmolality
Altered vascular endothelial permeability	Pain Inflammation Microthrombus formation	Hyperosmolality

angiography procedures will result in physiological effects on the kidney, the primary route of excretion of the angiographic media. Intravascular contrast media also exert general chemotoxic effects on the blood and vasculature regardless of their site of administration.

VASCULAR EFFECTS (TABLE 1.12):
GENERAL ANGIOGRAPHY

Blood Volume/Hematocrit. The intravascular administration of a hyperosmolar contrast medium produces an immediate increase in plasma osmolality, the extent of this increase being directly dependent on the dose and osmolality of the administered agent and inversely on the blood volume of the patient. In response to this increase in plasma osmolality there is a rapid shift of fluid from blood cells and the extravascular space into the plasma, resulting in a corresponding increase in blood volume with a fall in hematocrit (Figure 1.7). Maximum blood volume and hematocrit effects are observed at approximately two minutes following injection. After this peak, there is a rapid decrease in plasma volume associated with renal excretion of the contrast medium combined with a diuretic effect induced by the presence of the hyperosmolar medium in

the kidney. Hematocrit and blood volume return to normal at about 15–20 minutes and may actually demonstrate a reversal (i. e., decreased blood volume, increased hematocrit) due to the dehydrating effect of contrast-induced osmotic diuresis (Weigen JF, and Thomas SF, 1973).

The hypervolemia produced by a hyperosmolar contrast medium results in an increase in cardiac output and a rise in left ventricular end-diastolic and left atrial pressures. These factors may also be responsible for hydrostatic effects on the pulmonary circulation (see Pulmonary Effects) leading to an increase in pulmonary artery and venous pressures (Fischer HW, 1968).

As might be expected, there is almost a linear relationship between the osmolality of the injected contrast medium and the resulting effects on blood volume and hematocrit (Aspelin P, 1978a). Hence, at equivalent iodine concentrations, the ratio-3 low-osmolality media produce less hypervolemia than the ratio-1.5 ionic media; and meglumine salts of iothalamate, diatrizoate or metrizoate produce less effects than their respective sodium salts.

Electrolyte/pH Effects Dilution effects associated with the hypervolemia induced

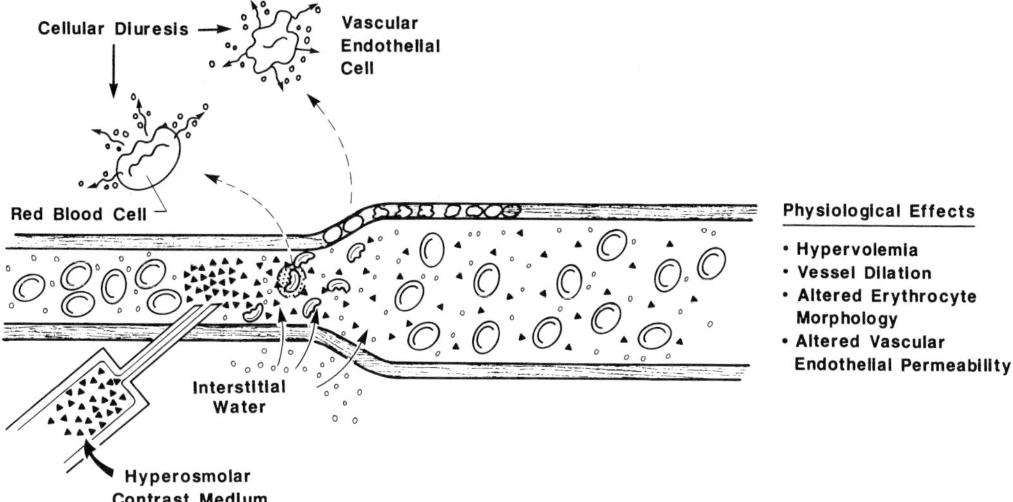

Figure 1.7   Diagram illustrating the immediate effects of a hyperosmolar contrast medium on vascular physiology. (Adopted from Weigen JF and Thomas SF, 1973, and Fischer HW, 1968).

by a hyperosmolar contrast medium should produce a net transient decrease in the plasma concentration of physiologic electrolytes (i. e., sodium, calcium, potassium, magnesium, etc.), but the relative ionic ratios and total quantities of available ions should remain unaltered. However, compared to these expected dilution effects, many angiographic media can produce a disproportionate decrease in the circulating levels of calcium (and possibly magnesium) cations as a result of direct calcium binding by the radiopaque anion moieties and the sequestering agents within the contrast formulation (Wolpers HG, et al, 1981). The ratio-3 nonionic contrast media do not demonstrate direct binding of calcium ions; however, the ratio-3 dimeric anion, ioxaglate, and the ratio-1.5 ionic media, iothalamate and diatrizoate, do bind calcium ions. As previously discussed (see Chemistry), the combination of sequestering agents, edetate disodium (0.04% w/v) and sodium citrate (0.32% w/v), can directly chelate 13 mMols of calcium ions per liter of contrast formulation (Thomson KR, et al, 1978), whereas the calcium-binding properties of the calcium edetate disodium additive are pre-neutralized.

In addition to their direct calcium-binding

effects, the ionic contrast media (ratio-1.5 ionic and ratio-3 dimeric agents) can also cause a decrease in blood pH due to a redistribution of anionic charges between the red cell and plasma. Depending on the radiopaque anion-to-blood ratio, the normal negative potential of 10 mV across the red cell membrane can be decreased, nullified, or reversed. As the red cell becomes more positive with respect to the plasma, it expels hydrogen ions, in a sense, via the generation and release of carbon dioxide. In the plasma, this carbon dioxide is rehydrated to form carbonic acid with the subsequent liberation of bicarbonate and the hydrogen ions responsible for acidemia. As expected, the ratio-3 nonionic coontrast media have little effect on the redistribution of anionic charges and blood pH (Lichtman MA, et al, 1975).

The disproportionate decrease in serum calcium concentration and the acidemia produced by ionic contrast media can have deleterious effects on the electrophysiology and contractility of the heart. These actions of angiographic contrast media will be discussed in greater detail under Cardiac Effects. At a given iodine concentration, the ratio-3 ionic-dimeric medium, ioxaglate meglumine-sodium, would be expected to produce less than 50% of the respective calcium-binding and pH effects of the conventional ratio-1.5 ionic media due to the corresponding reduced number of anionic molecules.

Within the ratio 1.5 contrast media group, meglumine salts of diatrizoate or iothalamate dissociate less in solution than sodium salts, resulting in a decreased number of distinct anionic molecules for calcium binding.

Red Cell Morphology/Aggregation/Blood Viscosity. Red blood cells exposed to intravascular contrast media undergo alterations in their morphology, changing from their normal disc shape into crenated spheres (echinocytes). This echinocyte formation occurs independent of the osmolality of the medium or the nature of its cations (if applicable), and thus appears to be due to direct molecular toxicity of the radiopaque organic moiety. Both the ratio-3 low-osmolality and ratio-1.5 ionic media are capable of producing echinocytes. That this physiological effect of intravascular contrast media is due to direct molecular toxicity is best illustrated by the greater degree of echinocyte formation observed with the ratio-3 nonionic agent, metrizamide, compared to the ratio-1.5 ionic agent, diatrizoate, at equal, isotonic osmolalities and contrast medium-to-blood concentration ratios (Aspelin P, 1978b)). Diatrizoate, in turn, demonstrates greater echinocyte formation than the ratio-3 media, ioxaglate meglumine-sodium, iopamidol, or iohexol (Stäubli M, et al, 1982; Dawson P, et al, 1983a). The respective effects of all agents increase in proportion to the contrast medium-to-blood concentration ratio. The mechanism of echinocyte formation may be related to the effects of charge (i. e., ratio-1.5 ionic, ratio-3 ionic-dimeric media) on the cellular membrane, the incorporation of the organic moiety (i. e., ratio-3 nonionics) into the membrane, or the inhibition of enzymes such as glucose-6-phosphatase (Aspelin P, 1978b; Lasser EC, 1971). Echinocyte formation does not, however, appear to be related to the degree of binding of the contrast medium to the erythrocyte membrane. The clinical importance of echinocyte formation, per se, is unclear since this phenomenon is rapidly reversible and

does not correlate with the intravenous toxicity (Table 1.5) of the angiographic media (Aspelin P, 1978b).

At high contrast media-to-blood concentration ratios (i. e., 90%), hyperosmolar contrast media cause a net transfer of fluid from the red cell into the plasma leading to the formation of desicocytes or shrunken red cells (Figure 1.7). In contradistinction to echinocyte induction, the formation of desicocytes is directly dependent on the osmolality of the contrast medium and its blood concentration ratio. That hyperosmolality is the primary factor in this physiological effect is evidenced by the formation of desicocytes by hypertonic saline and hyperosmolar ratio-1.5 ionic contrast media, but not by equal blood concentration ratios of the ratio-3 low-osmolality media or by less concentrated (i. e., decreased osmolality) solutions of the same ratio-1.5 ionic media (Aspelin P, 1978b; Stäubli M, et al, 1982). The clinical importance of desicocyte formation is related to the fact that red cells must be able to deform and bend in order to pass through the smaller diameter capillaries. Desicocyte formation, which may be induced by the high contrast medium-to-blood concentration ratios of rapid intravenous injections or selective angiographic procedures, results in rigidification of the erythrocytes and their decreased deformability. As such, these morphologically altered cells may obstruct the capillaries and be responsible for the diminished blood flow and the increased precapillary resistance observed in various angiographic procedures (see Pulmonary Effects, Renal Effects). Echinocytes produced by the ratio-3 low-osmolality media or reduced concentrations of the ratio-1.5 ionic media are less resistant to deformability than the desicocytes caused by hyperosmolar media (Aspelin P, 1979).

Both the ratio-3 and ratio-1.5 angiographic contrast media can decrease erythrocyte aggregation in a dose-dependent manner. This effect appears to be related to a combination of the direct molecular toxicity of the medium and its hyperosmolality. At isotonic concentrations, the nonionic agent, metrizamide, produces a greater disaggregation effect on red blood cells than the ratio-1.5 ionic medium, diatrizoate; whereas at hypertonic concentrations, the relative effects become equalized. Hypertonic saline is also known to produce disaggregation of erythrocytes, thus substantiating the effect of hyperosmolality. Apparently, the morphologically altered echinocytes and desicocytes produced by contrast media do not possess an appropriate binding surface to permit aggregation (Aspelin P, 1978b). In a recent in vitro study an increased degree (nonionic > ionic) of red cell aggregation was noted when blood was added to various contrast media (Raininko R, and Ylinen SL, 1987). However, this investigation did not take into account the high shear rates encountered with normal blood flow. With the inclusion of shear, the contrast media-induced red cell aggregates rapidly dissolve (Aspelin, P, 1988).

Following intravascular injection, both the ratio-1.5 ionic and the ratio-3 low-osmolality contrast media produce an immediate increase in the viscosity of the local blood. The resulting increase in plasma viscosity is directly proportional to the viscosity of the injected medium (Tables 1.2–1.4), whereas the increase in whole blood viscosity is also dependent on the degree of echinocyte and desicocyte formation. Hence, the acute increase in blood viscosity is dependent on both the chemical nature and osmolality of the injected medium. The hyperosmolality of the contrast medium is probably of primary importance since desicocytes are more resistant to flow than echinocytes. The reduced rate of blood flow associated with increased blood viscosity prolongs the time of exposure of the contrast medium to the vascular endothelial cells and may explain, in part, the increased vessel dilation, pain, and other physiological effects observed with the administration of hyperosmolar contrast media versus equiosmolar, hypertonic saline solutions or the ratio-3 low-osmolality contrast media (Aspelin P, 1978a).

Sickle Cell Disease. A specific hematologic contraindication may exist in regard to the administration of angiographic contrast media to patients who are homozygous for sickle cell hemoglobin. In vitro experiments have demonstrated the promotion of severe sickling when the blood of these patients is mixed with contrast media at blood concentrations (i.e., approximately 30%–35% by weight) approaching those obtained with rapid, high-dose angiographic procedures. This phenomenon appears to be related to hyperosmolarity-induced cellular diuresis resulting in an increase in the intracellular concentration of hemoglobin-S. Hence, the ratio-3 nonionic and ionic-dimeric media demonstrate less sickling potential than the ratio-1.5 ionic agents (Rao VM, et al, 1982).

Platelet Aggregation. In addition to their effects on erythrocyte morphology and aggregation, intravascular contrast media can also interfere with platelet function as demonstrated by an inhibition of normal aggregation. The effects of different contrast media on platelet aggregability appear to vary, however, depending on the nature of the aggregation-inducer used in the testing procedure. For example, at equivalent plasma iodine concentrations, the ratio-1.5 ionic-monomer, metrizoate meglumine, and the ratio-3 ionic-dimer, ioxaglate meglumine-sodium, produce substantially greater inhibition of collagen-induced platelet aggregation than the ratio-3 nonionic media, iohexol or iopamidol. In contrast, equal minor levels of inhibition are observed with each of these same agents if their antiplatelet effects are compared using an adenosine diphosphate (ADP)-inducer. The various inducers of platelet aggregation apparently exert their effects at different sites on the platelet membrane. The results of the previously described studies would therefore suggest that the ability of a contrast medium to inhibit platelet aggregation is dependent on the affinity of its inhibitory component for the platelet membrane site of the aggregation-inducer used in the respective testing procedure (Stormorken H, et al, 1986).

The role that the hyperosmolarity of a contrast medium plays in the induction of its antiplatelet activity is uncertain. Hyperosmolar control solutions have been shown to inhibit collagen-induced platelet aggregation but have a considerably lesser effect on ADP-induced and an opposite effect (i. e., increased aggregability) on AA-induced aggregation (Stormorken H, et al, 1986; Paajanen H, et al, 1984; Parvez Z, et al, 1984). Also, the inhibitory effects of contrast media on platelet function do not appear to be related to hyperosmolarity-induced disruption of the platelet cytoplasmic membrane (Paajanen H, et al, 1984). Direct binding of calcium ions by the radiopaque anions of ionic contrast media may contribute to their inhibition of platelet aggregation; however, the addition of calcium chloride to the test platelet-rich plasma does not ameliorate their respective antiplatelet effects (Parvez Z, et al, 1984). It has also been suggested that meglumine cations within ionic contrast medium formulations may be the primary factor responsible for their demonstrated platelet inhibitory activity (Parvez Z, et al, 1984).

Coagulation Factors. Intravascular, iodinated contrast media can also suppress coagulation factors of both the intrinsic and extrinsic pathways and inhibit fibrin formation as demonstrated by a prolongation of prothrombin, activated partial thromboplastin, and thrombin times. An in vitro study has shown that at equivalent plasma iodine concentrations, the ratio-1.5 ionic-monomer, metrizoate meglumine, and the ratio-3 ionic-dimer, ioxaglate meglumine-sodium, produce greater inhibition of clotting times than the ratio-3 nonionic media, iohexol and iopamidol (Stormorken H, et al, 1986). Based on these results and comparative studies using hyperosmolar control solutions it appears that contrast inhibition of coagulation is dependent on the direct molecular toxicity of the contrast medium rather than its hyperosmolarity.

An assay of fibrinmonomer formation has been used to evaluate the mechanism by which contrast media inhibit coagulation (Belleville J, et al, 1985). The results of this study indicate that contrast media interact with and/or denature the fibrinogen molecule, thereby preventing the access of thrombin to its respective catalytic binding sites. In the presence of a normal thrombin interaction, fibrinogen is converted to fibrin with subsequent clot formation. By interfering with the fibrin polymerization step, contrast media produce a prolongation of all global and specific assays of clotting time. Hence, although contrast media may also interact with a specific coagulation factor, the results of this interaction would be difficult to separate from the final fibrinogen effect. This study also confirmed that the inhibitory effect of a contrast medium on coagulation is not related to hyperosmolarity, nor is the presence of meglumine cations or calcium binding a responsible factor. It was futher suggested that the described interaction of contrast media with fibrinogen may explain, in part, their antiplatelet effects, since fibrinogen is an essential cofactor for platelet aggregation.

Human in vivo studies have demonstrated a significant inhibition of platelet aggregation and clotting times following the administration of routine angiographic dosages of the conventional, ratio-1.5 iodinated contrast media. The magnitude of these effects are dose dependent and reach a maximum at 15–30 minutes post injection with return to normal at 3 hours (Bjork L, 1968; Stein HL, et al, 1968; Parvez Z, et al, 1982). A prolongation of bleeding times, the most critical parameter of the effects of contrast media on clotting physiology, has not been routinely observed in the presence of these alterations in platelet aggregation and coagulation (Shapiro GA, et al, 1977). It must be noted, however, that these studies typically did not involve large numbers or excluded patients with preexisting bleeding disorders or those undergoing heparinization or chronic therapy with anticoagulants or antiplatelet drugs (e. g., aspirin, dipyridamole, nonsteroidal anti-inflammatory agents). The contrast-induced inhibition of clotting mechanisms has been experimentally shown to potentiate the anticoagulant effects of heparin and to be enhanced in plasma from patients with coagulation pathway deficiencies (Bjork L, 1968; Parvez Z, et al, 1982), and would therefore be expected to be additive to the in vivo effects of these conditions.

Vessel Dilation. The vessels of the peripheral arterial system dilate in response to their exposure to intravascular contrast media (Figure 1.7). This vasodilation is accompanied by a decrease in vascular resistance and a corresponding increase in arterial blood flow. The contrast media appear to exert these dilation effects via a direct action on the vascular smooth muscle. Experimental studies have shown that spinal anesthesia, vagotomy, and pharmacological manipulation (i. e., sympathetic agents, atropine, antihistamine) exert negligible effects on the vasodilating properties of angiographic contrast media, thus negating the possibility that their action is via a reflex neurogenic pathway or by direct inhibition or stimulation of adrenergic receptors, acetylcholine receptors, or the release of histamine (Hilal SK, 1966; Steiner RM, et al, 1980). The degree of vasodilation induced by an intravascular contrast medium is primarily dependent on its osmolality. It should be noted, however, that hypertonic saline solutions produce less dilation of a shorter duration than equiosmolar solutions of contrast media, thus implicating additional factors such as direct molecular toxicity of the contrast agent or viscosity-associated prolongation of vessel exposure (Nyman U, et al, 1980b). Meglumine salts of iothalamate, diatrizoate, or metrizoate produce less vasodilation and blood flow changes than equiiodine concentrations of their corresponding sodium salts, with relative differences between the radiopaque anions being minimal (Hilal SK, 1966; Holder JC and Dalrymple GV, 1981). As expected, the ratio-3 nonionic and ionic-dimeric media demon-

strate approximately one-third of the vasodilatation and blood flow effects exhibited by equiiodine concentrations of the ratio-1.5 ionic media (i. e., blood flow increase of 30% vs 90%, respectively) (Steiner RM, et al, 1980). Within the low osmolality group, the ionic-dimeric agent, ioxaglate meglumine-sodium, may produce slightly less vessel dilation than the nonionic media as a result of its lower osmolality per given iodine concentration (Table 1.10).

Blood Pressure/Heart Rate. The contrast-induced vasodilation and increase in blood flow is normally of short duration (1–2 minutes) unless additional complicating factors (e. g., cardiovascular disease, renal dysfunction) are present. Systemic hypotension, which may be expected with these effects, is usually neutralized or reversed by the previously described increase in blood volume. With arterial dilation and a reduction in blood pressure, there is often a reflex stimulation of heart rate (transient tachycardia) and cardiac output (Fishcer HW, 1968).

It should be noted that although hyperosmolar contrast media, in general, cause acute vasodilation, their overall effect on systemic blood pressure is dependent on a complex interaction of direct and reflex mechanisms that vary with the site of administration. Specific effects of angiographic contrast media on systemic blood pressure is therefore discussed under each organ system.

Vascular Endothelial Permeability. In addition to their dilation effects on vascular smooth muscle, intravascular contrast media can also elicit an increase in vascular endothelial permeability. The hyperosmolality of the injected contrast medium is the primary factor responsible for this effect (Zinner G and Gottlob P, 1959; Almén T, 1985). Hyperosmolarity induces osmotic cellular diuresis and shrinkage of the vascular endothelial cells with a corresponding widening of the intercellular junctions (Figure 1.7). However, similar to the effects on vessel dilation, hypertonic saline solutions produce less vascular endothelial disruption than equiosmolar solutions of contrast media, thus suggesting an additional role of direct molecular toxicity or viscosity. Microscopic examination of vessels exposed in vivo and in vitro indicate greater alterations of endothelial permeability with sodium salts of the ratio-1.5 ionic media than with equiiodine concentrations of their meglumine salts (Wiedeman MP, 1963; Fuju K, et al, 1963). Although experimental evidence suggests greater aortic endothelial disruption with the iothalamate versus diatrizoate anion (Raininko R, 1979), any conclusion of relative efficacy based on this single study is probably not warranted. Each of the ratio-3 nonionic or ionic-dimeric media demonstrate less endothelial damage than equiiodine concentrations of the ratio-1.5 ionic media, with minimal differences between the low-osmolality agents (Almén T, 1985; Laernum F, 1983; Morettin LB, et al, 1984.

The vascular endothelial disruption induced by intravascular contrast media is usually rapidly reversible unless preexisting stasis of blood flow (e. g., ischemia, thrombus) prolongs the duration of contrast medium exposure to the vessel (Bettman MA, et al, 1984). Under this condition, or in the presence of preexisting vascular damage, an increased endothelial leakage of plasma proteins can result in activation of the complement system with subsequent leukocyte localization and microthrombosis formation at the site of endothelial disruption (Richie W, et al, 1974).

Pain/Warmth. The acute pain that routinely accompanies angiographic procedures is thought to be primarily related to the degree of direct vasodilation induced by the contrast agent (Padayachee TS, et al, 1983). It has also been suggested that delayed pain may be due, as least in part, to the extent of contrast-induced vascular endothelial damage (Thomas ML, et al, 1983). Although the incidence and intensity of pain is greatest with arterial injections, it also occurs following the injection of contrast media into veins that have

minimal dilation capacity. The adjunctive administration of the anesthetic agent, lidocaine, significantly reduces the pain of angiographic procedures, but has no effect on the degree of vessel dilation induced by the contrast medium (Padayachee TS, 1983). This would suggest that pain is mediated via a nervous route. Hyperosmolarity is the underlying factor responsible for both the dilation and endothelial disruption responses of intravascular contrast media, and is therefore directly related to the degree of pain experienced by patients during angiography procedures (Holder JC and Dalrymple GV, 1981). Contrast media considerations aimed at reducing the blood flow and endothelial disruption effects (see previous discussion) will also result in a reduction in pain.

In contrast to pain, the heat sensation that normally accompanies angiographic procedures is not influenced by the adjunctive administration of lidocaine (Gordon IJ and Wescott JL, 1977). Hence, this reponse may be due to the degree of direct vasodilation induced by the contrast medium and the subsequent increase in blood flow to the muscles and skin. It should be noted, however, that warmth is also a common complaint following the intravascular administration of the less vasoactive low-osmolality media. It has therefore been speculated that this sensation may be related to contrast medium exposure of the median eminence, an area of the brain that lacks the protective effects of the blood-brain barrier (Kido DK, et al, 1985). Stimulation of this region is known to produce effects on body temperature and the release of vasopressin.

GASTROINTESTINAL EFFECTS (TABLE 1.13): GENERAL ANGIOGRAPHY

Nausea and vomiting are commonly observed following the intravascular administration of angiographic contrast media. These gastrointestinal side effects are usually mild and self-limited with

Table 1.13 GASTROINTESTINAL EFFECTS OF ANGIOGRAPHIC CONTRAST MEDIA

PHYSIOLOGICAL EFFECT(S)	RESPONSE(S)	RESPONSIBLE CHEMOTOXIC FACTORS(S)
Area postrema: Alteration of neuroelectrical activity	Nausea Vomiting	Presence/concentration of ions · Hyperosmolality

minimal clinical significance unless they occur in infants or in patients with preexisting fluid or electrolyte imbalance. It has been suggested that these adverse gastrointestinal effects are due to direct contrast medium exposure of the area postrema, a region of the brain devoid of the protective effects of the blood-brain barrier (Kido DK, et al, 1985). The diminished number or lack of electrically charged ions associated with the ratio-3 ionic-dimeric or nonionic media, respectively, may result in less alteration of the normal neuroelectrical activity of this region, and thus explain their respective incidences of nausea and vomiting compared to equiiodine concentrations of the ratio-1.5 ionic media.

PULMONARY EFFECTS (TABLE 1.14): BOLUS INTRAVENOUS, RIGHT HEART, PULMONARY ARTERY INJECTIONS

Pulmonary Artery Blood Flow/Pressure. Pulmonary blood flow and blood pressure both significantly increase following the rapid intravenous, right atrium, right ventricle, or pulmonary artery administration of angiographic contrast media. In this regard, the immediate (i. e., 0–3 heartbeats) peak increases in flow and pressure are apparently related to the rapidly injected volumes since they can be reproduced by similar rapid injections of normal saline or blood. Analogous to their physiological effects on peripheral arteries (see Vascular Effects), the sustained (i. e., 10–30 heartbeats) elevation of pulmonary artery blood flow produced by hyperosmolar contrast media (not observed with normal saline or blood) is probably due to direct vessel dilation. As expected, the more hyperosmolar ratio-1.5 ionic media produce a greater effect than equiiodine concentrations of the ratio-3 low-osmolality media. In contradistinction to their peripheral hemodynamic response, this dilation of the pulmonary

Table 1.14 PULMONARY EFFECTS OF ANGIOGRAPHIC CONTRAST MEDIA

PHYSIOLOGICAL EFFECTS(S)	RESPONSE(S)	RESPONSIBLE CHEMOTOXIC FACTOR(S)
Pulmonary artery dilation · ↓ Vascular resistance	↑ Pulmonary artery blood flow	Rapidly injected volume (acute) Hyperosmolality (sustained)
Hypervolemia (systemic) · ↑ L. atrial pressure · ↑ Cardiac output	↑ Pulmonary artery blood pressure	Rapidly injected volume (acute) Hyperosmolality (sustained)
Desicocyte formation · ↑ Pulmonary capillary resistance	↑ Pulmonary artery blood pressure	Hyperosmolality
↓ L. ventricular contractility · ↑ L. atrial pressure	↑ Pulmonary artery blood pressure	Calcium-binding · Radiopaque anions · Sequestrants
Bezold-Jarisch reflex stimulation	Bradycardia · Systemic hypotension Apnea (acute) Tachypnea (secondary)	Hyperosmolality (?)
Bronchospasm	↓ Forced expiratory volume ↓ Maximal expiratory force	Pseudo-allergic (?)
Alteration of pulmonary capillary permeability (?)	Pulmonary edema (acute)	Molecular toxicity

artery is accompanied by a prolonged increase in pulmonary artery pressure. These actions of contrast media on pulmonary artery blood flow and pressure are greatest with direct pulmonary artery injections, diminishing with more peripheral (i. e., right ventricle, right atrium, intravenous, respectively) sites of administration (Lange PE, et al, 1984; Peck WW, et al, 1983).

The increase in pulmonary artery pressure that is commonly observed following the intravascular administration of angiographic contrast media can be explained by the increase in blood volume, decrease in peripheral vascular resistance (i. e., reduced cardiac afterload), and the resulting increase in cardiac output induced by these agents (see Vascular Effects). The increase in pulmonary artery pressure can also occur as a result of an increase in pulmonary venous pressure associated with contrast-induced depression of left ventricular contractility (see Cardiac Effects: Coronary Angiography) and a corresponding increase in left atrial pressure (Peck WW, et al, 1983). In an animal model of embolic pulmonary hypertension, the early and late rises in pulmonary artery pressure induced by hypertonic contrast media were abolished (Rees, CR, et al, 1988a). Rather, pulmonary artery pressure decreased and there was a greater than normal fall in systemic blood pressure apparently due to an inability to increase cardiac output in the presence of right-sided hypertension.

As previously discussed (see Vascular Effects), high blood concentrations of hyperosmolar contrast media can induce desicocyte formation. These morphologically altered and rigid red blood cells substantially increase blood viscosity and may become trapped in the capillary bed of the lungs, thus resulting in an increase in precapillary resistance (Almén T, et al, 1980). However, in fact, a decrease in pulmonary vascular resistance is commonly observed with injection of contrast media into the pulmonary artery (Peck WW, et al, 1983). Moreover, since these contrast-induced desicocytes would be expected to become lodged in the first capillary bed they encounter, it is difficult to associate this mechanism with the increase in pulmonary artery pressure ob-

served following peripheral arteriography or aortography procedures. This mechanism may, however, partially explain the higher incidence of adverse reactions encountered with intravenous versus intraarterial routes of administration.

Based on this discussion of factors that may be responsible for the elevation of pulmonary artery blood pressure, it is not surprising that this physiological effect of angiographic contrast media can be decreased by reducing the osmolality of the injected agent. As previously discussed, the degree of hypervolemia, increase in cardiac output, and the extent of desicocyte formation induced by intravascular contrast media are directly dependent on their osmolalities. Furthermore, it is the calcium-binding property of the ratio-1.5 ionic contrast media and sequestering agents within their formulations that is responsible for the depressive effect on left ventricular contractility. This cardiodepression is greatly reduced or eliminated with use of the ratio-3 ionic-dimeric or nonionic agents, respectively (see Cardiac Effects: Coronary Angiography).

Heart Rate/Systemic Blood Pressure/Respiration. In addition to effects on pulmonary artery blood flow and pressure, the intravenous, right heart, or pulmonary artery administration of angiographic contrast media stimulate a Bezold-Jarisch reflex within the lungs, resulting in bradycardia, systemic hypotension, and respiratory apnea (30–40 seconds) followed by rapid, shallow tachypnea. This response is also observed with multiple pulmonary emboli and, hence, may be associated with contrast-induced desicocyte formation or with an increase in pulmonary artery or venous pressures. Bilateral vagotomy eliminates this respiratory reflex experimentally, whereas intravenous atropine has no effect, thus implicating the role of the vagus nerve as an afferent branch of this response. Since procaine blockage of both pulmonary hili abolishes the postinjection apnea, the receptors of this reflex are apparently localized within this region (Bernstein EF, 1965).

Although there are no definitive studies that evaluate the role of contrast media hyperosmolality or molecular toxicity on the stimulation of this respiratory reflex, the possible relationship to desicocyte formation or changes in pulmonary blood pressure suggest a reduction of reflex activation with the use of contrast media of lower osmolalities. As a further consideration, subsequent exposure of the aorta to the contrast medium bolus will produce an osmolality-dependent arterial dilation with systemic hypotension that is additive to the bradycardia and hypotensive responses of this reflex (see Cardiac Effects: Left Ventriculography/Aortography).

Subclinical Bronchospasm. Intravascular contrast media can exert effects on the pulmonary airways resulting in an alteration of pulmonary function as measured by a decrease in forced expiratory volume and maximal expiratory force. Although the exact mechanism associated with this adverse reaction is unknown and perhaps more closely related to the pseudoallergic rather than chemotoxic effects of angiographic contrast media, its relationship to pulmonary physiology warrants discussion under this section. Fortunately, these bronchospasm effects of angiographic contrast media are usually mild and rarely result in overt clinical symptoms.

Early retrospective studies suggested that meglumine salts of the ratio-1.5 ionic contrast media produced a greater incidence of bronchospasm than their corresponding sodium salts (Ansell G, 1970), possibly due to a greater degree of induced histamine release (Rockoff SD and Brasch R, 1971). However, clinical studies designed specifically to evaluate this parameter found no significant differences between meglumine and sodium salts of ratio-1.5 ionic media in regard to the prevalence or magnitude of pulmonary function alterations in either atopic or nonatopic patients (Littner MR, et al, 1981). Atopic patients did demonstrate significantly greater decreases in pulmonary function compared to nonatopic patients, regardless of the media injected. No changes in pulmonary function were observed with "sham" procedures (i. e., needle puncture, injections of 5% Dextrose in Water) or with the injection of hypertonic sodium chloride solution (Littner MR, et al, 1977). The role of hyperos-

molality cannot be completely discounted, however, since the ratio-3 nonionic media, iohexol and iopamidol, have been shown to produce a decreased magnitude of subclinical bronchospasm compared to the ratio-1.5 ionic media (Dawson P, et al, 1983b; Saeed, M, et al, 1987). The ratio-3 ionic dimer, ioxaglate meglumine-sodium, also appears to produce less bronchospasm effects than the conventional ratio-1.5 media as demonstrated by a significantly reduced incidence of coughing during pulmonary angiography (Smith DC, et al, 1987). In a comparison of ioxaglate meglumine-sodium and iopamidol, there was no significant difference in regard to post-administration changes in forced expiratory volume (Longstall AJ and Henson JHL, 1985).

Pulmonary Edema. Pulmonary edema occurs when the net filtration of fluid from the pulmonary capillaries into the extravascular, extracellular lung spaces exceeds the draining capacity of this interstitial tissue. Contrast media can produce pulmonary edema by increasing the microvasculature driving pressure (i. e., increased pulmonary venous pressure) or by inducing direct disruption of the pulmonary vascular endothelium with a resultant increase in capillary permeability. Although the incidence of contrast-induced pulmonary edema is rare, it is a common finding in severe reactions or death (Måre K, et al, 1984a).

Since it has been shown that hypertonic solution can disrupt vascular endothelial permeability and can increase pulmonary venous pressure, it would be expected that the hyperosmolarity of the injected contrast media would be responsible for the induction of acute pulmonary edema. However, in an animal model of contrast-induced pulmonary edema it was demonstrated that the degree of acute increase in interstitial fluid accumulation did not correlate with the osmolality of the injected agent (Måre K, et al, 1983). For example, hypertonic solutions of sodium chloride, mannitol, or urea produced no acute increase in lung weight, whereas an equiosmolar solution of diatrizoate meglumine-sodium resulted in a significant increase in pulmonary interstitial fluid accumulation. Moreover, equal total iodine doses of different concentrations and, hence, different osmolalities of the same diatrizoate medium produced equivalent effects on lung water accumulation (Måre K, et al, 1984b). Additional evidence that the intrinsic molecular toxicity of the contrast medium is responsible for acute pulmonary edema is based on the observation that the ratio-3 agent, ioxaglate meglumine-sodium, produces greater fluid accumulation in the lung than an equiiodine concentration of the ratio-1.5 ionic medium, diatrizoate meglumine-sodium (Måre K, et al, 1984a). In this same model, the ratio-3 nonionic media, iohexol and iopamidol, produced less acute pulmonary edema than the ionic agents. The finding that the pulmonary edema effects of angiographic contrast media are not osmolality-dependent argues against the increased microvascular driving pressure mechanism, thereby enhancing the concept of direct vascular endothelial disruption. Respective differences in the sodium ion concentrations of contrast media may provide another explanation for these effects, however hypertonic sodium chloride did not produce the same increase in lung fluid accumulation as equiosmolar contrast media in the previously described pulmonary edema model.

It is important, at this point, to differentiate between contrast-induced acute pulmonary edema and the relative physiological effects of angiographic contrast media as they relate to preexisting pulmonary edema. The high dose administration of sodium salts of ionic contrast media to patients with congestive heart failure and normal renal function should be an area of concern. In contrast to meglumine derivatives, the extensive extravascular distribution and tubular reabsorption of the administered sodium ions increase the extravascular and intravascular osmotic load and may thus exacerbate the patient's edematous state. However, in patients with congestive failure and concomitant renal dysfunction neither the meglumine nor the sodium cations would be excreted or reabsorbed to a great extent, and both would contribute equally to the osmotic challenge (Talner LB, 1972). The increased osmotic load of ratio-1.5 ionic media combined with their greater alterations of pulmonary artery and venous pressures, left ventricular contractility, and left atrial pressure would render these agents more likely to produce worsening of preexisting pulmonary edema than would equivalent use of the ratio-3 low-osmolality agents.

RENAL EFFECTS (TABLE 1.15): GENERAL ANGIOGRAPHY, RENAL ARTERIOGRAPHY, AORTOGRAPHY

The primary route of excretion of each of the angiographic contrast media is via the kidneys (see Pharmacokinetics). It is therefore not surprising that these agents

Table 1.15   RENAL EFFECTS OF ANGIOGRAPHIC CONTRAST MEDIA

PHYSIOLOGICAL EFFECT(S)	RESPONSE(S)	RESPONSIBLE CHEMOTOXIC FACTOR(S)
Renovascular dilation (transient) · ↓ Vascular resistance	↑ Renal blood flow (transient)	Hyperosmolality
Renovascular constriction (sustained) · ↑ Vascular resistance	↓ Renal blood flow (sustained)	Hyperosmolality · Renin release · Osmotic diuresis · Desicocyte formation
Alteration of glomerular permeability	Albuminuria	Hyperosmolality
Renal tubular toxicity	Enzymuria Osmotic nephrosis	Molecular toxicity (?)

can produce alterations in renal function as a result of their physiological effects on the renal vasculature, the glomerular tuft, and the renal tubules. These effects of angiographic contrast media on renal physiology may manifest as proteinuria, elevations in serum creatinine or blood urea nitrogen, or oliguria, which may persist for several days. The incidence and severity of these nephrotoxic effects of angiographic contrast media are greatest for radiographic procedures (e. g., renal arteriography, aortography) that directly expose the renal arteries to high doses and concentrations of the agent (Harkonen S and Kjellstrand C, 1981).

Renovascular Effects. Renal artery exposure to high concentrations of angiographic contrast media results initially in the expected hyperosmolality-induced vessel dilation and increase in renal blood flow. Unlike other peripheral vascular beds, however, this vasodilation is followed by sustained (i. e., up to 15 minutes) vasoconstriction and a substantial decrease in renal blood flow (Byrd L and Sherman RL, 1979; Golman K and Holtas S, 1980).

It has been suggested that the renovascular constrictive effect of angiographic contrast media may be related to an initial dilation-induced stimulation of the juxto-glomerular apparatus with subsequent activation of the renin-angiotensin system. The released vasoconstrictive products (i. e., renin, angiotensin) are known to exert pronounced effects on the renal vasculature. In this regard, increased renin release has been demonstrated but it is not a consistent finding post renal angiography. Moreover, converting enzyme inhibitors and angiotensin-II blockers do not completely abolish the renal vasoconstrictive response to intravascular contrast media (Larson, TS, et al, 1983), thus suggesting the involvement of (an) alternate mechanism(s).

The reduction in renal blood flow may be related to rapid glomerular excretion of the hypertonic contrast medium. Within the renal tubules, the nonreabsorbable contrast agent exerts an osmotic effect, thus preventing the reabsorption of water. The resulting osmotic diuresis leads to an increase in intratubular and, subsequently, intracapsular pressures, which may in turn cause compression of the glomerular capillary loops, an increase in total renal vascular resistance, and a decrease in renal perfusion.

A recent study (Arend LJ, et al, 1987) suggests that the decrease in renal blood flow produced by intravascular hypertonic, contrast media may be mediated by an increase in intrarenal adenosine levels. Systemic arterial and venous adenosine levels did not increase post contrast injection; however, the urinary concentration of adenosine significantly increased. Co-administration of the adenosine receptor antagonist, theophylline, reduced substantially the renal vasoconstrictive effects of the intravascular media.

Finally, the observed decrease in renal blood flow could be explained by contrast-induced desicocyte formation with subsequent blockage of renal capillary flow and an increase in renal capillary resistance. However, this mechanism cannot account for the renovascular constriction and decreased renal perfusion observed with intravenous procedures wherein the rigidified red cells would be expected to become trapped in the pulmonary capillaries.

The degree of initial dilation and subsequent constriction of the renal vascular bed is dependent on the hyperosmolality of the injected contrast medium (Byrd L and Sherman RL, 1979; Golman K and Holtas S, 1980). Hypertonic solutions of saline, urea, or dextrose produce qualitatively and quantitatively equivalent effects as equiosmolar concentrations of the angiographic contrast media. Moreover, equiiodine concentrations of the ratio-3 low osmolality media produce a diminished response in comparison to the ratio-1.5 ionic media. That hyperosmolality is the determining factor in these hemodynamic effects is consistent with each of the proposed mechanisms since reducing the osmolality of the injected contrast medium is known to produce less effects on direct vessel dilation and, hence, less stimulation of the juxtoglomerular apparatus; less osmotic diuresis; and less erythrocyte rigidification. Following an intravenous injection, the concentration and osmolality of the contrast medium reaching the renal artery would be considerably less than that associated with renal arteriography or aortography. Hence, the relationship between hyperosmolarity and the renovascular constrictive effects of angiographic contrast media is also consistent with the reduced incidence of nephrotoxic reactions observed with intravenous versus direct renal artery procedures.

Alterations in Glomerular Permeability. The renal artery injection of hyperosmolar contrast media is associated with a substantial increase in the concentration of urinary albumin, reflecting contrast-induced alterations in the glomerular permeability. Presumably, this physiological effect is related to hyperosmolarity-induced cellular diuresis and shrinkage of the endothelial cells of the capillaries comprising the glomerular tuft. However, the direct molecular toxicity of the contrast medium may also be a major factor (Golman K and Holtas S, 1980). The ratio-1.5 ionic media have been shown to produce significantly greater albuminuria than equiiodine concentrations of the ratio-3 low-osmolality agents (Törnquist C, et al, 1980).

It should be noted that a disruption of glomerular permeability can also be caused by a decrease in renal blood flow or by the infusion of renin (see preceding Renovascular Effects). Furthermore, an increase in urinary albumin concentration may not only indicate alterations in glomerular permeability, but may also reflect renal tubular damage and associated inhibition of the normal albumin reabsorption process (Golman K and Holtas S, 1980).

Renal Tubular Toxicity. Angiographic contrast media concentrated within the kidney can affect renal tubular physiology as demonstrated by an increase in the urinary excretion of various enzymes known to be present in the brush border of proximal tubular cells (e. g, alkaline phosphatase, leucinearylpeptidase, lactic dehydrogenase, SGOT, alanine aminopeptidase) or intracellularly within lysosomes (i. e., lysozyme, N-acetyl-beta-glucosamidase) (Byrd L, and Sherman RL, 1979; Golman K and Holtas S, 1980; Severini, G, et al, 1987). It has been shown that renal artery injections of equiiodine doses of the ratio-3 medium, metrizamide, and the ratio-1.5 ionic agent, iothalamate meglumine, resulted in equivalent levels of enzymuria (Golman K and Holtas S, 1980), thus suggesting a dependence on direct molecular toxicity rather than osmolality. A consideration in this regard, however, is the fact that the nonionic medium would achieve a urinary concentration approximately twice that of the meglumine salt of the ratio-1.5 ionic agent due to its reduced osmotic diuretic effects. It should be further noted that in addition to direct contrast-induced damage to the tubular cells, the observed enzymuria may also reflect the previously described alterations in glomerular permeability (Golman K and Holtas S, 1980).

Additional evidence of the renal tubular toxicity of angiographic contrast media is based on their induced reduction in the renal extraction of paraaminohippurate, a diagnostic agent that is primarily secreted via the renal tubules. This decrease in paraaminohippurate excretion could not be experimentally reproduced by equiosmolar control solutions, again suggesting a dependence on direct molecular toxicity rather than osmolality (Byrd L and Sherman RL, 1979).

The direct renal tubular toxicity of angiographic contrast media has also been implicated by the observation of an increased number of vacuoles within the cytoplasm of proximal tubular cells biopsied post renal arteriography and intravenous urography (Moreau J-F, et al, 1980). The exact cause of this "osmotic nephrosis" in uncertain. It is not related to hyperosmolality, per se, since the ratio-3 nonionic and ionic-dimeric media produce effects similar to both the meglumine and the sodium salts of ratio-1.5 ionic media. It does appear that an underlying nephropathy is a requirement for contrast-induced osmotic nephrosis; however, the intensity of subsequent vacuolization does not correlate with the severity of the preexisting disease, the dose of the medium, or the degree of eventual functional impairment. It has been speculated that this osmotic nephrosis may be related to increased tubular cell pinocytosis of protein-bound contrast medium as stimulated by the contrast-induced proteinuria.

In in vitro studies, the ratio-1.5 contrast media have been shown to directly inhibit metabolic processes (e. g., sodium transport, ATP-metabolism, respiratory rate) within proximal renal tubular segments (Humes HD, et al, 1987a). These effects appear to be potentiated by the presence of meglumine cations or hypoxia. The ratio-1.5 anions can also directly interact with the proximal tubular membranes to form a dense precipitate that may contribute to intraluminal obstruction. Preliminary investigations also suggest that the ratio-3 nonionic media may exhibit less metabolic toxicity and potential for precipitate formation (Humes HD, 1987b). It should be noted, however, that these in vitro comparisons were made using equal millimolar concentrations of the respective media. Following systemic administration of the same total iodine dose, differences in the osmotic diuretic activities of these agents would result in a urinary concentration of the ratio-1.5 media that is approximately one-half that of the ratio-3 media.

Summary. Based on this discussion, it is evident that the exact pathogenesis of contrast-induced nephrotoxicity is uncertain and may involve a combination of factors. It is interesting to note that each of the described physiological effects (i. e., renovascular effects, alterations in glomerular permeability, renal tubular toxicity) of angiographic contrast media can lead to an increase in the concentration of urinary proteins. Hence, the combination of these contrast-induced effects may result in significant proteinuria, and subsequent precipitation of these proteins

in the renal tubules may lead to obstruction and renal failure. The reduced level of proteinuria observed with intravenous versus renal artery or aortic injections of angiographic contrast media is consistent with respective differences in the incidence of acute renal failure (Golman K and Holtas S, 1980).

Note also that each of the undesirable physiological effects of angiographic contrast media may be enhanced by the presence of preexisting renal disease. For example, the renal vasoconstrictive effects of contrast media are further increased in the presence of diabetic vascular disease, renal hypertension, atherosclerotic disease, age-associated decreases in renal blood flow, and the previous physiological effects of multiple contrast injections. Similarly, contrast-induced alterations in glomerular permeability and tubular function can present an increased risk to patients with preexisting proteinuria (i. e., due to multiple myeloma, dehydration) or renal tubular dysfunction. Angiographic contrast media, ratio-1.5 ionic or ratio-3 low-osmolality, should be administered with caution to these at-risk patients (see Clinical Use/Contraindications).

CEREBRAL EFFECTS (TABLE 1.16): CEREBRAL ANGIOGRAPHY

Angiographic contrast media within the cerebral circulation can produce undesirable physiological effects on carotid blood flow, heart rate and systemic blood pressure, blood-brain barrier permeability, and central nervous system activity.

Frequently, the radiology literature combines these physiological effects in describing the "neurotoxicity" of intracarotid contrast media. It must be emphasized, however, that each of these effects of angiographic contrast media is due to a separate mechanism and may, therefore, be dependent on differing characteristics of the administered agent. Furthermore, each effect is manifested in a different clinical response. For example, the sensations of pain and discomfort that accompany cerebral angiography are associated

Table 1.16   CEREBRAL EFFECTS OF ANGIOGRAPHIC CONTRAST MEDIA

PHYSIOLOGICAL EFFECT(S)	RESPONSE(S)	RESPONSIBLE CHEMOTOXIC FACTOR(S)
External carotid artery dilation · ↓ Vascular resistance	↑ External carotid blood flow · Redistribution ICA-ECA flow Pain	Hyperosmolality
Carotid chemoreceptor stimulation · Carotid body · Internal carotid chemoreceptors · External carotid chemoreceptors	Tachypnea (general) · Bradycardia–hypotension · Tachycardia · Hypertension (systemic)	Hyperosmolality
Alteration of blood-brain barrier permeability	Potential CNS exposure · Neurotoxicity	Hyperosmolality
Alteration of neuroelectrical activity	CNS excitation/depression	Presence/concentration of ions · Hyperosmolality

with contrast-induced dilation of the external carotid artery, whereas the effects on systemic blood pressure, heart rate, and respirations are due to stimulation of carotid chemoreceptors. These hemodynamic effects occur independent of the degree of blood-brain barrier disruption or the central nervous system toxicity induced by the respective angiographic medium.

Carotid Artery Effects. Injection of an angiographic contrast medium into the common carotid artery results in the expected hyperosmolarity-induced increase in common carotid blood flow. This flow increase is primarily associated with contrast-induced dilation of the external carotid artery. The internal carotid arteries do not dilate in response to hyperosmolar contrast media as evidenced by a minimal rise of blood flow with selective injection into this branch of the cerebral circulation. Following common carotid administration of a contrast medium, these differing responses of the external and internal carotid arteries can result in a redistribution of the normal cerebral blood flow, favoring the vascular bed of the external carotid (Hilal SK, 1966).

As previously discussed (see Vascular Effects), the degree of pain and discomfort that accompany angiographic procedures are related to the extent of vessel dilation induced by the injected contrast medium. It is therefore not surprising that the common carotid or selective external carotid administration of a hyperosmolar contrast medium produces considerably more discomfort to the patient than selective angiography of the internal carotids.

Analogous to the physiological effects of angiographic media on the peripheral arteries (see Vascular Effects), the degree of external carotid dilation and the associated pain and discomfort of cerebral angiography procedures are primarily dependent on the osmolality of the injected agent (Morris TW, et al, 1979). Pure meglumine salts of the ratio-1.5 ionic media produce significantly less discomfort than equiiodine concentrations of pure sodium salts or combination meglumine/sodium derivatives (Shealy CN, 1963; Dempsey PJ, et al, 1975). There are minimal differences, in this regard, between the diatrizoate or iothalamate anions, provided cationic formulations of equivalent sodium content are compared (Kricheff II and Chase NE, 1967). As expected, equiiodine concentrations of the ratio-3 nonionic and ionic-dimeric media produce less dilation of the external carotid and less subjective discomfort than the ratio-1.5 ionic media (Norman D, et al, 1984; Cronqvist S, 1983; Bird CR, et al, 1984).

Systemic Blood Pressure, Heart Rate, Respiration. The injection of an angiographic contrast medium into the common carotid artery produces a complex series of reflex actions on heart rate, systemic blood pressure, and respiration resulting from the stimulation of various chemoreceptors within the cerebral circulation (Higgins CB and Schmidt WS, 1979). The principal components of this carotid chemoreflex are an initial phase (2–4 seconds) of bradycardia-induced hypotension and increased respirations followed by a secondary phase (5–10 seconds) of tachycardia, increased blood pressure, and increased respirations. The initial hypotensive phase is apparently associated with contrast stimulation of the carotid body and is mediated via the vagal nerve. Experimental denervation of the carotid body abolishes this bradycardia effect of intracarotid contrast media as does cholinergic blockage. The secondary increase in heart rate results from contrast stimulation of chemoreceptors within the internal carotid circulation, whereas the secondary increase in blood pressure is due to stimulation of chemoreceptors in the external carotid circulation. Experimental ligation of the internal carotids abolishes the secondary tachycardia, but has no effect on the secondary hypertension. This secondary increase in blood pressure is not related to carotid body or baroreceptor stimulation since it persists following elimination of the initial hypotensive phase. The chemoreceptor responses of this hypertensive phase are mediated via a sympathetic mechanism that can be interrupted by alpha or beta blockade.

The heart rate and blood pressure alterations actually observed following the intracarotid administration of angiographic contrast media are dependent on the nature of patient preparation for the procedure. As previously described, prior administration of the anticholinergic agent, atropine, will abolish the initial hypotensive phase, and tachycardia and hypertension will predominate. In contrast, the prior administration of anesthetic agents can abolish the adrenergically mediated tachycardia and hypertensive reflexes, and the initial bradycardia-induced hypotension will prevail. The tachypnea common to both phases will

occur regardless of the nature of patient preparation.

The degree of carotid chemoreflex stimulation and the incidence and severity of subsequent heart rate, blood pressure, and respiratory alterations also appear to be dependent on the osmolality of the injected contrast medium (Morris TW, et al, 1979). It should be noted, however, that sodium salts of the ratio-1.5 ionic media seem to produce chemoreceptor stimulation in excess of what would be expected based on relative differences in their osmolality compared to equiiodine concentrations of the meglumine media (Fischer HW and Rodman HC, 1971; Morris TW, et al, 1979). Again, there are no apparent differences between equivalent cationic formulations of the diatrizoate, iothalamate, or metrizoate anions. The changes in heart rate, blood pressure, and respirations produced by the ratio-3 nonionic or ionic-dimeric media are minimal and less than equiiodine concentrations of the ratio-1.5 ionic media (Morris TW, et al, 1979; Higgins CB and Schmidt WS, 1979).

Blood-Brain Barrier Alterations. Experimental animal studies have demonstrated that the intracarotid injection of supraclinical doses of angiographic contrast media can produce alterations in the blood-brain barrier as measured by an abnormal leakage of radioactive ions (e.g., P-32 sodium phosphate, Hg-197 mercuric chloride or acetate) or protein-bound dyes (e.g., Tryptan Blue, Evans Blue) into the extravascular spaces of the brain (Junck L and Marshall WH, 1983). It has been proposed that at least two mechanisms may be involved in this contrast-induced alteration of blood-brain barrier permeability: (1) as a result of its direct molecular toxicity the contrast medium stimulates pinocytotic activity within and the transport of ions through the vascular endothelial cells; and (2) the hypertonicity of the contrast medium produces cellular diuresis and shrinkage of the vascular endothelial cells with corresponding opening of the normally tight endothelial junctions that comprise the blood-brain barrier. The first mechanism is reflected by contrast-induced leakage of radioactive ions whereas the second mechanism permits the leakage of ions and the larger protein-bound dyes (Gonsette RE and Liesenborgh L, 1980).

That the molecular toxicity of a contrast medium is an important factor in blood-brain barrier physiology is evidenced by the significantly greater brain extravasation of radioactive ions induced by the ratio-3 nonionic agent, metrizamide, compared to other low-osmolality media (e. g., iohexol, ioxaglate meglumine-sodium) (Aulie A, 1980; Golman K, 1979). Similarly, the ratio-1.5 ionic contrast media produce greater alterations of blood-brain barrier permeability than equiosmolar solutions of hypertonic mannitol, glucose, or sodium fluoride (Junck L and Marshall WH, 1983; Sage MR, et al, 1983). The importance of hyperosmolarity on blood-brain barrier disruption is demonstrated by a greater leakage of protein-bound dyes with the ratio-1.5 ionic media versus equiiodine concentrations of the ratio-3 low-osmolality agents (Sage MR, et al, 1983; Golman K, 1979; Michelet AA, 1987). Based on animal studies, it has been suggested that the threshold for hyperosmolality-induced opening of the blood-brain barrier is approximately 1200 mOsm/kg; whereas below 800 mOsm/kg, there appears to be negligible disruption (Rapoport SI, et al, 1974). Contrast-induced alterations in the blood-brain barrier may also be dependent on dosage. For example, Zamani, et al (1982) found no induced abnormalities of the blood-brain barrier with intravenous contrast medium (i. e., diatrizoate meglumine 60% w/v) dosages of less than 3 mL/kg; however, leakage was observed at intravenous dosages of 4–6 mL/kg.

Within the ratio-1.5 ionic media group, sodium salts of the radiopaque anions demonstrate significantly greater potential for blood-brain barrier disruption than equiiodine concentrations of meglumine salts (Kodama JK, et al, 1963; Jeppsson PG and Olin T, 1970). Some experimental studies have demonstrated increased blood-brain barrier disruption with the diatrizoate versus iothalamate anion (Kodama JK, et al, 1963); whereas other studies have revealed the opposite effect (Jeppsson PG and Olin T, 1970; Cassady RL, et al, 1978). The actual difference between these anions in regard to induced blood-brain barrier alterations is probably negligible at routine clinical dosage levels.

To date, no experimental studies have specifically addressed the effect of contrast formulation sequestering agents (see Chemistry) on the degree of blood-brain barrier damage induced by intracarotid contrast media. It has been shown, however, that the addition of calcium ions to the ratio-1.5 ionic medium, metrizoate sodium, and to the ratio-3 nonionic media, iohexol and metrizamide, significantly reduces their respective alterations of blood-brain barrier permeability (Salvesen S, et al, 1967; Golman K, 1979). Apparently, the added calcium ions counteract the endothelial disruptive effects of sodium ions or hypertonicity, or prevent structural alterations of desmosomes. Based on these studies, one questions whether the increased calcium-binding effects of contrast media formulations that contain the edetate disodium/sodium citrate sequestering agents may have a greater potential for blood-brain barrier alterations than comparable media that contain the calcium edetate disodium sequestrant.

Neurotoxicity. The unaltered blood-brain barrier restricts the passage of intravascular ionic or nonionic contrast media into the extravascular spaces of the brain and their subsequent exposure to the cells of the central nervous system. Hence, the neurotoxic effects of angiographic contrast media become important primarily in the presence of preexisting (i. e., cerebral tumor, abscess, infarct) or contrast-induced alterations of the blood-brain barrier; the latter situation being unlikely at routine angiographic dosage levels. The neurotoxic effects of angiographic contrast media may also be important in procedures (i. e., vertebral arteriography) that expose the spinal cord to high doses and concentrations of the agent.

Experimental studies have demonstrated variable concentrations of intravenously administered contrast media within the cerebral spinal fluid (CSF) in the absence of blood-brain barrier disruption (Harnish PP, et al 1988). In this regard, the CSF may represent a reservoir for contrast that have diffused through the blood-brain barrier and localized within the interstitial spaces of the brain. It is also possible that intravascular contrast media may enter the CSF via regions of the brain that lack the protective vascular permeability barrier or directly through the choroid plexus. Ratio-1.5 ionic media are known to decrease CSF production by the choroid plexus (Harnish PP, et al, 1984; 1988a).

Central nervous system exposure to nonphysiological electrically charged ions can inhibit normal or elicit abnormal neuroelectrical activity. Thus the ionic nature and hyperosmolarity (i.e., concentration of ions) of the angiographic contrast medium are important factors in regard to its potential for induced neurotoxicity (Bryan RN and Hershkowitz N, 1984). In the presence of an altered blood-brain barrier, the ratio-1.5 ionic media would therefore be expected to exert more neurotoxic effects than an equiiodine concentration of the ratio-3 ionic-dimer, ioxaglate meglumine-sodium. The ratio-3 nonionic media would have the least neurotoxic potential because of their lack of electrical charges (Gonsette RE and Liesenborgh L, 1980; Bryan RN, et al, 1982). Within the ratio-1.5 ionic group, meglumine salts are less neurotoxic than equiiodine concentrations of their corresponding sodium salts (Kodama JK, et al, 1963; Hilal SK, 1966). Based on toxicological evaluations of the mean lethal dose following direct intracerebral injection and the mean least convulsive dose following spinal arteriography, the iothalamate anion appears to be approximately one-half as neurotoxic as the diatrizoate anion (Kodama JK, et al, 1963; Albertson KW, et al, 1973).

Several considerations must be borne in mind when extrapolating these findings to the potential neurotoxic effects of an angiographic contrast medium. First, the contrast medium will not normally come into contact with the central nervous tissue unless there is damage to the blood-brain barrier. Second, the total amount of the contrast medium that may be expected to penetrate through the altered blood-brain barrier and be present in the extravascular space of the brain is substantially less than the volumes and concentrations utilized in experimental toxicological studies. Finally, it is assumed that the extravasated contrast medium will primarily expose brain tissue that is already damaged or abnormal (i.e., tumor, abscess) and will have minimal contact with normal central nervous system tissue.

CARDIAC EFFECTS (TABLE 1.17): CORONARY ARTERIOGRAPHY

The selective injection of an angiographic contrast medium into the coronary arteries can produce profound hemodynamic and electrophysiologic effects due to a complex interaction of direct and reflex mechanisms. These physiological effects of contrast media on the myocardium are of primary importance in coronary angiography procedures but may also be observed to a lesser degree with injection into the cardiac chambers or great vessels.

Coronary Artery Dilation. Injection of an angiographic contrast medium into a coronary artery produces an immediate (i.e., 0–4 second) decrease in respective blood flow; the extent of this decrease being directly proportional to the volume of injection. Equivolume injections of ratio-1.5 ionic and ratio-3 nonionic media produce similar early reductions in blood flow, thus indicating that this transient hemodyanamic effect is not related to the hyperosmolality of the injected medium but rather the effects of the contrast agent on blood viscosity (Friedman HZ, et al, 1987).

Similar to the physiological effects of angiographic contrast media on peripheral arteries (see Vascular Effects), the selective injection of a hyperosmolar contrast medium into the coronary arteries results in an osmolality-dependent dilation of the

Table 1.17 CARDIAC EFFECTS OF ANGIOGRAPHIC CONTRAST MEDIA: CORONARY ANGIOGRAPHY

PHYSIOLOGICAL EFFECT(S)	RESPONSE(S)	RESPONSIBLE CHEMOTOXIC FACTOR(S)
Coronary artery dilation · ↓ Vascular resistance	↑ Coronary artery blood flow	Hyperosmolality
Coronary stretch receptor stimulation	Electrocardiographic alterations · Sinus bradycardia-hypotension · Conduction delays · Ventricular fibrillation	Hyperosmolality Sodium ion concentration
Hypocalcemia (coronary sinus)	Ventricular fibrillation ↓ L. ventricular contractility (initial) · ↓ Cardiac output · Hypotension (systemic)	Calcium binding · Radiopaque anions · Sequestrants
Adrenergic reflex stimulation	↑ L. ventricular contractility (secondary)	Hyperosmolality

vessel and a secondary increase in coronary blood flow (Hayward R and Dawson P, 1984; Gerber KH and Higgins CB, 1982a). Sodium salts of the ratio-1.5 ionic media induce a greater degree of direct arterial dilation than equiiodine concentrations of meglumine salts; the differences between equivalent cationic formulations of the radiopaque anions (i. e., diatrizoate, iothalamate, metrizoate) being negligible (Hilal SK, 1966). Per given iodine concentration, the ratio-3 nonionic and ionic-dimeric media produce less alteration of coronary blood flow than the ratio-1.5 ionic media; however, the respective coronary blood flow differences between these media groups are not as great as the blood flow differences observed with peripheral artery injections (Gerber KH and Higgins CB, 1982a). It is known that the coronary vascular bed can only dilate to a certain maximum degree. Hence an explanation for the diminished differences in coronary versus peripheral blood flow changes between the ratio-1.5 ionic and ratio-3 low-osmolality media may be that the former agents are inducing or approaching these maximum dilation effects within the coronary arteries.

Following selective coronary artery injection of a given hyperosmolar contrast medium, the percent increase in coronary blood flow is greater in patients with normal coronary arteries than in patients with cardiovascular disease (Bassan M, et al, 1975). This phenomenon occurs because the stenotic process has already produced maximal compensatory dilation of the resistant vessels. Such differences in the contrast-induced dilation of normal versus diseased coronary arteries may lead to a coronary steal phenomenon and the precipitation or worsening of an ischemic event in patients with preexisting cardiovascular disease (Emanuelsson H, et al, 1983).

Chronotropic Effects/Ventricular Fibrillation. Selective coronary artery injection of a hyperosmolar contrast medium produces a dose-dependent inhibition of impulse generation and conduction within the myocardium. These electrophysiologic effects occur independent of sinoartrial or artrioventricular node exposure to the contrast medium, and can be blocked by the prior administration of atropine or by experimental bilateral vagotomy. It thus appears that the sinus slowing and conduction delays (i. e., prolongation of P–R interval) observed in coronary angiography are related to a reflex vagal mechanism, perhaps vasodilation-induced stimulation of coronary stretch receptors (Abe S, et al, 1976).

The electrophysiological effects of intracoronary contrast media are primarily dependent on the osmolality of the injected agent and can be reproduced by hypertonic sodium chloride, meglumine chloride, glucose, and mannitol solutions. This finding is consistent with the reflex involvement of coronary stretch receptors, since, as previously discussed, the degree of direct coronary artery dilation induced by an angiographic contrast medium is also osmolality dependent. Therefore, as expected, the negative chronotropic effects of intracoronary contrast media can be reduced by utilizing equiiodine concentrations of the ratio-3 low-osmolality versus the ratio-1.5 ionic media (Higgins CB, 1984; Trägardh B, 1980). Within the latter groups of agents, there are no conclusive studies that demonstrate the superiority of the diatrizoate, iothalamate, or metrizoate anion for coronary angiography. Per given iodine concentration, meglumine salts of these radiopaque anions produce less inhibition of impulse generation and conduction than sodium salts; the electrophysiology of the myocardium being particularly sensitive to the sodium concentration of the injected medium (Gensini GG and DiGiorgi S, 1964; Brown TG, 1967). It must be emphasized, however, that the appropriate ratio-1.5 contrast medium for coronary angiography should not be a pure meglumine derivative; some sodium is required to prevent an increased incidence of ventricular fibrillation.

Ventricular fibrillation occurs as a result of the dyssnchronous conduction of premature impulses through an incompletely repolarized myocardium, thus allowing the formation of multiple reentrant pathways. As previously described, early experimental studies compared the myocardial toxicity of sodium and meglumine salts of ratio-1.5 ionic media and demonstrated that pure sodium salts produced a substantially greater incidence and duration of hemodynamic and negative chronotropic alterations following intracoronary administration. As the sodium concentration of the injected contrast medium decreased, so did its respective cardiotoxic effects. Based on these observations, the manufacturer of a combination meglumine-sodium (6.6:1 ratio, 4.48 mg sodium/mL) diatrizoate medium altered the cationic composition of this agent to make it a pure meglumine salt.

Subsequent clinical use of this pure meglumine medium for coronary angiography unexpectedly resulted in an increased incidence of ventricular fibrillation compared to previous use of the combination agent (Paulin S and Adams DF, 1971). Various experimental studies have since confirmed that the complete absence of sodium or its decrease to very low levels in ratio-1.5 ionic contrast media intended for intracoronary administration significantly increases the frequency of ventricular fibrillation (Snyder C, et al, 1971; Simon AL, et al, 1972; Almén T, 1973).

The observations that the presence of sodium in ratio-1.5 ionic media reduces the potential for ventricular fibrillation during coronary angiography raise an interesting question as to the mechanism involved in this protective effect. A possible explanation for this mechanism came from a study wherein the measurement of monophasic action potentials from the heart muscle revealed that both the combination meglumine/sodium (4.48 mg sodium/mL) and the pure meglumine (0.91 mg sodium/mL) derivatives of ratio-1.5 ionic media prolong the time of cardiac depolarization as a result of their osmolality-dependent, negative chronotropic effects. However, increasing the sodium concentration from 0.91 to 4.48 mg/mL resulted in greater prolongation of the repolarization phase (i.e., greater T-wave alterations) and lengthening of the refractory period. This lengthening of the refractory period displaces the vulnerable period of the myocardial cell temporally from the prolonged depolarization, and, in a manner, may serve to protect the myocardium from fibrillation (Simon AL, et al, 1972).

Based on strenuous experimental conditions involving prolonged (i.e., 25–30 seconds) coronary artery injections it has been shown that the ratio-3 nonionic media (i.e., iohexol, iopamidol), which lack substantial amounts of sodium, produce a significantly greater incidence of ventricular fibrillation than ratio-1.5 ionic or ratio-3 ionic-dimeric (i.e., ioxaglate meglumine-sodium) media, which do contain sodium (Morris TW, et al, 1986; Donadieu AM, et al, 1987; Morris TW, 1988). Moreover, in this same animal model, the addition of sodium to the nonionic media resulted in a significantly reduced propensity for fibrillatory effects (Morris TW, 1988). In contradistinction, with other experimental models it has been shown that the nonionic media (unmodified) have a very low potential to produce venticular fibrillation (Wolf GL, et al 1981a;

En Piao, Z, et al, 1987; Piao, ZE, et al, 1988), and that the addition of sodium to these agents increased significantly the frequency of fibrillatory effects (En Piao Z, et al, 1987). The discrepancy in these findings is most likely related to differences in the experimental conditions employed. Whether the results observed with any of these animal models can be directly extrapolated to conditions predisposing to ventricular fibrillation in the clinical setting also remains a question. Therefore final conclusions as to the relative fibrillatory propensities of the two categories of low-osmolality media (i. e., nonionic versus ionic-dimeric) awaits more extensive clinical evaluations or experience.

The exact concentration of sodium that should be present in a combination meglumine-sodium ratio-1.5 contrast medium for coronary angiography has not been determined. It is obvious, however, that very low or high concentrations will increase the incidence of undesirable physiological effects. It has been demonstrated that the coronary artery injection of ratio-1.5 ionic media containing less than 1.6 mg sodium/mL resulted in a high frequency of electrocardiographic abnormalities (Simon AL, et al, 1972), whereas combination salts of diatrizoate and iothalamate (Table 1.4) that contain 3.6–4.5 mg sodium/mL (6.6:1 meglumine-sodium ratio) or 9.4 mg sodium/mL (2:1 meglumine-sodium ratio) had considerably less fibrillatory potential (Paulin S and Adams DF, 1971; Snyder C, et al, 1971; Carter AM and Olin T, 1973).

Another important factor related to the fibrillatory propensity of an intracoronary contrast medium is the degree of direct calcium binding exhibited by the agent. That the hypocalcemic effects of intracoronary contrast media lead to further alterations of impulse generation and conduction is demonstrated by the fact that the addition of calcium ions to ratio-1.5 ionic media results in less electrocardiographic disturbances (Trägardh B, et al, 1974; Thomson KR, et al, 1978; Wolf GL, 1980). In addition, contrast-induced decreases in extracellular calcium and potassium concentrations accelerate the spontaneous firing rate of Purkinje fibers. This hypocalcemic effect combined with the osmolality-dependent sinus bradycardia can give rise to the formation of ectopic beats from latent pacemaker cells within the myocardium. The additional dyssynchronous effects of these hypocalcemia-induced ectopic beats and conduction delays further promote the development of reentry mechanisms and ventricular fibrillation (Wolpers HG, et al, 1984).

Angiographic contrast media can produce hypocalcemia by two mechanisms; direct binding of cationic calcium ions by the radiopaque anion, or by sequestrant chelating agents within the contrast media formulations (Wolpers HG, et al, 1981; Morris TW, et al, 1982). Since sodium salts of the ratio-1.5 ionic media dissociate in solution to a greater extent than meglumine salts, they present an increased number of distinct anions available for calcium binding. Compared to these ionic media, an equiiodine concentration of the ratio-3 ionic-dimeric agent, ioxaglate meglumine-sodium, yields 50%, or less, of the available calcium-binding anions (Wolpers HG, et al, 1981). Ratio-3 nonionic media are devoid of calcium-binding anions. These considerations describe and explain, in part, the respective fibrillatory propensities of these agents.

As previously described (see Chemistry), the combination of sequestering agents, edetate disodium (0.04% w/v) and sodium citrate (0.32% w/v), can directly chelate 13 mMols of calcium per liter of contrast formulation (Wolpers HG, et al, 1981). The alternative sequestrant, calcium edetate disodium, is devoid of calcium-binding activity. The significance of the respective calcium-binding properties of these routinely utilized sequestrants is demonstrated by the observation that the intracoronary injection of a saline solution containing edetate disodium (0.04% w/v) and sodium citrate (0.32% w/v) produced marked prolongation of the Q–T interval and ventricular fibrillation, whereas saline, alone, or a saline solution containing calcium edetate disodium (0.1% w/v) produced no chronotrophic effects (Murdock DK, et al, 1984a). Clinical and experimental studies have shown a significant reduction in the incidence of and potential for ventricular fibrillation with the intracoronary administration of ratio-1.5 ionic media containing the calcium edetate disodium sequestrant versus equivalent media (Table 1.4) that contain the combination edetate disodium and sodium citrate additives (Murdock DK, et al, 1985; Murdock DK, et al, 1984a; Violante MR, et al, 1978; Wolf GL, et al, 1981b; Morris TW, et al. 1984). Each of the ratio-3 low-osmolality media contain the calcium edetate disodium sequestrant (Table 1.11).

Inotropic Effects. Alterations in myocardial contractility are also observed with the intracoronary injection of angiographic contrast media. Hyperosmolar, ionic media (i. e., ratio-1.5 ionic or ratio-3 ionic-dimeric) produce an initial, transient (10–20 second) depression of myocardial contractility followed by a secondary increase in contractility. In contradistinction, hyperosmolar, ratio-3 nonionic contrast media or hypertonic solutions of glucose or mannitol produce only the secondary increase in contractility. Based on these observations it is apparent that hyperosmolarity, per se, is responsible for the observed positive inotropic effect, whereas the cardiodepressive effect is associated with a separate mechanism (Newell JD, et al, 1980; Higgins CB, 1980; Gerber KH, et al, 1982b).

Measurement of serum electrolyte concentrations within the coronary sinus following the intracoronary injection of ionic contrast media reveals that the negative inotropic effect coincides temporally with a maximum increase in the sodium-to-calcium ionic ratio (Higgins CB and Schmidt W, 1978a). Several factors may be involved in the alteration of these electrolyte concentrations.

Dilutional effects associated with the hypervolemia induced by hyperosmolar contrast media would be expected to decrease the extracellular concentrations of both sodium and calcium ions. This, however, would not explain the increase in the sodium-to-calcium ionic ratio, nor would it explain the varying degrees of cardiodepression produced by equiosmolar concentrations of the angiographic media (Higgins CB, 1980; Wolpers HG, et al, 1981).

The observed increase in the sodium-to-calcium ratio may result from the administration of excessive, nonphysiological concentrations of sodium ions in the contrast media formulations used for coronary angiography. The importance of administered sodium becomes apparent with the observation that the intracoronary injection of hypertonic sodium chloride produces a similar negative inotropic effect (Newell JD, et al, 1980). Although the differences in administered sodium concentration may explain, in part, the respective inotropic activities of the ratio-1.5 ionic and ratio-3 nonionic (i. e., no sodium cations) contrast media, it must be noted that significant increases in the coronary sinus sodium-to-calcium ionic ratio can occur in the presence of a negligible alteration of the normal coronary sinus sodium ion concentration (Gerber KH, et al, 1982b). The administered sodium concentration is therefore not the sole factor responsible for the cardiodepressive effects of ionic contrast media.

A decrease in the coronary sinus calcium concentration and a corresponding increase in the sodium-to-calcium ionic ratio can occur as a result of the direct calcium-binding properties of ionic contrast media and sequestrant chelating agents within their formulations. The importance of the calcium-binding effects of angiographic contrast media in the etiology of their cardiodepressive activity is indicated by the observation that the addition of calcium ions to ratio-1.5 or ratio-3 ionic contrast media significantly ameliorates or reverses the initial decrease in contractility with no effect on the secondary increase in contractility (Trägardh B., et al, 1982). As previously discussed, the anionic radiopaque moieties of ionic media are capable of directly binding calcium ions, whereas the nonionic media are devoid of this property and, hence, produce no alterations of the coronary sinus sodium-to-calcium ratio. This explains, in part, the observed differences between these media groups in regard to their production of negative inotropic effects. Similarly, the reduced anion concentration associated with the ratio-3 ionic-dimer, ioxaglate meglumine-sodium, is responsible for its decreased cardiodepressive activity compared to equiiodine concentrations of the ratio-1.5 ionic media (Trägardh B, et al, 1982; Higgins CB, 1980).

Ratio-1.5 contrast media formulations that contian the combination of additives, edetate disodium (0.04% w/v) and sodium citrate (0.32% w/v), bind significantly greater quantities of calcium within the coronary sinus than equivalent ratio-1.5 contrast media formulations (Table 1.4) that contain the calcium edetate disodium sequestrant (Wolpers HG, et al, 1981; Morris TW, et al, 1982). As expected, clinical and experimental studies have shown that the degree of initial cardiodepression produced by the former agents is significantly greater than the latter media wherein thc calcium-binding effects of the sequestrant have been pre-neutralized (Murdock DK, et al, 1984b). Each of the ratio-3 low-osmolality agents contain the calcium edetate disodium sequestrant (Table 1.11).

The secondary increase in myocardial contractility observed with the intracoronary injection of hyperosmolar contrast media may be associated with an adrenergically mediated reflex mechanism (Higgins CB and Schmidt WS, 1978b); Higgins CB, 1980). Combined alpha- and beta-receptor blockade abolishes the seconary positive inotropic effects of both the nonionic and ionic media without affecting the initial negative inotropic effect exhibited by the latter agents. This reflex response does not appear to be related to peripheral baroreceptor stimulation since it occurs in the absence of a significant decline in peripheral arterial pressure. The positive inotropic effects of the hyperosmolar media are also observed in isolated heart models, suggesting a local, rather than distal mechanism (Haberey M, et al, 1980; Serur JR, et al, 1980).

Hyperosmolar contrast media may exert this effect by inducing the direct release of catecholamine stores from the myocardium or by stimulating coronary artery mechanoreceptors, which are mediated by a sympathetic afferent limb. It has also been suggested that hyperosmolar contrast media may promote the contractility of myocardial fibers by increasing the intracellular concentration of calcium ions via their cellular diuretic effects (Newell JD, et al, 1980). This mechanism should not, however, be affected by adrenergic blockade. Finally, an increase in myocardial contractility could occur secondary to the hypervolemia (i. e., increased cardiac preload) induced by the injected medium and its osmotic diuretic actions. However, the relatively small volumes of contrast media utilized in coronary angiography render this mechanism unlikely (Higgins CB and Schmidt W, 1978b).

In the presence of myocardial ischemia, the initial negative inotropic effect of an ionic contrast media becomes more severe and prolonged and the secondary increase in contractility is not observed. Ischemia does not, however, alter the positive inotropic effect of a hyperosmolar, nonionic medium (Higgins CB, 1980; Deutsch AL, et al, 1982). The exact mechanism responsible for the ischemia-enhanced cardiodepressive activity is unknown. It may be related to the inherent decrease in blood flow that prolongs the time of exposure of the myocardial cells to the physiological effects of the ionic agent. Or it may be that coronary blood flow cannot increase sufficiently in ischemia to support reversal of the cardiodepressive effects. Regardless of the mechanism, the prolonged negative inotropic effects of ionic contrast media in ischemia may be problematic in patients with concomitant left ventricular dysfunction (i. e., cardiomyopathy, severe aortic valvular disease) or severe coronary artery disease. Conversely, the positive inotropic effects of hyperosmolar contrast media increase the oxygen demands of the myocardium resulting in dilation of the normal coronary arteries and, perhaps, worsening or precipitation of the ischemic event. In regard to this latter statement, it has been shown that the addition of calcium to ratio-1.5 ionic contrast media or the appropriate use of the calcium edetate disodium sequestrant can ameliorate the initial cardiodepressive effect of these agents with no further increase in their secondary positive inotropic effect (Trägardh B, et al, 1982).

Blood Pressure, Heart Rate Effects. The negative chronotropic (i.e., sinus bradycardia) and inotropic effects of angiographic contrast media produce a subsequent decrease in cardiac output and mean arterial pressure. That this blood pressure decrease occurs as a result of the contrast-induced heart rate and contractility changes rather than direct vessel dilation is evidenced by its temporal relationship (i.e., follows heart rate and contractility changes) and its attenuation following atropine premedication (i.e., abolishes chronotropic effects). As expected, the reduced chronotropic activity of the ratio-3 low-osmolality media, combined with their diminished or absent cardiodepressive effects, result in less heart rate and blood pressure alterations than equiiodine concentrations of the ratio-1.5 ionic media (Higgins CB, 1984; Hayward R and Dawson P, 1984).

Controversy exists as to whether the hypotensive effect of coronary angiography is accompanied by peripheral vasoconstriction or vasodilation. A compensatory increase in peripheral vascular resistance has been demonstrated to occur in response to the contrast-induced reduction in cardiac output and peripheral blood flow (Kurnick PB, et al, 1985). However in a separate study, peripheral vasodilation and an increase in peripheral blood flow was observed following coronary angiography (Zelis R, et al, 1976). This latter study implicated the involvement of a vagally mediated, myocardial reflex mechanism, perhaps ventricular epicardial or pressure receptors in the peripheral responses. Prior administration of atropine abolished the peripheral vasodilation and blood flow increase. The different findings of these studies may reflect varying times of observation or the inhibition of reflex mechanisms by patient preparation procedures.

CARDIAC EFFECTS (TABLE 1.18): LEFT VENTRICULOGRAPHY, AORTOGRAPHY

Injection of large volumes of angiographic contrast media into the left ventricle or proximal aorta results in direct and reflex alterations of myocardial contractility, systemic blood pressure, and heart rate. In addition to these specific hemodynamic responses, it must be remembered that a substantial percentage of the ventricular output or aortic outflow is distributed to the kidneys, brain, and coronary

Table 1.18　CARDIAC EFFECTS OF ANGIOGRAPHIC CONTRAST MEDIA: LEFT VENTRICULOGRAPHY

PHYSIOLOGICAL EFFECT(S)	RESPONSE(S)	RESPONSIBLE CHEMOTOXIC FACTOR(S)
Volume loading	↑ L. ventricular contractility (acute)	Rapidly injected volume
Hypocalcemia (coronary sinus)	↓ L. ventricular contractility Electrocardiographic abnormalities	Calcium-binding · Radiopaque anions · Sequestrants
Adrenergic reflex stimulation	↑ L. ventricular contractility	Hyperosmolality
Hypervolemia · ↑ Cardiac preload	↑ L. ventricular contractility	Hyperosmolality
Peripheral artery dilation · ↓ Vascular resistance	↑ Peripheral blood flow Hypotension (systemic) · Reflex tachycardia · ↓ Cardiac afterbad ↑ L.ventricular contractility	Hyperosmolality
Coronary stretch receptor stimulation	Electrocardiographic abnormalities · Sinus bradycardia · Conduction delays · Ventricular fibrillation	Hyperosmolality Sodium ion concentration

arteries. Hence, the contrast media effects previously described for selective angiography of these organs/vessels must also be incorporated into the selection of an appropriate contrast medium for left ventriculography or aortography.

As noted in the previous discussion of cerebral angiography and renal arteriography, the undesirable physiological effects of ratio-1.5 ionic contrast media can be minimized by using pure meglumine salts of diatrizoate, iothalamate, or metrizoate. In coronary angiography, however, a combination meglumine-sodium derivative of these radiopaque anions must be utilized to reduce the incidence of ventricular fibrillation. The appropriate contrast medium for left ventriculography or aortography must therefore have an acceptable (i.e., for coronary angiography), but minimal concentration of sodium. Based on this consideration, the combination meglumine-sodium contrast media that contain a 6.6:1 ratio of meglumine to sodium cations (3.6–4.5 mg sodium/mL) would be more appropriate for left ventriculography and aortography than media containing a 2:1 (9.4 mg sodium/mL) or lower ratio (Table 1.4).

Peripheral Artery Dilation. Large volumes of hyperosmolar contrast media injected into the left ventricle or aorta produce direct dilation of the peripheral arteries resulting in a decrease in peripheral vascular resistance and an increase in peripheral blood flow (see Vascular Effects). This physiological effect of angiographic contrast media is primarily dependent on the osmolality of the injected agent, and is diminished with equivalent use of the ratio-3 low-osmolality versus the ratio-1.5 ionic media (Hilal SK, et al, 1966).

Systemic Blood Pressure, Heart Rate Effects. In aortography or left ventriculography the systemic blood pressure transiently increases as a result of the injected volume of contrast media. This increase is rapidly followed by a decrease in systemic blood pressure in response to the contrast-induced peripheral artery dilation and decreased vascular resistance. With this fall in systemic blood pressure, there is a compensatory increase in heart rate (Fischer HW, 1968).

Inotropic Effects. Injection of a concentrated ionic contrast medium (i.e., ratio-1.5 ionic or ratio-3 ionic-dimer) into the left ventricle results initially in a volume-dependent increase in myocardial contractility in accordance with Starling's law. As expected, this initial positive inotropic effect of left ventriculography is not observed with selective injection into the aorta. Subsequent delivery (i.e., 5–10 seconds) of the somewhat diluted but still concentrated medium to the coronary arteries elicits the early negative and secondary positive inotropic effects that are characteristic of selective coronary artery injection of ionic contrast agents (see Cardiac Effects: Coronary Angiography). The secondary positive intropic effect is further enhanced with left ventriculography and aortography due to the significant decrease in arterial blood pressure (i.e., decreased afterload) and the expanded blood volume (i.e., increased preload) associated with the large volume of injected medium and its osmolality-dependent hypervolemic effects (see Vascular Effects). Return to a normal state of contractility occurs in approximately 10–15 minutes (Fischer HW, 1968; Hayward R and Dawson P, 1984).

The left ventricular or aortic administration of a ratio-3 *nonionic* contrast medium produces a different pattern of inotropic effects. The initial volume-dependent increase in contractility is maintained since exposure of the coronary arteries to a hyperosmolar nonionic contrast medium does not result in the early cardiodepressive effects observed with the ionic agents.

Compared to the ratio-1.5 ionic contrast media, left ventricular injection of equivalent volumes and iodine concentrations of the ratio-3 nonionic or ionic-dimeric media produce a similar degree of the initial volume-dependent increase in myocardial contractility. The secondary positive inotropic effects of left ventriculography or aortography are decreased with the low-osmolality agents, however, as a result of their reduced degree of arterial dilation, systemic hypotension, and hypervolemia.

Subsequent exposure of the coronary arteries to the hyperosmolar angiographic contrast medium used for ventriculography/aortography can also result in the previously described alterations in cardiac electrophysiology (see Cardiac Effects: Coronary Angiography). The complex interaction of the multiple inotropic and chronotropic effects of left ventriculography may lead to the formation of premature ventricular contractions. This adverse response can present a major problem in the evaluation of the associated ventriculogram.

IV. Precautions

PHYSICAL INCOMPATIBILITIES

Drugs. Table 1.19 lists several drugs that are known to be physically incompatible with ratio-1.5 ionic contrast media and the ratio-3 ionic-dimeric agent, ioxaglate meglumine-sodium. Although differences do appear to exist between the various angiographic contrast media in regard to their relative reactivities with each of these drugs, it is probably best to assume that the listed drugs are generally incompatible with ionic (i. e., ratio-1.5 or ratio-3) contrast agents. This incompatibility is most likely related to the acidic nature of the added drug that results in precipitation of the radiopaque anion (Marshall TR, et al, 1965). In general, the ratio-3 nonionic contrast media appear to be less prone to such an interaction (Fischer HW, 1987; Pilla TJ, et al, 1986).

As a rule, it is probably best to avoid the direct mixing of any drug with any intravascular iodinated contrast medium if possible. Catheters should be thoroughly flushed between drug and contrast medium injections. If the direct mixing of a drug with the contrast medium in unavoidable, the possibility of a physical incompatibility should be a constant consideration. At a minimum, the compatibility of the drug and the contrast medium should be visually evaluated (i. e., for precipitate formation) prior to patient administration (Fisher HW, 1987).

Syringes/Rubber. Hyperosmolar, intravascular contrast media are capable of leaching significant amounts of potent rubber allergens (e. g., mercaptobenzothiazole, hydroxyethylmercaptobenzothiazole) from the rubber plunger seals of disposable plastic syringes (Hamilton G and Fischer HW 1984). It is possible that this phenomenon may contribute to the etiology and incidence of pseudo-allergic reactions to water-soluble iodinated contrast agents. Therefore, intravascular contrast media should not be allowed to remain in contact with the rubber components of syringes for a prolonged period of time prior to their injection.

It is also possible that hyperosmolar contrast media may be capable of leaching allergens from the rubber stoppers of their bulk vial or bottle containers upon

Table 1.19   DRUGS KNOWN TO BE PHYSICALLY INCOMPATIBLE WITH ANGIOGRAPHIC CONTRAST MEDIA

DRUG	INVOLVED CONTRAST MEDIA[a]	REFERENCE(S)
Brompheniramine maleate (e.g., Dimetane®)	Conv.	Marshall TR, et al, 1965
Cimetidine hydrochloride	Iox.	Shah SJ and Gerlock AJ, 1987; Fischer HW, 1987
Diphenhydramine hydrochloride (e.g., Benadryl®)	Conv., Iox.	Marshall TR, et al, 1965; Fisher HW, 1987
Hyaluronidase (e.g., Wydase®)	Conv.	Marshall TR, et al, 1965
Papaverine hydrochloride	Conv., Iox.	Pilla TJ, et al, 1986; Shah SJ, et al, 1987; Zagoria RJ, et al, 1987
Promethazine hydrochloride (e.g., Phenergan®)	Conv.	Marshall TR, et al, 1965
Tolazoline hydrochloride	Iox.	Zagoria RJ, et al, 1987

[a] Conv. = Conventional ratio-1.5 media, Iox. = Ioxaglate meglumine-sodium

Table 1.20 KNOWN OR SUGGESTED INTRAVASCULAR CONTRAST MEDIUM-LABORATORY TEST/DIAGNOSTIC-PROCEDURE INTERACTIONS

LABORATORY TEST/DIAGNOSTIC PROCEDURE	RESULT OF CONTRAST MEDIUM INTERACTION	POSSIBLE MECHANISM OF CONTRAST MEDIUM INTERACTION	REFERENCES
Serum electrolytes, chemistry; Hematocrit, blood counts	· General decrease in values · Specific decrease in [Ca, Mg]	· Hypervolemia (hyperosmolality) · Direct cation binding (radiopague anion)	· Weigen JF and Thomas SF, 1973 · Wolpers HG, et al, 1981
Urinalysis	· General decrease in values · Aluminuria, proteinuria · False (+) for proteinuria (Ioxaglate)	· Osmotic diuresis (hyperosmolality) · Glomerular permeability alterations (hyperosmolality) · Precipitation complex	· Saxton HM, 1969 · Golman K and Holtas S, 1980 · Shanahan JC, et al, 1985
Platelet aggregation	Decreased	· Direct: Alteration of platelet morphology · Indirect: Fibrinogen-binding	· Parvey Z, et al, 1984 · Belleville J, et al, 1985
Clotting times (thrombin time, partial thromboplastin time, prothrombin time, etc.)	Increased	Fibrinogen-binding	Belleville J, et al, 1985
Erythrocyte sedimentation rate	Prolonged	Alteration of erythrocyte morphology	Aspelin P, et al, 1978c
Thyroid function tests · Radioactive iodine uptake · Protein-bound iodine	· Decreased[a] · Increased[a]	Free iodine component (chemical impurity or metabolic byproduct)	· Grayson RR, 1960 · Davis RJ, 1966
Nuclear medicine studies · ^{99m}Tc-PYP (MDP?) bone scans	· Increased renal, liver; decreased bone activity	· Hyperosmolality, chemical displacement of Tc-99m (?)	· Crawford JA, et al, 1978
· ^{99m}Tc-RBC labeling (in-vivo or syringe method) · ^{99m}Tc-DTPA, glucoheptonate brain scanning.	· Decreased labeling efficiency · Increased activity in normal brain and surrounding soft tissues	· Interference with cellular ion transport systems (?) · Blood-brain barrier alterations (hyperosmolality)	· Tatum JL, et al, 1983; Rao SA, et al, 1987 · Rosenthall L, et al, 1969
Bacterial cultures	Inhibition	Bacterocidal, bacterostatic activity	Dawson P, 1983; Kim KS and Lachman R, 1982

[a] May persist for several weeks

prolonged storage in an inverted position (Hamilton G, 1987; Hamilton G and Fisher HW, 1984). This could explain the observed nonrandom clustering of contrast-induced pseudo-allergic reactions (Winter J, 1982), which does not appear to be related to a specific lot or batch of the involved medium but may be associated with improper storage of a given box or carton. Although this latter consideration remains to be proved, it is currently advisable to ensure that containers of intravascular contrast media are stored in upright position.

CONTRAST MEDIUM-LABORATORY TEST/DIAGNOSTIC PROCEDURE INTERACTIONS

Intravascular, iodinated contrast media can interfere with simultaneous or subsequent laboratory tests or diagnostic procedures as a result of their chemical properties or effects on vascular and organ physiology. Although by no means conclusive, Table 1.20 lists several known or suggested intravascular contrast media-laboratory test or diagnostic procedure interactions. It can be speculated that several other interactions may exist based on the myriad of physiological effects induced by the angiographic contrast media and the extremely high vascular and renal concentrations achieved with their routine dosages. In general, however, the potential for these interactions is relatively short-lived due to the normal, rapid systemic elimination of the injected contrast agents and their single-dose use. Hence, the question of a contrast medium interaction should be considered with any unexpected laboratory test/diagnostic procedure finding occurring within 24–48 hours following contrast administration.

CONTRAST MEDIUM— DRUG INTERACTIONS

In recognition of the numerous effects of intravascular contrast media on vascular and organ physiology, it is not surprising that these agents can interact with tra-ditional drugs to produce an alteration of desired pharmacological activity or an enhancement of side effects. Table 1.21 provides a summary of reported known or possible contrast medium-drug interactions. In general, the indicated interactions involve a physiological effect of the intravascular contrast medium that is additive to the pharmacological effect of the therapeutic drug. Such interactions would be expected to be short-lived due to the normally rapid systemic elmination of the contrast medium. However, the duration of the interaction may bear no relationship to its severity and clinical outcome.

Unfortunately, the area of contrast medium-drug interactions has, to date, received little evaluative attention; therefore the presented table is by no means definitive or complete. Radiologists should be cognizant of the various physiological effects of intravascular contrast media on sensitive organ systems (e.g., cardiovascular, kidney) and be able to evaluate when these effects may be additive to the effects of concurrent drug therapy to the possible detriment of the patient. The radiologist should also be aware of what steps may be taken (e.g., alternate use of a low-osmolality contrast medium, discontinuance of drug therapy for an appropriate interval) to reduce the potential for a serious reaction. Conversely, in the event of an unexpected reaction to contrast medium administration or drug therapy, the possibility of a respective interaction should be taken into consideration. If possible, such an interaction should be documented with appropriate experimental or clinical studies.

PREGNANCY/BREAST FEEDING

Intravascular, iodinated contrast media cross the placenta and are excreted in the breast milk of lactating females. Distribution of these agents to the fetus or infant can result in alterations in thyroid function, and possibly, systemic pseudo-allergic reactions. The benefit-versus-risk

Table 1.21   REPORTED KNOWN OR POSSIBLE INTRAVASCULAR CONTRAST MEDIUM·DRUG INTERACTIONS

DRUG CLASSIFICATION	COMMON EXAMPLES	POSSIBLE MECHANISM(S) OF CONTRAST-DRUG INTERACTION	POTENTIAL OUTCOME(S) OF INTERACTION	REFERENCES(S)
Antiarrhythmics	Procainamide, quinidine	· Additive: Prolongation of Q-T interval · Additive: Negative inotropic, hypotensive effects	· Ventricular tachycardia · Accentuation and prolongation of hypotensive effects	· Duncan JS and Ramsay LE, 1985
Anticoagulants	Heparin, dicumarol, warfarin	Additive: Prolongation of clotting times	Prolongation of bleeding time	Parvez Z, et al, 1984 Belleville J, et al, 1985
Antiplatelet drugs	Aspirin, dipyridamole, NSAIA (ibuprofen, indomethacin, naproxen)	Additive: Inhibition of platelet aggregation	Prolongation of bleeding time	Parvez Z, et al, 1984
Beta-adrenergic receptor blocking agents	Propanolol, atenolol, metoprolol, nadolol, pindolol, timolol	· Additive: Negative inotropic, hypotensive effects · Inability to increase cardiac output to compensate for contrast-induced hypotension	Accentuation and prolongation of hypotensive effects	Hamilton G, 1985 Svenson RH, 1984
Calcium-channel blocking agents	Verapamil, diltiazem, nifedipine	· Additive: Negative chronotropic effects · Additive: Negative ionotropic effects, decrease in systemic vascular resistance	· Cardiac arrythmias, fibrillation, heart block · Accentuation and prolongation of hypotensive effects[a]	· Peck WW, et al, 1984; Higgins CB, et al, 1983 · Svenson RH, 1984; Morris DL, et al, 1985
Cardiac glycosides	Digitalis	Additive: Lowering of ventricular fibrillation threshold	Ventricular fibrillation	Fischer HW and Morris TW, 1980; Wolf GL, 1980 Mulry C, et al, 1980
Diuretics	Furosemide, thiazides, ethacrynic acid, triamterene[b], amiloride[b], spironolactone[b]	· Additive: Diuretic effects · Additive: Hypotensive effects · Hypokalemia (diuretics): Additive prolongation of Q-T interval	· Dehydration (increased risk of contrast nephropathy), electrolyte inbalance · Accentuation and prolongation of hypotensive effects · Ventricular tachcardia	· Berkseth RO and Kjellstrand C, 1984 Harkonen S and Kjellstrand C, 1981 · Duncan JS and Ramsay LE, 1985
Nephrotoxic drugs	Aminoglycosides, amphotericin, rifampin, lithium carbonate, antineoplastics	Additive: Nephrotoxic effects	Accentuation and prolongation of nephrotoxicity	—
Rauwolfia alkaloids	Reserpine	Additive: Prolongation of Q-T interval	Ventricular tachycardia	Duncan JS and Ramsay LE, 1985

[a] Proven clinically significant
[b] Potassium-sparing diuretics

of administering intravascular contrast media to pregnant or potentially pregnant patients should therefore be carefully considered. Breast feeding should be interrupted for a period of 24–48 hours following injection of these agents.

V. Clinical Considerations

CLINICAL INDICATIONS

Angiographic procedures are generally indicated for the diagnosis or evaluation of suspected or known neoplasms (Figure 1.8) or congenital or acquired vascular diseases (Figures 1.9–1.12) that may cause alterations in normal vascular anatomy or physiology (Table 1.22). Specific indications for the various selective angiographic procedures (Table 1.1) are numerous and beyond the scope or focus of this book. For a more complete discussion of the indications, techniques, and

risks of particular angiographic procedures, the reader is referred to more extensive, procedure-oriented reviews of this subject.

CONTRAST MEDIA CONSIDERATIONS

Ratio-1.5 Ionic Media. The selection of an intravascular contrast medium for a given angiography procedure should be based on an attempt to obtain adequate opacification while minimizing the number and intensity of undesirable physiological effects induced by the medium on the organ/vascular system under investigation. In this regard, product selection recommendations for the ratio-1.5 angiographic media are indicated in Table 1.23. These recommendations are based on the previously described organ-specific physiological effects of angiographic contrast media and the required iodine concentrations for adequate opacification (see Dosage). Note that the contrast media are

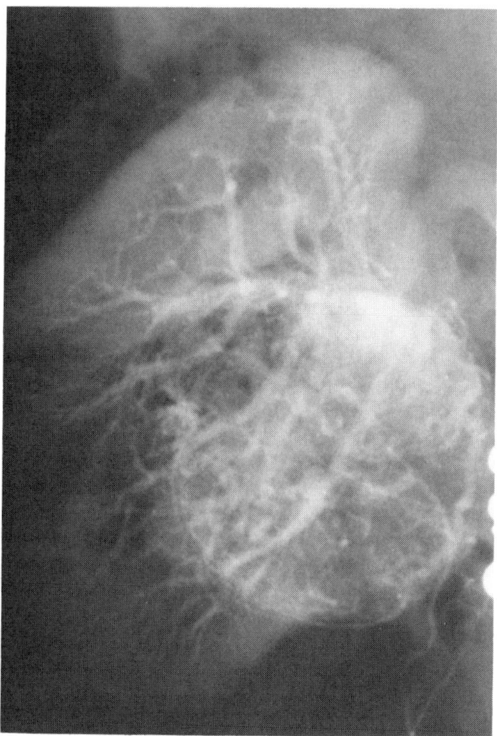

Figure 1.8 Selective right kidney arteriogram demonstrating large hypervascular mass involving the renal hilum. Pathologic diagnosis of renal cell carinoma.

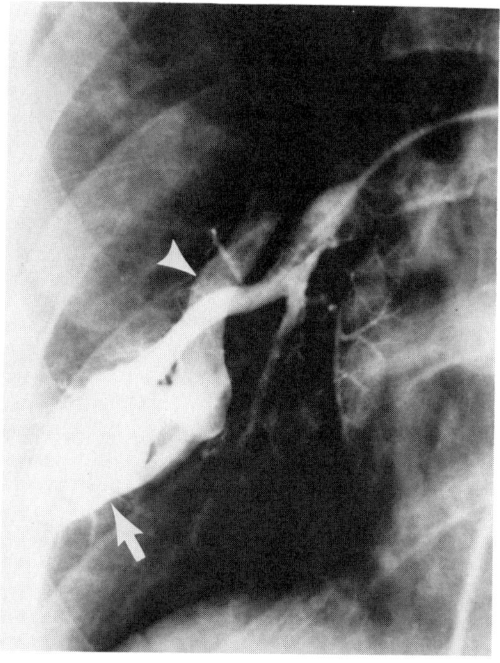

Figure 1.9 Selective pulmonary arteriogram demonstrating (arrow) large arteriovenous malformation. Note (arrowhead) large draining vein.

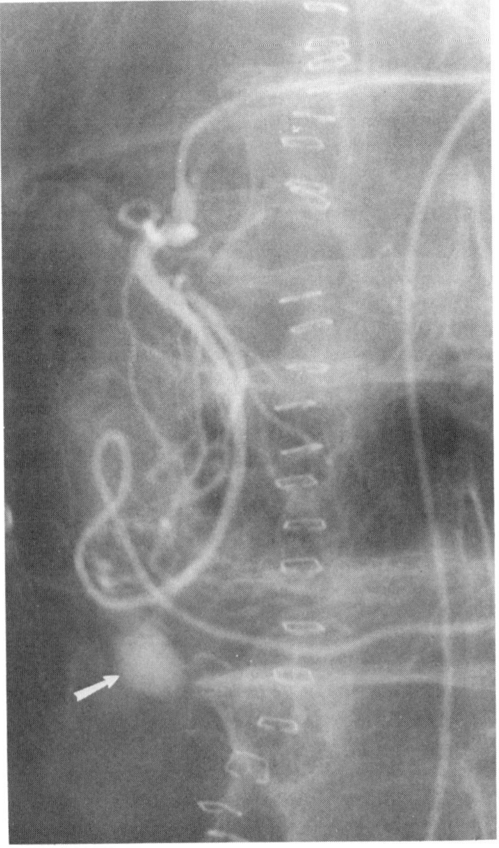

Figure 1.10 Selective gastroduoden-al arteriogram demonstrating (arrow) contrast extravasation associated with duodenal bleeding.

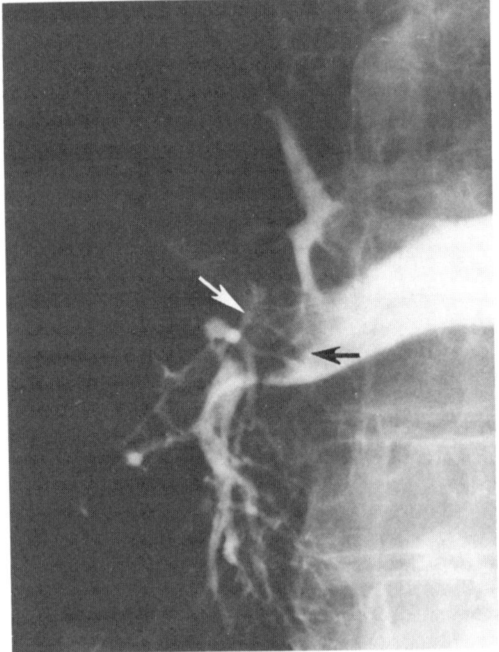

Figure 1.11 Selective right main pul-monary arteriogram demonstrating (arrows) a large intraluminal filling de-fect caused by a saddle embolus.

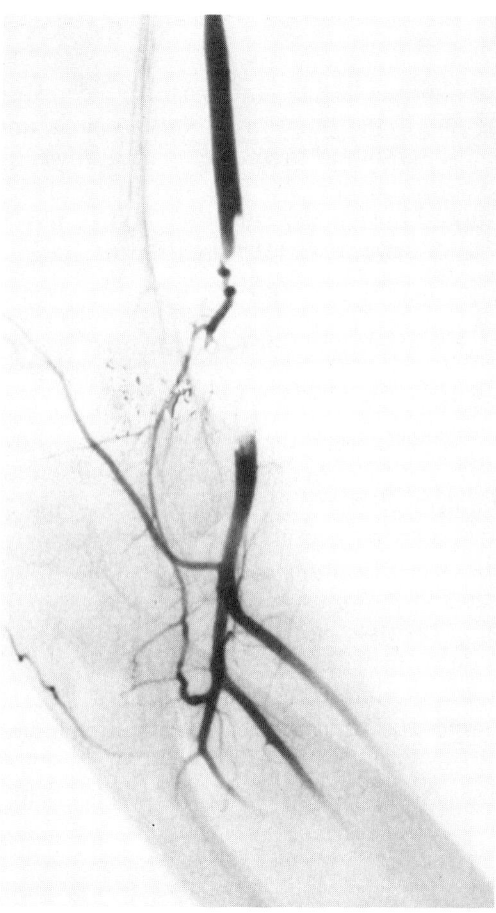

Figure 1.12 Selective brachial arter-iogram demonstrating respective distal transection and occlusion.

Table 1.22   GENERAL DIAGNOSTIC INDICATIONS FOR ANGIOGRAPHIC PROCEDURES

KNOWN OR SUSPECTED

Mass Lesions
  Trauma
  Infection
  Neoplasia (Figure 1.8)

Vascular Diseases
  Arteriovenous malformation (Figure 1.9)
  Aneurysm
  Vasculitis
  Internal bleeding (Figure 1.10)

Occlusive Processes
  Stenosis
  Thrombosis
  Embolism (Figure 1.11)
  Trauma (Figure 1.12)

Table 1.23   PRODUCT SELECTION RECOMMENDATIONS FOR RATIO-1.5 ANGIOGRAPHIC CONTRAST MEDIA

ANGIOGRAPHIC PROCEDURE	ANION	CATION(S)	SEQUESTRANT[a]	CONCENTRATION (%w/v)	MG IODINE ML
Aortic arch	Diatrizoate	meglumine (66%)–sodium (10%)	CaEDTA	76	370
Aortography (thoracic, lumbar, abdominal)	Diatrizoate	meglumine (66%)–sodium (10%)	CaEDTA	76	370
Cerebral angiography	Diatrizoate or Iothalamate	meglumine	CaEDTA	60	282
Peripheral arteriography Large, rapid-flow arteries	Diatrizoate	meglumine (66%)–sodium (10%)	CaEDTA[b]	76	370
· Celiac					
· Hepatic					
· Mesenteric					
· Pancreatic					
· Pelvic					
· Pulmonary					
· Renal					
Small, slow-flow arteries	Diatrizoate or Iothalamate	meglumine	CaEDTA[b]	60	282
· Adrenal					
· Brachial					
· Femoral					
· Subclavian					
· Vertebral					
Venography Adrenal vein	Diatrizoate or Iothalamate	meglumine	CaEDTA[b]	60	282
Peripheral	Diatrizoate or Iothalamate	meglumine	CaEDTA[b]	60	282
Splenoportography	Diatrizoate	meglumine (66%)–sodium (10%)	CaEDTA[b]	76	370
Vena cava (inferior, superior)	Diatrizoate	meglumine (66%)–sodium (10%)	CaEDTA[b]	76	370
Ventriculography	Diatrizoate	meglumine (66%)–sodium (10%)	CaEDTA	76	370

[a] CaEDTA = Calcium edetate disodium
[b] Not based on demonstrated physiological effect but an attempt to limit total number of inventory items. See previous and subsequent recommendations

listed by generic name and % w/v concentration. The reader should refer to Tables 1.2–1.4 for associated brand names and manufacturers. It is advised that the package insert for the specific product be consulted to ascertain that the respective indication is listed.

Ratio-3 Low Osmolality Media.   As a result of their substantially reduced osmolalities per given iodine concentration and degree of x-ray opacification, angiographic use of the ratio-3 low-osmolality media (Table 1.11) is generally associated with a reduced number and intensity of undesirable physiological effects compared to the ratio-1.5 ionic media (see Physiological Effects). However, at the time of this writing, the comparative costs of the low-osmolality agents exceed those of the conventional, ratio-1.5 media by

factors of 10–20 or greater. This latter consideration, combined with the cost-containment trends in medical economics, pose major limitations to routine clinical use of the better tolerated, ratio-3 media.

An approach to the cost-benefit issues surrounding low-osmolality contrast media is to use these agents in patients with preexisting conditions who are known to be at increased risk for conventional (i. e., ratio-1.5) contrast media reactions. This approach takes maximum advantage of the physiological advantages of the ratio-3 media while also incorporating the cost considerations. The authors' current recommendations for such use of the low-osmolality media are discussed under Risk Factors/Low Osmolality Contrast Media Recommendations and outlined in Table 1.24. It is recognized that, based on individual experience, controversy may exist in regard to the preexisting conditions that render a patient at increased risk for conventional contrast media reactions. Each institution or affiliated group

Table 1.24 CONSIDERATIONS FOR THE USE OF RATIO-3 (LOW-OSMOLALITY) ANGIOGRAPHIC MEDIA IN AT-RISK PATIENTS

CONSIDERATION SHOULD BE GIVEN TO USING A RATIO-3 LOW-OSMOLALITY CONTRAST MEDIUM IN PLACE OF THE CONVENTIONAL RATIO-1.5 MEDIUM IN PATIENTS WHO HAVE OR EXPERIENCE THE FOLLOWING CONDITION(S):

A. *Previous reactions to contrast media*
   1. Documented history of a major contrast medium reaction.
   2. Clinically significant BP or ECG alteration upon initial injection of the ratio-1.5 medium.
   3. Intolerable pain (precludes completion of study) upon initial injection of the ratio-1.5 medium.

B. *Renal considerations*
   1. Serum creatinine ≥ 4 mg/dL.
   2. Serum creatinine of 2 mg/dL–4 mg/dL with concomitant: Diabetes mellitus
                                       Hypertension (sustained)
                                       Multiple myeloma
                                       Single kidney/renal transplant

C. *Cerebral considerations*
   1. Cerebrovascular disease, cerebral tumor or abscess (known or suspected) with concomitant renal dysfunction (serum creatinine ≥ 2 mg/dL).
   2. Seizure history associated with cerebrovascular abnormality, cerebral tumor, or abscess.

D. *Cardiopulmonary considerations*
   1. Severe coronary artery disease/unstable angina.
   2. Severe aortic valvular stenosis.
   3. Severe congestive heart failure.
   4. Shock.

of radiologists should therefore develop its own guidelines for the use of these agents. The presented recommendations will, one hopes, provide a foundation for subsequent debate and modification. Of course, these recommendations are also subject to constant revision as increased clinical experience and new information related to the intravascular use of low-osmolality contrast media become available.

In the following discussion, the risk factors for angiographic contrast media injections are presented in relation to specific organ considerations. It must be emphasized, however, that the effects of an angiographic contrast medium on a given organ result not only from studies aimed at the direct angiographic evaluation of that organ, but also from any procedure that exposes the organ to a high dose and concentration of the contrast medium. For example, a high dose, bolus injection of a contrast medium for intravenous digital subtraction angiography (DSA) can result in contrast-induced physiological effects on the pulmonary and cardiac systems. Likewise, with ventriculography, the cerebral effects of the angiographic medium must be considered. Conversely, contrast-induced stimulation of the carotid chemoreceptors during cerebral angiography results in cardiac responses. All angiographic procedures can elicit physiological effects on the kidneys, the primary route of contrast excretion. Based on these considerations, the risk-factor-based recommendations regarding the use of low-osmolality agents should generally apply to all angiographic procedures.

As an alternative to the use of low-osmolality media, a similar reduction in the hyperosmolarity-induced physiological effects of ratio-1.5 angiographic media can be achieved by reducing the concentration and, hence, osmolality of the medium utilized to 50% of the routine concentration. Of course, this decrease in the contrast medium and, hence, iodine concentration will also result in a reduction in the degree of x-ray opacification. Although this approach would not be acceptable for conventional film-screen angiographic studies, it is feasible with many arterial DSA procedures. Based on this discussion, the low-osmolality recommendations (Table 1.24) should not apply to intra-arterial DSA procedures that incorporate a ratio-1.5 contrast medium concentration that is substantially (i. e., 50%) less than the concentration normally required for film-screen procedures. Although it may be argued that the use of a low-osmolality agent could further reduce the risks of such DSA procedures, this reasoning would have to be based primarily on molecular toxicity rather than hyperosmolarity considerations. The low-osmolality recommendations do apply, however, to DSA procedures that involve the administration of concentrated, ratio-1.5 ionic media.

Viscosity. The speed at which a viscous contrast medium can be injected is a major concern in radiological examinations that require a rapid rate of iodine delivery for adequate organ or vessel opacification. This problem can be overcome, to a certain degree, by preheating the medium to 37° C prior to injection, thus decreasing its viscosity.

The preheating step is particularly important with angiographic studies that require the high flow-rate delivery of concentrated, highly viscous (e. g., >10cps at 25 °C, Tables 1.4, 1.11) through small-bore (e. g., 4 or 5 French) catheters, which are being increasingly utilized for outpatient procedures (Halsell RD, 1987). However, with less concentrated media, the small decreases in viscosity achieved with heating (Tables 1.2–1.3, 1.11) result in only small improvements in their flow rate through high-pressure, high-flow catheters (Rees CR, et al, 1988b). It should also be noted, in this regard, that the manufacturer's specification of a maximum flow-rate limit for a given catheter is commonly based on preheating the contrast medium to 37° C (Grollman JH, 1984).

It has also been suggested that by prolonging the length of local vessel exposure the viscosity of an intravascular contrast medium may be an important factor in the degree of vessel dilation and associated pain, warmth, and subjective discomfort experienced by the patient (Nyman U, et al, 1980b). Preheating the contrast media to reduce viscosity does not, however, appear to alter the subsequent incidence of more severe adverse reactions (Turner E, et al, 1982).

PATIENT PREPARATION

Fasting. Patients should fast for 4–6 hours prior to the angiographic procedure in order to reduce the risk of aspiration pneumonitis associated with nausea and vomiting responses to the administered contrast medium. However, all patients should be well hydrated both before and after angiographic examinations. If the patient is prevented from receiving oral fluids, appropriate intravenous fluids should be administered to ensure adequate hydration.

Atropine/Analgesics/Sedatives. The intramuscular administration of atropine (0.4 mg [adult dose]) and a narcotic analgesic (e. g., meperidine, 50 mg [adult dose]; morphine, 10 mg [adult dose]) at approximately 30 minutes prior to the angiographic procedure is a standard practice in many institutions. Pretreatment with atropine may reduce the potential for vaso-vagal reactions. In addition, it will block the vagally mediated cardiovascular effects of the subsequently administered intravascular contrast medium (see Physiological Effects—Cerebral, Cardiac). Narcotic analgesics are included to alleviate the pain and discomfort commonly associated with angiographic procedures. Since there is evidence in the literature to suggest that anxiety may be associated with, at least, minor reactions or complications during angiography, the incorporation of a sedative (e. g., diazepam, 5–10 mg intramuscular [adult dose]) into the pretreatment regimen may also be considered. In many cases, the administration of a sedative will obviate the need for a narcotic analgesic. Recent attention in the radiology literature has been directed toward pretreatment use of the more recent narcotic analgesic and sedative agents, fentanyl and midazolam (Miller DL and Wall RT, 1987; Redmond RC and Krump DA, 1987; Ayre-Smith G, 1987). As a result of their increased lipid solubility and more rapid central nervous system kinetics, these agents exhibit a faster onset of action and shorter recovery time than the previously described agents.

A complete discussion of the relative advantages and disadvantages of the various currently available analgesic and sedative agents and precautions associated with their use is beyond the scope of this book. It must be emphasized, however, that narcotic analgesics and sedatives, in general, produce a dose-dependent depression of respiration, and additive effects must be considered with their coadministration. Prior to using any of the narcotic analgesics or sedatives, radiologists are advised to consult with an anesthesiologist to be certain of the appropriate use of these drugs. Once a specific pretreatment regimen has been adopted, the radiology staff should become thoroughly cognizant of the respective dosages, contraindications, and potential side effects. Patients must be closely monitored, and resusitative equipment and drugs must be readily available.

Previous Contrast Media Reactors. As discussed in Chapter 8, pretreatment with corticosteroids, antihistamines, and ephedrine has been shown to be effective in reducing the incidence and severity of subsequent contrast reactions in patients with a history of severe reactions to contrast media. To be effective, however, it is recommended that the pretreatment regimen be initiated at least 12 hours prior to the scheduled examination. In spite of its potential inconvenience, pretreatment of previous contrast media reactors should be considered unless it would adversely delay the performance of an emergent angiographic procedure.

Preexisting Renal Dysfunction. It has been suggested that the prophylactic intravenous infusion of the osmotic diuretic, mannitol (e. g., 20%, 250–500 mL), or the loop diuretic, furosemide, may be useful in preventing contrast medium-induced renal failure, especially in patients with preexisting renal disease (Berkseth RO, et al, 1984). These agents apparently protect against the renal vasoconstrictive effects of hyperosmolar contrast media and thereby maintain glomerular filtration driving pressure and prevent tubular obstruction (Burke TI, et al, 1980). It must be remembered, however, that the diuretic effects of these prophylactic agents will be additive to the osmotic diuretic effects of angiographic contrast media, therefore proper attention to the patient's hydration state and electrolyte values is required. Moreover, the administration of hyperosmolar mannitol solution or furosemide is not without inherent risks. Since the ratio-3, low-osmolality media produce substantially less renal vasoconstriction and glomerular permeability alterations than the conventional ratio-1.5 agents (see Physiological Effects—Renal), the alternate use of these ratio-3 media in patients with clinically significant renal dysfunction (see Clinical Considerations) may represent a more practical and efficacious approach than the prophylactic use of mannitol or furosemide; however, this remains to be substantiated.

Vasospasm. The exact etiology of angiography-associated vasospasm (Figure 1.13 is unknown. It may be related to catheter introduction and irritation of the vessel wall, physiological effects of

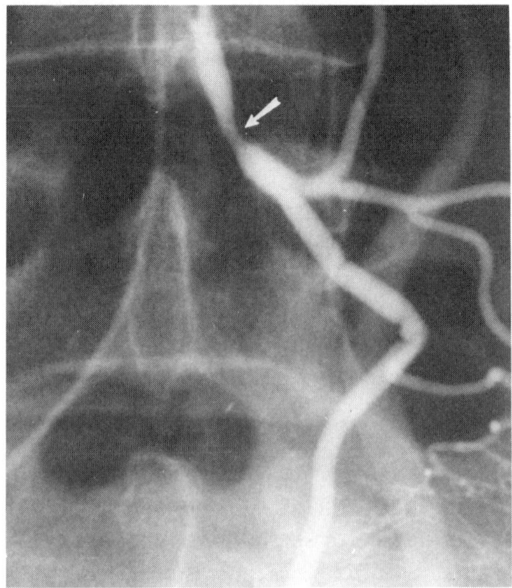

Figure 1.13   Selective inferior mesenteric arteriogram demonstrating (arrow) spasm adjacent to the catheter tip.

the contrast medium (see Physiological Effects—Vascular), or external injury to the vessel. The initial stimulation, regardless of its source, apparently causes a cascade effect involving neurogenic, chemical, and metabolic pathways (Dodek A, et al, 1984). Direct administration of the vasodilating agent, tolazoline (10–50 mg), is frequently employed to relieve peripheral vasospasm. Coronary vasospasm may be prevented or treated with sublingual nitroglycerin, or, if severe, with the direct arterial injection of nitroglycerin at progressively increasing doses of 0.1 mg–1 mg (Levin DC, 1983; Abrams HL, 1983b).

PHARMACOANGIOGRAPHY

Christopher K. Shier

The interventional administration of vasoactive drugs has been investigated experimentally and clinically as a potential method for increasing the diagnostic accuracy of angiographic procedures. Emphasis has historically been placed on using pharmacoangiographic techniques to improve the delineation of malignant tumors or to enhance the ability to distinguish between neoplastic, inflammatory, and normal vessels. Vasodilating and vasoconstricting agents have also been respectively utilized to increase the arterial delivery or venous retention of the contrast medium, resulting in enhanced vascular opacification.

The ideal vasoactive drug for pharmacoangiography should consistently produce an increase in diagnostic information with a negligible incidence of side effects. Its vasodilating or vasoconstricting response should occur rapidly and predictably at the dose utilized. In order to minimize the potential for systemic hemodynamic reactions, the vasoactive effects of the interventional drug should be limited to the specific vascular system under investigation. Such specificity can be achieved as a result of distinct pharmacological characteristics of the vasoactive drug or with its rapid in vivo metabolism. Depending on the administered dose, rapid degradation of the interventional agent can limit its effects to the vasculature at the site of administration. In the event of an adverse reaction, methods (i. e., antagonistic drugs) should be available to permit rapid reversal of the physiological effects of the intervention.

Vasoconstrictors. The angiographic diagnosis of malignant tumors is typically based on the demonstration of blood vessels that are atypical in appearance or profuse in number. Occasionally, however, it may be difficult to precisely delineate the extent of a tumor due to overlying normal vessels. This problem can be theoretically overcome with the incorporation of an interventional drug that would constrict normal vessels and thus reduce their contrast delivery and opacification but would have no effect on neoplastic vessels. The feasibility of this approach was originally suggested by the knowledge that malignant tumors are supplied by both normal and abnormal embryonic vessels, the latter being devoid of elastic tissue or a normal density of humoral receptors (Billing L and Lindgren AGH, 1944). Prelimi-

nary studies that indicated that neoplastic vessels may not respond in a normal fashion to vasoactive agents formed the basis for subsequent pharmacoangiography research and similar interventional studies aimed at the pharmacological enhancement of chemotherapy delivery to malignant tumors (Bierman HR, et al, 1951; Bierman HR, et al, 1952).

The first demonstration of the utility of a pharmacological intervention for the improved angiographic visualization of a malignant tumor involved the renal artery administration of *epinephrine*. This adrenergic neurohormone stimulates both alpha and beta receptors resulting in vessel constriction or dilation, respectively; its overall effect on a given vascular system being dependent on the relative number of beta-receptors present. Epinephrine is rapidly metabolized by endogenous enzymes (catechol-o-methyl transferase, monoamine oxidase) after its introduction into the vascular compartment. Following direct arterial or intravenous injection, epinephrine produces a decrease in blood flow to the normal renal vasculature. It appears that this effect is primarily related to constriction of the large extrarenal arteries (Abrams HL, et al, 1962). In a patient with malignant hypernephroma, epinephrine-augmented (25 micrograms, renal artery injection) renal arteriography resulted in reduced delivery of contrast to the normal renal parenchyma and a corresponding dense opacification of the tumor vessels (Abrams HL, 1964).

Subsequent investigations on the interventional renal artery administration of epinephrine for the enhanced angiographic visualization of renal malignancies (Figure 1.14) have shown similar results. It has been noted, however, that not all tumor vessels lack a vasoconstrictive response to epinephrine (Abrams HL, et al, 1971; Kahn PC, 1965). Lowering the dose (2–5 micrograms) of epinephrine appears to have overcome this problem (Ekelund L, et al, 1978; Bosniak MA, 1977), but extensive clinical studies to define the most efficacious dose of epinephrine for

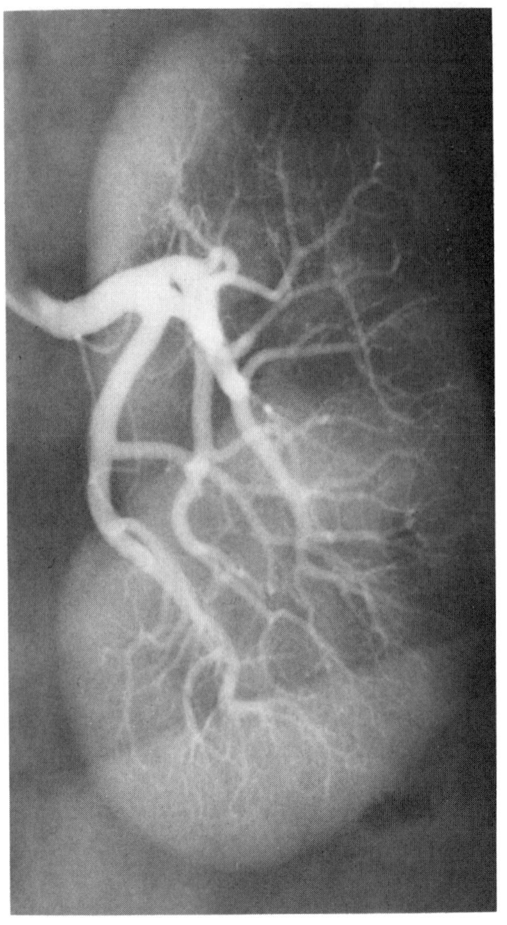

A

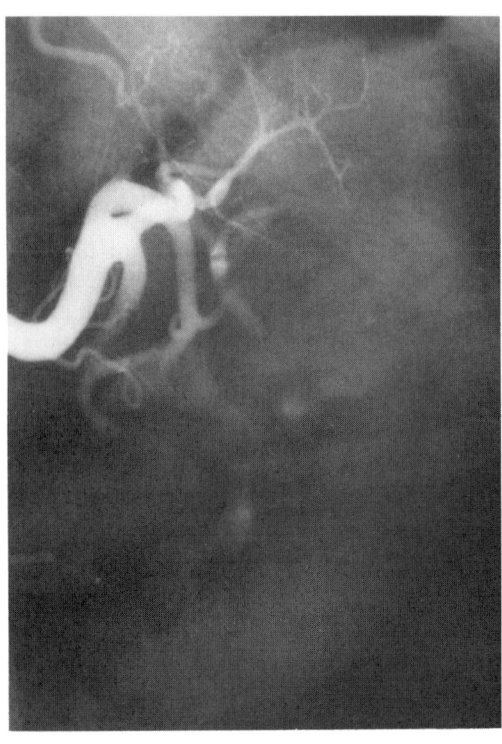

B

Figure 1.14 A. Selective left renal arteriogram demonstrating neovascularity and irregular opacification involving the upper pole of the kidney. B. Repeat left renal arteriogram, obtained following the injection of epinephrine (5 micrograms, left renal artery), demonstrates constriction of normal renal vasculature but no response by upper pole tumor vessel. Pathologic diagnosis of renal cell carcinoma.

optimal pharmacoangiographic demonstration of renal masses have not been performed.

Another potential problem associated with the pharmacoangiographic evaluation of renal masses is related to the fact that the neovasculature of inflammatory granulation tissue within the kidney constricts less consistently and to a reduced extent in response to epinephrine than does the normal vasculature (Cen M and Rosenbusch G, 1968). This variable response of inflammatory vessels may result in problems in differentiating neoplastic and inflammatory vessels and is the major factor limiting the current widespread use

of vasoconstrictor pharmacoangiography for tumor detection.

In contradistinction to the previous statements, the interventional renal artery administration of epinephrine can also permit improved differentiation of renal masses. For example, the angiographic appearance of renal hamartoma (angiomyolipoma) is often indistinguishable from hypernephroma. It has been shown that epinephrine may produce a vasoconstrictive response in benign hamartomas, thus permitting their angiographic differentiation from hypernephroma or hamartoma associated with tuberous sclerosis (Jander HP and Tonkin IL,

1979). The consistency of this vasoconstrictive response to epinephrine in benign hamartomas does, however, require more extensive evaluation. It has also been demonstrated that interventional epinephrine will produce constriction of the inflammatory hypervascularity of renal pelvic carcinoma invading the kidney and thus allow its angiographic differentiation from hypernephroma invading the pelvis, since the latter renal mass tends not to provoke an inflammatory response (Lagergren C and Ljungqvist A, 1969).

Epinephrine pharmacoangiography for the improved delineation of abnormal masses localized to other vascular beds has also been investigated with variable results. Optimization of this interventional procedure will apparently require extensive dose-response investigations for each vascular tumor system under consideration.

Renal artery constriction induced by the interventional injection of epinephrine results in the reflux of coadministered contrast medium into the adrenal artery. Hence, epinephrine pharmacoangiography can be used to enhance angiographic visualization of the adrenal vasculature. It is also possible to improve angiographic demonstration of renal veins if renal venography is performed in conjunction with epinephrine-induced constriction of the renal artery (Olin TB and Reuter SR, 1965). With this technique, the temporary decrease in renal blood flow diminishes contrast dilution and permits sufficient retrograde opacification to visualize the renal cortical veins (Ekelund L, 1980). Although epinephrine-enhanced renal venography has been found to be useful in the diagnosis and evaluation of a variety of renal parenchymal disorders, evidence suggests that the incorporation of epinephrine may result in an increased risk of nephrotoxic reactions (Cochran ST, et al, 1982).

Epinephrine and acetylcholine pharmacoangiography have been used to evaluate the hemodynamic significance of renal artery stenosis (Bookstein JJ, et al, 1976.

Renal artery injection of the vasodilating agent, acetylcholine, increases the transstenotic gradient and augments collateral blood flow to the affected kidney, whereas the vasoconstrictor, epinephrine, produces opposite effects. Surgical correction of the stenotic process in patients who demonstrate the previous responses to the vasoactive drugs was generally associated with a favorable outcome. Failure of the renal artery to dilate or constrict in response to such an intervention may, however, indicate a fixed lesion with replacement or destruction of the contractile elements of the vessel wall (Cen M and Rosenbusch G, 1968).

Epinephrine has also been used alone or in combination with other vasoactive drugs as an adjunct to intestinal angiography. Epinephrine (5–10 micrograms) injected into the celiac artery produces constriction of the hepatic and splenic arteries, but exerts minimal effects on the pancreatico- or gastroduodenal arterial beds (Pokieser H, 1975; Uden R, 1976). Epinephrine-enhanced celiacography has therefore been investigated as a method for improving visualization of the pancreatic vasculature. Epinephrine combined with a second vasoconstricting agent, angiotensin, were found to improve the angiographic demonstration of arterioles in the head and body of the pancreas while reducing the extent of opacification in the tail region (Pokieser H, 1975; Cen M, 1975). The hormone, secretin, is known to increase blood flow through the pancreas and duodenum. Pharmacoceliacography performed with the combination of epinephrine and secretin (90–150 "clinical" units) has permitted visualization of small pancreatic veins, and was found to be useful in the diagnosis of pancreatic carcinoma and pancreatitis (Uden R, 1976). The detection of insulinomas was not, however, improved with these techniques (Clouse M, et al, 1977). Superselective pancreatic arteriography is commonly performed for current evaluations of the pancreatic vasculature; the discussed pharmacoangiographic techniques being reserved for those conditions wherein catheterization of the pancreatic artery is not possible.

Hepatic neoplasms derive the majority of their blood flow from the hepatic artery, whereas the normal liver parenchyma is primarily supplied via the portal vein. The preferential arterial flow to hepatic tumors can be further augmented with the hepatic artery administration of epinephrine. Pharmacoangiography with epinephrine (5 micrograms) results in vasoconstriction and reduced delivery of contrast medium to normal hepatic tissue and shunting of blood flow with enhanced opacification of the unaffected tumor vasculature (Steckel RJ, et al, 1971).

The mesenteric arteries do not constrict in response to epinephrine. However, vasoconstriction does occur in arteries supplying an inflammatory lesion (i. e., Crohn's disease, ulcerative colitis). Both normal and inflammatory mesenteric vessels constrict if epinephrine (5 micrograms) is combined with propranolol (5 milligrams). The latter agent acts to block beta adrenergic vasodilation activity and thus increases the vasoconstriction response to epinephrine. Tumor neovascularity does not respond to epinephrine, alone, or in combination with propranolol. Hence, epinephrine-propranolol pharmacoangiography has been utilized to enhance the diagnosis and differentiation of inflammatory and malignant lesions of the bowel (Uden R, 1974).

The majority of pharmacoangiography investigations involving vasoconstrictors have incorporated the use of epinephrine. Other vasoconstricting agents have been utilized for similar purposes with varying degrees of success. The more common of these agents and their advantages/disadvantages relative to epinephrine are summarized below. The reader should refer to traditional pharmacology texts for more detailed discussion of the individual interventional drugs.

Angiotensin is an extremely potent vasoconstrictor that exerts its effects via a direct action on the vascular smooth muscle. It is rapidly degraded by tissue and plasma aminopeptidases resulting in a plasma half-life of approximately 20 seconds. Like epinephrine, angiotensin is a natural hormone; its endogenous occurrence being associated with stimulation of the renin system.

It has been shown that the renal vasoconstrictive effect of angiotensin is limited to the major arteries proximal to the interlobar arteries (Elkin M and Meng C–H, 1966). Hence, in comparison with epinephrine, the pharmacoangiographic use of angiotensin may decrease the risk of constricting the feeding, interlobar artery to a tumor and the associated potential for a "false-negative" diagnosis of renal neoplasm. For this reason, there has been considerable interest in the use of angiotensin for the evaluation of renal masses (Ekelund L, 1980). It has been determined that the optimal dose of angiotensin for pharmacoangiography of renal masses is 0.5–1 microgram administered 10–60 seconds prior to the injection of contrast medium (Ekelund L and Göthlen J, 1977a). Routine clinical use of this agent has been greatly restricted, however, due to the nonavailability of an FDA "approved" commercial product.

Similar to epinephrine, the adjunctive, selective arterial administration of angiotensin has been shown to enhance the angiographic visualization of malignant tumors localized in other vascular beds (Ekelund L, et al, 1977b; Laurin S, et al, 1980). Optimal results may, however, require the use of higher doses (e. g., 10–15 micrograms). Angiotensin (1–4 micrograms) injected into the celiac artery produces constriction of the hepatic, splenic, and gastric vessels with shunting of blood flow to the unaffected pancreatic artery. Hence, angiotensin pharmacoangiography has also been implicated for the improved visualization of the pancreatic vasculature (Kaplan JH and Bookstein JJ, 1972).

Vasopressin (antidiuretic hormone) is a natural pituitary hormone that is primarily responsible for maintaining serum osmolality by promoting the absorption of water from the renal tubules. At doses that exceed those required for its antidiuretic effect, vasopressin stimulates direct contraction of arteriole and capillary smooth muscle resulting in constriction of the splanchnic, pancreatic, coronary, and peripheral vasculature. With direct celiac or mesenteric artery administration, vasopressin produces constriction of the mesenteric, gastroduodenal, gastric, and splenic arteries but has no effect on the hepatic artery. Following its release or injection into the vascular compartment, vasopressin also undergoes rapid renal and hepatic degradation.

Vasopressin (0.2–0.4 Units/min.) has been shown to produce a biphasic response on renal blood flow consisting of a decrease followed by a compensatory increase. Renal tumor vessels may also demonstrate a varying degree of response to vasopressin, thus rendering this agent less attractive for pharmacoangiography of renal masses (Göthlin J, 1976).

Due to a resulting increase in blood flow to the unaffected hepatic artery, the adjunctive celiac artery injection of vasopressin (0.1–0.5 Units) has been shown to improve celiacographic visualization of hypervascular hepatic tumors (Boijsen E, 1974) and the identification of anomalous origins of the right hepatic artery (Kaneko M, 1974). It has been similarly used with wedged hepatic venography to both promote and maintain hepatic sinusoidal filling for a prolonged period of time. In general, however, the pharmacoangiographic use of vasopressin has been limited. A synthetic derivative of vasopressin, octapressin, may prove to be more acceptable for respective pharmacoangiographic and therapeutic procedures due to its greatly diminished antidiuretic activity per given degree of vasoconstriction (Kaneko M, 1974).

The natural neurohormone, *norepinephrine*, produces substantially greater pressor activity than epinephrine due to its lack of beta-receptor stimulation and vasodilating activity in peripheral blood vessels. On a molar basis, however, norepinephrine is less potent than epinephrine in causing renal artery constriction. Pharmacoangiography with norepinephrine (10–30 micrograms) does not appear to provide substantial advantages over epinephrine or angiotensin, and has not been extensively investigated.

Vasodilators. Numerous clinical and experimental studies have described the adjunctive use of various vasodilating agents for the enhancement of angiographic diagnoses (Hollenberg NK, et al, 1983). Vasodilator pharmacoangiography is primarily indicated to increase blood flow and the delivery of contrast medium to regions perfused by small or nonaccessible (i.e., for selective catheterization) arteries, thus permitting improved opacification and visualization of their respective vascular beds. The interventional administration of vasodilating drugs has also been utilized to differentiate functional vasospastic disorders from fixed organic lesions and to evaluate the dilation reserve capacity of blood vessels. Similar to vasoconstricting agents, vasodilators do produce a differing response in normal versus neoplastic vasculature. However, the use of vasodilator pharmacoangiography for the improved delineation of malignant tumors has, in general, not been as successful as the interventional use of vasoconstrictors. Vasodilation and increased opacification of the overlying normal vasculature often obscures visualization of the unaffected and, hence, less opacified tumor vessels.

The synthetic drug, *tolazoline*, is commonly used as an adjunct to angiographic procedures. This imidazoline derivative produces vasodilation via direct relaxation of vascular smooth muscle. It also produces alpha adrenergic receptor blockade. However at the doses routinely utilized for pharmacoangiography, its vasodilating effects are primarily related to its direct action. Following intravascular administration, tolazoline is rapidly eliminated, unchanged, in the urine.

The slow rate and low volume of blood flow in small arteries and their vascular beds often limits the quality of or diagnostic information available from respective angiograms, especially if hemodynamic or mechanical impairment of flow is present. Interventional incorporation of a vasodilator, such as tolazoline, into the angiography procedure permits more rapid injection of increased volumes of the radiopaque contrast medium into the vessel of interest. The ability to rapidly deliver a concentrated bolus of contrast results in diminished vascular dilution of opacification and improved angiographic demonstration of the respective arterial and venous beds (Figure 1.15). The adjunctive use of tolazoline (10–50 milligrams) has thus been shown to improve the diagnostic quality of both lower and upper extremity peripheral arteriography with substantial benefits in the evaluation of patients with preexisting peripheral vascular disorders (Kahn PC and Callow AD, 1965; Neubauer B, 1978).

Vasodilator pharmacoangiography is similarly used to improve or permit radiographic visualization of the portal and superior mesenteric veins in the related diagnosis of neoplasms, varices, or venous-systemic shunts. With the adjunctive administration of tolazoline (50 milligrams)

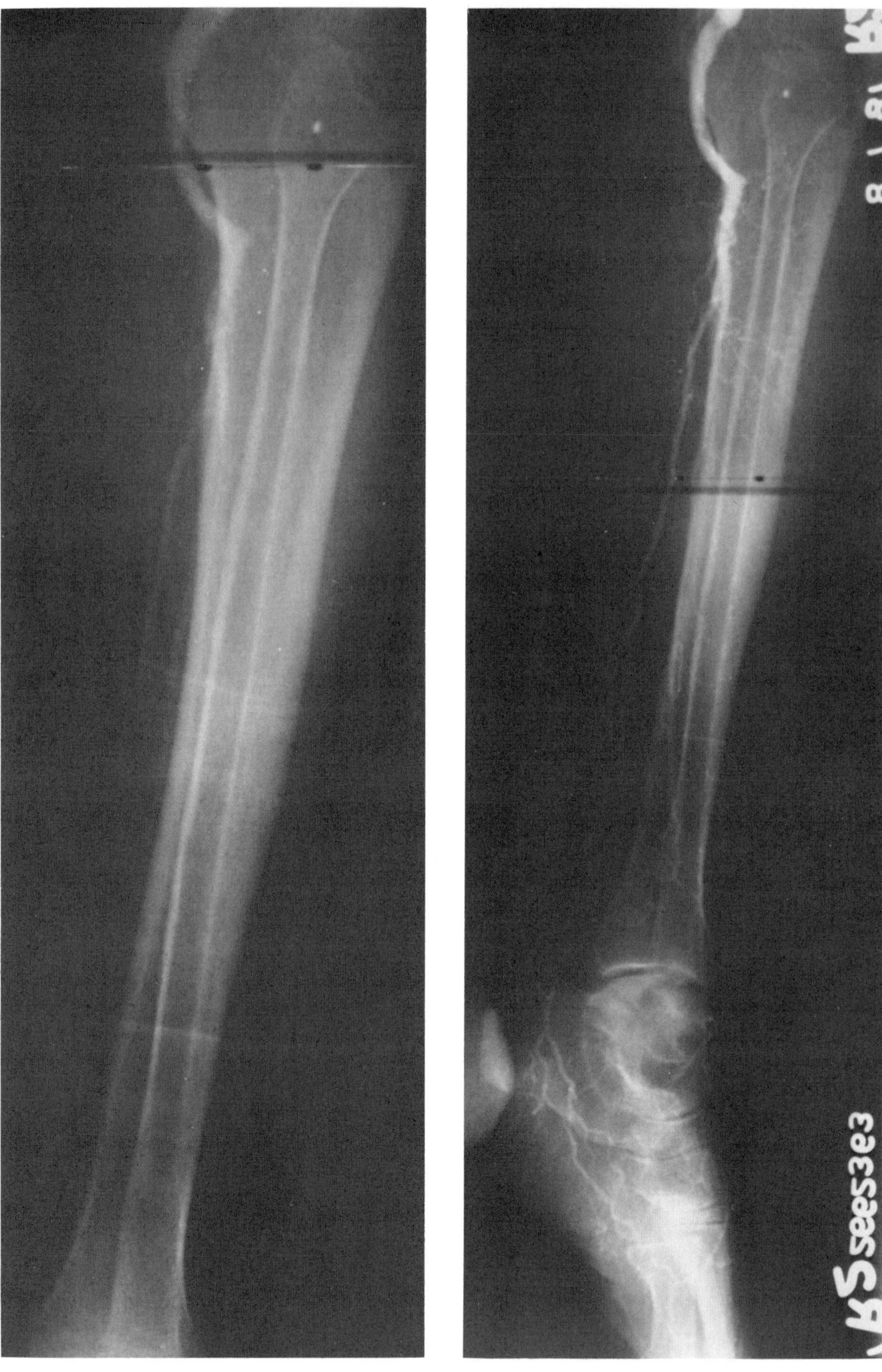

A   B

Figure 1.15 Selective right femoral arteriogram (lateral view) performed before (A) and after (B) the administration of tolazoline (25 mg, femoral artery). Note improved opacification of the peripheral vessels of the leg and foot in the dilator-augmented study.

in celiac or superior mesenteric arteriography there is often a reduction in opacification quality of the arterial phase relative to the noninterventional procedure. However, contrast enhancement on the venous side occurs earlier and is usually dramatically improved. Frequently, the superior mesenteric vein cannot be visualized unless a vasodilator is employed (Redman HC, et al, 1969). Tolazoline (10–40 milligrams) has also been combined with selective or superselective pancreatic arteriography to produce improved demonstration of intrapancreatic veins and pancreatic neoplasms (Schmarson R and Peters PE, 1975; Hawkins JF and Kaude J, 1975). The diagnostic quality of pancreatic examinations does not appear to be improved, however, with the interventional use of tolazoline in celiacography (Pokieser H, 1975). Use of tolazoline for these pharmacoangiographic procedures does not appear to be associated with any serious adverse reactions. Patients may, however, commonly experience abdominal pain or discomfort and tachycardia.

A second imidazoline derivative, *phentolamine*, also produces vasodilation by a direct action on vascular smooth muscle, but it demonstrates considerably greater alpha adrenergic blocking effects than tolazoline. Following intravascular administration, phentolamine undergoes rapid metabolic degradation with only 10% of the active drug being recovered in the urine.

Celiac and superior mesenteric arteriography incorporating phentolamine, alone, resulted in poor visualization of the portal or superior mesenteric veins. However, phentolamine (0.5–0.75 milligrams) combined with the beta adrenergic agonist, isoproterenol (15–40 micrograms), produced greater opacification of the portal and superior mesenteric venous systems than achieved with tolazoline (Cioffi CM, et al, 1973). Extensive studies on the adjunctive use of phentolamine have not been performed, and tolazoline remains preferable to the previous combination of agents for the enhancement of celiac and superior mesenteric arteriography.

The parasympathetic neurohormone, *acetylcholine*, exerts profound vasodilation activity (Ozer H and Hollenberg NK, 1974). Degradation via the action of endogenous cholinesterase enzymes occurs rapidly following its neuronal release or injection. Although acetylcholine pharmacoangiography has been extensively investigated in renal applications, routine interventional use of this agent has been limited by the nonavailability of a commercial preparation indicated for intravascular administration.

The infusion of acetylcholine (30–60 micrograms/min.) during renal arteriography produces a dose-dependent increase in renal arterial blood flow with greatest effects on the interlobar branches (Freed TA, et al, 1968). This vasodilation is accompanied by an increase in renal size, a more radiodense nephrogram with earlier nephrographic washout, and improved angiographic visualization of the renal veins. Acetylcholine augmented renal arteriography has therefore been found to be useful in assessing the renal contour and in demonstrating venous abnormalities such as varices and shunts (Vesin S, 1974). Pharmacoangiography with acetylcholine has been used somewhat less successfully in the investigation of renal tumors. High-dose acetylcholine infusion (500 microgram over 1 minute) combined with high-dose renal arteriography has been shown to improve the visualization of blood vessels associated with hypovascular renal cell carcinomas and to increase the density of the subsequent tumor stain (Chuang VP and Fried AM, 1978). Although these findings have not been consistently observed (Ekelund L, 1980), the increased renal vein opacification obtained with this technique does routinely permit an improved evaluation of collateral vessels associated with tumor infiltration of the renal veins and may obviate the need for renal venography and cavography.

Acetylcholine augmented renal arteriography is also an effective technique for differentiating permanently damaged renal vessels from functional abnormalities (Bookstein JJ, et al, 1976; Hollenberg NK, et al, 1974). As previously described, acetylcholine produces a dose-dependent increase in renal blood flow in patients with normal renal physiology. In patients with mild essential hypertension this response to acetylcholine is accentuated with substantially larger increases in blood flow occurring at lower doses. However, in the presence of advanced nephroschlerosis or parenchymal disease and secondary renal hypertension, the vasodilatory response to acetylcholine and the angiographic demonstration of the abnormality remain unaltered, thus suggesting a fixed, nonreversible lesion. A similar but less marked influence of increasing age on the renal vasodilatory response to acetylcholine is consistent with this latter finding.

The endogenous catecholamine, *dopamine*, is the biosynthetic precursor of norepinephrine. With the intravascular injection of low doses (0.5–2 microgram/kg/min), it primarily stimulates specific dopaminergic receptors in the renal, mesenteric, coronary, and intracerebral vascular beds to produce respective vasodilation. Larger doses (2–10 microgram/kg/min) result in general vasodilation responses associated with B_1-adrenergic stimulation, whereas further dose increases can lead to adrenergic stimulation and vasoconstriction. Like epinephrine and norepinephrine, intravascular dopamine is rapidly metabolized by the endogenous enzymes, catechol-o-methyl transferase and monoamine oxidase.

The adjunctive administration of dopamine (3 microgram/min/kg) in renal arteriography has been shown to produce renal artery dilation and arteriographic patterns that are qualitatively the same as those observed with acetylcholine, but less marked in degree (Ozer H and Hollenberg NK, 1974). As with acetylcholine, a potentiated vasodilator response to dopamine has been observed in functionally abnormal renal vessels. Likewise, nephrosclerosis produced a diminished dilatory response to dopamine (Borgensen A and Ayers CR, 1968; Hollenberg NK, et al, 1975). Hence, commercially available dopamine, indicated for intravascular administration, appears to provide an effective alternative to acetylcholine for renal pharmacoangiographic indications. Other interventional applications of dopamine have been limited.

The endogenous peptide, *bradykinin* (0.15–0.25 microgram/kg) has also been investigated as an interventional agent for renal arteriography based on its extremely potent vasodilation properties. In this regard, its effects on renal blood flow have been shown to be qualitatively and quantitatively similar to the respective effects of acetylcholine (Dollery CT, et al, 1965). Bradykinin apparently produces arterial dilation via a direct action on smooth muscle. Degradation occurs rapidly by several plasma and tissue proteolytic enzymes. Like acetylcholine, routine pharmacoangiographic use of bradykinin is limited by the nonavailability of a commercial product for intravascular administration.

Bradykinin has also been used in conjunction with superior mesenteric and celiac arteriography to improve the quality of the subsequent mesenteroportogram (Boijsen E and Redman HC, 1966). Maximum opacification of the portal venous system occurs following selective injection of bradykinin (5–10 micrograms) into the superior mesenteric artery with simultaneous injection of contrast medium into both the superior mesenteric artery and celiac axis (Boijsen E, 1974). Celiac

artery injection of bradykinin does not appear to improve respective venous opacification.

Prostaglandins are endogenous fatty acid arachiodonic acid substrates that exert a diverse range of vasoactive effects depending on their specific chemical structure or class, the vascular region-of-interest, and the dose administered. As a result of their rapid degradation by tissue-bound enzymes, the respective vascular effects of the prostaglandins are generally localized to the immediate region at their site of injection. Certain classes of the prostaglandins (e. g., F2-alpha, E2) are commercially available, but are indicated for their oxytocic properties following direct amniotic instillation rather than their vasoactive effects.

Prostaglandin E1 (1 microgram/min, not commercially available) has been shown to produce renal artery dilation and peak increases in renal blood flow that are essentially identical to the effects of acetylcholine but of shorter duration (Ozer H and Hollenberg NK, 1974). Prostaglandin E1 is also a potent dilator of the splancnic and peripheral arterial beds (Davis LJ, et al, 1975; Jonsson K, et al, 1978). When used as an intervention in superior mesenteric arteriography, prostaglandin E1 (7.5 micrograms) produced minimal alteration of arterial phase opacification; however, aortic reflux was decreased and the angiographic demonstration of the mesenteric and portal venous systems were markedly improved (Jonsson K, et al, 1977). The enhanced portal filling also resulted in increased opacification of the hepatic parenchyma. Hypo- and hypervascular hepatic tumor masses, which are only minimally perfused via the portal circulation, also appeared as more prominent filling defects following incorporation of prostaglandin E1 into the superior mesenteric arteriography procedure. Although similar results can be obtained with the vasodilator, tolazoline, a purported avantage of prostaglandin E1 is its more rapid rate of degradation and reduced risk of systemic hypotension and compensatory tachycardia.

Prostaglandin F2-alpha produces dilation of the normal splancnic vasculature at low doses (Denker H, et al, 1972). When used as an intervention in selective hepatic arteriography, the slow injection of prostaglandin F2-alpha (60 micrograms) resulted in improved opacification of the smaller intrahepatic and cystic arteries. The visualization of hypovascular hepatic metastases against a highly opacified liver parenchyma was improved as was the demonstration of tumor vessels associated with gallbladder carcinoma. Hypervascular hepatic masses were, however, better visualized with respective pharmacoangiographic use of a vasoconstrictor. It has therefore been suggested that selective hepatic arteriography for the evaluation of suspected hepatic masses may be optimized with interventional use of a short-acting vasoconstrictor, such as angiotensin, followed by a vasodilator, such as prostaglandin F2-alpha (Legge D, 1977).

The effects of prostaglandin F2-alpha on normal and diseased colonic vasculature have also been explored (Yuasa Y, et al, 1984; Kusano S, et al, 1983). In normal colonic vessels, prostaglandin F2-alpha (50–100 micrograms) produced dilation, whereas in the presence of both inflammatory (e. g., Crohn's disease, tuberculosis, abscess) and neoplastic (e. g., colon cancer, leiomyosarcoma, malignant lymphoma) colonic disease a vasoconstrictive effect was observed. The degree of vasoconstriction correlated with the hypervascularity of the colonic lesion and was localized to the affected site. No differences were noted in this vasoconstrictive effect between inflammatory and neoplastic lesions. The vasoconstrictive effect of prostaglandin F2-alpha (50–100 micrograms) has also been noted in various soft tissue tumors (i. e., liposarcoma, malignant fibrous histiocytoma, synovial sarcoma, malignant lymphoma) and has resulted in their improved angiographic demonstration relative to the increased opacification of normal surrounding tissue (Yuasa Y, et al, 1984). Prostaglandin F2-alpha does not, however, appear to produce vasoconstriction in renal tumors, hepatoma, osteosarcoma, or hemangioma.

The major physiological role of the endogenous polypeptide, *glucagon*, is the promotion of carbohydrate metabolism. In this regard, it is commercially available for the treatment of hypoglycemic crisis associated with insulin overdosage. The renovascular dilation properties of glucagon were first described using an indicator dye technique (Danford RO and Davidson AJ, 1969). Following injection into the renal artery, glucagon produced dilation of the renal arterial branches and a slow increase in renal blood flow occurring over a 30-minute period. Glucagon appears to exert this effect via a direct relaxation of smooth muscle. As with other endogenous polypeptides, the biological half-life of glucagon is short due to its degradation by proteolytic enzymes.

When investigated as an interventional agent in renal arteriography, glucagon (0.5 milligrams) demonstrated angiographic responses qualitatively equivalent to those of acetylcholine, despite producing much smaller blood flow increases (Ozer H, et al, 1974). Glucagon (0.025–0.05 milligram/kg) has also

been shown to produce greater arterial detail and increased portal venous opacification when combined with celiac and superior mesenteric arteriography (Danford RO, et al, 1969). Routine pharmacoangiographic use of glucagon has been limited, however, by the routine occurrence of nausea and vomiting at doses slightly larger than those required for a maximal vasodilator response (Ozer H, et al, 1974).

In addition to its vascular effects, glucagon also relaxes the smooth muscle of stomach, duodenum, small bowel, and colon, and inhibits gastric motility. Hence, intravenous glucagon (0.1–1 milligram) is routinely utilized to reduce peristalsis-induced artifacts in abdominal digital angiography and computed tomography procedures, and in gastrointestinal radiology studies.

Papaverine is a nonspecific smooth muscle relaxant that produces general dilation of large and small arteries and arterioles. Although intravascular papaverine is fairly rapidly metabolized by the liver, it is not totally degraded on a single pass. Subsequent dose accumulation and the general vasodilation properties of papaverine can lead to systemic hypotension (Hollenberg NK, et al, 1983), a major factor limiting routine interventional use of this commercially available agent.

The pharmacoangiographic use of papaverine (45 milligrams) has been evaluated in superior mesenteric and celiac arteriography (Widrich WC, et al, 1974). Similar to most other vasodilators, angiographic visualization of the arterial phase was somewhat degraded but opacification of the mesenteric and portal venous systems was greatly improved. Selective pharmacoarteriography with papaverine has also been proposed as a method for distinguishing reversible mesenteric vascular injury from irreversible infarction (Siegelman SS, et al, 1974). However, this interventional use of papaverine has only been investigated on a preliminary basis with controversial results (Bookstein JJ, et al, 1977).

Papaverine and other coronary artery dilators, including *nitroglycerin, dipyridamole and isoproterenol*, have also been used as interventional agents in various angiocardiography procedures. Coronary vasodilators are administered in conjunction with coronary angiography to permit the evaluation of dilation or coronary flow reserve capacity in the physiological assessment of obstructive coronary artery disease (Wilson RF and Pashayan AG, 1986). The ideal interventional agent for this purpose should produce maximum coronary vasodilation with minimal systemic effects, and should exhibit a short duration of action to permit multiple measurements. Both intravenous dipyridamole (0.56 mg/kg/4 min) and intracoronary papaverine (6–8 milligram R-coronary artery, 8–12 milligram L-coronary artery) produce near maximum elevations of coronary flow at doses that produce only minor decreases in systemic blood pressure; whereas isoproterenol infusion and intracoronary nitroglycerin are associated with submaximal flow increases. The duration of coronary dilation with intravenous dypyridamole does, however, appear to be slightly longer than that observed with intracoronary papaverine. The coronary vasodilator, nitroglycerin, has also been utilized in left ventriculography to identify regions of contractile reserve in the diagnosis of ischemic versus irreversibly damaged myocardium. Coronary artery dilation produces an unloading effect and an improvement in contractility in ischemic areas; whereas contractility is not improved in regions of infarct involvement (Hefant RH, et al, 1974).

RISK FACTORS/LOW-OSMOLALITY CONTRAST MEDIA RECOMMENDATIONS

For every angiographic request, the potential benefit to be gained from performing the procedure must be weighed against the risk of a possible reaction to the administrated contrast medium, catheter placement, or other aspects of the technique. With the exception of injecting an ionic contrast medium (ratio-1.5 or ratio-3 ionic-dimeric) agent into the subarachnoid space or into dorsal cysts or sinuses that may communicate with the subarachnoid space, there are, however, no absolute contraindications to the administration of angiographic contrast media. Based on extensive clinical experience, it is known that certain preexisting conditions may render the patient at an increased risk for conventional (i. e., ratio-1.5) intravascular contrast media reactions. Careful consideration should be given to such patients both prior to and after the indicated angiographic procedure. The use of special pretreatment regimens, the ratio-3 low-osmolality contrast media (Table 1.24), and prolonged monitoring may be warranted.

Previous Reactions to Contrast Media. Although pseudo-allergic reactions to angiographic contrast media occur unpredictably, it is known that a patient's history of allergies, asthma, or previous reactions to contrast media increases the relative risk of severe reactions to intravascular contrast media by factors of 2–4, 5, and 10, respectively (Wolf GL, 1986). As discussed in Chapter 8, clinical evidence indicates that the use of an appropriate pretreatment regimen (i. e., antihistamines, steroids, and ephedrine) may substantially reduce the expected incidence of pseudo-allergic reactions in patients who have experienced a previous contrast reaction. Experimental studies have also shown a diminished effect of the ratio-3 versus the ratio-1.5 angiographic media in regard to the proposed causative mechanisms for contrast-induced pseudo-allergic reactions (Swanson DP, et al, 1986). Based on these considerations, it is recommended that a low-osmolality contrast medium be utilized in patients with a documented history of a major reaction to an intravascular contrast medium (Table 1.24). Until more conclusive evidence is obtained, a pretreatment regimen should be continued with use of the low-osmolality agent unless its incorporation delays performance of an emergent radiographic procedure.

If a clinically significant blood pressure or electrocardiographic alteration is observed upon initial injection of a ratio-1.5 ionic medium, consideration should be given to completing the diagnostically required angiographic procedure using a ratio-3 low-osmolality agent (Table 1.24). Similarly, if the initial injection of a ratio-1.5 contrast medium produces intolerable pain and patient movement that preclude completion of the examination, substitution of a low-osmolality agent would increase the chance of obtaining a diagnostically useful study (Table 1.24).

Renal Considerations. In patients with normal renal function the incidence of contrast-induced acute renal failure is low, ranging from 0.6% for intravenous radiographic examinations to 2% for angiographic procedures (i. e., renal arteriography, aortography) that expose the renal artery to high concentrations of the ratio-1.5 media. However, this risk increases substantially in diabetic and hypertensive patients with a serum creatinine exceeding 2 mg/dL, or in otherwise "normal" patients with a serum creatinine greater than 5 mg/dL (Harkonen S and Kjellstrand C, 1981; Berkseth RO and Kjellstrand CM, 1984). Although the ratio-3 low-osmolality media have not been clinically proven (i. e., at the time of this writing) to produce less acute renal dysfunction than the conventional ratio-1.5 media, their demonstrated reduction in contrast-induced renal vaso-constriction and glomerular permeability alterations probably warrants consideration of their use in these at-risk patients (Table 1.24).

Multiple myeloma is commonly cited as a warning in the contrast media product literature, however the contribution of this disease to subsequent contrast-induced renal failure remains questionable (Harkonnen S and Kjellstrand C, 1981; Berkseth RO and Kjellstrand, CM, 1984). It is recommended (Table 1.24) that a ratio-3 low-osmolality contrast medium be utilized in patients with multiple myeloma and concomitant renal dysfunction (i. e., serum creatinine >2 mg/dL). This consideration is supported by a diminished potential for additive proteinuria with use of the ratio-3 versus the ratio-1.5 angiographic media (see Physiological Effects—Renal). The presence of an abnormally functioning (i. e., serum creatinine >2 mg/dL) single kidney represents another serious condition that necessitates special consideration and, if indicated, the use of a contrast medium (i. e., ratio-3 low osmolality agent) that exerts a minimum of effects on renal physiology (Table 1.24). Adequate hydration of the patient remains a primary concern with the administration of intravascular contrast media regardless of the nature of the agent utilized or the patient's renal function.

In addition to addressing the risk of preexisting renal dysfunction as it relates to contrast-induced renal failure, it is also important to consider the effect of renal dysfunction on delaying the rate of contrast media excretion and prolonging its exposure to the vasculature and sensitive organs. Although the acute hypersomolarity-induced effects of an angiographic contrast medium on vascular and organ physiology would be greatly diminished as a result of vascular dilution, the delayed excretion and retention of the agent in the vascular compartment would contribute to the intravascular osmotic load and increase or prolong its hypervolemic effects. This situation may precipitate a catastrophic worsening of borderline severe pulmonary edema or hypertension. Furthermore, a corresponding increase in left ventricular volume may elicit a detrimental effect in the presence of aortic valvular stenosis.

Cerebral Considerations. In a large prospective study of the complications of cerebral angiography performed using the conventional ratio-1.5 media, it was found that there is no statistically significant relationship between the incidence of reversible or permanent neurological reactions and the diagnosis of cerebrovascular disease, including tumors, subarachnoid hemorrhage, arteriovenous malformations, frequent transient ischemic attacks, and recent stroke (Earnest F, et al, 1984). There was a significant correlation, however, between the occurrence of these complications and the concomitant presence of renal dysfunction or an age greater than 60. In regard to concomitant renal dysfunction, the delayed excretion of an intravascular contrast medium may result in its prolonged exposure to the damaged blood-brain barrier and a corresponding increase in the amount of contrast medium exposed to and extravasated into the central nervous system tissue. Based on this consideration and the relative neurotoxic effects of ratio-1.5 ionic versus ratio-3 low-osmolality contrast media, the use of the latter agents should be considered in patients with known or suspected blood-brain-barrier disruption and preexisting, clinically significant renal dysfunction (Table 1.24). For maximum reduction in neurotoxic risk it is suggested that the nonionic media, iohexol and iopamidol, may be preferred to the ionic-dimer, ioxaglate meglumine-sodium (See Physiological Effects—Cerebral).

It has been speculated that the age-related risk factor may be associated with a diminished capacity for the development of collateral circulation to the regions of cerebrovascular abnormality. This risk of increased age could also be related to a general condition of atherosclerosis; however, this same study showed no significant correlation between the development of serious neurological complications and the concomitant presence of hypertension (Earnest F, et al, 1984). Recent studies have shown, however, that acute hypertension (>190 mm Hg) potentiates contrast-induced blood-brain-barrier opening in a rat model (Harnish PP and Hagberg DJ, 1988b).

Clinical experience also suggests that the risk of contrast-induced seizures increases in the presence of a seizure history associated with blood-brain-barrier disruption (Hayman LA and Hinck VC, 1985). It is therefore recommended (Table 1.24) that, if an angiographic procedure is indicated, the less neurotoxic ratio-3 nonionic media be utilized in these at-risk patients. Careful consideration should also be given to patients with a migraine history. If such a patient has experienced a previous major reaction to an intravascular contrast medium, or if intolerable pain occurs upon initial administration of a ratio-1.5 medium, an alternate diagnostic procedure or use of ratio-3 low-osmolality agent may be warranted.

Cardiopulmonary Considerations. As might be expected, there are multiple cardiac risk-factors associated with the administration of angiographic contrast media. Clinical experience suggests an increased potential for serious complications with severe coronary artery disease (i.e., left main stem disease, 3-vessel disease), severe aortic valvular stenosis, or left ventricular dysfunction with severe conges-

tive failure and pulmonary edema (Wolf GL, 1986; Cumberland DC, 1984; Adams DF, 1982). Problems arise, however, in attempting to identify these at-risk patients prior to performing the angiographic procedure that is indicated to make the respective diagnosis. Moreover, the severity of cardiac disease does not always correlate with patient symptoms or routine clinical or laboratory findings.

Although the natural history and pathogensis of unstable angine (i.e., angina at rest or upon minimal exertion, crescendo angina) are still under investigation, over 90% of patients with this condition have positive coronary arteriograms. Furthermore, there is a higher incidence of left main stem coronary artery stenosis and a less well-developed collateral circulation in patients with unstable versus stable angina (Braunwald E, 1980). Based on these considerations and the absence of a more definitive diagnosis, the presence of unstable angina may represent an indicator of severe coronary artery disease. Patients with aortic valvular stenosis usually have a characteristic midsystolic murmur and electocardiographic changes indicative of hypertrophy. In severe aortic stenosis the substantially reduced cardiac output and increased ventricular pressure can impair the blood supply to the myocardium (especially the subendocardium) and produce angina even in the presence of normal coronary arteries. Finally, severe congestive failure and pulmonary edema are generally recognizable clinically and would be expected to manifest as dyspnea at rest.

Based on their diminished hypervolemic effects, combined with their decreased or absent chronotropic, cardiodepressive, and vasodilatory effects, it is recommended that the ratio-3 low-osmolality agents be administered as an alternative to the ratio-1.5 ionic media in patients presenting with these severe cardiopulmonary conditions (Table 1.24). In recognition of the potential for hyerosmolarity-induced dilation of the peripheral arteries, it is also suggested that the ratio-

3 low-osmolality agents be utilized in the presence of circulatory collapse or shock syndrome (Table 1.24).

Procedure or Disease-Specific Considerations. The relative neurotoxic effects of angiographic contrast media become extremely important with procedures that expose the spinal cord to high doses and concentrations of the medium. Hence, use of the ratio-3 nonionic media should be considered for conventional (i. e., film-based) spinal arteriography.

In patients with known or suspected pheochromocytoma, the administration of angiographic contrast media can induce the release of stored catecholamines resulting in a hypertensive crisis. Since the exact mechanism responsible for this response is unknown, it is difficult to speculate if such a patient may be at less risk with use of a ratio-3 low-osmolality versus a ratio-1.5 ionic medium. If an angiographic procedure is required in this situation, it should be performed with a minimum dose of the contrast medium and the patient should be pretreated with appropriate alpha- and beta-receptor blocking agents.

The vascular endothelial effects of intravascular contrast media become especially important with direct injection into the peripheral veins, where the extremely slow blood flow and reduced vessel diameter result in delayed dilution of the contrast medium and prolonged vascular exposure. As a result, intense pain is a common complaint with phlebography of the legs. Phlebography-induced superficial phlebitis (1–2 hours post injection) and thrombosis (1–5 days post injection) are also recognized as rare, but reported, complications (Bettman MA and Paulin S, 1977). The thrombotic effects of intravascular contrast media are more evident following phlebography of the lower limbs than of the upper extremities (Laernum F, 1983). This may be related to differences in the respective rates of blood flow or the fact that ratio-1.5 ionic contrast agents have been shown to significantly depress the normal fibrinolytic activity of the vein intima (Whitehouse WM, et al, 1981). The initial fibrinolytic activity of arm veins is 3–4 times greater than that of the lower extremity veins (Nilsson IM, 1971).

Since the degree of endothelial damage induced by a contrast medium is directly dependent on its osmolality, it is obvious that the risk of phlebography complications can be reduced by utilizing a ratio-3 low-osmolality medium or a reduced concentration (i. e., < 45% w/v, 200 mg iodine/mL) of a meglumine salt of a ratio-1.5 ionic medium (Bettman MA, et al, 1984). The latter approach may present problems, however, since subsequent vascular dilution of the contrast medium following its injection into the peripheral foot vein may result in an inadequate iodine concentration for suitable opacification of the more central pelvic veins and inferior vena cava. Whether or not to substitute a low-osmolality agent for this procedure should be based on an evaluation of the observed rates of complications and success in obtaining diagnostically adequate studies. The thrombotic risk of phlebography using the hyperosmolar ratio-1.5 ionic media may also be reduced by elevating the limb and by incorporating a heparinized-saline flush to minimize the duration of contact between the medium and vessel walls. Such routine use of anticoagulants in phlebography procedures does necessitate caution in regard to preexisting and postprocedure bleeding disorders (Enge I, 1983).

VI. Dosage

The dosages (volumes and iodine concentrations) of intravascular contrast media used for the various angiographic procedures can vary considerably depending on the respective vascular region under investigation, the site of injection, the radiographic technique employed, and the age and condition of the patient. In general, the dose is based on an attempt to achieve adequate opacification for a

Table 1.25 COMMONLY UTILIZED DOSAGES OF INTRAVASCULAR CONTRAST MEDIA FOR ROUTINELY PERFORMED, CONVENTIONAL (I.E., FILM-SCREEN BASED) ANGIOGRAPHY PROCEDURES

STUDY/VESSEL INJECTED	ANATOMICAL LOCATION	IODINE CONC. (MG./ML.)	INJECTION RATE[a] (ML./SEC.)	SINGLE DOSE		TOTAL DOSE
				mL^a	$Range\ (mL)^b$	$(Range\ mL)^b$
Angiocardiography						
· Right coronary artery		370	2	4		
· Left coronary artery		370	3–4	7	5–10	40–225
· Left ventriculography		370	13–15	40	30–60	70–220
Cerebral angiography						
· Internal carotid	C2–3	280	7	10		30–100
· External carotid	C2–3	280	4	6		12–30
· Common carotid	C4–5	280	8–9	14	8–12	100–200
· Vertebral	Clavicle or C7	280	6–7	8–9	6–10	
· Four-vessel arch		280	25	35	40–80	
Subclavian artery	Clavicle	280	8	20		
Brachial artery		280	5	15		
Aorta						
· Thoracic		370	25–30	40–45	40–60	90–225
· Abdominal	L2	370	25	35	30–60	80–225
· Abdominal with runoff	L2	370	12–15	60–75		
Pulmonary artery		370	30–35	35–45	30–60	100–200
Celiac artery	T12–L1	370	8–10	40	30–60	80–225
Hepatic artery	T12–L1	370	6–7	25	20–50	70–225
Splenic artery	T12–L1	370	6–7	25	20–70	70–225
Mesenteric artery						
· Superior	L1	370	6–7	35		
· Inferior	L3	370	3–5	15–20		
Renal artery	L2	370	7	14	8–15	20–45
Femoral artery		280	6	15		
· with runoff		280	4–5	35–45	20–80	120–240

[a] Author's recommendations
[b] Based on Committee on Safety of Contrast Media, International Society of Radiology, survey of dosages commonly utilized. (Adapted from Shehadi WH, 1977)

quality study while minimizing the quantity of medium injected and, hence, the potential for organ or vessel toxicity. Table 1.25 lists commonly utilized dosages for routinely performed angiographic procedures. It must be emphasized, however, that individual patient and study conditions must be considered in determining the final dose for any given examination. Frequently, repeat doses of the contrast medium may be required for complete examination of the region under investigation.

Concentration Considerations. A primary determinant of the iodine and, hence, contrast medium concentration required for a given angiographic procedure is the diameter of the respective vasculature under investigation and its corresponding rate of blood flow. Injection of a contrast medium into a large, rapid-flow vessel will result in more rapid dilution of the iodine concentration and reduction in angiographic opacification than will injection into a smaller, slower flow vessel. Hence, the former situation requires the use of a contrast medium of higher initial iodine concentration than the latter.

The iodine concentration of the injected contrast medium may be limited by the ability of the organ being directly perfused by the medium to tolerate its chemotoxic effects. As previously discussed (see Physiological Effects), the chemotoxic effects of a given angiographic contrast medium increase as a function of its % w/v and iodine concentration. Some organs, such as the brain, are particularly sensitive to the chemotoxic effects of angiographic media resulting in generally recognized restrictions on the concentration of the contrast medium used for the respective angiographic procedure (e. g., 60% w/v diatrizoate meglumine or iothalamate meglumine for cerebral angiography). A similar consideration may apply to reducing the concentration of the contrast medium when examining a severely diseased versus "normal" organ.

Problems can arise, however, in maintaining a sufficient iodine concentration to achieve adequate vascular opacification for a quality examination. Under these circumstances, use of a ratio-3 low-osmolality agent in place of a conventional ratio-1.5 medium provides a method of maintaining the required iodine concentration while reducing the potential for chemotoxic effects. Alternatively, an advantage of the digital subtraction radiographic technique is the ability to obtain a quality angiographic examination using lower concentrations of the conventional ratio-1.5 media administered intraarterially.

Volume Considerations. The total volume of contrast medium injected in a given angiographic study is determined by the injection rate (mL/sec) and duration of injection (seconds). The rate at which the contrast medium should be injected is determined by the rate of vascular blood flow at the site of injection. If the rate of blood flow in the respective vessel is 6 mL/second then the contrast medium must also be injected at a rate of 6 mL/second to achieve complete opacification of that vessel. Incomplete opacification can result in a nondiagnostic study that must be repeated. Hence, the net result of injecting the contrast medium at a suboptimal rate is a requirement for additional injections per angiographic examination and excessive exposure to radiation and the contrast medium.

The appropriate volume of contrast medium to be injected per second into a visceral artery-of-interest can usually be determined by injecting the medium briskly and forcefully by hand while fluoroscopically observing for reflux of the medium out of the vessel into the artery from which it originates. The angiographer knows the volume that was contained in the syringe before and after injection and can judge an appropriate injection rate for maximum opacification of the artery without excessive reflux.

Certain guidelines exist for injection rates into the aorta. Adequate opacification of the ascending and transverse portions of the aorta typically require an injection rate of 25–30 mL/second for a duration of 2 seconds (i. e., total volume of 50–60 mL). As a general rule, aortic blood flow decreases by a factor of 30–50% after each location where a major set of arteries arise. Thus, 20–25 mL/second is an appropriate aortic injection rate after takeoff of the brachiocephalic arteries (i. e., proximal descending aorta), 10–12 mL/sec after takeoff of the visceral arteries (infrarenal abdominal aorta), and 6–7 mL/sec for the ilio-femoral arteries. The duration of aortic injections is usually 2 seconds unless opacification of the lower extremities is required, wherein the duration of injection must be prolonged to 8–10 seconds. Patients with larger arteries will, of course, require the injection of higher volumes of the contrast per second.

The duration of the contrast medium injection is dependent on the site of administration and the relative location and vascular volume of the region under investigation. For example, due to the larger volume of distribution of the injected contrast medium, an angiographic examination of the lower extremities following an intraaortic injection requires a longer duration of injection than is required with a selective femoral artery injection. Similarly, assuming equivalent rates of blood flow (i. e., injection rates) at the arterial site of injection, organ systems containing large vascular volumes require longer injection durations for a complete arterial and venous phase examination than do organ systems with small vascular volumes. Indeed, high volumes of the contrast medium are required to adequately visualize the venous systems of large visceral organs. When neoplastic involvement of the liver, spleen, or pancreas is a consideration, optimal opacification of the respective organ parenchyma is essential, especially for the demonstration of hypovascular lesions. Hence, a typical duration of contrast injection into the hepatic artery may involve 10 seconds or more in order to obtain a satisfactory parenchymal phase. Since the rate of injection is limited by the rate of arterial blood flow at the injection site, it is the duration of the injection that becomes a critical factor in ensuring a sufficient volume of contrast medium for adequate parenchymal opacification.

The duration of injection may also be limited by the ability of the organ being directly perfused by medium to tolerate its chemotoxic effects. The brain, kidney, and heart are particularly sensitive to the chemotoxic effects of angiographic contrast media; thus the duration of respective selective arterial injections is usually limited to 1 second or less. The limited time during which the arteries are opacified following such injections requires a very rapid filming sequence (i.e., 3–4 films/ sec) in order to acquire diagnostic information during the arterial phase of the study. Fortunately, the large visceral organs with their increased vascular volumes can generally tolerate more prolonged contrast medium injections. Prolongation of the duration of injection may also be considered if the organ to be studied lacks function or is to be resected. Such is the case with a kidney harboring a renal carcinoma wherein preoperative visualization of the renal vein is required to assess for tumor extrusion into the venous system. Under such circumstances, the duration of the selective renal artery injection is commonly increased to 5 seconds to permit optimal opacification of the renal draining vein.

Digital Subtraction Angiography Considerations. As previously discussed (see General Considerations), the increased contrast sensitivity of digital substraction angiography (DSA) can permit the intravenous administration of an intravascular contrast medium for many angiographic examinations that would normally require an arterial injection if the conventional film-based technique were utilized. Similarly, if an arterial route of administration is employed, the w/v or iodine concentration of the contrast medium required

for DSA is often lower than the corresponding requirement for conventional angiography. As with the conventional radiographic techniques, the total volume of the dilute contrast medium utilized for DSA must be sufficient to ensure complete filling and adequate opacification of the vascular region under investigation.

The rapid, direct intraarterial or intravenous injection of a contrast medium into the vessel-of-interest produces an

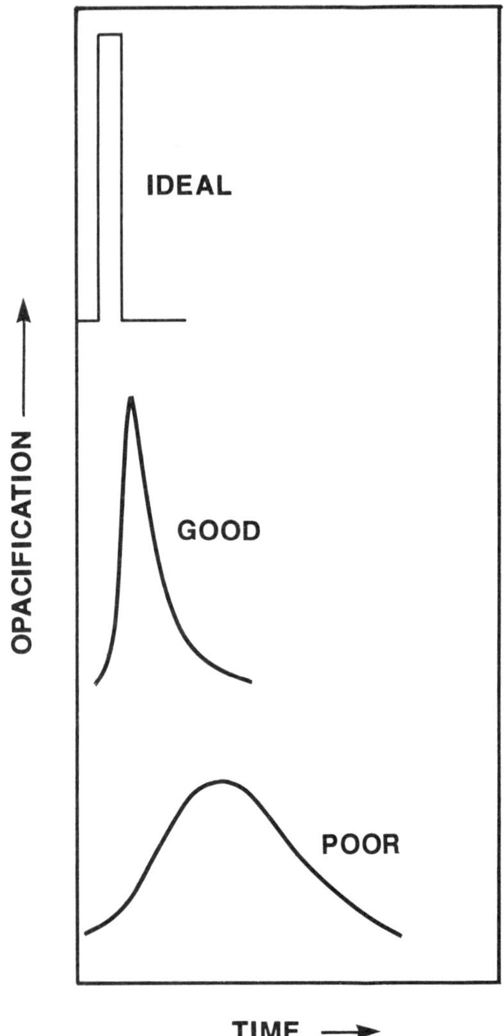

Figure 1.16 Illustration of ideal (high peak, narrow width), good (approximation of ideal), and poor (low peak, broad width) time-vascular opacification curves for digital subtraction angiography. (From Burbank FH, 1983; with permission.)

ideal "time-iodine concentration" curve of high peak and narrow width at a short distance from the catheter tip (Figure 1.16). For both conventional film-based and DSA procedures, a high peak iodine concentration maximizes vascular enhancement and image quality. Of special importance for DSA is the curve's shape. A narrow curve maximizes the iodine difference between the contrast-enhanced image and closely spaced (no or low iodine) mask images and reduces the potential for misregistration (patient movement) artifacts. Unfortunately, the intravenous injection of a contrast medium cannot produce an ideal arterial time-concentration curve due to dilution and mixing of the contrast in the lungs and heart. It is possible, however, to optimize the arterial time-concentration curve of intravenous DSA procedures if certain factors such as concentration and volume

of the injected medium, the site of injection, and contrast osmolality are considered (Burbank FH, 1983).

With a peripheral (i. e., cephalic) intravenous injection, the arterial curve peak is directly proportional to the total quantity (i. e., product of volume and concentration) of administered iodine. Hence, increasing the contrast medium volume at a given iodine concentration or increasing the iodine concentration at a given volume increases the height of the curve peak with little effect on curve width. Injection into a peripheral vein is associated with greater dilution of the contrast in a large central volume (i. e., decreased curve peak, increased curve width) compared to injection into a more central location, such as the subclavian vein, vena cava, or right heart (Figure 1.17). With central injections, however, the osmolality of the medium becomes an

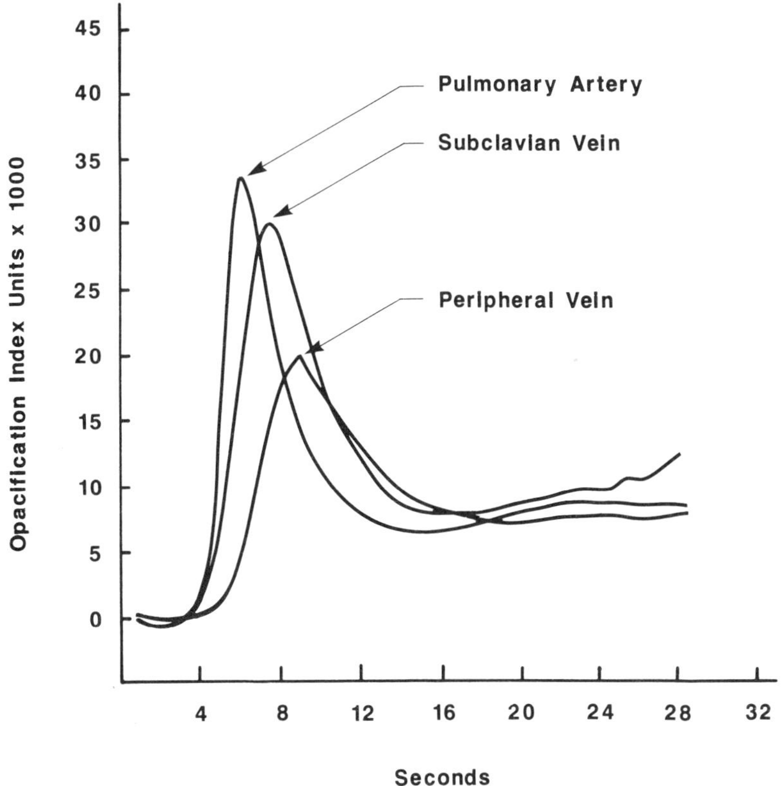

Figure 1.17   Time-vascular opacification curves as a function of site of contrast injection. Central injections yield more ideal curves for DSA than peripheral injections. (From Rubin DL, et al, 1984; with permission.)

important factor. Central injection of a hyperosmolar contrast medium produces a substantial osmotic diuretic effect in the lungs with a corresponding significant increase in central blood volume and cardiac output. These increases are associated with a detrimental effect on the peak of the subsequent arterial time-concentration curve (Burbank FH and Thompson WM, 1986). Increasing the iodine concentration of the administered contrast medium is associated with an increase in its osmolality. Therefore, the arterial curves of intravenous-DSA are optimized by a central injection of appropriate total iodine doses (e. g., 14–15 gm) using increased volumes of less concentrated ratio-1.5 ionic media or ratio-3 low-osmolality media (Burbank FH, 1983; Rubin DL, et al, 1984, Burbank FH, et al, 1986). High rates of injection are not required for intravenous-DSA procedures, the rate of injection having negligible influence on curve peak, width, or central blood volume.

The volumes and rates of injection used for intraarterial DSA studies are essentially the same as those utilized for the respective conventional angiography procedures (Table 1.25). However, with intraarterial DSA, the required (i. e., for equivalent angiographic resolution) % w/v and iodine concentrations of the injected contrast medium are substantially less (e. g., 50%) due to the increased contrast sensitivity of DSA versus standard techniques (Flynn MJ, et al, 1985). Frequently, intraarterial DSA studies employ a contrast medium of similar or slightly lower concentration (e. g., 280 mg iodine/mL for intraarterial-DSA versus 370 mg iodine/mL for conventional angiography) than that required for the conventional procedure to permit the im-

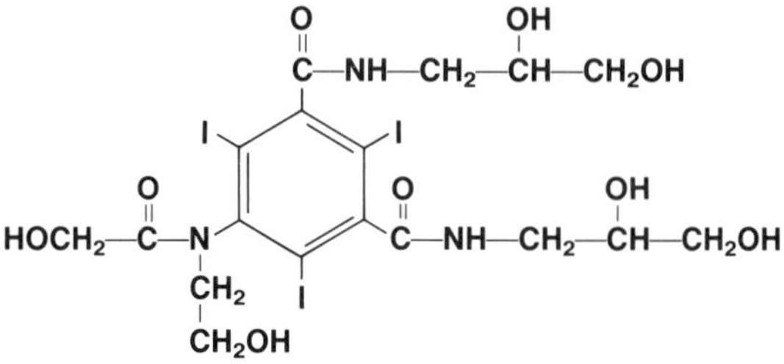

Figure 1.18 Chemical structure of ioversol.

proved demonstration of vascular anatomy.

Ioversol. Ioversol (Optiray®, Figure 1.18 is a ratio-3, nonionic contrast medium currently under development by Mallinckrodt, Inc. It has a molecular weight of 807 and an organically bound iodine content of 47.2%. Solutions of ioversol are buffered to pH 6–7.4 using tromethamine (3.6 mg/mL) and contain calcium edetate disodium (0.2 mg/mL) as a sequestering-stabilizing agent. Ioversol solutions are sensitive to light and should therefore be protected from prolonged exposure.

Ioversol will be available in multiple formulations (Table 1.26) indicated for angiography throughout the entire cardiovascular system including cerebral, coronary, peripheral, visceral, and renal arteriography, aortography, and left ventriculography. It will also be indicated for contrast enhanced computed tomography procedures (head and body) and for excretory urography. Unlike the other available ratio-3 nonionic media (e. g., iohexol, iopamidol), ioversol will not be initially indicated for myelography procedures.

Although little comparative data is available at this time, it is anticipated that ioversol, as a result of its substantially lower osmolality, will demonstrate a reduction (i. e., similar to the currently available ratio-3 media) in the number and severity of undesirable physiological effects compared to equiiodine concentrations of the conventional ratio-1.5 media. A discussion of the relative advantages and disadvantages of ioversol compared to the currently available ratio-3 nonionic and ionic-dimeric media awaits more extensive use of this new agent.

Table 1.26 **CHARACTERISTICS OF PROPOSED IOVERSOL FORMULATIONS (COURTESY OF RW JURGENS, PHD., MALLINCKRODT, INC., ST. LOUIS, MO.)**

BRAND NAME	IOVERSOL CONC. (% w/v)	IODINE CONC. (MG./ML.)	OSMOLALITY (MOSM/KG.)	VISCOSITY (CPS) 25°C	VISCOSITY (CPS) 37°C
Optiray-160	34	160	355	2.7	1.9
Optiray-240	51	240	502	4.6	3.0
Optiray-320	68	320	702	9.9	5.8

References

Abe, S, Ioh M, Unakami H, et al. Sinus slowing produced by intracoronary arterial injections of hyperosmotic solutions in man. *Am Heart J* 1976, 91:339–345.

Abrams HL, Boijsen E, Borgström K. Effect of epinephrine on the renal circulation. Angiographic observations. *Radiology* 1962, 79:911–922.

Abrams HL. The response of neoplastic renal vessels to epinephrine in man. *Radiology* 1964, 82:217–224.

Abrams HL, Obrez I, Hollenberg KN, et al. Pharmacoangiography of the renal vascular bed. *Curr Prob Diag Radiol* 1971, 1:1–50.

Abrams HL. Introduction and historical notes. *In Abrams Angiography: Vascular and Interventional Radiology*, Third Edition, (Abrams HL, ed.), Little, Brown and Co., Boston, 1983a, Vol. 1, pp. 3–14.

Abrams HL. Angiography in coronary disease. In *Abrams Angiography: Vascular and Interventional Radiology*, Third edition, (Abrams HL, ed.) Little, Brown and Co., Boston, 1983b, pp. 616–618.

Adams DF. How safe is the coronary angiogram? *Cardiovasc Intervent Radiol* 1982, 5:168–173.

Albertson KW, Doppman JL, Ramsey R. Spinal seizures induced by contrast media. *Radiology* 1973, 107:349–351.

Almén T. Effects of metrizamide and other contrast media on the isolated rabbit heart. *Acta Radiol* 1973, 335 (Suppl):216–222.

Almén T, Aspelin P, Nilsson P. Aortic and pulmonary arterial pressure after injection of contrast media into the right atrium of the rabbit. *Acta Radiol* 1980, 362 (Suppl):37–40.

Almén T. Development of nonionic contrast media. *Invest Radiol* 1985, 20 (Suppl):52–59.

Ansell G. Adverse reactions to contrast agents. *Invest Radiol* 1970, 5:374–391.

Arend LJ, Bakris GL, Burnette JC, et al. Role for intrarenal adenosine in the renal hemodynamic response to contrast media. *J Lab Clin Med* 1987, 110:406–411.

Aspelin P, Nylander G, Petterson H. Bradykinin-induced changes in caliber of portal vein during splanchnic angiography. *Invest Radiol* 1975, 11:10–19.

Aspelin P. Effect of ionic and non-ionic contrast media on whole blood viscosity, plasma viscosity, and hematocrit in vitro. *Acta Radiol Diag* 1978a, 19:977–989.

Aspelin P. Effect of ionic and non-ionic contrast media on morphology of human erythrocytes. *Acta Radiol* 1978b, 19:675–687.

Aspelin P, Schmid-Schönbein H. Effect of ionic and non-ionic contrast media on red cell aggregation in vitro. *Acta Radiol Diag* 1978c 19:766–784.

Aspelin P. Effect of ionic and non-ionic contrast media on red cell deformability in vitro. *Acta Radiol Diag* 1979, 20:1–12.

Aspelin P. Nonionic contrast media and red blood cell aggregation. *Clin Courier* 1988, 6:6.

Aulie A. Effect of iohexol, metrizamide and ioxaglate on the blood-brain barrier. *Acta Radiol* 1980, 362 (Suppl):13–16.

Ayre-Smith G. Fentanil and midazolam: An alternative to diazepam. (Letter to Editor). *Radiology* 1987, 164:285.

Bassan M, Ganz W, Marcus HS, et al. The effect of intracoronary injection of contrast-medium upon coronary blood flow. *Circulation* 1975, 51:442–452.

Belleville J, Baguet J, Paul J, et al. In vitro study of the inhibition of coagulation induced by different radiocontrast molecules. *Thrombosis Res* 1985, 38:149–162.

Berkseth RO, Kjellstrand CM. Radiologic contrast-induced nephropathy. *Med Clin North Am* 1984, 68:351–370.

Bernstein EF. The respiratory factor in angiographic media toxicity. *Radiology* 1965, 84:670–676.

Bettman MA, Paulin S. Leg phlebography: The incidence, nature, and modification of undesirable side effects. *Radiology* 1977, 122:101–104.

Bettman MA, Finkelstein J, Geller S. The

use of iopamidol, a new non-ionic contrast agent, in lower limb phlebography. *Invest Radiol* 1984, 19 (Suppl): S225–S228.

Bierman HR, Byron RL, Jr., Kelly KH, et al. Studies of the blood supply of tumors in man. III. Vascular patterns of the liver by hepatic arteriography in vivo. *J Nat Cancer Inst* 1951, 12:107–131.

Bierman HR, Kelly KH, Singer G. Studies on the blood supply of tumors in man. IV. The increased oxygen content of venous blood draining neoplasms. *J Nat Cancer Inst* 1952, 12:701–707.

Billing L, Lindgren AGH. Die pathologisch-anatomische unterlage der geschwalst-arteriographie; eine untersuchung der arteriellen gefässe des hypernephroms und des magenkarzinoms. *Acta Radiol* 1944, 25:625–640.

Bird CR, Drayer BP, Velaj R, et al. Safety of contrast media in cerebral angiography. Iopamidol versus methylglucamine iothalamate. *AJNR* 1984, 5:801–803.

Bjork L. The effect of cardiac catheterization and angiocardiology in the coagulation activity of blood. *AJR* 1968, 102:441–445.

Boijsen E, Redman HC. Effect of bradykinin on celiac and superior mesenteric angiography. *Invest Radiol* 1966, 1:422–430.

Boijsen E. Pharmacoangiography of the gastrointestinal tract. In *Radiology* Vol. 1 (Gomes-Lopez J, Bonmati J, eds.) Exerpta Medica, Amsterdam 1974, 247–252.

Bookstein JJ, Walter JF, Stanley JC, et al. Pharmacoangiographic manipulation of renal collateral blood flow. *Circulation* 1976, 53:328–334.

Bookstein JJ, Goldberger L, Niwayama G, et al. Angiographic aspects of experimental nonocclusive intestinal ischemic injury. *AJR* 1977, 128:923–930.

Borgensen A, Ayers CR. Effect of dopamine on renal vasculature of dogs with experimental renovascular hypertension. *Invest Radiol* 1968, 3:1–5.

Bosniak MA, Ambos MA, Madayag MA, et al. Epinephrine-enhanced renal angiography in renal mass lesions: Is it worth performing? *AJR* 1977, 129:647–652.

Brunwald E. *Heart Disease*, Vol. 2, W.B. Saunders Co., Philadelphia, 1980, pp. 1408–1410.

Brown TG. Cardiovascular actions of angiographic media. *Angiology* 1967, 18:273–281.

Bryan RN, Centino RS, Hershkowitz N, et al. Neurotoxicity of iohexol: A new non-ionic contrast medium. *Radiology* 1982, 145:379–382.

Bryan RN, Hershkowitz N. Neuronal effects of water-soluble contrast agents. *Invest Radiol* 1984, 19:329–332.

Burbank FH. Determinants of contrast enhancement for intravenous digital subtraction angiography. *Invest Radiol* 1983, 18:308–316.

Burbank FH, Thompson WM. Contrast media toxicity. Part I. Effects upon IV-DAS time-concentration curve peak and width. *Invest Radiol* 1986, 21:240–247.

Burke TI, Cronin RE, Duchin KL, et al. Ischemia in tubule obstruction during acute renal failure in dogs: Mannitol protection. *Am J Physiol* 1980, 238:F305–F314.

Byrd L, Sherman RL. Radiocontrast-induced acute renal failure: A clinical and pathophysiolgic review. *Medicine* 1979, 58:270–279.

Caldicott WJH, Hollenberg NK, Abrams HL. Characteristics of response of renal vascular bed to contrast media. *Invest Radiol* 1970, 5:539–547.

Carter AM, Olin T. Toxicity of roentgen contrast media at selective injection into the coronary artery in the rabbit. *Invest Radiol* 1973, 10:73–78.

Cassady RL, Kitten GL, Bradley IM, et al. Sites of cerebrovascular injury induced by radiographic contrast media. *Am J Anat* 1978, 153:477–482.

Cattell WR, Fry IK, Spencer AG, et al. Excretion urography. I. Factors determining the excretion of Hypaque. *Br J Radiol* 1967, 40:561–580.

Cen M, Rosenbusch G. Nierenangiographie mit adrenalin (möglich keiten der pharmakoangiographie). *Fortschi Geb Rontgenstr* 1968, 169:702–711.

Cen M. Pharmacoangiography of the pancreas. In *Efficiency and Limit of Radiologic Examination of the Pancreas*, (Anacker H, ed.) Stuttgart, Thieme, 1975, p. 180.

Chuang VP, Fried AM. High-dose renal pharmacoangiography in the assessment of hypovascular renal neoplasms. *AJR* 1978, 131:807–811.

Cioffi CM, Ruzicka FF, Jr., Carillo FJ, et al Enchanced visualization of the portal system using phentolamine and isoproterenol in combination. *Radiology* 1973, 108:43–49.

Clouse M, Costello P, Legg MA, et al. Subselective angiography in localizing insulinomas of the pancreas. *AJR* 1977, 128:741–746.

Cochran ST, Waisman J, Pagani JJ, et al. Nephrotoxicity of epinephrine-associated venography. *Invest Radiol* 1982, 17:583–592.

Crawford JA, Gumerman LW. Alteration of the body distribution of ^{99m}Tc-pyrophosphate by radiographic contrast material. *Clin Nucl Med* 1978, 3:305–307.

Cronqvist S. Iohexol in cerebral angiography. Survey and present state. *Acta Radiol* 1983, 366 (Suppl):135–139.

Cumberland DC. Low-osmolality contrast media in cardiac radiology. *Invest Radiol* 1984, 19 (Suppl):S301–S305.

Danford RO, Davidson AJ. The use of glucagon as a vasodilator in visceral angiography. *Radiology* 1969, 93:173–175.

Davis LJ, Anderson JH, Wallace S, et al. The use of prostaglanding E1 to enhance the angiographic visualization of the splanchnic circulation. *Radiology* 1975, 114:281–286.

Davis RJ. Factors affecting the determination of the serum protein-bound iodine. *Am J Med* 1966, 40:918–940.

Dawson P. Some aspects of contrast medium chemotoxicity. *Acta Radiol* 1983c, 366 (Suppl):174–179.

Dawson P, Harrison MJG, Weisblatt E. Effect of contrast media on red cell filtrability and morphology. *Br J Radiol* 1983a, 56:707–710.

Dawson P, Pitfield J, Button J. Contrast media and bronchospasm: A study with iopamidol. *Clin Radiol* 1983b 34:227–230.

Dawson P. New contrast agents. Chemistry and pharmacology. *Invest Radiol* 1984a, 19 (Suppl):S298–S300.

Dawson P, Heron C, Marshall J. Intravenous urography with low-osmolality contrast agents: Theoretical considerations and clinical findings. *Clin Radiol* 1984b, 35:173–175.

Dempsey PJ. Goree JA, Jimenez JP, et al. The effect of contrast media on patient motion during cerebral angiography. *Radiology* 1975, 115:207–209.

Dencker H, Göthlin J, Hedner P, et al. Superior mesenteric angiography and blood flow following intra-arterial injection of prostaglandin F2α. *AJR* 1972, 125:111–118.

Deutsch AL, Gerber KH, Haigler FH, et al. Effects of low-osmolality contrast materials on coronary hemodynamics, myocardial function, and coronary sinus osmolality in normal and ischemic states. *Invest Radiol* 1982, 17:284–291.

Dodek A, Hooper RO. Coronary spasm provoked by angiography. *Am Heart J* 1984, 107:781–784.

Dollery CT, Goldberg LI, Pentecost BL. Effects of intrarenal infusions of bradykinin and acetylcholine on renal blood flow in man. *Clin Sci Mol Med* 1965, 29:433–441.

Donadieu AM, Hartl C, Cardinal A, et al. Incidence of ventricular fibrillation during coronary angiography in the rabbit. A comparative study of isotonic ioxaglate and iohexol. *Invest Radiol* 1987, 22:106–110.

Duncan JS, Ramsay LE. Ventricular tachycardia precipitated by sodium iothalamate (Conray 420) injection during prenylamine treatment; a predictable adverse drug interaction. *Postgrad Med J* 1985, 61:415–417.

Earnest F, Forbes G, Sandok BA, et al.

Complications of cerebral angio-graphy: A prospective assessment of risk. *AJR* 1984, 142:247–253.

Ekelund L, Göthlen J. Effect of angiotensin on normal renal circulation by angiography and a dye dilution technique. *Acta Radiol Diag* 1977a, 18:39–48.

Ekelund L, Laurin S, Lunderqvist A. Comparison of a vasoconstrictor and a vasodilator in pharmacoangiography of bone and soft tissue tumors. *Radiology* 1977b, 122:95–99.

Ekelund L, Gerlock J Jr, Goncharenko V. The epinephrine effect in renal angiography revisited. *Clin Radiol* 1978, 29:387–392.

Ekelund L. Pharmacoangiography of the kidney: An overview. *Urol Radiol* 1980, 2:9–15.

Elkin M, Meng C-H. The effects of angiotensin on renal vascularity in dogs. *AJR* 1966, 98:927–934.

Emanuelsson H, Holmberg S, Selin K, et al. Effects of iohexol and metrizoate on myocardial blood flow and metabolism. *Acta Radiol* 1983, 466 (Suppl):121–125.

En Piao Z, Murdock DK, Hwang MH, et al. The effect of sodium on the fibrillatory propensity of non-ionic contrast media. *Invest Radiol* 1987, 22:895–900.

Enge I. Phlebography. Survey and present state. *Acta Radiol* 1983, 366 (Suppl):50–53.

Felder E. Chemistry of iopamidol. *Invest Radiol* 1984, 19 (Suppl):S164–S167.

Fisher HW. Hemodynamic reactions to angiographic media. A survey and commentary. *Radiology* 1968, 91:66–73.

Fisher HW, Redman HC. Comparison of sodium methylglucamine diatrizoate contrast media of minimal sodium content with a pure methylglucamine preparation. *Invest Radiol* 1971, 6:115–118.

Fischer HW, Morris TW. Possible factors in intravascular contrast media toxicity. *Invest Radiol* 1980, 15 (Suppl):S232–S238.

Fischer HW. Incompatibilities between contrast media and pharmacologic agents. *Radiology* 1987, 162:875.

Flynn MJ, Patel S, Zerwekh J, et al. Subtraction angiography: Comparative performance and cost of digital vs. film subtraction methods. In *Medical Imaging and Instrumentation '85: Practical Applications of Conventional and New Imaging Technologies*, Vol. 555, S.P.I.E., Bellingham, WA, 1985, pp. 230–245.

Freed TA, Hager H, Venik M. Effects of intraarterial acetylcholine on renal arteriography in normal humans. *AJR* 1968, 104:312–318.

Friedman HZ, De Boe SF, McGillen MJ, et al. Immediate effects of graded ionic and nonionic contrast injections on coronary blood flow and myocardial function. *Invest Radiol* 1987, 22:722–727.

Fuju K, Grayson T, Margulis AR, et al. The effects of intraarterial injection of contrast media on canine intestine. *AJR* 1963, 89:730–733.

Gensini GG, DiGiorgi S. Myocardial toxicity of contrast agents used in angiography. *Radiology* 1964, 82:24–34.

Gerber KH, Higgins CB. Comparative effects of ionic and non-ionic contrast materials on coronary and peripheral blood flow. *Invest Radiol* 1982a, 17:292–298.

Gerber KH, Higgins CB, Yuk Y-S, et al. Regional myocardial hemodynamic and metabolic effects of ionic and non-ionic contrast media in normal and ischemic states. *Circulation* 1982b, 65:1307–1314.

Golman K. The blood-brain barrier: Effects of non-ionic contrast media with and without addition of Ca^{2+} and Mg^{2+}. *Invest Radiol* 1979, 14:305–308.

Golman K, Holtas S. Proteinuria produced by urographic contrast media. *Invest Radiol* 1980, 15 (Suppl):S61–S66.

Gonsette RE, Liesenborgh L. New contrast media in cerebral angiography. Animal experiments and preliminary clinical studies. *Invest Radiol* 1980, 15 (Suppl):S270–S274.

Gordon IJ, Wescott JL. Intra-arterial lidocaine: An effective analgesic for peripheral angiography. *Radiology* 1977, 124:43–45.

Göthlin J. Effects of vasopressin on human renal circulation investigated by angiography and dye dilution technique. *Acta Radiol Diag* 1976, 17:763–772.

Grainger RG. Intravascular contrast media—The past, the present and the future. *Br J Radiol* 1982, 55:1–18.

Grayson RR. Factors which influence the radioactive iodine uptake test. *Am J Med* 1960, 28:397–415.

Grollman JH. The importance of preheating contrast media. *AJR* 1984, 142:391–392.

Haberey M, Schröder G, Mannesmann G. Cardiovascular effects of iohexol in the rat and the isolated rabbit heart. *Acta Radiol* 1980, 362 (Suppl):29–35.

Halsell RD. Heating contrast media: Role in contemporary angiography. *Radiology* 1987, 164:276–278.

Hamilton G, Fischer HW. Re: Contamination of contrast agents by rubber components of 50 ml disposable syringes. *AJR* 1984, 143:(Letter) 199–200.

Hamilton G. Severe reactions to urography in patients taking B-adrenergic blocking drugs. *Can Med Assoc J* 1985, 133:122.

Hamilton G. Contamination of contrast agent by MBT in rubber seals. *Can Med Assoc J* 1987, 136:(Letter) 1020–1021.

Harkonen S, Kjellstrand C. Contrast nephropathy. *Am J Nephrol* 1981, 1:69–77.

Harnish PP, DiStefano V. Decreased cerebrospinal fluid production by intravenous sodium diatrizoate. *Invest Radiol* 1984, 19:318–323.

Harnish PP, Northington FK, Samuel KA. Diatrizoate levels in cerebrospinal fluid following intravenous administration. Role of fluid production rate. *Invest Radiol* 1988a 23:377–380.

Harnish PP, Hagberg DJ. Contrast-media induced blood-brain barrier damage potentiation by hypertension. *Invest Radiol* 1988b, 23:463–465.

Hawkins JF Jr., Kaude J. Selective pancreatic angiography enhanced by tolazoline and using geometric magnifica-tion. In *Efficiency and Limit of Radiologic Examination of the Pancreas.* Stuttgart, Thieme 1975, pp. 174–179.

Hayman LA, Hinck VC. Water-soluble iodinated contrast media. In *Computed Tomography of the Head, Neck and Spine.* (Latchaw RE, ed.) Year Book Medical, Chicago, 1985, pp. 3–25.

Hayward R, Dawson P. Contrast agents in angiocardiography. *Br Heart J* 1984, 52:361–368.

Hefant RH, Pine R, Meister SG, et al. Nitroglycerin to unmask reversible asynergy: Correlation with post coronary bypass ventriculography. *Circulation* 1974, 50:108–113.

Higgins CB, Schmidt W. Alterations in calcium levels of coronary sinus blood during coronary angiography in the dog. *Circulation* 1978a, 58:512–519.

Higgins CB, Schmidt W .Direct and reflex myocardial effects of intracoronary administered contrast materials in the anesthetized and conscious dog: Comparison of standard and newer contrast materials. *Invest Radiol* 1978b, 13:205–216.

Higgins CB, Schmidt WS. Identification and evaluation of the contribution of the chemoreflex in the hemodynamic response to intracarotid administration of contrast materials in the conscious dog: Comparison with the response to nicotine. *Invest Radiol* 1979, 14:438–446.

Higgins CB. Effects of contrast materials on left ventricular function. *Invest Radiol* 1980, 15 (Suppl):S220–S231.

Higgins CB, Kuber M, Slutsky RA. Interaction between verapamil and contrast media in coronary arteriography: Comparison of standard ionic and new nonionic media. *Circulation* 1983, 68:628–635.

Higgins CB. Overview of cardiovascular effects of contrast media. Comparison of ionic and nonionic media. *Invest Radiol* 1984, 19 (Suppl):S187–S190.

Hilal SK. Hemodynamic changes associated with the intraarterial injection of contrast media. *Radiology* 1966, 86:615–633.

Holder JC, Dalrymple GV. Pain and

aortofemoral arteriography: The importance of chemical structure and osmolality of contrast agents. *Invest Radiol* 1981, 16:508–512.

Hollenberg NK, Adams DF, Solomon HS, et al. Senescence and the renal vasculature in normal man. *Circ Res* 1974, 34:309–316.

Hollengerg NK, Adams DF, Solomon H, et al. Renal vascular tone in essential and secondary hypotension: Hemodynamic and angiographic responses to vasodilators. *Medicine* 1975, 54:29–44.

Hollenberg NK, Garnic JD. Harrington DP. Pharmacoangiography. In *Abrams Angiography*, Third Edition (Abrams HL, ed.) Little, Brown and Co., Boston, 1983, pp. 95–104.

Hoppe JO. Some pharmacological aspects of radiopaque compounds. *Ann NY Acad Sci* 1959, 78:727–739.

Humes HD, Hunt DA, White MD. Direct toxic effect of the radiocontrast agent diatrizoate on renal proximal tubule cells. *Am J Physiol* 1987a, 252:F246–F255.

Humes HD, Cieslinski DA, Messana JM. Pathogenesis of radiocontrast-induced acute renal failure: Comparative nephrotoxicity of diatrizoate and iopamidol. *Diag Imaging* 1987b, May (Suppl): 12–18.

Jander HP, Tonkin IL. Epinephrine enhanced renal angiography in the diagnosis of hamartoma (angiomyolipoma): A reevaluation. *Radiology* 1979, 132:61–66.

Jeppsson PG, Olin T. Neurotoxicity of roentgen contrast media. *Acta Radiol Diag* 1970, 10:17–34.

Jonsson K, DeSantos LA, Wallace S, et al. Prostaglandin E1 (PGE) in angiography of tumors of the extremities. *AJR* 1978, 130:7–11.

Jonsson K, Wallace S, Jacobson ED, et al. The use of prostaglandin E1 for enhanced visualization of the splanchnic circulation. *Radiology* 1977, 125:373–378.

Junck L, Marshall WH. Neurotoxicity of radiological contrast agents. *Ann Neurol* 1983, 13:469–484.

Kahn PC. The epinephrine effect in selective renal angiography. *Radiology* 1965, 85:301–305.

Kahn PC, Callow AD. Selective vasodilatation as an aid in angiography. *AJR* 1965, 94:213–220.

Kaneko M. Pharmacoangiography with vasopressin and its mimetics. In *Radiology* Vol. 1, (Gomez-Lopez J, Bonmati J, eds.) Exerpta Medica, Amsterdam 1974, pp. 262–266.

Kaplan JH, Bookstein JJ. Abdominal visceral pharmacoangiography with angiotensin. *Radiology* 1972, 103:79–83.

Kaude J, Wirtanen G. Celiac epinephrine enhanced angiography. *AJR* 1970, 110:818–826.

Kido DK, Potts DG, Bryan RN, et al. Iohexol in cerebral angiography. Multicenter clinical trial. *Invest Radiol* 1985, 20 (Suppl): 555–557.

Kim KS, Lachman R. In vitro effects of iodinated contrast media on the growth of staphylococci. *Invest Radiol* 1982, 17:305–309.

Kodama JK, Butler WM, Tusing TW, et al. Iothalamate: A new intravascular radiopaque medium with unusual pharmacotoxic inertness. *Expt Mol Pathol* 1963, 2 (Suppl):65–80.

Kricheff II, Chase NE. Evaluation of complication rates of meglumine diatrizoate and meglumine iothalamate in cerebral angiography. *Radiology* 1967, 101:220–223.

Kurnick PB, Tiefenbrunn AJ, Ludbrook PA, et al. Peripheral hemodynamic effects of intraventricular and intracoronary contrast media in man. *Invest Radiol* 1985, 20:203–211.

Kusano S, Murata K, Tominaga S, et al. The response of neoplastic intestinal vessels to prostaglandin F2α: Angiographic observations with emphasis on therapeutic applications. *Cardiovasc Intervent Radiol* 1983, 6:97–103.

Laernum F. Injurious effects of contrast media on human vascular endothelium. *Acta Radiol* 1983, 366 (Suppl): 70–71.

Lagergren G, Ljungqvist A. Radiography in the differential diagnosis between carcinoma of the kidney and of the renal pelvis. *Scan J Urol Nephrol* 1969, 3:111–115.

Lange PE, Neubert D, Onnasch GW, et al. Effects of angiographic contrast media on the pulmonary circulation in pigs. *Am J Cardiol* 1984, 54:1125–1130.

Lasser EC, Farr RS, Fugimagari T, et al. The significance of protein binding of contrast media in roentgen diagnosis. *AJR* 1962, 87:338–360.

Lasser EC. Metabolic basis of contrast material toxicity—Status. *AJR* 1971, 113:415–422.

Laurin S, Ekelund L, Persson B. Late recurrence of giant-cell tumor of bone: Pharmacoangiographic evaluation. *Skeletal Radiol* 1980, 5:227–231.

Legge D. The use of prostagladin F2-alpha in selective hepatic angiography. *Radiology* 1977, 124:331–335.

Levin DC. Pitfalls in coronary arteriography. In *Abrams Angiography*, Third Edition (Abrams HL, ed.), Little, Brown and Co., Boston, 1983, pp. 664–666.

Lichtman MA, Murphy MS, Whitlock AA, et al. Acidification of plasma by the red cell due to radiographic contrast materials. *Circulation* 1975, 52:943–950.

Littner MR, Rosenfeld AT, Ulreich S, et al. Evaluation of bronchospasm during excretory urography. *Radiology* 1977, 124:17–21.

Littner MR, Ulreich S, Putnam CE, et al. Bronchospasm during excretory urography. Lack of specificity for the methyl-glucamine cation. *AJR* 1981, 137:377–381.

Longstaff AJ, Henson JHL. Bronchospasm following intravenous injection of ionic and nonionic contrast media. *Clin Radiol* 1985, 36:651–653.

Måre K, Violante M. Pulmonary edema following high intravenous dose of di-atrizoate. A study in the rat. *Acta Radiol Diag* 1983, 24:419–424.

Måre K, Violante M, Zack A. Contrast media induced pulmonary edema. Comparison of ionic and nonionic agents in an animal model. *Invest Radiol* 1984a, 19:566–569.

Måre K, Violante M, Fischer HW. Pulmonary edema following high in-travenous doses of ionic contrast media. Effect of the anion composition and concentration. *Invest Radiol* 1984b, 19:188–191.

Marshall TR, Ling JT, Follis G, et al. Pharmacological incompatibility of contrast media with various drugs and agents. *Radiology* 1965, 84:536–539.

Michelet AA. Effects of intravascular contrast media on the blood-brain barrier. *Acta Radiol* 1987; 28:329–333.

Miller DL, Wall RT. Fentanyl and diazepam for analgesia and sedation during radiologic special procedures. *Radiology* 1987, 162:195–198.

Moreau J-F, Droz D, Noel LH, et al. Tubular nephrotoxicity of water-soluble iodinated contrast media. *Invest Radiol* 1980, 15 (Suppl):S54–S60.

Morettin LB, Olifant DM, Brown RW. Comparative evaluation of the effects of an ionic vs. a nonionic contrast medium on the venous endothelium. *Invest Radiol* 1984, 19:593–596.

Morris DL, Wisneski JA, Gertz EW, et al. Potentiation by nifedipine and diltiazem of the hypotensive response after contrast angiography. *J. Am Coll Cardiol*, 1985, 6:785–791.

Morris TW, Francis M, Fischer HW. A comparison of the cardiovascular responses to carotid injections of ionic and nonionic contrast media. *Invest Radiol* 1979, 14:217–223.

Morris TW, Sahler LG, Fischer HW. Calcium binding by radiopaque media. *Invest Radiol* 1982; 17:501–505.

Morris TW, Sahler LG, Whynot LK, et al. Contrast media induced fibrillation. Comparison of Angiovist 370 and Re-nografin 76. *Radiology* 1984, 152:203–204.

Morris TW, Haya kawa K, Sahler LG, et al. Incidence of fibrillation with isotonic contrast media for intraarterial DSA. *Diag Imag Clin Med* 1986; 55:109–113.

Morris TW. Ventricular fibrillation during right coronary arteriography with iox-aglate, iohexol, and iopamidol in dogs. *Invest Radiol* 1988, 23:205–208.

Mulry C, Wolf GL, Kilzer K. The effect of cardiac glycosides on the ventricular fibrillation threshold in the ischemic and non-ischemic dog heart. *Invest Radiol* 1980, 15 (Abstract):417.

Murdock DK, Euler DE, Kozeny G, et al. Ventricular fibrillation during coronary angiography in dogs: The role of calcium-binding additives. *Am J Cardiol* 1984a, 54:897–901.

Murdock DK, Walsh J, Euler DE, et al. Inotropic effects of ionic contrast media: The role of calcium binding additives. *Cath Cardiovasc Diag* 1984b, 10:455–463.

Murdock DK, Johnson SA, Loeb HS, et al. Ventricular fibrillation during coronary angiography: Reduced incidence in man with contrast media lacking calcium binding additives. *Cath Cardiovasc Diag* 1985, 11:153–159.

Neubauer B. Intraarterial tolazoline in angiography of the foot. *Acta Radiol Diag* 1978, 19:793–798.

Newell JD, Higgins CB, Kelley MJ, et al. The influence of hyperosmolarity on left ventricular contractile state. Disparate effect of nonionic and ionic solutions. *Invest Radiol* 1980, 15:363–370.

Nilsson IM. Trombos och trombosbehandling. In *Blödnings-och Trombossjukdomar*. Stockholm, Kabi, Almgvist and Wiksell, 1971, p. 169.

Norman D, Brant-Zawadzki M, Sobel D. Tolerability and efficacy of Hexabrix in cerebral angiography. *Invest Radiol* 1984, 19 (Suppl):S306–S307.

Nyman U, Almén T, Landtman S. Effect of pH, buffer, and osmolality of different contrast media on aortic blood pressure in the rabbit. *Acta Radiol Diag* 1980a, 21:679–684.

Nyman U, Almén T, Landtman M. Effect of contrast media on femoral blood flow. *Acta Radiol* 1980b, 362 (Suppl): 43–48.

Olin TB, Reuter SR. A pharmacologic method for improving nephrophlebography. *Radiology* 1965, 85:1036–1042.

Ozer H, Hollenberg NK. Renal angiographic and hemodynamic responses to vasodilators. A comparison of five agents in the dog. *Invest Radiol* 1974, 9:473–478.

Paajanen H, Kormano M, Uotila P. Modification of platelet aggregation and thromboxane synthesis by intravascular contrast media. *Invest Radiol* 1984, 19:333–337.

Padayachee TS, Reidy JF, King DH, et al. Femoral artery blood flow and pain during lumbar aortography. *Clin Radiol* 1983, 34:79–85.

Parvez Z, Moncoda R, Messmore HL, et al. Ionic and nonionic contrast media interaction with anticoagulant drugs. *Acta Radiol Diag* 1982, 23:401–404.

Parvez Z, Moncoda R, Fareed J, et al. Antiplatelet action of intravascular contrast media. *Invest Radiol* 1984, 19: 208–211.

Paulin S, Adams DF. Increased ventricular fibrillation during coronary angiography with a new contrast medium preparation. *Radiology* 1971, 101:45–50.

Peck WW, Slutsky RA, Hackney DB, et al. Effects of contrast media on pulmonary hemodynamics: Comparison of ionic and nonionic agents. *Radiology* 1983, 149:371–374.

Peck WW, Slutsky RA, Mancini GBJ, et al. Combined actions of verapamil and contrast media on atrioventricular conduction. *Invest Radiol* 1984, 19:202–207.

Piao ZE, Murdock DK, Hwang MH, et al. Combined actions of verapamil and contrast media on atrioventricular fibrillation. A comparison of Hypaque 76, Herabrix, and Omnipaque. *Invest Radiol* 1988, 23:466–470.

Pilla TJ, Beshany SE, Shields JB. Incompatibility of Hexabrix and paraverine. *AJR* 1986, 146:1300–1301.

Pokieser H. Pharmacoangiography. In *Efficiency and Limit of Radiologic Examination of the Pancreas*, (Anacher H, ed.) Stuttgart, Thieme, 1975 pp. 167–174.

Ranges HA, Bradley SE. Systemic and renal circulatory changes following administration of adrenin, ephedrine and paredrinol to normal man. *J Clin Invest* 1943, 22:687–693.

Raininko R. Endothelial permeability increase produced by angiographic contrast media. *Fortschr Röntgenstr* 1979, 4:433–438.

Raininko R, Ylinen SL. Effect of ionic and nonionic contrast media on aggregation of red blood cells in vitro. *Acta Radiol* 1987 28:887–892.

Rao SA, Trembath LA, Collier BD. Effect of ionic and nonionic iodinated contrast agents on red blood cell labeling with Tc-99m. *J Nucl Med* 1987, 28 (Abstract):574.

Rao VM, Rao AK, Steiner RM, et al. The effect of ionic and nonionic contrast media on the sickling phenomenon. *Radiology* 1982, 144:291–293.

Rapoport SI, Thompson HK, Bidinger JM. Equi-osmolal opening of the blood-brain barrier in the rabbit by different contrast media. *Acta Radiol* 1974; 15:21–32.

Redman HC, Reuter SR, Miller WJ. Improvement of superior mesenteric and portal vein visualization with tolazoline. *Invest Radiol* 1969, 4:24–27.

Redmond RL, Kumpe DA. Fentanyl and diazepam for analgesia and sedation during radiologic special procedures. (Letter to Editor) *Radiology* 1987, 164:284.

Rees CR, Palmaz JC, Garcia O, et al. The hemodynamic effects of the administration of ionic and nonionic contrast materials into the pulmonary arteries of a canine model of acute pulmonary hypertension. *Invest Radiol* 1988a, 23:184–189.

Rees CR, Merchun G, Becker GJ, et al. In vitro study of high pressure catheters and various contrast agents. *Radiology* 1988b, 166:53–56.

Richie W, Lynch P, Stewart G. The effect of contrast media on normal and inflamed canine veins. *Invest Radiol* 1974, 19:593–596.

Rockoff SD, Brasch R. Contrast media as histamine liberators. III. Histamine release and some associated hemodynamic effects during pulmonary angiography in dogs. *Invest Radiol* 1971, 6:110–114.

Rosenthall L, Ambhanwong S, Stratford J. Observations on the effect of contrast material on normal and abnormal brain tissue using radiopertechnetate. *Radiology* 1969, 92:1467–1472.

Rubin DL, Burbank FH, Bradley BR, et al. An experimental evaluation of central vs. peripheral injection of intravenous digital subtraction angiography (IV-DSA). *Invest Radiol* 1984, 19:30–35.

Saeed M, Braun SD, Cohan RH, et al. Pulmonary angiography with iopamidol: Patient comfort, image quality, and hemodynamics. *Radiology* 1987; 165:345–349.

Sage MR, Wilcox J, Evill CA, et al. Comparison of blood-brain barrier disruption by intracarotid iopamidol and methylglucamine iothalamate. *AJNR* 1983, 4:893–895.

Salvesen S, Nilsen PL, Holtermann H. Effects of calcium and magnesium ions on the systemic and local toxicities of the N-methylglucamine (meglumine) salt of metrizoic acid (Isopaque). *Acta Radiol* 1967, 270 (Suppl):180–193.

Saxton HM. Urography. *Br J Radiol* 1969, 42:321–396.

Schmarson R, Peters PE. The pancreatographic effect during pharmacoangiography of the pancreas. *Acta Radiol Diag* 1975, 16:73–80.

Serur JR, Als AV, Miner-Green N, et al. Comparative effects of three radiographic contrast agents in isolated normal and ischemic canine hearts. *Invest Radiol* 1980, 15 (Suppl):S196–S202.

Severini G, Aliberti LM. Variation of urinary enzymes N-acetyl-beta-glucosamidase, alanine-aminopeptidase, and lysozyme in patients receiving radiocontrast agents. *Clin Biochem* 1987, 20:339–341.

Shah SJ, Gerlock AJ. Incompability of Hexabrix and papaverine in peripheral arteriography. *Radiology* 1987, 162:619–620.

Shanahan JC, Palmer C, Egginton J: Misleading urine tests after Hexabrix I.V.U. *Br. J. Radiol* 1985, 58:389.

Shapiro GA, Loeb PM, Bern RN, et al. Influence of Cholografin and Renografin-76 on platelet function. *Radiology* 1977, 124:641–643.

Shapiro JR, Xie F, Meltzer RS. Myocardial contrast two-dimensional echocardiography: Dose-myocardial effect relations of intracoronary microbubbles. *J Am Coll Cardiol* 1988, 12:765–771.

Shaw DD, Potts DG. Toxicology of iohexol. *Invest Radiol* 1985, 20 (Suppl): S10–S13.

Shealy CN. A comparison of Renografin and Hypaque for carotid arteriography. *J Neurosurg* 1963, 20:137–138.

Shehadi WH. Contrast media in diagnostic radiology. Recommendation for labels, package inserts, and dosage determination. *AJR* 1977, 129:167–170.

Siegelman SS, Sprayregan S, Boley SJ. Angiographic diagnoses of mesenteric arterial vasoconstriction. *Radiology* 1974, 112:533–542.

Simon AL, Shabetai R, Lang JH, et al. The mechanism of production of ventricular fibrillation in coronary angiography. *AJR* 1972, 114:810–815.

Smith DC, Lois JF, Gomes AS, et al. Pulmonary arteriography. Comparison of cough stimulation effects of diatrizoate and ioxaglate. *Radiology* 1987, 162:617–618.

Snyder C, Cramer R, Amplatz K. Isolation of sodium as a cause of ventricular fibrillation. *Invest Radiol* 1971, 6:245–248.

Staübli M, Braunschweig J, Tillman U. Changes in the rheological properties of blood as induced by sodium/meglumine diatrizoate and metrizamide. *Acta Radiol Diag* 1982, 23:71–78.

Steckel RJ, Rosch J, Ross G, et al. New developments in pharmacoangiography (and arterial pharmacotherapy) of the gastrointestinal tract. *Invest Radiol* 1971, 6:199–211.

Stein HL, Hilgartner MW. Alteration of coagulation mechanism of blood by contrast media. *AJR* 1968, 104:458–463.

Steiner RM, Grainger RG, Memon N, et al. The effect of contrast media of low-osmolality on the peripheral arterial blood flow in the dog. *Clin Radiol* 1980, 31:621–627.

Stormorken H, Skalpe IO, Testart MC. Effects of various contrast media on coagulation, fibrinolysis, and platelet function: An in vitro and in vivo study. *Invest Radiol* 1986, 21:348–354.

Svenson RH. Comparison of the hemodynamic effects of Hexabrix and Renografin-76 following left ventriculography and coronary arteriography. *Invest Radiol* 1984, 19 (Suppl):S333–S334.

Swanson DP, Thrall JH, Shetty PC. Evaluation of intravascular low-osmolality contrast agents. *Clin Pharm* 1986, 5:877–891.

Talner LB. Urographic contrast media in uremia. *Radiol Clin North Am* 1972, 10:421–432.

Tatum JL, Burke TS, Hirsch JI, et al. Pitfall to modified in vivo method of technetium-99m red blood cell labeling. *Clin Nucl Med* 1983, 8:585–586.

Thomas ML, Briggs GM, Keeling FP. Iohexol and meglumine iothalamate in phlebography of the leg. *Acta Radiol* 1983, 366 (Suppl):54–57.

Thomson KR, Violante MR, Kenyon T, et al. Reduction of ventricular fibrillation using calcium-enriched Renografin-76. *Invest Radiol* 1978, 13:238–240.

Tornquist C, Almén T, Golman K, et al. Proteinuria following nephroangiography. VII. Comparison between ionic monomeric, monoacidic dimeric and nonionic contrast media in the dog. *Acta Radiol* 1980, 362 (Suppl):49–52.

Trägårdh B, Bove AA, Lynch PR. Cardiac conduction abnormalities during coronary arteriography in dogs. Reduced effects of a new contrast medium. *Invest Radiol* 1974, 9:340–345.

Trägårdh B. Coronary angiography with iohexol and other contrast media in the dog. I. Electrocardiographic alterations. *Acta Radiol* 1980, 362 (Suppl): 17–20.

Trägårdh B, Heckman JL, Lynch PR. Coronary arteriography in canines with calcium-enriched ioxaglate and diatrizoate. *Invest Radiol* 1982, 17:66–69.

Turner E, Kentor P, Melamed JL, et al. Frequency of anaphylactoid reactions during intravenous urography with radiographic contrast media. *Radiology* 1982, 143:327–329.

Uden R. Effects of epinephrine and β-receptor blocker in intestinal angiography. In *Radiology*, Vol. 1 (Gomez-Lopez J, Bonmati J, eds.), Exerpta Medica, Amsterdam, 1974, pp. 80–83.

Uden R. Secretin and epinephrine combined in celiac angiography. *Acta Radiol Diag* 1976, 17:17–40.

Vesin S. Diagnostic value of noradrenaline and acetylcholine in pharmacodynamic renal angiography. In *Radiology*, Vol. 1 (Gomez-Lopez J, Bonmati J, eds.), Exerpta Medica, Amsterdam, 1974, pp. 267–272.

Violante MR, Thomson KR, Fischer HW, et al. Ventricular fibrillation from diatrizoate with and without chelating agents. *Radiology* 1978, 128:497–498.

Wang YJ. Deiodination kinetics of water-soluble radiopaques. *J Pharm Sci* 1980, 69:671–675.

Weigen JF, Thomas SF. *Complications of Diagnostic Radiology*, Springfield, IL, Charles C Thomas, 1973, pp. 5–10.

Whitehouse WM Jr., Queral LA, Flinn WR. The effect of sodium diatrizoate on the fibrinolytic activity of saphenous vein intima. *J Surg Res* 1981, 30:391–397.

Widrich WC, Nordahl DL, Robbins AH. Contrast enhancement of the mesenteric and portal veins using intra-arterial papaverine. *AJR* 1974, 121:374–379.

Wiedeman MP. Vascular and intravascular responses to various contrast media. *Angiology* 1963, 14:107–109.

Wilson RF, White CW. Intracoronary papaverine: An ideal coronary vasodilator for studies of the coronary circulation in conscious humans. *Circulation* 1986; 73:444–451.

Winter J. Nonrandom clustering of adverse reactions of iodinated radiographic contrast media used for computed tomography. *JCAT* 1982, 6:109–112.

Wolf GL. The fibrillation propensities of contrast agents. *Invest Radiol* 1980, 15 (Suppl):S208–S214.

Wolf GL, Mulry SC, Kilzer K, et al. New angiographic agents with less fibrillatory propensity. *Invest Radiol* 1981a; 16:320–323.

Wolf GL, LeVeen RF, Mulry C, et al. The influence of contrast media additives upon ventricular fibrillation thresholds during coronary angiography in ischemic and normal canine hearts. *Cardiovasc Intervent Radiol* 1981b, 4:145–147.

Wolf GL. Safer, more expensive iodinated contrast agents: How do we decide? *Radiology* 1986, 159:557–558.

Wolpers HG, Baller D, Ensink FBM, et al. Influence of arteriographic contrast media on the Na^+/Ca^{++} ratio in blood. *Cardiovasc Intervent Radiol* 1981, 4:8–13.

Wolpers HG, Baller D, Hoeft A, et al. The effect of ion composition on cellular membrane potentials during selective coronary arteriography. *Invest Radiol* 1984, 19:291–295.

Yuasa Y, Kohda E, Ido K, et al. Vasoconstrictive effects of prostaglandin F2-alpha angiography on colonic lesions. *Radiology* 1984, 151:305–309.

Zagoria RJ, D'Souza VJ, Baker HL. Recommended precautions when using low-osmolality or non-ionic contrast agents with vasodilators. *Invest Radiol* 1987, 22:513–514.

Zamani AA, Kido DK, Morris JH, et al. Permeability of the blood-brain barrier to intravenous high doses of diatrizoate meglumine-60. *AJNR* 1982; 3:631–634.

Zelis R, Caudill CC, Baggette K, et al. Reflex vasodilation induced by coronary angiography in human subjects. *Circulation* 1976, 53:490–493.

Zinner G, Gottlob P. Vessel morphologic changes in endothelia caused by contrast media. *Angiology* 1959, 10:207–213.

Urographic Contrast Media: Excretory and Retrograde

Dennis P. Swanson
Mark Weingarden

I. Excretory Urography

Radiographic examinations of the renal parenchyma, calyces and pelves, ureters and bladder are commonly performed following the intravenous administration of water-soluble, iodinated contrast media. As a result of their rapid renal excretion and nephron kinetics, these agents produce selective opacification and delineation of the kidneys and permit visualization of the terminal structures of the collecting system of the urinary tract.

CHEMISTRY

Development of the water-soluble, angiographic contrast media described in Chapter 1 was originally based on their rapid and extensive renal excretion and their potential use for radiographic examinations of the kidney. Hence, the intravascular iodinated contrast media currently utilized for angiographic procedures (Figures 2.1–2.3) are also indicated for intravenous urography. In addition to the agents described in Chapter 1, a ratio-1.5 ionic medium, iodamide meglumine (Figure 2.4) is also commercially available and indicated for urographic procedures.

PHARMACOKINETICS

The urinary iodine concentration and degree of renal opacification achieved with an intravascular urographic contrast medium is, in general, directly dependent on the initial plasma iodine concentration and inherent glomerular filtration rate of the kidney and inversely dependent on the degree of osmotic diuresis induced by the excreted medium (see Cattell WR, et al, 1967; Cattell WR, 1970a; Dure-Smith P, 1977; Golman K and Almén T, 1984; Saxton HM, 1969; Talner LB, 1972; Thompson WM, 1984).

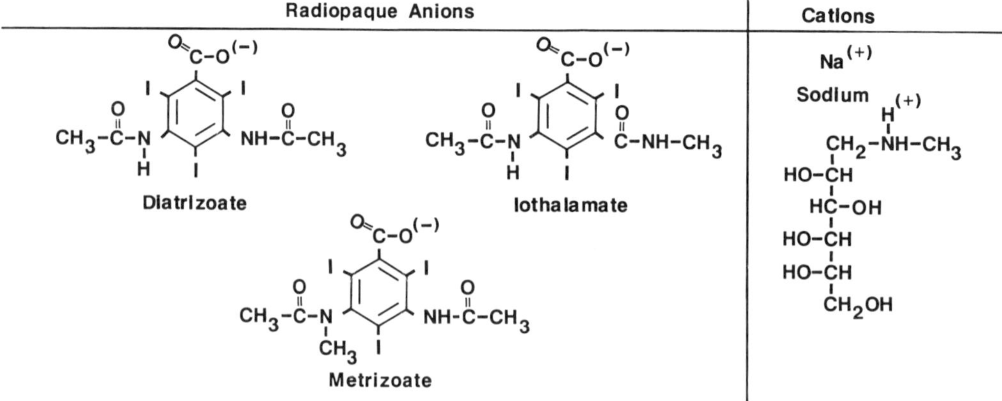

Figure 2.1 Chemical structures of ratio-1.5 contrast media commonly used for excretory urography.

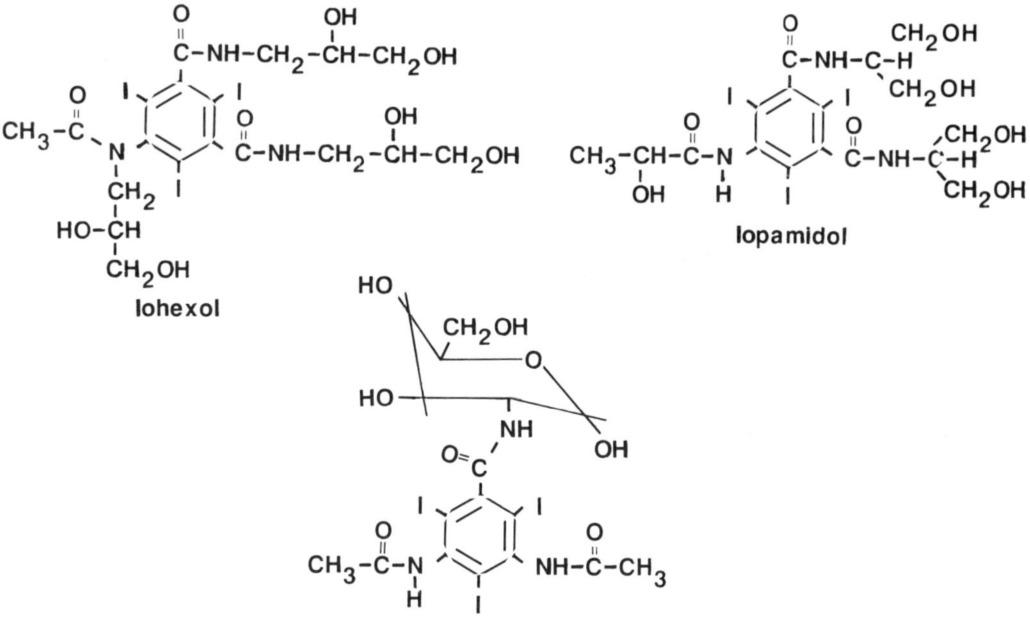

Iohexol

Iopamidol

Metrizamide

Figure 2.2 Chemical structures of ratio-3 nonionic contrast media indicated for excretory urography.

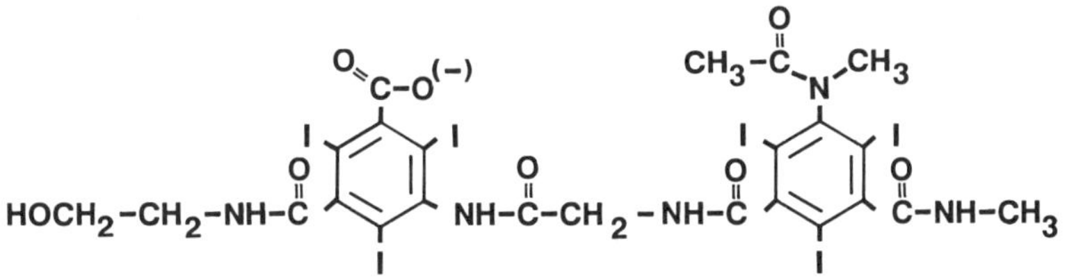

Ioxaglate

Figure 2.3 Chemical structure of ioxaglate (meglumine-sodium), a ratio-3 ionic-dimeric contrast medium indicated for excretory urography.

Iodamide

Meglumine

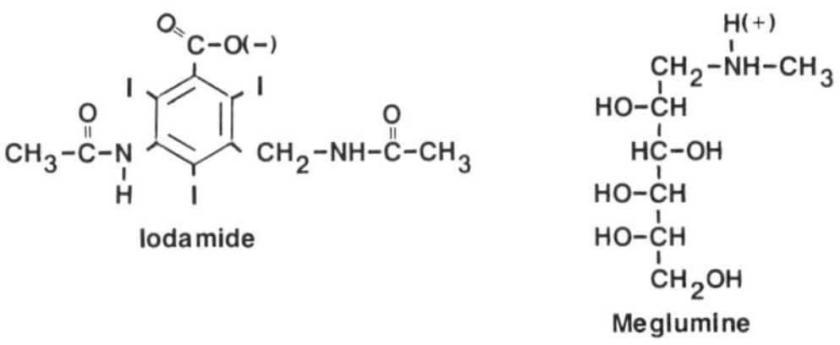

Figure 2.4 Chemical structure of iodamide meglumine.

Plasma Kinetics

General. Urographic contrast media achieve a peak plasma iodine concentration immediately following their bolus, intravenous administration (Figure 2.5). This plasma concentration decreases rapidly with dilution of the bolus in the total volume of the vascular compartment combined with the hypervolemic effects of hyperosmolarity-induced cellular diuresis. Due to the presence of a concentration gradient, the urographic media passively diffuse into and mix with the extravascular, extracellular fluid of the interstitial space, resulting in a further, but slower, decrease in their plasma concentration. Based solely on diffusion kinetics, approximately 2 hours would be required for equilibrium to be established between the

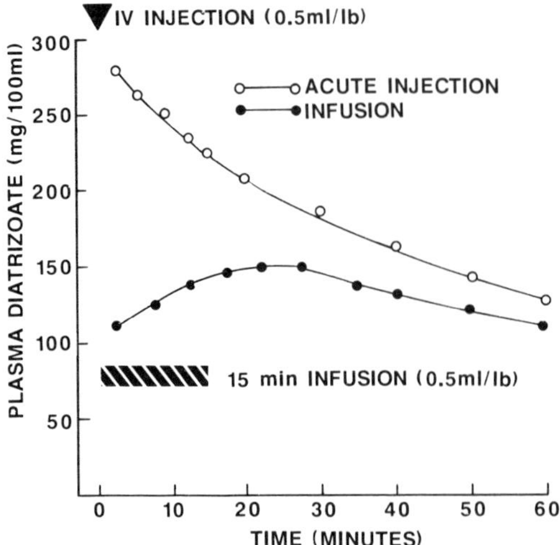

Figure 2.5 Plasma concentrations of diatrizoate (sodium) following bolus intravenous injection and slow intravenous infusion. (From Cattell WR, 1970a; with permission.)

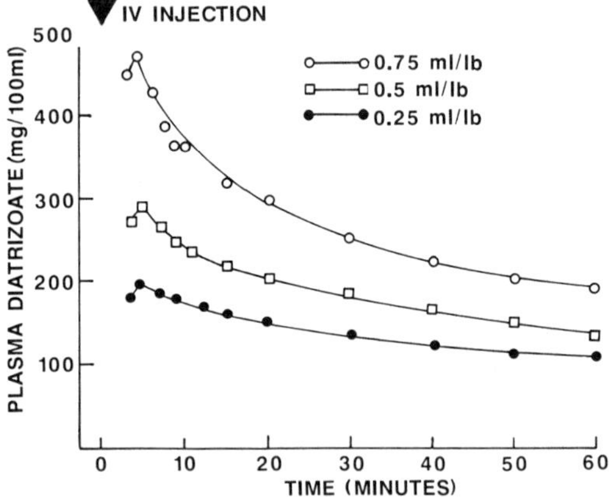

Figure 2.6 Plasma concentrations of diatrizoate (sodium) following single injections of increasing volumes at a constant iodine concentration. (From Cattell WR, 1970a; with permission.)

intravascular and interstitial concentrations of the media. However, this process is effectively completed within 10 minutes as a result of concomitant glomerular filtration and renal elimination of the intravascular contrast agents. As urinary excretion continues, the plasma concentration becomes less than the interstitial concentration, and reverse diffusion of the media occurs. With normal renal function, 50% of the administered dose of urographic media is eliminated from the body within approximately 2 hours; 100% within 24 hours. The normal plasma half-life is approximately 30–60 minutes (Cattell WR, et al, 1967; Talner LB, 1972; Dawson P, et al, 1984).

Factors Affecting Plasma Iodine Concentration. Increasing the administered volume of a urographic contrast medium at a fixed % weight/volume (w/v) iodine concentration or increasing the % w/v iodine concentration at a fixed volume results in an increase in the plasma iodine concentration throughout the kinetic profile of the medium (Figure 2.6). As previously described, bolus injection produces an immediate peak plasma iodine concentration that is greater than that achieved by infus-

ing the same dose over a longer period (Figure 2.5). Also with slower infusion of the dose, the peak plasma iodine concentration occurs at a later time and is sustained for a longer interval.

The total volume of the interstitial space increases as a function of increasing body size. Hence, at a given contrast medium dose and rate of administration, the plasma contrast medium and, hence, iodine concentration decrease as the body size increases (Figure 2.7). Interstitial volume also varies with age. The percent of extracellular water per kilogram of body weight is higher in children (i. e., 45%—newborn, 25%—one year) than in adults (i. e., 17%) (Gardeur D, et al, 1980). It is for these reasons that intravascular contrast media dosages for urographic studies are routinely based on body weight and patient age (see Dosage). The patient's state of hydration can also produce changes in the volume of interstitial space. Dehydration and salt depletion reduce the interstitial volume, whereas hydration and salt-loading increase the volume. The differences in plasma iodine concentrations achieved by a given dose of a contrast medium under various states of hydration are, however, small (Figure 2.8) and of minimal clinical significance (Cattell WR, 1970a).

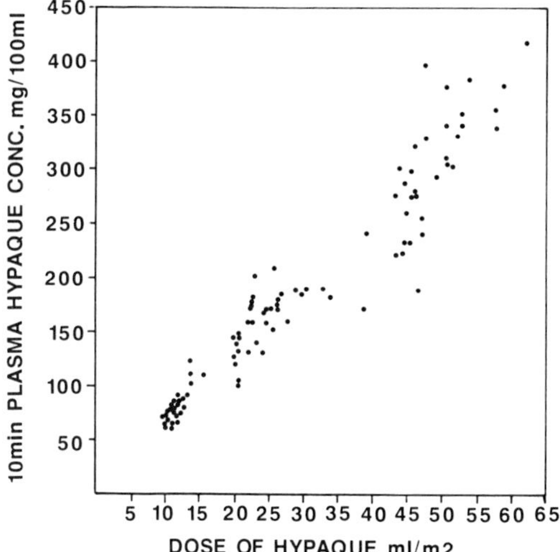

Figure 2.7 Plasma contrast medium (Hypaque®, diatrizoate sodium) concentration as a function of the intravenous dose/m² of body surface area. (From Cattell WR, et al, 1967; with permission.)

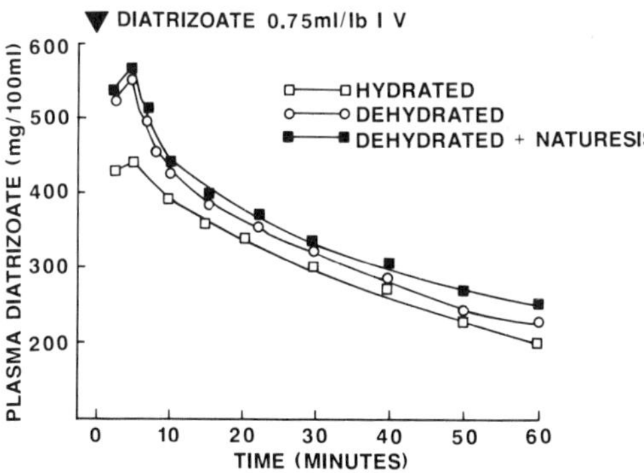

Figure 2.8 Effects of dehydration and salt depletion on the plasma contrast medium concentration. (From Cattell WR, 1970a; with permission.)

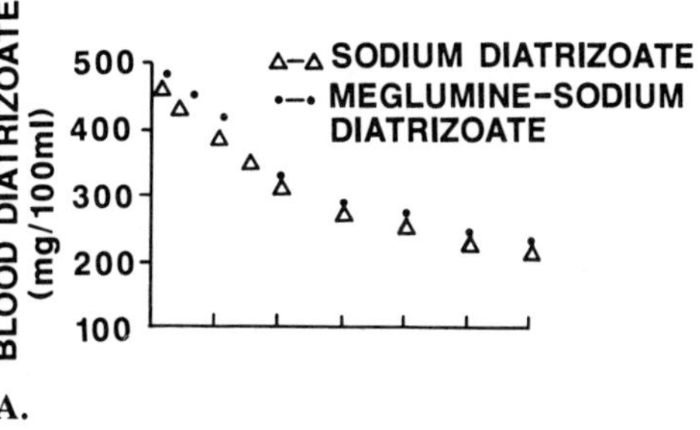

A.

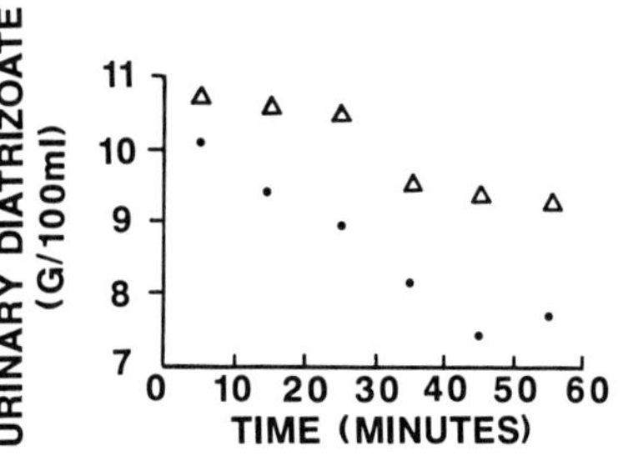

B.

Figure 2.9 Plasma (A) and urinary (B) diatrizoate (i. e., iodine) concentrations following equiiodine doses of pure sodium versus meglumine (52%)-sodium (8%) diatrizoate. (From Cattell WR, et al, 1970b; with permission.)

The various radiopaque anions (e. g., diatrizoate, iothalamate) of the ratio-1.5 ionic media demonstrate similar plasma kinetics regardless of whether they are administered as a sodium or meglumine salt (Figure 2.9A) (Taenzer V, et al, 1973; Cattell WR, et al, 1970b). Compared to the ratio-1.5 media, equivalent iodine doses and rates of administration of the ratio-3 low-osmolality agents may produce slightly greater immediate plasma iodine concentrations (Figure 2.10) as a result of their diminished degree of hyperosmolarity-induced cellular diuresis and hypervolemic effects (Spataro RF, et al, 1982; Spataro RF, et al, 1984). However, the advantages of ratio-3 low-osmolality versus ratio-1.5 ionic media in regard to plasma iodine concentration per administered dose may be offset by their higher viscosity (Table 2.1). High viscosity limits the rate of injection and, hence, the peak plasma iodine concentration obtainable with the urographic medium (Golman K and Almén T, 1984). A similar consideration may also apply to the use of the more viscous meglumine versus sodium salts of the ratio-1.5 media (Table 2.1).

RENAL KINETICS

The use of water-soluble, iodinated contrast media for intravenous urography is based on the fact that these agents are predominantly and rapidly eliminated

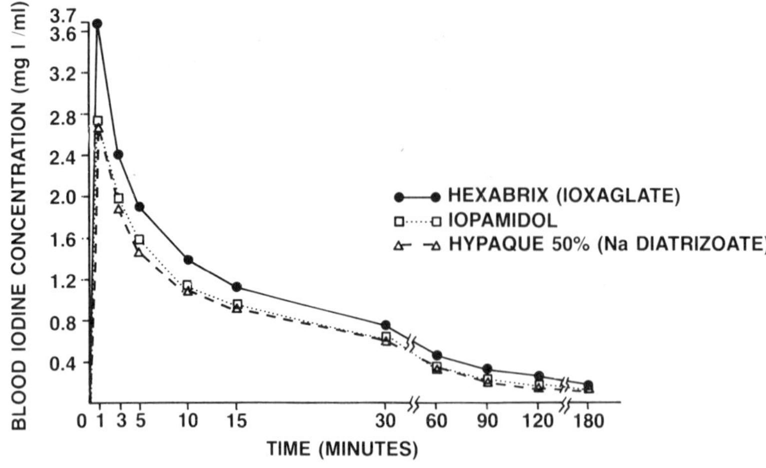

Figure 2.10 Comparative blood iodine concentrations following the bolus, intravenous injection of equiiodine doses of ratio-3 (Hexabrix®, iopamidol) and ratio-1.5 (Hypaque 50%®) contrast media. (From Spataro RF, et al, 1982; with permission.)

Table 2.1 VISCOSITIES OF SELECTED RATIO-1.5 IONIC AND RATIO-3 LOW OSMOLALITY CONTRAST MEDIA AT EQUIVALENT IODINE CONCENTRATIONS

| | | MG IODINE | VISCOSITY (CPS)[a] | |
| | CONCENTRATION | | | |
CONTRAST MEDIUM	(% w/v)	ML	25°C	37°C
Diatrizoate sodium	50	300	3.3[b]	2.4[b]
Diatrizoate meglumine	60	282	5.6[b]	4.1[b]
Ioxaglate meglumine (39.3%)-sodium (19.6%)	58.9	320	15.7	7.5
Iohexol	64.7	300	10.4	6.8
Iopamidol	61	300	8.8[c]	4.7

[a] From Fischer HW Catalog of intravascular contrast media *Radiology* 1986, 159: 561–563.
[b] Average of available products
[c] Determined at 20°C

from the body by the kidneys. With normal renal function, only approximately 1% of the administered dose of these agents is excreted by the alternate hepatic pathway (see Cattell WR, 1970a). Renal excretion of the urographic contrast media is primarily a passive glomerular filtration process. The radiopaque moieties demonstrate negligible active tubular secretion with the exception of iodamide. Animal and clinical studies have shown that iodamide is excreted at a faster rate than inulin or the conventional ratio-1.5 radiopaque anions, thus suggesting an active tubular component in addition to its renal excretion by glomerular filtration. However, at the high contrast media doses utilized for urography, this active tubular process for iodamide excretion becomes saturated and, as such, represents only a small fraction of the total urinary excretion of this agent (Bollerup AC, et al, 1975).

Glomerular Filtration. The amount of a substance undergoing glomerular excretion during any period, or the filtered load, is determined by the product of its "freely filterable" plasma concentration and the glomerular filtration rate (GFR). Whether or not a substance is "freely filterable" is dependent on its degree of binding to plasma proteins. Urographic contrast media exhibit minimal protein binding, hence their total plasma concentration is considered "freely filterable." Based on these considerations, it is not surprising that peak excretion (i.e.,

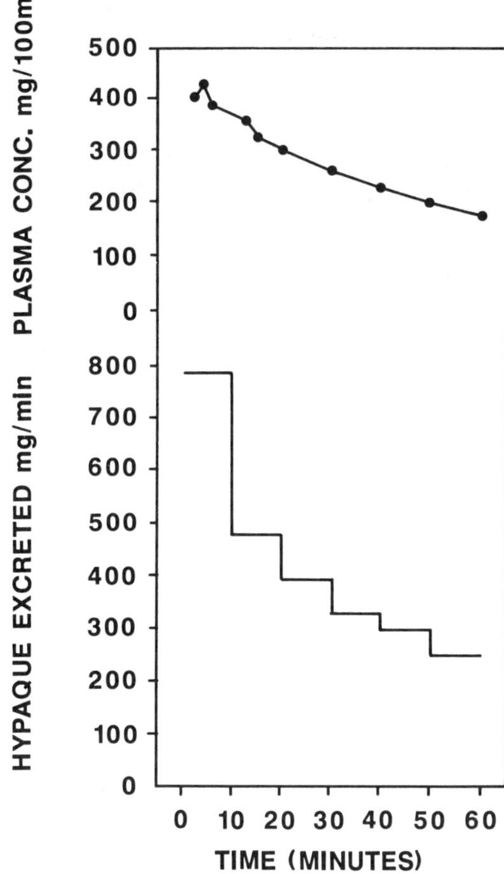

Figure 2.11 Relationship between plasma concentration and urinary excretion of diatrizoate sodium (Hypaque® 45% w/v, 270 mg I/mL.) following a bolus intravenous injection of 0.75 mL/lb. (Adapted from Cattell WR, et al, 1967.)

approximately 12% of the administered dose) of the urographic contrast media occurs during the first 10 minutes following a bolus injection (Cattell WR, et al, 1967), since this is the period of their peak plasma concentration (Figure 2.11). Peak excretion occurs at a later time with slower rates of administration.

Small differences do exist between urographic contrast media in regard to their degree of plasma protein binding and the freely filterable plasma concentration. For example, the mean percent of protein binding for the iodamide anion (8%) is greater than that of the diatrizoate or iothalamate anions (2%) (Bollerup AC, et al, 1975). Protein binding of the low-osmolality ionic-dimer, ioxaglate, is equivalent to iothalamate, and slightly greater

than the nonionic media, iohexol and iopamidol (Dawson P, 1985). As a result of their extremely low values, these differences in protein binding between the urographic media are clinically insignificant in regard to their respective filtered loads following intravenous administration.

Glomerular filtration is a passive diffusion process based on a gradient between the plasma and glomerular filtrate concentrations of the filterable solute. Thus, at any given point in time, the concentration of the solute (e. g., radiopaque moiety) in the glomerular filtrate is equal to its plasma concentration. The osmolality of the glomerular filtrate and the plasma are also similar since the capillaries of the glomerular tuft are freely permeable to all plasma solutes with the exception of proteins. Due to their large molecular weight, the colligative properties or osmotic activities of proteins are insignificant compared to those of small molecules or ions.

The filtered load or rate of glomerular excretion of a urographic contrast medium is dependent on its plasma concentration and the inherent GFR of the patient (Figure 2.12). The various factors

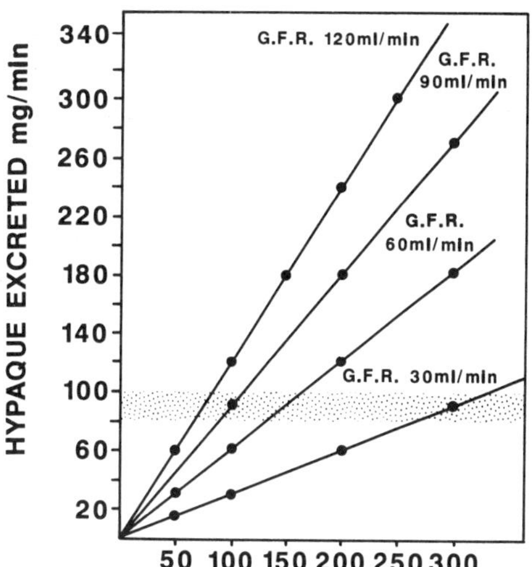

PLASMA HYPAQUE CONC. mg/100ml

Figure 2.12 Relationship between plasma concentration and urinary excretion rate of diatrizoate sodium (Hypaque® 45% w/v) at different rates of glomerular filtration. (From Cattell WR, et al, 1967; with permission.)

that affect the plasma concentration of a urographic contrast medium have been discussed previously. Glomerular filtration rate is a physiologic process that varies with body size, age, and sex, and with various pathological conditions. Glomerulonephritis and other intrinsic diseases of the kidney are commonly associated with a decrease in the number of functional nephrons and, hence, a decrease in GFR. An abnormally depressed GFR is also commonly observed in the presence of systemic hypotension or renal vasoconstriction. In patients with diminished GFR, it is necessary to increase the dose (i. e., plasma concentration) of the urographic constrast medium in order to maintian and adequate filtered load. It is interesting to note that serum creatinine values may be normal in the presence of a 60% or greater reduction in the GFR. The possibility of such "hidden renal failure" is one reason for the contemporary use of high doses (see Dosage) of contrast media in urography procedures (Saxton HM, 1969; Cattell WR, et al, 1967; Talner LB, 1972).

Proximal Tubular Events. Sodium salts of physiological anions represent the major solutes normally found in the glomerular filtrate. In the proximal renal tubule, sodium cations are reabsorbed from the filtrate by an active transport mechanism (Figure 2.13A). Since the proximal tubular membranes are freely permeable to water, this active reabsorption of sodium is accompanied by the passive diffusion of water. Via this process, over 80% of the water in the original glomerular filtrate is reabsorbed without producing a significant change in the sodium concentration or osmolality of the fluid that remains. This proximal tubular concentrating mechanism, called "iso-osmotic reabsorption," occurs independent of the patient's state of hydration.

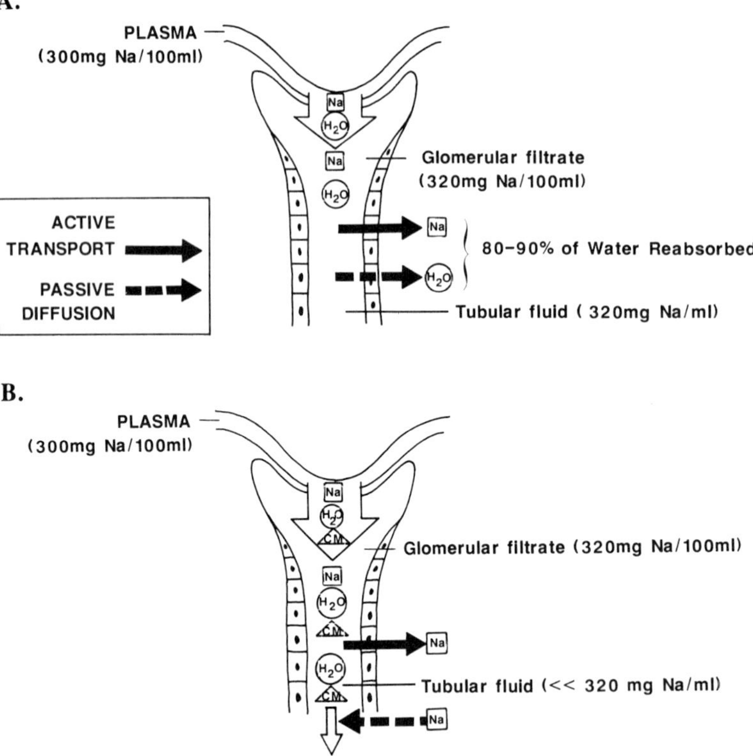

Figure 2.13 Proximal and renal tubular events in the absence (A) or presence (B) of a urographic contrast medium (Na = sodium ions, H_2O = water, CM = contrast medium).

The radiopaque moieties (anionic or nonionic) of urographic contrast media are not reabsorbed from the glomerular filtrate. In the presence of the inherent osmotic pressure of a nonreabsorbable solute, such as the radiopaque moiety, the diffusion of water from the proximal renal tubule is reduced relative to the active transport of sodium (Figure 2.13B). As a result of this contrast medium-induced retention of water, the volume of urine increases (osmotic diuresis) and the urinary concentrations of iodine and sodium rapidly decrease. In the face of an abnormally low sodium concentration, it becomes increasingly difficult for the tubule to actively reabsorb further sodium, thus enhancing the osmotic diuretic effect of the nonreabsorbable radiopaque moiety. The efficiency of the proximal tubular concentrating mechanism decreases with increasing concentrations of nonreabsorbable solutes in the renal tubule. Hence, it is not surprising that peak osmotic diuresis occurs during the period of maximum filtered load of the contrast medium, or immediately following its bolus administration. The increased rate of urine flow associated with osmotic diuresis interferes with reabsorption processes and urine concentrating mechanisms throughout the nephron. It is also common for urographic contrast media to produce naturesis as a result of a net flux of sodium back into the proximal tubule once the urinary sodium concentration falls below that of the peritubular interstitium Figure 2.13B).

The filtered load of a contrast medium is dependent on its plasma concentration and, hence, on the administered dose. Increasing the total administered dose (i. e., volume and concentration) of the contrast medium increases the filtered load and the subsequent degree of contrast-induced osmotic diuresis within the proximal tubule (Figure 2.14). Based on the fact that the efficiency of the proximal tubular concentrating mechanism decreases with an increasing intratubular concentration of nonreabsorbable solutes, it is evident that an optimal contrast medium dosage

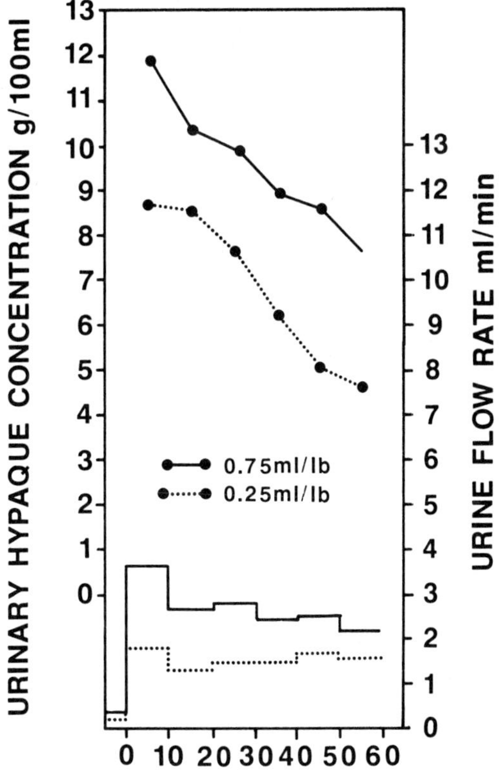

Figure 2.14 Urinary concentrations (closed circles) of diatrizoate and urine flow rates (histogram) following bolus intravenous injection of different doses of diatrizoate sodium (Hypaque® 45% w/v). (Adapted from Cattell WR, et al. 1967.)

must exist at which any further increase in the dose will result in no further increase in the urinary contrast medium or iodine concentration. Although the exact value of this "optimal dose" is subject to several variables (e. g., nature of the contrast medium utilized, rate of administration), it is currently felt that maximum urinary concentrations of conventional ratio-1.5 media are obtained with doses in the range of 200–500 mg Iodine/kg body weight (see Saxton HM, 1969; Fischer HW, et al, 1971; Golman K and Almén T, 1984).

Bolus administration of a urographic contrast medium produces an immediate peak plasma concentration and filtered load. In comparison, infusion of the same dose would result in a lower peak plasma concentration and filtered load. Hence, the degree of proximal tubular diuresis produced by a bolus injection would be greater than that of an infusion, resulting in a greater urinary iodine concentration with the infusion technique. The improvement in urinary iodine concentration with infusion versus bolus injection is offset, however, by the initially lower amount of contrast medium in the glomerular filtrate. Drip infusion urography therefore provides no significant opacification advantages over bolus administration, provided the "optimal dose" has not been exceeded in the bolus procedure (Dure-Smith P, 1970).

Since glomerular filtration is a concentration-dependent, passive diffusion process, a decrease in the number of functional nephrons with intrinsic kidney disease does not affect the initial concentration of the urographic contrast medium in the glomerular filtrate of surviving nephrons. The associated decrease in GFR does, however, result in a decrease in the total filtered load and a reduction in the proximal tubular diuretic effects of a given dose of the contrast medium. The corresponding improvement in urinary iodine concentration is again offset by the initial reduction in filtered load. With intrinsic kidney disease there is also an increase in the tubular concentration of urea. Urea is a nonreabsorable solute that exerts osmotic diuretic effects that are additive to those of the urographic contrast medium. Hence, uremia results in a further decrease in the concentrating capacity of the proximal tubule and a corresponding reduction in urinary iodine concentration. Dialysis, performed prior to urography, will reduce the tubular concentration and diuretic effects of urea, and permit an improvement in urinary iodine concentration in patients with intrinsic kidney disease (Saxton HM, 1969; Talner LB, 1972).

As previously described, the radiopaque moieties of urographic contrast media are excreted by glomerular filtration and are not reabsorbed from the renal tubules. Similarly, the nonphysiological meglumine cations of ionic (e. g., ratio-1.5 or ratio-3 ionic-dimeric) contrast media formulations also undergo rapid glomerular filtration with no reabsorption. The excreted, nonopaque meglumine cations therefore act to increase the filtered load of nonreabsorbable solutes and produce an additive effect on proximal tubular diuresis. This results in a further decrease in the urinary concentration of the radiopaque anion and the urinary iodine concentration. Compared to meglumine, the sodium cations of contrast medium formulations have a greater volume of distribution and, hence, a diminished initial filtered load. In addition, administered sodium ions appearing in the glomerular filtrate are capable of being reabsorbed and, as such, do not contribute to the osmotic diuretic effects of nonreabsorbable solutes. However, with very high filtrate concentrations of sodium, the sodium transport system of the proximal tubule can become saturated and any sodium cations remaining in the proximal tubule will exert osmotic diuretic effects. Based on these factors, sodium salts of ionic contrast media have been shown (Benness GT, 1970; Cattell WR, et al, 1970b) to produce less osmotic diuresis and greater urinary iodine concentrations than equiiodine doses of meglumine salts (Figure 2.9B). Sodium salts would also be expected to have a greater "optimal dose" than meglumine salts. An exception to this statement is associated with the urographic medium, iodamide meglumine. This agent appears to produce urinary iodine concentrations equivalent to sodium salts of diatrizoate due to its direct tubular secretion component (Bollerup AC, et al, 1975).

The ratio-3 nonionic media are devoid of sodium and meglumine cations and the respective additive effects of these nonreabsorbable solutes on osmotic diuresis. Hence, equiiodine doses of the nonionic agents produce less proximal tubular diuresis and greater urinary iodine concentrations (Figure 2.15) than meglumine or, with high-dose urography, sodium

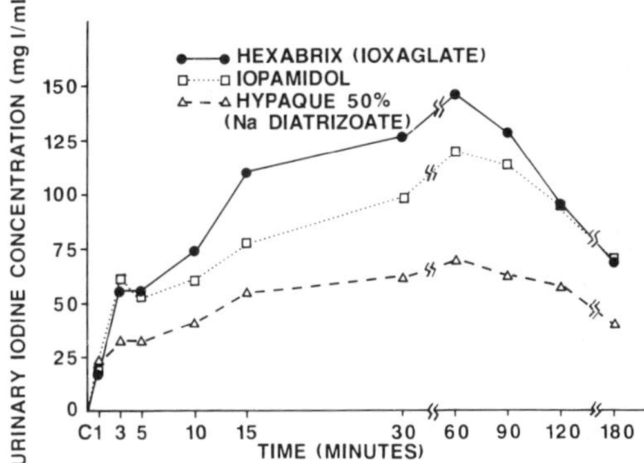

Figure 2.15 Comparative urinary iodine concentrations following the bolus, intravenous injection of equiiodine doses of ratio-3 nonionic (iopamidol), ratio-3 ionic-dimeric (Hexabrix®) and ratio-1.5 (Hypaque® 50%) contrast media. (From Spataro RF, et al, 1982; with permission.)

salts of the ratio-1.5 ionic media (Spataro RF, et al, 1982; Thompson WM, 1984). Since the sodium cations of the ratio-3 ionic-dimeric agent, ioxaglate meglumine-sodium, are reabsorbed and therefore contribute minimally to the filtered load of nonreabsorbable solutes, this medium (6 iodine atoms/1.67 nonreabsorbable solute "particles") produces less osmotic diuresis and greater urinary iodine con-

centrations (Figure 2.15) than even the nonionic media (3 iodine atoms/1 non-reabsorbable solute "particle") (Brennan RE, et al, 1982). It may also be concluded that the "optimal dose" for the ratio-3 low-osmolality media is greater than for the ratio-1.5 ionic media.

Distal Tubule and Collecting Duct Events. Active reabsorption of sodium, accompanied by the passive diffusion of water, also occurs in the distal tubule of the nephron (Figure 2.16). The rate of sodium reabsorption in the distal tubule is under the direct, positive control of the adrenal cortical hormone, aldosterone. An increase in aldosterone synthesis and release occurs in response to hyponatremia-, hypotension-, or hypovolemia-induced stimulation of the renin-angiotensin system. The release of renin by the juxtoglomerular apparatus and a subsequent increase in plasma aldosterone is also induced by a high concentration of sodium or a diminished rate of urinary flow in the distal tubule, as sensed by tubular cells comprising the macula densa. Hence the osmotic diuretic effects exerted by urographic contrast media in the proximal tubule would act to decrease the macula densa stimulation of aldosterone release,

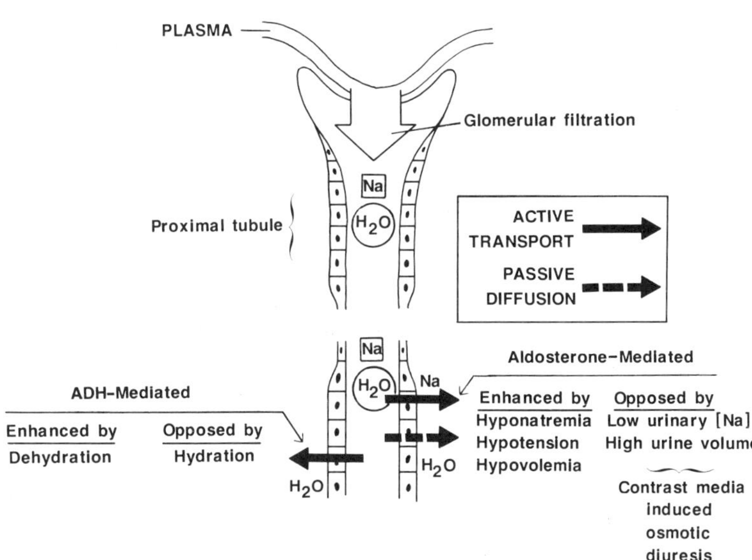

Figure 2.16 Distal tubule and collecting duct events (Na = sodium ions, H₂O = water).

and thus reduce the corresponding reabsorption of sodium and water from the distal tubules (Figure 2.16). The net effect of a high concentration of nonreabsorbable solutes in the initial filtered load is therefore a reduction in the aldosterone-stimulated concentrating capacity of the distal tubule.

The rate of water reabsorption in the distal tubule and collecting ducts is also under the control (Figure 2.16) of anti-diuretic hormone (ADH or vasopressin). This hormone is released from the pituitary in response to an increase in plasma osmolality (as detected by hypothalamic osmolreceptors) or by a fall in vascular volume (via stimulation of baroreceptors). The released ADH acts to increase the permeability of distal tubular and collecting-duct membranes, thus permitting greater reabsorption of water and a further increase in the concentration of the final urine.

The patient's state of hydration is a primary factor governing the urinary concentrating mechanisms of the distal tubule and collecting duct. Dehydration stimulates the release of ADH and aldosterone resulting in an increase in the reabsorption of water and the final urinary concentration of the urographic contrast medium. This dehydration-induced increase in urinary iodine concentration will occur regardless of the dose, rate of administration, or nature of the urographic medium. The extent of this increase will continue to be determined, however, by the osmotic effects produced by the initial filtered load of nonreabsorbable solutes.

The patient's state of hydration is an extremely difficult variable to control and is a primary factor responsible for the controversy surrounding the determination of "optimal doses" and the comparative evaluations of various urographic media (Cattell WR, et al, 1967; Saxton HM, 1969). It must also be stressed that dehydration has been recognized as a risk factor for contrast-induced nephrotoxicity, especially in patients with preexisting renal dysfunction. If an increased urinary iodine concentration is required for adequate interpretation of urographic procedures, it is probably safer to increase the dose of the contrast medium than it is to dehydrate the patient.

PHYSIOLOGICAL EFFECTS/PRECAUTIONS

Physiological effects and precautions associated with the intravascular administration of the water-soluble, iodinated contrast media commonly utilized for urographic procedures are discussed in detail in Chapter 1. With regard to the intravenous bolus injection or infusion of these agents for urography, particular attention should be directed at their Vascular, Pulmonary, and Renal Effects. It is important to note that although sodium salts of the ratio-1.5 ionic media produce greater pyelogram opacification than equivalent doses of meglumine salts; their intravenous administration is associated with a higher incidence and severity of undesirable effects, especially arm pain and general subjective discomfort.

Although specific comparative data is limited, the overall incidence of observable adverse reactions with iodamide meglumine is equivalent to or slightly greater than meglumine salts of diatrizoate or iothalamate (Product information: Renovue®; Squibb Diagnostics). Iodamide meglumine is a ratio-1.5 ionic medium and, as such, would be expected to produce the same nature and degree of hyperosmolarity-induced physiological effects as equiiodine concentrations of the meglumine salts of diatrizoate or iothalamate. The small increase in the incidence of adverse effects observed with iodamide may be associated with its slightly greater degree of plasma protein-binding relative to the conventional anions.

As a result of their reduced osmolality per given iodine concentration, intravenous administration of the ratio-3 intravascular media results in less arm pain and subjective discomfort than observed with the conventional ratio-1.5 media. Use of the low-osmolality media is also generally associated with a reduced number and in-

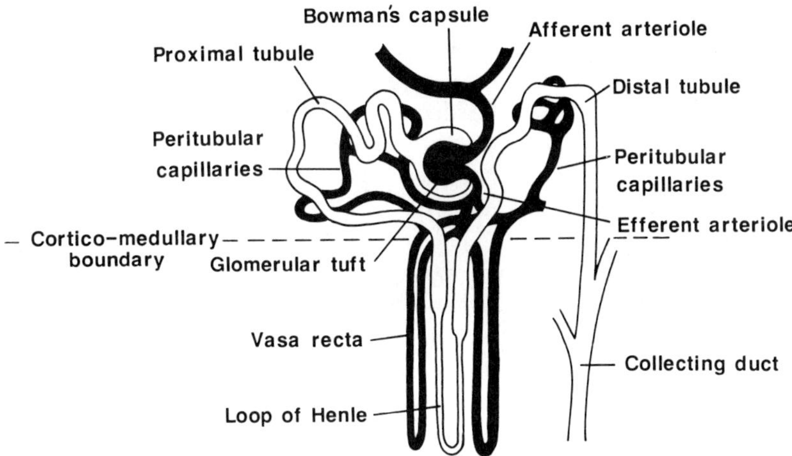

Figure 2.17　Anatomical configuration of a nephron within the renal parenchyma.

tensity of physiological effects on other organ systems (see Chapter 1, Physiological Effects). The improved efficacy of these ratio-3 media must, however, be weighed against their substantially increased costs compared to the conventional ratio-1.5 agents. It is therefore recommended that the use of low-osmolality contrast media be directed at patients known to be at increased risk for conventional contrast media reactions (see Chapter 1, Clinical Considerations).

CLINICAL CONSIDERATIONS

Nephrogram Opacification.　A nephrogram is a radiograph of the renal parenchyma including the renal cortex and medulla. The renal cortex contains the renal corpuscle (i.e., Bowman's capsule and glomerular tuft) and the proximal and distal tubular components of the nephron, whereas the medulla includes the loop of Henle and the collecting ducts (Figure 2.17).

The most intense nephrogram opacification occurs at approximately 1 minute following rapid injection of the urographic contrast media (Figure 2.18). The density of nephrogram opacification is dependent on the peak plasma concentration of the administered agent and the patient's glomerular filtration rate. These factors determine the initial filtered load of the medium and the tubular iodine concentration. The concentrating activity of the renal tubules has little affect on overall nephrogram density in comparison to the plasma and initial glomerular filtrate concentrations of the medium.

Nephrogram quality improves with increasing doses (volume or iodine concentrations) of the urographic contrast media, and with bolus versus infusion methods of administration. The degree of nephrogram opacification occurs independent of the nature of the urographic contrast medium, provided that differences in viscosity do not preclude similar rates of

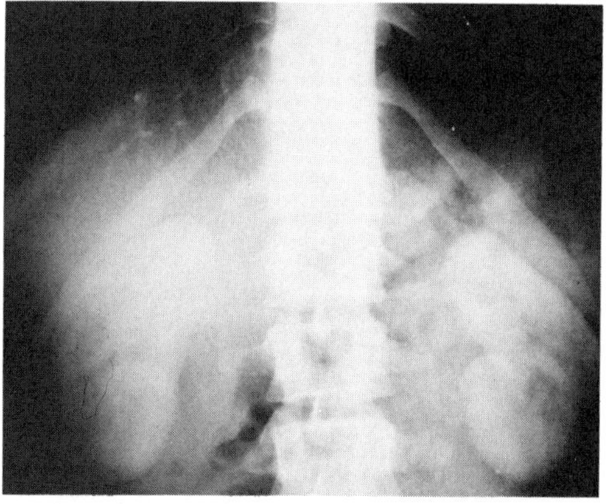

Figure 2.18　Normal nephrogram phase obtained at 1 minute following rapid injection of a urographic contrast medium.

injection. Since the distal tubules and collecting ducts represent only a small percentage of total nephron volume within the renal parenchyma, the density of the nephrogram is not dependent on the patient's state of hydration (see Cattell WR, et al, 1967; Saxton HM, 1969; Dure-Smith P, 1970; Thompson WM, 1984; Golman K and Almén T, 1984).

Nephrogram density progressively increases in the presence of post-renal obstruction, because continued glomerular filtration with limited tubular excretion results in an increase in tubular volume and distension. This factor is combined with an elevation in urinary iodine concentration produced by increased reabsorption of sodium and water in the presence of a slow rate of urine flow. Systemic hypotension also results in a marked reabsorption of sodium and water and a corresponding increase in the proximal tubular concentration of the non-reabsorbable radiopaque moiety (Saxton HM, 1969).

The nephrogram phase of an excretory urography study is often used for the demonstration and differentiation of intrarenal masses, including tumors and cysts (Figure 2.19) and extra-renal masses impinging on the renal parenchyma. Other indications do exist for this segment of the excretory urography study; however, their complete listing and discussion is beyond the scope of this text. The deter-

mination of absolute renal function from urography studies is usually not attempted due to problems associated with the standardization of dosages, the maintainence of a consistent state of hydration, and the accurate quantification of opacification density.

Pyelogram Opacification. The pyelographic phase of an excretory urography study is defined as a radiographic examination of the terminal renal collecting system, including the calyces, pelves, and ureters (Figure 2.20). Pyelogram opacification reaches a maximum at approximately 10–15 minutes after bolus injection, and is dependent on both the final urinary iodine concentration and the volume of urine within the respective regions of the urinary tract.

The extent to which an x-ray beam is attenuated by a urographic contrast medium is determined by the total number of iodine atoms in its path. The degree of urinary tract opacification may therefore be dependent not only on the urinary iodine concentration but also on the volume of urine within the region under investigation. As previously described, renal tubular concentrating efficiency decreases with contrast media factors that produce an increase in the filtered load of

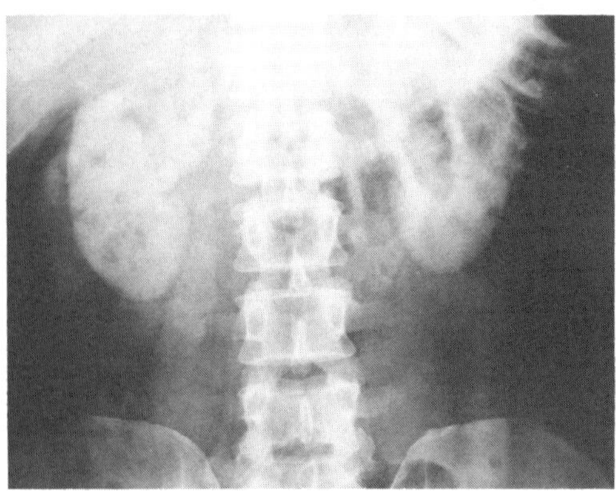

Figure 2.19 Nephrogram demonstrates large mass defect (simple cyst) in upper pole of right kidney.

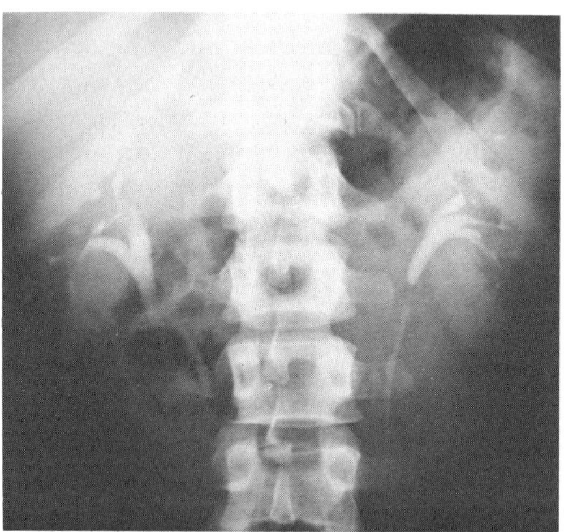

Figure 2.20 Normal pyelogram phase obtained at 8 minutes following rapid injection of a urographic contrast medium.

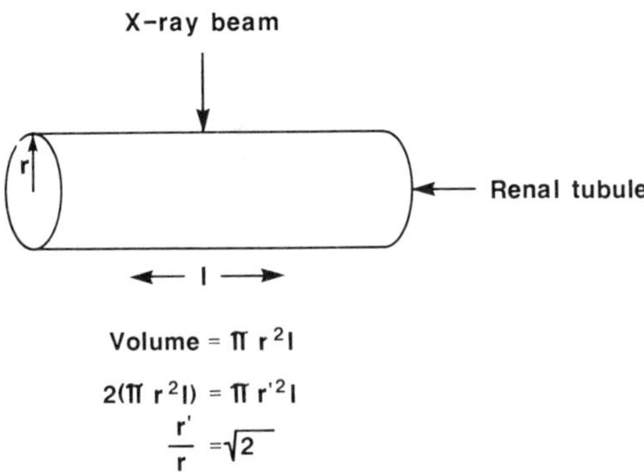

Figure 2.21 Pyelogram opacification: relationship between renal tubular volume and x-ray path length. (Adapted from Golman K and Almén T, 1984.)

Table 2.2 **FACTORS THAT AFFECT THE DEGREE OF PYELOGRAPHIC OPACIFICATION**

Factors that increase *pyelographic opacification:*
 1. Increasing the contrast medium dosage. (*Unless optimal dose has been exceeded*)
   · ↑ injected volume
   · ↑ injected iodine concentration
 2. Chemical nature of injected contrast medium
   · Sodium salts > meglumine salts (Ratio-1.5 media)
   · Ratio-3 media > ratio-1.5 media
 3. Abdominal compression
 4. Patient dehydration
Factors that decrease *pyelographic opacification:*
 1. Renal disease with diminished GFR
 2. Uremia

nonreabsorbable solutes. These contrast-media factors decrease the urinary iodine concentration by inducing osmotic diuresis and an increase in urinary volume. The overall result of these osmotic diuresis effects (i. e., decreased urinary iodine concentration versus increased urinary volume) is to produce an equivalent amount (i. e., product of volume and concentration) of total iodine atoms in the terminal collecting system. Pyelogram opacification is, however, slightly more dependent on urinary iodine concentration that it is on urine volume. This occurs due to the three-dimensional nature of the renal tubules. For example, if a cylindrical configuration (Figure 2.21) is assumed for the pelvic-calyceal system, the x-ray path length increases by only a factor of 1.4 (i. e., $\sqrt{2}$) with a factor of 2 increase in volume. Thus, doubling the urinary iodine concentration at constant urinary volume would increase x-ray opacification by a factor of 1.4 (i. e., $2/\sqrt{2}$) over doubling the urinary volume at a constant urinary iodine concentration (Golman K and Almén T, 1984; Thompson WM, 1984).

Several factors can affect the degree of pyelographic opacification (Table 2.2). Pyelogram density increases with the dose (volume of iodine concentration) of the administered contrast medium unless the "optimal dose" has been exceeded. Sodium salts of the ratio-1.5 urographic media produce greater urinary iodine con-

centrations and pyelogram opacification than equiiodine doses of meglumine salts, and would be expected to have an increased "optimal dose". The ratio-3 ionic-dimeric and nonionic media result in improved pyelogram opacification and increased "optimal doses" compared to sodium and meglumine salts of the ratio-1.5 ionic media. These differences between the urographic contrast media are further accentuated with the incorporation of abdominal compression. By producing partial mechanical obstruction, this adjunctive procedure produces an increase in the urinary volume and maximum distention of the pelvic-calyceal collecting systems and ureters. Thus, abdominal compression effectively eliminates the differences in urinary volume and tubular distention produced by the different contrast agents and makes opacification differences primarily dependent on their urinary concentrating effects only. Pyelogram density can also be improved by inducing a state of dehydration, regardless of the nature of the contrast medium or dose. This latter maneuver may, however, place the patient at increased risk and should be avoided (see Cattell WR, et al, 1967; Saxton HM, 1969; Dure-Smith P, et al, 1971; Golman K and Almén T, 1984; Thompson WM, 1984).

There is a reduction in the density of pyelogram opacification in the presence of certain renal diseases. This occurs as a result of the diminished GFR and initial filtered load of the contrast medium and the additional osmotic diuretic effects of nonreabsorbable uric acid in those patients with uremia. Pyelogram opacification increases with the hindered elimination and associated pelvi-calyceal distention of acute post-renal obstruction. However, the pyelographic accumulation of unopacified urine in prolonged or chronic obstruction will act to dilute the excreted contrast medium and produce a decrease in pyelogram opacification. Prerenal obstruction results in delayed renal excretion of the injected contrast medium and a slower filling of the pelvi-calyceal system, thus also leading to decreased pyelogram opacification at routine imaging times (Saxton HM, 1969).

Excretory urography is routinely indicated for the evaluation of hematuria or for known or suspected obstructive lesions (e. g., tumors, calculi) of the renal calyces, pelves, or ureters (Figure 2.22–2.25). Additional indications for radiographic evaluation of the urinary tract may include chronic urinary tract infections, trauma, or prostatic hypertrophy.

Patient Preparation. All patients should be well hydrated prior to the urography procedure. An appropriate bowel cleansing regimen should be utilized to eliminate potential renal opacification artifacts associated with overlying fecal matter or gas. Since most bowel cleansing regimens tend to produce dehydration, it is essential that respective patient instructions include information regarding adequate hydration.

It has been suggested that intravascular infusion of the osmotic diuretic, mannitol, or the loop diuretic, furosemide, may be useful in preventing contrast medium-

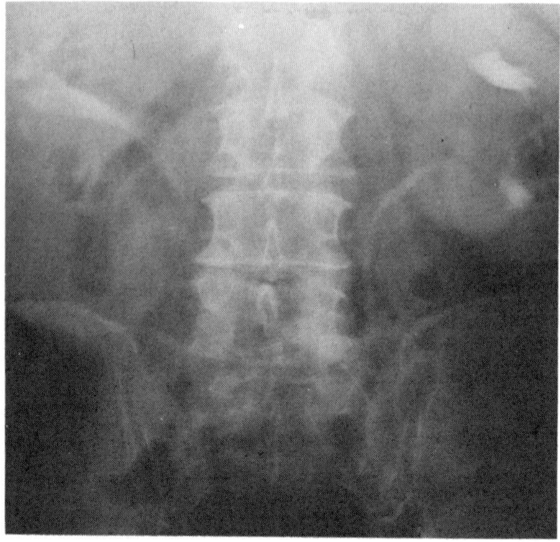

Figure 2.23 Pyelogram demonstrates bilateral hypernephromas involving the lower pole of the right kidney and the medial aspect of the left kidney.

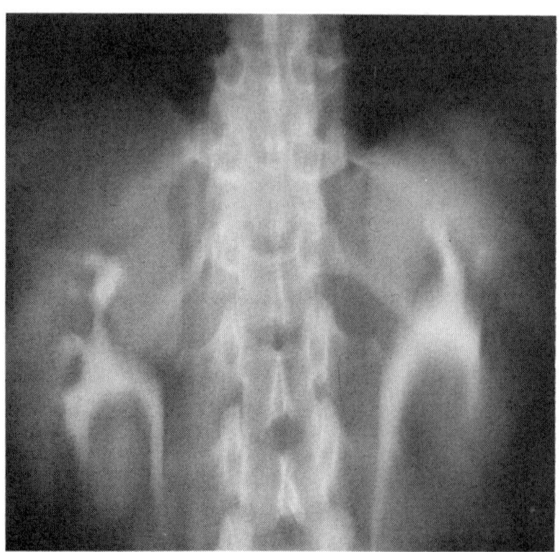

Figure 2.22 Pyelogram demonstrates large mass defect (simple cyst) in upper pole of right kidney. (Same patient as Figure 2.19.)

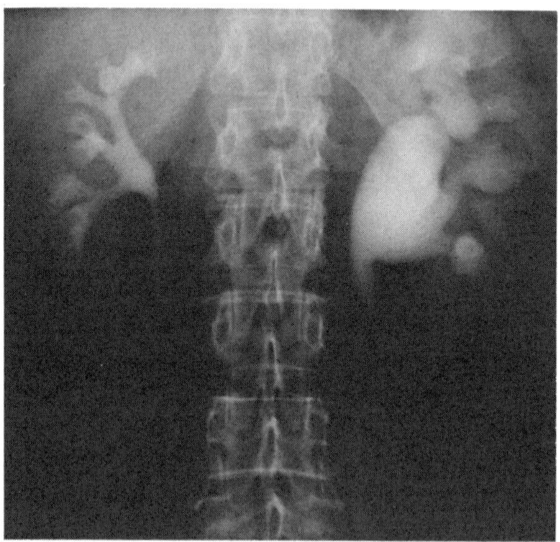

Figure 2.24 Pyelogram demonstrates hydronephrosis of the left kidney. Note dilatation of the left renal pelvis and calyces compared to the normal right kidney.

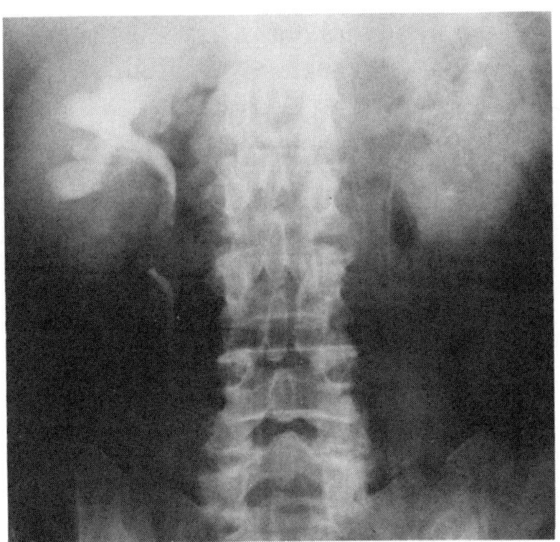

Figure 2.25   Pyelogram demonstrates transitional cell carcinoma involving the right renal pelvis and proximal ureter. Note hydronephrosis of renal collecting system proximal to tumor.

induced renal failure, especially in patients with preexisting renal insufficiency (see Berkseth RO and Kjellstrand CM, 1984). The agents apparently protect against the renal vasoconstrictive effects of hyperosmolar contrast media and thereby maintain glomerular filtration driving pressure and prevent tubular obstruction (Burke TJ, et al, 1980). It must be remembered, however, that the diuretic effects of these interventions will be additive to the osmotic diuretic effects of urographic contrast media, therefore proper attention to the patient's hydration state and electrolyte levels is required. Moreover, the administration of hyperosmolar mannitol solutions or furosemide is not without inherent risks. Since the ratio-3 low-osmolality media produce substantially less renal vasoconstriction and glomerular permeability effects than the conventional ratio-1.5 agents (see Chapter 1, Physiological Effects), the alternate use of these ratio-3 agents in patients with clinically significant renal dysfunction may represent a more practical approach than the interventional use of mannitol or furosemide.

Adjunctive techniques.   As previously discussed, abdominal compression pro-

duces partial mechanical obstruction and thereby increases the volume of urine (and excreted contrast medium) in the terminal collecting system and ureters and results in their maximum distention. By increasing the total amount of contrast medium iodine in the x-ray path, compression often improves the quality of pyelograhic opacification. This maneuver is obviously contraindicated in the presence of preexisting post-renal obstruction or conditions such as abdominal aortic aneurysm, recent abdominal surgery, or in patients with ostomy devices.

An alternative approach to obtaining improved pyeloureteral vizualization that has received limited attention is the interventional administration of glucagon. Following intravenous injection of a 1 mg dose, this agent has been shown to inhibit ureteral peristalsis for a duration of approximately 20 minutes; producing radiographic results similar to abdominal compression (Hillman BJ, et al, 1980). The risks associated with the use of glucagon are minimal. It can produce hypersensitivity reactions and is contraindicated in patients insulinoma or pheochromocytoma.

Contraindications.   There are no absolute contraindications to the intravascular administration of water-soluble iodinated contrast media for excretory urography. Ultrasound is currently recognized as the procedure-of-choice for evaluating the kidneys in patients with renal failure. Excretory urography performed on such patients will require higher initial doses and/or delayed imaging for adequate renal opacification (Talner LB, 1972). There is probably a certain level of renal failure above which adequate pyelographic opacification cannot be achieved. Defining this level by a specific serum creatinine or BUN value may be impossible or inappropriate. However, if adequate visualization of the collecting system has not been obtained with a total dose of 35–40 grams of iodine, it may be assumed that any further increase in dosage will not result in significant pyelographic advantages (Saxton HM, 1969).

The incidence of contrast medium-induced renal failure is low in patients with normal renal function. However, this risk may increase substantially in patients with diabetes or hypertension and concomitant renal dysfunction (i. e., serum creatinine >1.5 mg/dL), or in otherwise "normal" patients whose serum creatinine concentrations exceed 5 mg/dL (Harkonen S and Kjellstrand C, 1981). Product literature also commonly cites multiple myeloma as a warning for intravascular contrast-media procedures, however the contribution of this disease to contrast-induced renal failure remains questionable (Harkonen S and Kjellstrand C, 1981). In addition, patients with severe heart disease may be at increased risk for electrocardiographic alterations produced by bolus intravenous injection of the hyperosmolar contrast media (Stadalnik RC, et al, 1977; Heron CW, et al, 1984). As a result of their reduced effects on renal and cardiac physiology, use of the ratio-3 low-osmolality media in place of the conventional ratio-1.5 agents should be considered in these at-risk patients (see Chapter 1, Physiological Effects, Clinical Considerations).

DOSAGE

Early studies indicated that a dose of 300 mg iodine/kg. of a sodium salt of a ratio-1.5 medium (i. e., diatrizoate, iothalamate, metrizoate) would produce a maximum urinary iodine concentration in patients with normal renal function. Doses above this level did not significantly improve pyelogram opacification (Saxton HM, 1969; Fischer HW, et al, 1971). It should be noted, however, that these early studies were performed with the patient dehydrated for a 12-hour period. As previously discussed, patient dehydration stimulates the urine-concentrating mechanisms of the distal renal tubules resulting in a higher urinary contrast medium and iodine concentration in the terminal collecting systems. It has been subsequently recognized, however, that dehydration may place the patient at increased risk for contrast medium-induced renal failure. Thus, with the elimination

of patient dehydration as a routine preparation for the urography procedure, the use of somewhat higher doses (i. e., 300–500 mg iodine/kg.) of the ratio-1.5 media has become an accepted practice for maintaining adequate pyelographic opacification. The routine use of this increased dose also helps to ensure adequate urographic opacification in the face of "hidden renal failure." It is known that serum creatinine or blood urea nitrogen values may remain within a normal range with up to a 60% decrease in glomerular filtration rate (GFR). Such a decrease in the GFR will substantially reduce the filtered load of the intravascular contrast medium and the degree of renal opacification per administered dose. To overcome this problem, the routine use of higher doses has been suggested, especially in older adults, since it is known that GFR progressively decreases with age (Saxton HM, 1969; Dure-Smith P, 1977).

The GFR of premature and newborn patients is also considerably lower than that of the normal adult. Even when corrected for body surface area, pediatric GFR values do not approach adult values until the age 1–3 years. Also, the renal tubular concentrating mechanisms are not fully developed in the newborn. These factors, combined with the relatively increased interstitial volume of pediatric patients (see Pharmacokinetics), form the basis for the routine use of higher contrast medium doses in this patient category (Dure-Smith P, 1977). Typically, doses of 800–900 mg iodine/kg are used in infants, 500–600 mg iodine/kg in children, and 400–500 mg iodine/kg in adolescents (Dure-Smith P, 1977).

Contrast medium doses for urography are administered rapidly (i. e., over 20–40 seconds) to obtain a peak plasma concentration for optimal nephrographic opacification. There are no nephrogram or pyelogram opacification advantages associated with slower infusion of the same dose. Studies have indicated that the slow, intravenous infusion of urographic contrast media may be associated with a higher incidence of reactions than rapid, bolus injection (Ansell G, et al, 1980; Shehadi WH, 1975). Other studies have shown a higher incidence of electrocardiographic changes with more rapid rates of intravenous injection (Stadalnik RC, et al, 1977).

As previously discussed, sodium salts of the ratio-1.5 ionic media produce greater urinary iodine concentrations than equiiodine doses of corresponding meglumine salts. Use of meglumine media should be considered, however, in patients on sodium restriction. Following intravascular administration, meglumine ions are rapidly excreted by the kidney and not reabsorbed. In the presence of congestive heart failure, the increased volume of distribution and tubular reabsorption of the more physiological sodium ions may precipitate a worsening of the patient's condition. The use of meglumine salts of the ratio-1.5 media should also be considered in pediatric patients. At equiiodine concentrations, meglumine salts are less hyperosmolar than sodium salts and produce less pain and subjective discomfort upon intravenous injection.

As a result of their reduced osmotic diuresis effects, the ratio-3 low-osmolality agents will produce greater urinary iodine concentrations than the ratio-1.5 media. However, the primary advantage of these low-osmolality agents is probably more related to their general reduction in the number and severity of undesirable effects on vascular and organ physiology than it is to their improved pyelographic opacification. It is therefore recommended that use of the considerably more expensive ratio-3 media be reserved for those patients known to be at increased risk for reactions to the conventional, ratio-1.5 agents (see Chapter 1, Physiological Effects, Clinical Considerations).

II. Direct Urography

Radiographic examinations of the renal collecting system (e. g., calyces and pelves) and the lower urinary tract (e. g., ureters, bladder, urethra) can be per-

Table 2.3 COMMON NOMENCLATURE FOR DIRECT UROGRAPHY STUDIES

DIRECT UROGRAPHY PROCEDURE	SPECIFIC URINARY TRACT REGION(S) UNDER RADIOGRAPHIC INVESTIGATION
Retrograde pyelography	Calyces, pelvis, (ureter)
Ureterography	Ureter
Voiding cystourethrography	Bladder, bladder neck, posterior urethra
Retrograde urethrography	Anterior urethra

formed following retrograde instillation of a radiopaque contrast medium into the region of interest using catheter techniques. Nomenclature associated with these direct urography procedures varies and is dependent on the specific region(s) under investigation (Table 2.3).

Clinical Indications. In general, direct urography procedures are performed when detailed evaluation of a specific region of the urinary tract is indicated. For example, retrograde pyelography and ureterography are commonly performed in patients with persistent, unexplained hematuria in which the calyces and ureters have been inadequately or suboptimally visualized on a prior excretory urography study. Direct urography procedures may also be utilized to localize the exact site or extent of a urinary tract laceration, fistula, or sinus tract. Direct urography procedures become particularly important in the face of severe renal insufficiency and the associated inability to obtain an adequate excretory study.

Although the bladder is routinely demonstrated during excretory urography, its definitive radiographic evaluation requires the complete filling and adequate opacification provided by direct retrograde instillation of the contrast medium. Voiding cystourethrography, which evaluates the bladder and urethra as a functioning unit, is commonly utilized to investigate persistent or frequent urinary tract infections. Radiographic imaging performed concomitant with voiding of the contrast medium permits detection of the vesicourethral influx commonly associated with chronic infections. Obstructive lesions of the posterior urethra may also be demonstrated during this procedure. Urethral strictures, valves, and polyps that are often difficult to observe with endoscopy may also be evaluated with direct urography techniques. The posterior urethra becomes distended only during patient voiding and is therefore best evaluated during a voiding cystourethrography procedure. The anterior urethra (i.e., the portion of the urethra distal to the urogenital diaphragm) is, however, often poorly visualized in the voiding cystourethrogram. Its selective evaluation usually requires retrograde instillation of the contrast medium using specialized catheters.

Contrast Media Considerations. The water-soluble, iodinated contrast media routinely utilized for excretory urography and angiography are also the primary contrast agents used for direct urography (Table 2.4). The urinary tract is routinely exposed to hyperosmolar urine containing high concentrations of physiological and nonphysiological substrates. Hence, considerations regarding the appropriateness of meglumine versus sodium cations, the nature of the radiopaque anion, or the use of conventional ratio-1.5 ionic versus ratio-3 low-osmolality media are probably of minimal importance with direct urography procedures. As a result of their aqueous solubility, these agents mix readily with the urine and present minimal risks in the event of their extravasation or backflow into the renal tubules. It is not unusual for small amounts (i.e., $< 1\%$) of these water-soluble, iodinated media to be systemically absorbed via the high vascularized pericalyceal plexus. The amount of this absorption may increase dramatically in the presence of pyelorenal backflow or increased intraureteric pressure. Therefore, there is always a small but possible risk of pseudo-hypersensitivity reactions associated with direct urography procedures (see Weigen JF and Thomas SF, 1973).

Contraindications/Precautions. The majority of the complications associated with direct urography are procedure-related rather than contrast medium-related. Catheterization of the renal collecting system, ureters, or bladder can produce

Table 2.4 IODINATED CONTRAST MEDIA INDICATED FOR DIRECT UROGRAPHY PROCEDURES[a]

| | | | MG IODINE | | INDICATIONS | |
GENERIC NAME	CONCENTRATION (%w/v)	BRAND NAME[®][b]	ML	ANTIBACTERIAL ADDITIVE	Cystourethrography	Retrograde Pyelography
Diatrizoate meglumine	18	Cystografin Dilute (S)	85	No	√	
Diatrizoate meglumine	30	Cystografin (S)	141	No	√	
Diatrizoate meglumine	30	Urovist-Cysto Pediatric (B)	141	No	√	
Diatrizoate meglumine	30	Urovist-Cysto (B)	141	No	√	
Diatrizoate meglumine	30	Hypaque Cysto (W)	141	No	√	
Diatrizoate sodium	20	Hypaque Sodium (W)	120	Yes		√
Diatrizoate meglumine	30	Reno-M-30 (S)	141	Yes		√
Iothalamate meglumine	17.2	Cysto-Conray II (M)	81	No	√	
Iothalamate meglumine	43	Cysto-Conray (M)	202	No	√	√

[a] U.S. market only
[b] (B) Berlex Imaging
(M) Mallinckrodt
(S) Squibb Diagnostics
(W) Winthrop-Breon Laboratories

transient anuria. There is also always the potential for catheter-induced perforation of the urinary tract. Strict aseptic technique is a requirement to reduce the risk of bacteremia. Some of the contrast media indicated for direct urography procedures contain antibacterial agents (Table 2.4); however, the inclusion of these additives is primarily to permit multiple-dose use of the respective vials rather than to prevent or limit bacteremia.

Direct urography procedures are contraindicated in the presence of acute urinary tract infection. The performance of these studies may also be limited by conditions (e. g., urinary tuberculosis, prostatic hypertrophy, urinary tract tumors) that prevent catheter introduction. Due to the potential for or the presence of procedure-induced transient anuria, caution should be observed in performing bilateral or repeat studies within 48 hours. It should also be noted that the presence of iodinated contrast medium in the urine can interfere with respective laboratory testing. Therefore, urinalysis evaluations should be performed on urine collected prior to the direct urography procedure or delayed until 48 hours following the procedure.

DOSAGE

The iodine concentration of the contrast medium utilized for a direct urography procedure is dependent on the thickness (i. e., x-ray path length) of the region under radiographic investigation. Retrograde pyelography, ureterography, and urethrography are typically performed using ratio-1.5 contrast media containing 120–200 mg of iodine/mL (Table 2.4). Contrast media with equal or slightly lower iodine concentrations (i. e., 80–140 mg/mL) may be used for cystography or voiding cystourethrocystography (Table 2.4).

The volume of the contrast medium administered is also dependent on the region under investigation and can vary considerably between patients due to ana-tomical variations and differences in the sensitivity of the micturation stimulus. It is recommended that instillation of the contrast medium be monitored fluoroscopically to ensure adequate filling of the region of interest and to prevent overfilling. The latter situation can result in inflammatory reactions associated with extravasation or renal tubular backflow of the contrast-laden urine. In retrograde pyelography and ureterography, the excessive distention produced by overfilling may mimic the radiographic pattern observed with obstructive disease.

References

Ansell G, Tweedie MCK, West CR, et al. The current status of reactions to intravenous contrast media. *Invest Radiol* 1980, 15:532–539.

Benness GT. Urographic contrast agents. A comparison of sodium and methylglucamine salts. *Clin Radiol* 1970, 21: 150–156.

Berkseth RO, Kjellstrand CM. Radiologic contrast-induced nephropathy. *Med Clin North Am* 1984, 68:351–370.

Bollerup AC, Hesse B, Steiness E. Renal handling of iodamide and diatrizoate. Evidence of active tubular secretion of iodamide. *Eur J Clin Pharmacol* 1975, 9:63–67.

Brennan RE, Rapoport S, Weinberg I, et al. CT-determined canine kidney and urine iodine concentration following intravenous administration of sodium diatrizoate, metrizamide, iopamidol, and sodium ioxaglate. *Invest Radiol* 1982, 17:95–100.

Burke TI, Cronin RE, Duchin KL, et al. Ischemia and tubule obstruction during acute renal failure in dogs: Mannitol in protection. *Am J Physiol*, 1980, 238: F305–F314.

Cattell WR, Fry IK, Spencer AG, et al. Excretion urography. I. Factors determining the excretion of Hypaque. *Br J Radiol* 1967, 40:561–580.

Cattell WR, Excretory pathways for contrast media. *Invest Radiol*, 1970a 5: 473–487.

Cattell WR, Fry IK, Lane R, et al. Comparison of the renal excretion of Hypaque 45% and Urografin 60%. *Br J Radiol* 1970b, 43:309–313.

Dawson P. Chemotoxicity of contrast media and clinical adverse effects. A review. *Invest Radiol* 1985, 20 (Suppl.): S84–S91.

Dawson P, Heron C, Marshall J: Intravenous urography with low-osmolality contrast agents. Theoretical considerations and clinical findings. *Clin Radiology* 1984, 35:173–175.

Dure-Smith P. The dose of contrast medium in intravenous urography. A physiological assessment. *AJR* 1970, 108:691–697.

Dure-Smith P, Simenhoff M, Zimskind PD, et al. The bolus effect on excretory urography. *Radiology* 1971, 101:29–34.

Dure-Smith P. Urographic agents. In *Radiographic Contrast Agents* (Miller RE, Skucas J, eds.). Baltimore, University Park Press, 1977, pp. 273–306.

Fischer HW, Rothfield NJB Carr JD. Optimum dose in excretory urography. *AJR* 1971, 113:423–426.

Gardeur D, Lautrow J, Millard JC, et al. Pharmacokinetics of contrast media: Experimental results in dog and man with CT implications. *J Compt Assist Tomog* 1980, 4:178–185.

Golman K, Almén T. Urographic contrast media and methods of investigative uroradiology. In *Radiocontrast Agents* (Sovak M, ed.). New York, Springer-Verlag, 1984, pp. 127–191.

Harkonen S, Kjellstrand C. Contrast nephropathy. *Am J Nephrol* 1981, 1: 69–77.

Heron CW, Underwood SR, Dawson P. Electrocardiographic changes during intravenous urography: A study with sodium iothalamate and iohexol. *Clin Radiology* 1984, 35:137–141.

Hillman BJ, Ovitt TW, Doering RT. Intravenous glucagon as an alternative to abdominal compression. Experimental urograms in dogs. *Invest Radiol* 1980, 15:419.

Saxton HM. Urography. *Br J Radiol* 1969, 42:321–346.

Shehadi WH. Adverse reactions to intravenously administered contrast media. AJR 1975, 124:145–152.

Spataro RF, Fischer HW, Boylan L. Urography with low-osmolality contrast media. Comparative urinary excretion of iopamidol, Hexabrix, and diatrizoate. *Invest Radiol* 1982, 17:494–500.

Spataro RF, Fischer HW, Kormano M. Clinical comparison of Hexabrix, iopamidol and Urografin-60 in whole body computed tomography. *Invest Radiol* 1984, 19 (Suppl.): S372–S375.

Stadalnik RC, Vera Z, DaSilva O, et al. Electrocardiographic response to intravenous urography: A prospective evaluation of 275 patients. *AJR* 1977, 129:825–830.

Taenzer V, Koeppe P, Samwer KF, et al. Comparative pharmacokinetics of sodium- and methylglucamine diatrizoate in urography. *Eur J Clin Pharmacol* 1973, 6:137–140.

Talner LB. Urographic contrast media in uremia. Physiology and pharmacology. *Radiol Clin North Am* 1972, X: 421–431.

Thompson WM. Excretory urography. A comparison of iopamidol and meglumine diatrizoate. *Invest Radiol* 1984, 19 (Suppl.): S229–S233.

Weigen JF, Thomas SF. Urinary tract. Excretory urography. In *Complications of Diagnostic Radiology* (Weigen, JF, Thomas SF, eds.). Springfield, IL, Charles C Thomas Publishers, 1973, pp. 288–313.

▼▼▼

Contrast Media for Computed Tomography: Intravascular, Intracavitary, Xenon, Reticuloendothelial

Dennis P. Swanson
Michael B. Alpern

In computed tomography (CT), a collimated x-ray beam is directed at the patient from several angles (projections) within a plane that lies perpendicular to the longitudinal axis of the patient's body (Figure 3.1). As these x-rays pass through the body, they are decreased in intensity or attenuated in proportion to the density of the tissues with which they interact. Transmitted x-rays emerging from the patient interact with radiation detectors to produce an electrical current that is proportional to the energy of the transmitted beam (i.e., inversely proportional to the density of the interacting body structures). This electrical current is quantitated numerically (digitized) and stored in a computer; the respective attenuation data for each projection representing an individual element in the complex set of mathematical equations used for image reconstruction. This latter process involves the formation of a matrix consisting of a finite number of picture elements (pixels). Each pixel value corresponds to the respective summation of attenuation data from multiple projections. These numerical values are subsequently converted into shades of grey to produce a cross-sectional image (i.e., computed tomogram) of the area-of-interest. Body structures within this area-of-interest can be differentiated due to their varying densities and, hence, differential x-ray absorption. Standard attenuation values of various body structures (Table 3.1) are frequently expressed in Hounsfield Units

(HU) according to an arbitrary scale obtained by internally calibrating the

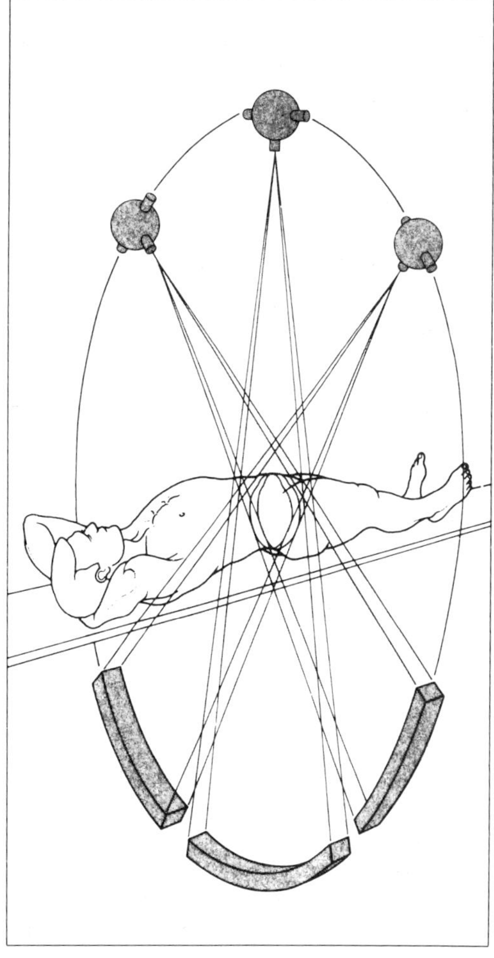

Figure 3.1 Illustration of computed tomography technique. (From Wegener OH, 1983; with permission.)

**Table 3.1 STANDARD CT ATTENUATION VALUES
FOR SELECTED BODY TISSUES AND FLUIDS**[a]

CALIBRATION STANDARD	BODY TISSUE	BODY FLUID	STANDARD ATTENUATION VALUE (HOUNSFIELD UNITS)
	Bone (compact)		>250
	Bone (spongy)		130 ± 100
		Blood (coagulated)	80 ± 10
	Thyroid		70 ± 10
	Liver		65 ± 5
		Blood (venous, whole)	55 ± 5
	Muscle		45 ± 5
	Spleen		45 ± 5
	Lymphoma		45 ± 10
	Pancreas		40 ± 10
	Kidney		30 ± 10
		Exudate/Transudate	18 ± 2
Water			0
	Fatty tissue		-90 ± 10
	Lung		< -300
Air			-1000

[a] Adapted from Wegener OH, 1983, with permission.

scanner such that the density value of water, air, and mineral (metal) are equal to 0, -1000 and $+1000$ HU respectively (Wegener OH, 1983).

Compared to film-based radiographic techniques, CT is more sensitive to small differences or changes (e. g., contrast media-induced) in tissue contrast. The increased contrast resolution of CT occurs as a result of the digitization of data, the increased sensitivity of digital versus film-based detectors, and the axial tomographic acquisition and presentation of data that eliminate superimposition of densities from body parts above or below the area-of-interest. However, the finite number of pixels within a computed tomographic image limits one's ability to resolve extremely small structures. Thus, the spatial resolution of computed tomograms is diminished relative to film-based techniques. Problems can also be encountered in computed tomography as a result of the length of time required for data acquisition. Any patient motion during the scanning interval may lead to substantial image degradation. Modern scanners have lessened this concern by reducing data acquisition time to 1–10 seconds; however, the problem of image degradation due to patient motion has not been totally eliminated.

Contrast enhancement in CT involves the administration of a radiopaque contrast medium to increase the degree of contrast between normal body structures and to improve the differentiation of pathological processes from normal tissues. Despite the obvious advantages that could be gained with the development and routine use of organ- (see Reticuloendothelial Contrast Media), tumor-, or function- (see Xenon) specific radiopaque contrast media, contrast-enhanced computed tomography is currently primarily limited to the intravascular administration of water-soluble iodinated contrast media and the direct instillation of radiopaque media into the gastrointestinal tract, cerebrospinal fluid space, or urinary tract (retrograde).

I. Intravascular Contrast Media

The water-soluble, iodinated contrast media routinely utilized for angiography (see Chapter 1) are also administered intravascularly to enhance CT visualization of major blood vessels and the urinary tract or to improve the CT delineation and differentiation of normal and pathological tissues. Use of these media for the latter indication is based on specific tissue characteristics related to blood flow, capillary integrity, and the volume of the extravascular, extracellular (i. e., intersti-

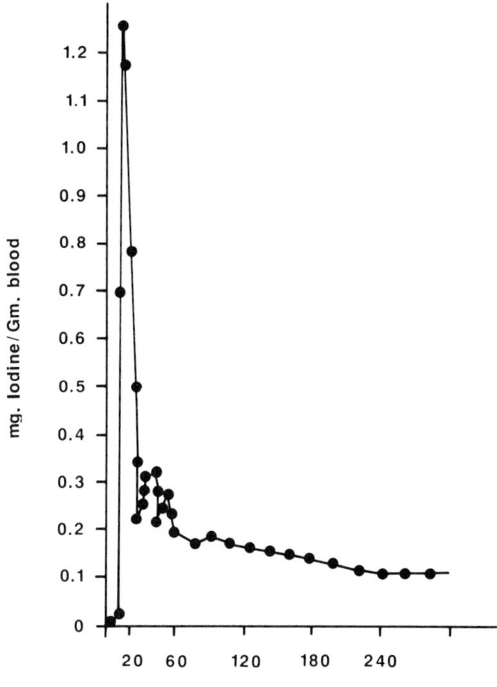

Figure 3.2 Blood (external iliac artery) iodine concentration following bolus intravenous injection of a water-soluble, iodinated contrast medium. Small peaks are due to first and second recirculation. (From Wegener OH, 1983; with permission.)

tial) fluid space. Inherent differences in these physiological features between normal and abnormal tissues result in differing contrast medium kinetics and temporal differences in their respective degrees of contrast enhancement.

CHEMISTRY

See Chapter 1 for a discussion of the chemistry of angiographic contrast media.

In addition to the agents described, infusion of the ratio-1.5 urographic contrast medium, iodamide meglumine, 24% weight/volume (w/v) (see Chapter 2, Urographic Contrast Media—Chemistry), is also indicated for CT of the brain.

PHARMACOKINETICS

Following bolus injection, the plasma concentration of an intravascular contrast medium decreases rapidly (Figure 3.2) as a result of vascular mixing, transcapillary diffusion of the medium from the circulation into the interstitial spaces, and renal excretion. Once the plasma concentration of the contrast medium falls below its interstitial concentration, the direction of this transcapillary diffusion reverses and the medium returns to the circulation with continuing renal excretion. CT density measurements obtained over the aorta and inferior vena cava have described three phases of respective vascular enhancement following bolus intravenous injection of a water-soluble, iodinated contrast medium (Table 3.2). The initial phase, or bolus effect, commences immediately after injection and is defined by a density difference of greater than 30 HU between the artery and veins. This phase, which typically lasts for less than 1 minute, is followed by a nonequilibrium phase of approximately 1-minute duration, wherein the arteriovenous density difference decreases to between 10 and 30 HU. Further diffusion of the contrast medium into the interstitial spaces and its renal excretion subsequently (i.e., at approximately 2 minutes post injection) result in an arteriovenous density difference of less than 10 HU. This is referred

Table 3.2   PHASES OF VASCULAR ENHANCEMENT FOLLOWING THE INTRAVENOUS INFUSION OR BOLUS INJECTION OF A RADIOPAQUE CONTRAST MEDIUM[a]

PHASE	AORTA-VENA CAVA ENHANCEMENT DIFFERENCE (HOUNSFIELD UNITS)	TIME OF APPEARANCE	
		BOLUS INJECTION	INFUSION
Bolus effect	30	Immediately post	—
Nonequilibrium	10–30	1–2 min.	During
Equilibrium	<10	>2 min.	Immediately post

[a] Adapted from Burgener FA and Hamlin DJ, 1981.

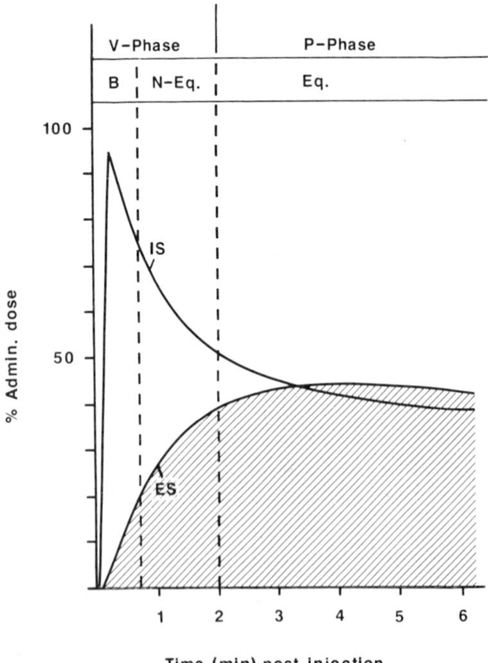

Figure 3.3 Relative distribution of a water-soluble, iodinated contrast medium in the intravascular space (IV) and the easily accessible extravascular, extracellular space (EC) following bolus intravenous injection. The vascular phase (V-phase) of opacification can be distinguished from the parenchymal phase (P-phase). B = bolus effect, Non-Eq. = nonequilibrium phase, Equil. = equilibrium phase. (Adapted from Wegener OH, 1983.)

to as the equilibrium phase. There is no bolus effect with an intravenous infusion of the contrast medium (Table 3.2). The nonequilibrium phase persists throughout the infusion, with the equilibrium phase commencing immediately following the termination of injection (Burgener FA and Hamlin DJ, 1981). The bolus and nonequilibrium phases may be collectively described as the vascular phase; the equilibrium phase is also known as the parenchymal phase (Figure 3.3).

The contrast enhancement of body (i. e., thoracic, abdominal) organs is primarily dependent on their blood flow and to a lesser extent on their interstitial volume. It is therefore not surprising that

maximum enhancement of major blood vessels and body organs (except the renal tubular collecting system) occurs during the vascular phase of contrast medium kinetics. Computed tomography during this phase thus provides optimal visualization of vascular structures and the optimal delineation and differentiation of normal and pathological tissues (Figure 3.4) (Burgener FA and Hamlin DJ 1981; Dean PB, 1980; Halvorsen RA, et al, 1984).

During the vascular phase, contrast enhancement differences between normal and pathological tissues occur as a result of differences in the time required for the contrast medium to pass from the site of injection to the respective tissues (i. e., circulation time), their rates of blood flow, and the volumes of their vascular beds. For example, differences in circulation time allow the differentiation of liver tumors, which are perfused via the hepatic artery, from the normal liver, which receives the majority of its blood flow from the portal vein. Differences between the inherent rate of blood flow to normal organs and hypovascular (i. e., cysts, many tumors, abscesses, or areas of necrosis) or hypervascular (i. e., tumor angiogenesis, inflammatory hyperemia) masses can also result in differing degrees of contrast enhancement. Finally, an area of infarction or ischemia can be identified due to its relative lack of blood flow or the prolonged circulation time associated with the presence of collateral pathways.

Differences in contrast enhancement between normal and abnormal tissues can also be observed in the parenchymal phase of contrast kinetics. This may again be related to differences in tissue blood flow since the interstitial concentration of a contrast medium at any given time is dependent on its relative rate of delivery to and clearance from the tissue. Other factors, such as capillary integrity and the associated rate of contrast diffusion into and out of the interstitial space, also contribute to temporal differences in the degree of contrast enhancement between these tissues. Furthermore, differences in the relative volume of the interstitial

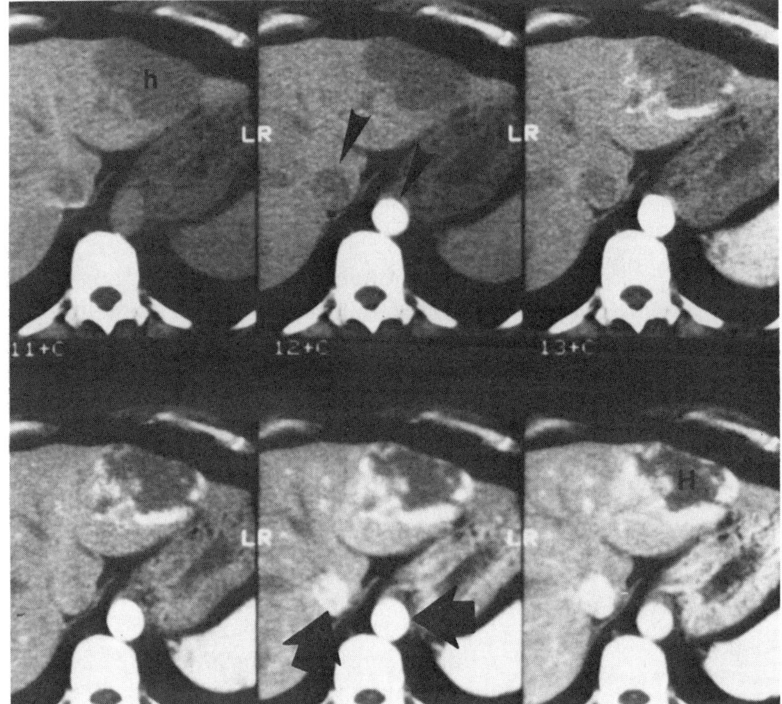

A

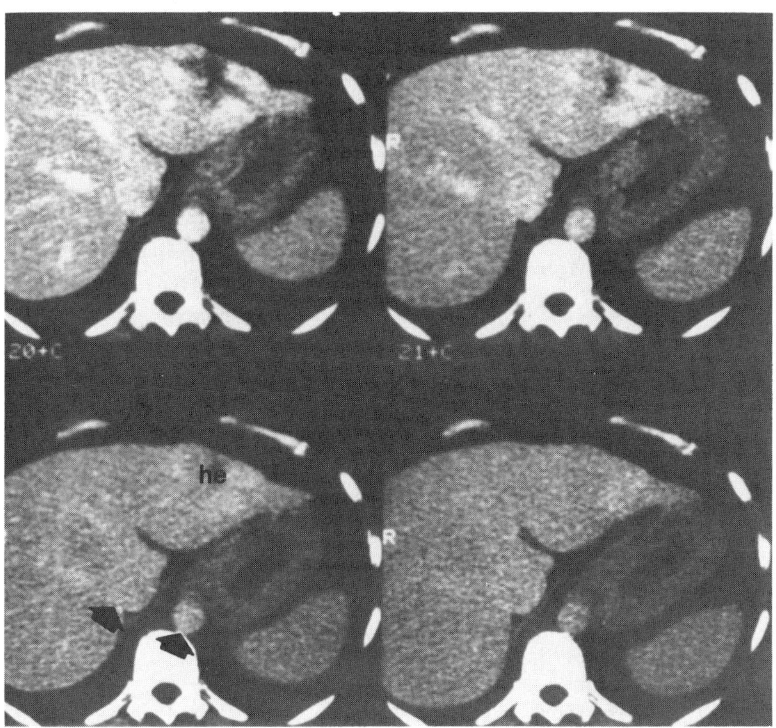

B

Figures 3.4 A,B Single-level dynamic study of liver hemangioma demonstrating characteristic CT features: low-density appearance (h) pre-contrast enhancement, hyperdense peripheral lakes (H) during maximum enhancement, persistent hyperdensity (he) on delayed images. Aorto-caval density differences correspond to the three phases of contrast medium kinetics: bolus effect (arrowheads), nonequilibrium phase (large arrows), and equilibrium phase (small arrows).

space in various tissues may lead to differences in contrast enhancement in the presence of equivalent rates of contrast delivery or diffusion. However, with the important exception of CT of the brain, scanning during the parenchymal phase of contrast medium kinetics generally provides less sensitivity for the differentiation of normal and abnormal processes than scanning during the vascular phase (Halvorsen RA, et al, 1984; Young SW, et al, 1980).

The diffusion of intravascular contrast media into the interstitial space of the brain is normally restricted by the limited capillary permeability of the intact blood-brain barrier. Pathological conditions (e. g., tumors, abscesses, cerebrovascular disorders) can lead to alterations in blood-brain barrier permeability with substantially increased diffusion of contrast media and subsequent enhancement relative to surrounding normal brain tissue (Zatz LM, 1980). As with the enhancement of body organs, the interstitial concentration of contrast at the locus of blood-brain barrier disruption is dependent on the blood supply to the associated lesion. For example, in the early stages, cerebrovascular infarcts may not demonstrate abnormal contrast enhancement due to the lack of a vascular delivery mechanism (Hayman LA and Hinck VC, 1985).

The use of intravascular contrast media for contrast enhancement of various regions of the urinary tract is based on renal blood flow and the normal glomerular filtration and renal tubular excretion of these agents. Computed tomography scanning during the vascular phase of contrast medium kinetics can readily differentiate the highly perfused renal cortex from the renal medulla and pelvis. In the later phases of contrast kinetics, enhancement of the renal cortex decreases relative to the medulla and pelvis due to accumulation of excreted contrast medium in the renal tubular collecting system. Maximum contrast enhancement of the urinary bladder is normally achieved at 10–15 minutes following intravenous administration of the contrast agent, although some enhancement may be seen as early as 2–4 minutes.

PHYSIOLOGICAL EFFECTS

The various effects of intravascular contrast media on vascular and organ physiology are discussed in detail in Chapter 1. In regard to the intravenous bolus injection or infusion of these agents for contrast enhancement in computed tomography, particular attention should be directed at their Vascular, Pulmonary, and Renal Effects (see Chapter 1). Pseudo-allergic reactions (see Chapter 8) to these contrast media also warrant consideration.

PRECAUTIONS

Precautions (i. e., physical incompatibilities, drug-, or laboratory test-contrast medium interactions) to be observed with the administration of intravascular contrast media for computed tomography are outlined in Chapter 1.

CLINICAL CONSIDERATIONS/ CONTRAINDICATIONS

Computed tomography, with or without contrast enhancement, is valuable in the diagnosis, evaluation, and staging of a variety of pathological processes. A complete discussion of the clinical indications for contrast-enhanced CT is beyond the scope or focus of this book, and the reader is referred to more extensive, procedure-oriented reviews of this subject for additional information.

Optimal use of an intravascular contrast medium for contrast enhancement in CT demands constant consideration of its pharmacokinetic characteristics. Nonmeticulous scanning techniques or imprecise use of the contrast medium can easily result in missed diagnoses (Dean PB, 1980).

Body CT. As previously discussed, maximum enhancement of major blood vessels and body (e. g., thoracic, abdominal) organs occurs during the vascular phase of contrast media kinetics. Contrast-enhanced CT of a particular vascular system or body organ can be optimized if the commencement of scanning is correlated with the time required for the contrast medium bolus to pass from the injection

Table 3.3 CIRCULATION TIMES FOR SELECTED ORGAN SYSTEMS FOLLOWING INTRAVENOUS INJECTION OF AN INDICATOR SUBSTANCE (E.G., RADIOPAQUE CONTRAST MEDIUM) INTO A HEALTHY PERSON[a]

ORGAN SYSTEM	TIME (SECS.) OF INDICATOR APPEARANCE POST START OF INJECTION
Heart	
R. ventricle	4
L. ventricle	11
Aorta	
Thoracic	12
Abdominal	13
Iliac Arteries	15
Liver	
Arterial circulation	20
Portal venous circulation	35
Abdominal organs	20
Brain	22
Kidney	
Cortex (renal artery)	20

[a] Adapted from Wegener OH, 1983.

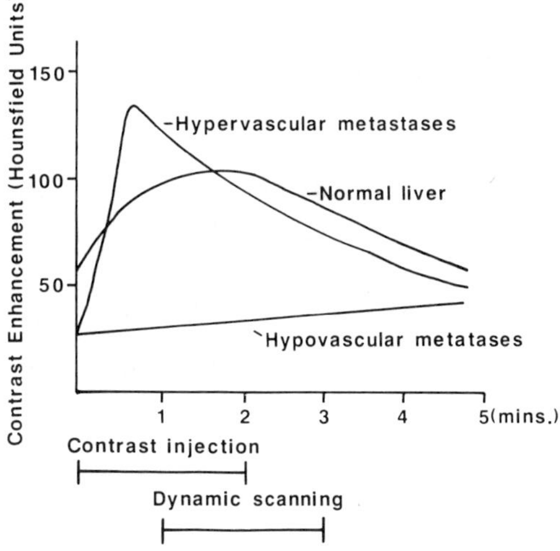

Figure 3.5 Enhancement characteristics of the normal liver and hepatic metastases following the bolus, intravenous injection of a water-soluble iodinated contrast media.

site to the area-of-interest (i. e., circulation time). As expected, circulation times can vary significantly depending on the location of the organ and the primary source of its perfusion (Table 3.3).

Computed tomography evaluation of the liver for metastatic disease is best performed following the intravascular administration of contrast agents. In most cases, contrast-enhanced scans of the liver are timed to coincide with the circulation time of portal venous blood flow (Table 3.3), the predominant source of hepatic perfusion. Using this technique, most abnormalities appear as foci of decreased x-ray attenuation against the contrast-enhanced liver parenchyma. Conversely, if the commencement of CT scanning is correlated with the circulation time of hepatic artery blood flow (Table 3.3), preferential enhancement of hepatic tumors may be observed. This phenomenon occurs since liver tumors usually derive the majority of their perfusion via hepatic arterial flow.

The time-density graph in Figure 3.5 illustrates the utility of dynamic scanning during the bolus injection of an intravascular contrast medium for the demonstration of hepatic lesions. The common metastases to the liver (e. g., colon, liver, breast tumors) are usually hypovascular, and therefore are less radiodense than the enhanced liver parenchyma during the period of 1–3 minutes after a bolus injec-

tion (Figure 3.6A, B). As the contrast washes out of the normal liver, there is a concurrent gradual increase in enhancement of the tumor due to contrast accumulation in its interstitial spaces. Hence, a delay of more than 3–5 minutes between contrast administration and CT scanning increases the likelihood that a metastasis will appear isodense relative to the surrounding normal liver. This isodense phenomenon is therefore more likely to occur with drip infusion techniques coupled with slower image acquisition rates.

In the smaller subgroup of patients with hypervascular hepatic metastases (e. g., renal cell carcinomas, pancreatic islet-cell tumors, carcinoids, pheochromocytomas), scanning during the 1–3 minutes following a bolus injection of contrast can also result in the lesion appearing isodense relative to the normal liver (Bressler EL, et al, 1987). In this circumstance, the hypervascular tumor rapidly enhances during the hepatic arterial phase. The contrast begins to wash out of the tumor as the normal liver parenchyma approaches maximal enhancement, thus resulting in isodensity (Figures 3.7A–C). It is for this reason that non-contrast-enhanced scans should be performed in this subgroup of patients prior to the performance of enhanced scans.

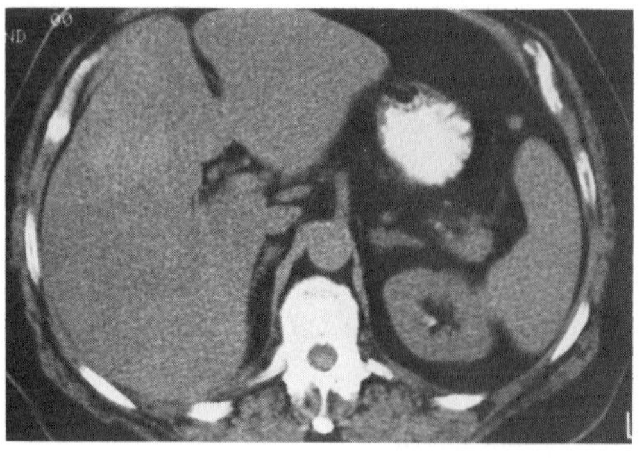

A

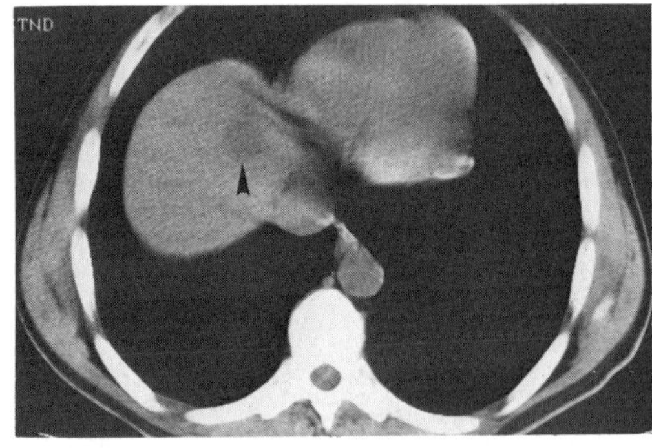

A

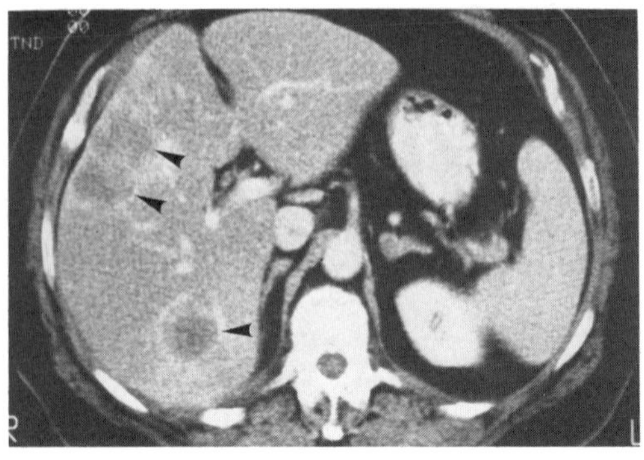

B

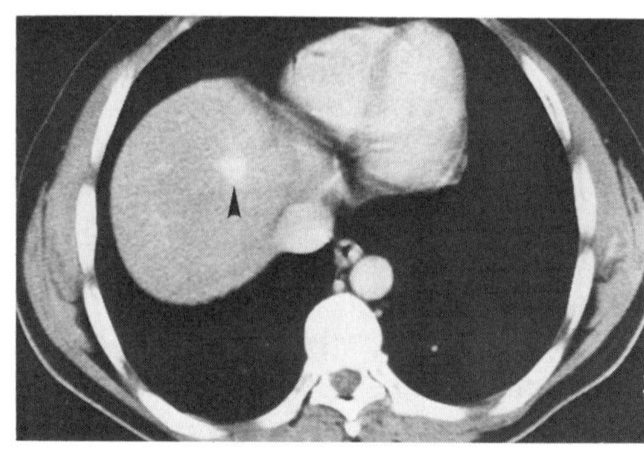

B

Figures 3.6 A,B Liver metastases from a colon carcinoma are isodense with normal liver parenchyma on the non–contrast-enhanced study (A), and of lower attenuation (arrowheads) than normal liver on the contrast-enhanced image (B). (From Alpern, MB, et al, 1986; with permission.)

In summary, incremental dynamic scanning 1–3 minutes after the onset of a prolonged (90–120 second) bolus injection of the contrast medium is the most efficient method of assessing the liver for focal abnormalities. The small subset of patients with suspected hypervascular liver metastases should be scanned without contrast prior to the enhanced study.

It has been suggested that CT images of the liver obtained at 4–6 hours after intravascular contrast administration may depict lesions not identifiable with the routine dynamic scanning protocol (Bernardino ME, et al, 1986). It has also been claimed that dynamic CT scanning during the direct injection of contrast into the celiac axis or superior mesenteric artery will demonstrate additional foci of tumor involvement (Takashima T and Matsui O, 1980; Matsui O, et al, 1985). Although these procedures

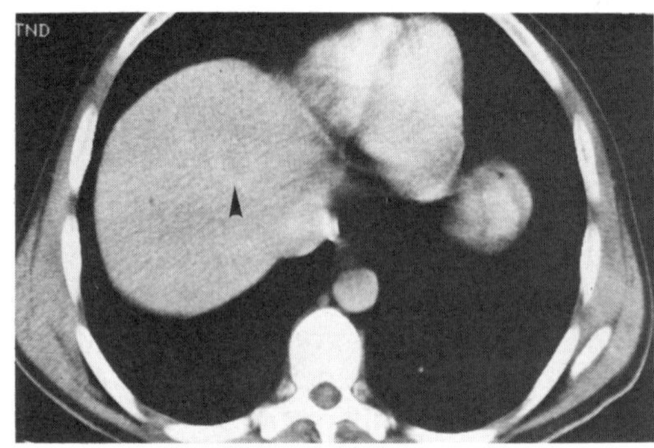

C

Figures 3.7 A–C Carcinoid metastasis demonstrating low attenuation on the non–contrast-enhanced study (A), hyperdensity (at 30 seconds post contrast injection) during the hepatic arterial phase (B), and isodensity late (2 minutes post contrast injection) in the nonequilibrium phase (C). (From Bressler, EL., et al, 1987; with permission.)

are considered impractical for routine imaging, they may prove of value in selected cases (e.g., determination of surgical resectability for solitary metastasis).

The diagnosis of hemangioma may be made when a lesion appears less dense than the liver on a nonenhanced image, and demonstrates "puddling" and hyperdense lakes during the parenchymal phase of the enhanced study (Figures 3.4A, B). Hyperdensity will persist for 5–60 minutes as the lesion gradually enhances in a centripetal manner. Approximately 50% of hemangiomas will demonstrate this classic pattern (Freeny PC and Marks WM, 1986).

For other body organs (except the kidney), the commencement of CT scanning is generally timed to correlate with the circulation time of their respective arterial blood flow. For example, thin-section dynamic imaging of the pancreas during maximal aortic and pancreatic arterial concentration of the contrast medium facilitates the visualization of islet-cell tumors, which are usually hypervascular (Figure 3.8). Other tumors such as some soft-tissue sarcomas (e. g., liposarcoma) or lymphomas tend to demonstrate significantly less dramatic contrast enhancement. Inflammatory masses, such as abscesses, occasionally demonstrate hyperemia-associated peripheral enhancement with rapid scanning techniques.

Brain CT. The CT demonstration of cerebral tumors and inflammatory disorders is usually dependent on an associated disruption of blood-brain barrier

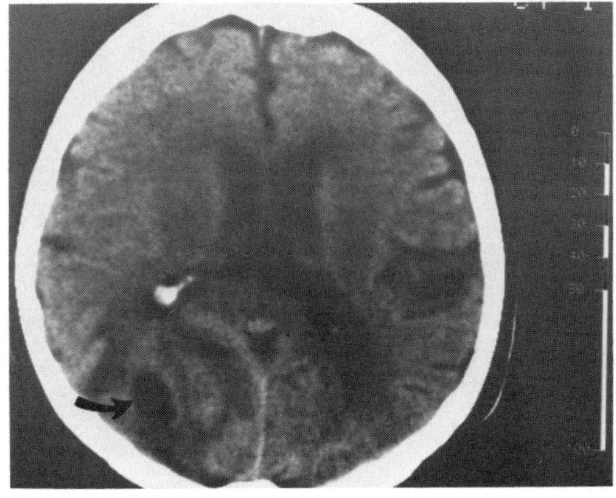

A

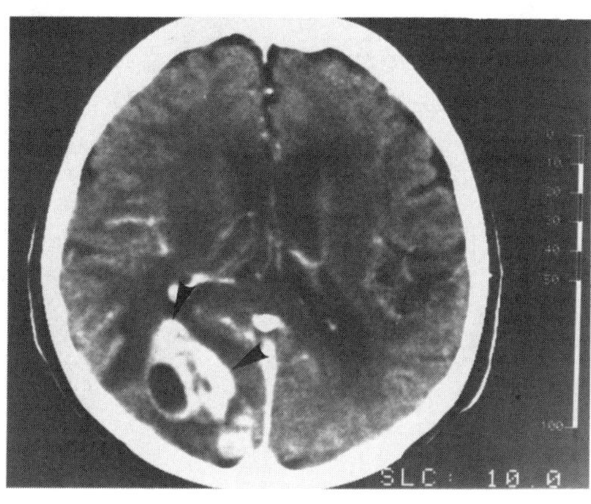

B

Figure 3.9 A,B This non-contrast-enhanced brain scan (A) reveals a cystic area (arrow). Contrast-enhancement (B) demonstrates the solid enhancing component (arrowheads) of the cystic astrocytoma.

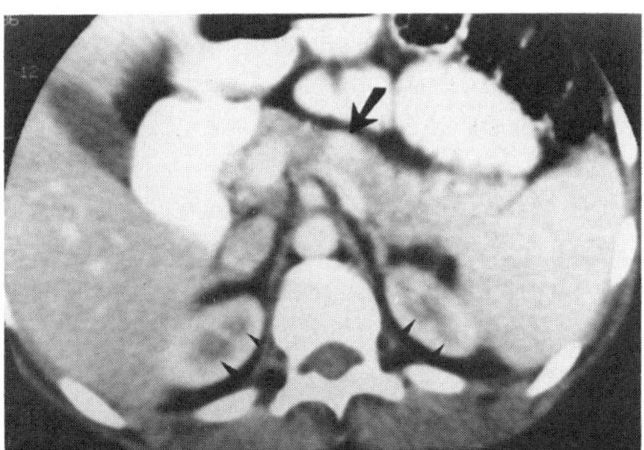

Figure 3.8 Contrast enhancement of an insulin-producing islet-cell tumor (arrow) within the pancreas. Note the cortical-medullary differentiation (arrowheads) in the kidneys during the bolus phase of contrast kinetics.

permeability and an abnormal diffusion of the intravascular contrast medium into the brain. Hence, cerebral tumors and abscesses demonstrate selective contrast enhancement in comparison to relatively nonenhanced normal brain tissues (Figure 3.9). As might be expected, the CT visualization of these enhancing cerebral abnormalities is best achieved during the parenchymal phase of contrast medium kinetics.

Cerebral vascular infarcts may also be diagnosed using contrast-enhanced CT. However, enhancement of an infarct is dependent on the length of time that has elapsed since the infarct event. Therefore,

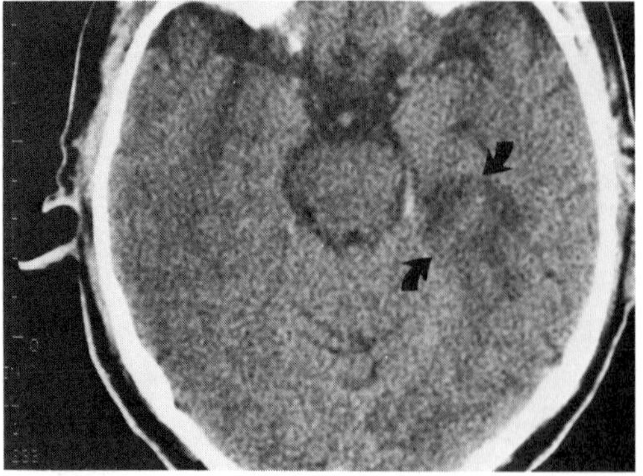

A

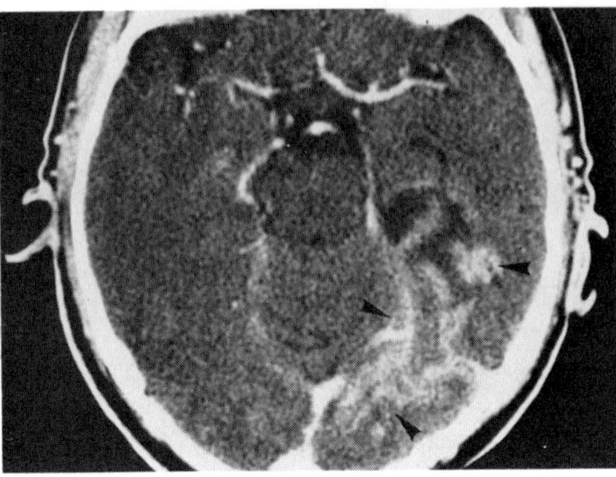

B

Figures 3.10 A,B Non–contrast-enhanced brain scan (A) shows an infarct as a low-attenuation zone (arrow). Contrast-enhanced image (B) demonstrates intense diffusion of contrast medium into the abnormal region (arrowheads) via collateral flow.

the optimal CT technique is also dependent on the length of time post infarction. In the early stages, cerebrovascular infarction does not demonstrate contrast enhancement during either the vascular or parenchymal phase of contrast medium kinetics due to the lack of primary or collateral perfusion. However, during the vascular phase of contrast kinetics, early cerebral infarcts can be distinguished as regions that lack the normal CT enhancement associated with the presence of concentrated contrast medium in the normal cerebral vasculature. Approximately 4 days post infarction, selective enhancement results from abnormal diffusion of

the contrast medium into the involved area of the brain (Figures 3.10 A, B) via immature collateral capillaries that initially lack a blood-brain barrier. This abnormal contrast diffusion will continue until the vascular endothelial cells of these capillaries form the tight junctions that comprise the normal blood-brain barrier. Contrast enhancement prior to 4 days following an ischemic event may be associated with the abnormal diffusion of contrast medium from compromised vessels surrounding the infarct zone. The abnormal diffusion of contrast medium into boundary zones surrounding cerebral infections (i. e., cerebritis, abscesses) or into areas of resolving cerebral hemorrhage also appears to be associated with the formation and presence of immature blood vessels that initially lack blood-brain barrier properties. On the other hand, contrast enhancement of neoplasms may be due to transcapillary diffusion of the contrast medium through mature vessels that are histologically devoid of or have a defective blood-brain barrier (Hayman LA and Hinck VC, 1985).

In addition to their relative perfusion, the degree of contrast enhancement of various cerebral neoplasms is also dependent on the extent of blood-brain barrier deficiency and the volume of their interstitial space. In certain cerebral neoplasms, transcapillary diffusion of the contrast medium proceeds at a slower rate, or via a different mechanism than that observed in other brain lesions. Hence, maximum enhancement of some brain tumors or the visualization of small lesions may require high doses of the contrast medium and/or scanning as late as 1–2 hours after injection (Hayman LA and Hinck VC, 1985). In most cases, however, brain lesions can be sufficiently differentiated at 5–10 minutes post injection due to the negligible enhancement of normal brain tissue. It should be noted that high-dose steroid therapy may result in a reduction in the degree of contrast enhancement of cerebral lesions (Crocker EF, et al, 1976; Whelan M and Hilal SK, 1980). This phenomenon appears to be related to a pharmacologically induced decrease in capillary permeability and perilesion edema, and hence a decrease in the extent of abnormal contrast medium diffusion. An increase in the contrast enhancement of apparently normal central nervous system tissue may also occur as a result of subclinical blood-brain barrier damage induced by associated radiation therapy (Hayman LA and Hinck VC, 1985). In contradistinction, capillary destruction produced by high-radiation doses would be expected to inhibit the delivery of an intravascular contrast medium and reduce the degree of contrast enhancement observed during the vascular phase.

Renal CT. Dynamic CT imaging during the vascular and parenchymal phases of contrast kinetics permits differentiation of the renal cortex from medulla due to differential blood flow and renal tubular contrast medium kinetics (Figure 3.8). In addition to the administered dose, the final concentration of a contrast medium within the renal parenchyma is dependent on the patients's renal function and state of hydration. It should be emphasized, however, that absolute renal function cannot be inferred from the degree of renal contrast enhancement achieved post intravenous administration of an intravascular contrast medium. Marked decreases in creatinine clearance may be required before evidence of diminished renal function manifests radiographically. Furthermore, post renal obstruction may significantly alter the rate at which the contrast medium is cleared from the renal parenchyma.

A renal mass that does not demonstrate contrast enhancement, has an imperceptible wall, and is of homogeneous water density (i. e., 0–15 HU) is a cyst. If these criteria are not met, one cannot confidently exclude a neoplasm. With the exception of a fat-containing angiomyolipoma, other renal masses cannot be reliably distinguished from each other, with most demonstrating enhancement following contrast administration. If a good bolus technique and dynamic scanning is

employed, contrast-enhanced CT can reliably diagnose the presence of thrombus in the renal vein or inferior vena cava in patients with renal cell carcinoma. Although the identification of a vascular thrombus does not significantly affect staging of the neoplasm, it is important for surgical planning.

Contrast Media Considerations. With the exception of renal opacification, there is no conclusive evidence, to date, to suggest that any of the various chemical forms of the ratio-1.5 ionic or ratio-3 low-osmolality contrast media produce clinically superior enhancement of any specific organ or improved differentiation of normal versus pathological processes. (Skalpe IO, 1983; Halvorsen RA, et al, 1984; Dean PB, et al, 1983; Fike JR, et al, 1984; Robins AH, et al, 1984).

Compared to equiiodine doses of the ratio-1.5 ionic media, the ratio-3 low-osmolality agents do demonstrate greater peak enhancement of the vascular blood pool immediately following bolus injection (Figure 3.11). This may be associated with a decrease in the degree of cellular diuresis and hypervolemia induced by the low-osmolality agents, or with differences between the ratio-1.5 ionic and low-osmolality media in regard to their rates of transcapillary diffusion (Spataro RF, et al, 1984). However, blood concentrations of the ratio-3 low-osmolality media rapidly approach those of the ratio-1.5 ionic media during the nonequilibrium and equilibrium phases (Figure 3.11), thus explaining the minimal differences in organ or lesion enhancement observed with these agents.

Assuming equiiodine doses and constant renal function, the concentration that an intravascular contrast medium achieves in the renal tubules is primarily dependent on the degree of osmotic diuresis that it induces (see Chapter 2, Urographic Contrast Media). Sodium salts of the conventional ratio-1.5 ionic media (e. g., diatrizoate, iothalamate, metrizoate) produce less osmotic diuresis and greater urinary iodine concentrations than

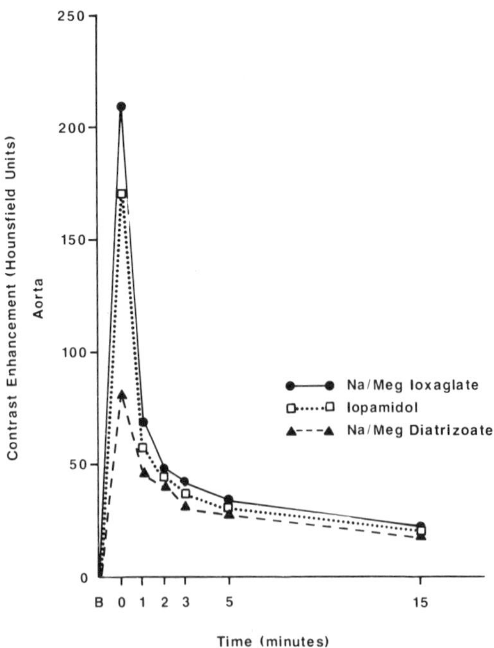

Figure 3.11 Contrast enhancement of aorta following the bolus, intravenous injection of equiiodine doses of ratio-1.5 ionic (Na/Meg Diatrizoate) and ratio-3 low-osmolality (Na/Meg Ioxaglate, Iopamidol) contrast media. (From Spataro RF, et al, 1984; with permission.)

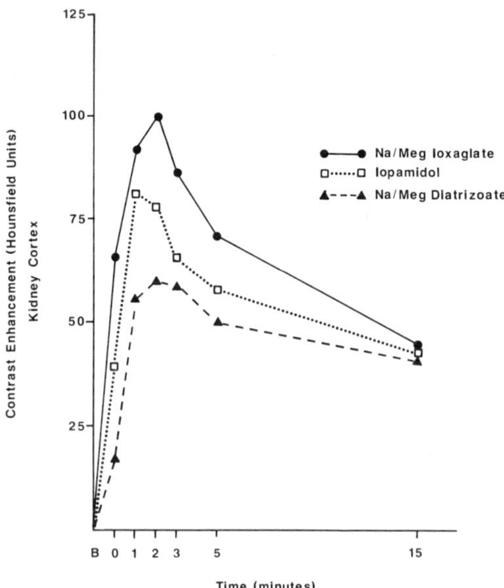

Figure 3.12 Contrast enhancement of the renal cortex following the bolus, intravenous injection of equiiodine doses of ratio-1.5 ionic (Na/Meg Diatrizoate) and ratio-3 low-osmolality (Na/Meg Ioxaglate, Iopamidol) contrast media. (From Spataro RF, et al, 1984: with permission.)

meglumine salts. This occurs because, unlike meglumine, the sodium cations are capable of being reabsorbed from the renal tubules, thus resulting in a reduced tubular concentration of osmotically active particles. Similarly, contrast enhancement of the kidney is greater with the ratio-3 low-osmolality versus ratio-1.5 ionic media as a result of the decreased osmotic diuresis and dilution effects induced by the former agents (Figure 3.12). In consideration of the contrast sensitivity of CT and the already high renal concentration achieved with each of the intravascular contrast media, the relative renal tubular opacification differences between these groups of agents are probably of minimal importance in clinical practice.

Attention should be given, however, to the relative incidence and severity of undesirable physiological effects produced by various formulations of ratio-1.5 ionic and ratio-3 low-osmolality media (See

Chapter 1, Physiological Effects, Clinical Considerations). Compared to equiiodine concentrations of the sodium salts of diatrizoate, iothalamate, and metrizoate, meglumine salts produce less pain and subjective discomfort upon intravenous administration. The incidence and severity of these responses and of other undesirable physiological effects can be further reduced with equivalent use of ratio-3 low-osmolality agents. The improved tolerability of these low-osmolality media must, however, be weighed against their substantially increased costs compared to the ratio-1.5 agents. It is therefore recommended that use of the ratio-3 low osmolality media be directed at patients known to be at increased risk for reactions to the ratio-1.5 media (See Chapter 1, Clinical Considerations).

DOSAGE

Depending on the body part to be studied and the pathologic process to be excluded, different rates of contrast medium administration may be employed to attain the desired diagnostic objective. Both bolus and drip infusion methods are therefore commonly utilized. As previously discussed, imaging during the vascular phase of contrast medium kinetics is useful for evaluations of the chest and abdomen, particularly when interest centers about the mediastinum or solid viscera such as the liver. The shorter the injection time of a given dose (i. e., product of volume and concentration) of a contrast medium, the greater the maximum iodine concentration and degree of contrast enhancement. Bolus administration of large doses of intravascular contrast media does, however, have certain limitations. Depending on the sophistication of the scanner used, it may not be possible to scan rapidly enough to encompass a large area of interest. Fortunately, most third- and fourth-generation CT scanners have overcome this problem.

Body CT. Incremental dynamic imaging combined with a sustained, bolus injection of an intravascular contrast medium is an example of an imaging technique that finds particular utility in evaluations of the liver and mediastinum. In this technique, the region to be examined is determined from a scout digital radiograph performed by the CT scanner prior to the contrast-enhancement study. This allows the monitoring radiologist to program the scanner to obtain images from a desired anatomic location (e. g., when imaging the liver, images would be obtained from dome of right hemidiaphragm through the tip of the right hepatic lobe). Usually, 10 mm-thick, contiguous images are obtained. Imaging is performed during suspended respiration using 2–3-second scan times when possible. Breathing is allowed during an interscan delay of approximately 6–7 seconds. An intravascular contrast medium is injected intravenously (e. g., 150–180 mL at 280–300 I/mL; total 42–50 g iodine) over approximately a 2-minute period with imaging commencing 30–60 seconds after

the onset of injection. For pediatric patients, 2 mL/kg of an intravascular contrast medium containing 280–300 mg iodine/mL is injected as an intravenous bolus, with dynamic scanning beginning when one-half of the total dose has been delivered. The above technique depends upon a cooperative patient, but gives reproducible results with consistent contrast enhancement.

Intravascular drip infusion of contrast agents lacks the vessel opacification advantages of the bolus effect. The non-equilibrium phase of contrast kinetics does persist throughout the infusion; however, the respective degree of enhancement is less than that observed with a bolus injection. As expected, the equilibrium phase of contrast kinetics commences immediately following termination of the infusion.

A biphasic approach (e. g., 50 mL intravenous bolus (followed by 100 mL infusion) may be utilized to achieve opacification of the major blood vessels and prolonged organ enhancement. Conversely, a pathological process or region-of-interest recognized during the infusion can be specifically examined using a subsequent bolus injection. Contrast enhancement of a particular organ can be further optimized if the contrast medium is injected directly into the arterial supply of the organ. This method of administration may lead to immediate and pronounced (i. e., "overloading") interstitial opacification; however, the required catheterization procedure is technically demanding and adds an additional risk to the procedure. Details concerning the use of CT arteriography will not be discussed.

Brain CT. The recommended adult dosage for cranial computed tomography is 28–42 g of iodine (e. g., 100–150 mL at 280–300 mg iodine/mL or 200–300 mL at 140–150 mg iodine/mL) administered over a 5–10-minute period with CT scanning commencing immediately following completion of the contrast injection. Contrast dosages significantly below this level have been shown to be considerably less reliable in the demonstration of cerebral tumors (Norman D, et al, 1978). Pediatric patients receive a total iodine dosage of 0.4–0.6 g/kg with CT scanning commencing once the complete dose has been delivered.

It has been suggested that expanded high-dose CT, involving an additional bolus injection of 30–40 g iodine (e. g., 100–150 mL at 280–300 mg iodine/mL) following the routine infusion, may be useful in detecting multiple brain lesions, resolving equivocal areas of abnormal enhancement, or in differentiating solid histologically microcystic from macrocystic neoplasms (Davis JM, et al, 1979). Improvements in lesion enhancement can also be realized with delayed scanning (e. g., at 1–2 hours) following routine dosages.

II. Intracavitary Opacification

Computed tomography procedures may incorporate the direct instillation of dilute solutions of radiopaque contrast media into enclosed compartments (e. g., gastrointestinal tract, bladder, cerebrospinal fluid space) to permit accurate delineation of the compartment and to improve the differentiation of intra- from extraluminal pathologies. The instilled contrast medium mixes with fluid present within the compartment. The final degree of opacification is determined by the instilled iodine dose (volume and concentration) and the total volume of distribution.

GASTROINTESTINAL OPACIFICATION (See Chapter 5, Gastrointestinal Contrast Media)

Unopacified bowel presents a problem in the accurate CT evaluation of the abdomen since bowel contents often simulate soft-tissue densities that may be misinterpreted as abnormal masses (e. g., tumors, abscesses). Air normally present within the bowel does provide negative contrast and may permit bowel delineation; however, not all bowel loops contain air, or isolated regions of bowel air may be confused with air within the necrotic centers of tumors or abscesses. Opacification of the gastrointestinal tract following the oral administration of dilute barium sulfate or iodinated contrast media solutions is therefore desirable, especially in evaluation of the pancreatic or pelvis area. It is felt to be essential when CT is used to search the abdomen for abscesses.

Bowel opacification for CT may be accomplished using the oral barium sulfate or water-soluble, iodinated contrast media routinely indicated for standard fluoroscopic and film-based studies of the gastrointestinal tract. However, the significantly increased contrast resolution of computed tomography and the potential for formation of unacceptable imaging artifacts (Figure 3.13) demands the use of very dilute concentrations of these media. Hence, the commercially available, concentrated (41.7% w/v, 76% w/v) oral solutions of iodinated contrast media (Table 3.4) must be diluted with sufficient water to yield an iodine concentration of 5–15 mg/mL (e. g., 1.1–3.3% w/v) for appropriate CT bowel opacification. Similar dilution of the concentrated barium sulfate preparations routinely utilized for conventional gastrointestinal studies has resulted in problems associated with subsequent product instability and in vivo flocculation. The recent development and introduction of dilute (i. e., 1–3% w/v) barium sulfate preparations designed specifically for CT bowel opacification (Table 3.5) has obviated these problems. Both the diluted iodine preparation and dilute barium sulfate suspensions produce column opacification with negligible coating properties. Since both preparations are hypotonic at the dilute concentrations administered, systemic absorption of water during their passage through the gastrointestinal tract may result in concentrating effects and an observed increase in opacification of distal segments of the bowel.

Small quantities (i. e., 1% of administered dose, product information, Hypaque sodium, Winthrop-Breon Labs.) of the iodinated contrast media may be

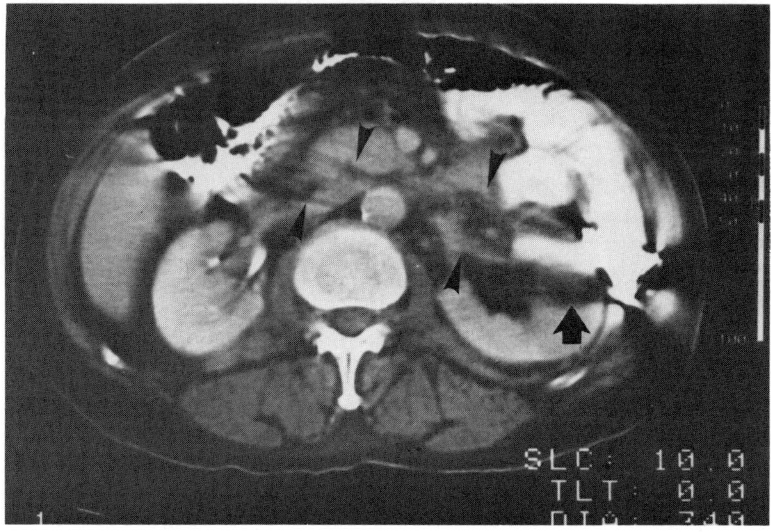

Figure 3.13 Streak artifacts (arrowheads) from excessive barium within the gastrointestinal tract degrade the CT image; in particular, evaluation of the left kidney (arrow).

Table 3.4 IODINATED CONTRAST MEDIA FOR ENHANCEMENT OF THE GASTROINTESTINAL TRACT IN CT EXAMINATIONS[a]

GENERIC NAME	CONCENTRATION (% w/v)	BRAND NAMES®[b]	MG IODINE / ML.
Diatrizoate meglumine-sodium solution (oral)	76	Gastrovist (B) MD-Gastroview (M) Gastrografin (S)	370
Diatrizoate sodium solution (oral)	41.7	Hypaque Liquid (W)	249
Diatrizoate sodium powder (oral)	Variable	Hypaque Powder (W)	(600 mg I/g. powder)

[a] Must be diluted to contain 5–15 mg. Iodine/mL. for use in CT examinations.

[b] (B) Berlex Imaging
(M) Mallinckrodt, Inc.
(S) Squibb Diagnostics
(w) Winthrop-Breon Laboratories

Table 3.5 BARIUM SULFATE MEDIA (1–3% w/v) INDICATED FOR ENHANCEMENT OF THE GASTROINTESTINAL TRACT IN CT EXAMINATIONS

BRAND NAME®	MANUFACTURER
E-Z-CAT	E-Z-EM, Inc.
Redi-CAT	E-Z-EM, Inc.
TomoCat (EneCat)	Lafayette-Pharmacal, Inc.
PrepCAT	Lafayette-Pharmacal, Inc.
Baro-CAT	Mallinckrodt, Inc.

absorbed from the gastrointestinal tract, therefore the possibility of unpredictable, pseudo-allergic reactions (i. e., dose and concentration independent) in susceptible individuals must be considered. Hypersensitivity reactions to the nonabsorbable barium sulfate preparations are rare. As discussed in Chapter 5, oral or rectal administration of barium sulfate is contraindicated in the presence of known or suspected acute gastrointestinal perforation or imminent gastrointestinal surgery. In these latter situations, the water-soluble, and hence, absorbable iodinated contrast media are preferred. The iodinated contrast media do, however, produce greater insult to the lung in the event of contrast aspiration. Therefore, in patients prone to aspiration or in those with suspected tracheoesophageal or bronchoesophageal fistulae or other lack of airway control, iodinated contrast agents should be avoided. Since adequate total bowel opacification requires oral doses to be administered 1–4 hours prior to CT examination, outpatient use of the premixed, dilute barium sulfate preparations tends to be more convenient, less confusing, and presents less risk of an unattended allergic reaction. Such unit dose, outpatient preparation of the bowel can greatly facilitate patient throughput.

The choice of which oral contrast agent (i. e., barium sulfate or iodinated agent) to utilize for bowel opacification in CT is probably not as critical as the timing of its administration. Adequate opacification of the colon and distal small bowel requires the oral administration of 500 mL of dilute media approximately 12 hours prior to scanning. Colon opacification can also be accomplished with rectal administration of the same dose of dilute media. Examinations of the pancreas and epigastric region are facilitated by opacification of the upper gastrointestinal tract using additional oral doses (300–500 mL) of contrast at 30–60 minutes and immediately prior to scanning.

Since opacification of adjacent loops of bowel may present difficulties in the identification of biliary calculi, the oral administration of dilute contrast media should be avoided if this is the primary purpose of the CT examination. Due to the potential for density artifacts associated with the concentrated oral contrast media used for routine gastrointestinal radiology studies, subsequent CT evaluation of the abdomen may require delay. Laxatives and adequate patient hydration should be utilized to promote evacuation of the concentrated media in such circumstances.

BLADDER OPACIFICATION (See Chapter 2, Urographic Contrast Media)

The intravascular administration of iodinated contrast media can result in significant enhancement of the urinary bladder as a result of the normal renal excretion of these agents. This route of administration may be suboptimal for specific computed tomographic evaluations of the bladder wall or lumen due to problems associated with incomplete bladder filling, layering of high specific gravity contrast media within the bladder contents, and "hardening" artifacts resulting from an excessively concentrated, excreted medium.

Computed tomographic examination of the bladder for the sole purpose of identifying primary bladder pathology is performed infrequently in light of the availability of cystoscopy and other diagnostic procedures. Since the apparent thickness of the bladder wall is dependent on its extent of filling, the evaluation of suspected pathological wall thickening requires complete bladder filling in order to identify focal abnormalities.

Retrograde catheter-instillation of a dilute solution of the water-soluble iodinated contrast media utilizing a sufficient volume to elicit a sensation of pressure (e. g., generally 200–400 mL for adults; 50–300 mL for children depending on age) ensures complete bladder filling and uniform opacification of the bladder contents. Commercially available iodinated contrast media, indicated for retrograde cystourethrography, must be diluted with sterile water, 5% dextrose, or 0.9% sodium chloride for injection to a final concentration of 1–3.5% w/v (5–15 mg iodine/mL) to avoid "hardening" artifacts on the computed tomography scans. Sterile techniques should be employed during the catheterization and instillation procedures, and care should be taken to avoid excessive filling or trauma. Intravasation of the iodinated contrast media may occur; hence, the risk of unpredictable pseudo-allergic reactions must be considered. If catheterization is impossible or impractical, bladder filling and opacification may be accomplished by intravascular infusion of 300 mL of a 30% w/v (140 mg iodine/mL) solution of iodinated contrast media.

INTRATHECAL OPACIFICATION (see Chapter 4, Myelographic Contrast Media)

Computed tomography examinations of the spinal canal may require opacification of the subarachnoid space using the direct instillation of a water-soluble, nonionic contrast medium. Such opacification facilitates differentiation of intradural from extradural processes and intradural,

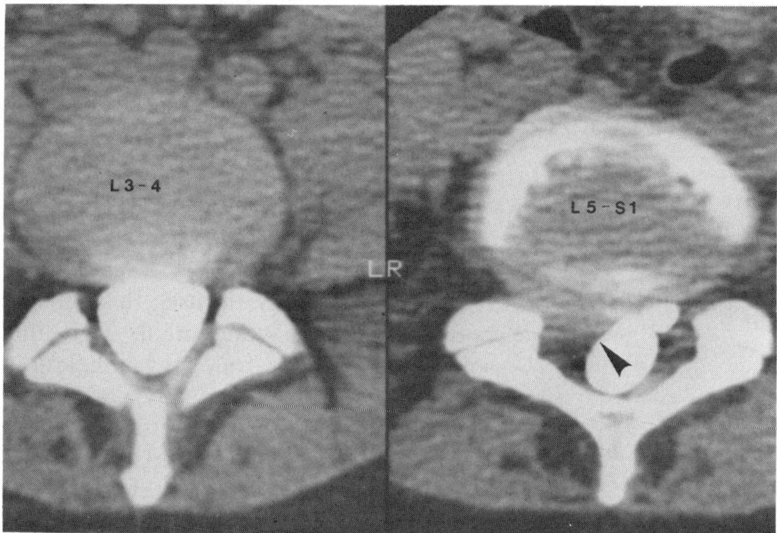

Figure 3.14 The normal disc at L3-4 does not compress the dural sac, whereas the herniated disc at L5-S1 does produce compression of the sac (arrowhead) and nerve root.

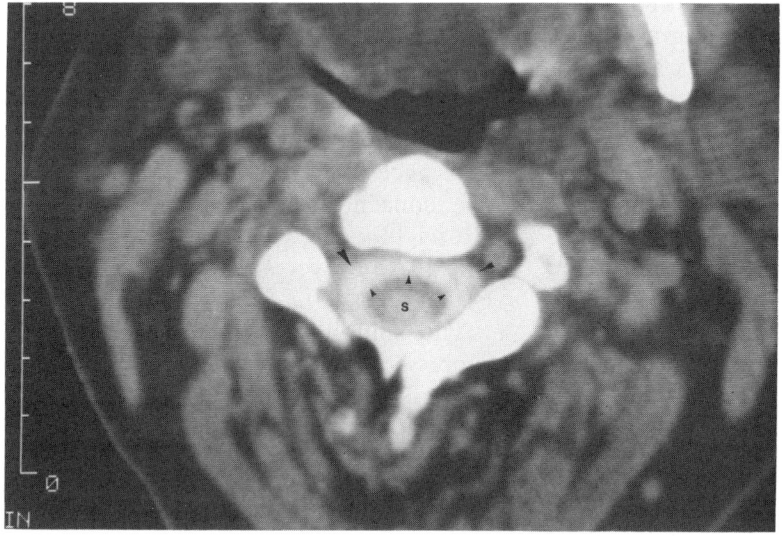

Figure 3.15 Myelographic contrast medium enhancement of the subarachnoid space (arrowheads) and the central syrinx (s).

extramedullary abnormalities from intramedullary lesions (Figure 3.14). This technique is also used to exclude the presence of syringomyelia, the latter diagnosis being made with visualization of the myelographic contrast medium within the central portion of the spinal cord substance (Figure 3.15). Computed tomography evaluations of the ventricles and basal cisterns may also be performed following the subarachnoid administration of a nonionic contrast medium. Magnetic resonance imaging (MRI) is rapidly changing the indications for use of post-myelography CT. For example, visualization of syrinx is now easily made with MRI, thus obviating the use of myelography and subsequent CT.

Table 3.6 CONTRAST MEDIA INDICATED SPECIFICALLY FOR ENHANCEMENT OF CEREBROSPINAL FLUID SPACES IN CT EXAMINATIONS[a]

GENERIC NAME	BRAND NAME(S)®[b]	IODINE CONCENTRATION MG./ML.
Iohexol	Omnipaque-180 (W)	180
	Omnipaque-240 (W)	240
Iopamidol	Isovue-M 200 (S)	200
Metrizamide	Amipaque (W)	170–220

[a] See also Chapter 4, Myelographic Contrast Media.
[b] (W) Winthrop-Breon Laboratories
　(S) Squibb Diagnostics

Myelographic CT procedures are generally performed subsequent to standard myelography, thus negating the requirement to readminister an additional dose of contrast medium. A delay of 1 or more hours is usually required prior to performing CT in order to permit subarachnoid excretion of the myelographic medium and an adequate reduction in contrast concentration to avoid beam-hardening artifacts. Computed tomography of the cisterns or ventricles requires a delay of 3–4 hours following lumbar administration to permit adequate contrast agent entry into these regions. Computed tomography evaluations of the spinal canal and/or cerebrovascular fluid spaces are performed following the lumbar subarachnoid administration of 4–6 mL of water-soluble, nonionic contrast media (Table 3.6) containing approximately 170–200 mg iodine/mL.

III. Xenon

Computed tomography of the brain, performed during and after the inhalation of stable xenon gas, has demonstrated clinical utility for the noninvasive evaluation and quantification of local cerebral blood flow and the characterization of cerebral tissues based on their xenon extraction fraction (i. e., tissue-blood partition coefficient).

CHEMISTRY

Elemental xenon is a chemically inert, noble gas that is slightly soluble in water but highly soluble in lipids. The high elec-

tion density (atomic number = 54) of xenon and its k-edge of 34.6 keV make it similar to iodine in providing a large cross-sectional area for x-ray absorption. This makes xenon a suitable contrast agent for use in CT.

PHARMACOKINETICS

Xenon gas freely diffuses through the body tissues as a result of its high lipid solubility. Hence, following inhalation, xenon is efficiently transferred across normal alveolar membranes into the blood, where it is transported bound to hemoglobin. The arterial concentration of xenon achieved during inhalation is proportional to the concentration of xenon in the inspired gas, the rate of pulmonary blood flow, and the solubility of xenon in blood. Xenon, delivered to the brain via arterial blood, rapidly diffuses across the intact blood-brain barrier. It concentrates in cerebral tissues as a function of its solubility in the respective cerebral tissue (i. e., tissue lipid content), the rate at which the xenon is delivered to the tissue (i. e., rate of local cerebral blood flow), and the relative concentration of xenon within the arterial blood and cerebral tissue (Kendall BE, 1980; Meyer JS, et al, 1980; Drayer BP, et al, 1980).

The solubility of xenon in tissues is expressed as the tissue : blood partition coefficient or extraction fraction. During inhalation the concentration of xenon in cerebral tissues increases until the tissue becomes saturated and an equilibrium is established between the tissue and arterial concentration of xenon. Computed tomography density measurements obtained at equilibrium over a cerebral region-of-interest can be utilized in conjunction with corresponding CT density measurements of known volumes of arterial blood to derive an extraction fraction for specific cerebral tissues within the region-of-interest. (In the absence of pulmonary disease, end-tidal measurements of xenon concentration during inhalation are in equilibrium with arterial blood concentrations and can be utilized to provide a noninvasive method of determining the arterial xenon concentration.) As might be expected, the xenon extraction fraction is greater for cerebral tissues with high lipid content due to the increased solubility of xenon in these tissues. Thus, at equilibrium, the xenon extraction fraction is greater for cerebral white matter (e. g., 1.2–1.3) than it is for gray matter (e. g., 0.8–1.0). In addition to the differentiation of normal cerebral tissues, the xenon extraction fraction can also provide a quantitative measurement of physical and chemical changes in tissue composition that may occur in cerebral pathologies. The xenon extraction fraction is also a necessary parameter for the accurate quantification of local cerebral blood flow (Meyer JS, et al, 1980).

Cerebral tissues with a high rate of blood flow will demonstrate a faster rate of xenon delivery and tissue saturation. Hence, the rate of xenon uptake into more highly perfused cerebral gray matter (blood flow = 65–100 mL/100 g/min) is faster than its uptake into white matter (blood flow = 15–30 mL/100 g/min). The rate at which xenon diffuses from arterial blood into tissue is also dependent on the respective concentration gradient at any given time. Therefore, the rate of xenon uptake into cerebral tissues is more rapid in the early phases of inhalation and gradually slows as equilibrium is approached (Meyer JS, et al, 1980; Drayer BP, et al, 1980; Haughton V, et al, 1980).

The factors that affect the clearance of xenon following inhalation are the same as those that govern its uptake (i. e., pulmonary ventilation, blood flow rates, and tissue:blood partition coefficients). Ventilation with room air or xenon-free gas results first in the elimination of xenon from the lungs followed by a decrease in its arterial concentration and a subsequent reversal of tissue concentrations. The rate of xenon washout is rapid from highly perfused tissues (i. e., cerebral gray matter) and slower from tissues with a reduced rate of blood flow or high lipid content (i. e., cerebral white matter). The overall clearance of xenon from the brain is more rapid (i. e., complete at 7–10 minutes) than other body tissues due to the relatively high rate of cerebral blood flow (Meyer JS, et al, 1980).

PHYSIOLOGIC EFFECTS

Because xenon is an inert gas with lack of biotransformation, it should demonstrate minimal physiological effects. However, the inhalation of xenon at high concentrations (e. g., > 70%) for prolonged periods can induce general anesthesia (Kendall BE and Moseley IF, 1981; Meyer JS, et al, 1980) similar to that observed with the routinely utilized inhalational anesthetics (e. g., halothane, cyclopropane, ethers, nitrous oxide). The anesthetic effect of xenon (and the inhalational anesthetics) is apparently related to its lipophilicity and associated solubilization in and local disordering of the lipid matrix of central nervous membranes. This process leads to alterations in the normal membrane flux of physiological ions with subsequent effects on neuronal-excitability and the production of anesthesia.

The anesthetic effects of xenon limit the concentration utilized for the enhancement of CT procedures to 30–40%. Inhalation of a xenon-oxygen mixture at this concentration for brief intervals (i. e., 6–10 minutes) will not normally produce true anesthesia (i. e., loss of feeling, consciousness); however preanesthesia side effects including disorientation, paraesthesia, and respiratory depression, may be observed (Latchaw RE, et al, 1987). Xenon-induced slowing of respiratory rate is accompanied by a compensatory increase in end-tidal volume, a factor that must be considered in the accurate timing and determination of arterial xenon concentrations and tissue:blood partition coefficients. Although the brain-localization and anesthetic effects of xenon are rapidly reversible, subjects have reported a prolonged "hangover" sensation following inhalation of a 35–40% concentration (Yonas H, et al, 1981; Meyer JS, et al, 1980).

Xenon is also known to produce physiological effects on cerebral blood flow, the parameter being evaluated in xenon-enhanced CT. Production of anesthesia is generally associated with a 10–20% decrease in global cerebral blood flow. This phenomenon has been described with the inhalation of 30–40% xenon for 2–6 minutes (Gur D, et al, 1982; Meyer JS, et al, 1980), as has a 10–20% increase in global cerebral blood flow (Gur D, et al, 1985). Such a relatively small decrease or increase in global cerebral blood flow may not detract from the xenon-enhanced CT evaluation of local cerebral blood flow provided the alterations are uniform across all brain regions. Animal studies have, however, demonstrated localized increases in cerebral blood flow of up to 70% in neocortical regions (Junck L, et al, 1985). Whether or not similar xenon-induced alterations in local cerebral blood flow occur in humans has not been firmly established. These findings remain a subject of considerable debate in the unequivocal acceptance of xenon-enhanced CT for the determination of local cerebral blood flow. It is also not without reason to expect that xenon-induced disorientation, hallucinations, or depression will elicit corresponding alterations in the metabolic and blood flow demands of involved brain regions.

CLINICAL USE/ CONTRAINDICATIONS

Although xenon-enhanced CT evaluations of local cerebral blood flow are in a preliminary, if not investigative, clinical stage, they have provided useful information in a variety of cerebral pathologies secondary to stroke, atherosclerosis, and trauma, and in the evaluation of associated therapeutic interventions (e. g., angioplasty, carotid artery bypass, etc.). This procedure may also provide useful information in the evaluation of cerebral disorders (e. g., Alzheimer's disease, seizures) that involve an increase or decrease in regional metabolic demands with corresponding changes in local blood flow re-

quirements. In addition, xenon-enhanced CT has found use in the diagnosis and evaluation of cerebral abnormalities (e. g., multiple sclerosis, infarct, tumors) based on alterations in the normal xenon extraction fraction (Meyer JS, et al, 1980; Haughton V, et al, 1980).

Patient Preparation. Due to potential side effects from xenon inhalation, it is advisable that patients fast for approximately 10 hours before the procedure. Patients should be continually monitored during the procedure and oxygen and appropriate resuscitative eqiupment should be available (Winkler S and Turski P, 1985).

Xenon enhancement of cerebral regions is more rapid and efficient if the patient's blood is denitrogenated by breathing pure oxygen for 10 minutes prior to the initiation of xenon inhalation. With this procedure, the partial pressure of oxygen in the blood exceeds that of the alveoli at the commencement of xenon inhalation. In the absence of nitrogen, the xenon diffuses rapidly across alveolo-capillary membranes into the pulmonary venous circulation to displace oxygen. As a result, the partial pressure of oxygen within the brain exceeds that of blood, and a similar rapid influx of xenon into brain tissues occurs (Meyer JS, et al, 1980).

Contraindications. Contraindications to xenon-enhanced CT include patients with both restrictive and obstructive airway disease as well as other forms of chronic or acute lung disease. In addition to increasing the anesthetic dangers of xenon by reducing its rate of clearance, reduced respiratory function delays the buildup of xenon in arterial blood and obviates the use of end-tidal measurements of xenon concentration as a noninvasive measure of its arterial concentration. These latter factors may significantly affect the accuracy of local cerebral blood flow determinations if not taken into consideration (Winkler S and Turski P, 1985; Meyer JS, et al, 1980). As a result of its potential neurological effects, xenon-enhanced CT should also be performed with extreme caution on patients with preexisting dementia or seizure disorders.

DOSAGE

The concentration of xenon utilized for the CT evaluation of local cerebral blood flow should be below the concentrations known to produce anesthesia and preanesthesia side effects, but high enough to ensure density changes sufficient for accurate and reproducible data. Reliable partition coefficient values have been obtained using a 27% concentration of xenon in oxygen or air. Most clinical investigations have been performed using a 30–40% concentration inhaled via a face mask or mouthpiece for 3–10 minutes (Meyer JS, et al, 1986; Latchaw RE, et al, 1987). In view of the anesthetic potential of inhaled xenon, it is extremely important that an appropriate gas-monitoring system (e. g., thermal conductivity meter) be incorporated into the administration procedure (Winkler S and Turski P, 1985).

Xenon-enhanced CT for the evaluation of local cerebral blood flow is based on the Fick principle. Determination of temporal changes in the arterial and tissue concentration of a highly diffusable inert tracer (i. e., xenon) combined with a knowledge of the respective blood:tissue partition coefficient permit an accurate quantification of local tissue blood flow as defined by the Kety-Schmidt equation. The high-contrast sensitivity and three-dimensional properties of CT permit the serial quantification of density changes in various brain regions associated with the uptake or washout of xenon gas and the determination of corresponding blood:brain partition coefficients during equilibrium or tissue saturation. These data may be subsequently applied to the Kety-Schmidt equation for the noninvasive quantification of local cerebral blood flow. Controversy remains as to whether the CT measurements of tissue xenon concentration should be performed during the uptake or washout phase. Advantages of the former approach include reduced patient immobilization time and decreased exposure to the anesthetic effects of xenon and the radiation exposure of multiple CT scans. However, errors can occur with the buildup technique due to limited density data and the extrapolation of tissue:blood partition coefficients from a single uptake scan rather than a direct measurement at equilibrium. The washout method involves the direct measurement of the partition coefficient at equilibrium but requires a longer inhalation period. If the washout procedure is utilized, serial analysis should not commence until 1 minute following the termination of xenon inhalation to allow for the recirculation of xenon that occurs during this period (Drayer BP, et al, 1980; Meyer JS, et al, 1980).

IV. Reticuloendothelial Contrast Media

Colloidal particles injected into the blood are phagocytized and removed from the circulation by cells of the reticuloendothelial system (RES). The majority of these RES cells are located in the liver (Kupffer's cells) with additional phagocytic cells found in decreasing quantities in the spleen, bone marrow, and lungs. The development of a colloidal radiopaque contrast medium for intravascular administration would therefore permit selective enhancement of the liver and spleen based on its RES accumulation. Moreover, significant CT density differences between normal hepatic or splenic tissue and pathological lesions can be achieved with this approach, since tumors or abscesses are devoid of RES cells and would therefore demonstrate minimal enhancement. The radiopaque colloid must, however, exhibit eventual metabolic clearance from the RES and, of course, be nontoxic in its original and metabolized forms.

Thoratrast, a 25% colloidal suspension of thorium dioxide, was introduced in the early

1930s for selective opacification and evaluation of the liver and spleen using standard radiographic techniques. A purported advantage of this agent was its lack of metabolism and clearance from the RES cells, thus permitting multiple radiographic examinations over an extended time period without the need for contrast readministration. Unfortunately, this retention factor combined with the radioactive properties of "stable" thorium-232 (physical half-life of 1.41×10^{10} years, alpha particle emissions) led to the induction of hepatic and splenic neoplasms and fibrosis and the eventual disuse of this agent.

Subsequent approaches to the development of colloidal radiopaque contrast media have included the synthesis and experimental evaluation of radiopaque liposomes (i. e., liposomes containing meglumine-sodium diatrizoate) (Havron A, et al, 1981), iodinated starch particles (Cohen Z, et al, 1981), iodipamide ethylester (Violante MR, et al, 1981), and sterol-esters of iopanoic acid (Seevers RH, et al, 1982). Agents that have realized some clinical investigation include emulsions of iodinated esters of poppyseed oil (EOE-13) and of perfluoroctylbromide. These emulsions are formed by the interaction of the radiopaque moiety with surfacants, resulting in micellar particles of colloidal dimension suspended in an aqueous medium.

EOE-13

Preliminary clinical investigations have demonstrated the potential utility of this aqueous emulsion of iodinated esters of poppyseed oil (with surfactants and buffers) for selective liver and spleen enhancement and the improved CT detection of hepatic and splenic lesions. Optimal RES localization of EOE-13 is dependent on colloid particle size. A medium having a mean particle diameter of 1.7 microns, with 75% of the particles in the 1–4 micron range, has been utilized clinically (Miller DL, et al, 1984).

Following intravascular infusion, EOE-13 clears rapidly from the blood with less than 5% of the administered dose remaining in the vascular compartment at 5 minutes following injection. Colloidal EOE-13 emulsion accumulates in RES cells of the liver (approximately 80% of administered dose), spleen, bone marrow, and lungs (2–3% of the dose in each organ) (Vermess M, 1984). It is retained for a sufficient period to permit selective CT of the liver and spleen for up to 3 hours after administration. Metabolism of the phagocytized EOE-13 does occur with virtually all of the liver and spleen concentration being eliminated within 48 hours (Vermess M, et al, 1982). The metabolic by-products are primarily excreted via the kidney; however, some deiodination with the liberation of free iodine does occur (Vermess M, 1984).

Limited clinical experience with EOE-13 has revealed a 3.6% incidence of severe reactions. Common side effects include headache, fever, and rigor (i. e., shaking chills), usually occurring at 2–4 hours post infusion.

Clinical studies have utilized a dose of 0.25 mL of a 53% w/v emulsion of EOE-13 per kilogram of body weight (i.e., 17 mL/70 kg), diluted with 100 mL of 5% Dextrose in Water for Injection, U.S.P., and infused over a 1 hour period. This dose provides approximately 50 mg of iodide per kilogram, resulting in an increase in liver and spleen densities of approximately 35 HU and 55 HU, respectively. As previously discussed, hepatic or splenic lesions exhibit minimal contrast enhancement (i. e., < 3 HU) following the administration of EOE-13 (Miller DL, et al, 1984).

The major problems limiting the routine clinical use of EOE-13, to date, are its relatively high incidence of severe reactions and its lack of specificity in differentiating the nature of demonstrated space-occupying lesions. In addition, the rapid blood clearance of EOE-13 results in the visualization of intrahepatic vascular structures as low-density areas on subsequent CT studies. Although this may be advantageous in demonstrating the relationship of vessels to hepatic lesions, it may also present problems in differentiating small masses from vascular structures (Patronas N, et al, 1984).

PERFLUOROCTYLBROMIDE

Perfluorocarbons, organic compounds in which the hydrogen atoms are replaced by fluorine atoms, are capable of dissolving oxygen and are therefore being investigated as potential oncotic agents, drugs capable of providing increased oxygen-carrying capacity relative to blood. Perfluoroctylbromide ($C_8 F_{17} Br$), a monobrominated perfluorocarbon derivative, has experimentally demonstrated the potential to produce selective contrast enhancement of the liver and spleen for CT examinations (Long DM, et al, 1980). The property of radiopacification is provided by the bromide atom (atomic number = 35, k-edge = 12.4 keV), and selective localization in the liver and spleen by the RES accumulation of emulsified colloidal particles of a diameter of 0.5 micron or less.

Following intravenous administration, the perfluoroctylbromide remains within the vascular compartment for an extended period of time, thus providing relatively constant vascular enhancement for selective CT evaluations of the cardiovascular blood pool for up to 5 hours after administration. The material is gradually phagocytized by RES cells to produce significant enhancement of the liver and spleen at 2 hours post injection. As expected, hepatic or splenic lesions demonstrate minimal enhancement. The phagocytized perfluoroctylbromide emulsion is slowly metabolized (liver and spleen half-life of 5.7 days [rabbit data]) with elimination via the lungs (Mattrey RF, et al, 1982).

In addition to demonstrating specific and prolonged enhancement of the vascular compartment, liver, and spleen, perfluoroctylbromide has also been shown to nonspecifically activate and become incorporated into circulating macrophages. These activated, radiopaque macrophages retain their normal physiological function and accumulate at sites of abnormal immunologic activity. Hence, perfluoroctyl bromide has experimentally demonstrated intense rim enhancement in tumors, abscesses, and myocardial infarcts at 2 days post administration. It has also produced a similar enhancement of nonliquified areas of inflammation including the early stages of abscess formation that are difficult to detect using standard CT techniques (Mattrey RF, et al, 1984a).

Human data on the physiological and adverse effects of perfluorocarbons is currently limited. Early studies did reveal an incidence of allergic reactions approaching 5%, apparently related to complement activation induced by the Pluronic-F68 surfacant used in the emulsification process. Substitution of yolk phospholipids appears to alleviate this problem and provides a stable emulsion. No acute hemodynamic effects were observed in dogs following bolus injection of 60 mL of a 50% w/v emulsion of perfluoroctylbromide (Peck WW, et al, 1984). A median lethal dose (LD50) of 40 g of perfluoroctylbromide per kilogram has been determined using a rat model (Mattrey RF, 1984b). This value represents a factor of 10 or greater margin of safety based on the proposed human dose.

The proposed human dose of perfluoroctylbromide is 6 mL of a 50% w/v emulsion (i. e., 3 g perfluorocarbon) per kilogram of body weight administered by rapid intravenous injection. Based on equivalent dose-to-organ weight animal studies, this dosage should produce an initial density increase of 100 HU for the vascular space (Peck WW, et al, 1984), and a selective increase in liver enhancement of approximately 50 HU at 2 hours post injection (Patronas N, et al, 1984).

Although no extensive clinical experience with perfluoroctylbromide has been reported, this reticuloendothelial contrast medium may provide advantages over the previously described EOE-13. As a result of the vascular retention of perfluoroctylbromide, intrahepatic vascular structures will appear hyperdense or isodense relative to the normal hepatic tissue at 2 hours following injection. This factor will obviate problems associated with the accurate differentiation of small hepatic masses and hypodense vascular structures (Patronas N, et al, 1984). The rim-enhancement characteristics of perfluoroctylbromide may facilitate the differentiation of space-occupying lesions within the liver or spleen, although this phenomenon has been observed with both tumors and abscesses (Mattrey RF, et al, 1984a). Whether the prolonged vascular retention of perfluorocytlbromide will present problems in the detection of vascularized masses, or whether macrophage-incorporated perfluoroctylbromide may render nonencapsulated sites of inflammation isodense with normal hepatic or splenic tissue awaits more extensive clinical experience with this agent.

References

Alpern MB, Lawson TL, Foley WD, et al. Focal hepatic masses and fatty infiltration detected by enhanced dynamic CT. *Radiology* 1986, 158:45–49.

Bernardino ME, Erwin BC, Steinberg HV, et al. Delayed hepatic CT scanning: Increased confidence and improved detection of hepatic metastases. *Radiology* 1986, 159:71–74.

Bressler EL, Alpern MB, Glazer GM, et al. Hypervascular hepatic metastases: CT evaluation. *Radiology* 1987, 162:49–52.

Burgener FA, Hamlin DJ. Contrast enhancement in abdominal CT: Bolus vs. infusion. *AJR* 1981, 137:351–358.

Cohen Z, Seltzer SE, Davis MA, et al. Iodinated starch particles: New contrast material for computed tomography of the liver. *JCAT* 1981, 5:843–846.

Crocker EF, Zimmerman RA, Phelps ME, et al. The effects of steroids on the extravascular distribution of radiographic contrast material and technetium pertechnetate in brain tumors as determined by computed tomography. *Radiology* 1976, 119:373–380.

Davis JM, Davis KR, Newhouse J, et al. Expanded high dose in computed cranial tomography: A preliminary report. *Radiology* 1979, 131:373–380.

Dean PB. Contrast media in body computed tomography. Experimental and theoretical background, present limitations, and proposals for improved diagnostic efficacy. *Invest Radiol* 1980, 15 (Suppl.): S164–S170.

Dean PB, Kivisaari L, Kormano M. Contrast enhancement pharmacokinetics of six ionic and non-ionic contrast media. *Invest Radiol* 1983, 18:368–374.

Drayer BP, Gur D, Wolfson SK, et al. Experimental xenon enhancement with CT imaging: Cerebral applications. *AJR* 1980, 134:39–44.

Fike JR, Cann CE, Norman D, et al. Relative uptake of low- and high-osmolality contrast media in CT of brain tumors. *AJNR* 1984, 5:413–417.

Freeny PC, Marks WM. Hepatic hemangioma: Dynamic bolus CT. *AJR* 1986, 147:711–719.

Gur D, Wolfson SK, Yonas H, et al. Progress in cerebral vascular disease. Local cerebral blood flow by xenon enhanced CT. *Stroke* 1982, 12:750–758.

Gur D, Yonas H, Jackson DL, et al. Measurement of cerebral blood flow during xenon inhalation as measured by the microspheres method. *Stroke* 1985, 16:871–874.

Halvorsen RA, Dunnick NR, Thompson WM. Contrast agent enhancement in abdominal computed tomography. *Invest Radiol* 1984, 19 (Suppl.): S239–S243.

Haughton V, Donegan J, Walsh P, et al. Clinical cerebral blood flow measurement with inhaled xenon and CT. *AJR* 1980, 134:281–283.

Havron A, Seltzer SE, Davis MA, et al. Radiopaque liposomes: A promising new contrast material for computed tomography of the spleen. *Radiology*, 1981, 140:507–511.

Hayman LA, Hinck VC. Water-soluble iodinated contrast media. In *Computed Tomography of the Head, Neck, and Spine*. (Latchaw RE, ed.) Chicago, Year Book Medical Publishers, 1985, pp. 3–25.

Junck L, Dhawan V, Thaler HT, et al. Effects of xenon and krypton on regional cerebral blood flow in the rat. *J Cereb Blood Flow Metabol* 1985, 5:126–132.

Kendall BE. Development in contrast

media applied to neuroradiology. *Br Med Bull* 1980, 36:273–278.

Kendall BE, Moseley IF. Xenon as a contrast agent for computed tomography. *J Neuroradiol*, 1981, 8:3–12.

Latchaw RE, Yonas H, Pentheny SL, et al. Adverse reactions to xenon-enhanced CT cerebral blood flow determinations. *Radiology* 1987, 163:251–254.

Long DM, Lasser BC, Shorts CM, et al. Experiments with radiopaque perfluorocarbon emulsions for selective opacification of organs and total body angiography. *Invest Radiol* 1980, 15:242–247.

Matsui O, Takashima T, Kadoya M, et al. Dynamic computed tomography during arterial portography. Most sensitive examination for small hepatocellular carcinomas. *JCAT* 1985, 9:19–24.

Mattrey RF, Long DM, Multer F, et al. Perfluoroctylbromide: A reticuloendothelial-specific and tumor-imaging agent for computed tomography. *Radiology* 1982, 145:755–758.

Mattrey RF, Andre M, Campbell J, et al. Specific enhancement of intraabdominal abscesses with perfluoroctylbromide for CT imaging. *Invest Radiol* 1984a, 19, 438–446.

Mattrey RF. Perfluorocarbons in computed tomography. *Invest Radiol* 1984b, 19 (Suppl.): S129–S130.

Meyer JS, Hayman LA, Yamamoto M, et al. Local cerebral blood flow measured by CT after stable xenon inhalation. *AJR* 1980, 135:239–251.

Meyer JS, Hata T, Imai A, et al. Xenon CT helps reveal blood flow disorders. *Diag Imaging* 1986, May, 92–97.

Miller DL, Verness M, Doppman JL, et al. CT of the liver and spleen with EOE-13: Review of 225 examinations. *AJR* 1984, 143:235–243.

Norman D, Enzmann DR, Newton TH. Optimal contrast dosage in cranial computed tomography. *AJR* 1978, 13:687–689

Patronas N, Miller DL, Girton M. Experimental comparison of EOE-13 and perfluoroctylbromide for the CT detection of hepatic metastases. *Invest Radiol* 1984, 19:570–573.

Peck WW, Mattrey RF, Slutsky RA, et al. Perfluoroctylbromide. Acute hemodynamic effects, in pigs, of intravenous administration compared with the standard ionic contrast media. *Invest Radiol* 1984, 19:129–132.

Robins AH, Thurm RH, Yeh T. Computed body tomography with iopamidol. *Invest Radiol* 1984, 19 (Suppl.): S234–S238.

Seevers RH, Groziak MP, Weichert JP, et al. Potential tumor- or organ-imaging agents, 23. Sterol esters of iopanoic acid. *J Med Chem* 1982, 25: 1500–1503.

Skalpe IO. Enhancement with water-soluble contrast media in computed tomography of the brain and abdomen. Survey and present state. *Acta Radiol* 1983, 366 (Suppl.): 72–75.

Spataro RF, Fischer HW, Kormano M. Clinical comparison of Hexabrix, iopamidol, and Urografin-60 in whole body computed tomography. *Invest Radiol* 1984, 19 (Suppl.): S372–S375.

Takashima T, Matsui O. Infusion hepatic angiography in the detection of small hepatocellular carcinomas. *Radiology* 1980, 136:321–325.

Vermess M, Doppman JL, Sugarbaker PH, et al. Computed tomography of liver and spleen with intravenous lipoid contrast material. Review of 60 examinations. *AJR* 1982, 138:1063–1071.

Vermess M. Biodistribution study of intravenous lipoid contrast material—EOE-13. *Invest Radiol* 1984, 19 (Suppl.): S130.

Violante MR, Mare K, Fischer HW. Biodistribution of a hepatolienographic CT contrast agent: A study of iodipamide ethyl ester in the rat. *Invest Radiol* 1981, 16:40–45.

Wegener OH. Technique of computerized tomography. In *Whole Body Computerized Tomography* (Wegener OH., ed.) West Germany, Schering AG, 1983, pp 1-00–1-50.

Whelan MA, Hilal SK. Computed tomography as a guide in the diagnosis and followup of brain abscesses. *Radiology* 1980, 135:663–671.

Winkler S, Turski P. Potential hazards of xenon inhalation. Editorial. *AJNR* 1985, 6:974–975.

Yonas H, Grundy B, Gur D, et al. Side effects of xenon inhalation. *JCAT,* 1981, 5:591–592.

Young SW, Turner RJ, Castellino RA. A strategy for the contrast enhancement of malignant tumors using dynamic computed tomography and intravascular pharmacokinetics. *Radiology* 1980, 137:137–147.

Zatz LM. Iodinated contrast media in cranial tomography. *Invest Radiol* 1980, 15 (Suppl.): S155–S159.

Myelographic Contrast Media

Dennis P. Swanson
Roushdy S. Boulos

The term *myelography* may be generally defined as a radiographic examination of the spinal cord and cerebrospinal fluid compartment following the subarachnoid administration of a radiographic (positive or negative) contrast medium. This diagnostic procedure is indicated for a variety of symptoms and conditions associated with diseases or abnormalities of the spinal column, spinal canal, and nervous system.

The subarachnoid administration of a contrast medium is required in myelography to permit adequate delineation of the spinal cord and nerve roots from the surrounding cerebrospinal fluid and the covering meninges and to define the contours of the spinal theca relative to the epidural tissues and the encompassing bony spinal column. The ideal myelographic contrast medium (Table 4.1) should demonstrate thorough mixing in the cerebrospinal fluid to permit its entry into the fine structures and crevices of the subarachnoid space. Of course, it must also produce an acceptable level of x-ray opacification after this mixing has occurred. The medium should exhibit complete absorption from the cerebrospinal fluid compartment within a short but examination-dependent time period, followed by rapid systemic excretion. The myelographic medium should be devoid of

Table 4.1   CHARACTERISTICS OF THE IDEAL MYELOGRAPHIC CONTRAST MEDIUM

1. Thorough mixing with cerebrospinal fluid
2. Satisfactory opacification of the total subarachnoid space
3. Rapid and complete absorption from the subarachnoid space upon completion of the procedure
4. Rapid systemic excretion
5. No undesirable physiological effects or observable adverse reactions

physiological effects, and there should be no acute or chronic, local or systemic toxicity associated with its use.

I. Negative Contrast Myelography

The use of a gas for radiographic visualization of the spinal cord was initially suggested by Dandy (Dandy WE, 1919) after he conceived the idea of performing pneumoencephalography following a spinal rather than a direct ventricular puncture. The spinal arachnoid space was first defined radiographically in the early 1920s using air as the negative contrast agent (Jacobaeus HC, 1921). Contrary to pneumoencephalography, which remained a vogue for about 50 years, air myelography did not achieve wide acceptance and use in the United States. This latter situation can be traced to several factors. First, since air and the other gases (e. g., oxygen, carbon dioxide, helium, nitrogen) that were utilized for this procedure are only minimally miscible with the cerebrospinal fluid, large volumes of the fluid had to be removed for replacement by the gas. As might be expected, this procedure resulted in marked disturbances of cerebrospinal fluid pressure and kinetics with a high incidence of acute headache, nausea, vomiting, and vertigo. In addition to these acute reactions, the instillation of a gas into the subarachnoid space also resulted in transient mild inflammatory reactions with pleocytosis and an elevation of glucose and protein levels. Severe complications to air myelography, such as tonsilar herniation or ventricular decompression, were rare but extremely serious events (Batnitsky S, 1977a; Chrzanowski R, 1982). A second limitation of gas myelography was a virtual requirement for tomography in order to eliminate the dense overlying bony structures. Third, while the degree of radiographic contrast was usually sufficient to produce adequate and reliable delineation of the spinal cord from the subarachnoid space, the interspace between the epidural tissues and the subarachnoid space was poorly defined. Therefore, it was often difficult to detect small contour defects produced by epidural lesions with air myelography. Finally, evaluation of the nerve root sheaths and the fine crevices of the subarachnoid space were always inadequate due to the inability of the gas to completely permeate these regions of the subarachnoid compartment.

For the above mentioned reasons, air myelography was usually reserved for specific indications (e. g., evaluation of spinal cord atrophy, intramedullary masses). Compared to myelography performed with the early positive contrast agents, Lipiodol® and Pantopaque®, air myelography provided advantages related to the improved detection of small lesions obscured by the excessive radiodensity of these agents. However, with the introduction of water-soluble, nonionic contrast media and the advances of computed tomography, there is currently no indication for gas myelography.

II. Positive Contrast Myelography

IOPHENDYLATE (PANTOPAQUE®) HISTORY

Early attempts to produce positive opacification of the spinal subarachnoid space centered on the direct administration of water-insoluble, radiopaque substances including bismuth subnitrate, colloidal silver, and thorium dioxide. These colloidal agents demonstrated negligible absorption from the subarachnoid space, and, due to their dispersion in the cerebrospinal fluid, could not be easily or completely removed by aspiration following the examination. Retention of these agents in the subarachnoid space resulted in the subsequent production of severe inflammation of the meningeal membranes. In addition, clinical use of thorium dioxide became associated with an iatrogenic induction of neoplasms due to the alpha particle emissions of the weakly radioactive, retained thorium.

During this same era (1920–1930), iodinated poppyseed oil (Lipiodol) was being injected into the epidural space for the treatment of sciatica and endemic encephalitis; a therapy based on its gradual release of germicidal iodine. The inadvertent, but uneventful, administration of this iodinated oil into the subarachnoid space eventually led to its routine use as a myelographic contrast medium (Sicard JA and Forestier JE, 1922). As such, Lipiodol was immiscible with the cerebrospinal fluid and demonstrated no, or extremely slow, absorption from the subarachnoid space. Its extremely high viscosity and surface tension resulted in the formation of large, noncohesive globules that often prevented delineation of the narrow spaces (i. e., nerve root sheaths, fine crevices) of the subarachnoid space, rendered positioning and postprocedure aspiration of the agent difficult, and produced excessive radiodensity that often obscured small masses. In addition to these problems, the subarachnoid administration of Lipiodol became generally recognized to cause headaches, fever, and more severe inflammatory reactions including chronic arachnoiditis, lower extremity pain, and paresthesia. Since many of the adverse effects of Lipiodol were felt to be related to its continual release of free iodine, subsequent research focused on developing an oily medium with both increased stability and decreased viscosity. These effects led to the availability and clinical use of iophendylate (Ramsey GH, et al, 1944; Steinhausen TB, et al, 1944). This radiopaque medium was the agent of choice for myelography until its use was superseded by the water-soluble, nonionic media (see Batnitsky S, 1977b; Sovak M, 1984).

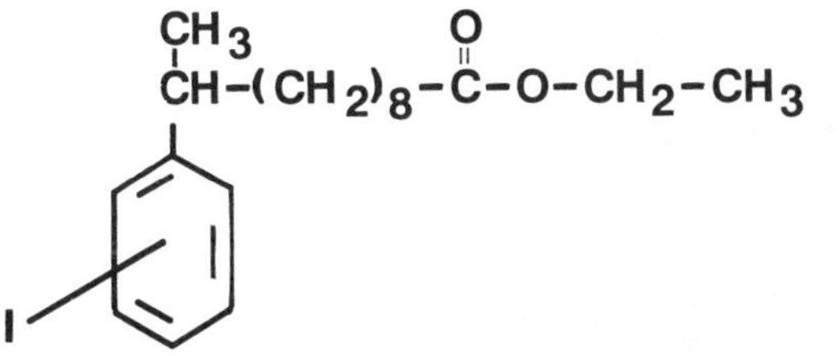

$$CH_3 \quad\quad O$$
$$CH-(CH_2)_8-C-O-CH_2-CH_3$$

Figure 4.1 Chemical structure of iophendylate (Pantopaque ®).

CHEMISTRY

The myelographic contrast medium, iophendylate (Pantopaque®), is a mixture of isomers of ethyl iodophenylundecanoate (Figure 4.1) containing 30.5%, by weight, of iodine (305 mg iodine/mL). This viscous contrast agent is only slightly soluble in water, and has a specific gravity of 1.25 at 25°C.

PHARMACOKINETICS

Following subarachnoid administration, iophendylate demonstrates virtually no mixing with the cerebrospinal fluid. As a result of its immiscibility, viscosity, and surface tension, iophendylate forms a relatively cohesive, continuous radiopaque column within the subarachnoid space (Figure 4.2). Since the specific gravity of iophendylate (1.25) is greater than that of the cerebrospinal fluid (1.09), this radiopaque column can be readily moved and repositioned under the influence of gravity. The degree of myelographic detail that can be obtained with iophendylate is limited, however, by the inability of this radiopaque column to completely penetrate the nerve root sheaths and the narrow crevices of the subarachnoid space. In addition, excessive radiodensity associated with the cohesive column and iodine concentration of iophendylate often obscures radiographic demonstration of small intramedullary or intradural masses (Kieffer SA, et al, 1978).

Iophendylate is very slowly absorbed from the subarachnoid space at an estimated rate of approximately 1 ml per year (Ramsey GH, et al, 1944). The cohesive-

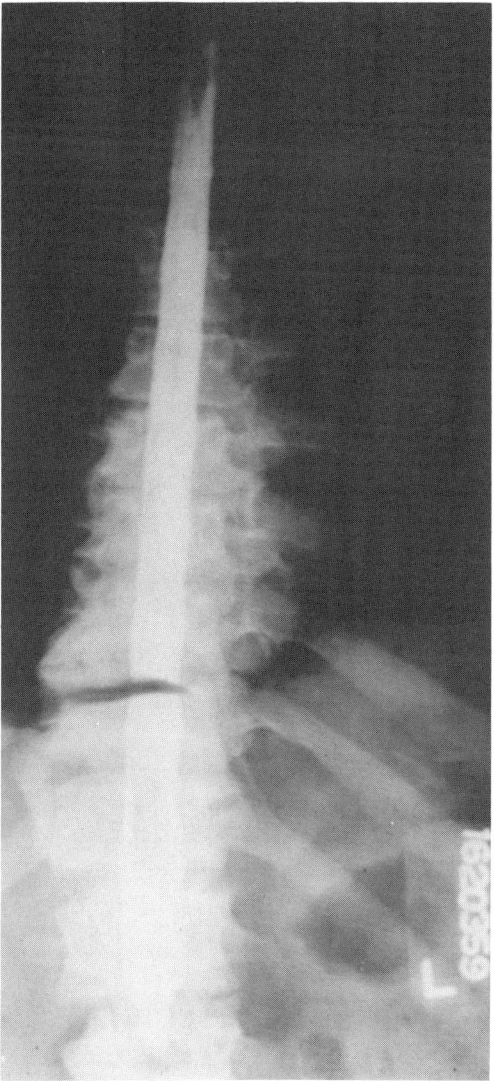

Figure 4.2 Myelogram obtained following the lumbar subarachnoid administration of iophendylate (Pantopaque®). Note the lack of definition of the spinal cord shadow and nerve root sheaths due to the excessive density and viscosity of this contrast medium, respectively.

ness of the iophendylate column does, however, permit most of the administered dose to be aspirated from the spinal canal following completion of the examination. Any iophendylate remaining within the subarachnoid space demonstrates a tendency to become fixed in position (Figure 4.3) apparently due to its incorpora-

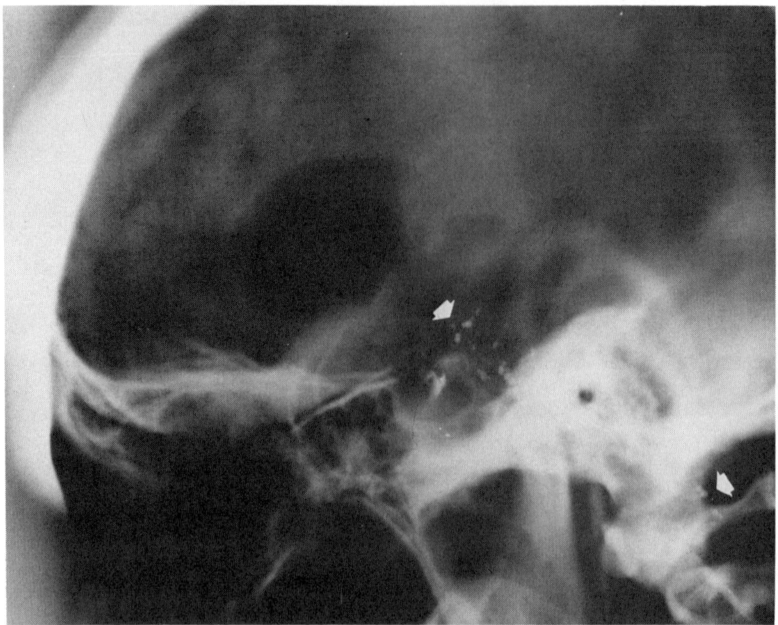

Figure 4.3 Skull radiograph demonstrating (arrows) incomplete removal and retention of iophendylate (Pantopaque®) in the cranium and spinal canal.

tion into cellular macrophages (Gjerris A, et al, 1978) and/or its loculation between adhesions associated with its induction of chronic arachnoiditis (see Physiological Effects).

PHYSIOLOGICAL EFFECTS

As a result of its insolubility in the cerebrospinal fluid, its limited kinetics, and its nonionic nature; iophendylate is virtually devoid of acute physiologic, neurotoxic, or other adverse effects. Hence, the reported 10–30% incidence of nausea, vomiting, and headaches observed with iophendylate myelography correlates with and is felt to be primarily attributable to the spinal puncture procedure and its complications rather than the administered contrast agent (Kieffer SA, et al, 1978). As expected, aspiration of iophendylate from the subarachnoid space following the myelography procedure significantly decreases the likelihood of late adverse reactions. It has been demonstrated experimentally, however, that the retention of iophendylate in the subarach-

noid space at concentrations corresponding to less than 10% of the routine clinical dose can result in a severe cellular inflammatory reaction (Haughton VM and Ho K-C, 1982a). This acute arachnoiditis may account for the more severe headaches, fever, and backaches occasionally observed post iophendylate myelography.

The subarachnoid administration of iophendylate, with post-procedure aspiration, has also been associated with a high incidence of chronic arachnoiditis (Burton CV, 1978). This adverse reaction is typically without clinical symptoms unless it is severe. Chronic arachnoiditis may be demonstrated on subsequent myelograms as a narrowing of the arachnoid sac, obliteration of the nerve root sleeves, and a loss of the striated appearance of the intrathecal nerve roots (Figure 4.4). The clinical significance of this iophendylate-induced, chronic arachnoiditis is related to the decreased diagnostic value of subsequent myelographic procedures, a delayed rate of cerebrospinal fluid and water-soluble contrast media absorption

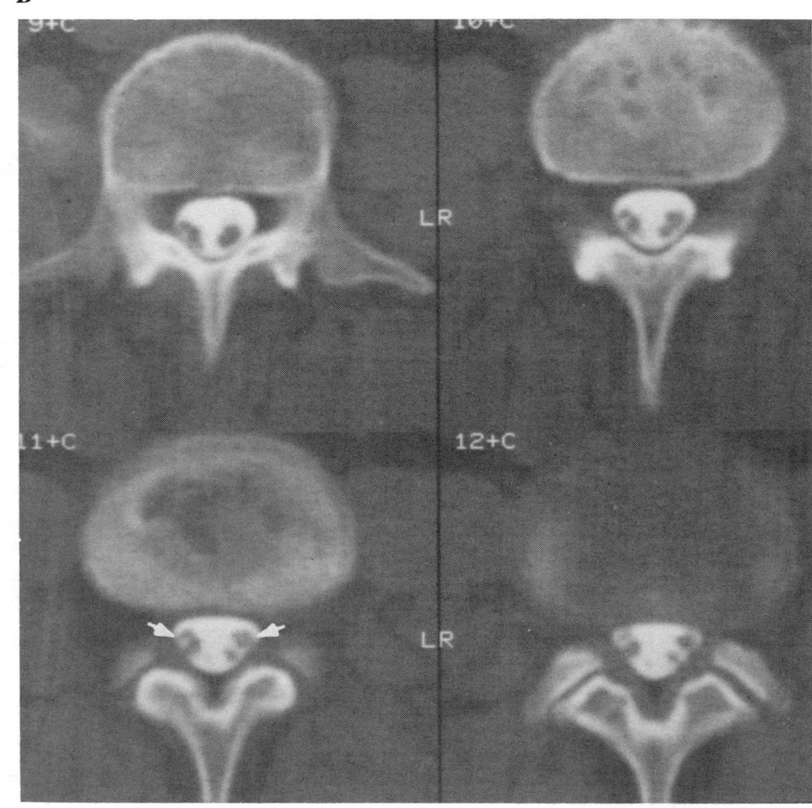

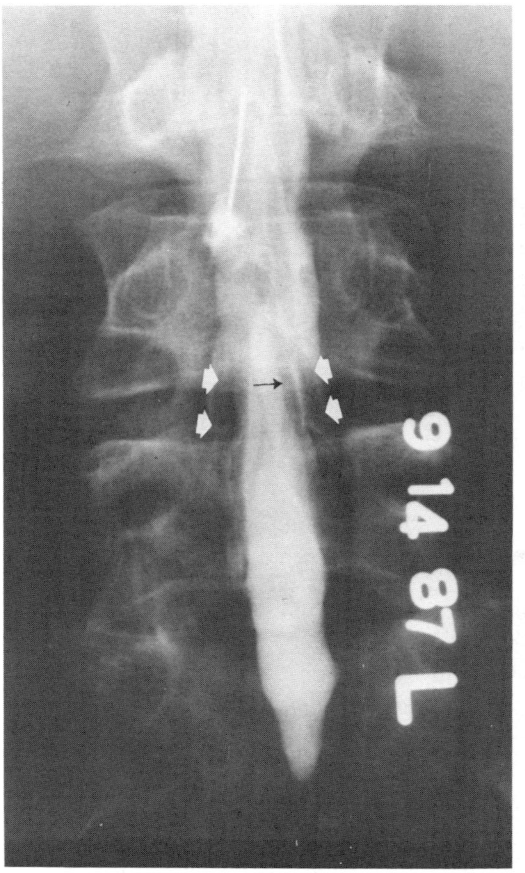

Figure 4.4 A. Myelogram obtained with a water-soluble, nonionic contrast medium demonstrates arachnoiditis caused by the prior subarachnoid administration of iophendylate (Pantopaque®). Note the homogenous appearance of the contrast in the lower dural sac, thickening and clumping of the nerve roots (arrows), and obliteration of the nerve root sheaths. B. Postmyelogram computed tomography on the same patient demonstrates (arrows) clumping of the nerve roots.

from the subarachnoid space (see II. Water-soluble Nonionic Contrast Media, Physiological Effects), and the possible development of late clinical symptoms including back or radicular pain and weakness (Haughton VM and Ho K-C, 1982a). It has been suggested that this chronic arachnoiditis may result from the inadvertent injection of glass fragments from the iophendylate ampule (Siegle RS, et al, 1982) or to the direct chemical toxicity or decomposition of any retained iophendylate (Sovak M, 1984). Although the iodine-aromatic bond of iophendylate is more stable than the iodine-carbon bond of Lipiodol, in vivo decomposition does occur as evidenced by iophendylate's interference with diagnostic thyroid function tests that involve the quantitation of systemic iodine (White AG, 1972).

PRECAUTIONS

Physical Incompatibilities. Iophendylate is incompatible with rubber and certain plastic polymers (e. g., styrene), thus necessitating its packaging in glass ampules (Marshall TR, et al, 1965). As with any parenteral agent packaged in a glass ampule, there is a risk associated with product contamination by glass fragments produced during ampule opening. In recognition of this risk, a sterile filter needle or filter disk of a pore size of 5 microns, or less, should be used for withdrawing iophendylate from the ampule. The rubber and plastic incompatibilities of iophendylate also suggest the use of glass syringes with non–rubber-sealed plungers, especially if the time period between agent withdrawal and administration is prolonged. In addition, iophendylate should be protected from direct exposure to light (Siegle RS, et al, 1982; product information, Pantopaque®, Alcon, Inc., Puerto Rico).

Iophendylate-Laboratory Test/Diagnostic Procedure Interactions. As mentioned previously, iophendylate within the subarachnoid space undergoes slow decomposition with the release of free iodine into the systemic circulation. Thyroid function tests based on the quantification of iodine (i. e., protein-bound iodine, thyroid iodine uptake) may therefore be altered for several months to years following myelography with incomplete iophendylate aspiration (White AG, 1972).

Pantopaque has been shown to exhibit a short T1 relaxation time on magnetic resonance images. Hence, its presence in the subarachnoid space should not be mistaken for fat or hemorrhage (Mamourian AC and Briggs RW, 1986).

Contraindications. Regardless of the contrast medium utilized, intrathecal puncture is contraindicated in the presence of significant bacteremia. Since a prior myelography or lumbar puncture procedure can result in leakage and extravasation of cerebrospinal fluid into extradural spaces and collapse of the subarachnoid space, the manufacturer of iophendylate suggests that a repeat myelography procedure be separated by at least 10 days to avoid inadvertent extra-arachnoid administration of the agent (product information, Pantopaque®, Alcon, Inc., Puerto Rico). Misadministration of water-insoluble iophendylate into the intravascular compartment can result in its embolic localization within the pulmonary circulation (i. e., with intravenous injection) or peripheral vasculature (i. e., with arterial injection).

Preliminary evidence indicates that acute inflammatory reactions to iophendylate may be potentiated by the presence of blood within the cerebrospinal fluid (see Siegle RS, et al, 1982). Likewise, the chemotoxic effects of this medium appear to be particularly pronounced in the presence of demyelating diseases, such as multiple sclerosis (Kaufman P and Jeans WD, 1976). Administration of an alternative myelographic contrast medium should be considered in these situations.

WATER-SOLUBLE NONIONIC CONTRAST MEDIA

Although iophendylate represents a reasonably safe and efficacious contrast agent for myelography, its immiscibility with the cerebrospinal fluid and extremely slow absorption from the spinal canal present problems in regard to the delineation of fine structures of the subarachnoid space and a requirement for postprocedure aspiration. Hence, in an attempt to develop a more optimal myelographic contrast medium, attention was directed toward the use of water-soluble agents in the cerebrospinal fluid greatly spinal fluid and be absorbed from the subarachnoid space within a short time period. It was soon to be recognized, however, that the solubilization of such agents in the cerebrospinal fluid greatly enhanced their potential for subsequent exposure to the sensitive cells of the central nervous system. Thus, the neurotoxic effects of water-soluble contrast agents became an important consideration in regard to their subarachnoid administration for myelography. Subsequent development of a safe and acceptable water-soluble medium for myelography proceeded through several evolutionary stages (see Amundsen P, 1977; Sovak, M, 1984; Skalpe IO, 1977).

One of the first water-soluble contrast media to be utilized for myelography was the ionic agent, methiodal sodium (Figure 4.5). Clinical use of this medium was, however, frequently associated with violent tonic and clonic spasms of the ex-

Table 4.2 SUBARACHNOID TOXICITY OF EARLY MYELOGRAPHIC CONTRAST MEDIA

CONTRAST MEDIUM	LD_{50} [MOUSE] (MG IODINE/KG)
Ratio-1.5 ionic (monomeric)	
Diatrizoate meglumine	50
Iothalamate sodium	160
Methiodal sodium	195
Iothalamate meglumine	205
Ratio-2 ionic (dimeric)	
Iocarmate meglumine	350
Ratio-3 nonionic	
Metrizamide	>1500

[a] Adapted from Almén T, 1980.

tremities, convulsions, and epileptogenic activity. These adverse reactions were apparently due to neurotoxic effects of this agent on the cells of the spinal cord and brain. Hence, myelographic studies with methiodal sodium were limited to the lumbar region and required the coapplication of spinal or general anesthesia. In addition, although methiodal sodium was rapidly absorbed from the subarachnoid space, it produced a high incidence of chronic arachnoiditis.

Upon recognition that meglumine salts of ionic contrast media produced less neurotoxic effects and local cellular irritation than sodium salts, and that the neurotoxicity of the iothalamate anion was less than that of the other available radiopaque anions (Table 4.2); the ionic contrast medium, iothalamate meglumine

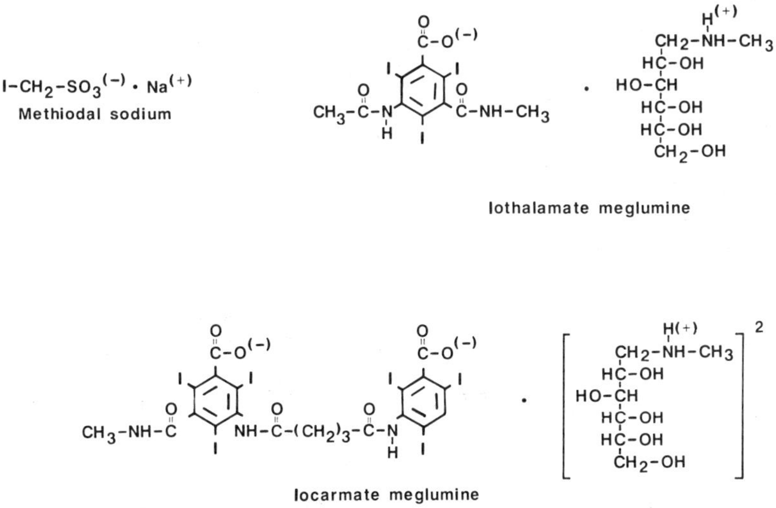

Figure 4.5 Early water-soluble, ionic contrast media used for myelography.

(Figure 4.5), replaced methiodal sodium for myelographic procedures. Although this water-soluble, ionic contrast medium did produce less spasmotic and convulsant activity relative to methiodal sodium, its potential for the production of epileptogenic reactions and arachnoiditis remained a problem.

Since preliminary investigations suggested that the neurotoxic effects and arachnoiditis produced by water-soluble, ionic media may be related to their hyperosmolarity, the manufacturer of iothalamate meglumine developed a dimeric derivative of this agent that possessed a lower number of osmotically active particles (i. e., 3 osmotic particles per 6 iodine atoms, ratio-2 medium) per equivalent iodine concentration. This ionic-dimeric contrast medium, iocarmate meglumine (Figure 4.5), did demonstrate a decreased frequency and severity of neurotoxic effects (Table 4.2) compared to the ratio-1.5 medium, iothalamate meglumine, and was used extensively for clinical myelography during the 1970s. The hazards of muscle spasms, convulsions, and arachnoiditis did not, however, completely resolve with the use of this dimeric agent. More recent experimental studies have, in fact, revealed an increase in the incidence of radiographically detected chronic arachnoiditis with iocarmate meglumine versus equiiodine doses of iothalamate meglumine or methiodal sodium (Ahlgren P, 1980). This suggests that the arachnoiditis produced by myelographic contrast media is related to their direct molecular toxicity rather than their hyperosmolarity (Haughton VM, et al, 1977).

As another method to reduce the osmolality-related, physiological effects of ionic contrast media, Almén proposed the development of a nonionic contrast agent that would retain water solubility, but would consist of only one osmotically active particle in solution per three iodine atoms (i. e., ratio-3 medium) rather than the two osmotically active particles (cation and anion) per three iodine atoms of conventional ratio-1.5 ionic media (Almén T, 1969). Although originally

proposed to reduce the number and intensity of undesirable physiological effects associated with the intravascular administration of ratio-1.5 media, it soon became recognized that the ratio-3 nonionic media also produced less subarachnoid toxicity (Almén T, 1980). This phenomenon is apparently related to the fact that the electrical charges of ionic contrast media (conventional-monomeric or dimeric) alter the ionic balance of the cerebral spinal fluid and interfere with the normal conduction of impulses in the central nervous system. An advantage of the nonionic versus ionic-dimeric (i. e., iocarmate meglumine) approach to reduced osmolality is the complete elimination of electrically charged ions. These considerations led to the development and routine myelographic use of water-soluble, nonionic contrast media.

CHEMISTRY

The first commercially available nonionic contrast agent, metrizamide (Figure 4.6), is a derivative of the ratio-1.5 ionic medium, metrizoate, wherein the carboxyl group of metrizoate is covalently attached to the glucose derivative, glucosamine, to confer water solubility without ionic dissociation. Hence, ideal solutions of metrizamide consist of three iodine atoms per one osmotically active,

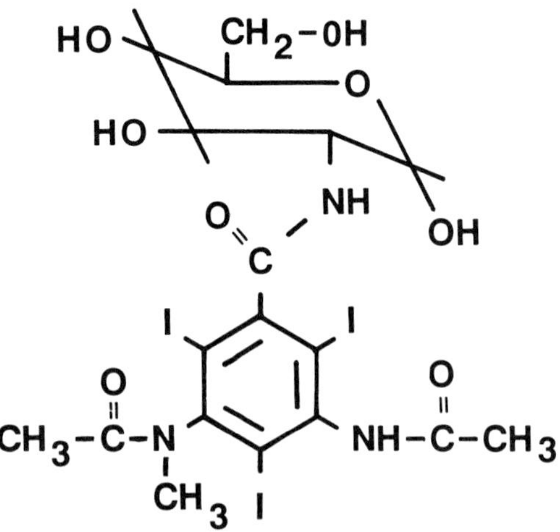

Figure 4.6 Chemical structure of metrizamide.

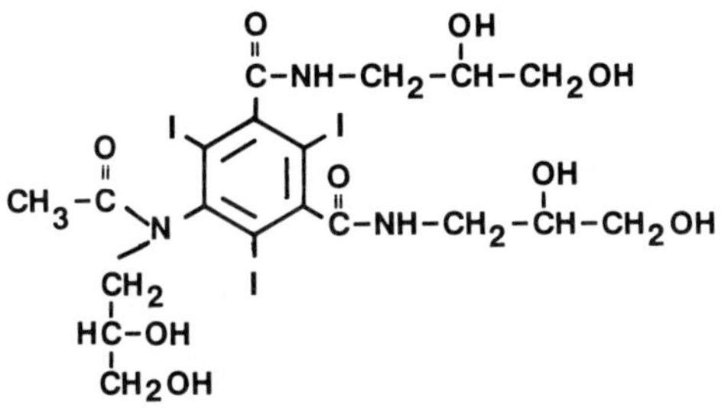

Iohexol

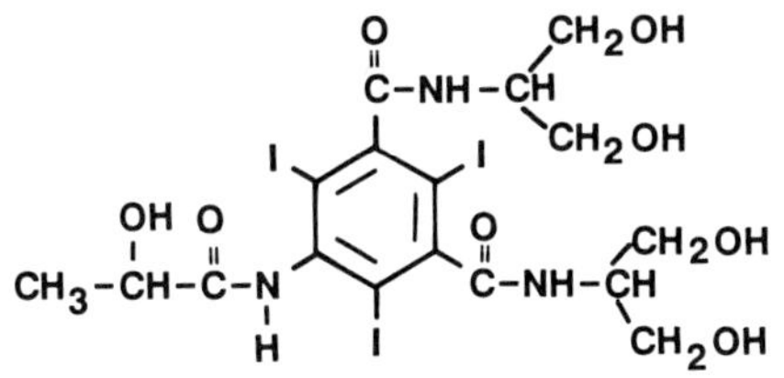

Iopamidol

Figure 4.7 Chemical structures of iohexol and iopamidol.

non-electrically charged particle (i.e., a ratio-3 nonionic medium). As a result of its reduced osmolality and absence of charge, the neurotoxicity of subarachnoid metrizamide was considerably less than that of the previously utilized ionic media (Table 4.2) resulting in a reduced incidence and severity of spasms, convulsions, and epileptogenic activity. Furthermore, routine myelographic use of metrizamide was not associated with the production of chronic arachnoiditis as was observed with iophendylate and the water-soluble, ionic media (Skalpe IO, 1977). Based on these advantages, metrizamide became recognized as the optimal contrast medium for myelography from its date of clinical introduction in the mid-1970s until recent development of the second-generation nonionic media.

Although more efficacious than previous myelographic agents, the routine use of metrizamide was associated with problems related to its high cost of production and price, its instability to heat and sterilization by autoclaving, and its instability in solution, the latter factor necessitating on-site reconstitution of lypophilized metrizamide powder immediately prior to administration. Subsequent research on nonionic contrast media, aimed primarily at the development of agents with improved stability and reduced cost, has resulted in the recent availability of iohexol and iopamidol (Figure 4.7). These second-generation, nonionic contrast media can be heat sterilized and are stable in solution, thereby decreasing their cost of production and price and increasing their convenience of use. Moreover, recent experimental and clinical studies suggest that the subarachnoid administration of either iohexol or iopamidol results in fewer neurologic effects compared to metrizamide. Based on these considerations, iohexol and iopamidol have or will soon replace metrizamide for myelography procedures. For comparative purposes, however, a discussion of metrizamide will be included in the following presentation of nonionic, myelographic contrast media (Table 4.3).

Table 4.3 CHEMICAL PROPERTIES OF WATER-SOLUBLE, NONIONIC CONTRAST MEDIA INDICATED FOR MYELOGRAPHY[a]

GENERIC NAME	BRAND NAME®[b]	CONCENTRATION (%w/v)	MG IODINE / ML	OSMOLALITY (mOsm/kg)	VISCOSITY (cps) 20° C	VISCOSITY (cps) 37° C
Iohexol	Omnipaque (W)	38.8	180	408	3.1	2.0
		51.8	240	520	5.8	3.4
Iopamidol	Isovue-M (S)	40.8	200	413	3.3	2.0
		61.0	300	616	8.8	3.3
Metrizamide	Amipaque (W)	35.2–62.5[c]	170–300	300–484	2.9–12.7	1.8–6.2

Adapted from respective product insert information.
[a] U.S. market only
[b] (S) Squibb Diagnostics
   (W) Winthrop-Breon Laboratories
[c] Lyophilized powder for reconstitution

Iodine Concentration. On a per molecular weight basis, iopamidol contains a slightly greater percentage of iodine (49%) than metrizamide (48.3%) or iohexol (46.4%) (Table 4.3). Based on the quantity of administered iodine, the intracisternal toxicity (i. e., LD_{50}-mouse) of all three nonionic media are similar and low (i. e., >2000 mg I/kg) (Shaw DD and Potts DG, 1985).

Viscosity. At equal iodine concentrations and room temperature (20°C), the viscosity of metrizamide is greater than that of iohexol (Table 4.4). Under these same conditions, the viscosity of iopamidol is less than that of iohexol. Reducing the concentration (Table 4.3) or increasing the temperature of the media to 37°C significantly reduces their respective viscosities and decreases the relative differences between agents (Table 4.4).

Osmolality. The ratio-3 nonionic contrast media should theoretically demonstrate a 50% decrease in the osmolality exhibited by equiiodine concentrations of the ratio-1.5 ionic media. However, the actual reduction in osmolality achieved by these ratio-3 media is greater than 50% (Table 4.4) due to aggregation of the nonionic molecules in solution. Molecular aggregation further reduces the osmolality of a contrast medium by both decreasing the total number of osmotically active particles in solution and increasing their molecular weight (Dawson P, 1984).

Within the nonionic contrast media group, the osmolality of iopamidol is less than that of an equiiodine concentration of iohexol, but greater than metrizamide (Table 4.4). These differences probably reflect the respective degrees of molecular aggregation of these agents.

PHARMACOKINETICS

Water-soluble, nonionic contrast media injected into the subarachnoid space mix readily with the cerebrospinal fluid and freely penetrate into the nerve root sheaths and fine crevices (Figures 4.8, 4.9). These agents are subsequently absorbed from the spinal canal into the systemic circulation via the same mechanisms that are responsible for cerebrospinal fluid absorption (see Potts DG, et al, 1985; Sage MR, 1983a).

Subarachnoid Absorption. Cerebrospinal fluid is normally produced primarily within the choroid plexus and actively secreted into the ventricles at a rate of approximately 20 mL/hour. It is subsequently absorbed from the subarachnoid space via arachnoid villi or granulations found in relation to the major dural venous sinuses of the cranium and, to a lesser extent, the epidural veins of the spinal canal. These arachnoid granulations are proliferations of arachnoid stroma covered by endothelium that is continuous with the endothelium of the related veins (Figure 4.10). Endothelial-lined tubules that directly link the subarachnoid space with the venous system are also frequently found in association with these arachnoid granulations. Cerebrospinal fluid passes from the subarachnoid space to the systemic circulation via

Table 4.4 COMPARATIVE VISCOSITIES AND OSMOLALITIES OF SELECTED WATER-SOLUBLE, NONIONIC CONTRAST MEDIA AT EQUAL IODINE CONCENTRATIONS

CONTRAST MEDIUM	MG IODINE / ML	VISCOSITY (CPS) 20° C	VISCOSITY (CPS) 37° C	OSMOLALITY (mOsm/kg)
Iohexol	300[a]	11.8	6.3	672
Iopamidol	300	8.8	4.7	616
Metrizamide	300	12.7	6.2	484
(Iothalamate meglumine)[b]	(282)			(1500)

Adapted from respective product insert information.

[a] Not indicated for myelography.

[b] Ratio-1.5 ionic medium, Conray®–60, Mallinckrodt.

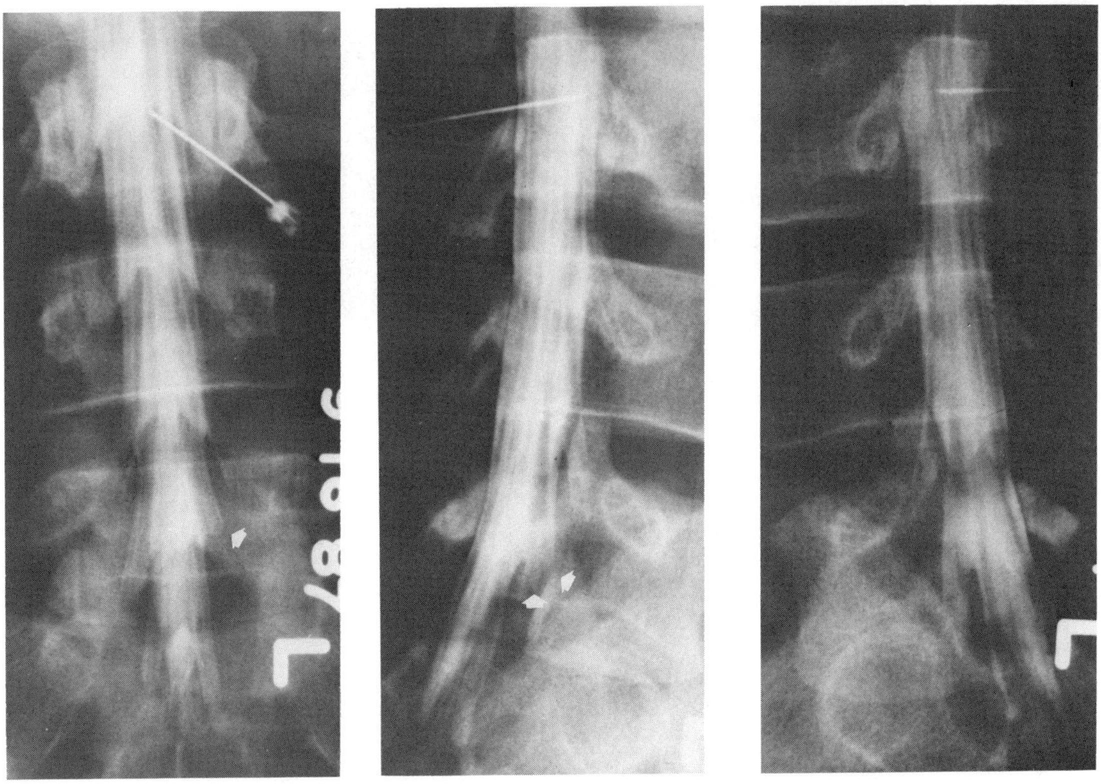

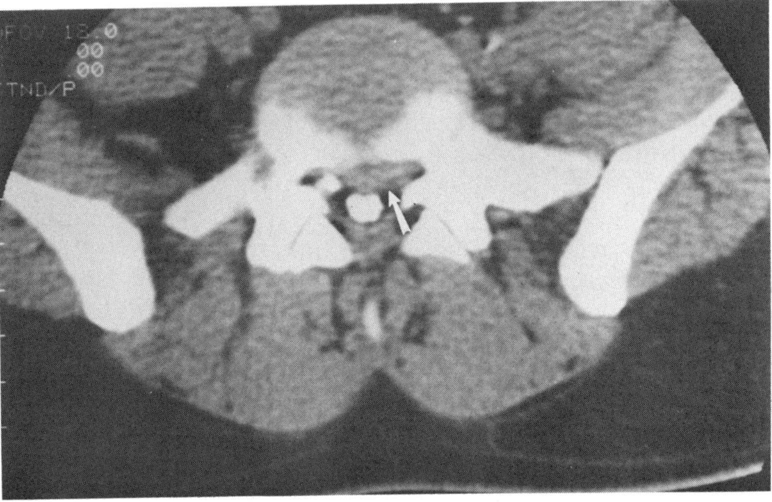

Figure 4.8   A–C. Frontal and oblique myelograms demonstrating excellent visualization of the cauda equina and nerve root sheaths following the lumbar subarachnoid injection of a water-soluble, nonionic contrast medium. Note (arrows) amputation of the left S_1 nerve root sheath by a herniated disc. D. Diagnosis of herniated disc confirmed (arrow) by postmyelogram computed tomography.

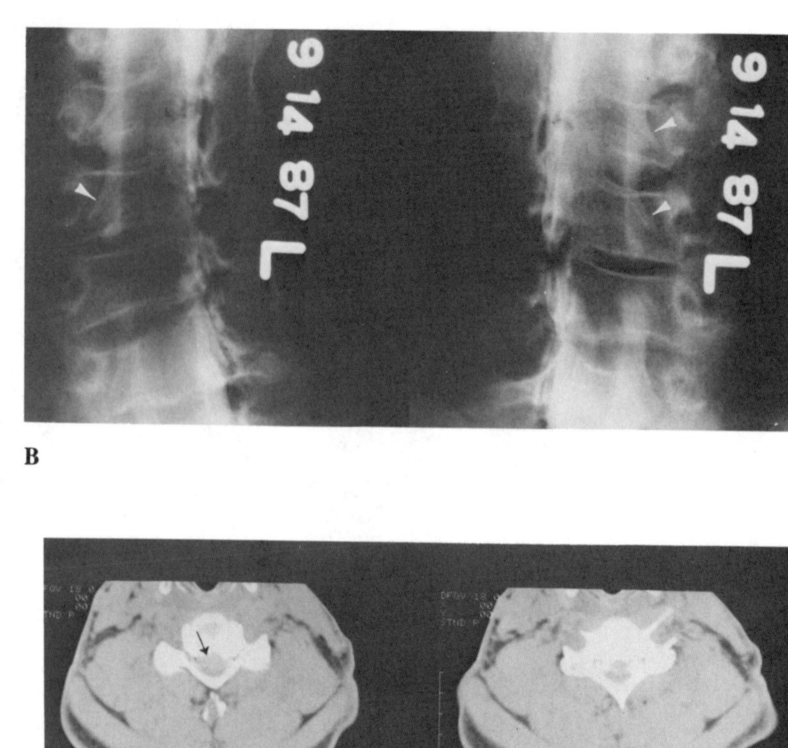

A   C

Figure 4.9 **A.** Myelogram demonstrating (closed arrow) a high-grade extradural block resulting from a posttraumatic, centrally herniated C5-6 disc. **B.** Note (arrowheads) excellent visualization of the exiting cervical nerve routes in this study. **C.** Diagnosis of herniated disc confirmed (arrow) by postmyelogram computed tomography.

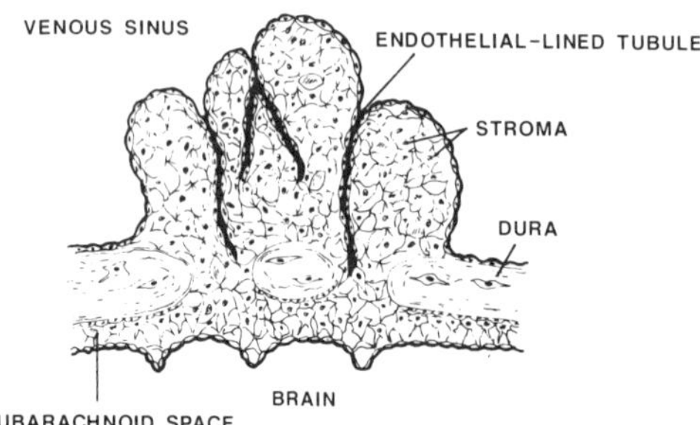

Figure 4.10 Diagram of arachnoid granulation. (From Potts DG, et al, 1985; with permission.)

these tubules or by simple diffusion through the cellular junctions of the endothelium of the arachnoid granulation. Since these pathways through the arach-noid granulations are sufficiently large to permit the passage of cerebrospinal fluid proteins, they will also readily permit the passage of water-soluble, nonionic contrast media.

The previously described, continuous, and active secretion of cerebrospinal fluid into the limited volume (i. e., 140 mL) of the cerebrospinal fluid space creates a cerebrospinal fluid pressure that normally exceeds the pressure of adjacent veins by approximately 6 cm H_2O. It is this pressure difference that produces the driving force for cerebrospinal fluid and contrast-media absorption from the subarachnoid space into the blood. The arachnoid granulations function as unidirectional valves that permit the flow of cerebrospinal fluid from the subarachnoid space into the vein, provided that the cerebrospinal fluid–venous pressure difference exceeds 2.5 cm H_2O. At pressure differences below this level, or at venous pressures that exceed the cerebrospinal fluid pressure, the arachnoid granulations collapse and the absorption process ceases. Factors that produce a decrease in the rate of cerebrospinal fluid formation and/or a drop in cerebrospinal fluid pressure (Table 4.5) can therefore cause a reduction in the rate of cerebrospinal fluid and, hence, nonionic contrast media absorption from the subarachnoid space. Patient positioning does not have an effect on the cerebrospinal fluid–venous pressure difference.

Cerebrospinal fluid is normally absorbed predominantly by the cranial arachnoid granulations with minimal absorption occurring at the spinal level. In contrast, water-soluble, nonionic myelographic media injected into the spinal space are primarily absorbed at the spinal arachnoid granulations with passage into the epidural veins. This most likely occurs because there is an absence of active cerebrospinal fluid circulation in the spinal subarachnoid space. Since the nonionic contrast media have specific gravities (1.2–1.3) in excess of the specific gravity of cerebrospinal fluid (1.09), there is a tendency for their gravitational diffusion in a downward direction, especially when the patient is placed in the traditional, semi-sitting position following the myelography procedure. It should be noted that horizontal (i. e., recumbent) positioning of the patient (with the head elevated) results in more rapid contrast-media absorption than a totally erect position by increasing the exposure of the agent to the total distribution of arachnoid granulations within the spinal canal (Sage MR, 1983a).

The previous statements should not be interpreted to mean that movement of the water-soluble, nonionic contrast media proceeds only in a caudal direction. Cephalad migration of the nonionic contrast media does occur regardless of the site of intrathecal administration or patient positioning. In fact, computerized tomography has demonstrated the diffusion of nonionic contrast media into the intracranial subarchnoid spaces and ventricles in 30% of patients at 6 hours post lumbar myelography (Galle G, et al, 1984). Hence, in addition to the cerebrospinal fluid–venous pressure difference, the rate of absorption of a water-soluble, nonionic contrast medium from the subarachnoid space is dependent on its rate of mixing and diffusion in the cerebrospinal fluid.

Studies to date indicate that iohexol, iopamidol, and metrizamide are absorbed from the subarachnoid space at similar rates (Drayer BP, et al, 1984; Haughton VW, 1982b; Sage MR and Wilcox J, et al, 1983b). Computed tomography quantification of density changes over the lumbar thecal sac reveals a subarachnoid half-life of approximately 6 hours (Drayer BP, et al, 1984); whereas direct measurements of the contrast medium (metrizamide) concentration in the cerebral spinal fluid of normal human subjects suggest a slightly longer half-life of 11 hours (Golman K, 1975).

Table 4.5 FACTORS THAT CAN PRODUCE A DECREASE IN THE RATE OF CEREBROSPINAL FLUID FORMATION AND/OR A DECREASE IN CEREBROSPINAL FLUID PRESSURE[a]

Alkalosis
Cerebrospinal fluid removal (without volume replacement)
Dehydration
Drugs
  · Acetazolamide ⎱ Diuretics
  · Furosemide   ⎰
  · Spironolactone
  · Amphotericin
  · Ouabain
  · Vasopressin
Hypothermia

[a] See Sage MR, 1983a, Potts DG, et al, 1985.

Systemic Excretion. Once these nonionic contrast media are absorbed into the systemic circulation, they are rapidly excreted, unmetabolized, via glomerular filtration. Following subarachnoid administration, peak serum concentrations of the nonionic contrast media are observed at 2–3 hours, with a plasma half-life of approximately 3 hours. Between 70–85% of the subarachnoid dose of these non-ionic media is recovered in the urine at 24 hours; elimination is virtually complete by 48 hours. None of the nonionic contrast media demonstrates significant binding to plasma, serum, or cerebrospinal fluid proteins (Drayer BP, et al, 1984; Golman K, 1975; Hindmarsh T, 1975a).

Brain Penetration. Unlike the blood-brain barrier that limits the diffusion of intravascularly administered, water-soluble contrast media into the brain, there is no diffusion barrier between the cerebrospinal fluid space and the extra cellular fluid space of the brain. Hence, small water-soluble molecules and ions in the subarachnoid space can freely enter the brain parenchyma via a simple diffusion process. As previously described, both ionic and nonionic myelographic media demonstrate penetration into the brain following subarachnoid administration (Sage MR and Wilcox J, 1983b; Galle G, et al, 1984). The extent of this penetration reflects a simple diffusion process with primary involvement of the superficial brain cortex and lesser involvement of the white matter and basal ganglia. The concentration that a contrast medium achieves in the extracellular spaces of the brain is dependent on several factors including the dose and concentration of the administered agent, the site of administration, the duration of contrast medium retention within the subarachnoid space (i. e., cerebrospinal fluid–venous pressure difference and rate of contrast-medium absorption), and patient positioning and degree of activity. Maximum concentration of water-soluble contrast media in the brain typically occurs by 6 hours following lumbar myelography with more rapid appearance following more cephalad sites of administration (Drayer BP, et al, 1984; Hindmarsh T, 1975a).

Studies have shown that the rate and depth of brain penetration associated with use of the earlier ionic media and the cur-rent nonionic media are similar. This would suggest that noted differences in the respective neurotoxic effects of these agents are not due to differing degrees of brain penetration but to the direct molecular toxicities of the agents (Sage MR and Wilcox J, 1983b). On the other hand, the incidence and severity of central nervous system side effects (i. e., EEG changes, depression, excitation) observed with a given ionic or nonionic contrast medium does appear to correlate with the extent of its brain penetration as determined by the aforementioned factors (see Ekholm SE, et al, 1983).

Experimental and preliminary clinical studies indicate that some variability may exist in regard to the persistence of myelographic contrast media within the gray matter of the central nervous system (Kerber, CW, et al, 1983; Hammer B and Deisenhammer E, 1985). Metrizamide appears to be retained in the gray matter for a longer duration than iopamidol, which in turn persists for a longer period than iohexol. The prolonged retention of metrizamide may be related to its binding to the membrane carrier responsible for glucose entry into the brain (see Physiological Effects). The duration of central nervous system exposure to the administered contrast medium may also play a role in regard to the relative neurotoxicities of myelographic media.

PHYSIOLOGICAL EFFECTS

The subarachnoid administration of a water-soluble, nonionic contrast medium can result in undesirable physiological effects and adverse reactions related to procedure-induced alterations in cerebrospinal fluid pressure, medium-induced local irritation of the spinal membranes, or direct central nervous system toxicity. Frequently the radiology literature combines these undesirable physiological effects in describing the complications of myelography. It must be noted, however, that the medium-induced effects are each associated with a separate causal mechanism and may therefore vary with the chemical characteristics of the administered agent. For example, the hyperosmolarity of the injected contrast medium is primarily responsible for central nervous system depression, whereas central nervous system excitation is associated with direct molecular toxicity of the medium. Adverse reactions related to the spinal puncture procedure are observed regardless of the chemical nature of the injected agent.

As previously discussed, the water-soluble, nonionic contrast media are absorbed from the subarachnoid space into the systemic circulation. Thus, there is a possibility that these iodinated agents can elicit reactions of a pseudo-allergic nature. Unpredictable, pseudo-allergic reactions to intravascular, iodinated contrast media are discussed in detail in Chapter 8.

Procedure-Induced Reactions. The most common complications of myelography are acute transient headaches and nausea that occur in approximately 30–40% and 10% of the procedures, respectively. The nature and frequency of these reactions suggest that they are directly related to the subarachnoid injection procedure, the incidence of acute headaches following simple lumbar puncture without contrast administration being 36% (Tourtellotte WW, et al, 1972). These reactions apparently occur due to increased pressure or tension on the meningeal membranes resulting from the leakage or removal of cerebrospinal fluid and the alteration of normal cerebrospinal fluid pressure and/or kinetics. Early headaches and nausea occur more frequently in females than in males and may be related to the size of the spinal needle utilized or the length of the procedure (Hauge O and Falkenberg H, 1982; Skalpe IO, 1977).

The frequency of these early reactions appears to be the same regardless of the chemical nature (i. e., ionic, nonionic, water-insoluble) of the myelographic medium utilized (Skalpe IO, 1977) or the site (i. e., lumbar vs. cervical) of injection (Nakstad P, et al, 1984). Further evidence that these acute reactions are procedure- rather than contrast-medium-related is based on a lack of correlation between their frequency and the central nervous

system concentration of the injected agent (Nakstad P, et al, 1984). It has been noted, however, that the duration and severity of headaches may increase if, during or after the procedure, a significant volume of contrast medium is allowed to enter the cranial subarachnoid space at a fast rate (e. g., with failure to maintain an extended head position during cervical or total myelography, assumption of a flat recumbent position with head lowered post myelography, or undue patient activity post myelography). This observation suggests that the delayed (i. e., >24-hours duration), severe headaches occasionally observed following myelography may be related to diffusion of the injected medium into the extracellular spaces of the brain and its chemotoxic induction of central nervous system excitation or depression (Meador K, et al, 1984). For similar reasons, the incidence of delayed headache may also be increased with more cephalad sites of administration.

Local Irritation of the Spinal Canal. Prior extensive use of metrizamide for myelography was associated with a 5–10% incidence of back or leg pain, paresthesia, or stiffness (Hanus PM, 1980; Hauge O and Falkenberg H, 1982). It is felt that these spino-radicular syndromes are related to metrizamide-induced local irritation of the nerve roots or inflammation of the spinal membranes, as suggested by an increase in their severity with patients in a sitting position (DeVilliers PD, et al, 1984) and by minor elevations of the cerebrospinal fluid white cell count (Skalpe IO, 1977). Whether these adverse inflammatory effects will appear with the same frequency with the myelographic use of iohexol or iopamidol awaits more extensive clinical experience. However, preliminary evidence suggests less local irritation with the second-generation nonionic media.

As previously discussed, a high incidence of acute and chronic arachnoiditis was associated with early myelographic use of the water-soluble, ionic contrast media. This suggested a possible relationship between the hyperosmolarity and/or concentration of these agents and the incidence and severity of this inflammatory response. Subsequent studies have, however, demonstrated a lack of acute arachnoiditis with the subarachnoid administration of hypertonic saline, thus indicating that local irritation or inflammation of the spinal membranes is not due to hyperomolarity per se, but is related to direct molecular toxicity of the injected medium (Haughton VM, et al, 1977). Subarachnoid metrizamide does not produce severe, acute arachnoiditis or chronic arachnoiditis at routine clinical dosage levels (i. e., $\leq$ 3 g total iodine). This agent has been shown, however, to produce arachnoiditis at very high doses in an animal model that involved suboptimal positioning (Haughton VM and Ho KC, 1982a). Similar experimental studies indicate that the more recent nonionic agents, iohexol and iopamidol, induce even less local inflammation than metrizamide (Haughton VM, et al, 1982b; Thevenin P, 1983).

Central Nervous System Effects—General Statement. The subarachnoid administration of water-soluble, nonionic contrast media can produce alterations of central nervous system function as evidenced by transient electroencephalographic (EEG) changes and by clinical symptoms of excitation, depression, and, in the case of metrizamide, psycho-organic syndromes. These central nervous system effects appear to be directly related to the molecular toxicity or hyperosmolarity of the injected medium, since their incidence and severity correlate with the concentration of the contrast medium in the extracellular space of the brain and differ depending on the chemical characteristics of the nonionic medium utilized. These central nervous system effects tend to be more pronounced with more cephalad sites of injection, improper patient positioning, and with factors (Table 4.5) that delay the rate of contrast-medium absorption from the subarachnoid space (Drayer

BP, et al, 1984; Hauge O and Falkenberg H, 1982).

Although post-injection EEG changes provide an objective method to evaluate the central nervous system toxicity of myelographic contrast media, evidence indicates that there is no strong correlation between these EEG changes and the eventual appearance of clinical symptoms (Bertoni JM, et al, 1981; Nau HE, 1981; Maly P, et al, 1986). Hence, this discussion of the central nervous system effects of water-soluble, nonionic contrast media focuses on observable (clinical or experimental) central nervous system reactions (e. g., convulsions, evoked corticospinal responses, etc.) rather than changes in brain wave activity.

Central Nervous System Excitation. Water-soluble, nonionic contrast media injected into the subarachnoid space can elicit an increase in the spontaneous activity of nerve cells of the spinal cord roots and brain resulting in muscle twitching, spasms, or convulsive seizures of an epileptogenic nature. In regard to the latter severe complication of myelography, the incidence of convulsions with extensive use of metrizamide was approximately 0.4% (Nickle AR and Salem JJ, 1977).

Since it has been determined that hyperosmolarity, per se, produces a depression of electrical activity, it is felt that the excitatory effects of nonionic myelographic media are related to their direct molecular toxicity (Maly P, et al, 1984a). This conclusion is substantiated by the fact that equivalent doses of the various nonionic media produce differing degrees of excitation. Metrizamide demonstrates greater excitatory responses in a high dose animal model than does iopamidol, with iohexol being virtually devoid of excitatory effects (Golman K, et al, 1980). Whether the respective excitatory differences between the second-generation nonionic media will be reflected clinically at routine dosage levels remains a question at this time. The results of a clinical study evaluating the incidence of spike or epileptiform EEG changes following iohexol and iopamidol administration showed no differences (Macpherson P, et al, 1985). However, preliminary clinical studies have shown that, compared to iopamidol, iohexol produced significantly less alteration of visual evoked responses and a reduced incidence and severity of post-procedure headaches (Broadbridge AT, et al, 1987).

A factor that has been proposed as a causative mechanism for the convulsive activity of nonionic contrast media is their ability to inhibit acetylcholinesterase or antagonize cholinergic activity (Marder E, et al, 1983). Direct exposure of the brain to acetylcholinesterase inhibitors or to cholinergic agonists or antagonists does result in convulsive actions. In vitro studies on the degree of acetylcholinesterase inhibition exhibited by the water-soluble contrast media (Dawson P, 1985) correlate, in general, with their respective epileptogenic activities following subarachnoid administration.

Central Nervous System Depression. The subarachnoid administration of nonionic contrast media has been shown to produce diffuse slowing of brain wave activity and a suppression of corticospinal-evoked responses. These depressive effects of nonionic contrast media may account for the general lassitude, malaise, weakness, and dizziness observed post myelography procedures. These relatively mild depressive responses should be considered separate from the psycho-organic events (i. e., dysphoria, aphasia, psychotic disturbances, hallucinations) that are occasionally observed following myelography with metrizamide.

The subarachnoid administration of hypertonic saline produces depressive effects consistent with those observed following the subarachnoid administration of hypertonic contrast media, thus implicating the role of hyperosmolarity as a causative factor for central nervous system depression. Metrizamide demonstrates less suppression of evoked corticospinal responses than equiosmolar, hypertonic saline. This observation would suggest that the overall response to subarachnoid contrast media reflects the combined effects of central nervous system excitation due to molecular toxicity and depression due to hyperosmolarity (Hilal SK, et al, 1978).

If hyperosmolarity is the primary factor responsible for the depressive activity of a myelographic contrast medium, then one would expect similar responses to equivalent doses of the various nonionic agents. In a high-dose animal model, iohexol and iopamidol did demonstrate similar degrees of central nervous system depression, however the depressive activity of metrizamide was significantly greater (Golman K, et al, 1980). This indicates that metrizamide must possess an additional chemotoxic factor that results in its relative increase in central nervous system depression.

Psycho-organic Syndromes. Various psycho-organic symptoms including dysphoria, dysphasia, confusion, psychotic disturbances, and hallucinations have been observed in a small percentage of patients following myelography with metrizamide. As with other central nervous system effects, the incidence and severity of these mental disturbances correlate with the extent of diffusion and the intracranial concentration of metrizamide but not with associated EEG changes (Galle G, et al, 1984; Richert S, et al, 1979).

It has been suggested that these psycho-organic syndromes reflect a metabolic encephalopathy resulting from metrizamide's ability to interfere with the normal brain utilization of glucose, its primary metabolic substrate. The metrizamide molecule (Figure 4.6) contains the deoxyglucose analog, glucosamine, and has been shown, in vitro, to competitively inhibit both yeast and mammalian hexokinase at concentrations typically found in the extracellular fluid of the brain following routine myelography (Bertoni JM and Steinman CG, 1982). Similar in vivo inhibition of glucose metabolism at the hexokinase level would require intracellular transport of the intact metrizamide molecule or its dissociation and release of the deoxyglucose moiety. Neither of these processes has been shown to occur. However, glucose is transported into brain cells via a facilitated membrane carrier that can also be inhibited by structural glucose analogues. Since it is known that metrizamide does inhibit glucose metabolism in rat hippocampal slices (Ekholm SE, et al, 1983). It is currently felt that it must exert this effect by binding to or distorting the membrane carrier responsible for glucose transport into brain cells. Since the brain is unable to store large amounts of glucose or glycogen, this inhibition of the glucose transport mechanism would be expected to produce significant metabolic disturbances (Ekholm SE, 1985).

Neither iohexol nor iopamidol contain deoxyglucose analogs in their molecular structures. As such, these agents do not inhibit glucose metabolism in the rat hippocampal-slice model (Ekholm SE, 1985; Ekholm SE, et al, 1986). It is therefore anticipated that extensive clinical use of these second-generation nonionic agents will not be associated with the severe depressive effects and psycho-organic syndromes previously observed with metrizamide myelography.

PRECAUTIONS

Formulation considerations. The instability of metrizamide in solution requires that it be reconstituted with the supplied 0.005% sodium bicarbonate diluent prior to patient administration. Complete dissolution of the metrizamide powder must be assured since the presence of undissolved metrizamide has been associated with an increased incidence of serious adverse reactions (Legre J, et al, 1981). Aqueous solutions of the second generation nonionic agents, iohexol and iopamidol, are stable. Thus, these media are commercially available in fixed-concentration formulations suitable for direct subarachnoid administration (Table 4.3). If necessary, dilution of iohexol and iopamidol formulations can be performed using Sodium Chloride for Injection, U.S.P.

None of the nonionic, myelographic contrast media contain bacteriostatic or preservative agents in their formulation. Hence, vials of these agents are intended for a single administration and should be discarded after such use.

Physical Incompatibilities. Each of the nonionic, myelographic contrast media should be stored at room temperature and protected from direct light. In general, the direct addition of drugs or other additives to radiopaque contrast media is to be avoided. Since it has been demonstrated that hypertonic contrast media can leach various chemicals and allergens from the rubber plunger seals of disposable syringes, the length of contact between nonionic contrast media and disposable syringes used for agent withdrawal and injection should be minimized (Hamilton G and Fischer WH, 1984).

Contrast Media–Drug Interactions. Perhaps the most recognized and cited contrast media-drug interaction is the possible potentiation of seizure activity associated with the coadministration of drugs that lower the seizure threshold, especially phenothiazine derivatives, and the myelographic agent, metrizamide. This concern originally developed from a case report (Hindmarsh T, et al, 1975b) of seizure occurrence in a patient receiving oral chlorpromazine (75 mg/day), who had undergone a full-column, prolonged myelography procedure using metrizamide (17 mL, 170 mg iodine/mL). Various animal studies have demonstrated that the central nervous system excitatory effect of large, subarachnoid doses of metrizamide is potentiated by high doses of phenothiazine or meperidine derivatives administered in conjunction with or immediately prior to the myelography procedure (Grepe A and Widen L, 1973; Gonsette RE and Bracher JM, 1977; Maly P, et al, 1984b). Although not documented, these observations have also implicated a potential interaction between subarachnoid metrizamide and other drugs known to lower the seizure threshold (Table 4.6).

Table 4.6 DRUGS, BY GENERAL CLASS, KNOWN TO LOWER THE SEIZURE THRESHOLD

DRUG CLASSIFICATION	COMMON EXAMPLES
Phenothiazines (antipsychotic)	Chlorpromazine, perfenazine, prochlorperazine, thioridazine
Phenothiazines (antihistamines)	Promethazine, trimeperazine
Antipsychotics (nonphenothiazine)	Haloperidol, chlorprothixene, thiothixene
Tricyclic antidepressants	Amitriptyline, desipramine, doxepin, imipramine, protriplyline
CNS stimulants (analeptics)	Amphetamine, methamphetamine, cocaine, methylphenidate
MAO inhibitors	Isocarboxazid, phenelzine, tranylcypromine
Anesthetics (specific)[a]	Enflurane, methohexital, Ketamine[a]

[a] From Pyles ST et al, 1983.

Based on these considerations and product literature recommendations, it is generally recognized and accepted that drugs known to lower the seizure threshold, especially phenothiazine derivatives, should be discontinued at 48 hours prior to the myelography procedure, with reinstatement delayed until 24 hours following the procedure. These time periods permit adequate serum clearance of the long half-life phenothiazines and the subarachnoid clearance of metrizamide, respectively (Hanus PM, 1980).

Although high-dose experimental studies and limited clinical experience suggest that this interaction is real, its actual significance at clinical dosage levels remains uncertain. In fact, some authors have reported no increase in myelographic complications in patients receiving simultaneous phenothiazine therapy (Hauge O and Falkenberg H, 1982; Nau HE, 1981), while others have even suggested a decrease in the severity of myelographic side effects with the coadministration of phenothiazine derivatives (Ahlgren P, 1980; Standes B, et al, 1982). This latter observation may be explained by a phenothiazine-induced decrease in the severity of vomiting, a condition that promotes cephalad migration of the contrast media with increased intracranial concentration and central nervous system effects.

It is interesting to note that this phenothiazine-myelographic contrast-medium precaution was carried over to the product literature of both iohexol and iopamidol regardless of the controversy surrounding its clinical significance and the demonstrated decrease in excitatory effects elicited by these second-generation nonionic agents versus metrizamide. This is especially true for iohexol, since a high-dose experimental study failed to demonstrate excitatory effects with or without the coadministration of a phenothiazine derivative (Maly P, et al, 1984b). The depressive effects of iohexol were, however, potentiated by simultaneous phenothiazine administration. Obviously, more conclusive studies are required to document the clinical significance of this potential drug–contrast media interaction, especially in regard to the recent nonionic agents. However, in view of current product literature recommendations, it is probably advisable to discontinue phenothiazine derivatives and other drugs that lower the seizure threshold if this action will not significantly effect the care or comfort of the patient.

Another potential myelographic contrast medium–drug interaction involves the coadministration of drugs that reduce the rate of cerebrospinal fluid formation and cerebrospinal fluid pressure (Table 4.5). As previously discussed (see Pharmacokinetics), the rate at which a contrast medium is absorbed from the subarachnoid space is directly dependent on the cerebrospinal fluid–venous pressure difference. A reduction of cerebrospinal fluid pressure decreases the normal rate of contrast-medium absorption and increases its subsequent distribution into the extracellular fluid of the brain. This is an important consideration in regard to the adverse reactions of myelography, since the more severe central nervous system effects appear to correlate with the intracerebral concentration of the injected medium. Again, the clinical significance of this potential drug interaction is uncertain; however it should be considered in evaluating the occurrence of unexpected adverse reactions post myelography. Moreover, it represents an additional consideration for ensuring adequate patient hydration both before and after the procedure (see Clinical Considerations).

Contrast Media–Laboratory Test/Diagnostic Procedure Interactions. The parenteral (intravascular, intrathecal) administration of iodinated contrast media can interfere with thyroid function tests based on the quantitation of iodine (i. e., protein-bound iodine, thyroid iodine uptake). Alternate assays of thyroid function should be utilized if testing is requested within 2–3 weeks following myelography with the nonionic media.

Since the water-soluble, nonionic contrast media undergo eventual renal clearance following their subarachnoid administration, they can also interfere with urinalysis. Such examinations should be performed prior to or delayed for at least 2 days following the administration of nonionic, myelographic media. Myelographic contrast media can also produce false elevations of cerebrospinal fluid protein content as determined using the Lowry method (Ericson K, et al, 1983).

CLINICAL CONSIDERATIONS

Clinical Indications. Myelography is currently indicated for the evaluation of a wide variety of neurological and neurosurgical problems where the signs and symptoms are attributed to spinal cord or nerve root involvement resulting from a congenital, traumatic, inflammatory, degenerative, metabolic, or neoplastic condition. The frequency of its use varies greatly from one center to another; two competing considerations being a concern about its invasiveness and safety on one hand versus its ability to outline the details of intraspinal pathology on the other. It is therefore difficult to be dogmatic in setting specific indications for myelography. However, with extensive procedural experience, it is possible to establish certain general principles and to outline specific indications where myelography can be of definite value.

Although advances of the last decade in the areas of water-soluble, nonionic contrast media and high-resolution computed tomography have combined to decrease the problems and improve the diagnostic yield of myelography; it remains that the diagnostic performance of this procedure requires access to the cerebrospinal fluid compartment and the injection of a foreign material, and therefore carries a slight but definite risk. It follows that myelography should not be resorted to as the first diagnostic method undertaken, but rather reserved for those cases where the diagnosis based on the findings of a thorough neurological evaluation and the results of other noninvasive testing needs confirmation, elucidation, or elaboration. Furthermore, every myelography examination should be tailored to address the specific clinical problem at hand. Based on these considerations, Table 4.7 outlines several situations where myelography may be indicated.

As previously discussed (see Pharmacokinetics), water-soluble, nonionic contrast media demonstrate rapid absorption from the subarachnoid space. Therefore, unlike iophendylate (Pantopaque®), there is not a requirement to aspirate these media fol-

Table 4.7 COMMON INDICATIONS FOR MYELOGRAPHY

1. To confirm or rule out an intraspinal lesion in the presence of equivocal clinical or diagnostic findings
2. To exclude the presence of a surgically treatable condition in patients with an inconclusive or atypical presentation and a working diagnosis of a degenerative or demyelinating condition (e. g., amyotrophic lateral sclerosis or multiple sclerosis)
3. To accurately localize the level of herniated disc(s) prior to surgical correction of untreatable lumbar radiculopathy. (It is well known that clinical determination of the level of compression is not entirely reliable and can be misleading)
4. To exclude the presence of a lesion that can mimic the clinical presentation at hand (e. g., some spinal tumors may be clinically misdiagnosed as disc herniation)
5. To accurately determine the location (i. e., extradural, intradural, extramedullary, intramedullary) of an intraspinal lesion relative to the spinal meninges and spinal cord
6. To demonstrate the extent or spread of a known intraspinal lesion
7. To prevent the missed diagnosis of multiple lesions (e. g., multiple spinal tumors or herniated discs)
8. To determine the cause of residual or recurrent symptoms after prior surgery
9. To provide diagnostic confirmation for medicolegal considerations

Table 4.8 COMMON INDICATIONS FOR CT CISTERNOGRAPHY

1. Cerebello-pontine angle (CPA), quadrigeminal, or suprasellar cistern masses
2. Cystic lesions suspected of communicating with the subarachnoid space
3. Empty sella syndrome
4. Suspected cerebrospinal fluid leak, meningocele, or meningoencephalocele
5. Evaluation of normal pressure hydrocephalus

lowing completion of the myelography procedure. By making use of the retained nonionic media, it is possible to perform subsequent (i. e., at 4–6 hours) computed tomography (CT) evaluations of regions of the spinal subarachnoid space in order to corroborate or augment the findings of the conventional myelography study. A major advantage of this approach is that it retains the ability to evaluate large areas of the spine using the conventional procedure and to concentrate on specific areas with CT, thereby combining the attributes of both techniques. Moreover, the performance of CT myelography is often critical in cases of a noncooperative patient, high-grade subarachnoid block, or partial extravasation of the contrast-medium dose. In these situations, the degree of contrast density on conventional films may not be adequate for an accurate interpretation, whereas the increased contrast sensitivity of CT overcomes this problem.

Nonionic contrast medium retained within the subarachnoid space post-myelography can, with proper patient positioning (i. e., table tilted with head down, neck flexed), also permit CT cisternography by providing adequate opacification of the intracranial subarachnoid spaces. This extends the utility of these agents beyond myelography to include several intracranial indications (Table 4.8).

Contrast Media Considerations. For many years, iophendylate (Pantopaque®) was the most widely used contrast medium for myelography due to the lack of a better agent. However, based on multiple advantages related to myelogram quality (Table 4.9) and patient safety, comfort, and convenience (Table 4.10),

myelographic use of water-soluble, nonionic media has almost totally replaced iophendylate. Of the nonionic media currently available for myelography, the second-generation agents, iohexol and iopamidol, are less costly and more convenient to use than metrizamide (see Chemistry) and are associated with a reduced

Table 4.9 ADVANTAGES OF WATER-SOLUBLE, NONIONIC CONTRAST MEDIA VERSUS IOPHENDYLATE (PANTOPAQUE®) IN REGARD TO IMPROVED MYELOGRAM QUALITY

1. Nonionic media distribute uniformly in the subarachnoid space as a single, continuous radiopaque column.
2. Nonionic media demonstrate better penetration into the narrow regions and crevices (e. g., nerve root sleeves) of the subarachnoid space.
3. Decreased radiodensity (initially or with time) of nonionic media avoids masking of small lesions and provides unobscured demonstration of fine details (Figure 4.11).
4. Significantly more rapid absorption of nonionic media from sites of epidural or subdural extravasation (Figure 4.12) permits acceptable completion of respective study without requirement for repeat examination at later date.

Table 4.10 ADVANTAGES OF WATER-SOLUBLE, NONIONIC CONTRAST MEDIA VERSUS IOPHENDYLATE (PANTOPAQUE®) IN REGARD TO INCREASED PATIENT SAFETY, COMFORT, AND CONVENIENCE

1. Risk of acute or chronic arachnoiditis is significantly lower with nonionic media.
2. Inadvertent intravascular administration of nonionic media does not pose embolic risk.
   - Administration of nonionic media is not contraindicated in the presence of bloody cerebrospinal fluid (e. g., post trauma)
3. Nonionic media demonstrate rapid absorption from subarachnoid space thereby obviating the requirement for postmyelography contrast aspiration (i. e., as with iophendylate).
   - Reduces potential for complications associated with second puncture or aspiration procedure.
   - Ability to remove needle immediately after injection facilitates subsequent patient positioning.
   - Permits performance of myelography in cases of severe spinal stenosis or adhesive arachnoiditis with "dry tap."
   - Retained nonionic media permits subsequent performance of computed tomography evaluations of spinal or cisternal subarachnoid space.
4. Lower viscosity of nonionic media allows use of small-bore needles (e. g., 20 or 22 gauge) for subarachnoid puncture.
   - Results in less trauma to meninges and pain.
   - Reduces the potential for CSF leakage from puncture site.
5. Free or facilitated (e. g., saline push) diffusion of nonionic media around all but total blocks of the subarachnoid space eliminates requirement for reinjection of contrast at puncture site cephalad to region of blockage (Figures 4.13, 4.14).

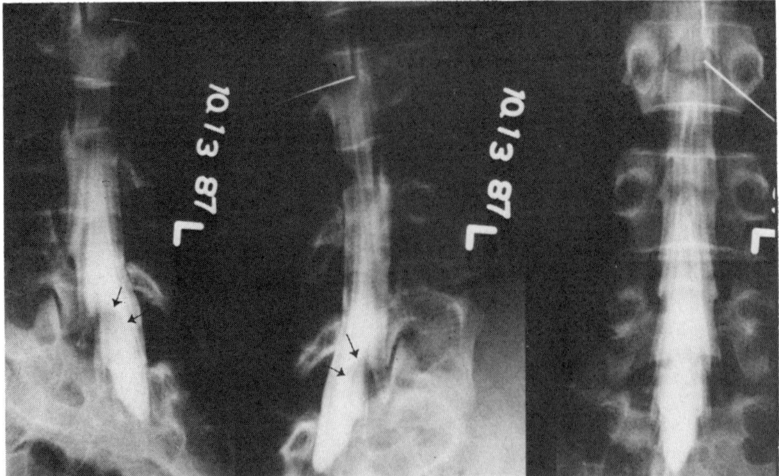

A

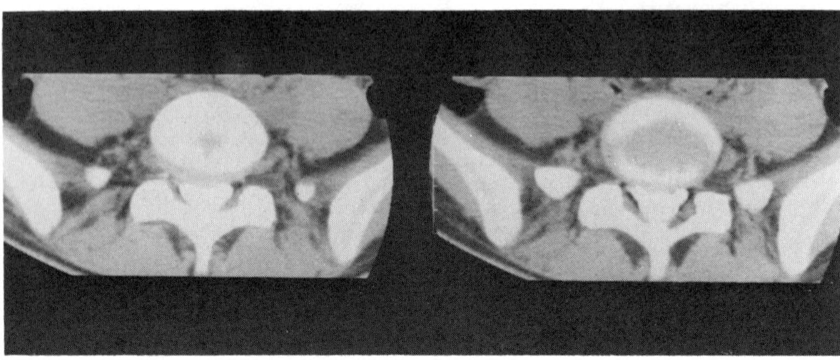

B

Figure 4.11 A. Oblique and frontal myelograms obtained on a patient with central herniation of the L5-S1 disc following the lumbar subarachnoid administration of a water-soluble, nonionic contrast medium. Note (arrows) the extradural impressions on the oblique projections which may have been obliterated by the high density of iophendylate (Pantopaque®). B. Postmyelogram computed tomography confirms the diagnosis of a centrally herniated L5-S1 disc.

number and intensity of undesirable neurological effects (see Physiological Effects).

Pre-myelography Patient Preparation. Solid foods should be withheld from the patient on the day of the scheduled examination. However, patients should be well hydrated, oral liquids being permitted and encouraged until up to the time of the procedure. It has been shown clinically that dehydration can result in an increase in the incidence and severity of side effects to myelography (Eldevik OP, et al, 1980). Apparently, dehydration causes a decrease in the rate of cerebrospinal fluid formation and an increase in the volume of the subarachnoid space (i. e., due to brain shrinkage); both processes leading to a decrease in the normal cerebrospinal fluid–venous pressure difference. This factor decreases the rate of contrast-medium absorption from the subarachnoid space, and increases and prolongs its central nervous system exposure.

Patients who have previously experienced a major reaction to an iodinated contrast medium should be pretreated

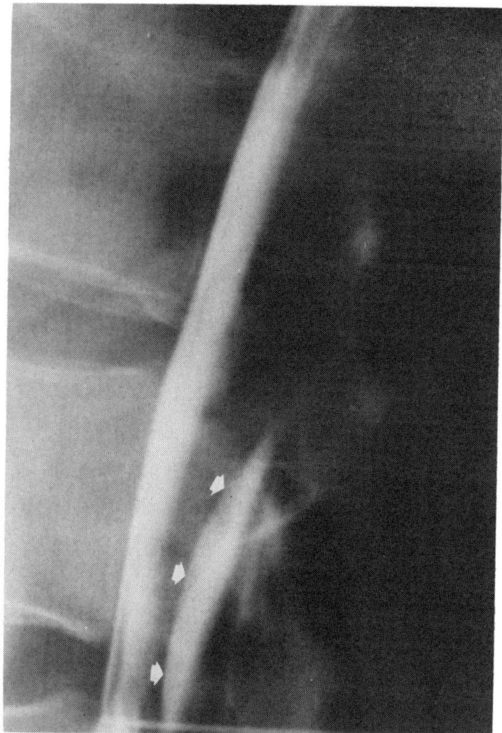

Figure 4.12. Myelogram demonstrating (arrows) partial extra-arachnoid, subdural extravasation of a water-soluble, nonionic contrast medium.

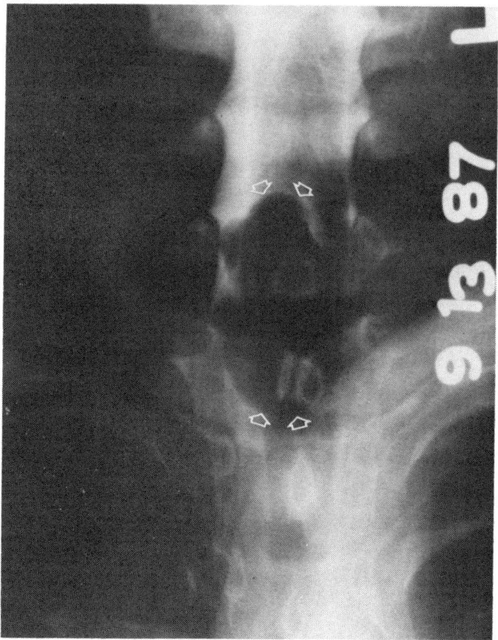

Figure 4.13 Single lumbar subarachnoid administration of a water-soluble, nonionic contrast medium permits myelographic delineation (arrows) of both the upper and lower borders of an intradural, extramedurally mass lesion.

with an appropriate corticosteroid-antihistamine regimen (see Chapter 8). Pretreatment with atropine may also be considered to prevent vasovagal-mediated cardiovascular reactions occasionally observed during myelographic procedures (McCormick CC, et al, 1981).

Post-myelography Patient Care. The patient should be placed in a semi-upright position (30°–45° angle) for the first 8 hours post myelography so as to limit cranial migration of the subarachnoid

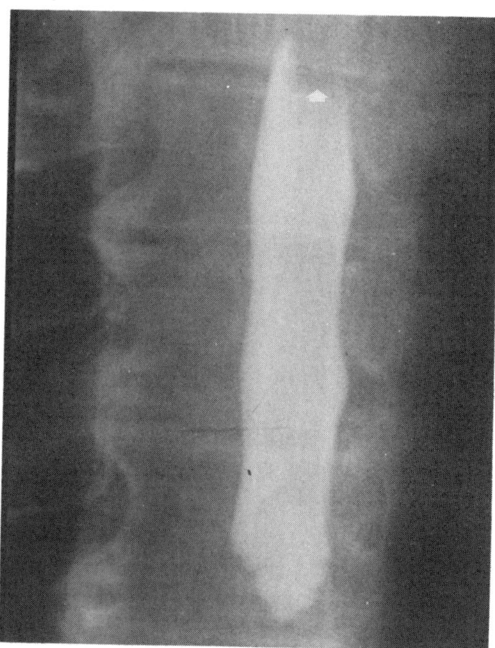

Figure 4.14 Single lumbar subarachnoid injection of iophendylate (Pantopaque®) demonstrates (arrow) only the lower border of a complete extradural block in the thoracic region. Visualization of the total extent of the block (i.e., upper border) requires a second puncture and injection of contrast at C1-C2 level.

nonionic contrast medium and reduce the potential for adverse reactions (see Physiological Effects). After 8 hours, the patient may assume a recumbent position, if desired. A full 24 hours of bed rest is recommended.

Fluid intake should be encouraged to minimize the side effects of myelography. In the absence of nausea and vomiting, the patient's previous diet may be resumed. Bathroom privileges can be permitted at 8 hours following the procedure; however, the patient should be cautioned against bending over, straining during bowel movements, or coughing and belching.

The single-dose administration of a phenothiazine antiemetic agent may be required to alleviate *severe* and *potentially harmful* nausea and vomiting post myelography. Such use of phenothiazine derivative probably represents a minimal increase in risk to the patient especially with the less neurotoxic, second-generation nonionic media. Postmyelography administration of phenothiazine antiemetics should not be routinely given for relatively mild nausea or vomiting and definitely avoided if concomitant behavioral disturbances are present. Nonphenothiazine antiemetics (i. e., cyclizine, buclizine, meclizine, trimethobenzamide) may be attempted; however, these agents are generally minimally effective or may also possess seizure activity (e. g., trimethobenzamide). Parenteral benzquinamide (Emete-Con®) does appear to be effective for the control of mild nausea and vomiting in the inpatient setting, but this agent is not available in an oral dosage form. Metoclopramide does not appear to lower the seizure threshold and has been used at high dosage levels (i. e., 1–2 mg/kg) to prevent nausea and vomiting associated with chemotherapy. However, its use (i. e., 20 mg IV at 30 min. pre and 3, 7, and 12 hours post myelography) as an antiemetic for myelography is of questionable effectiveness (Goldsmith TL, et al, 1987).

Postmyelography convulsive activity may be ameliorated with diazepam or phenobarbitol. The latter agent should also be considered for anesthesia or for pretreatment of patients (i. e., epileptics, multiple sclerosis, psychiatric disorders) predisposed to central nervous system excitation (Gonsette RE and Bracher JM, 1977).

Contraindications. Myelography procedures, in general, are contraindicated in the presence of systemic infections or bacteremia. The subarachnoid administration of the water-soluble, nonionic contrast media should be performed with caution in patients with a history of epilepsy, psychiatric disorders, multiple sclerosis, and drug or alcohol abuse. Epileptic or psychiatric patients should be maintained on their respective therapeutic regimens if myelography remains indicated.

DOSAGE

Subarachnoid Puncture Considerations. The introduction of a myelographic contrast medium into the subarachnoid space is commonly achieved via a lumbar or high cervical (i. e., C_1 or C_2) puncture. The cisternal route has been almost totally replaced by the easier and safer cervical approach. As previously mentioned, myelography procedures, including selection of the puncture site, should be tailored to the clinical problem at hand. Therefore, myelography performed for a suspected herniated lumbar disc would typically incorporate a lumbar puncture at the appropriate level unless this procedure is contraindicated or difficult to accomplish (Table 4.11). On the other hand, myelography performed for cervical myelopathy or radiculopathy may employ either the lumbar or cervical route with equally good results in most cases. However, if hyperextension of the neck is contraindicated (e. g., trauma cases) or impractical (e. g., kyphotic deformity of the cervical spine), the C_1-C_2 puncture may offer distinct advantages to the lumbar approach. Table 4.11 lists several additional indications for cervical puncture. If performed, familiarity with the

Table 4.11 INDICATIONS FOR EMPLOYING A HIGH CERVICAL (C$_1$-C$_2$) PUNCTURE SITE FOR MYELOGRAPHIC CONTRAST MEDIUM ADMINISTRATION

1. Known or suspected cervical myelopathy and/or radiculopathy
2. Determinations of the upper level of a spinal subarachnoid block (especially if level of block delineated by prior lumbar injection does not correlate with clinical level, thus suggesting the presence of a second or higher lesion)
3. When lumbar puncture is contraindicated, for example:
   · Skin infection in lumbar area
   · Suspected mass lesion involving the cauda equina
   · Recent lumbar puncture (i. e., within 5–7 days)
4. When lumbar puncture is difficult or impossible to accomplish, for example:
   · Severe scoliosis
   · Severe degenerative disease
   · Lumbar spinal stenosis
   · Adhesive arachnoiditis
   · Extreme obesity

procedure is essential. Biplane fluoroscopy to guide needle introduction is especially helpful, otherwise a C-arm configuration or repeated-check radiographs are required. High cervical (i. e., C$_1$-C$_2$) puncture is contraindicated in the presence of respective skin infections or known or suspected high cervical cord or craniovertebral junction lesions (e. g., tumors or tonsilar herniation).

Puncture of the spinal canal and the introduction of contrast media must be performed with extreme aseptic precautions since the subarachnoid space is extremely sensitive to the introduction of bacteria and pyrogens. Moreover, as a result of the blood-brain barrier, meningeal infections and inflammation are extremely difficult to treat systemically. Delayed onset reactions resembling aseptic meningitis have been reported as rare occurrences following myelography with the nonionic contrast media. Although these reactions may be due to some chemotoxic property of the injected agent, they are usually effectively treated with systemic steroids; thus suggesting an immune mechanism (Weissman BM, 1984). Other factors that may be responsible for these delayed meningitis reactions include the inadvertent introduction of glove powder, contrast medium particulates, and rubber chemicals or allergens (Siegle RS, et al, 1982).

Contrast Medium Dosage. The volume and iodine concentration of the water-soluble, nonionic contrast medium used for myelography depend on the type of study (e. g., lumbar, thoracic, cervical, total columnar) being performed, the puncture site location, and the specific clinical indication at hand. Table 4.12 outlines recommended adult dosages for various myelographic procedures and routes of injection. However, as a general rule, the most appropriate dosage is the minimum volume and iodine concentration required for adequate opacification. With lumbar administration, the total iodine dose should not exceed 3 g; and with high cervical instillation, the total iodine dose should be limited to approximately 2 g, or less. The use of lower dosages should be considered in the presence of adhesive arachnoiditis and spinal stenosis. In cases of suspected spinal block, a small volume of the contrast medium may be injected first and advanced to the presumed level,

Table 4.12 RECOMMENDED DOSAGES OF WATER-SOLUBLE, NONIONIC CONTRAST MEDIA FOR VARIOUS MYELOGRAPHIC PROCEDURES

	LUMBAR PUNCTURE		CERVICAL PUNCTURE	
MYELOGRAPHIC STUDY	Volume[a] (mL)	Iodine Conc. (mg I/mL)	Volume[a] (mL)	Iodine Conc. (mg I/mL)
Lumbar	10–15	180–200	—	—
Thoracic	10–15	200–240	—	—
Cervical	10	240–300	8–10	200–240
Total columnar	10–12	240–300	—	—

[a] Adult dosage. Pediatric dosage incorporates volumes of 20–30% (age <3 years), 40–50% (3–7 years), 60–70% (8–12 years), and 80–90% (13–18 years) adult dosage at equivalent iodine concentrations.

followed by administration of the remaining volume.

Regardless of the nature of the myelography study or the administration site, it is important that the contrast medium be injected slowly over 1–2 minutes to avoid excessive mixing and dilution in the cerebrospinal fluid. Similarly, positioning of the radiopaque column by tilting the examination table and patient manipulation should be performed slowly under fluoroscopic control in an attempt to maintain the contrast bolus. Patients should be advised against active or abrupt movements. To prevent intracranial entry of the contrast medium, excessive cephalad tilting of the examination table should be avoided and the patient's head maintained at a higher elevation than the spine via hyperextension of the neck.

With appropriate dosage and technique, an adequate level of subarachnoid opacification for conventional myelography should persist for up to 30–60 minutes. As a result of its substantially greater contrast sensitivity, postmyelography CT examination of the spinal column should be delayed for approximately 4 hours to permit subarachnoid dilution and clearance of excessive contrast. If subarachnoid instillation of a nonionic contrast medium is performed specifically for CT myelography, a smaller volume (e. g., approximately 50% of conventional procedure recommendations) of a low iodine concentration (e. g., 180–200 mg iodine/ml) should be utilized with scanning performed within 4 hours. For CT cisternography, 4–6 ml (3–5 ml pediatric dose) of a water-soluble, nonionic contrast medium containing 180–200 mg iodine/mL is injected via lumbar puncture and permitted to migrate intracranially as facilitated by cephalad tilting of the examination table and patient positioning.

IOTROL

Iotrol is a highly water-soluble, nonionic dimer (Figure 4.15) currently under investigation for use as a myelographic contrast medium. Based on its iodine atom-to-osmotic particle ratio of 6 (i. e., ratio-6 medium) and molecular iodine concentration of 46.8%, iotrol can be formulated so as to contain up to 300 mg iodine/mL while remaining virtually isoosmotic (360 mOsm/kg) with the cerebrospinal fluid. At the iodine concentrations (i. e., 180–300 mg iodine/mL) routinely used for myelography procedures, the current ratio-3 nonionic media (e. g., iohexol, iopamidol, metrizamide) are each hyperosmolar relative to the cerebrospinal fluid.

Following subarachnoid administration, iotrol readily mixes with the cerebrospinal fluid. Its rate of absorption from the subarachnoid space and systemic clearance is similar to that of the ratio-3 nonionic agents (Skutta T, et al, 1983). Excretion occurs almost exclusively by glomerular filtration with no demonstrated metabolism. Some variability may exist in regard to the differential distribution of myelographic media within the cerebrospinal fluid compartment. Iotrol has demonstrated less penetration into the central nervous system and substantially less persistence in the gray matter than metrizamide. Its gray matter persistence is also less than iopamidol, but equivalent to iohexol (Kerber CW, et al, 1983; Hammer B and Deisenhammer E, 1985). Since the incidence and severity of certain of the adverse effects (e. g., depression, excitation, seizures) of myelography appear to be related to the degree and duration of central nervous system exposure to the injected contrast medium, these pharmacokinetic characteristics of iotrol may prove advantageous.

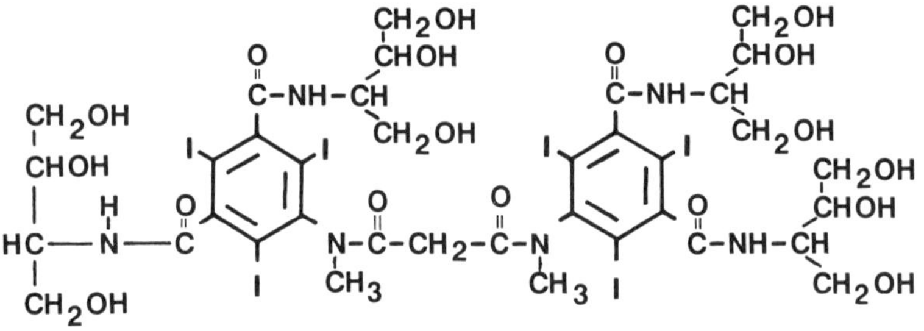

Figure 4.15 Chemical structure of iotrol.

As previously discussed (see Physiological Effects), the depressive effects of myelographic contrast media on the central nervous system appear to occur as a result of their hyperosmolar nature, whereas excitatory effects are related to direct molecular toxicity. As might be expected, isotonic iotrol has been experimentally shown to produce less EEG and behavorial evidence of central nervous system depression than equiiodine doses of iohexol, iopamidol, or metrizamide (Caille J-M, 1983; Sovak M, et al, 1984). In animal studies, it has also been shown to elicit less excitatory potential than iohexol (Sovak M, et al, 1984), the least neurotoxic of the current ratio-3 nonionic media. Preliminary clinical studies have shown that iotrol produces fewer adverse effects than metrizamide (Hammer B and Deisenhammer E, 1985; Malnor MO, et al, 1986). Whether this ratio-6 myelographic medium will demonstrate significant clinical advantages over the second-generation nonionic media, iohexol and iopamidol, remains in question (Hammer B and Deisenhammer E, 1985).

References

Ahlgren P. Early and late side effects of water-soluble contrast media for myelography and cisternography: A short review. *Invest Radiol* 1980, 15 (Suppl.): S264–S266.

Almén T. Contrast agent design. *J Theor Biol* 1969, 24:216–226.

Almén T. Experience from 10 years of development of water-soluble nonionic contrast media. *Invest Radiol* 1980, 15 (Suppl.): S283–S288.

Amundsen P. Water-soluble myelographic agents. In *Radiographic Contrast Agents* (Miller RE and Skucas J, eds.) Baltimore, University Park Press, 1977, pp. 437–448.

Batnitsky S. Negative contrast myelographic agents. In *Radiographic Contrast Agents* (Miller RE and Skucas J, eds.) Baltimore, University Park Press, 1977a, pp. 419–427.

Batnitsky S. Positive contrast myelography: Water-soluble iodinated organic agents. In *Radiographic Contrast Agents* (Miller RE and Skucas, J, eds.) Baltimore, University Park Press, 1977b, pp. 429–436.

Bertoni JM, Schwartzman RJ, VanHorn G, et al. Asterixis and encephalography following metrizamide myelography. Investigations into possible mechanisms and review of the literature. *Ann Neurol* 1981, 9:366–370.

Bertoni JM, Steinman CG. Competitive inhibition of brain hexokinase by metrizamide. *Neurology* 1982, 32:320–323.

Broadbridge AT, Bayliss SG, Brayshaw CI. The effect of intrathecal iohexol on visual evoked response latency: A comparison including incidence of headache with iopamidol and metrizamide in myeloradiculography. *Clin Radiol* 1987, 38:71–74.

Burton CV. Lumbosacral arachnoiditis. *Spine* 1978, 3:24–30.

Caille J-M, Gious M, Arne P, et al. Neurotoxicity of nonionic iodinated water-soluble contrast media in myelography: Experimental study. *AJNR* 1983, 4:1185–1189.

Chrzanowski R. The contrast media used for myelography. *Eur Neurol* 1982, 21:194–197.

Dandy WE. Roentgenography of the brain after the injection of air into the spinal canal. *Ann Surg* 1919, 70:397–400.

Dawson P. New contrast agents. Chemistry and pharmacology. *Invest Radiol* 1984, 19 (Suppl.): S298–S300.

Dawson P. Chemistry of contrast media and clinical adverse effects. A review. *Invest Radiol* 1985, 20 (Suppl.): S84–S92.

DeVilliers PD, Snyman PJNH, VanRensburg MNJ, et al. Iopamidol for myelography—practical implications. *SA Med J* 1984, 66:697–698.

Drayer BP, Allen S, Vassallo C, et al. Comparative safety of intrathecal iopamidol vs. metrizamide for myelography and cisternography. *Invest Radiol* 1984, 19 (Suppl.): S259–S267.

Ekholm SE, Reece K, Coleman JR, et al. Metrizamide—a potential in vivo inhibitor of glucose metabolism. *Radiology* 1983, 147:119–121.

Ekholm SE. Iohexol versus metrizamide in studies of glucose metabolism. A survey. *Invest Radiol* 1985, 20:518–521.

Ekholm SE, Morris TW, Fonte D, et al. Iopamidol and neural tissue metabolism. A comparative in vitro study. *Invest Radiol* 1986, 21:798–801.

Eldevik OP, Haughton VM, Sasse EA. The effect of dehydration on the elimination of aqueous contrast media from the subarachnoid space. *Invest Radiol* 1980, 15:155–157.

Ericson K, Hindmarsh T, Hannez J. Experience with iohexol in lumbar myelography. *Acta Radiol Diag* 1983, 24:503–505.

Galle G, Huk W, Arnold K. Psychopathometric demonstration and quantification of mental disturbances following myelography with metrizamide and iopamidol. *Neuroradiol* 1984, 26:229–233.

Gjerris A, Praestholm J, Klinken L. Comparison of metrizamide and iodophendylate for cerebral ventriculography. *Neuroradiol* 1978, 15:79–84.

Goldsmith TL, Norton JA, Young AB, et al. Safety and antiemetic effects of metoclopramide in metrizamide myelography. *Clin Pharm* 1987, 6:807–810.

Golman K. Absorption of metrizamide from cerebrospinal fluid to blood: Pharmacokinetics in humans. *J. Pharm Sci* 1975, 64:405–407.

Golman K, Olivecrona H, Gustafson C, et al. Excitation and depression of nonanesthetized rabbits following injection of contrast media into the subarachnoid space. *Acta Radiol* 1980, 362 (Suppl.): 83–86.

Gonsette RE, Bracher JM. Potentiation of Amipaque. *Neuroradiol* 1977, 14:27–30.

Grepe A, Widen L. Neurotoxic effect of intracranial subarachnoid application of metrizamide and meglumine iocarmate. An experimental investigation in dogs in neurol-analgesia. *Acta Radiol* 1973, 335 (Suppl.): 102.

Hamilton G, Fischer HW. (reply) Re: Contamination of contrast agents by rubber components of 50 ml disposal syringes. *AJR*, 1984, 143:199–200.

Hammer B, Deisenhammer E. Iotrol, a new water-soluble non-ionic dimeric contrast medium for intrathecal use. *Neuroradiology* 1985, 27:337–341.

Hanus PM. Metrizamide: A review with emphasis on drug interactions. *Am J Hosp Pharm* 1980, 37:510–513.

Hauge O, Falkenberg H. Neuropsychologic reactions and other side effects after metrizamide myelography. *AJR*, 1982, 139:357–360.

Haughton VM, Ho K-C, Unger GF. Arachnoiditis following myelography with water-soluble agents. *Radiology*, 1977, 125:731–733.

Haughton VM, Ho K-C. Arachnoid response to contrast media: A comparison of iophendylate and metrizamide in experimental animals. *Radiology* 1982a, 143:699–702.

Haughton VM, Ho K-C, Lipman BT Experimental study of arachnoiditis from iohexol, an investigational non-ionic aqueous contrast medium. *AJNR* 1982b, 3:375–377.

Hilal SK, Dauth GW, Hess KH, et al. Development and evaluation of a new water-soluble iodinated myelographic contrast medium with markedly reduced convulsive effects. *Radiology* 1978, 126:417–422.

Hindmarsh T. Elimination of water-soluble contrast media from the subarachnoid space. *Acta Radiol* 1975a, 346 (Suppl.): 45–50.

Hindmarsh T, Grepe A, Widen L. Metrizamide-phenothiazine interaction. *Acta Radiol Diag* 1975b, 16:129–133.

Jacobaeus HC. On insufflation of air into the spinal canal for diagnostic purposes in cases of tumors in the spinal canal. *Acta Med Scand* 1921, 55:555–564.

Kaufman P, Jeans WD. Reactions to iophendylate in relation to multiple sclerosis. *Lancet*, 1976, 2:1000.

Kerber CW, Sovak M, Ranganathan RS, et al. Iotrol, a new myelographic agent. Radiography, CT, CSF clearance, and brain penetration. *AJNR* 1983, 4:317–318.

Kieffer SA, Binet EF, Esquerra JV, et al. Contrast agents for myelography:

Clinical and radiological evaluation of Amipaque and Pantopaque. *Radiology* 1978, 129:695–705.

Legre J, Lauieille J, Debaene A, et al. Prevention of adverse reactions to Amipaque in cervical myelography. *J Neuroradiol* 1981, 8:353–361.

Macpherson P, Teasdale E, Coutinho MB, et al. Iohexol versus iopamidol for cervical myelography: A randomized double-blind study. *Br J Radiol* 1985, 58:849–851.

Malnor MD, Houston LW, Strother CM, et al. Iotrol versus metrizamide in lumbar myelography. A double-blind study. *Radiology* 1986, 158:845–847.

Maly P, Almén T, Golman K, et al. Excitative effects in anesthetized rabbits from subarachnoidally injected iso- and hyperosmolar solutions of iohexol and metrizamide. *Neuroradiol* 1984a, 26:131–136.

Maly P, Olivecrona H, Almén T, et al. Interaction between chlorpromazine and intrathecally injected non-ionic contrast media in non-anesthetized rabbits. *Neuroradiol* 1984b, 26:235–240.

Maly P, Elmquist D, Almén T, et al. Comparison between EEG and observation of animal behavior in evaluation of subarachnoid neurotoxicity of metrizamide. *Acta Radiol Diag* 1986, 27:235–240.

Mamourian AC, Briggs RW. Appearance of Pantopaque on MR images. *Radiology* 1986, 158:457–460.

Marder E, O'Neill M, Grossman RI, et al. Cholinergic actions of metrizamide *AJNR* 1983, 4:61–65.

Marshall TR, Ling JT, Follis G, et al. Pharmacological incompatability of contrast media with various drugs and agents. *Radiology* 1965, 84:536–539.

McCormick CC, ApSimon HT, Chakera TMH. Myelography with metrizamide: An analysis of the complications encountered in cervical, thoracic, and lumbar myelography. *Aust NE J Med*, 1981, 11:645–650.

Meador K, Hamilton WJ, Taher AM, et al. Irreversible neurologic complications of metrizamide myelography. *Neurology* 1984, 34:817–821.

Nakstad P, Helgetveit A, Aaserud O, et al. Iohexol compared to metrizamide in cervical and thoracic myelography. *Neuroradiol* 1984, 26:479–484.

Nau H-E. Electroencephalography (EEG) after introduction of water-soluble contrast media into cerebral spinal fluid (CSF). *Acta Neurochir* 1981, 57:75–82.

Nickle AR, Salem JJ. Clinical experience in North America with metrizamide. *Acta Radiol* 1977, 355 (Suppl.): 409–416.

Potts DG, Gomez DG, Shaw DD. Cranial and spinal cerebrospinal fluid absorption and the clearance of water-soluble myelographic contrast media. *Invest Radiol* 1985, 20 (Suppl.): S51–S54.

Pyles ST, Pashayan AG: Anesthesia and neuroradiology: Considerations regarding metrizamide, *Anesthesiology* 1983; 58:590–591.

Ramsey GH, French JD, Strain WH. Iodinated organic compounds as contrast media for radiographic diagnosis. IV. Pantopaque myelography. *Radiology* 1944, 43:236–240.

Richert S, Sartor K, Holl B. Subclinical organic psychosyndromes on intrathecal injection of metrizamide for lumbar myelography. *Neuroradial* 1979, 18:177–184.

Sage MR. Kinetics of water-soluble contrast media in the central nervous system. *AJR* 1983a, 141:815–824.

Sage MR, Wilcox J. Brain parenchyma penetration by intrathecal nonionic iopamidol. *AJR* 1983b, 4:1181–1183.

Shaw DD, Potts DG. Toxicology of iohexol. *Invest Radiol* 1985, 20 (Suppl.): S10–S13.

Sicard JA, Forestier JE. Methode generale d'exploration radiologique par l'huile iodee (Lipiodol). *Bull Soc Med Hp* Paris, 1922, 46:463–468.

Siegel RS, Williams AG, Waterman RE. Potential complications in myelography: I. Technical considerations. *AJR* 1982, 138:705–708.

Skalpe IO. Adverse effects of water-soluble contrast media in myelography, cisternography, and ventriculography. *Acta Radiol* 1977, 355 (Suppl.): 359–370.

Skutta T, Vogelsang H, Galanski M, et al. Clinical trial of iotrol for lumbar myelography. *AJNR* 1983, 4:302–303.

Sovak M. Contrast media for imaging of the central nervous system. In *Radiocontrast Agents* (Sovak, M., ed.). New York, Springer-Verlag, 1984, pp. 295–340.

Sovak M, Ranganathan R, Hammer B. Early experience with iotrol, a nonionic isotonic dimer for intrathecal space. *Invest Radiol* 1984, 19 (Suppl.): S140.

Standes B, Oftedal SI, Weber H. Effect of levomepromazine on EEG and on clinical side effects after lumbar myelography with metrizamide. *Acta Radiol Diag* 1982, 23:111–113.

Steinhausen TB, Dungan CE, Furst JB, et al. Iodinated organic compounds as contrast media for radiographic diagnoses. III. Experimental and clinical myelography with ethyl iodophenylundecylate (Pantopaque). *Radiology* 1944, 43:230–235.

Thevenin P. First European seminar: Contrast media in radiology. *Neuroradiol* 1983, 24:133–137.

Tourtellotte WW, Henderson WG, Tucker RP, et al. A randomized, double-blind clinical trial comparing the 22 versus 26 gauge needle in the production of the post-lumbar puncture syndrome in normal individuals. *Headache* 1972, 12:73–78.

Weissman BM. Delayed onset of dexamethasone dependent cerebral dysfunction following metrizamide myelography. *Arch Neurol* 1984, 41:569–570.

White AG. Prolonged elevation of serum protein-bound iodine following myelography with Myodil. *Br J Radiol* 1972, 45:21.

Gastrointestinal Contrast Media: Barium Sulfate and Water-Soluble Iodinated Agents

Dennis P. Swanson
Robert D. Halpert

Radiological examinations of the alimentary tract are indicated for a variety of gastrointestinal conditions, including digestive disorders, distinct changes in bowel habit, abdominal pain, and gastrointestinal bleeding. These procedures are generally classified according to the gastrointestinal segment or segments being evaluated and require the administration of a radiopaque contrast medium to permit adequate delineation of the respective lumen or mucosal surface from surrounding soft tissues. Hence, barium sulfate or iodinated contrast media are administered orally to evaluate abnormalities of the mouth, pharynx, and esophagus (i.e., esophagram); and the stomach, duodenum, and proximal small intestine (i.e., upper gastrointestinal examination). These contrast media are also administered rectally for retrograde examinations of the colon and distal small intestine (i.e., lower gastrointestinal examination). A specific, antegrade examination of the small intestine may also be performed following ingestion (small bowel follow-through) or the direct-infusion of these contrast media into the distal duodenum via an intubation tube (i.e., small bowel enteroclysis).

I. Barium Sulfate

Soon after the discovery and introduction of roentgen diagnostic techniques, it became apparent that administration of a radiopaque contrast medium was often required to permit the delineation and differentiation of soft tissue structures. Early studies centered on the oral administration of encapsulated iron, bismuth, and lead solutions for evaluations of the esophagus and stomach, (Miller RE and Skucas J, 1977a). Subsequent gastrointestinal radiology studies primarily utilized oral bismuth subnitrate or subcarbonate suspensions or meals (e.g., bismuth subnitrate or subcarbonate mixed with bread or gruel) due to the availability of these nontoxic, insoluble compounds in a relatively purified form and their high degree of x-ray attenuation. In 1910, Bachem and Gunter proposed the routine use of barium sulfate suspensions for radiographic examinations of the gastrointestinal tract (Bachem C and Gunther H 1910). This radiopaque, insoluble compound of barium was less expensive to manufacture than bismuth subnitrate or subcarbonate. Moreover, it could be purified to a high degree, and was not associated with the production of toxic metabolites as were the bismuth preparations (Miller RE and Skucas J, 1977a).

Barium sulfate contrast media continue to be the preferred agents for opacification of the gastrointestinal tract. Depending on the patient's history and suspected clinical problem, gastrointestinal radiology examinations using barium sulfate may be performed following its oral or rectal administration and using either a single-contrast or double-contrast technique. In a single-contrast examination, a large volume of low-density barium sulfate preparation is administered to produce full-column opacification and distension of the segmental lumen under investigation. A double-contrast examination involves the administration of a relatively small volume of a barium sulfate preparation of high density and low viscosity for the purpose of coating the mucosal surface of the area being studied. Distension of the lumen is achieved with a gas (i. e., negative-contrast agent), resulting in specific mucosal opacification and delineation of fine surface detail.

The product-selection criteria, advantages, disadvantages, and indications for the single- versus double-contrast technique will be discussed in greater detail under Clinical Considerations; however, this brief introduction clearly indicates that no one single barium sulfate formulation can totally satisfy the requirements of gastrointestinal radiology. Furthermore, the pH of the gastrointestinal tract can vary between 1 and 8.5 with distinct regional differences in the chemical composition of the intestinal fluid. Hence, a particular barium sulfate formulation that demonstrates good single- or double-contrast characteristics in one region of the gastrointestinal tract may be inappropriate for use in a different region (Ott DJ and Gelfand DW, 1982).

Several preparations of barium sulfate are currently available from commercial manufacturers (see Tables 5.1–5.5).

Table 5.1 SELECTED BARIUM SULFATE CONTRAST MEDIA FOR SINGLE-CONTRAST EXAMINATIONS: UPPER AND/OR LOWER GASTROINTESTINAL TRACT

BRAND NAME®	MANUFACTURER	AVAILABLE FORM(S)[a]	POWDER CONCENTRATION (% w/w)	SUSPENSION (% w/v)	CONCENTRATION (% w/w)
Barotrast	Armour	BP	92.5		
E-Z-Paque	E-Z-EM	BP, UP	95		
Polibar	E-Z-EM	BP, UP	96		
Sol-O-Pake	E-Z-EM	BP, UP	97		
Ultra-R	E-Z-EM	UP	95		
Liquid E-Z-Paque	E-Z-EM	BS		56	37.5
Liquid Polibar	E-Z-EM	BS		100	56
Polibar-Plus	E-Z-EM	BS		105	58
Liquid Sol-O-Pake	E-Z-EM	BS		72	45
Barobag	Lafayette-Pharmacal	UP	98		
Barodense	Lafayette-Pharmacal	BP	97		
Baroloid	Lafayette-Pharmacal	BP	96		
Intropaque	Lafayette-Pharmacal	BP	91		
Tonopaque	Lafayette-Pharmacal	BP, UP	96		
HD-85	Lafayette-Pharmacal	BS, US		85	50
Liquid Intropaque	Lafayette-Pharmacal	BS		60	40
Liquipake	Lafayette-Pharmacal	BS		100	56
Preview	Lafayette-Pharmacal	BS, US		60	40
Barosperse	Mallinckrodt	BP, UP	95		
Micropaque	Picker	BP	92		
Mixture III	Picker	UP	96		
Novopaque	Picker	BS, US		60	40

[a] BP = Bulk powder
UP = Unit dose powder
BS = Bulk/concentrated suspension
US = Unit-dose suspension

Table 5.2 SELECTED BARIUM SULFATE CONTRAST MEDIA FOR ENTEROCLYSIS

BRAND NAME®	MANUFACTURER	AVAILABLE FORM(S)[a]	SUSPENSION (% w/v)	CONCENTRATION (% w/w)
Entero-H	E-Z-EM	BS	80	—
Liquid Polibar	E-Z-EM	BS	100	56
Liquid Sol-O-Pake	E-Z-EM	BS	72	45
Entrobar	Lafayette-Pharmacal	US	50	35.7
EpiStat-57	Mallinckrodt	BS, US	103	57

[a] BS = Bulk/concentrated suspension
US = Unit-dose suspension

Table 5.3   BARIUM SULFATE PASTE FOR ESOPHOGRAM PROCEDURES

| | | CONCENTRATION | |
BRAND NAME[®]	MANUFACTURER	(% w/v)	(% w/w)
Esophatrast	Armour	100	56
E-Z-Paste	E-Z-EM	120	60
Microtrast	Picker	150	70

These products include bulk and unit-dose containers of barium sulfate powder that require reconstitution to the desired or recommended concentration prior to administration, or barium sulfate liquid suspensions in a concentrated form for subsequent dilution or a unit-dose form for direct use. The physical properties of the final formulations of these barium sulfate products can vary considerably in regard to density, viscosity, and regional gastrointestinal stability, these properties being dependent on several factors including the size, uniformity, and concentration of the barium sulfate particles and the nature and concentration of various additives (i.e., suspending agents, dispersing agents, antifoaming agents, etc.) used in

their formulation (Miller RE and Skucas J, 1977b; 1977c).

CHEMISTRY

Purified barium sulfate is a white, radiopaque (atomic number of barium = 56, k-edge = 32 keV), crystalline powder that is practically insoluble in water. Although commercially available barium sulfate contrast media exhibit "colloidal" properties (i.e., resistance to settling and aggregation), they often contain barium sulfate particles with dimensions in the suspension (i.e., > 0.1 micron diameter) rather than colloidal (i.e., 0.001–0.1 micron diameter) size range (Miller RE and Skucas J, 1977b). The colloidal properties of barium sulfate suspensions are conferred by the addition of various surface-active substances that coat the barium sulfate particles. The relative size, shape, and uniformity of the barium sulfate particles within a barium contrast medium play a significant role in regard to its density and stability.

Table 5.4   SELECTED BARIUM SULFATE CONTRAST MEDIA FOR DOUBLE-CONTRAST EXAMINATIONS: UPPER GASTROINTESTINAL TRACT

BRAND NAME[®]	MANUFACTURER	AVAILABLE FORM(S)[a]	POWDER CONCENTRATION (% w/w)
E-Z-HD	E-Z-EM	UP	98
HD-200 Plus	Lafayette-Pharmacal	BP, UP	98
Baricon	Mallinckrodt	BP, UP	95

[a] BP = Bulk powder
UP = Unit-dose powder

Table 5.5   SELECTED BARIUM SULFATE CONTRAST MEDIA FOR DOUBLE-CONTRAST EXAMINATIONS: COLON

BRAND NAME[®]	MANUFACTURER	AVAILABLE FORM(S)[a]	SUSPENSION (% w/v)	CONCENTRATION (% w/w)
E-Z-AC	E-Z-EM	BS	100	56
Polibar Plus	E-Z-EM	BS	105	58
Liquid Polibar	E-Z-EM	BS	100	56
Flow-Coat	Lafayette-Pharmacal	BS	100	56
HD-85	Lafayette-Pharmacal	BS, US	85	50
Hi Tone	Lafayette-Pharmacal	BS	125	62
Liquipake	Lafayette-Pharmacal	BS	100	56
Epi-C	Mallinckrodt	BS	150	70
EpiStat-57	Mallinckrodt	BS, US	103	57
EpiStat-61	Mallinckrodt	BS, US	116	61

[a] BS = Bulk suspension
US = Unit-dose suspension

Concentration. The concentrations of commercially available barium sulfate suspensions are typically expressed in terms of percent by weight (% w/w) and/or percent weight-in-volume (% w/v). Percent by weight signifies the number of grams of barium sulfate per 100 grams of final suspension. Hence, a 60% w/w barium sulfate preparation contains 60 grams of barium sulfate powder added to sufficient water (i. e., 40 grams) to make 100 grams of final suspension. Percent by weight concentrations are also applied frequently to barium sulfate powders. In this context, % w/w refers to the proportion of the total powder weight that is due to pure barium sulfate, the remainder of the weight associated with solid additives. (A 100% w/w barium sulfate preparation represents pure powder with no solute or additives.) Percent weight-in volume indicates the number of grams of barium sulfate per 100 mL of final suspension. In a 60% w/v barium sulfate preparation, 60 grams of barium sulfate are suspended in a sufficient volume of water to make 100 mL of final suspension.

In the radiology literature, the concentration expressions of % w/v and %w/w are often used inappropriately to represent the density of the barium sulfate suspension. The density (g/mL) of a barium sulfate preparation is defined as the mass (grams) represented by a unit volume (mL) of the *final suspension*, as determined at a fixed temperature and pressure. The term *specific gravity* may also be used as an indication of the density of a barium sulfate preparation. Specific gravity, an expression void of units, is-defined as the ratio of the density of the barium sulfate suspension to the density of water; the density values for both substances being determined at the same temperature and pressure. Since the density of water, at room temperature and ambient pressure, is approximately equal to 1g/mL, the specific gravity of a given barium sulfate suspension is approximately equal to its density. The density (and specific gravity) of barium sulfate preparations can be estimated by dividing the % w/v concentration of the agent by its % w/w concentration.

Density. The density of a barium sulfate preparation may also be considered in terms of the proportion of the measured volume that is occupied by barium sulfate particles versus the proportion that is occupied by "voids" (i. e., air, water, additives, or combinations thereof). As might be expected, barium sulfate preparations with a high percentage of "voids" have a relatively low density (Miller RE and Skucas J, 1977b).

The percentage of "voids" and, hence, the density of barium sulfate media are highly dependent on the size and uniformity of the barium sulfate particles in suspension. Particles of a uniform size demonstrate the fewest points of contact and the greatest percentage of "voids." As the particle size decreases, the percentage of "voids" increases further due to the increased surface area provided by the smaller particles and the associated increased surface adsorption of air and water. In summary, the densest barium sulfate preparations comprise large particles of nonuniform size.

The degree of radiopacification produced by a barium sulfate contrast medium is directly proportional to the density of the medium and the total volume of medium within the path of the x-ray beam (i. e., the thickness of the barium sulfate coating or column). Hence, in order to achieve adequate opacification in a double-contrast examination, the barium sulfate preparation that thinly coats the mucosal surface must have a high density. The increased thickness of a full-column, single-contrast examination necessitates the use of a low-density barium sulfate preparation. Use of a barium sulfate medium of excessive density for a single-contrast examination may not permit adequate x-ray penetration of the barium column, resulting in potential obscuring of lesions oriented *en face.*

Viscosity. The viscosity of a barium sulfate contrast medium is a measure of its resistance to flow. Measurements of the viscosity of barium sulfate preparations are usually performed using a Ford cup viscometer wherein the amount of time required for 100 ml of the agent to pass through a 0.4 cm diameter hole is determined (at 37° C). Such measurements of kinematic viscosity reflect the effects of both viscosity and specific gravity and are expressed in seconds; longer flow times indicate greater viscosity.

If only the barium sulfate-related properties are considered, the viscosity of a barium contrast medium is directly dependent on the concentration of barium sulfate in suspension, and inversely proportional to the temperature of the medium (Miller RE and Skucas J, 1977c). Particle size has little influence on viscosity; however, very small particles will lead to an increase in viscosity as a result of their increased surface area and adsorption of air and water. Many barium sulfate contrast media demonstrate thixotropic behavior. This phenomenon is characterized by a marked decrease in viscosity when the medium is agitated or made to flow rapidly. Following the cessation of agitation or rapid flow, the medium will rapidly assume its initial state of increased viscosity.

The viscosity of barium sulfate preparations is also dependent on the concentration, chemical nature (i. e., molecular weight, chain-length, degree of cross-linking), and spacial configuration of surface-active additives used in their formulation (Miller RE and Skucas J, 1977c). Hence, a preparation that incorporates low-molecular-weight sodium citrate as a surface-active agent will have a lower viscosity than a preparation that utilizes a high-molecular-weight, linear colloid additive, such as carboxymethylcellulose. The addition of or exposure to salts or acids can further increase the viscosity of the latter linear colloid formulations by inducing changes in their shape (i. e., coiling) with a resulting increase in their bulkiness.

The viscosity of a barium sulfate contrast medium is an important factor in regard to its stability and suitability for use. Virtually all suspensions of high specific gravity, such as barium sulfate, will settle out with time due to the influence of gravity. Barium sulfate contrast media for single- or double-contrast examinations must be relatively stable against settling in order to provide uniform opacification and to avoid the obscuring of lesions.

The rate of settling of a barium sulfate suspension is dependent on several factors including the concentration of barium sulfate, its particle size, and the viscosity of the medium (Miller RE and Skucas J, 1977b) In general, increasing the concentration of barium sulfate in suspension retards the rate of settling as a result of particle–particle interference. As might be expected, large particles of barium sulfate do exhibit a tendency to settle out at a faster rate than small particles. Finally, the rate of particle settling is slower for barium sulfate formulations of increased viscosity. Based on these brief statements, it is apparent that viscosity is the critical factor in maintaining the stability of both single- and double-contrast barium preparations. As previously discussed, barium sulfate contrast media for single-contrast examinations require a relatively low density (i. e., low barium sulfate concentration), thus increasing their susceptibility to settling. Similarly, the high density of double-contrast barium sulfate preparations is achieved by using nonuniform particles of a large size. The increased tendency of these low barium sulfate concentrations or large particles toward settling is prevented by incorporating adtives to increase the viscosity of the media.

Although the exact reason that certain barium sulfate contrast media demonstrate better coating characteristics for double-contrast examinations is not completely understood, it appears that the viscosity and/or the thixotrophy of the media play a significant role in the extent and degree (i. e., thickness) of film formation. If the viscosity of a preparation is too low, only a very thin coating will be deposited and retained on the mucosal surface, resulting in inadequate opacification

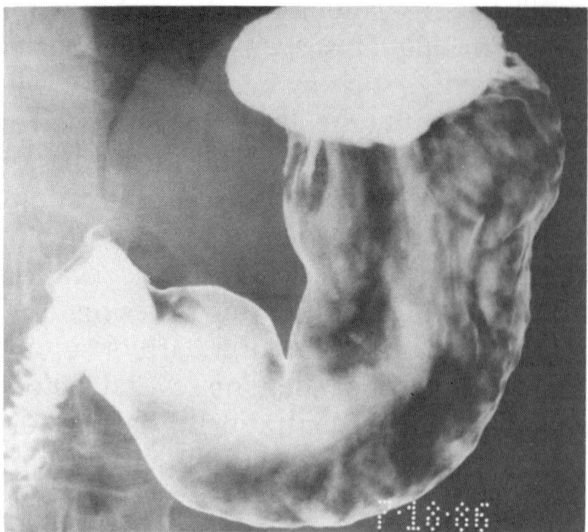

Figure 5.1 The barium film coating of the gastric mucosa is excessive, resulting in the possible obscuring of superficial mucosal lesions.

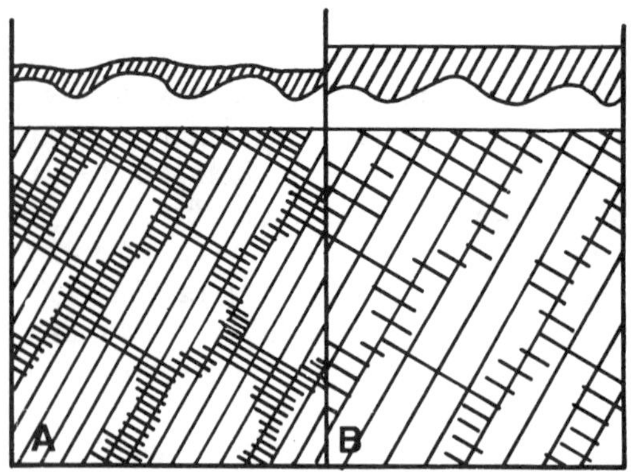

Figure 5.2 Diagram illustrating greater mucosal surface detail obtainable with low-viscosity, high-density barium sulfate suspension. A. Thin coating of low-viscosity, high-density preparation permits radiographic demonstration of surface contours and irregularities. B. Thick coating of high-viscosity, low-density preparation partially obscures structural details, since the depth of contour variations is considerably less·than the coating thickness. (From Gelfand, DW, 1978; with permission.)

and a tendency to "weak spot" formation and rapid film breakdown. Conversely, if the medium is too viscous, it will not flow readily and the mucosa may not be coated completely or uniformly. In addition, if the film deposited on the mucosal surface is too thick, the demonstration of lesions may be masked as a result of excessive opacification (Figure 5.1). Fine irregularities of the mucosal surface may also be obscured if the thick coating produced by a highly viscous preparation cannot readily conform to the surface characteristics (Figure 5.2), or if the flow lines, bubble craters, or defects produced by mucosal contact are unable to level out (Gelfand DW, 1978; Miller RE and Skucas J, 1977c).

Additives. Commercially available barium sulfate preparations incorporate a variety of additives for multiple purposes. In general, these additives include suspending and dispersing agents, antifoam agents, flavoring and coloring agents, and antibacterial preservatives. As previously discussed, the exact chemical nature and concentration of these additives within a given barium sulfate preparation are usually kept secret; however, the reasons for their introduction are relatively standard.

The most important class of additive substances are the suspending and dispersing agents. The stability of colloidal solutions and suspensions is determined by the presence of electrical charges adsorbed on the surface of the suspended particles and by the particles' affinity for the suspending medium. Pure barium sulfate particles suspended in an aqueous medium represent an example of a hydrophobic (i. e., "water-hating") system. As such, the pure barium sulfate particles are stabilized only by their surface adsorption of electrical charges (e. g., hydrogen, hydroxyl, electrolyte ions), resulting in particles with like charges that repel each other to maintain suspension stability. If these charges are neutralized by the addition of substrates of an opposite charge or by a change in pH, the stability of the suspension no longer exists and the barium sulfate particles will coagulate to form large masses that rapidly settle out (Miller RE and Skucas J, 1977b). This chemical process, termed *flocculation*, can deleteriously affect the uniformity of opacification or the coating characteristics of barium sulfate suspensions, resulting in a loss of diagnostic accuracy. Considering the variable electrolyte and pH environment of the gastrointestinal tract, flocculation of barium sulfate preparations can be a problem unless protective, surface-active hydrophilic substances (i. e., protective colloids) are incorporated into their formulations.

With aqueous suspensions of a hydrophilic (i. e., "water-loving") colloid, neutralization of the surface charge does not necessarily result in particle coagulation due to the colloid's affinity for water (i. e., its ability to hydrate). Hydrophobic particles, such as barium sulfate, can be coated with hydrophilic colloids, such as gelatin, albumin, bentonite, dextran, pectin, gum arabic, sodium carboxymethylcellulose, and so on, the resulting surface of the hydrophobic colloid assuming hydrophilic characteristics. Hence, the addition of such surface-active suspending agents protect the barium sulfate suspensions against the flocculating effects of electrolyte or pH changes. In addition, the electrical charges associated with these or additional surface-active substances tend to increase the viscosity of barium sulfate preparations, thus acting as dispersing agents to further increase suspension stability. The coating characteristics (e. g., flow, thickness, film flexibility) are also markedly influenced by the viscosity and hydrating effects of these surface-active additives (Miller RE and Skucas J, 1977c).

Solutions containing surface-active substances, including barium sulfate preparations, can readily form bubbles or foam. The presence of foam or bubbles in a barium sulfate contrast medium is an undesirable property that can result in lesion-resembling artifacts, coating irregularities, or "weak spot" formation and rapid film breakdown (Figure 5.3). It should be noted that the formation and stability of bubbles or foam in double-contrast examinations is primarily dependent on the type of barium sulfate utilized and not on the nature of the negative-

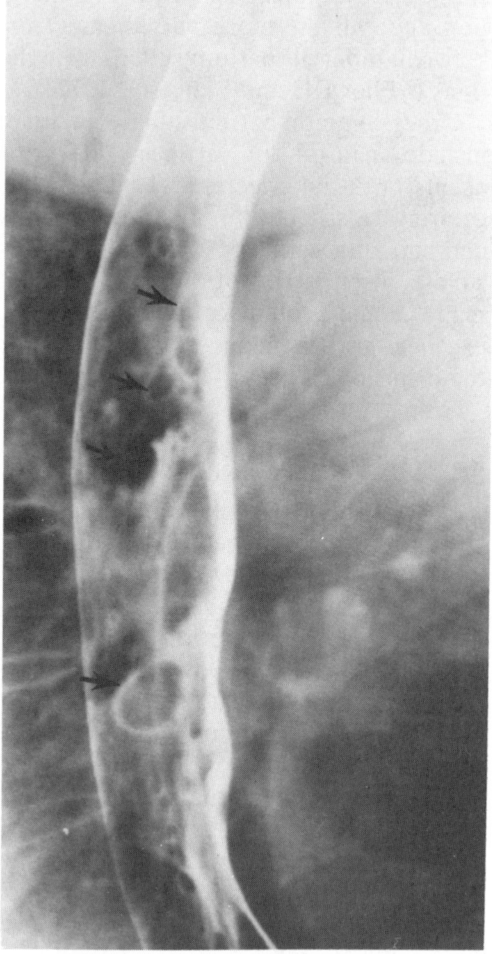

Figure 5.3 Air bubbles on the barium-coated mucosal surface appear as rounded lucencies, simulating the appearance of polyps.

contrast gas (e. g., air, carbon dioxide, or nitrogen).

The stability of foams is markedly influenced by the amount and type of dissolved ions. Hence, water-soluble salts are often incorporated into barium sulfate formulations as antifoam agents. In addition to dissolved salts, various oily substances (e. g., vegetable oils, castor oil, alcohols of fatty acids) also have anti foam properties. Silicone oils of very low surface tension (e. g., simethicone) are particularly effective at breaking bubbles and are frequently added to barium sulfate preparations. The antifoam effectiveness of a given additive is highly dependent on the nature of the foam-producing surface-active substances in the preparation and can therefore vary significantly between different barium sulfate formulations (Miller RE and Skucas J, 1977c).

Other common barium sulfate additives include natural or artificial flavoring agents, artificial sweeteners, and artificial coloring agents to improve palatability and patient acceptance. Although barium sulfate, itself, will not support bacteria, many of the proteinaceous additives are excellent growth media, thus necessitating the inclusion of preservatives.

PHARMACOKINETICS

Barium sulfate demonstrates negligible absorption from the gastrointestinal tract following either oral or rectal administration. It is excreted, unchanged, in the feces, the rate of excretion being dependent on the route of administration and the status of the patient's normal peristaltic activity and gastrointestinal motility. In normal subjects, orally administered barium sulfate is generally excreted within 24 hours. Rectally administered barium sulfate is eliminated with evacuation of the enema. Colonic retention and delayed excretion of barium sulfate may be evident following oral or rectal administration in the presence of decreased intestinal motility.

The time post administration required for the barium sulfate to produce adequate opacification of the various segments of the gastrointestinal tract is dependent on the route and rate of administration and the dose, concentration, and viscosity of the administered medium. In general, maximum opacification of the esophagus, stomach, and duodenum occur almost immediately following oral administration; whereas antegrade opacification of the small intestine is dependent on the patient's gastric emptying rate and the rate of flow or viscosity of the administered medium and may be delayed for 15–90 minutes. With enteroclysis procedures, the desired degree of small bowel opacification is achieved immediately following direct instillation of the barium sulfate medium. The rate and degree of retrograde colon and distal small intestine opacification is highly dependent on the patient positioning technique and hydrostatic pressure, with fluoroscopic monitoring commencing at the time of instillation of the barium sulfate enema.

PHYSIOLOGICAL EFFECTS/PRECAUTIONS

Barium sulfate, being chemically inert and relatively nonabsorbable, produces few physiological effects in patients with normal gastrointestinal anatomy and physiology. Hypersensitivity reactions to barium sulfate, itself, are unlikely, however, allergic reactions can occur to the various proteinaceous and flavoring additives used in the barium sulfate formulations.

Impaction of orally administered barium sulfate has been observed proximal to complete or high-grade obstructions of the colon. However, impaction is never a problem with obstruction of the upper gastrointestinal tract or small bowel. In the latter situations, the barium sulfate remains in suspension and is, in fact, diluted by the large amount of fluid that accumulates proximal to the obstruction. The normal reabsorptive processes of the colon can, however, lead to dehydration of the retained barium sulfate and the formation of barium fecaliths that are capable of inducing intestinal obstruction. Although known or suspected colonic obstruction was recognized as a contraindication to the oral administration of early barium sulfate preparations, the improved suspension characteristics and stability of the more recent barium sulfate formulations have greatly decreased the respective potential for a serious problem (Ott DJ and Gelfand DW, 1983).

Intestinal distension produced by large volumes of barium sulfate suspension may result in intestinal cramping and diarrhea. Colon distension has also been reported to cause ECG changes, primarily in elderly patients with a history of cardiac disease (Berman CZ, et al, 1965; Eastwood GL, 1972). Transient bacteremia has also been associated with the increased intracolonic pressures of barium sulfate enema procedures (LeFrock J, et al, 1975).

Aspiration of small amounts of barium sulfate into the tracheobronchial tree usually has negligible effects on pulmonary anatomy or physiology. In fact, barium sulfate suspensions (50% w/v) have been utilized for bronchography in a large number of patients with few acute reactions and no chronic pulmonary effects or fibrosis (Nelson SW, et al, 1964). Although pneumonitis and nodular granulomas of the interstitial lung tissue and lymph nodes may be rarely observed following the aspiration of barium sulfate (Zakova N and Svoboda M, 1965), barium sulfate aspiration is a relatively frequent occurrence in a busy gastrointestinal radiology department and is considered innocuous.

Extravasation of barium sulfate into the peritoneal cavity via a perforated stomach, duodenum, or colon can produce adverse effects ranging from mild peritonitis to fibrogranulomatous reactions, dense adhesion formation, and death. The severity of the reaction associated with this peritoneal extravasation is dependent on the extent of leakage and the nature and degree of bacterial contamination that accompanies the barium sulfate. As expected, colon perforation typically produces the most severe complications due to the presence of fecal material. Perforation of the segments of the gastrointestinal tract may occur as a result of the increased intraluminal pressure of barium sulfate administration combined with preexisting disease states (e. g., inflammation, ulceration, malignancy) or iatrogenic weakening of the mucosa (e. g., sigmoidoscopy, endoscopy, biopsy). Perforation of the colon at the level of the rectum is also associated with improper insertion of enema tips or repositioning of balloon-retention devices during the barium enema examination. Peritoneal contamination, should it occur, requires immediate treatment with intravenous fluids and appropriate antibiotics, and may require surgery to repair the perforation and remove contaminating barium sulfate and bacteria. Extra-peritoneal leakage of barium sulfate is usually associated with mild inflammatory reactions only, but should be avoided if possible (Ott DJ and Gelfand DW, 1983).

Intravasation of barium sulfate into the venous system is an extremely infrequent but serious complication of gastrointestinal examinations. This event has been associated with the presence of mucosal ulcerations, and with inappropriate administration of barium sulfate into the vagina. Outcomes include granulomatous liver abscesses and severe or fatal pulmonary and cardiac embolization (Ott DJ and Gelfand DW, 1983).

Barium Sulfate—Drug Interactions. Although no extensive studies have been reported in the literature, it should be noted that barium sulfate suspensions are unstable adsorption complexes that are capable of binding many chemical entities including drugs. Hence, the potential interaction of oral barium sulfate contrast media with oral drugs of narrow therapeutic margin should be considered.

Barium Sulfate—Diagnostic Procedure Interactions. The normal distribution or retention of radiopaque barium sulfate in the gastrointestinal tract can interfere with the interpretation of other diagnostic procedures including endoscopy or angiography for the diagnosis of gastrointestinal bleeding, abdominal CT procedures, and various nuclear medicine examinations involving organs localized to the abdominal region.

II. Iodinated Contrast Media

Based on the knowledge that they demonstrate minimal absorption from the gastrointestinal tract, the water-soluble, iodinated contrast media developed initially for intravascular, urographic use were investigated as potential contrast agents for gastrointestinal opacification.

Although these iodinated agents produce adequate full-column opacification of most segments of the alimentary tract following oral or rectal administration, barium sulfate preparations provide greater delineation of mucosal detail, cause fewer local effects, and are less expensive. Hence, the current use of iodinated contrast media for gastrointestinal examinations is primarily limited to those situations (e.g., known or suspected intestinal perforation) where the oral or rectal administration of barium sulfate is contraindicated (see Clinical Indications).

CHEMISTRY

The water-soluble, iodinated contrast media currently indicated for gastrointestinal opacification following oral or rectal administration include sodium or combination meglumine-sodium salts (Table 5.6) of the radiopaque anion, diatrizoate (Figure 5.4). The degree of gastrointestinal opacification produced by these agents is directly proportional to the total quantity of iodine (i.e., product of iodine concentration and volume) administered. At the available and utilized concentrations, these media are hyperosmotic.

The 76% w/v concentration of the combination meglumine-sodium (6.6:1 ratio) salts of diatrizoate (Table 5.6) have an osmolality of approximately 2000 mOs/kg and provide 370 mg iodine/mL. Dilution to approximately 16% w/v (78 mg I/mL)

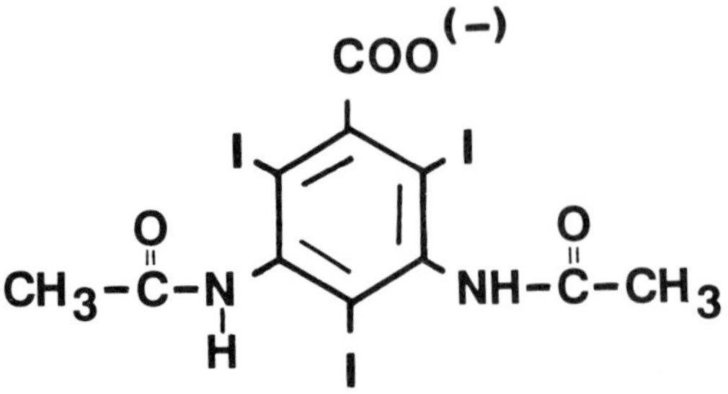

Figure 5.4   Chemical structure of diatrizoate anion.

is required for isotonicity; however, this degree of dilution results in very unsatisfactory radiopacification of the bowel. The 41.7% w/v concentration of sodium diatrizoate (Table 5.6) has an osmolality of approximately 1100 mOs/kg and an iodine concentration of 250 mg/mL. Sodium diatrizoate is also available as a bulk powder for on-site preparation of radiopaque solutions of desired concentration, each gram of powder containing approximately 600 mg of iodine. Isotonic solutions of sodium diatrizoate have a concentration of approximately 11% w/v (66 mg I/mL). Unlike barium sulfate preparations, the viscosity of the iodinated contrast media is relatively unimportant since these latter media do not demonstrate mucosal-coating properties. Various flavoring agents may be added to improve palatability and patient acceptance. The commercially available preparations of diatrizoate for oral or rectal administration are not guaranteed sterile or pyrogen free, and, therefore, must not be utilized for parenteral administration.

Table 5.6   WATER-SOLUBLE, IODINATED CONTRAST MEDIA FOR GASTROINTESTINAL OPACIFICATION

GENERIC NAME	BRAND NAME[®a]	CONCENTRATION (% w/v)	MG IODINE ML
Diatrizoate meglumine(66%)-sodium (10%)	Gastrografin (S)	76	367
Diatrizoate meglumine(66%)-sodium (10%)	Gastroview (M)	76	367
Diatrizoate meglumine(66%)-sodium (10%)	Gastrovist (B)	76	367
Diatrizoate sodium	Hypaque Oral Solution (W)	41.7	249
Diatrizoate sodium	Hypaque Oral Powder (W)	[b]	600[c]

[a] (B) Berlex Imaging
  (M) Mallinckrodt, Inc.
  (S) Squibb Diagnostics
  (W) Winthrop-Breon Laboratories
[b] Powder for reconstitution
[c] mg Iodine/g

PHARMACOKINETICS

The radiopaque diatrizoate anion demonstrates minimal (i. e., <1% of administered dose) absorption from the intact gastrointestinal tract following oral or rectal administration (Product information, Hypaque® sodium Oral Solution, Winthrop-Breon Laboratories). Systemic absorption may be substantially increased in the presence of intestinal perforation (see Physiological Effects/Precautions). The rate of gastrointestinal transit and excretion of orally administered iodinated contrast media is more rapid than barium sulfate preparations as a result of their saline cathartic effects. The hyperosmolar nature of an oral iodinated contrast medium results in a net influx of interstitial fluid into the gastrointestinal tract in a compensatory attempt to render the medium isotonic. The subsequent increase in intestinal volume stimulates peristaltic activity that propels the medium through the gastrointestinal tract (Margulis AR, 1977). Following oral administration, opacification of the esophagus and stomach occurs immediately with diluted opacification of the small bowel observed at 30–90 minutes. The presence of contrast in the colon is evident as early as 4 hours after oral administration, with rapid elimination occurring as a result of the increased intestinal volume.

Colonic opacification is immediate following rectal administration of the iodinated contrast media. Elimination occurs with evacuation of the enema. As mentioned previously, opacification of the small bowel may be inadequate following oral or rectal administration of these agents due to their progressive osmotic dilution as they transit through the respective segments of the gastrointestinal tract.

PHYSIOLOGICAL EFFECTS/PRECAUTIONS

As a result of their minimal absorption from the alimentary tract, the iodinated contrast media for gastrointestinal examinations elicit virtually none of the physiological effects associated with the intravascular use of these same agents (see Chapter 1, Angiographic Contrast Media). It must be noted, however, that pseudo-allergic reactions to iodinated contrast media can occur with extremely low systemic levels. Hence, the possibility of an unexpected pseudo-allergic reaction following the oral administration of these agents must be a constant consideration.

The oral or rectal administration of hyperosmolar concentrations of these iodinated contrast media results in a net diffusion of interstitial fluid across the intestinal mucosa into the lumen of the gastrointestinal tract. This osmotic activity typically results in cramping, diarrhea, and systemic dehydration. The latter condition may be dangerous in infants or debilitated patients with preexisting fluid and electrolyte disturbances unless adequate hydration is maintained.

Compared to barium sulfate preparations, the primary physiological advantage of iodinated contrast media is the fact that they are absorbed from the peritoneal cavity and soft tissues in the event of their extravasation from a perforated or weakened gastrointestinal tract. Thus, the iodinated agents do not produce the same incidence of peritonitis, fibrogranulomatous reactions, or adhesion formation that is observed with peritoneal extravasation of barium sulfate. Serious complications can occur, however, if hyperosmolar, iodinated contrast media are administered orally in the presence of an esophago-tracheal fistula, or are inadvertently aspirated into the lungs. Even though these media may be rapidly absorbed or expectorated, significant osmotic-induced effusion and retention of water in the pulmonary tissue can result in severe pneumonitis, pulmonary edema, and death (Margulis AR, 1977; Ott DJ and Gelfand DW, 1983).

Precipitation of the diatrizoate anion has been demonstrated at pH values below 2.3. Should it occur, gastrointestinal precipitation of the oral iodinated media can lead to false positive diagnoses of intragastric or gastric calcifications or foreign bodies, and may induce mucosal irritation. Although the average pH of the fasting stomach is in the range of 2–3, it may become substantially lower with stress, postoperative fasting, or a food stimulus. Thus, in the presence of a hyperacidity condition (especially with concomitant obstruction) it is advisable to pretreat the patient with antacids or to utilize a buffer solution (e. g., sodium bicarbonate) for dilution of the iodinated media (Ball DS, et al, 1986).

Drug/Laboratory Test Interactions. The results of thyroid-function tests based on measurements of iodine (i. e., radioactive iodine uptake studies, protein-bound iodine) may be altered for several weeks following the gastrointestinal administration of iodinated contrast media. If indicated, alternate tests of thyroid function (i. e., T3-resin uptake, total and free thyroxin) should be utilized following the administration of iodinated contrast media.

Pancreatic function tests involving the spectrophotometric assay of trypsin may yield invalid low values in the presence of small amounts of intestinal contrast media. Such studies should be performed prior to or several days following gastrointestinal radiology procedures (Drug Information, 1987).

III. Clinical Considerations/ Dosage

SINGLE-CONTRAST BARIUM EVALUATION OF THE GASTROINTESTINAL TRACT

The single-contrast method has until recently been the most widely used technique for radiological examination of the gastrointestinal tract. The object of this type of examination is to adequately fill the lumen of the gut with a relatively low-density barium preparation (Figure 5.5). Films are obtained at a high kilovoltage, and the examination is necessarily supplemented with compression of the

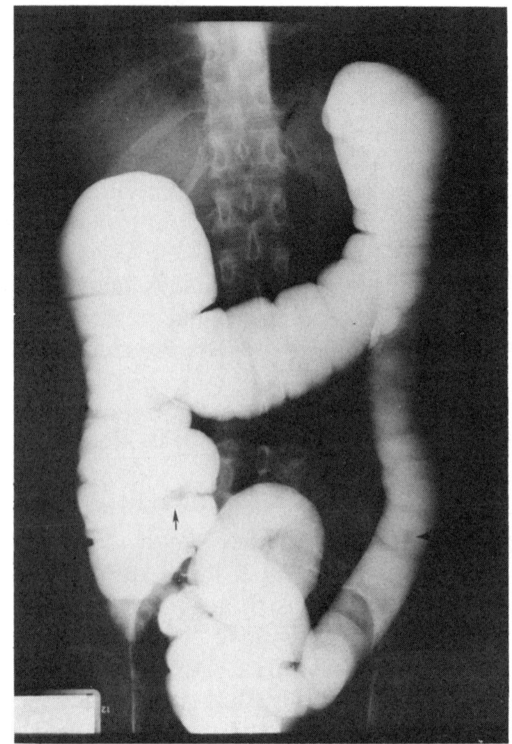

Figure 5.5 An overhead film from a single-contrast barium enema is demonstrated. The combination of high-kilovoltage technique and sufficiently low-density barium preparation results in the ability to detect filling defects in the barium column. The arrow on the right demonstrates a small rounded polyp in the distal descending colon. This is confirmed with compression spot films of the area. On the left the iliocecal valve is demonstrated.

barium-filled bowel. Evaluation of the bowel margin in degrees of obliquity (obtained by moving the patient) results in the display of contour abnormalities that form the basis for diagnosis (Figure 5.6). The fact that the lumen is barium filled means that lesions that are not displayed on the bowel contours could be easily missed. This drawback is addressed by the use of compression and manipulation techniques wherever possible. When the bowel is compressed, lesions hidden in the barium pool may become more evident (Figure 5.7).

Single-contrast examinations of the gastrointestinal tract have fallen into clinical

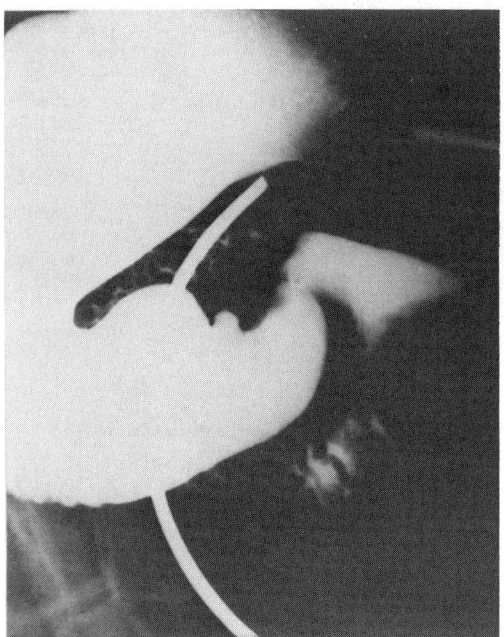

Figure 5.6 A benign gastric ulcer demonstrated in this single-contrast upper GI Study is shown to advantage using compression technique.

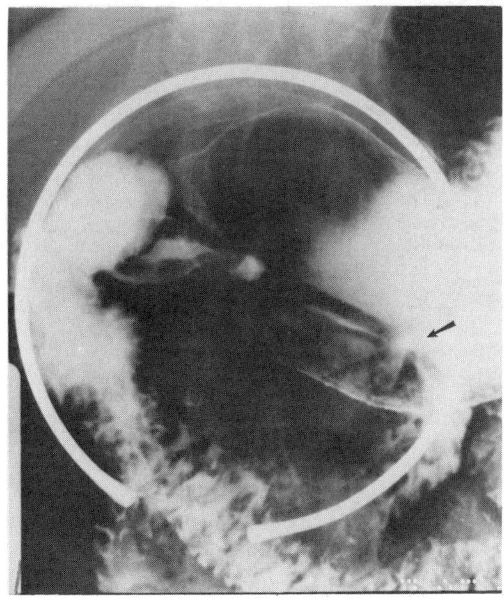

Figure 5.7 A single-contrast upper GI examination is demonstrated. Compression technique of the distal stomach has displaced the barium from the lumen and two gastric ulcers (arrows) are demonstrated.

disrepute for two reasons. First, meticulous and careful compression and manipulation of the bowel are absolute requirements for a successful single-contrast examination. In the opinion of many gastrointestinal radiologists, sufficient attention to technique has not been properly observed in the general performance of single-contrast examinations. As a result, numerous diagnostic errors surrounding the single-contrast technique were observed and reported in the literature. This observable error and the ensuing pressure from endoscopists to have the primary role in gastrointestinal diagnosis spurred the rediscovery and the accelerated development of high-quality double-contrast examinations, which, in many centers, have subsequently replaced the single-contrast technique for routine work.

The single-contrast examination does, however, remain quite common, and indeed, probably continues to be more utilized today than the double-contrast technique. It should not be considered an obsolete procedure. When performed properly with careful attention to patient preparation and technique, it can yield very good results. The obvious shortcoming of the single-contrast examination is that not all parts of the bowel can be compressed or manipulated. Those parts of the colon that are under the rib cage and protected by the diaphragm, and some loops of bowel within the lower pelvis cannot be compressed. The esophagus, which cannot be compressed, is also clearly a problem area for the single-contrast procedure.

Nevertheless, there is still a well-defined place for properly performed single-contrast examinations in the radiology department. Table 5.7 outlines the clinical situations wherein the use of a single-contrast versus double-contrast technique is recommended. In general, a bad single-contrast examination of the colon or upper gastrointestinal tract will often yield more information than a bad double-contrast examination.

Single-contrast examinations of the gastrointestinal tract are performed using various concentrations of low-density

Table 5.7 CLINICAL SITUATIONS WHEREIN A SINGLE-CONTRAST EXAMINATION MAY BE PREFERABLE TO THE DOUBLE-CONTRAST TECHNIQUE

1. Suspicion of high-grade obstructing process in either the upper or lower gastrointestinal tract
2. Suspected diverticulitis without perforation. (Single-contrast barium tends to diffuse into pericolic or intramural tracts more readily than barium sulfate used for double-contrast examinations.)
3. Known diverticulous coli. (Single-contrast examination with compression better demonstrates polypoid lesions in presence of numerous diverticular changes.)
4. Patients (e. g., debilitated, handicapped) who are unable to cooperate with the extensive on-table positioning required for the double-contrast procedure
5. Patients who are examined in an emergency situation to rule out bowel obstruction and who have not had the benefit of an adequate bowel-cleansing preparation

Table 5.8 CONCENTRATIONS AND VOLUMES OF BARIUM SULFATE COMMONLY USED FOR SINGLE-CONTRAST EXAMINATIONS

GASTROINTESTINAL REGION-OF-INTEREST	CONCENTRATION ($\%$ w/v)	CONCENTRATION ($\%$ w/w)	VOLUME (ML)
Esophagus	60–170	40–75	5–60
Stomach, duodenum	40–120	30–60	200–400
Small bowel (follow-through)	40–120	30–60	400–600
Colon (enema)	15–40	15–30	1500–2500

barium sulfate preparations (Table 5.1). Since radiographic opacification is dependent on the total amount of barium in the path of the x-ray, the relative $\%$ w/v concentration of barium sulfate utilized for a given procedure is, in general, inversely related to the diameter of the lumen under investigation. Hence, the $\%$ w/v concentration of barium sulfate required for a single-contrast examination of the esophagus is substantially higher than that required for the colon. Table 5.8 lists concentrations and volumes of low-density barium sulfate preparations commonly used for single-contrast examinations of various regions of the gastrointestinal tract. It should be noted, however, that considerable variation exists within the

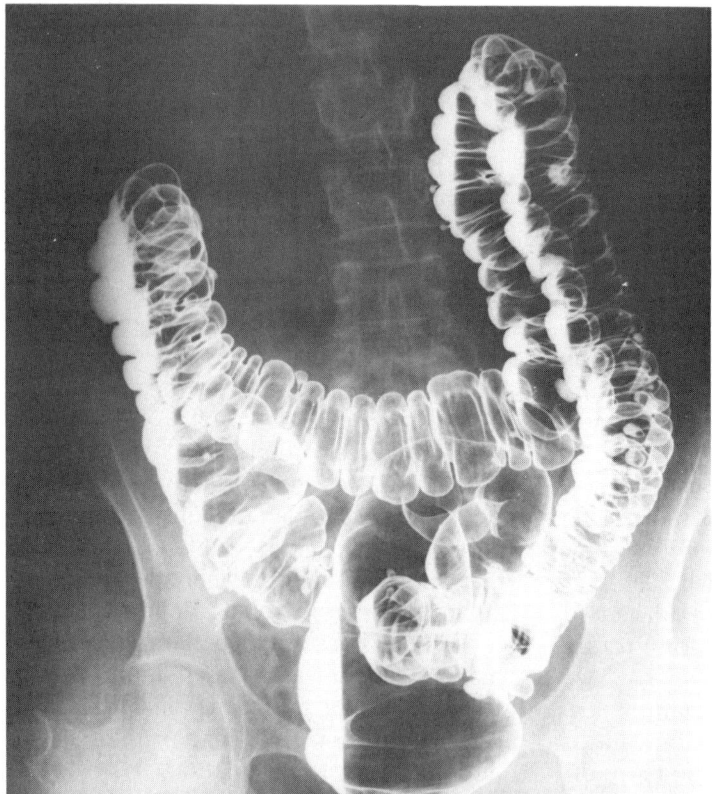

Figure 5.8 A right decubitus film from a double-contrast barium enema demonstrates uniform barium coating throughout the colon and well-defined contours.

gastrointestinal radiology community regarding the preferred barium sulfate preparation and concentration. Moreover, adequate filling of the region under investigation is usually monitored fluoroscopically, and the required volume may vary greatly from patient to patient.

DOUBLE-CONTRAST EXAMINATIONS OF THE GASTROINTESTINAL TRACT

Double-contrast examinations of the gastrointestinal tract have been utilized since the early part of the century and were extremely popular in parts of Europe and Japan prior to coming into wider recognition in North America. A well-performed double-contrast procedure involves distension of the bowel combined with uniform barium coating of the mucosal surface. This requires the use of air or other gases to produce distension and a high-density, low-viscosity barium sulfate preparation to properly flow over and coat the mucosal surface. In a prop-

erly prepared patient, the results can be an elegant demonstration of both the mucosal surface and bowel margin (Figures 5.8–5.11).

Whereas diagnostic principles are related to contour evaluation and compression technique in the single-contrast study, the double-contrast examination relies not only on detection of contour abnormalities but also on the *en face* evaluation of the mucosal surface (Figures 5.12 and 5.13). This latter characteristic has resulted in a newer and more complex set of diagnostic principles that in turn has led to some resistance in the acceptance of double-contrast technique. Clearly this procedure requires a significant commitment of time and interest in learning and understanding not only the new technique but also the new diagnostic principles. Double-contrast examinations may initially be more time consuming to perform and

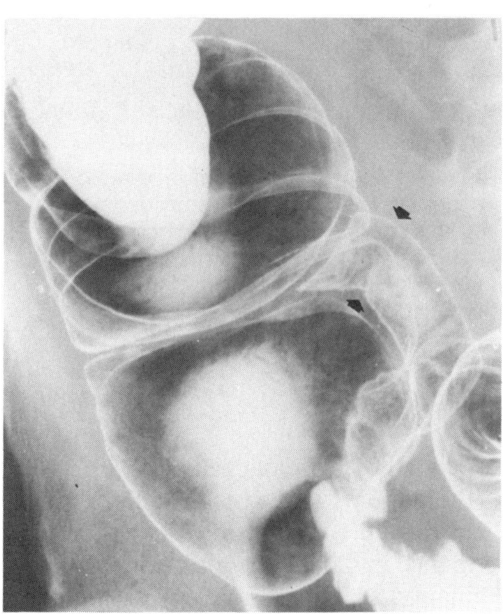

Figure 5.9 A spot film from a double-contrast barium enema demonstrates an excellent evaluation of both the cecal contours and mucosal surface. Also note the ileocecal valve and the air contrast display of the terminal ileum (arrows).

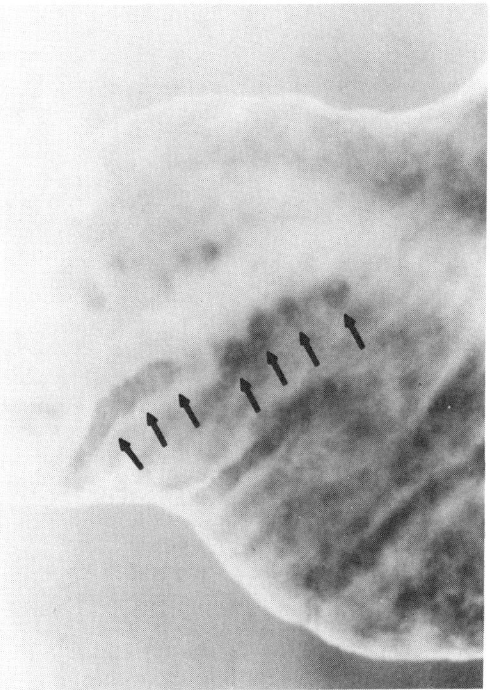

Figure 5.10 By utilizing "flow technique" in which barium is washed over the mucosal surface and allowed to thin out, subtle mucosal abnormalities can be demonstrated. This spot film from a double-contrast upper GI demonstrates a line of superficial erosions (arrows) in the gastric antrum.

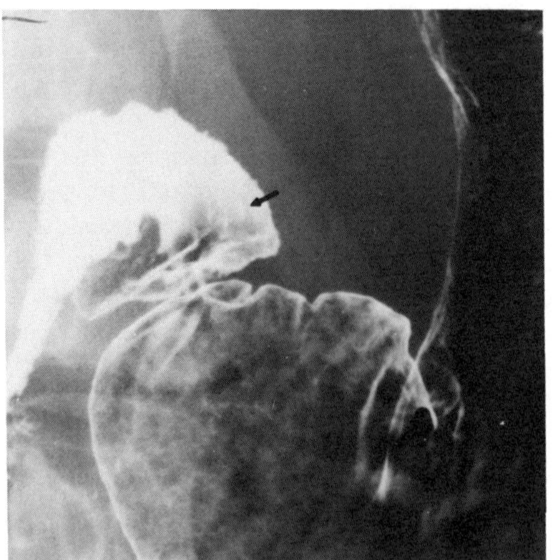

Figure 5.11 A spot film from a double-contrast upper GI examination demonstrates tiny superficial duodenal erosions (arrow) of erosive duodenitis.

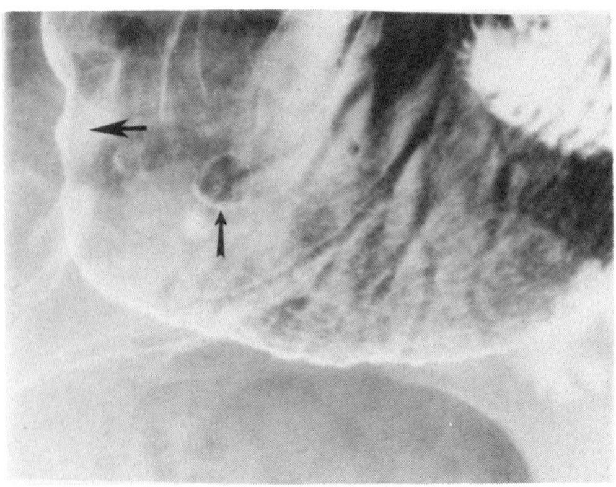

Figure 5.12 A film from a double-contrast upper GI examination demonstrates both contour and *en face* abnormalities produced by two benign gastric ulcers. The ulcer at the junction of the antrum and body is demonstrated *en face* (lower arrow) and is observed as a shallow mucosal excavation. The outline in white represents barium that is coating but not filling the ulcer. The upper arrow demonstrates the contour abnormalities associated with a gastric ulcer along the greater curvature. A shallow barium collection is visible in the center of an edematous mound.

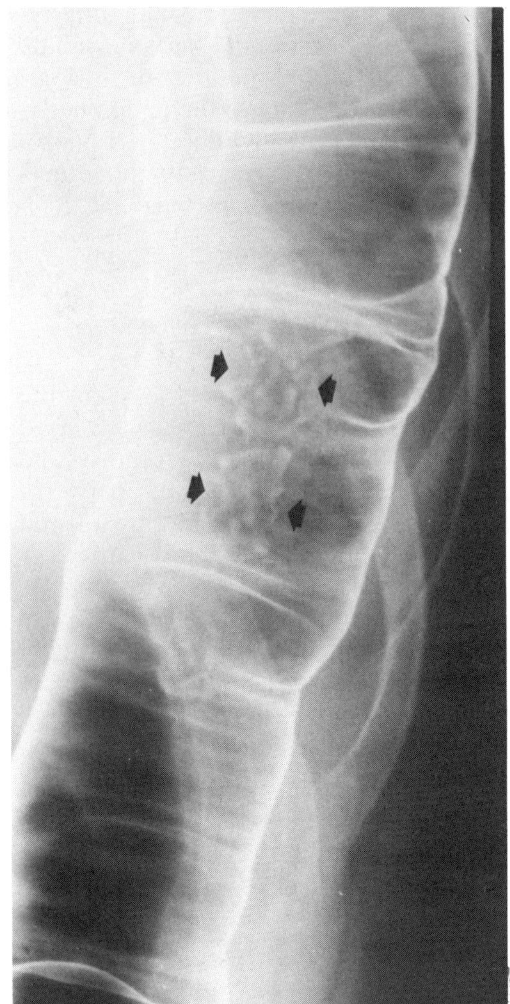

Figure 5.13 A film from a double-contrast colon examination demonstrates a wide, shallow, vertical area of ulceration in the descending colon. The ulcer is seen *en face*. This type and configuration of superficial ulceration is typically seen in Crohn's disease.

associated with greater radiation exposure to the patient. However, familiarity with the procedure and expertise in its performance invariably result in a routine examination that should take no more time than a good single-contrast study.

In most large diagnostic centers, double-contrast examinations of the gastrointestinal tract are common. Although there is still ongoing argument, it is currently felt that a good double-contrast technique

Table 5.9 CONCENTRATIONS AND VOLUMES OF BARIUM SULFATE COMMONLY USED FOR DOUBLE-CONTRAST EXAMINATIONS

GASTROINTESTINAL REGION-OF-INTEREST	CONCENTRATION (% w/v)	(% w/w)	VOLUME (mL)
Esophagus	60–250	40–85	15–60
Stomach, duodenum	200–250	80–85	75–90
Small bowel (enteroclysis)	85	50	150–400
Colon (enema)	85–125	50–65	350–600

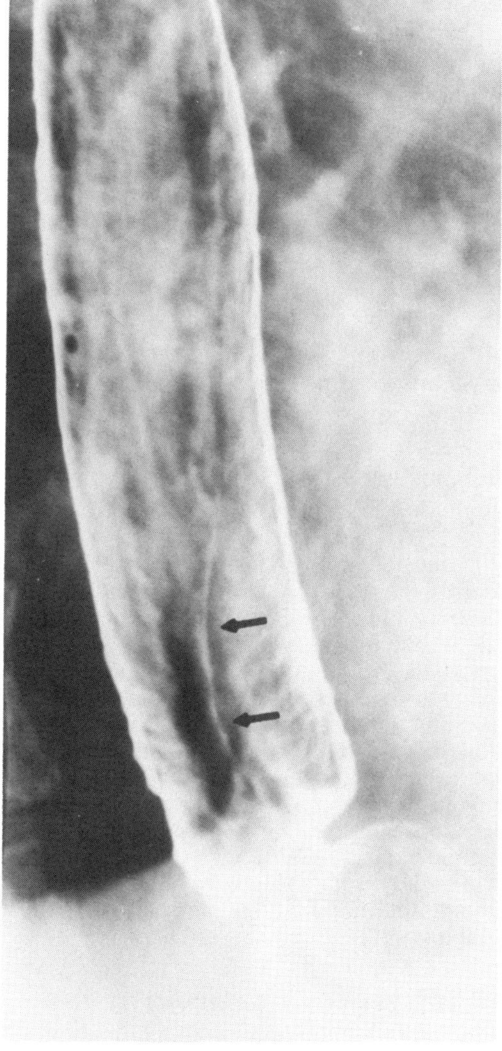

Figure 5.14 Adequate distention achieved by the use of gas-producing granules is essential for the demonstration of subtle, superficial abnormalities. This spot film from an air contrast esophagram demonstrates a long, shallow, linear ulcer (arrows) in the distal esophagus above a hiatal hernia.

increases the diagnostic accuracy of polyp and cancer detection and provides a significant improvement in the evaluation of mucosal changes associated with inflammatory bowel disease.

As previously discussed, the use of a barium sulfate preparation for a double-contrast procedure is dependent on its mucosal coating characteristics. The viscosity of the agent must be low to permit its flow over and to provide conformity with the irregularities of the mucosal surface. Yet, the viscosity must be sufficient to result in a uniform coating that is retained for the period of time required for completion of the examination. Since the thickness of the mucosal coating is limited, the density of the double contrast barium sulfate preparation must be necessarily high to yield adequate x-ray opacification.

Table 5.9 outlines the concentrations and volumes of high-density, low-viscosity barium sulfate preparations (Tables 5.4 and 5.5) commonly used for double-contrast examinations of various regions of the gastrointestinal tract. As with the single-contrast agents, personal experience dictates the specific barium sulfate preparation and concentration utilized for a given procedure. Mucosal coating is monitored using fluoroscopy.

In a double-contrast examination, distension of the gastrointestinal lumen and negative contrast are produced by the introduction of air or carbon dioxide (Figure 5.14). Upper gastrointestinal procedures routinely incorporate the use of commercially available sodium bicarbonate preparations (Table 5.10) that have been specifically designed for this purpose. Following oral administration, these agents interact with the stomach acid to

Table 5.10 ORAL SODIUM BICARBONATE PREPARATIONS FOR USE IN DOUBLE-CONTRAST EXAMINATIONS OF THE UPPER GASTROINTESTINAL TRACT

BRAND NAME®	MANUFACTURER
Baros	Mallinckrodt, Inc.
E-Z-GAS	E-Z-EM Co., Inc.
Sparkles	Lafayette-Pharmacal, Inc.

produce a sufficient volume (300–500 mL) of carbon dioxide for adequate distension. The barium sulfate is administered immediately following the effervescent agent, which may also include simethicone to prevent foaming. Double-contrast examinations of the colon routinely involve the insufflation of air (approximately 2000 mL) via a specially designed enema tip. This procedure is performed following administration of the barium, with distension monitored fluoroscopically. It has been shown that patients experience less discomfort if carbon dioxide versus air is used for the double-contrast colon study. (Coblentz CL, et al, 1985). This appears to be related to a more rapid absorption of carbon dioxide from the bowel and, hence, more rapid relief from gaseous distension. Although the maintenance of a carbon dioxide gas delivery system may be inconvenient, recent studies have shown that a carbon dioxide-producing effervescent powder (i. e., containing sodium bicarbonate/sodium citrate) can be directly mixed with barium sulfate to produce an acceptable double-contrast colon examination (Pochaczevsky R, 1987).

BIPHASIC EXAMINATION

Biphasic examinations of the upper gastrointestinal tract represent an attempt to incorporate the advantages of both the single- and double-contrast techniques. Double-contrast views of the esophagus, stomach, and duodenum are initially obtained to evaluate the respective mucosal surfaces. However, since the value of barium-filled views of the esophagus, stomach, and duodenum cannot be underestimated, the double-contrast study is routinely followed by a single-contrast procedure. *For example*, demonstration of hiatal hernia is best seen in the recumbent barium-filled esophagus. In addition, esophageal motility cannot be studied using a double-contrast technique, and again, the examiner must resort to a single-contrast study. Prone compression views of the barium-filled gastric an-

trum and duodenum are often required for adequate evaluation of the upper gastrointestinal tract.

In radiographic examinations of the colon, the double-contrast technique is routinely used except in those patients for whom it is either not indicated or not preferred (Table 5.7). However, as described previously, there is still a significant place for a properly performed single-contrast study of the colon. Few radiologists will attempt to routinely undertake a so-called biphasic examination of the colon, where a proper double-contrast examination is followed by a full-column, single-contrast examination. It is too arduous an undertaking for the patient, results in a prolonged procedure with increased radiation exposure, and is usually not required for an adequate diagnosis. Occasionally following evacuation of the low-density barium used for a single-contrast study, the colon is inflated with air and "air contrast views" are obtained. This is a most unsatisfactory way of performing a double-contrast examination of the colon and is prone to error due to the suboptimal mucosal-coating characteristics of the single-contrast barium preparation.

During the undertaking of a routine double-contrast study of the colon, manipulation and compression of the bowel have an important role. Although many had felt this to be obsolete with the advent of the double-contrast technique, we have found it extremely helpful in evaluation of the sigmoid colon. Compression of the sigmoid will not only push the loops apart, but when dealing with severe diverticulosis in this region, it can be helpful in polyp detection (Figure 5.15). Manipulation and compression are also utilized during evaluation of the medial ascending colon, an area of known difficulty in obtaining a satisfactory double-contrast examination.

SMALL BOWEL EXAMINATIONS

The traditional radiographic evaluation of the small bowel has depended upon the small bowel follow-through study performed following the antegrade administration of a low-density barium sulfate preparation. A multipurpose barium sulfate suspension (Table 5.1) of approx-

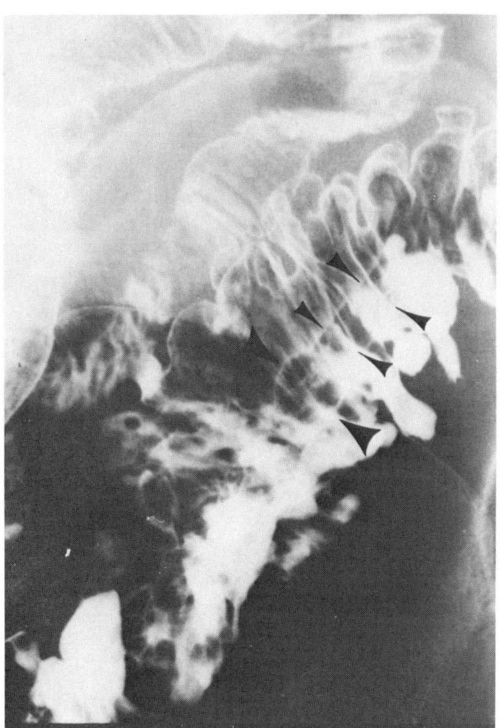

Figure 5.15 A compression spot film obtained during a double-contrast barium enema demonstrates numerous diverticula in the sigmoid colon resulting in significant distortion of the bowel margins. However, with compression a polyp on a long stalk (arrows) is demonstrated.

imately 50% w/v (20–30% w/w) is utilized in a dosage range of 300–500 mL. Films of the small bowel are obtained according to a predetermined schedule (e. g., at 15–30 minute intervals until the total small bowel is visualized). In the evaluation of small bowel obstruction, diffuse small bowel disease and potential malabsorption, the small bowel follow-through is an adequate examinations (Figures 5.16A, 5.16B). However, the effectiveness of this method is limited by the relative inaccessibility of the small bowel and by its low diagnostic yield.

An alternative method of examining the small bowel radiologically, small bowel enteroclysis, is rapidly gaining acceptance. This method requires the use of a polyvinyl enterostomy tube, which is passed through the patient's mouth into the stomach and eventually positioned in the jejunum with the tip of the tube at or beyond the ligament of Treitz (Figure 5.17). Barium sulfate is infused at a constant flow rate through the tube and the loops of bowel are examined using compression technique as they are filled and distended (Figures 5.18 and 5.19). The examination is complete when the terminal ileum and cecum are displayed.

The enteroclysis examination is associated with some degree of patient discomfort, even in the best hands, and is probably best utilized in certain restricted clinical situations. Although it is recognized that some controversy may exist, Table 5.11 lists recommended clinical indications for an enteroclysis examination.

Enteroclysis may be performed as a single-contrast or as a double-contrast study. When done using a single-contrast technique, a 25% w/v (approximately 20% w/w) low-density barium sulfate preparation (Tables 5.1, 5.2) is most useful. However, it should be noted that the barium sulfate suspension will rapidly become diluted in the presence of dilated, fluid-filled loops of the small bowel, thus severely limiting the quality of the examination. When faced with a clinical situation where increased small bowel secretions may be encountered, such as mechanical obstruction or ileus, a 50% w/v (20–30% w/w) barium sulfate preparation is therefore recommended. Filling of the small bowel is monitored fluoroscopically; total volumes of 1–2 liters may be required for a complete examination.

Enteroclysis may also be performed as a double-contrast study using methylcellulose as the negative contrast agent. A volume of approximately 200–400 mL of a 50% w/v (35–60% w/w) barium sulfate preparation (Table 5.2) is infused into the proximal small bowel via the enterostomy tube. This is followed by 1–2 liters of 0.5% methylcellulose solution. The double-contrast technique does not appear to substantially improve examinations of the small bowel. On the contrary, the examination tends to be prolonged

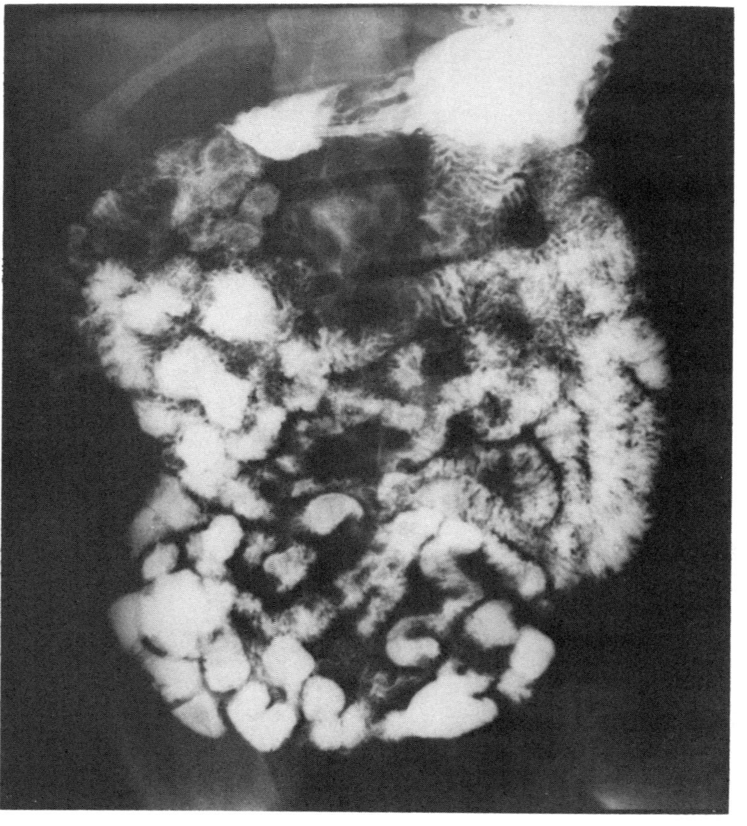

Figure 5.16A An overhead film obtained during a small bowel follow-through examination is demonstrated. Although there is barium seen throughout the entire small bowel, the bowel loops are inadequately filled and distended with barium for detailed analysis.

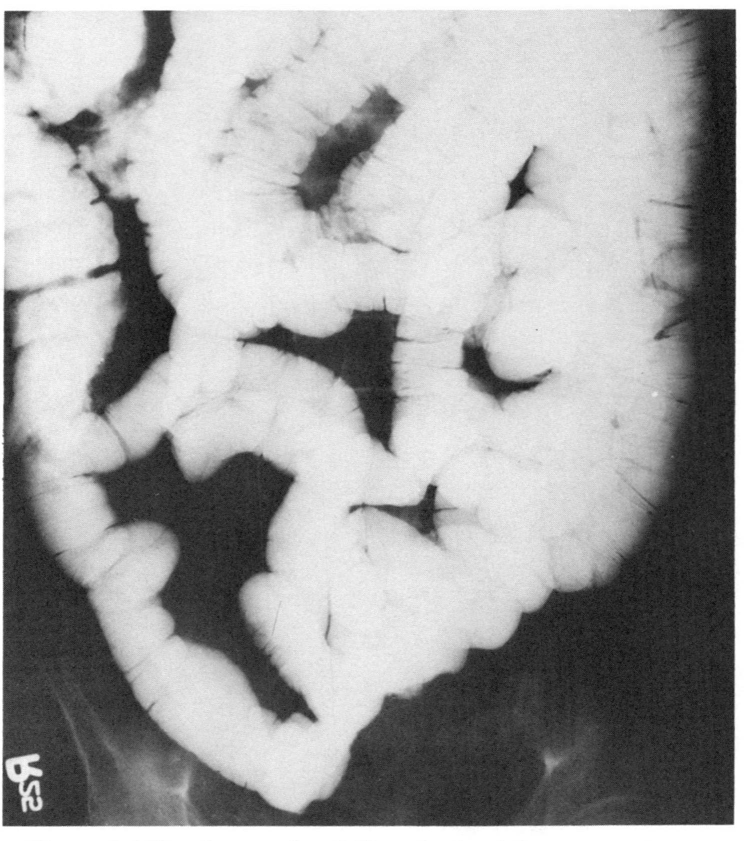

Figure 5.16B An overhead film obtained from a small bowel enteroclysis examination shows complete and adequate distention throughout the entire small bowel. Individual segments of the small bowel are examined using compression technique.

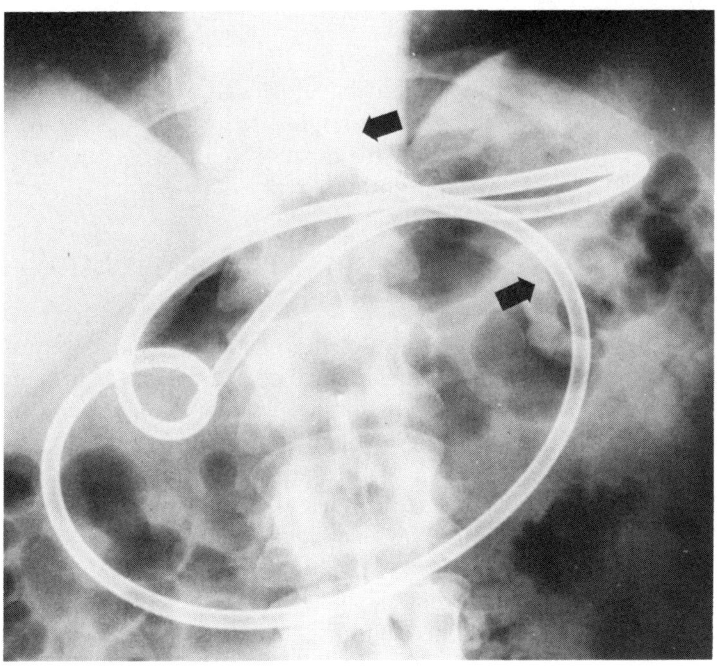

Figure 5.17 A positioned enteroclysis tube is demonstrated. The upper arrow indicates the gastroesophageal junction. The lower arrow shows the termination of the duodenal sweep at the ligament of Treitz. The tip of the enteroclysis tube is placed in the jejunum just beyond the ligament of Treitz. The course of the tube relates to the patient's individual anatomy and can be variable.

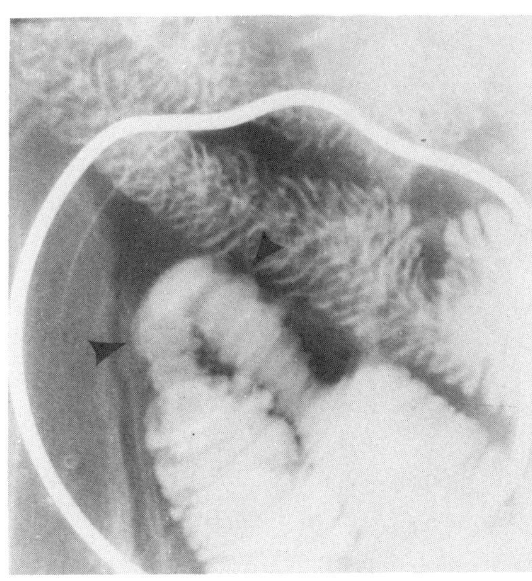

Figure 5.18 A compression spot film obtained during a small bowel enteroclysis examination demonstrates an area of focal narrowing, fold thickening, and intact mucosa. At surgery this was found to be an area of ischemic stricture.

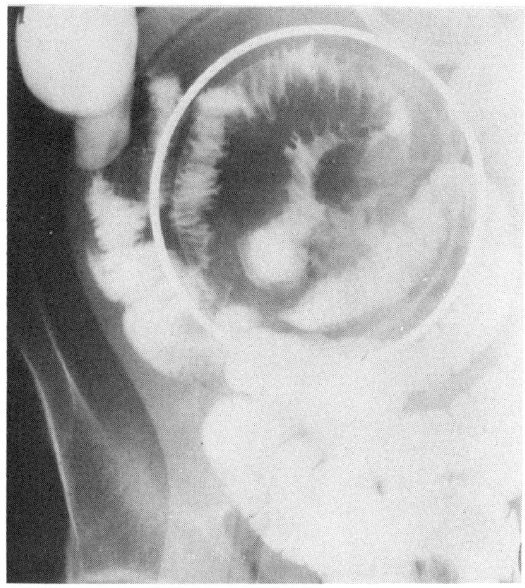

Figure 5.19 Spot film from an enteroclysis examination of the small bowel taken at the distal ileum demonstrates at least two loops of small bowel in which there is significant fold and wall thickening and distortion of the lumen. At least two previous small bowel follow-throughs had been interpreted as normal. The findings are consistent with carcinoid tumor.

1. Chronic abdominal pain in which no source can be identified in the upper or lower gastrointestinal tract
2. Gastrointestinal bleeding in which the site cannot be identified in the upper or lower gastrointestinal tract
3. Inconclusive small bowel follow-through examination in which questions of abnormality are raised
4. Patients with known or suspected inflammatory disease of the small bowel

without any demonstrable benefit. Although the double-contrast views of the proximal small bowel are dramatic, they probably represent little improvement in the ability to demonstrate lesions in this region of the bowel as compared with the single-contrast compression technique. In addition, by the time the barium and methylcellulose have reached the deep ileal loops localized to pelvic area, mixing has occurred with dilution of barium opacification (Figure 5.20). In a region of the bowel where a double-contrast techni-

que would be most valuable, namely the non-compressible deep ileo loops surrounded by the pelvis, it gives the most disappointing results.

BARIUM SULFATE FORMULATION CONSIDERATIONS

Generally, the particle-size distribution and exact nature of the additives a given barium sulfate product comprises are proprietary information and therefore unknown to the radiology user. Even if the concentration and chemical nature of all additives were known, the in vivo behavior of the final product could not be predicted, since the order of their addition in the manufacturing process can greatly influence the physical properties of the final preparation. Although in vitro comparisons of various barium sulfate products have appeared in literature, it is difficult to directly extrapolate these studies

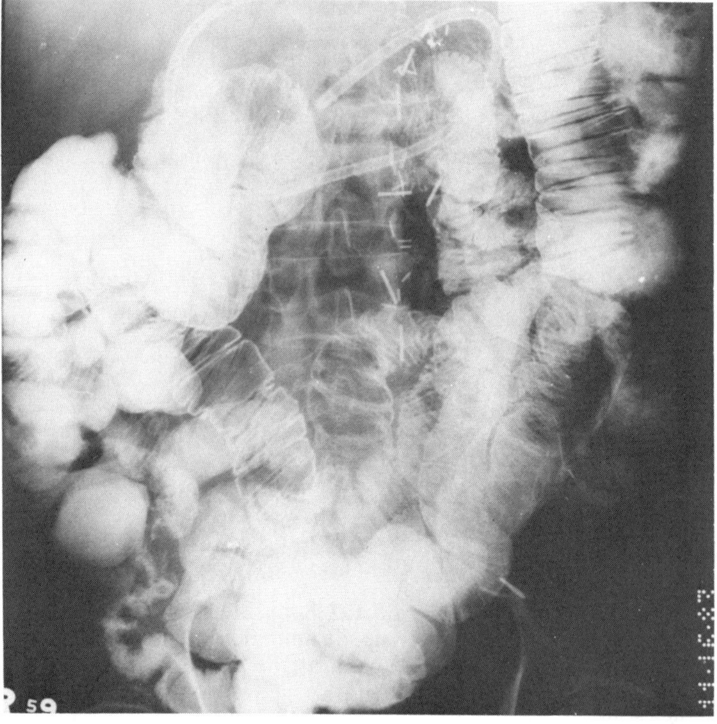

Figure 5.20 A double-contrast small bowel enteroclysis examination using methylcellulose. The upper proximal small bowel loops are well demonstrated. However, it can be seen in the lower pelvic ilial loops that there is mixture of the barium and methylcellulose.

to the heterogeneity of gastrointestinal conditions found in the human gastrointestinal tract. Hence, selection of a barium sulfate product for a particular gastrointestinal examination is dependent on the manufacturers' recommendations, knowledge of the desired physical properties, and previous clinical experience with the product. Additional product selection considerations include relative cost, ease of preparation and use, and palatability.

The correct application and interpretation of barium sulfate examinations requires constant uniformity of the barium sulfate products used for the various procedures. Maintaining such uniformity with bulk powders that require measurement and reconstitution prior to their use can be problematic (Miller RE and Skucas J, 1977d). Volumetric measurements of barium sulfate powders are highly inaccurate due to their dependence on the degree of packing, whereas weight measurements are time consuming and require additional equipment. Variability in the ion content of tap water can significantly affect the stability and foaming characteristics of barium sulfate suspensions, thus necessitating a constant source of deionized water to alleviate these concerns. Lastly, the characteristics and uniformity of the final barium sulfate suspension are highly dependent on the method and degree of mixing; factors that can vary considerably between personnel and varying department demands. Based on the previously outlined considerations and increased convenience, the preweighed, unit-dose packages of barium sulfate powder for suspension and the various preformulated barium sulfate suspensions (Tables 5.1–5.5) have properly gained increased popularity in recent years, even though their unit-of-use cost may be somewhat greater than that of the bulk powders.

A fundamental characteristic of almost all colloidal systems is their lack of stability. Hence, it is not surprising that the properties (e.g., viscosity, coating characteristics, suspension stability, etc.) of barium sulfate preparations can change after prolonged standing or aging (Miller RE and Skucas J, 1977b). Since the use of a barium sulfate contrast medium is based upon uniformity of its properties, it is extremely important that the expiration dating (i.e., preformulated products) or recommended time-of-use post reconstitution be adhered to carefully.

GASTROINTESTINAL USE OF IODINATED CONTRAST MEDIA

The gastrointestinal use of water-soluble, iodinated contrast media is indicated where there is known or suspected perforation of the gut. Barium sulfate is contraindicated in such incidences due to the potential for peritoneal extravasation and associated granulomatous reactions (see Physiological Effects/Precautions). However, the site and extent of the perforation may be demonstrated using an oral iodinated contrast medium, since its water solubility will result in rapid absorption should it escape into body cavities. In addition, barium sulfate administration should not be performed until 1 week following deep biopsy of the gastrointestinal mucosa, polypectomy, or polyp biopsy using electrosurgery (Harned RK, et al, 1982; Harned RK, et al, 1985). If a gastrointestinal examination is required during this interval, a water-soluble, iodinated medium should be substituted. Barium sulfate may be utilized if there is histological confirmation that the biopsy is superficial.

There continues to be some confusion as to appropriate indications for the oral administration of water-soluble, iodinated contrast media. In terms of their use as gastrointestinal contrast agents, the iodinated media are far inferior to barium sulfate. As a result, the most important indication for their use is suspected perforation of the gut (Figure 5.21). Obstruction anywhere in the alimentary canal is not an indication for the use of an iodinated contrast medium. Indeed, obstruction proximal to the ligament of Trietz should preclude the use of a water-soluble agent.

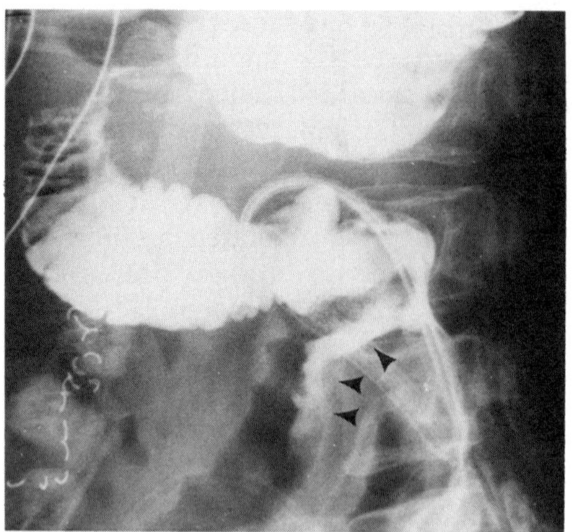

Figure 5.21 A film obtained during an upper GI examination utilizing water-soluble contrast is demonstrated. Perforation and leakage of contrast (arrows) is seen in the distal duodenal sweep.

This is an important consideration in light of the fact that high upper gastrointestinal obstructions are associated with vomiting. Although the aspiration of barium sulfate is relatively innocuous, the aspiration of a hypertonic, iodinated contrast medium is dangerous and may induce chemical pneumonitis or contrast-induced pulmonary edema. Distal to the ligament of Treitz, obstructions are best demonstrated using barium sulfate. Again, there is some confusion concerning the use of iodinated contrast media in the presence of small bowel obstruction. The very high osmolality of the water-soluble preparations results in an osmotic diffusion of water into the gut. This factor combined with the frequent presence of fluid accumulation proximal to the obstruction results in a degree of contrast dilution that renders administration of the iodinated contrast medium relatively useless. Barium sulfate preparations will undergo dilution in accumulated bowel fluid, but they do not exert osmotic effects. There is also no particular use for water-soluble, iodinated contrast media in evaluation of colonic obstruction. Indeed, barium sulfate will give more detailed information concerning the level and the nature of the obstructing process.

As a result of its saline cathartic effect, the rectal administration of a hyperosmolar, iodinated contrast medium may be useful in promoting the elimination of inspissated meconium (Frech RS, et al, 1970) or fecal matter and the reversal of meconium ileus or fecal impaction. As a result of their hygroscopic, distension and peristaltic activities, the oral administration of water-soluble contrast agents may provide relief of postoperative adynamic ileus (Margulis AR, 1977) or adhesive obstructions. It must be remembered, however, that these potential therapeutic effects of water-soluble, iodinated media may be gained at the expense of diagnostic information. Similar treatment can be initiated with the rectal or oral administration of saline laxatives following radiographic diagnosis using a more appropriate barium sulfate preparation.

Upper gastrointestinal examinations typically involve the oral administration of a total of 20–40 grams of iodine (e. g., 60–100 mL at 367 mg iodine/mL, 90–180 mL at 249 mg iodine/mL). The hyperosmolar nature of the concentrated water-soluble contrast media necessitates special precautions when they are administered to pediatric or debilitated patients. In addition to ensuring adequate patient hydration, it is often advised that the media be diluted to a concentration of 100–150 mg iodine/mL prior to administration. Pediatric patients also require lower volumes. These steps may, however, lead to problems in providing an acceptable level of gastrointestinal opacification. Although not indicated in the respective product literature, an alternate approach in these at-risk patients with suspected perforation may be the oral administration of the lower osmolality (i. e., ratio-3) water-soluble, iodinated media (see Chapter 1, Angiographic Contrast Media). Compared to the conventional (i. e., ratio-1.5) iodinated media indicated for oral administration, use of the low-osmolality media would alleviate the concerns associated with hyperosmolarity while maintaining an adequate iodine concentration for gastrointestinal opacification.

Colon examinations are performed following the rectal administration of 1000–1500 mL of the conventional (i. e., ratio-1.5) iodinated media following their dilution to an iodine concentration of approximately 60–100 mg/mL. Pediatric patients will again require lower volumes. The water-soluble iodinated contrast media do not pose significant hyperosmolarity-related considerations at these dilute concentrations.

PATIENT PREPARATION

Esophagus Examinations. Evaluation of the esophagus requires only a limited amount of patient preparation. Generally, patients are advised to avoid ingestion of liquid or food on the day of their examination. Overhydration of the esophagus can result in diminished mucosal coating during a double-contrast technique. In addition, such patient preparation usually results in a relatively clear stomach, thus if an evaluation of the stomach is required in addition to the esophagus, this can be accomplished at the same time.

Stomach and Duodenum Examinations. For evaluation of the stomach and duodenum, patients are advised to avoid taking anything by mouth after midnight before their examination.

Small Bowel Enteroclysis Examinations. In most cases, the primary aim of bowel preparation for an enteroclysis examination is to achieve a collapsed, empty right colon. Experience has shown that a stool-filled right colon will result in a hypotonic ileum and slow progression of the barium sulfate through the ileo loops, resulting in increased distension of proximal loops and increased patient discomfort. The examination is lengthened considerably. In addition, residual debris in the distal ileum results in numerous filling defects. Conversely, an empty right colon will achieve a faster examination with more rapid flow of contrast through the ileo loops, as well as decreased patient discomfort. This can be accomplished by prescribing the same bowel preparation for the enteroclysis examination as is prescribed for the barium enema-colon examination, the only difference being that

on the day of the enteroclysis examination nothing is permitted by mouth. The avoidance of liquids prior to enteroclysis helps to prevent the accumulation of fluid within hypotonic or obstructed loops of the small bowel and associated contrast dilution. It also ensures better mucosal coating with a double-contrast technique. However, in patients with small bowel obstruction or known inflammatory bowel disease, the full-bowel preparation for enteroclysis should be avoided.

Barium Enema-Colon Examinations. Diagnostic evaluation of the colon requires that it be clean and empty. Residual food, secretions, or fecal material will result in a less than optimum display of the bowel, possible false-negative or false-positive diagnoses of lesions, and a potential requirement for a repeat examination (Figure 5.22).

Although there is considerable controversy regarding the best bowel-preparation regimen for barium enema-colon examinations, the most successful procedures have certain common steps. The patient's diet should be restricted to clear liquids for a minimum of 24 hours prior to the scheduled examination. Clear liquids may include nonpulpy fruit juices, clear soup, plain gelatin, tea, or coffee. Dairy products and carbonated beverages should be avoided. Due to the dehydrating effects of many prescribed laxatives, adequate fluid intake is required and should be encouraged to further promote bowel cleansing. The patient should drink a minimum of 6–8 glasses (8-ounce-size) of water on the day preceding the examination, assuming there are no medical contraindications. In addition, clear liquids are permitted until 1 hour before a barium enema study.

The laxatives employed in preparing the bowel for a barium enema-colon examination should produce cleansing of both the small and large intestines. Commonly utilized bowel-preparation kits typically include a saline laxative, such as magnesium citrate or a sodium phosphate-biphosphate solution, to promote cleansing mainly of the small bowel. As a

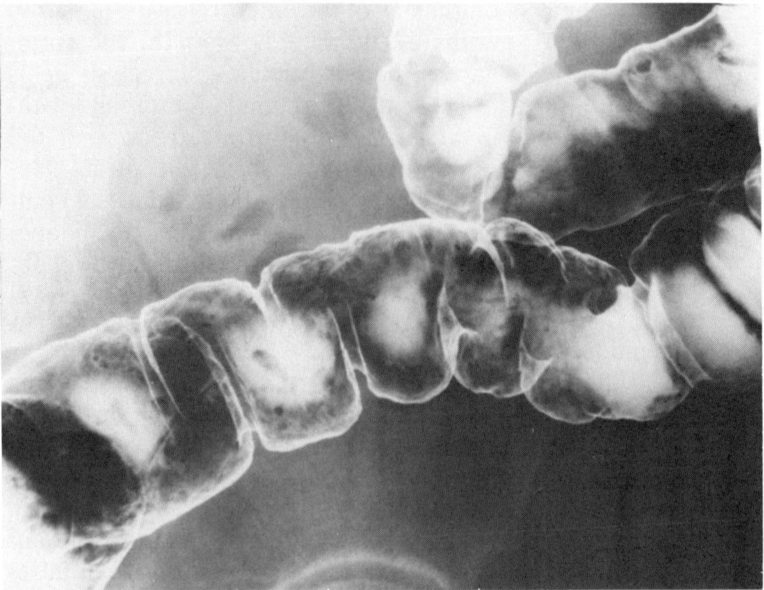

Figure 5.22   Retained fecal material can result in filling defects and lucencies that resemble lesions and can present difficulty in the interpretation of the examination. Often subsequent films obtained in different positions can be helpful in observing the movement of these filling defects. However, fecal material adherent to the mucosa can result in the false diagnosis of polyps.

result of the poor intestinal absorption of magnesium and phosphate ions, these agents exert a hyperosmolar effect, resulting in the retention or accumulation of water in the small intestine and the stimulation of respective peristaltic activity. Saline laxatives exert their effects best on an empty stomach and should be administered approximately 1 hour prior to the evening meal (clear liquids only) preceding the scheduled examination. In the presence of impaired renal function, the small amount of absorbed magnesium or phosphate ions may accumulate in the serum to produce electrolyte disturbances and toxic reactions. However, this usually presents a problem only in the presence of long-term use or overdosage. Caution should be observed in administering the sodium phosphate-biphosphate preparations to patients on a sodium-restricted diet.

Most bowel-preparation kits also incorporate an oral stimulant-type laxative. These agents exert an irritating effect on the bowel mucosa to stimulate peristaltic activity. They may also alter fluid and electrolyte absorption to produce a net accumulation of water and stimulation of evacuation. Commonly utilized stimulant laxatives include castor oil, phenolphthalein, and bisacodyl. The main site of action of castor oil is on the small intestine with somewhat less stimulation of the large intestine. Conversely, phenolphthalein acts to primarily increase peristaltic activity of the colon with decreased effects on small bowel. The direct irritant action of bisacodyl (Dulcolax®) is limited to the lower intestine as a result of the enteric coating routinely utilized in its tablet formulation. For cleansing of the small intestine, the previously described saline laxatives are generally better tolerated and accepted by patients than castor oil preparations. The diphenylmethane derivatives, phenolphthalein and bisacodyl, are both available in tablet formulations and acceptable for cleansing of the large intestine. Evacuation normally occurs at approximately 6–8 hours following their oral administration; therefore they can and should be taken at bedtime prior to the scheduled barium enema-colon examination. Phenolphthalein (normal cleansing dose = 130–270 mg adult) does demonstrate some absorption from the gastrointestinal tract and has been associated with hypersensitivity reactions. Bisacodyl is not absorbed from the gastrointestinal tract. Based on the latter consideration, oral bisacodyl (20 mg) is preferred for cleansing of the colon. To avoid irritation of the upper gastrointestinal tract, the bisacodyl tablets should not be chewed or crushed prior to administration. Milk or antacids will degrade the enteric coating of bisacodyl tablets and also lead to upper gastrointestinal irritation.

Cleansing of the colon is usually augmented by the rectal administration of a saline enema or a stimulant suppository at 1–2 hours prior to the scheduled examination. Although effective, cleansing enemas tend to be difficult to self-administer correctly and are not well accepted by the patient. Use of a 10-mg bisacodyl rectal suppository is therefore recommended. It is important to advise the patient to lie on his or her left side and to rectally insert the suppository as far as possible. The urge to evacuate should be resisted for at least 15 minutes if possible.

Recently, oral whole-gut lavage using large volumes of an isosmotic, electrolyte solution (e. g., Golytely®, Braintree Laboratories) has been promoted for bowel cleansing prior to barium enema colon examinations. Although this method does have advantages related to the avoidance of dehydrating effects, adequate bowel cleansing and barium sulfate mucosal coating require the concomitant oral administration of bisacodyl (Girard CM, et al, 1984). Moreover, the expense of this preparation is considerably greater than that associated with the previously described regimens.

Patients who have clinical or radiological suspicion of gastrointestinal obstruction or significant inflammatory bowel disease should not receive the routine bowel preparation regimen. Although each case must be considered separately, such patients may require nothing more than diet restrictions prior to the examination.

Pediatric patients also require special consideration. Essentially, the same bowel preparation may be utilized; however, the dosages should be adjusted downward accordingly.

Postexamination Laxatives. With the improved suspension stability of recent barium sulfate preparations, the routine postprocedure administration of a laxative is no longer required to avoid potential problems associated with barium sulfate inspissation and obstruction. Patients should be advised to maintain adequate levels of hydration. A laxative may be required in the event of constipation or abnormally hard stools (Miller RE, 1978).

Patient Compliance. The exact nature of the laxatives utilized for bowel cleansing is probably not as important as ensuring patient compliance with the diet restrictions, hydration requirements, and recommended bowel-preparation procedure. To this end, patients should be clearly advised as to the importance of adequate bowel preparation and the necessity for strict adherence to the respective instructions. To assist in compliance, the instructions should be given to the patient in the form of a readily understandable check list. In addition, it is advisable to contact all patients the day before the scheduled barium enema colon study to reemphasize the importance of adequate bowel cleansing and to answer any questions.

ADJUNCTIVE DRUGS

Glucagon. Traditionally glucagon is used to increase blood glucose concentrations in the emergency treatment of severe hypoglycemia associated with insulin overdosage. However, it is routinely utilized as an adjunct agent in radiology departments due to its secondary ability to inhibit gastric motility. Many gastrointestinal radiologists use glucagon routinely when performing a double-contrast esophagram or upper gastrointestinal examination. Experience has indicated that glucagon is most valuable in improving demonstration of the duodenum. In addition, glucagon-induced relaxation of the lower esophageal sphincter at the gastroesophageal junction may contribute to a better double-contrast display of the esophagus by permitting the reflux of air or gas that was initially instilled or produced in the stomach. The use of glucagon in barium enema examinations may be of benefit in reducing peristalsis and spasms, resulting in improved patient comfort, procedural continence, and diagnostic quality.

In dosages of 0.1–0.2 mg intravenously, side effects to glucagon are rare. It is known that there is an increased incidence of mild reflux during upper gastrointestinal examinations when glucagon is utilized. Since glucagon is a foreign protein, the potential for a hypersensitivity reaction does exist. In patients with insulin-dependent diabetes, use of glucagon for an upper gastrointestinal examination is probably of no particular value. These patients often demonstrate degrees of intestinal hypotonicity as a result of their disease. The use of glucagon in patients with the history of insulinoma may lead to subsequent hypoglycemia. Patients receiving glucagon in the presence of pheochromocytoma may develop a sudden and marked increase in blood pressure. In both these latter situations, the use of glucagon should be avoided.

Phentolamine. This short-acting vasodilater should be maintained in the fluoroscopic area at all times. For a patient who has received glucagon and subsequently develops a sudden increase in blood pressure (i.e., as a result of the stimulation and release of catecholamines from a previously unknown pheochromocytoma), 5–10 mg of phentolamine may be administered intravenously to counteract the hypertensive reaction.

Metoclopramide. This drug is used primarily in enteroclysis examinations of the small bowel. At intravenous dosages of 10 mg (metoclopramide base) it acts to increase gastric tone and contractions, stimulate peristaltic activity of the duodenum and jejunum, and promote relaxation of the pyloric sphincter. These effects of metoclopramide not only facilitate passage of the enterostomy tube for enteroclysis, but also result in a faster transit of the administered barium sulfate through the small bowel and a reduced examination time. The stimulated peristaltic activity appears to occur distal to the head of the barium column. Behind the head of the barium column, lumenal distension and physiological hypotonia occur, resulting in optimal conditions for compression and evaluation of the small bowel.

Metoclopramide is contraindicated in any situation where stimulated gastrointestinal activity might be deleterious, such as gastrointestinal hemorrhage, mechanical obstruction, or perforation. It is also contraindicated in patients with pheochromocytoma, as the drug may also result in increased secretion of catecholamines and possibly hypertensive crisis. Phentolamine may again be used to control hypertensive reactions in these situations.

References

Bachem C, Gunther H. Barium sulfat als schattenbildendes Kontrastmittel bei Rontgenunter such ungen. *Z Rontgenk Rad Forschr* 1910, 12:369–376.

Ball DS, Radecki PD, Friedman AC, et al. Contrast medium precipitation during abdominal CT. *Radiology* 1986, 158:258–260.

Berman CZ, Jacobs MG, Bernstein A. Hazards of the barium enema examination as studied by electrocardiographic telemetry: Preliminary report. *J Am Geriat Soc* 1965, 13:672–686.

Coblentz CL, Frost RA, Molinaro V, et al. Pain after barium enema: Effect of CO_2 and air on double-contrast study. *Radiology* 1985, 157:35–36.

Drug Information. American Hospital Formulary Service, American Society of Hospital Pharmacists, Bethesda, 1987, pp 1230–1247.

Eastwood GL. ECG abnormalities associated with the barium enema. *JAMA* 1972, 219:719–721.

Frech RS, McAlister WH, Ternberg J, et al. Meconium ileus relieved by 40 percent water-soluble contrast enemas. *Radiology* 1970, 94:341–342.

Gelfand DW. High-density, low-viscosity barium for fine mucosal detail on double-contrast upper gastrointestinal examinations. *AJR* 1978, 130:831-833.

Girard CM, Rugh KS, DiPalma JA, et al. Comparison of Golytely® lavage with standard diet/cathartic preparation for double-contrast barium enema. *AJR* 1984, 142:1147–1149.

Harned RK, Consigny PM, Cooper NB. Barium enema examination following biopsy of the rectum or colon. *Radiology* 1982, 145:11–16.

Harned RK, Williams SM, Maglinck DDT, et al. Clinical application of in vitro studies for barium enema examination following colorectal biopsy. *Radiology* 1985, 154:319–321.

LeFrock J, Ellis CA, Klainer AS, et al. Transient bacteremia associated with barium enema. *Arch Intern Med* 1975, 135:835–837.

Margulis AR. Water-soluble radiographic contrast agents in the gastrointestinal tract. In *Radiographic Contrast Agents* (Miller RE, Skucas, J, eds.), Baltimore, University Park Press, 1977, pp 169–191.

Miller RE. Laxative should not be routinely ordered after barium enema examination. *JAMA* 1978, 239:970–971.

Miller RE, Skucas J. Barium sulfate: Radiologists' control factors. In *Radiographic Contrast Agents* (Miller RE, Skucas J, eds.), Baltimore, University Park Press, 1977a, pp 65–84.

Miller RE, Skucas J. Barium sulfate: Basic properties. In *Radiographic Contrast Agents* (Miller RE, Skucas J, eds.), Baltimore, University Park Press, 1977b, pp 9–37.

Miller RE, Skucas, J. Barium sulfate: Clinical properties. In *Radiographic Contrast Agents* (Miller RE, Skucas J, eds.), Baltimore, University Park Press, 1977c, pp 85–141.

Miller RE, Skucas J. Introduction to gastrointestinal agents. In *Radiographic Contrast Agents* (Miller RE, Skucas J, eds.), Baltimore, University Park Press, 1977d, pp 3–8.

Nelson SW, Christoforidis AJ, Pratt PC. Further experience with barium sulfate as a bronchographic contrast medium. *AJR* 1964, 92:595–614.

Ott DJ, Gelfand DW. Barium sulfate suspensions. An evaluation of available products. *AJR* 1982, 138:935–941.

Ott DJ, Gelfand DW. Gastrointestinal contrast agents. Indications, uses and risks. *JAMA* 1983, 249:2380–2384.

Pochaczevsky R. Double contrast examination of the colon with carbon dioxide. The use of effervescent powder. *AJR* 1987, 149:502–504.

Zakova N, Svoboda M. Morphological changes in the lungs following bronchography with barium sulfate. *Acta Univ Carol* [*Med*] 1965, 11:125–136.

Cholecystographic and Cholangiographic Contrast Media

Dennis P. Swanson
Stuart M. Simms

Contrast media-based studies of the hepatobiliary system have been largely superseded by sonographic, computed tomography, and radionuclide techniques. They are still valuable for selected patients but are less commonly performed in current practice.

Cholecystographic contrast media are administered orally for the purpose of producing radiographic opacification of the gallbladder (Figure 6.1). Hence, cholecystography procedures are indicated for the direct demonstration of gallbladder stones or the evaluation of chronic cholecystitis. Oral cholecystographic agents are of limited value in the direct demonstration and evaluation of the bile ducts.

The primary objective of administering an intravenous cholangiographic contrast medium is the radiographic opacification and demonstration of the cystic and common bile ducts. The cholangiographic contrast media will opacify the gallbladder if the cystic duct is patent; however, due to their increased potential for serious adverse reactions, these agents should not be used as a substitute for the oral cholecystographic media.

Based on their differing diagnostic indications and routes of administration, it is not surprising that cholecystographic and cholangiographic contrast media have different chemical properties and pharmacokinetic characteristics. In general, cholecystographic agents require properties that permit adequate absorption from the intestinal tract following oral administration, preferential hepatic up-take with biliary excretion, and eventual concentration within the gallbladder. The rate of hepatobiliary excretion of the oral cholecystographic media and the concentration that they achieve in the bile ducts are not critical factors in regard to final visualization of the gallbladder. Cholangiographic contrast media must, however, achieve high concentrations within the bile ducts, requiring their rapid and efficient hepatocyte uptake and biliary excretion. These factors necessitate that cholangiographic media have chemical properties that permit intravenous administration and direct hepatobiliary excretion, thus avoiding the rate-limiting steps of intestinal absorption and hepatic metabolism (see Berk RN, et al, 1977a; Loeb PM, et al, 1977; Hatfield PM, et al, 1976; Barnhart JL, 1984).

HISTORY

The development of cholecystographic and cholangiographic contrast media originated with early studies that investigated the potential use of intravenous tetrachlorophenophthalein as a long-acting cathartic. Based on the observation that this agent was almost entirely excreted in the bile, combined with the knowledge that the normal gallbladder could concentrate bile by a factor of 8–10 through electrolyte and water reabsorption, Graham and Cole theorized that a bromo- or iodo-derivative of tetrachlorophenophthalein may permit radiographic

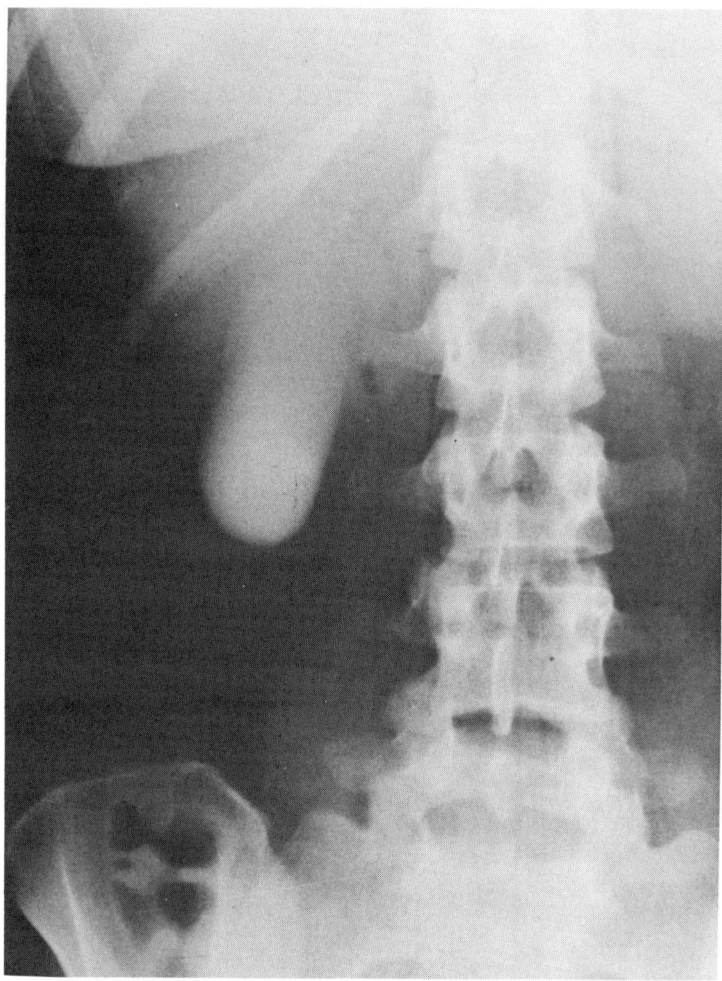

Figure 6.1 Cholecystogram (prone view) demonstrating well-opacified, normal gallbladder.

opacification of the gallbladder (Graham EA, et al, 1924). These investigators subsequently produced successful cholecystograms in dogs and humans following the intravenous administration of tetrabromophenolphthalein (Figure 6.2). The more radiodense tetraiodophenolphthalein derivative, initially restricted by the presence of toxic impurities, was eventually distributed commercially as Iodeikon (Figure 6.2). Although the intravenous injection of Iodeikon produced more reproducible gallbladder opacification, it was also possible to obtain adequate cholecystograms following its oral administration. Oral Iodeikon frequently produced gastrointestinal side effects of nausea, vomiting, and diarrhea, but of a less severe nature than the side effects encountered with its intravenous injection.

In 1940, iodoaliphonic acid (Priodax, Figure 6.2) was introduced as an oral cholecystographic medium. Compared to Iodeikon, this diiodinated agent produced more reliable gallbladder opacification with a decreased incidence of side effects. Subsequent research efforts were aimed at increasing the number of iodine atoms per molecule for improved opacification and at decreasing the frequency and severity of associated adverse reactions. These efforts led to the current chemical classes of cholecystographic and cholangiographic media.

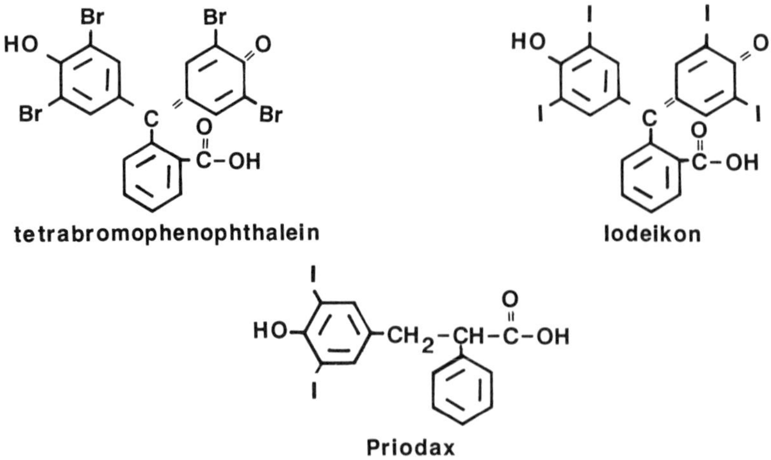

tetrabromophenophthalein

Iodeikon

Priodax

Figure 6.2 Historical cholecystographic and cholangiographic contrast media.

I. Cholecystographic Contrast Media

CHEMISTRY

Iopanoic acid, developed in the early 1950s (Hoppe JO and Archer S, 1953), represents the first of a series of aromatic triiodoalkanoic acid derivatives currently available for opacification of the gallbladder following oral administration (Figure 6.3, Table 6.1). Each of these cholecystographic agents can be described as a weak organic acid containing approximately 60% iodine by weight (Table 6.1). The agents differ in regard to the nature of the chemical substituents at positions 1 and 3 on the aromatic ring (Figure 6.3). The balance between the respective hydrophilic and lipophilic groups determines the relative aqueous and lipid solubility of each agent and its rate of absorption from the gastrointestinal tract. The different physical forms (i.e., salt versus acid; granular suspension, powdered capsule versus compressed tablet) of the agents (Table 6.1) also play an important role in regard to their rate of intestinal dissolution and absorption. Each of the derivatives is devoid of a substituent at position 5 of the aromatic ring (Figure 6.3). This important feature of cholecystographic media accounts for the preferential hepatobiliary versus renal elimination of these agents.

PHARMACOKINETICS

The appropriate use and efficacy of an oral cholecystographic agent is dependent on its pharmacokinetic properties. Following oral administration, a cholecystographic medium must undergo several distinct pharmacokinetic steps before its final concentration in the gallbladder. Differences between the various cholecystographic media in regard to any of these steps can result in differences in the final degree of gallbladder opacification and differing requirements for patient dosage and preparation.

Intestinal Absorption. Following oral administration, cholecystographic contrast media are absorbed from the gastrointestinal tract by a passive diffusion process occurring primarily in the small bowel. Absorption from the colon is also possible; however, it proceeds at a slower rate (Nelson J, et al, 1973).

Initial solubilization of the cholecystographic agents in the bulk-water phase of the intestinal lumen is the rate-limiting step in their gastrointestinal absorption. The cholecystographic media are weak organic acids that, depending on their pKa values, exhibit wide variations in aqueous solubility at a given pH value (Table 6.2). At the extremely low pH of the stomach, each of the media is virtually

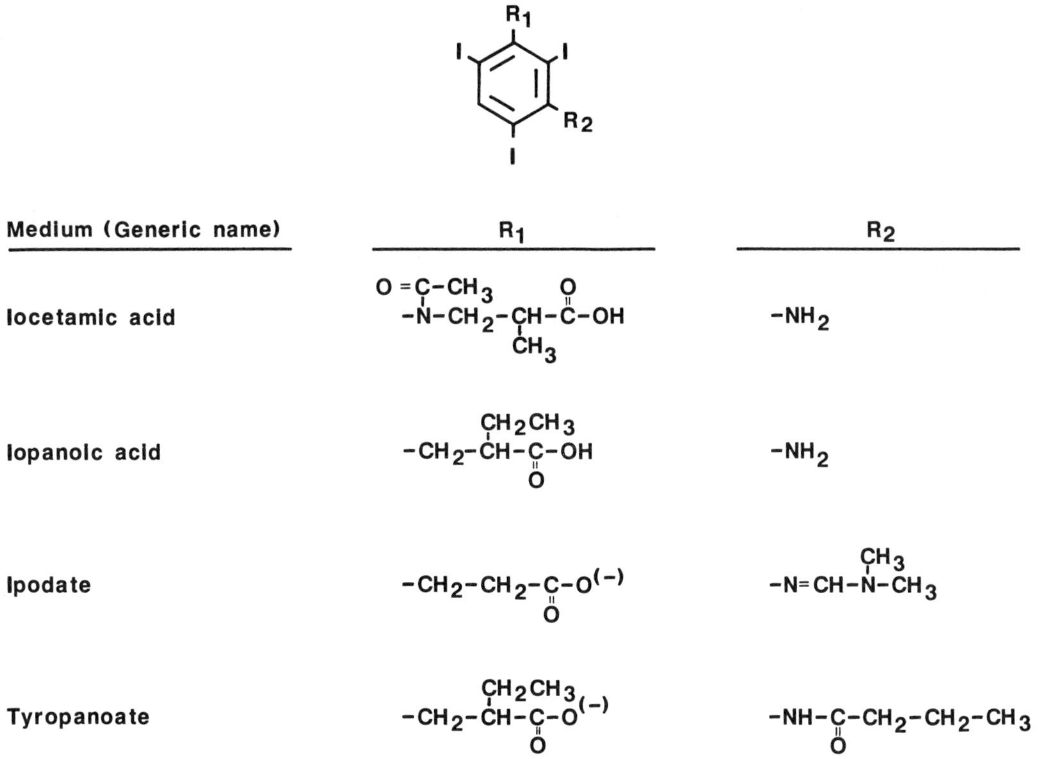

Medium (Generic name)	R_1	R_2
Iocetamic acid	$O=\overset{\displaystyle}{C}-CH_3$ $-N-CH_2-CH-\overset{O}{\overset{\|}{C}}-OH$ CH_3	$-NH_2$
Iopanoic acid	$\overset{CH_2CH_3}{\overset{\|}{-CH_2-CH-C-OH}}$ O	$-NH_2$
Ipodate	$-CH_2-CH_2-\overset{}{\underset{O}{C}}-O^{(-)}$	$\overset{CH_3}{-N=CH-\overset{\|}{N}-CH_3}$
Tyropanoate	$\overset{CH_2CH_3}{-CH_2-CH-\overset{}{\underset{O}{C}}-O^{(-)}}$	$-NH-\overset{}{\underset{O}{C}}-CH_2-CH_2-CH_3$

Figure 6.3 Chemical structures of commercially available (U.S. market) cholecystographic contrast media.

Table 6.1 PHYSICOCHEMICAL PROPERTIES OF COMMERCIALLY AVAILABLE CHOLECYSTOGRAPHIC MEDIA[a]

GENERIC NAME	BRAND NAME(S)[b]	IODINE CONCENTRATION (% w/w)	UNIT FORMULATION	MG CONTRAST / UNIT
Iocetamic acid	Cholebrine (M)	62.0	Tablet	750
Iopanoic acid	Telepaque (W)	66.7	Tablet	500
Ipodate calcium	Oragrafin Calcium(s)	61.7	Granules[c]	3000
Ipodate sodium	Bilivist (B); Oragrafin Sodium(S)	61.4	Capsule	500
Tyropanoate sodium	Bilopaque (W)	57.4	Capsule	750

[a] U.S. market only
[b] (B) Berlex Imaging
    (M) Mallinckrodt
    (S) Squibb Diagnostics
    (W) Winthrop-Breon Laboratories
[c] For suspension

Table 6.2 MAXIMUM AQUEOUS SOLUBILITY OF CHOLECYSTOGRAPHIC MEDIA AT pH 7.4, 37°C[a]

CONTRAST MEDIUM	AQUEOUS SOLUBILITY (MMOL/LITER)
Iopanoic acid	0.61
Ipodate calcium	1.87
Ipodate sodium	3.75
Iocetamic acid	8.61
Tyropanoate sodium	26.48

[a] Adapted from Janes JO, et al, 1979.

insoluble, thus restricting their absorption from this site. However, in the more alkaline environment (pH = 6.5) of the small intestine, the degree of ionization and the water solubility of the cholecystographic agents increase. Iopanoic acid remains poorly soluble within the small bowel, the principle advantage of the other cholecystographic media being their increased solubility in the bulk-water phase of the small intestine and hence their increased rate and degree of gastrointestinal absorption.

The pH of the gastrointestinal contents can also be affected by the patient's dietary state. Fasting increases the pH of the stomach and small intestine and, hence, the degree of ionization and water solubility of the cholecystographic agents. Conversely, a protein meal can significantly decrease the pH of the gastrointestinal contents and the water solubility of the cholecystographic media (Taketa RM, et al, 1972; Nelson J, et al, 1973; Goldberger LE, et al, 1974).

Another factor that can affect the solubility of a cholecystographic agent in the bulk-water phase of the intestinal lumen is its formulation state (Table 6.1). The sodium or calcium salts of ipodate and tyropanoate rapidly precipitate upon their contact with the low pH of the stomach. Colloidal particles formed during this precipitation process are of an extremely small size compared to the particles formed by simple dispersion of tablet formulations of the respective cholecystographic media. A reduction in particle size is generally associated with an increase in surface area and a faster rate of subsequent aqueous dissolution within the small bowel (Goldberger, LE, et al, 1974; Lasser EC, 1966a).

The presence of bile salts within the lumen of the small bowel significantly enhances the water solubility and intestinal absorption of lipophilic physiological substrates (e. g., cholesterol, fatty acids) via micelle formation. Bile salt micelles are composed of multiple bile salt molecules aligned in a radial fashion such that the lipophilic portions of the molecules are on the inside and the polar portions at the periphery of the colloidal micelle particle (Figure 6.4). Lipophilic substrates dissolve within the lipophilic center of the micelle, whereas the polar periphery confers water solubility. The gallbladder functions as a reservoir for bile salts. The stored bile salts are emptied into the duodenum when the gallbladder is stimulated to contract via the action of cholecystokinin, a hormone released following ingestion of a fatty meal. Intestinal bile salt micelles are absorbed from the terminal ileum into the portal venous blood, whereupon they undergo first-pass hepatic extraction and hepatobiliary excretion with subsequent restorage in the gallbladder.

As previously discussed, the solubility of iopanoic acid in the bulk-water phase of the gastrointestinal tract is extremely low, resulting in slow and erratic intestinal absorption. As with lipophilic physiological substrates, the presence of bile salts within the small bowel has been shown to significantly increase the water solubility and rate of intestinal absorption of iopanoic acid (Goldberger LE, et al, 1974; Berk RN, et al, 1974a). Bile salts also increase the aqueous solubility of the other cholecystographic agents. Thus, in the presence of similar intestinal environments, iopanoic acid still remains the least water soluble of the cholecystographic media. Although a fatty meal will induce bile salt release and enhance the water solubility and absorption of iopanoic acid, it should be noted that the meal can interfere with gastrointestinal absorption of other cholecystographic agents by delaying the rate of gastric emptying, altering gastrointestinal pH, or by direct binding of the agent (Stanley RJ, et al, 1974).

Once dissolved in the bulk water phase of the gastrointestinal lumen, the cholecystographic agent must diffuse across an "unstirred water layer" that lies adjacent to the intestinal mucosa. Although it does represent an additional barrier to the intestinal absorption of the cholecystographic agents, little is known about the physicochemical factors that affect the rate of diffusion across this "layer".

Ultimately, a cholecystographic agent must be able to dissolve in, and passively diffuse through, the lipid membrane of the gastrointestinal mucosa. Hence, the orally administered cholecystographic media must possess lipophilic properties in addition to their requirement for initial water solubility. The relative rate of movement of a cholecystographic agent through the intestinal mucosa (in the absence of bile salts) has been described in

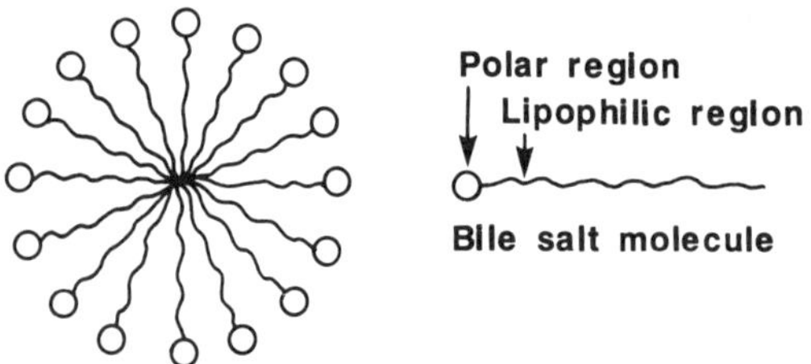

Figure 6.4 Diagram of the bile salt micelle.

Table 6.3 PASSIVE PERMEABILITY COEFFICIENTS AND BENZENE/WATER PARTITION RATIOS FOR CHOLECYSTOGRAPHIC MEDIA[a]

CONTRAST MEDIUM	PASSIVE PERMEABILITY COEFFICIENT[b]	BENZENE/WATER PARTITION RATIO[c]
Iopanoic acid	0.264	31.96
Ipodate sodium	0.225	8.23
Ipodate calcium	0.115	4.93
Tyropanoate sodium	0.143	0.49
Iocetamic acid	0.133	0.14

[a] Adapted from Janes JO, et al. 1979

[b] μmol/min/loop/mM

[c] Determined at 37°C in 0.15 M aqueous phosphate buffer (pH = 7.4)

terms of a passive permeability coefficient (Janes JO, et al, 1979). It has been shown that this permeability coefficient varies directly as a function of the relative solubility of the agent in lipid (e. g., benzene) versus water (Table 6.3), and inversely as a function of its polarity or water solubility (Table 6.2). This would suggest that cholecystographic agents that demonstrate excellent dissolution in the bulk-water phase of the gastrointestinal tract would have correspondingly slow rates of movement across the intestinal mucosa. However, relative differences in the permeability coefficients of cholecystographic media are considerably less than the corresponding differences in their benzene:water partition ratios (Table 6.3). This apparently occurs as a result of the fact that the rate-limiting membranes of the gastric mucosa do possess some polar properties. Thus, in the absence of bile salts, the initial water solubility of the cholecystographic agent remains the most important factor in regard to its rate of gastrointestinal absorption (Loeb PM and Berk RN, 1977; Barnhart JL, 1984).

Poor intestinal absorption of an oral cholecystographic agent can result in non-visualization of the gallbladder and a high degree of colonic retention of the medium. The latter factor may explain the higher incidence of gastrointestinal side effects and the residual bowel opacification commonly observed with the less water-soluble iopanoic acid versus the other cholecystographic media. Moreover, even at equivalent degrees of intestinal retention, the more water-soluble agents would demonstrate greater dispersion within the colonic contents and, hence, a reduced density of residual opacification (Berk RN and Loeb PM, 1977a).

Blood Transport. Cholecystographic agents, absorbed across the gastrointestinal mucosa, enter the systemic circulation via the portal venous system (Reinke RT and Berk RN, 1971), the vasculature responsible for draining the digestive tract, pancreas, gallbladder, and spleen. The cholecystographic agents are transported in blood extensively bound to serum albumin. They demonstrate negligible binding to other plasma proteins. The binding of the cholecystographic agents to albumin occurs primarily via the formation of hydrophobic bonds, and involves the vacant position 5 on their aromatic rings (Figure 6.3). Iopanoic acid demonstrates greater albumin binding (> 97% of plasma concentration) than the other cholecystographic media; differences between the agents being related to the number and nature of hydrophilic groups at positions 1 and 3 of the aromatic ring (Lang JH and Lasser EC, 1967).

The binding of the cholecystographic agents to serum albumin plays an important role in regard to their hepatic excretion and eventual gallbladder localization. Albumin binding increases the plasma solubility of the poorly soluble cholecystographic media and prevents phagocytosis of respective micelles or insoluble colloid by cells of the reticuloendothelial system. The albumin binding also appears to be responsible for preferential hepatic versus renal elimination of the cholecystographic media. Disse's spaces within the liver are freely permeable to albumin, whereas the renal glomerular membrane is albumin impermeable. Finally, albumin binding of these agents may also have important effects in regard to the rate or the specific mechanism of their hepatocyte uptake (Song CS, et al, 1976).

Hepatocyte Uptake. Hepatocyte uptake of the cholecystographic media occurs across the sinusoidal-hepatic cell membrane. The systemic blood levels of orally administered cholecystographic agents can be significant, indicating that their first-pass extraction from the portal blood is incomplete (Barnhart JL, 1984).

In vitro studies utilizing isolated rat hepatocytes have shown that, in the absence of albumin, the hepatocyte uptake of free iopanoic acid appears to occur by a passive diffusion process. Under physiological conditions, however, it must be assumed that virtually all of the absorbed iopanoic acid would be bound to serum albumin. In the presence of albumin, the hepatocyte uptake of iopanoic acid appears to occur primarily by a saturable carrier- or receptor-mediated mechanism (Barnhart JL, et al, 1983).

It has been suggested that the albumin-mediated hepatocyte uptake of cholecystographic media is related to their selective binding to cytoplasmic anion-binding proteins, Y and Z, found within the hepatocyte (Sokoloff J, et al, 1973). This mechanism has also been proposed for the hepatocyte uptake of bilirubin and Bromsulphalen® (Song CS, et al, 1976). The function of the hepatocyte cell membrane in this proposed mechanism is uncertain. It may simply act as a barrier to prevent passive diffusion of the albumin-bound cholecystographic media, thus forcing their hepatocyte uptake via the saturable mechanism. The binding of the cholecystographic agents to albumin appears to play no direct role in this mechanism other than providing competition for the cytoplasmic protein binding. Such competitive protein binding would be expected to result in the formation of an equilibrium across the hepatic cell membrane (Song CS, et al, 1976). Although no comparative studies on the rate of hepatocyte uptake of the cholecystographic agents have been performed, one can speculate that the more extensive albumin binding of iopanoic acid may decrease its rate of uptake compared to the other derivatives. In contradistinction, iopanoic acid may demonstrate stronger binding to the cytoplasmic proteins resulting in an enhanced rate of uptake.

Other mechanims have been proposed for the hepatocyte uptake of cholecystographic media, including the existence of a specific plasma membrane receptor for organic anions. Facilitated hepatocyte entry of the albumin-bound cholecystographic agent may also occur via plasma membrane receptors for albumin (Barnhart JL, 1984). However, this latter mechanism is unlikely based on the observation that the rate of hepatocyte uptake of iopanoic acid is actually diminished in the presence of albumin (Barnhart JL, et al, 1983).

Hepatic Metabolism. Following their hepatocyte uptake, the cholecystographic media are metabolized to form a monoglucuronide derivative. This process presumably occurs in the endoplasmic reticulum of the hepatocyte and involves the catalytic transfer of glucuronic acid from uridine diphosphate glucuronide via the enzyme, glucuronyl transferase. Bilirubin undergoes a similar biotransformation within the hepatocyte; however, bilirubin is excreted into bile as a diglucuronide derivative. It is theorized that the second glucuronide group is added to bilirubin at its canalicular membrane excretion site (Loeb PM and Berk RN, 1977).

Glucuronide conjugation of the cholecystographic media appears to play an important role in regard to their hepatobiliary excretion. The formation of the glucuronide derivative effectively decreases the concentration of the unmodified cholecystographic agent in the cytoplasm of the hepatocyte and may thus promote further uptake of the agent from the space of Disse by establishing a positive concentration gradient. Glucuronide metabolism also results in the formation of a derivative of increased molecular weight and water solubility, characteristics associated with more optimal biliary excretion. In fact, the formation of a glucuronide conjugate may be a structural requirement for the active-transport mechanism involved in the biliary excretion of the cholecystographic agents. The observation that iopanoate-glucuronide is excreted at a faster rate than the iopanoic acid base following intravenous injection suggests that glucuronide conjugation may be the rate-limiting step in the hepatobiliary excretion process (McChesney EW and Hoppe JO, 1956). Glucuronide conjugation may further promote the biliary excretion of cholecystographic agents by increasing their polarity and preventing their reverse diffusion from the bile ducts into the hepatocytes (Berk RN and Loeb PM, 1977a; Loeb PM and Berk RN, 1977).

Biliary Excretion and Bile Concentration. Excretion of the conjugated cholecystographic media from the hepatocytes into the bile ducts appears to involve an active-transport, carrier-mediated mechanism located at the canalicular membrane. Analysis of the kinetics of hepatobiliary excretion of cholecystographic agents indicates that the overall process is saturable. As the concentration of the cholecystographic agent in plasma increases, its rate of excretion in the bile also increases (Figure 6.5). Eventually, however, the rate of biliary excretion of the conjugated agent slows and reaches a

maximum (i.e., transport maximum), whereupon any further increase in the plasma concentration has no further effect on the rate of biliary excretion (Berk RN, et al, 1977b; Loeb PM and Berk RN, 1977; Barnhart JL, 1984). The specific rate-limiting step (or steps) responsible for this transport maximum may involve the hepatocyte uptake process, the requirement for glucuronide conjugation, or the carrier-mediated transport mechanism at the canalicular membrane. It has been suggested that the known renal excretion of glucuronide conjugates of the cholecystographic agents occurs as a result of reverse diffusion of the conjugated agent from the hepatocyte into the blood (Cooke WJ and Mudge GH, 1975). This would indicate that the hepatic capacity for uptake and conjugation of the cholecystographic agents exceeds the net capacity for their excretion into the bile, thus suggesting that the transport mechanism at the canalicular membrane is the rate-limiting step.

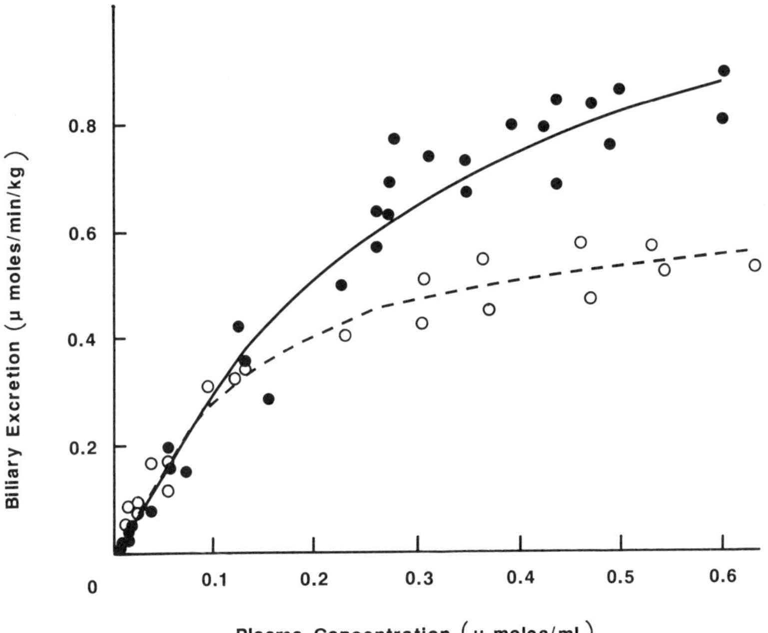

Figure 6.5 Relationship between plasma concentration of iopanoic acid and its biliary excretion rate. Data obtained in dogs at two rates of continuous bile salt (taurocholate sodium) infusion, 0.5 μmol/min/kg (open circles) and 2 μmol/min/kg (closed circles). (From Berk RN, et al, 1976; with permission.)

Table 6.4 MAXIMUM BILIARY EXCRETION RATES (EM) OF CHOLECYSTOGRAPHIC MEDIA AT DIFFERENT RATES OF BILE SALT (TAUROCHOLATE) INFUSION (DATA DERIVED) FROM CHRONIC BILE FISTULA DOGS)

	EM[a]	
	Tauroholate Infusion Rate[a]	
CONTRAST MEDIUM	*0.5*	*2.0*
Iopanoic acid[b]	0.67	1.33
Tyropanoate[b]	0.96	1.12
Iocetamic acid[c]	1.07	1.24
Ipodate[b]	1.47	1.42

[a] μmol/min/kg
[b] Adapted from Loeb PM and Berk RN, 1977
[c] Adapted from Barnhart JL, 1984

The cholecystographic agents do exhibit different rates of maximum biliary excretion (Table 6.4). In addition, the rates of biliary excretion of iopanoic (Cooke WJ and Mudge, GH, 1975; Berk RN, et al, 1974b; Moss AA, et al, 1972) and iocetamic acid (Barnhart JL, et al, 1979a) have been shown to increase in the presence of bile salt-induced choleresis (increased bile flow), whereas the rates of biliary excretion of tyropanoate and ipodate are either not affected (Berk RN, et al, 1976), or are affected significantly less (Barnhart JL, 1984), by the presence of bile salts (Table 6.4). Several mechanisms have been proposed to explain this bile salt enhancement of iopanoic and iocetamic acid excretion (Loeb PM and Berk RN, 1977; Barnhart JL, 1984).

Due to osmotic forces created by their active biliary excretion, bile salts increase bile flow by promoting the passive transport of water into the bile canaliculi. The choleresis produced by bile salts dilutes the bile concentration of the excreted cholecystographic agent and may thus enhance their hepatocyte excretion by establishing a positive concentration gradient. It has been shown, however, that the induction of choleresis in the absence of bile salts has no effect on the biliary excretion of iopanoic acid (Berk RN, et al, 1974b). Hence, the bile salt itself is the key component responsible for the increased biliary excretion of the involved cholecystographic agents. This enhancing effect of bile salts has been demonstrated to occur independent of changes in the plasma-to-liver concentration ratio or in the hepatic subcellular distribution of the cholecystographic agent (Barnhart JL, et al,

1980), thus negating the possibility that bile salts influence the rate of hepatic uptake or conjugation of the involved agents. Bile salts may promote biliary excretion of the involved cholecystographic media by forming micelles to prevent reverse diffusion of the agent from the bile duct to the hepatocyte. However, as previously discussed, glucuronide conjugates of the cholecystographic agents are polar and, as such, are already resistant to reverse diffusion. Moreover, the bile salt, dehydrocholate, is minimally capable of forming micelles, but it does enhance the biliary excretion of iopanoic acid (Berk RN, et al, 1974b). All low rates of bile salt infusion, the canalicular excretion of bile salts occur primarily in the periphery of the hepatic lobule, whereas at higher infusion rates the centrilobular canaliculi also become involved. Hence, bile salts may increase biliary excretion of the involved cholecystographic agents via recruitment of the centrilobular bile canaliculi. This mechanism should, however, be relatively nonspecific and promote increased biliary excretion of each of the cholecystographic agents. Finally, it has been suggested that the bile salts may elicit a change in the structure and activity of the carrier enzyme responsible for active transport of the conjugated cholecystographic agent at the site of the canalicular membrane. This allosteric interaction may involve the carrier's affinity for the chemical group at position 3 of the aromatic ring of the cholecystographic agents. Iocetamic acid and iopanoic acid commonly possess a single amino group at this position, whereas ipodate and tyropanoate have extended chemical substituents (Figure 6.3).

The concentration that a cholecystographic agent achieves in the bile is dependent on several factors including its rate of biliary excretion, the basal rate of bile flow, and the degree to which the contrast agent itself induces choleresis. As previously described, the basal rate of bile flow is primarily influenced by the osmotic effects of excreted bile salts. In addition, basal flow may also be affected by a bile salt independent, active sodium transport mechanism. The excreted glucuronide conjugates of the cholecystographic agents are also capable of exerting osmotic effects and producing choleresis (Table 6.5). The choleretic activities of conjugated tyropanoate and iocetamic acid are relatively equivalent and slightly greater than ipodate. Conjugated iopanoic acid is virtually devoid of choleretic effects. Each of the oral cholecystographic media produce significantly less choleresis than the intravenous cholangiographic agents (Barnhart JL, 1984). Increased rates of basal bile flow or agent-induced choleresis act to reduce the bile duct concentration of the ex-

Table 6.5 CHOLERETIC ACTIVITY OF GLUCURONIDE DERIVATIVES OF CHOLECYSTOGRAPHIC CONTRAST MEDIA[a]

CONTRAST MEDIUM	INDUCED CHOLERESIS[b]
Iopanoic acid	1
Ipodate	8
Tyropanoate	10
Iocetamic acid	10

[a] Adapted from Barnhart JL, 1984

[b] mL/mmol contrast excreted

creted media. The bile duct concentration of iodine achieved with the oral administration of the cholecystographic media is extremely low regardless of their induced choleretic effects, the clinical use of these oral media being primarily based on their concentration in the gallbladder.

Gallbladder Concentration. Although 40–70% of an oral dose of a cholecystographic medium is normally excreted by the hepatobiliary route, the rate of biliary excretion following oral administration is slow, thus limiting the concentration of iodine in the bile at any given point in time. Hence, the ability of these agents to produce adequate opacification of gallbladder is based on the fact that during the interdigestive phase the majority of bile (and excreted cholecystographic media) produced by the hepatocytes is diverted to the gallbladder where it is stored until the gallbladder is stimulated to contract via the physiological effects (i. e., cholecystokinin release) of a subsequent meal. Since the capacity of the gallbladder is only approximately 50–60 mL, the bile must be concentrated significantly to permit its storage. The gallbladder concentrates bile by a process that initially involves the active reabsorption of sodium, chloride, and bicarbonate ions. In order to maintain an isoosmotic environment, this reabsorption of physiological ions is accompanied by the passive diffusion of water. By way of this mechanism, the concentration of biliary solutes retained within the gallbladder can increase by a factor of 8–10 (Rous P and McMaster PD, 1921).

The glucuronide conjugates of the cholecystographic media are not reabsorbed

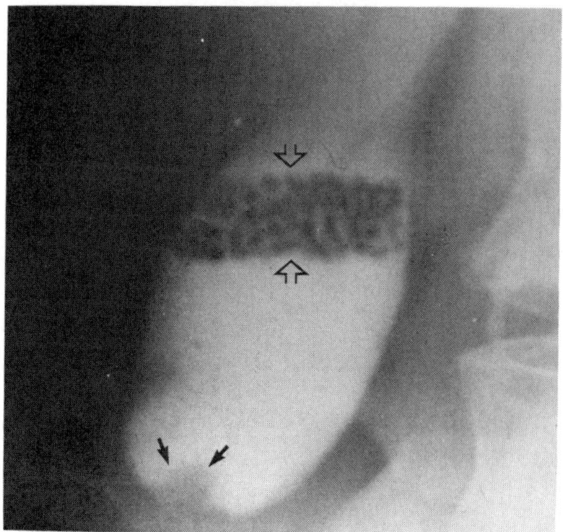

Figure 6.6 Multiple small stones form a broad layer (open black arrows) in the body of the upright gallbladder due to their lower specific gravity relative to the bile-contrast medium mixture. The filling defect at the apex of the fundus (closed black arrows) was due to focal fibrosis.

from the normal gallbladder, hence their gallbladder concentration and the associated degree of opacification increase substantially with time. Glucuronide conjugation acts to increase the aqueous solubility of the cholecystographic agents and thus prevents their precipitation within the gallbladder lumen. However, the glucuronidase activity of bacteria present within a diseased gallbladder can lead, in rare instances, to deconjugation and precipitation of the cholecystographic media (Berk RN, et al, 1974a). The specific gravity of the concentrated contrast-bile mixture commonly exceeds that of gallstones resulting in the layering of stones within the opacified gallbladder contents (Figure 6.6).

An iodine concentration of 0.25–1% is required for adequate radiographic visualization of the gallbladder (Edholm P and Jacobson B, 1959; Joffe H and Wachowski TJ, 1942). Depending on their relative rates of intestinal absorption and biliary excretion, the various cholecystographic agents may require different time intervals post oral administration in order to achieve an adequate

Table 6.6 TIME INTERVALS POST ORAL ADMINISTRATION OF CHOLECYSTOGRAPHIC MEDIA FOR OPTIMUM GALLBLADDER OPACIFICATION

CONTRAST MEDIUM	OPTIMUM TIME INTERVAL (HRS)
Iocetamic acid	10–15
Iopanoic acid	14–19
Ipodate calcium, sodium	10
Tyropanoate sodium	10–12

[a] Adapted from respective product insert information

gallbladder concentration and optimal gallbladder visualization (Table 6.6). Radiographic imaging performed prior to the appropriate time interval post administration may result in a false-positive study for gallbladder disease.

Several physiological factors may alter the normal kinetics of cholecystographic media and result in nonvisualization of the gallbladder. Since bilirubin competes for the same transport mechanisms, the rate of hepatocyte uptake and biliary excretion of the cholecystographic media may be substantially restricted in the presence of hepatic dysfunction and hyperbilirubinemia. Of course, cystic duct obstruction will result in gallbladder nonopacification by preventing respective entry of the cholecystographic medium. Stasis of bile flow associated with prolonged hyperalimentation or fasting can produce a similar effect in the presence of a patent cystic duct. This latter situation can be alleviated by including (e. g., fatty meal, exogenous cholecystokinin-derivative) gallbladder contraction and elimination of the viscous bile prior to administration of the cholecystographic medium.

Cholecystographic nonvisualization of the gallbladder in the presence of a patent cystic duct can also occur due to alterations in the normal resorptive processes of the gallbladder. As previously described, glucuronide conjugates of the cholecystographic agents are not reabsorbed from the normal gallbladder. It has been shown, however, that iopanoate-glucuronide is rapidly absorbed from an inflammed gallbladder, resulting in a reduction in its luminal concentration and

a decrease in gallbladder opacification (Berk RN and Lasser EC, 1964).

Gallbladder Excretion and Enterohepatic Circulation. The presence of fat within the small intestine stimulates the release of cholecystokinin from the intestinal mucosa. This hormone acts directly on the smooth muscle of the biliary system to produce contraction of the gallbladder and relaxation of the sphincter of Oddi. The concentrated bile and conjugated cholecystographic agent stored within the gallbladder are thus excreted into the duodenum via the common bile duct. Most of the conjugated contrast agent subsequently passes into the colon and is eliminated in the feces. For example, studies indicate that 65–75% of an oral dose of iopanoic acid is recovered in the feces within 5 days post administration (Schroder JS and Rooney D, 1953).

Cholecystographic agents excreted into the duodenum are capable of undergoing intestinal reabsorption with reentry into the blood. Such enterohepatic circulation of a cholecystographic medium may occur in the form of its excreted glucuronide conjugate or its free base. Although the lipid solubility and, hence, passive permeability coefficient of a glucuronide conjugate may be less than that of the free base by a factor of 3–4, its solubility in the bulk-water phase of the intestinal lumen may be a factor of 25–40 times greater. As previously discussed (see Intestinal Absorption), the initial water solubility of a cholecystographic agent has a greater effect on its rate of intestinal absorption than its passive permeability coefficient. It is therefore not surprising that the glucuronide conjugates of cholecystographic media are capable of direct intestinal absorption (Barnhart JL, et al, 1980; Barnhart JL, 1984). It is also possible for the excreted glucuronide conjugates of cholecystographic media to undergo deconjugation to the free base via the action of beta-glucuronidase, an enzyme produced by normal bacteria (especially anaerobic coliforms) within the intestinal tract. Enterohepatic circulation of the cholecys-

Table 6.7 APPROXIMATE DEGREE OF RENAL EXCRETION OF THE CHOLECYSTOGRAPHIC MEDIA[a]

CONTRAST MEDIUM	RENAL EXCRETION (% ADMINISTERED DOSE)
Iopanoic acid	33[b]
Ipodate calcium, sodium	45[c]
Tyropanoate sodium	45[b]
Iocetamic acid	62[d]

[a] Assuming normal liver function
[b] From McChesney E W and Hoppe JO, 1965
[c] From Heckster R E M, 1968
[d] From *Drug Information*, 1985

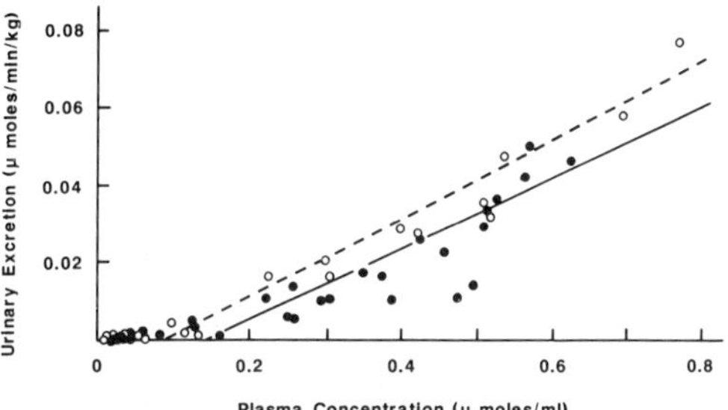

Figure 6.7 Relationship between urinary excretion rate of iopanoic acid and plasma concentration. Data obtained in dogs at two rates of continuous bile salt (taurocholate sodium) infusion, 0.5 μmol/min/kg (open circles) and 2.0 μmol/min/kg (closed circles). (From Berk RN, et al, 1976; with permission.)

tographic media by this process would be expected to be delayed since the conjugated agent must first pass from the duodenum to the colon where the bacteria reside (Goldberg HI, et al, 1977).

Renal Excretion. The various cholecystographic media can exhibit significant renal excretion following their oral administration (Table 6.7). Analysis of the chemical nature of the urinary cholecystographic agents indicates that they are excreted primarily in the form of their glucuronide conjugates (McChesney EW and Hoppe JO, 1956; McChesney EW and Banks WF, 1965). This would suggest that hepatic metabolism of the oral cholecystographic agents must occur prior to their renal excretion. The kidney is capable of directly forming glucuronide derivatives of certain drugs; however, this process appears to occur to a negligible extent with the cholecystographic media (Berndt WO, et al, 1971). The source of the conjugated cholecystographic agents for renal excretion may therefore be associated with their previously described direct enterohepatic circulation. It appears more likely, however, that urinary excretion of the conjugated cholecystographic agents occurs as a result of their reverse diffusion from the hepatocytes into the blood. This could occur if the hepatic capacity for uptake and conjugation of a cholecystographic agent exceeds the capacity for biliary excretion of the conjugated derivative at the active transport site of the canalicular membrane (Cooke WJ and Mudge GH, 1975).

An evaluation of the renal clearance kinetics of the cholecystographic agents reveals that, above a minimum plasma concentration, their rate of renal excretion is linearly related to their plasma concentration (Figure 6.7). This would suggest that a passive diffusion mechanism, most likely glomerular filtration, is involved in the renal excretion of the conjugated derivatives. The lack of significant renal excretion of the conjugated media below a minimum plasma concentration probably reflects a requirement for saturation of the hepatobiliary transport mechanism prior to their elimination by the alternate renal pathway. As might be expected, hepatic dysfunction further increases the extent of renal excretion of the cholecystographic media (Loeb PM and Berk RN, 1977; Barnhart JL, 1984).

PHYSIOLOGICAL EFFECTS

In the early 1960s, Lasser and others demonstrated direct correlation between the systemic toxicity (LD_{50}) of radiopaque contrast media and their degree of protein binding (Lasser EC, et al, 1962). Based on this observation and the knowledge that cholecystographic media are transported in blood extensively bound to serum albumin, it may be expected that the clinical use of these agents would be associated with a high incidence of adverse reactions. However, as a result of their slow and often incomplete absorption from the intestinal tract, the incidence of major adverse reactions with the oral cholecystographic media is relatively low. Intestinal retention of these oral media and their excreted metabolites does, however, result in a high incidence of gastrointestinal disturbances.

Unpredictable pseudo-allergic reactions to iodinated contrast media can occur independent of the dose or plasma concentration of the administered agent (see Chapter 8). Thus, reactions of a hypersensitivity nature can occur with the slow intestinal absorption and low plasma concentrations of the cholecystographic agents. Moreover, as a result of their enterohepatic circulation and prolonged blood levels, the occurrence of a pseudo-allergic reaction to an oral cholecystographic agent may be delayed for several days following its administration. Cross-sensitivity reactions between iodinated intravascular and cholecystographic media have been known to occur, therefore cholecystography should be performed with caution and pretreatment regimens instituted in patients who have previously experienced a major pseudo-allergic reaction to any iodinated contrast medium.

Gastrointestinal Effects. Approximately 50% of the patients who receive oral cholecystographic media will experience gastrointestinal side effects including nausea, vomiting, and diarrhea (White WW and Fischer HW, 1962). It is felt that these gastrointestinal disturbances are primarily related to direct molecular toxicity of the administered agent and are therefore dose dependent. In view of its lower solubility in the bulk-water phase of the intestinal tract and its diminished intestinal absorption, the incidence of gastrointestinal side effects, especially diarrhea, are greater for iopanoic acid versus equivalent diagnostic doses of the other cholecystographic media.

The gastrointestinal disturbances and various systemic side effects of cholecystographic media may also be associated with their ability to inhibit the enzyme acetylcholinesterase (Lasser EC and Lang JH, 1966b). An associated increase in systemic levels of acetylcholine may be responsible for the increase in gastrointestinal activity and diarrhea, the vasodilation and decrease in systemic blood pressure, and the increase in depth and rate of respirations commonly observed following the administration of cholecystographic media.

Renal Effects. Renal impairment, evidenced by an increase in blood urea nitrogen or serum creatinine levels or a decrease in creatinine clearance, may occur following administration of the oral cholecystographic media. The nephrotoxic effects produced by these agents are usually mild and transient, however complete renal failure has been reported. Animal toxicology studies have revealed microscopic changes consistent with diffuse renal tubular degeneration. Albumin and bile casts or albuminous interstitial exudate may or may not be present (Fink HE, et al, 1964).

Several mechanisms (Table 6.8) have been proposed to explain the renal toxicity of cholecystographic media (Mudge GH, 1970). It has been suggested that the nephrotoxic effects of these agents may be related to their high degree of protein binding and interference with tubular enzyme systems. Although there is no direct evidence that the associated renal tubular toxicity is due to obstructive uric acid crystallization, it is known that iopanoic acid and ipodate are potent uricosuric agents (Postlethwaite AE and Kelley WH, 1971). This effect appears to be related to the ability of these media to displace uric acid from its albumin-binding sites and thus promote its tubular secretion. The uricosuric effect of these cholecystographic media commences at 3–7 hours post administration and may persist

Table 6.8 POSSIBLE MECHANISMS RESPONSIBLE FOR THE NEPHROTOXIC EFFECTS OF CHOLECYSTOGRAPHIC MEDIA

Interference with renotubular enzymes
Obstructive crystaluria
  · Uricosuria
  · Contrast medium precipitation
Renovascular constriction
Idiosyncratic

for 5–6 days. It is unlikely that the cholecystographic media themselves form obstructive crystals, since they are slowly excreted in the form of their highly water-soluble glucuronide conjugates. It is known that the cholecystographic agents can produce direct dilation of blood vessels and systemic hypotension (Fink HE, et al, 1964). It has therefore been speculated that the nephrotoxic effects of these agents may be related to the compensatory renin-mediated renovascular constriction that normally accompanies systemic hypotension.

The incidence of renal impairment with the cholecystographic media does not appear to correlate with the presence of preexisting renal diesease (Harrow BR and Winslow OP, 1966). There is, however, an increased incidence of contrast-induced renal dysfunction with any factor that results in elevated renal excretion of the cholecystographic agents (Teplick JG, et al, 1965). For example, excessively large or multiple doses of a cholecystographic medium may produce plasma levels that exceed its hepatic transport capacity, thus resulting in an increase in the extent of its renal excretion and potential for renal toxicity. Preexisting liver disease can be expected to decrease the hepatic transport capacity for a cholecystographic medium and lead to an increase in renal clearance even at normal dosage levels. This latter condition may also result in diminished glucuronide conjugation of the cholecystographic agent resulting in a greater potential for its precipitation in the renal tubules and an increase in plasma half-life and hypotensive effects. Hence, the oral cholecystographic agents should be administered with caution to patients with elevated serum bilirubin levels. The dosage of the cholecystographic medium should not be increased above routine levels in an attempt to obtain a satisfactory cholecystogram in the face of its decreased hepatic excretion.

Hepatic Effects. The oral cholecystographic media can demonstrate mild hepatotoxic effects as evidenced by an asymptomatic elevation of alkaline phosphatase or other liver enzymes. Total serum bilirubin levels may also increase with these agents; however, this finding may be related to competition for the same hepatobility-excretion mechanisms rather than a toxic effect on the liver cells.

PRECAUTIONS

Drug–Contrast Media Interactions. Cholestyramine resins, administered orally, bind bile salts in the gastrointestinal tract and promote their fecal elimination. This results in diminished enterohepatic circulation of bile salts and decreased gastrointestinal absorption of lipid-soluble substrates (i. e., cholesterol, fatty acids) incorporated into bile salt micelles. Hence, cholestyramine resins are commonly used therapeutically to reduce plasma cholesterol levels and to control pruritis associated with high plasma concentration of bile salts. It has been shown that the gastrointestinal absorption of oral cholecystographic agents is reduced if they are administered concurrently with cholestyramine resins (Nelson JA, 1974; Lindgren I, 1976). This may be related to direct cholestyramine binding of the contrast agent, or to cholestyramine binding of bile salts with a corresponding decrease in micelle-facilitated gastrointestinal absorption of the cholecystographic media. It is therefore advisable that cholestyramine therapy be discontinued during the interval of cholecystographic agent administration and associated imaging.

In recognition of the extensive albumin binding of the cholecystographic agents, consideration must be given to their respective effects on the competitive displacement and pharmacological enhancement of other albumin-bound drugs. For example, experimental studies have shown that the oral cholecystographic media can displace warfarin and diazepam from their albumin-binding sites and may thus induce an increase in the respective anticoagulant and sedative activities of these drugs (Wosilait WD and Ryan MP,

1980; Fehske EJ and Miller WE, 1981). However, the low plasma concentrations associated with slow intestinal absorption of oral cholecystographic media make it unlikely that such competitive displacement of albumin-bound drugs would result in clinically significant effects.

Iopanoic acid, administered intravenously in concurrence with iodipamide, results in diminished hepatic excretion of the latter agent (Goergen T, et al, 1974). Such competition of the cholecystographic and cholangiographic media for the same hepatobiliary-excretion mechanisms could result in a prolongation of their plasma concentrations and an increase in their degree of renal excretion and potential for nephrotoxic effects. However, iopanoic acid administered orally at 14 hours prior to iodipamide had no effects on respective hepatic or renal kinetics. Therefore, if cholecystography and cholangiography are indicated for the same patient, it is generally suggested that administration of the cholangiographic medium should be delayed until 24 hours following administration of the cholecystographic agent. A similar consideration would apply to the performance of hepatobiliary scintigraphy procedures following the oral administration of cholecystographic media, since the involved radiopharmaceuticals (Tc-99m disofenin, merbrofenin, or alternate HIDA derivatives), are also excreted by the same hepatobiliary mechanisms.

Contrast Media–Laboratory Test Interactions. The hepatobiliary excretion of oral cholecystographic media involves the same mechanisms that are responsible for the excretion of a variety of organic anions including bilirubin and Bromsulphalein®. Hence, it is possible that the administration of oral cholecystographic media can lead to an elevation in the serum concentration of bilirubin and Bromsulphalein® in the absence of hepatic disease. Normal oral doses of the cholecystographic agents do not, however, result in sufficient plasma concentration to routinely produce clinically significant alterations in the serum levels of

these diagnostic indicators (Johnson RA and Mora LO, 1968; Reiner RG, et al, 1980).

As previously discussed (see Physiological Effects), the mild hepatoxic effects of oral cholecystographic agents can lead to an elevation of serum transaminase or alkaline phosphatase enzymes (Heckster REM, 1968). These alterations in hepatic enzyme levels are usually clinically insignificant but may be observed as late as 22 days post administration of the radiopaque contrast media (Reiner RG, et al, 1980).

Iopanoic acid and sodium ipodate have been shown to produce alterations in thyroid function tests in the absence of thyroid disease (Reiner RG, et al, 1980; Kleinman RE, et al, 1980; Beng CG, et al, 1980; Burghi H, et al, 1976). These interactions, which include a depression of total T_3 and an elevation of total T_4 and TSH values, appear to occur as a result of contrast inhibition of the enzyme responsible for 5-monodeiodination of T_4, or contrast-induced displacement of T_4 from its hepatic binding sites. (Felicetta JV, et al, 1980). Significant abnormalities in these thyroid function tests may persist for as long as 3 weeks following contrast administration. In addition, thyroid function tests based on iodine measurements (i e., radioactive iodine uptake, serum protein-bound iodine) can be altered for several weeks to months following cholecystography (Clark RE and Shipley RA, 1957).

Iopanoic acid and sodium ipodate are known to be potent uricosuric agents, with effects that persist for 5–6 days post administration (Postlethwaite AE and Kelly WH, 1971). Hence, the oral administration of these agents can invalidate serum or urinary measurements of urate levels performed during this interval. In addition, oral cholecystographic media can produce false-positive findings of albuminuria based on urinary protein precipitation tests (Holonbek JE, et al, 1953). This laboratory test interaction may be observed for up to 3 days after contrast administration.

CLINICAL INDICATIONS

Study Indications. Cholecystography, performed following the oral administration of a cholecystographic medium, is primarily indicated for the demonstration of gallbladder calculi in patients with symptoms of chronic cholecystitis (Table 6.9) or with acute pancreatitis. The radiographic diagnosis of cholelithiasis is commonly based on the direct visualization of gallstones within the opacified gallbladder (Figures 6.6, 6.8). Nonvisualization of the gallbladder following two consecutive daily doses (see Dosage) of an oral cholecystographic contrast medium is strongly suggestive of obstruction of the cystic duct or gallbladder neck and gallbladder inflammation, provided that extrabiliary causes of gallbladder nonvisualization have been excluded. Several factors (Table 6.10) associated with altered gastrointestinal or hepatic kinetics of the cholecystographic medium can result in nonvisualization of the gallbladder in the absence of respective disease. These factors must be excluded prior to adequate interpretation of the examination (Berk RN, 1977c). Benign processes (eg., tumors, polyps), carcinomas, or metastases can also appear as fixed defects within the opacified gallbladder (Figure 6.9) or be associated with its nonvisualization.

Cholecystography is less commonly indicated for the diagnosis or evaluation of hyperplastic cholecystic syndromes. Included in this category are the noninflammatory pathological processes of adenomyomatosis, which involves proliferation of the gallbladder mucosa with muscle wall thickening, protrusion, and compartmentalization (Figure 6.10), and cholesterosis. Alterations in gallbladder anatomy (Figures 6.11, 6.12) or location (Figure 6.13) may also be demonstrated with cholecystography. The adjunct administration of a fatty meal or cholecystokinin analog (see Adjunctive Drugs) to stimulate gallblader contraction has been utilized for the cholecystographic evaluation of gallbladder dysfunction in suspected acalculous cholecystitis or biliary dyskinesis (Berk RN, 1977c).

Contrast Media Considerations. The choice of which of the commercially available agents to utilize for cholecystography is probably not as critical as being fully aware of the respective pharmacokinetic properties of the agent selected. As noted, depending on their relative rates of gastrointestinal absorption and biliary excretion, the various cholecystographic media require different time intervals post administration for optimal gallbladder visualization (Table 6.6). Certain of the available agents require the concomitant administration of a fatty meal for associated bile salt enhancement of their intestinal aborption (i. e., iopanoic acid) or biliary excretion (i. e., iopanoic acid, iocetamic acid), whereas with alternate agents the concomitant administration of a fatty meal can decrease their ability to opacify the gallbladder. Although several comparison studies have appeared in the literature, a conclusion regarding the most efficacious agent for cholecystography is difficult due to lack of study attention to the aforementioned pharmacokinetic parameters and the nonavailability of a single, controlled study comparing all four of the available agents. The majority of clinical comparisons involving iopanoic acid have noted that this agent is associated with an increased incidence of gastrointestinal side effects, especially diarrhea, in comparison with the other media (Juhl JH, 1963; White WW and Fischer HW, 1962; Heckster REM, 1968). In addition, iopanoic acid generally produces less gallbladder opacification than the other agents if administered in the absence of a fatty meal (Stanley RJ, 1974).

Table 6.9 INDICATIONS FOR CHOLECYSTOGRAPHY

Cholelithiasis (gallstones)
Hyperplastic cholecystosis syndromes
  · Adenomyomatosis
  · Cholesterolosis
Anatomical abnormalities
Abnormal gallbladder function
  · Acalculous cholecystitis
  · Biliary dyskinesis

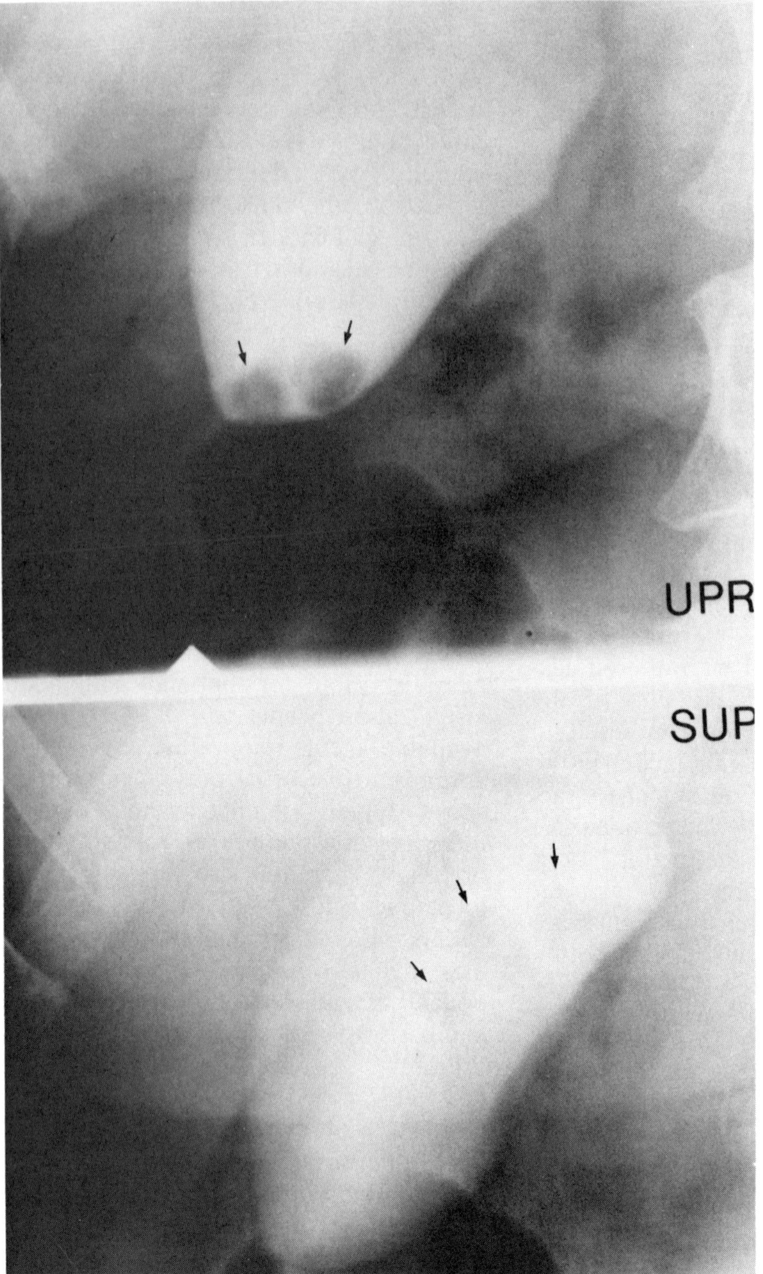

Figure 6.8   Mobile gallstones (black arrows) accumulate at the dependent fundus with the patient in an upright (UPR) position. With supine (SUP) positioning, the stones gravitate proximally.

Patient Preparation. It is advised that the patient ingest a fatty meal on the day preceding the initial oral dose of the cholecystographic medium, regardless of the nature of the agent. The purpose of this procedure is to induce gallbladder contraction and elimination of its contents. In the absence of this maneuver, the gallbladder may be distended with thick or stagnated bile that can greatly diminish subsequent entry of the cholecystographic medium into, and its concentration within, the gallbladder.

Whether or not a fatty meal should be administered with the cholecystographic medium is dependent on which agent is

Table 6.10   EXTRABILIARY CAUSES OF GALLBLADDER NONVISUALIZATION[a]

Patient noncompliance re contrast dosing
Altered gastrointestinal kinetics
  · Vomiting
  · Esophageal disease/obstruction
  · Gastric retention
  · Nasogastric suctioning
  · Postoperative ileus
  · Gastrocolonic fistula
  · Pyloric obstruction
Altered gastrointestinal absorption
  · Decreased intestinal pH
  · Inadequate bile salt concentration (iopanoic acid)
  · Crohn's disease
  · Ileal resection
Altered hepatic kinetics
  · Liver disease
  · Hyperbilirubinemia
  · Inadequate bile salt excretion (iopanoic, iocetamic acids)
Stagnation of bile in gallbladder
  · Fasting
  · Hyperalimentation
Cholecystectomy
Acute pancreatitis/peritonitis
Trauma
Pernicious anemia

[a] Adapted from Berk RN, 1977c

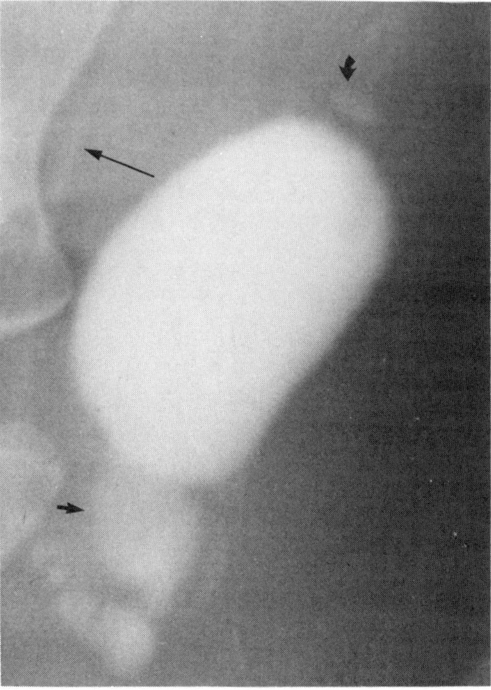

Figure 6.10 Cholecystographic (incorporating cholecystokinin-induced gallbladder contraction) demonstration of adenomyomatosis of the gallbladder. Note the deformity at the fundus (curved black arrow) and the focal contraction of the gallbladder neck (short black arrow). Contrast has been excreted into the common bile duct (long black arrow).

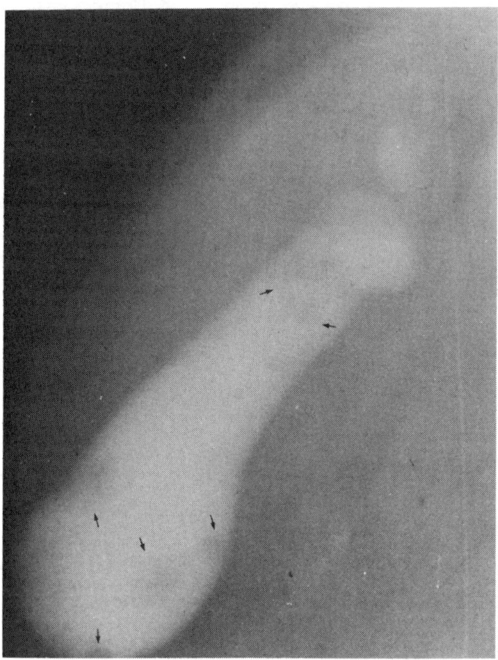

Figure 6.9 Multiple benign polyps appear as filling defects (black arrows) scattered throughout the gallbladder.

being utilized (Berk RN, 1977c). The enterohepatic circulation of bile salts induced by the ingestion of a fatty meal is a requirement for adequate intestinal absorption of iopanoic acid and enhances the biliary excretion of both iopanoic and iocetamic acids. Conversely, the ingestion of a fatty meal can interfere with intestinal absorption of the other cholecystographic media. Fatty meals ingested following administration of the cholecystographic media will promote gallbladder contraction and elimination of the slowly accumulating contrast. In general, it has been shown that the concomitant administration of a fatty meal improves gallbladder opacification with iopanoic acid, but decreases opacification with other cholecystographic agents (Stanley RJ, 1974). Hence, patients should be maintained on a fat-free diet during the 2-day interval associated with the administration of ipodate sodium or calcium, tyropanoate sodium, or iocetamic acid.

As a result of their renal-excretion and potential uricosuric effect, dehydration

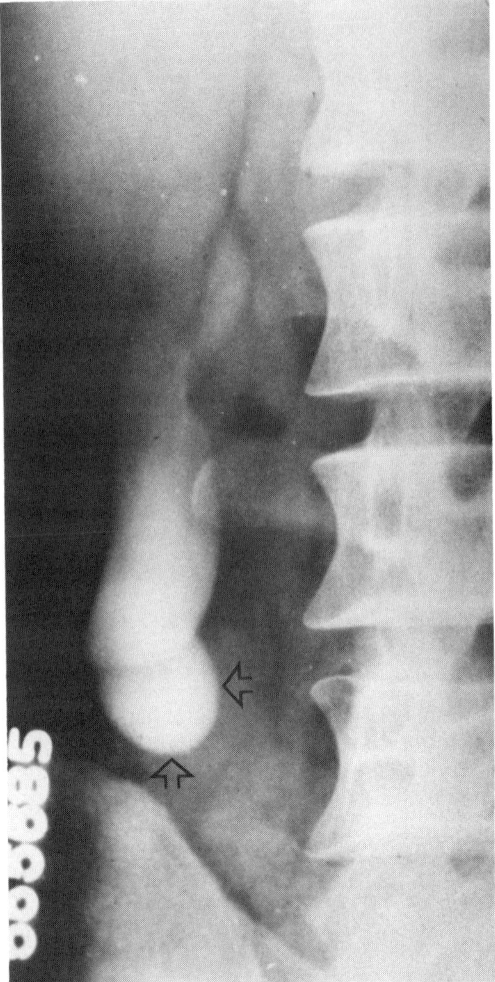

Figure 6.11 Cholecystogram demonstrating a "phrygian cap," an anatomical variant of no clinical significance.

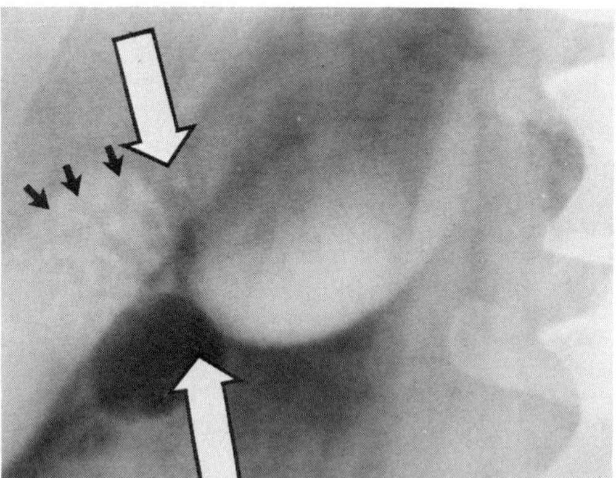

Figure 6.12 Cholecystogram demonstrating gallbladder duplication. The large white arrows denote the separation between the normal medial gallbladder and the stone-filled (black arrows) lateral gallbaldder.

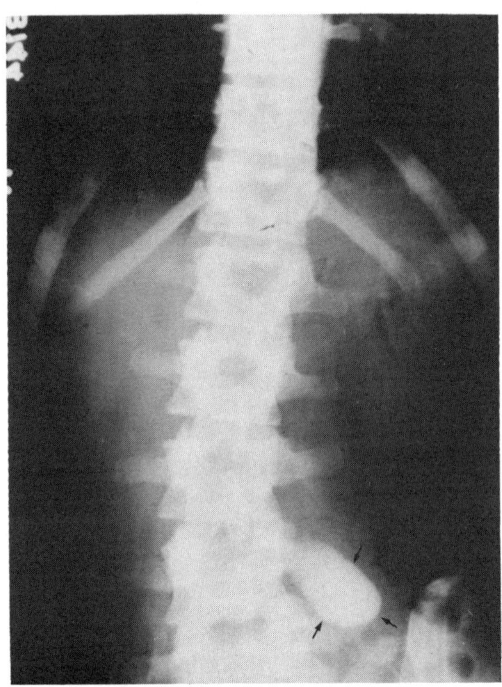

Figure 6.13 Cholecystogram demonstrating the gallbladder (black arrows) localized to the left lower quadrant. Since the liver is not enlarged, this finding suggests an elongated gallbladder mesentery.

should be avoided in patients receiving the oral cholecystographic media. In patients with a history of gout, it may be advisable to prescribe a specific hydration regimen and to alkalinize the urine. As an additional note, the concomitant administration of aspirin, 600 mg every 2 hours, has been shown to decrease the uricosuric activity of cholecystographic media (Postlethwaite AE and Kelly WH, 1972).

Laxatives or cleansing enemas are commonly administered prior to the cholecystographic imaging procedure in order to eliminate overlying fecal material or intestinal gas which might interfere with gall-bladder visualization or interpretation of the examination (Figure 6.14).

Adjunctive Drugs. Cholecystographic evaluations of gallbladder function and

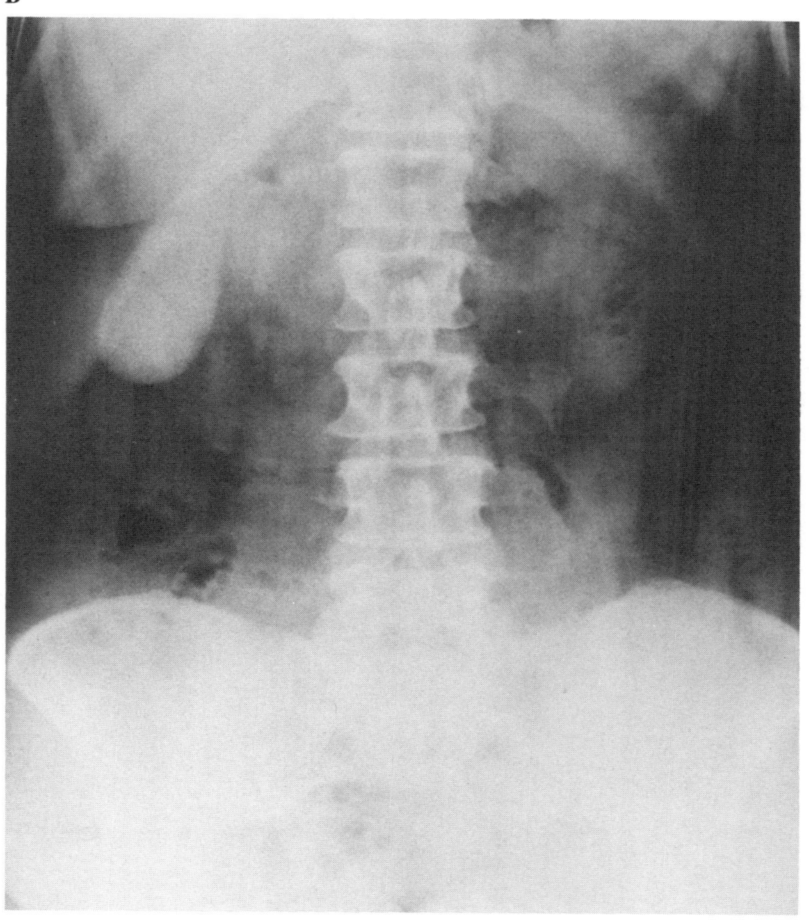

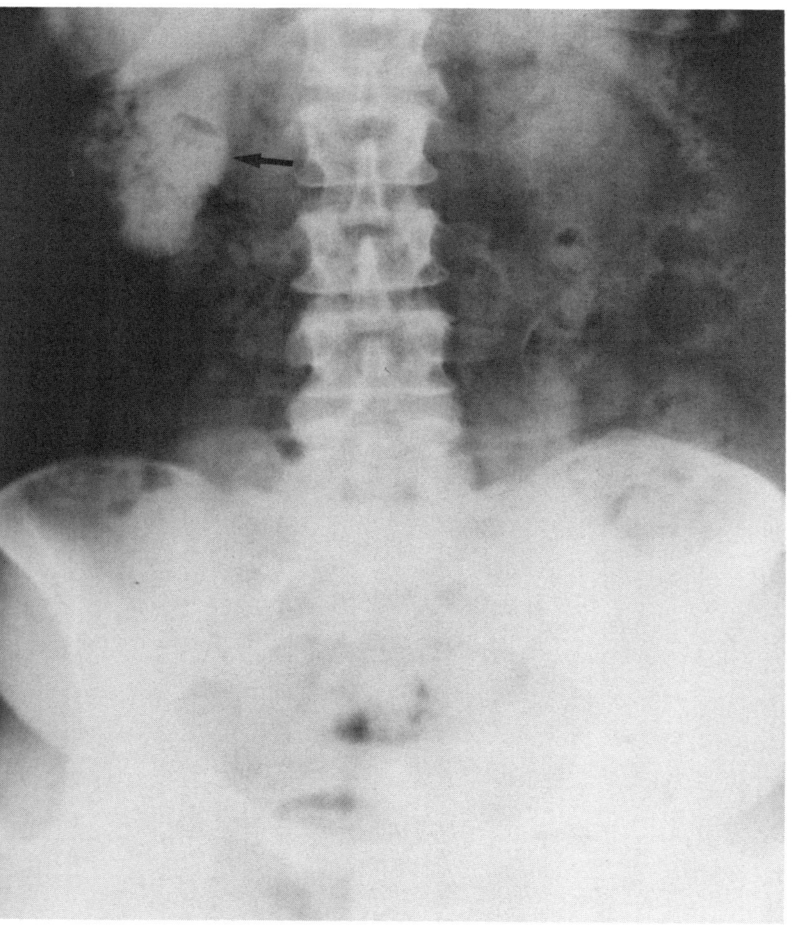

Figure 6.14   A. Cholecystogram demonstrating a well-opacified gallbladder (black arrow) partially obscured by colonic contents. B. Following bowel cleansing, the gallbladder is diagnosed as normal.

contractility involve the adjunctive administration of a fatty meal or cholecystokinin analog to stimulate gallbladder contraction and emptying of the stored radiopaque medium. The diagnosis of biliary dyskinesis is based on a demonstration of incomplete emptying (i. e., volume reduction of less than 20–50%) or spasm of the gallbladder in the absence of calculi or other causative pathologies. These techniques to induce gallbladder contraction may also prove useful for differentiating freely moving gallstones from fixed-wall defects (e. g., polyps, tumors), although a similar effect can usually be achieved with simple patient repositioning (Figure 6.8). Gallbladder contraction with elimination of some or all of the contrast-laden bile can result in the improved demonstration of adenomyomatosis (Figure 6.10), cholesterosis, or small calculi in the gallbladder neck, and permit the diagnosis of common bile duct obstruction (Berk RN, 1977c).

Although the administration of a fatty meal represents the most physiological approach to the stimulation of gallbladder contraction, the response is extremely variable in regard to both time and intensity. The reliable and rapid gallbladder contraction produced by intravenous cholecystokinin analogs, such as sincalide (20 ng/kg, IV), overcome the variabilities in response associated with a fatty meal and result in a less time-consuming examination.

Contraindications. Diminished and often inadequate opacification of the gallbladder will occur in the presence of hepatic disease and elevated serum bilirubin levels. This situation is due to both a disease-associated impairment of the hepatic transport capacity for the administered cholecystographic agent and a corresponding hyperbilirubinemia-associated increase in competition for the hepatobiliary-excretion mechanisms. Hence, the feasibility of obtaining an adequate oral cholecystogram decreases greatly with serum bilirubin levels above 2 mg % (Berk RN and Loeb PM, 1977a). More-

over, with diminished hepatobiliary excretion of the contrast medium, there is an increase in its plasma half-life and degree of renal excretion, thus increasing the potential for systemic or renal adverse effects. These agents should therefore be administered with caution to jaundiced patients, especially infants.

Patients with chronic renal disease have been shown to have an abnormally high frequency of gallbladder nonvisualization following a single 3.0 g dose of the cholecystographic media (Perrillo RP, et al, 1978). Such diminished or inadequate opacification of the gallbladder in the presence of renal failure may be associated with retained organic metabolites and their competition for the hepatobiliary-excretion mechanisms or the albumin-binding sites of cholecystographic media. Based on these considerations, the oral administration of cholecystographic agents is contraindicated in the presence of concomitant hepatic and renal disease.

DOSAGE

It has been shown that 10–20% of the cholecystograms that demonstrate no gallbladder visualization following a single 3.0 g dose of a cholecystographic medium will convert to a normal study after a second 3.0 g dose. Similarly, 65–75% of studies with faint gallbladder visualization after a single dose will demonstrate normal opacification after a second dose. Hence, nonvisualization or faint visualization of the gallbladder following a single 3.0 g dose of a cholecystographic medium cannot be considered a sensitive indicator of gallbladder disease even if extrabiliary causes of impaired opacification have been excluded (Berk RN, 1970).

Based on these considerations and a desire to avoid the expense and inconvenience of nondiagnostic single-dose examinations, the currently accepted procedure for cholecystography involves the oral administration of a 3.0 g dose of the cholecystographic medium on each of two consecutive evenings prior to radiographic examination (Burhenne HJ and Obata WG, 1975). This dosage regimen has been shown to produce reliable gallbladder opacification in normal subjects. It appears to overcome any problems associated with inadequate intestinal absorption of the administered agent and provides additional time for the hepatobiliary excretion and gallbladder concentrating mechanisms. Compared to a single 6.0 g "double" dose, this consecutive dosing method is less likely to exceed the hepatic transport capacity for the administered agent and is thus associated with a decreased potential for systemic or renal toxicity. The administration of more than two consecutive 3.0 gm doses of the cholecystographic medium has not been shown to produce a further increase in the frequency of gallbladder visualization (Berk RN, 1977c).

It has been suggested that fractionating the administration of the cholecystographic medium over a 5–6 hour period (i. e., 500 mg every hour for 6 hours) may decrease the percentage of false-positive gallbladder nonvisualizations observed with a single 3.0 g dose (Koehler PR and Kyaw MM, 1973). However, the reliability of this technique is questionable (Nehen AM and Kruse V, 1978), and in view of the limited toxicity and expense of the oral cholecystographic media, administration of the second 3.0 g dose remains advisable.

II. Cholangiographic Contrast Media

CHEMISTRY

The only cholangiographic contrast medium currently available commercially in the United States is the meglumine salt of iodipamide (Figure 6.15). This relatively strong dibasic acid is ionic at physiological pH values and is therefore soluble in sterile, pyrogen-free aqueous solutions suitable for intravenous administration. The commercially available formulations (Table 6.11) incorporate low concentrations of edetate disodium and sodium citrate as sequestering and buffering agents to enhance the aqueous stability of the medium. Two concentrations of the agent are available, the 52% w/v formulation being indicated for slow intravenous administration and the 10.3% w/v formulation for drip infusion. Iodipamide meglumine contains 49.4% iodine on a per weight basis. The medium is stable to mild heating, but should not be heated excessively or exposed directly to light for a prolonged period of time.

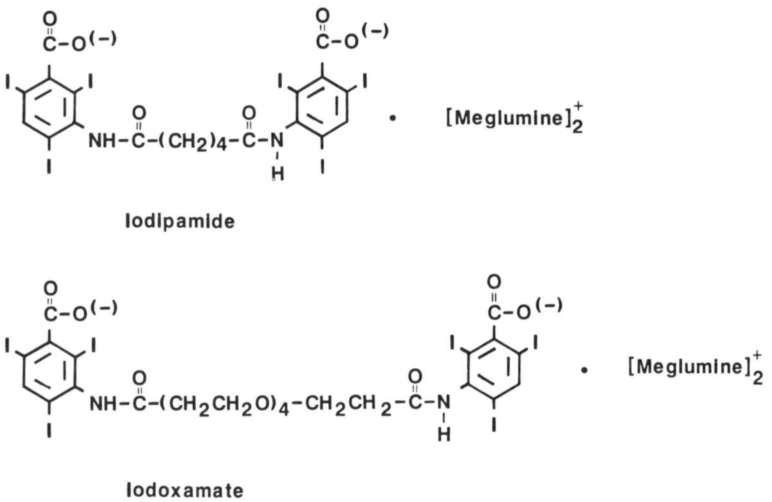

Figure 6.15 Chemical structures of cholangiographic contrast media.

Table 6.11   COMMERCIALLY AVAILABLE CHOLANGIOGRAPHIC MEDIA[a]

GENERIC NAME	BRAND NAME[®][b]	CONCENTRATION (% w/v)	MG IODINE ML
Iodipamide meglumine	Cholografin (S)	52	25.7
Iodipamide meglumine	Cholografin for Infusion (S)	10.3	5.1

[a] U.S. market only
[b] (S) Squibb Diagnostics

A second cholangiographic contrast medium, iodoxamate meglumine (Figure 6.15), was commercially available until just prior to this writing. This dimeric agent was similar in structure to iodipamide; however, it possessed a long polyether chain between the benzene rings. As a result of its increased molecular weight, iodoxamate meglumine contained slightly less iodine (i. e., 45%) on a per weight basis than iodipamide. Although it did provide some advantages to iodipamide meglumine in regard to its more rapid rate of hepatobiliary excretion (see Biliary Excretion and Bile Concentration), iodoxamate meglumine was removed from the market apparently as a result of its limited use.

PHARMACOKINETICS

As previously indicated, certain of the pharmacokinetic characteristics of cholangiographic contrast media are the same, whereas others differ from those of the oral cholecystographic agents. It is the differences that result in the high bile concentrations achieved by the cholangiographic agents and, hence, their specific indication for radiographic opacification and visualization of the bile ducts (Loeb PM and Berk RN, 1977; Berk RN, et al, 1977d; Barnhart, JL, 1984).

A primary difference between cholecystographic and cholangiographic media is associated with their respective routes of administration. The chemical properties of iodipamide meglumine are such that it is virtually completely ionized at physiological pH values. This agent is therefore readily soluble in aqueous solutions suitable for intravenous injection. This route of administration results in immediately high and relatively controllable plasma *and bile duct* concentrations, unlike the situation that occurs with the slow and often erratic intestinal absorption of the oral cholecystographic media. However,

such high plasma concentrations are also associated with an increased potential for adverse reactions, a factor that limits the use of cholangiographic media to bile-duct visualization.

Blood Transport. Like the cholecystographic media, iodipamide demonstrates extensive binding to plasma albumin. Although species differences do exist, evidence suggests that, in humans, the albumin binding of iodipamide exceeds 90% of the administered dose and involves more than one class of binding sites (Lasser EC, et al, 1962). The albumin-binding of cholecystographic and cholangiographic contrast media plays an important role in preventing their renal excretion by glomerular filtration, and may thus be responsible for their preferential elimination by the hepatic route. As will be discussed, the albumin binding of iodipamide also appears to effect its rate of hepatocyte uptake.

Iodipamide exhibits a biphasic pattern of blood clearance following intravenous injection. A major percentage of the administered dose is eliminated in the initial phase with a half-life of 10–15 minutes. The half-life of the second phase approaches 2 hours (Shames DM and Moss AA, 1974).

Hepatocyte Uptake. Iopanoic acid, administered intravenously and in conjunction with iodipamide, results in delayed hepatobiliary excretion of the latter agent (Goergen T, et al, 1974). This would suggest that iodipamide shares the same mechanism for hepatic uptake and biliary excretion as the cholecystographic media (see Cholecystographic Media—Hepatocyte Uptake). This mechanism appears to involve the competitive protein binding of albumin-bound iodipamide by cytoplasmic proteins, Y and Z, found within the hepatocyte. It has been suggested that the hepatic uptake of iodipamide may also involve specific cell membrane receptors for organic anions or albumin. The latter mechanism does not appear likely, however, since in vitro studies have shown that the rate of hepatocyte uptake of iodipamide actually proceeds at a faster rate in the absence of albumin (Song CS, et al, 1976).

The normally functioning liver excretes approximately 80% of an injected dose of iodipamide, with a net hepatic extraction fraction of 12% (Shames DM and Moss AA, 1974). It has been shown that the rate of reflux of iodipamide from the hepatocytes to blood greatly exceeds its rate of biliary excretion. Hence, the hepatocyte uptake mechanism does not appear to be the rate-limiting step in the hepatobiliary excretion of this agent.

Hepatic Metabolism. Unlike the oral cholecystographic media, iodipamide is excreted into the bile unchanged (Loeb PM, et al, 1975). Hence, the potentially rate-limiting step of glucuronide conjugation, or an alternative form of hepatic metabolism, is not a requirement for the biliary excretion of this cholangiographic agent. This factor may also contribute to the rapid hepatobiliary excretion and relatively high bile-duct concentration achieved by iodipamide compared to the oral cholecystographic media.

Biliary Excretion and Bile Concentration. The hepatobiliary excretion of cholangiographic media demonstrates a kinetic pattern consistent with the involvement of a saturable, active-transport mechanism (Berk RN, et al, 1976; Shames DM and Moss AA, 1974; Rosati G and Schiantarell P, 1970). Initially, the rate of biliary excretion of iodipamide increases rapidly as a function of its rate of injection and plasma concentration (Figure 6.16). This increase in the rate of biliary excretion gradually slows, however, as the plasma

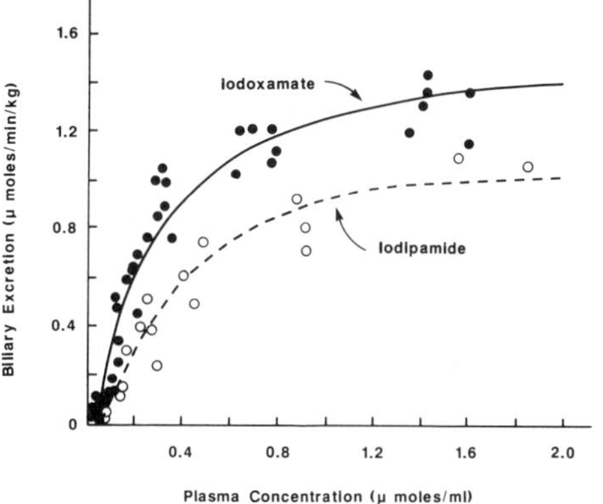

Figure 6.16 Relationship between the plasma concentration and biliary excretion rate of iodipamide and iodoxamate. (From Berk RN, 1976; with permission.)

concentration continues to increase. Eventually, the rate of biliary excretion of iodipamide reaches a maximum; whereupon any further increase in its plasma concentration has no effect on the rate of biliary excretion.

Hepatobiliary excretion of the oral cholecystographic media also involves an active transport mechanism. The fact that the simultaneous, intravenous injection of iopanoic acid delays the hepatobiliary excretion of iodipamide suggests that the biliary-excretion mechanism for cholecystographic and cholangiographic media may be identical. It should be noted, however, that competition between these agents may also occur at the hepatocyte uptake site. In contrast to the cholecystographic media, the biliary transport mechanism for the cholangiographic media does not require their prior glucuronide conjugation. Furthermore, the transport maximum of iodipamide is not affected by the presence or absence of bile salts, as is the case with iopanoic and iocetamic acid (Barnhart JL, 1984).

As noted previously (see Chemistry), a second cholangiographic medium, iodoxamate meglumine, was commercially available until just prior to this writing. Compared to iodipamide, the rate of biliary excretion of iodoxamate was approximately 25% greater for all equivalent plasma concentrations (Figure 6.16). It was suggested that as a result of its

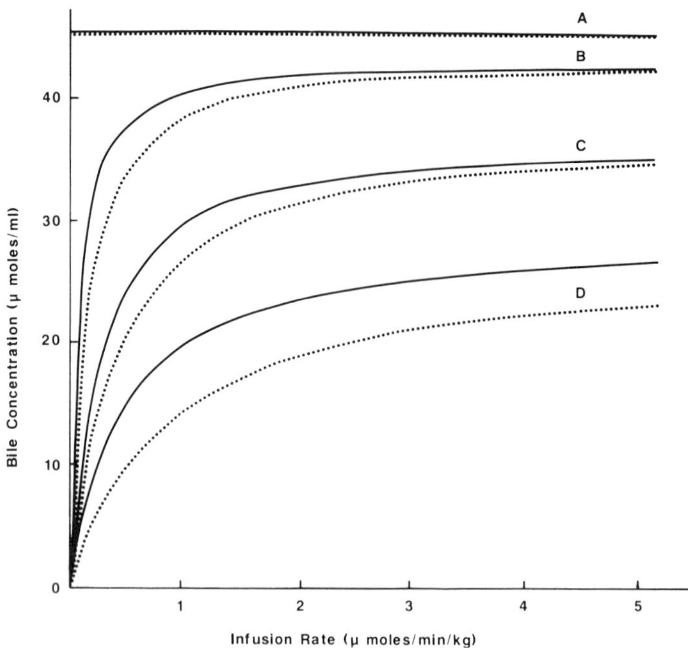

Figure 6.17 Theoretical relationship between the infusion rate and the final bile concentration of iodipamide (dashed lines) and iodoxamate (solid lines). A assumes no basal bile flow. B, C, and D assume basal bile flow rates of 0.002, 0.0068, and 0.02 mL/min/kg, respectively. (From Berk RN, 1976; with permission.)

increased rate of biliary excretion, iodoxamate would provide improved opacification of the bile ducts, especially in patients with preexisting liver dysfunction (Berk RN, et al, 1976).

The concentration that a cholangiographic medium achieves in the bile is dependent on its rate of biliary excretion, the amount of choleresis induced by its excretion and the basal rate of bile flow. The cholangiographic media are potent choleretic agents, their excretion across the canalicular membrane of the hepatocyte being accompanied by the excretion of a fixed amount (i.e., 22 mL/mmol) of water and, hence, a stimulation of bile flow. As a result of this choleretic relationship, the volume of bile produced per amount of cholangiographic agent excreted is the same (i.e., 22 mL/mmol), regardless of the rate of excretion. If there is no basal rate of bile flow, the cholangiographic media would thus achieve a constant (i.e., 1 mmol/22 mL = 45.5 μmol/mL) and equal molar, and hence, iodine concentration within the bile independent of their rate of biliary excretion (Figure 6.17). This would indicate that the faster rate of biliary excretion of iodoxamate would provide no opacification advantages in regard to the final bile concentration of iodine. It must be emphasized, however, that the attenuation of an x-ray beam is dependent on the total amount (i.e., volume and concentration) of

iodine in its path. Thus, the increased volume of bile produced by the more rapid excretion of iodoxamate may result in ductular distension and improve opacification even though the biliary iodine concentration is constant (Berk RN, et al, 1976).

Basal bile flow is defined as the respective flow rate that is present independent of the choleretic effects of the cholangiographic medium. Basal bile flow may be induced by the excretion of bile salts and other solutes across the canalicular membrane, or by the action of secretin or vagal stimulation. As might be expected, basal bile flow acts to dilute the bile concentration of a cholangiographic medium (Figure 6.17). The higher the rate of basal bile flow, the greater its dilutional effects regardless of the rate of infusion and biliary excretion of the cholangiographic medium. At low rates of contrast-medium infusion and biliary excretion, the basal bile flow would represent a high percentage of the total bile flow (i.e., basal flow plus media-induced flow), resulting in substantial dilutional effects. As a result of its more rapid rate of biliary excretion and associated increase in choleretic effects, basal bile flow would produce less dilution of iodoxamate versus iodipamide at equivalent low infusion rates. The dilutional effects of basal bile flow and the differences between cholangiographic media become less significant at high rates of contrast media infusion and biliary excretion (Berk RN, et al, 1976).

These dilutional effects of basal bile flow suggest that it is advantageous to eliminate fatty foods prior to the administration of cholangiographic media. A fatty meal stimulates the gallbladder release and enterohepatic circulation of bile salts with a corresponding increase in basal bile flow (Berk RN and Loeb PM, 1977a).

Iodipamide appears in the bile at 10–15 minutes following slow (i. e., over 10 minutes) intravenous administration of the concentrated (52% w/v) formulation. Radiographic demonstration of the hepatic and common bile ducts is possible at approximately 20–30 minutes after injection. Drip infusion (i. e., 2–3 mL/min) of the 10.3% w/v formulation delays optimal demonstration of the biliary ducts until 40–80 minutes following initiation of the injection (Product information, Cholografin®, Squibb Diagnostics).

Several disease factors can interfere with the kinetics of cholangiographic media and delay or diminish the bile concentration. Liver damage can significantly impair the hepatocyte uptake and hepatobiliary excretion mechanisms. With common bile-duct obstruction, the intraductal pressure increases and may exceed the maximum secretory pressure of the liver. In this event, the cholangiographic media appear in the bile, but their concentration is never sufficient to permit adequate radiographic opacification. Further increasing the dose does not obviate this problem (Burgener FA, 1975).

Gallbladder Concentration. During the interdigestive phase a majority of the bile produced by the hepatocytes is concentrated by and stored within the gallbladder. Therefore, if the cystic duct is patent, the cholangiographic media will also be transported to and concentrated within the gallbladder. The cholangiographic media can be used for the radiographic evaluation of gallbladder disease; however, they should not be substituted for the less toxic oral cholecystographic agents if this is the sole purpose of the examination.

Iodipamide appears in the gallbladder within 1 hour following "bolus" administration of the concentrated (52% w/v) formulation. Maximum opacification occurs at approximately 2 hours. Slow infusion of the 10.3% w/v formulation delays maximum opacification of the gallbladder until approximately 3 hours (Product information, Cholografin®, Squibb Diagnostics).

Gallbladder Excretion/Enterohepatic Circulation. The stored cholangiographic medium is excreted from the gallbladder into the duodenum upon gallbladder contraction. Unlike the oral cholecystographic agents, the cholangiographic media do not undergo enterohepatic recirculation (Loeb PM and Berk RN, 1977). Approximately 80–95% of an injected dose of iodipamide can be recovered in the feces at 24 hours following administration (Product information, Cholografin®, Squibb Diagnostics).

Renal Excretion. Between 5–20% of an intravenous dose of iodipamide is excreted, unchanged, by the kidneys within 24 hours following administration. Similar to the glucuronide derivatives of the cholecystographic agents, the renal excretion of iodipamide appears to occur by a passive diffusion process, most likely glomerular filtration. The rate of renal excretion of iodipamide is linearly related to its plasma concentration once a minimum plasma concentration has been exceeded (Figure 6.18). The lack of substantial renal excretion below this minimum plasma concentration probably reflects a requirement for saturation of the hepatic transport mechanism prior to elimination by the alternate renal pathway. Hence, the degree of renal excretion of iodipamide may be expected to increase in the presence of liver disease due to a corresponding impairment of hepatobiliary transport mechanisms. Also, saturation of the hepatic transport mechanisms and a higher percentage of renal excretion are more likely to occur with rapid injection of the concentrated (i. e., 52% w/v) formulation

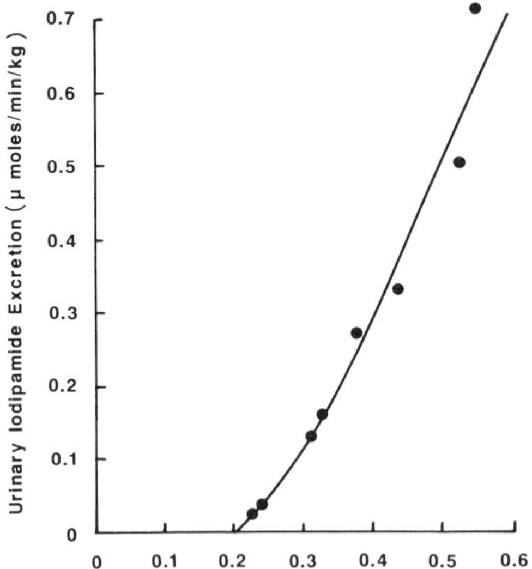

Figure 6.18 Relationship between the plasma concentration and urinary excretion rate of iodipamide. (From Loeb PM, et al, 1975; with permission.)

of iodipamide than it is with slower rates of injection or with infusion of the dilute (10.3% w/v) formulation (Loeb PM, 1975; Berndt WO, 1968).

PHYSIOLOGICAL EFFECTS

Intravenous cholangiographic media produce a higher incidence of moderate to severe adverse reactions than either the intravascular angiographic or urographic media or the oral cholecystographic agents (Ansell G, 1970). Common side effects associated with the injection of iodipamide include pseudo-allergic reactions, hypotension, and acute renal dysfunction. As with other contrast media, these reactions may occur as a result of direct chemical toxicity of the agent, or they may be of an unknown origin. Compared to the angiographic and urographic media, the chemical toxicity of iodipamide may be enhanced as a result of its extensive binding to proteins, perhaps including enzyme systems. In comparison to the highly protein-bound oral cholecystographic agents, the increased toxicity of iodipamide may be related to the substan-

tially higher plasma concentrations achieved with intravenous versus oral administration. Cross-sensitivity reactions between the angiographic, urographic, cholecystographic, and cholangiographic media can occur; therefore, caution should be observed in administering any of these agents to patients who have experienced a previous contrast media reaction.

Hypotension. The rapid, intravenous injection of a large dose of iodipamide can produce a transient, dramatic decrease in blood pressure accompanied by pallor, dizziness, nausea, and, rarely, circulatory collapse. This effect may result from a combination of factors including hyperosmolality induced vasodilation (osmolality of 52% w/v iodipamide $\cong$ 600 mOsm/kg) or direct molecular toxicity. Iodipamide is a moderate inhibitor of the enzyme, acetylcholinesterase (Lasser EC and Lang JH, 1966b). Hence, the observed responses of vasodilation, hypotension, and respiratory alterations following iodipamide administration may be mediated by increased systemic levels of acetylcholine.

Renal Effects. Intravenous iodipamide can produce alterations in renal function as evidenced by an acute increase in serum creatinine and blood urea nitrogen levels or a decrease in creatinine clearance, and by proteinuria and crystalluria (Mudge GH, 1970). As with the oral cholecystographic agents, these nephrotoxic effects of iodipamide may be related to its high degree of protein binding and inhibition of renal tubular enzyme systems. Iodipamide also possesses uricosuric activity resulting from its ability to displace albumin-bound uric acid (Postlethwaite AE and Kelley WH, 1971). The uricosuric effect of iodipamide persists for approximately 24 hours and is therefore of substantially less duration than the respective effects of iopanoic acid and ipodate sodium. The rapid and potentially extensive renal excretion of iodipamide can result in a high urinary concentration and the possibility of its renal tubular precipitation, especially in the presence of dehydration and an acidic environment. Based on these considerations, it is possible that the nephrotoxic effects of iodipamide may be related to obstructive uric acid and contrast medium crystallization within the renal tubules (Mudge GH, 1971). Finally, the systemic hypotensive effects of iodipamide can produce a compensatory, renin-mediated constriction of the renal vasculature. Hence, contrast-induced renal ischemia may represent an additional causative factor for the observed proteinuria and alterations of renal function following iodipamide administration.

The nephrotoxic effects of iodipamide appear to be dose-rate dependent. This is most likely related to the linear increase in renal excretion that occurs once the plasma concentration of iodipamide exceeds its hepatic transport capacity. This factor represents a potential advantage associated with slow infusion of the less concentrated formulation of this agent (Lindgren P, et al, 1966). As expected, the nephrotoxic effects of a given dose of iodipamide also increase in the presence of the reduced transport capacity of hepatic dysfunction. The incidence and severity of iodipamide-induced nephrotoxicity do not, however, appear to correlate with the presence or absence of pre-existing renal disease.

Hepatic Effects. Intravenous iodipamide can produce mild hepatotoxic effects as evidenced by an acute elevation of serum transaminase or alkaline phosphatase levels (Sutherland LR, et al, 1977; Burk RF and Barnhart JL, 1979). A return to normal values usually occurs within 1 week. This effect of iodipamide appears to be dose related; approximately 9% of patients demonstrate elevated transaminase levels at a total dose of 10.4 g compared to 17% at a total dose of 20.8 g (Scholz FJ, et al, 1975). Iodipamide also commonly produces an increase in the serum bilirubin level; however, this effect may be more related to competition for the same hepatobiliary excretion mechanisms than direct hepatic toxicity. Symp-

toms of severe hepatotoxicity, including abdominal pain, fever, and liver tenderness, occur rarely following iodipamide administration.

Animal studies have demonstrated that hepatotoxic doses of iodipamide produce centrizonal necrosis and fatty infiltration of the liver with minimal inflammation (Burk RF and Barnhart JL, 1979). Additional studies suggest that the hepatotoxic effects of iodipamide may increase with age due to a corresponding decrease in the rate of its biliary excretion and, thus, prolonged exposure to the hepatocytes (Barnhart JL and Berk RN, 1979b).

PRECAUTIONS

Physical Incompatibilities. Iodipamide meglumine precipitates in the presence of gentamicin sulfate and the hydrochloride or maleate salts of a variety (Table 6.12) of tertiary amines (Stevens JS, 1975; *Drug Information*, 1985); Marshall TR, et al, 1965). Hence, these pharmacological agents (or drugs of similar **chemical structure should not be mixed** with the cholangiographic medium prior to injection and care should be taken to avoid their direct contact in administration devices.

Drug–Contrast Medium Interactions. In recognition of the extensive albumin binding of iodipamide, consideration must be given to its ability to displace other albumin-bound drugs from their respective binding sites. For example, the albumin binding of iodipamide appears to involve the same site as albumin-bound warfarin (Fehske EJ and Miller WE, 1981). Hence, the administration of iodipamide could lead to a displacement of warfarin and a potentiation of its anticoagulant activity.

Table 6.12   DRUGS KNOWN TO BE PHYSICALLY INCOMPATIBLE WITH IODIPAMIDE MEGLUMINE

Brompheniramine maleate
Chlorpheniramine maleate
Chlortrimeton
Dimenhydrinate
Diphenhydramine hydrochloride
Gentamicin sulfate
Hyaluronidase
Promethazine hydrochloride

The clinical significance of these competitive displacement interactions of iodipamide is limited by its rapid rate of blood clearance. However, the presence of hepatic and renal dysfunction can substantially prolong the plasma half-life of iodipamide, rendering such interactions of increased importance.

Conversely, it should be noted that certain drugs with extremely high albumin-binding affinities can competitively displace iodipamide from its albumin-binding site. This consideration may explain the decreased biliary concentration and increased renal excretion of iodipamide observed in patients receiving probenecid (Berndt WO and Mudge GH, 1968). Since progesterone can also displace albumin-bound cholangiographic media, patients may be at an increased risk for contrast-induced side effects during certain stages of their menstrual cycle or if they are undergoing progesterone-associated therapy or contraception (Wirell S, 1978; Lindgren P, et al, 1974).

Any drug that is excreted in high quantities via the same hepatobiliary transport mechanisms can competitively decrease the biliary concentration of iodipamide. This explains the diminished biliary excretion of iodipamide when administered concurrently with intravenous or oral doses of the cholecystographic media (Goergen T, et al, 1974). Inadequate iodipamide demonstration of the bile ducts has also been associated with the simultaneous administration of methyltestosterone.

The various opiate-agonists (e. g., codeine, morphine, meperidine, fentanyl, etc.) can elicit spasm of the sphincter of Oddi and can produce an increase in biliary-tract pressure as a side effect to their analgesic indication. Choleretic effects and increased biliary pressure associated with the concomitant administration of iodipamide meglumine can result in acute abdominal pain (*Drug Information*, 1985).

Contrast Media–Laboratory-Test Interactions. The intravenous administration and albumin binding of iodipamide results in the competitive displacement of albumin-bound uric acid and an increase in its renal tubular secretion. This uricosuric effect of iodipamide persists for approximately 24 hours and would invalidate any serum or urinary measurements of uric acid performed during this period (Postlethwaite AE and Kelley WH, 1971).

At routinely obtained serum concentrations (i. e., 2 μm/mL), iodipamide has been shown to produce moderate inhibition of platelet aggregation. This in vivo effect on platelet function is not, however, associated with an alteration in bleeding time and rapidly returns to normal with excretion of the medium (Shapiro GA, 1977).

As a direct result of its hepatoxic effects, iodipamide produces an acute elevation in serum transaminase and alkaline phosphatase levels. Return to normal values usually occurs within a week. Serum bilirubin levels may also demonstrate a transient increase following iodipamide meglumine injection due to competition for the same hepatobiliary-excretion mechanisms. Thus, an evaluation of hepatic disease based on serum bilirubin or enzyme levels must take into account the respective effects of recently administered iodipamide.

As with other iodinated contrast media, iodipamide meglumine can invalidate thyroid function tests based on iodine measurements (i. e., radioactive iodine uptake, protein-bound iodine) for several days to weeks following its intravascular administration. Hence, these tests, if indicated, should be performed prior to cholangiography or alternate tests of thyroid function utilized. Iodipamide excreted by the kidneys can also interfere with laboratory tests performed on the urine. For example, iodipamide will interact with cupric sulfate glucose tests to produce a black coloration suggestive of alkaptouria. Therefore, testing should be performed on urine collected prior to the cholangiography procedure or delayed until at least 2 days after iodipamide administration (*Drug Information*, 1985).

CLINICAL CONSIDERATIONS

Clinical Indications. With the advent of ultrasound, computed tomography, and hepatobiliary scintigraphy for the evaluation of biliary anatomy and patency, the clinical use of cholangiography has become extremely limited. Intravenous cholangiography may be indicated if a strong suspicion of bile-duct obstruction remains following negative ultrasound and scintigraphy studies; or if ultrasound or computed tomography demonstrates dilated ducts, but fails to define the cause of obstruction. However, as a result of its greater potential for systemic toxicity, intravenous cholangiography should not be utilized for these indications if direct cholangiographic procedures (i. e., endoscopic retrograde cholangiopancreatography, percutaneous transhepatic cholangiography) are available. Intravenous cholangiography should not be performed as an alternative to oral cholecystography for the evaluation of cholelithiasis. In addition to its increased potential for adverse effects, iodipamide produces relatively poor opacification of the gallbladder and fails to demonstrate gallstones in a high percentage of patients with proven cholelithiasis.

Contrast Media Considerations. The only intravenous cholangiographic contrast medium currently marketed is iodipamide meglumine. Two formulations of this agent are available, a 52% w/v concentration (20-mL vial) for slow, intravenous injection and a 10.3% w/v concentration (100-mL bottle) for drip infusion.

Patient Preparation. Patients should be on a fat-free diet for 12 hours prior to the cholangiographic procedure. Fatty foods promote gallbladder contraction and the enterohepatic circulation of bile salts. The biliary excretion and associated choleretic activity of these bile salts increases the rate of basal bile flow, resulting in a dilutional effect on the bile-duct concentration and degree of opacification achieved by the administered iodipamide.

Laxatives should be appropriately administered prior to the examination to eliminate fecal material and intestinal gas that may interfere with adequate visualization of the biliary tree. Due to the uricosuric effect and direct renal excretion of iodipamide, patients should be well hydrated prior to and for at least 24 hours following cholangiography.

Adjunctive Drugs. Orally administered cholestyramine resin binds bile salts and prevents their intestinal absorption. Hence, it has been suggested that the administration of this agent prior to cholangiography might improve biliary-tract opacification by decreasing the rate of basal bile flow associated with the biliary excretion and choleretic activity of absorbed bile salts. The adjunctive use of anticholinergic agents would similarly inhibit the component of basal bile flow mediated via the vagal mechanism (Berk RN, et al, 1977d).

Contraction of the sphincter of Oddi during the cholangiography procedure can result in a radiographic pattern consistent with mechanical obstruction of the common bile duct. This physiological process can be differentiated from an obstructing gallstone by a lack of associated ductular dilation or by incorporating the adjunct administration of glucagon (1 mg, intravenous) which acts to relax the sphincter of Oddi. Conversely, morphine has been used as an adjunct agent to induce contraction of the sphincter of Oddi in an attempt to increase the degree of bile-duct opacification following iodipamide administration (Berk RN, 1977e). Caution must be observed, however, in distinguishing between the resulting pharmacological versus true mechanical obstruction of the common duct.

Intravenous glucagon has also been shown to produce a transient increase in the biliary concentration of cholangiographic contrast media (Jarrett LN and Bell GD, 1980). This action of glucagon occurs within 2–3 minutes of injection and persists for only approximately 5 minutes, appearing to be related to a glucagon-induced increase in hepatic blood flow or bile salt excretion.

Contraindications. The transport mechanism involved in the hepatobiliary excretion of iodipamide becomes impaired in the presence of liver disease. Moreover, elevated serum bilirubin levels result in increased competition for the hepatobiliary-excretion mechanisms. Hence, the intravenous administration of iodipamide meglumine rarely produces adequate visualization of the bile ducts if the serum bilirubin is greater than 2–3 mg % (Berk RN, 1977e).

As a result of reduced hepatic transport capacity, the degree of renal excretion of iodipamide and its potential for nephrotoxic effects also increases in the presence of liver disease. The intravenous administration of iodipamide is therefore contraindicated in the presence of concomitant hepatic and renal diseases.

DOSAGE

Considerable controversy exists regarding the optimal dosage regimen for iodipamide meglumine (Loeb PM and Berk RN, 1977). The slow intravenous injection of 0.3 mL/kg of the 52% w/v formulation over a 10–15 minute interval appears to provide consistent and adequate bile-duct visualization while maintaining an acceptable level of side effects. If nausea occurs during the administration procedure, the rate of injection should be decreased. With this dosage regimen, the bile ducts are typically visualized within 20–30 minutes after the injection is completed unless hepatic disease is present. Further increasing the mL/kg dose or the rate of injection does not substantially improve bile-duct opacification, but it does increase the incidence of systemic side effects and the degree of renal excretion and potential for nephrotoxic effects.

The 10.3% w/v formulation of iodipamide is intended for drip infusion at a rate of 2–3 mL/minute. With slow infusion of the less concentrated formulation there is less chance that the hepatic transport capacity for iodipamide will be exceeded. Hence, this dosage regimen should result in less potential for renal excretion of the contrast medium and associated nephro-

toxic effects. A slower rate of iodipamide injection also produces a lower peak plasma concentration and a decreased risk of systemic side effects. Once adequate radiographic opacification of the biliary tree is achieved, the infusion can be immediately terminated.

As previously discussed (see Pharmacokinetics), in the absence of any basal bile flow, the concentration that iodipamide achieves in the bile is constant regardless of its rate of biliary excretion. This would suggest that the degree of biliary-tree opacification would be the same with slow injection of the 52% w/v formulation or drip infusion of the 10.3% w/v formulation. However, this consideration neglects the fact that radiographic opacification is dependent on the total quantity (i.e., volume and iodine concentration) of iodine atoms in the path of the x-ray, not just the iodine concentration. Hence, the more rapid rate of biliary excretion of iodipamide achieved with the concentrated versus dilute formulation would be associated with a greater amount of iodine in the biliary ducts at an earlier time period and hence improved opacification (Berk RN, et al, 1977d). Furthermore, basal bile flow, if present, produces less dilutional effects with higher rates of iodipamide injection and biliary excretion (see Pharmacokinetics).

III. DIRECT CHOLANGIOGRAPHY

The direct instillation of a radiopaque contrast medium into the bile ducts provides a method for the radiographic evaluation of biliary obstruction in the presence of elevated serum bilirubin levels (Figure 6.19). Direct cholangiography techniques include percutaneous transhepatic cholangiography, endoscopic retrograde cholangiopancreatography, and operative or post operative (i.e., T-tube) cholangiography.

Procedure Indications. In percutaneous transhepatic cholangiography (PTC), a thin needle is passed through the abdo-

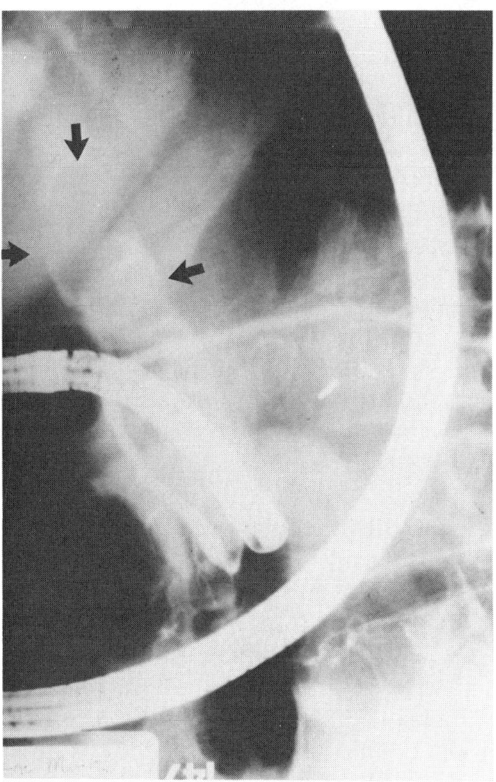

Figure 6.19 Endoscopic retrograde cholangiopancreatography (ERCP) demonstrating multiple large stones (black arrows) within a markedly enlarged common bile duct.

also increases the likelihood of a successful examination. In addition, with ERCP both the common bile duct and the pancreatic duct may be opacified, resulting in an increase in available diagnostic information. Based on these considerations, the performance of PTC is generally limited to situations wherein ERCP is not available or has failed, or occasionally to supplement ERCP in demonstrating the proximal aspects of biliary obstruction. Cholangitis, a possible complication of both procedures, may be avoided with prophylactic antibiotics and careful technique. A transient elevation in serum amylase and the rare occurrence of pancreatitis may also be observed with ERCP, whereas bile peritonitis represents an additional complication of PTC.

The clinical indications for ERCP or PTC are limited. If ultrasound demonstrates dilated biliary ducts, but it or subsequent computed tomography fails to identify the cause of obstruction, ERCP or PTC should be considered. Another possible indication for performing direct cholangiography is a strong suspicion of a moving and intermittently obstructing biliary stone in the face of normal ultrasound and hepatobiliary scintigraphy.

Direct cholangiography may also be indicated during cholecystectomy procedures to exclude the presence of concomitant common bile duct stones or other ductular pathology. Operative cholangiography typically involves the injection of contrast medium into the catheterized cystic duct. It should be performed prior to extensive manipulation of the ductal system to avoid artifacts associated with ductal spasm or contraction of the sphincter of Oddi. For postoperative evaluations of biliary patency, the contrast medium may be injected via the indwelling T-tube or cholecystostomy tube, or into associated fistula tracts.

Contrast Media Considerations. Direct cholangiography does not require the use of a contrast medium that demonstrates selective hepatobiliary excretion kinetics. Hence, the more commonly available and less expensive intravascular iodinated media can and should be utilized for these procedures rather than the cholangiographic agent, iodipamide meglumine.

Although studies evaluating the relative effects of intravascular iodinated media for direct cholangiography are limited, it is obvious that the agent utilized should

minal wall into the liver. Under fluoroscopic guidance, the needle is advanced toward the hilum of the liver where the major segmental bile ducts converge. Once entry into a bile duct has been confirmed by successful bile aspiration or the injection of a small amount of a radiopaque contrast medium, a suitable volume of the contrast medium is injected to obtain an adequate cholangiogram. Endoscopic retrograde cholangiopancreatography (ERCP) involves the passage of a fiberoptic scope into the duodenum with subsequent identification and cannulation of the common bile duct and pancreatic duct. The radiopaque contrast medium is subsequently instilled into the ducts to obtain a retrograde cholangiogram and/or pancreatogram.

ERCP is a much less invasive procedure compared to PTC. Cannulation of the common bile duct under direct endoscopic control produce a minimum of damage to the epithelial cells of the ductal or gallbladder walls or to the acinar cells of the pancreas if respective exposure should occur. Compared to equiiodine concentrations of the corresponding sodium derivatives, meglumine salts of the radiopaque anions, diatrizoate and iothalamate, demonstrate less damage to cells of the vascular endothelium (Penry JB and Livingston A, 1972; Wiedeman MP, 1963). Hence, it has been suggested that the use of meglumine salts for direct cholangiography may also be associated with less epithelial damage than sodium salts. (Kasugai T, et al, 1972). Since epithelial damage may be directly related to the hyperosomolarity of the instilled contrast medium, use of a ratio-3, low-osmolality agent may be expected to produce less irritation than a ratio-1.5 medium. Various experimental histological studies have confirmed this expectation (Kivisaari L, 1979; Bub H, et al, 1983). In a clinical ERCP study, the ratio-3 nonionic medium, metrizamide, was also shown to produce a lower level of hyperamylassemia compared to equivalent use of the ratio-1.5 medium, metrizoate sodium (Osnes M, 1977). However, this latter finding could not be reproduced in a separate study comparing metrizamide with diatrizoate meglumine (Hamilton I, et al, 1982), or in an experimental study comparing metrizamide with a ratio-1.5 metrizoate medium (Lilleas F and Swenson T, 1977).

Direct cholangiography procedures should be performed utilizing a contrast-medium formulation that contains approximately 300 mg Iodine/mL. Based on the previous considerations, a 60% w/v concentration (282 mg Iodine/mL) of diatrizoate or iothalamate meglumine should be the routine agent of choice for direct cholangiography. It should be noted that significant (i. e., 20% of administered dose) systemic absorption of the instilled contrast medium can occur with exposure of the pancreatic duct, and to a considerably lesser degree (i. e., < 1% of administered dose) with biliary-tract exposure and subsequent emptying of the medium into the intestinal tract (Sable RA, et al, 1983). Hence, there is a potential for unpredictable pseudo-allergic reactions following direct cholangiography procedures.

Dosage. The volume of the contrast medium utilized for direct cholangiography procedures can vary considerably, depending on the nature of the examination, the presence and location of biliary obstruction, the extent of surgical intervention, and so forth. Fluoroscopic monitoring should be incorporated to ensure adequate filling of the biliary tree. With ERCP, the incidence of postprocedure pancreatitis (0.7–1.3%) appears to be related to the injection of excessive volumes of the contrast medium and associated exposure of the acinar cells (Hamilton I, et al, 1983). Therefore, the instillation of excessive volumes of the contrast medium should be avoided, as should the injection of bubbles. If possible, bile is aspirated prior to the injection of the contrast medium. With the proximal techniques (i. e., PTC, operative cholangiography) and biliary obstruction, the contrast medium can also be aspirated following completion of the procedure. In the presence of a patent biliary tract or with ERCP, the administered contrast medium rapidly drains into the intestinal tract.

References

Ansell G. Adverse reactions to contrast agents. *Invest Radiol* 1970, 5:374–384.

Barnhart JL, Berk RN, Czuleger PC. Biliary excretion of three cholecystographic agents in dogs: iocetamic acid, iopronic acid and iosametic acid. *Invest Radiol* 1979a, 14:79–87.

Barnhart JL, Berk RN. Reduction in biliary transport of bile salts, iodipamide, and iopanoic acid in aging rats. *Gastroenterology* 1979; 77:A4.

Barnhart JL, Berk RN, Janes JO, et al. Isolation, hepatic distribution and intestinal absorption of the glucuronide metabolite of iopanoic acid. *Invest Radiol* 1980, 15:5109–5115.

Barnhart JL, Witt BL, Hardison WG, et al. Uptake of iopanoic acid by isolated rat hepatocytes in primary culture. *Am J Physiol* 1983, 244:G630–G636.

Barnhart JL. Hepatic disposition and elimination of biliary contrast media. In *Radiocontrast Agents* (M Sovak, ed.), New York, Springer-Verlag, 1984, pp 367–418.

Beng CG, Wellby ML, Symons RG, et al. The effects of ipodate on the serum iodothyronine pattern in normal subjects. *Acta Endocrinol* (*Copenh*), 1980, 93:175–178.

Berk RN, Lasser EC: Altered concepts of the mechanism of non-visualization of the gallbladder. *Radiology* 1964, 82:296–302.

Berk RN. Consecutive dose phenomenon in oral cholecystography. *AJR* 1970, 110:230–244.

Berk RN, Loeb PM, Goldberger LE, et al. Oral cholecystography with iopanoic acid. *N Engl J Med* 1974a, 290:204–210.

Berk RN, Goldberger LE, Loeb PM. The role of bile salts in the hepatic excretion of iopanoic acid. *Invest Radiol* 1974b, 9:7–15.

Berk RN, Loeb PM, Cobo-Frenkel A, et al. Saturation kinetics and choleretic effects of iodoxamate and iodipamide—an experimental study in dogs. *Radiology* 1976, 119:529–535.

Berk RN, Loeb PM. Contrast materials for oral cholecystography. In *Radiographic Contrast Agents* (RE Miller, J Skucas, eds.), Baltimore, University Park Press, 1977, pp 195–221.

Berk RN, Loeb PM, Cobo-Frenkel A, et al. The biliary excretion of sodium tyropanoate and sodium ipodate in dogs. *Invest Radiol* 1977b, 12:85–95.

Berk RN. Oral cholecystography. In *Radiology of the Gallbladder and Bile Ducts* (RN Berk, AR Clemett, eds.), Philadelphia, W.B. Saunders Co., 1977c, pp 101–199.

Berk RN, Loeb PM, Ellzey BA. Contrast materials for intravenous cholangiography. In *Radiographic Contrast Agents* (RE Miller, J Skucas, eds.), Baltimore, University Park Press, 1977d, pp 223–250.

Berk RN. Intravenous cholangiography. In *Radiology of the Gallbladder and Bile Ducts* (RN Berk, Clemett AR, eds.), Philadelphia, W.B. Saunders Co., 1977e, pp 200–240.

Berndt WO, Mudge GH. Renal excretion of iodipamide. *Invest Radiol* 1968, 3:414–426.

Berndt WO, Wade DN, Mudge GH. Renal cortical slice accumulation of iopanoic and iophenoxic acids. *J Pharm Exp Ther* 1971, 179:74–84.

Bub H, Bürner W, Riemann JF, et al. Morphology of the pancreatic ductal epithelium after traumatization of the papilla of vater or endoscopic retrograde pancreatography with various contrast media in cats. *Scan J Gastroenterol* 1983, 18:581–592.

Burgener FA, Fischer HW, Adams JT. Intravenous cholangiography in different degrees of common bile duct obstruction. *Invest Radiol* 1975, 10:342–350.

Burghi H, Wimpfheimer C, Burger A, et al. Change in circulating thyroxine, triiodothyronine and reverse triiodothyronine after radiopaque contrast agents. *J Clin Endocrinol Metab* 1976, 43:1203–1210.

Burhenne HJ, Obata WG. Single visit oral cholecystography. *N Engl J Med* 1975, 292:627–628.

Burk RF, Barnhart JL. Iodipamide hepatotoxicity in the rat. *Gastroenterology* 1979, 76:1363–1367.

Clark RE, Shipley RA. Thyroidal uptake of ^{131}I after iopanoic acid (Telepaque) in 74 subjects. *J Clin Endocrinol Metab* 1957, 17:1008–1010.

Cooke WJ, Mudge GH. Biliary and urinary excretion of iopanoic acid in the dog. *Invest Radiol* 1975, 10:25–34.

Drug Information, American Hospital Formulary Service, American Society of Hospital Pharmacists, Inc., Bethesda, 1985; pp 1005–1062.

Edholm P, Jacobson B. Quantitative determination of iodine in vivo. *Acta Radiol* 1959, 52:337–346.

Fehske EJ, Miller WE. Optimal studies on interaction of biliary contrast agents with native and modified human serum albumin. *J Pharm Sci* 1981, 70:549–554.

Felicetta JV, Green WL, Nelp WB. Inhibition of hepatic binding of thyroxine by cholecystographic agents. *J Clin Invest* 1980, 65:1032–1040.

Fink HE, Roenigk WJ, Wilson GP. An experimental investigation of the nephrotoxic effects of oral cholecystographic agents. *Am J Med Sci* 1964, 247:201–216.

Goergen T, Goldberger LE, Berk RN. The combined use of oral cholecystographic media and iodipamide. *Radiology* 1974, 111:543–546.

Goldberg HI, Lin SK, Thoeni RF, et al. Recirculation of iopanoic acid after conjugation in the liver. *Invest Radiol* 1977, 12:537–541.

Goldberger LE, Berk RN, Lang JH, et al. Biopharmaceutical factors influencing the intestinal absorption of iopanoic acid. *Invest Radiol* 1974; 9:16–23.

Graham EA, Cole WH, Copher GH. Visualization of the gallbladder by the sodium salt of tetrabromophthalein. *JAMA* 1924, 82:1777–1778.

Hamilton I, Lintott DJ, Rothwell J, et al. Metrizamide as contrast medium in endoscopic retrograde cholangiopancreatography. *Clin Radiol* 1982, 33:293–295.

Hamilton I, Lintott DJ, Rothwell J, et al. Acute pancreatitis following endoscopic retrograde cholangiopancreatography. *Clin Radiol* 1983, 34:543–546.

Harrow BR, Winslow OP. Renal toxicity following oral cholecystography with Oragrafin. *Radiology* 1966, 87:721–724.

Hatfield PM, Wise RE. Indirect methods of visualizing the gallbladder and bile ducts. In *Radiology of the Gallbladder and Bile Ducts*, Section 22, Golden's Diagnostic Radiology (LL Robbins, ed.), Baltimore, Williams and Wilkins Co., 1976, pp 40–76.

Heckster REM. Results obtained in comparative radiographic, clinical, and clinical-chemical studies on iocetamic acid (DRC 1201) and iopanoic acid. *Radiol Clin Biol* 1968, 37:338–352.

Holonbek JE, Carroll WH, Riley GM, et al. Evaluation of pseudoalbuminuria following cholecystography in 76 cases. *JAMA* 1953, 153:1018.

Hoppe JO, Archer S. Observations on a series of aryltriiodoalkanoic acid derivatives with particular reference to a new cholecystographic medium, Telepaque. *AJR* 1953, 69:631–637.

Janes JO, Dietschy JM, Berk RN, et al. Determination of the rate of intestinal absorption of oral cholecystographic agents in the dog jejunum. *Gastroenterology* 1979, 76:970–977.

Jarrett LN, Bell GD, Effect of intravenous glucagon on the biliary secretion of cholangiographic contrast media. *Clin Radiology* 1980, 31:657–661.

Joffe H, Wachowski TJ. Relation of density of cholecystographic shadows on the gallbladder to the iodine content. *Radiology* 1942, 38:43–46.

Johnson RA, Mora LO. Unaltered bromosulfphthalein retention following oral cholecystography. *Postgrad Med J* 1968, Oct:108–113.

Juhl JH, Cooperman LR, Crummy AB: Oragrafin, a new cholecystographic medium. *Radiology* 1963, 80:87–91.

Kasugai T, Kuno N, Kobayashi S, et al. Endoscopic pancreatocholangiography. I. The normal endoscopic pancreatocholangiogram. *Gastroenterology* 1972, 63:217–226.

Kivisaari L. Contrast absorption and pancreatic inflammation following experimental ERCP. *Invest Radiol* 1979, 14:493–497.

Kleinman RE, Vagenakis AG, Braverman LE. The effect of iopanoic acid on the regulation of thyrotropin secretion in euthyroid subjects. *J Clin Endocrinol Metab* 1980, 51:399–403.

Koehler PR, Kyaw MM. Effect of fractionated administration of Telepaque on gallbladder visualization. *Radiology* 1973, 108:517–519.

Lang JH, Lasser EC. Binding of roentgenographic contrast media to serum albumin. *Invest Radiol* 1967, 2:396–400.

Lasser EC, Farr RS, Fujimargari T, et al. The significance of protein binding of contrast media in roentgen diagnosis. *AJR* 1962, 87:338–360.

Lasser EC, Saunders AM. Gallbladder mucosa in cholecystography. *JAMA* 1965, 193:427–431.

Lasser EC. Pharmacodynamics of biliary contrast media. *Radiol Clin North Am* 1966a, 4:511–519.

Lasser EC, Lang JH. Inhibition of acetylcholinesterase by some organic contrast media. *Invest Radiol* 1966b, 1:237–242.

Lillias F, Swenson T. Retrograde pancreatography in the pig. Comparison of Isopaque and Amipaque. *Acta Radiol Diagn (Stockh)* 1977, 6:621–624.

Lindgren I. A cause of non-opacification of the gallbladder. Treatment with Secholex. *Br J Radiol* 1976, 49:734.

Lindgren P, Nordenstam H, Saltzman GF. Effects of iodipamide on the kidneys. *Acta Radiol Diagn (Stockh)* 1966, 4:129–138.

Lindgren P, Salzman FG, Zeuchner E. Intravenous cholegraphy and per oral contraceptives. A preliminary report. *Acta Radiol Diagn (Stockh)* 1974, 15:217–224.

Loeb PM, Berk RN, Feld GH, et al. Biliary excretion of iodipamide. *Gastroenterology* 1975, 68:554–562.

Loeb PM, Berk RN. Biliary contrast materials. In *Radiology of the Gallbladder and Bile Ducts*. (RN Berk, AR Clemett eds.) Philadelphia, W.B. Saunders Co., 1977, pp 71–100.

Marshall TR, Ling JT, Follis G, et al. Pharmacological incompatibility of contrast media with various drugs and agents. *Radiology* 1965, 84:536–539.

McChesney EW, Hoppe JO. Observations on the absorption and excretion of the glucuronide of iopanoic acid in the cat. *Arch Int Pharmacodyn Ther* 1956, 105:306–312.

McChesney EW, Banks WF. Urinary excretion of three oral cholecystographic agents in man. *Proc Soc Exp Biol Med* 1965, 119:1027–1030.

Moss AA, Amberg JR, Jones PS. Relationship of bile salts and bile flow to biliary excretion of iopanoic acid. *Invest Radiol* 1972, 7:11–15.

Mudge GH. Some questions of nephrotoxicity. *Invest Radiol* 1970, 50:407–421.

Mudge GH. Uricosuric action of cholecystographic agents. A possible factor in nephrotoxicity. *N Eng J Med* 1971, 284:929–933.

Nehen AM, Kruse V. The effect on nonfractionated and fractionated administration of iopanoic acid on gallbladder visualization. *Radiology* 1978, 128:605–607.

Nelson J, Moss AA, Goldberg HI, et al. Gastrointestinal absorption of iopanoic acid. *Invest Radiol* 1973, 8:1–8.

Nelson JA. Effect of cholestyramine on Telephaque oral cholecystography. *AJR* 1974, 122:333–334.

Osnes M, Skjennald A, Larsen S. A comparison of a new non-ionic (metrizamide) and a dissociable (metrizoate) contrast medium in endoscopic retrograde pancreatography (ERP). *Scand J Gastroenterol* 1977, 12:821–825.

Penry JB, Livingston A: A comparison of the diagnostic effectiveness and vascular side effects of various diatrizoate salts used for intravenous pyelography. *Clin Radiol* 1972, 23:362–369.

Perrillo RP, Zuckerman GR, Koehler R, et al. Oral cholecystography in chornic renal insufficiency. *Dig Dis* 1978, 23:829–832.

Postlethwaite AE, Kelley WH. Uricosuric effect of radiocontrast agents, a study in man of four commonly used preparations. *Ann Intern Med* 1971, 74:845–852.

Postlethwaite AE, Kelley WH. Radiocontrast agents and aspirin. *JAMA* 1972, 219:1479.

Reiner RG, Lawson MJ, Marshall J, et al. Thyroid, renal and hepatic function tests following cholecystography with high-dose contrast agents. *Dig Dis Sci* 1980, 25:379–383.

Reinke RT, Berk RN. The mode of Telepaque absorption from the intestine. *AJR* 1971, 113:578–581.

Rosati G, Schiantarell P. Biliary excretion of contrast media. *Invest Radiol* 1970, 5:232–243.

Rous P, McMaster PD. The concentrating activity of the gallbladder. *J Exp Med* 1921, 34:47–73.

Sable RA, Rosenthal WS, Siegel J, et al. Absorption of contrast medium during ERCP. *Dig Dis Sci.* 1983, 28:801–806.

Scholz FJ, Johnston DO, Wise RE. Intravenous cholangiography. *Radiology* 1975, 114:513–518.

Schroder JS, Rooney D. Excretion of 3-(3-amino-2,4,6-triiodophenyl)-2-ethyl-proprionic acid (Telepaque) by man. *Proc. Soc Exp Biol Med* 1953; 83:544–546.

Shames DM, Moss AA. Iodipamide kinetics in the dog. A multicompartmental analysis. *Invest Radiol* 1974, 9:141–148.

Shapiro GA, Loeb PM, Berk RN, et al. Influence of Cholografin and Renografin-76 on platelet function. *Radiology* 1977, 124:641–643.

Sokoloff J, Berk RN, Lang JH, et al. The role of the Y and Z hepatic proteins in the excretion of radiographic contrast materials. *Radiology* 1973, 106:519–523.

Song CS, Beranbaum ER, Rothchild MA. The role of serum albumin in the hepatic excretion of iodipamide. *Invest Radiol* 1976, 11:39–44.

Stanley RJ, Melson GL, Cubillo E, et al. A comparison of three cholecystographic agents. A double-blind study with and without a prior fatty meal. *Radiology* 1974, 112:513–517.

Stevens JS. Incompatibility of diphenhydramine hydrochloride (Benadryl) and meglumine iodipamide (Cholografin). *Radiology* 1975, 117:224–225.

Sutherland LR, Edwards LA, Medline A, et al. Meglumine iodipamide hepatotoxicity. *Ann Intern Med* 1977, 86:437–439.

Taketa RM, Berk RN, Lang JH, et al. The effect of pH on the intestinal absorption of Telepaque. *AJR* 1972, 114:767–772.

Teplick JH, Myerson RM, Sanen FJ. Acute renal failure following oral cholecystography. *Acta Radiol Diagn (Stockh)* 1965, 3:353–368.

White WW, Fischer HW. A double-blind study of Oragrafin and Telepaque. *AJR* 1962, 87:745–748.

Wiedeman MP. Vascular and intravascular responses to various contrast media. *Angiology* 1963, 14:107–109.

Wirell S. Effects of steroid hormones on the binding of ioglycamide (Bilivistan) to human blood serum. *Acta Radiol Diagn (Stockh)* 1978, 19:289–296.

Wosilait WD, Ryan MP. Multiple competitive displacement interactions involving human serum albumin, anticoagulants, oleic acid, and various drugs. *Gen Pharmacol* 1980, 11:387–394.

Miscellaneous Radiopaque Contrast Media

I. Arthrographic Contrast Media

Dennis P. Swanson
Burton I. Ellis

Arthrography involves a radiological examination of a joint cavity, including the articulations and surrounding tissues, following the direct instillation of a negative-and/or positive-contrast medium. Based on contrast-medium considerations, three types of arthrographic procedures can be described. Pneumoarthrography utilizes a negative-contrast agent, such as filtered air or carbon dioxide, to permit improved visualization of the more radiopaque intraarticular structures from the surrounding fluid space. In a positive, single-contrast arthrography procedure, a water-soluble iodinated contrast medium is injected to render the fluid space radiodense relative to the intraarticular structures (Figure 7.1). Double-contrast arthrography examinations involve the aspiration of joint fluid followed by the injection of a small amount of an iodinated contrast medium for the purpose of thinly coating the surfaces of the cartilaginous and other intraarticular structures. Subsequent instillation of a negative-contrast agent results in improved delineation of the coated structures and a method for evaluating their surface contours and irregularities (Figure 7.2).

HISTORY

Arthrograms were first obtained in the early 1900s following the injection of air into the knee joint (Werndorff R and Robinson I, 1905). Pneumoarthrography did not gain widespread acceptance, however, primarily because of problems associated with its low diagnostic accuracy. Radiodensity differences between the instilled gas and certain of the more radiolucent intraarticular structures (e. g., cartilage) were not great. Since air (and other utilized gases) is not miscible with the joint fluid, failure to completely aspirate the joint prior to gas introduction

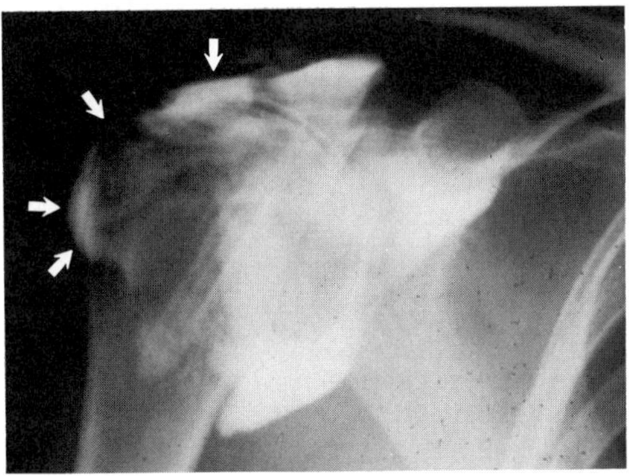

Figure 7.1 Single-contrast right shoulder arthrogram demonstrating (arrows) abnormal collection of contrast media due to a tear in the shoulder capsule.

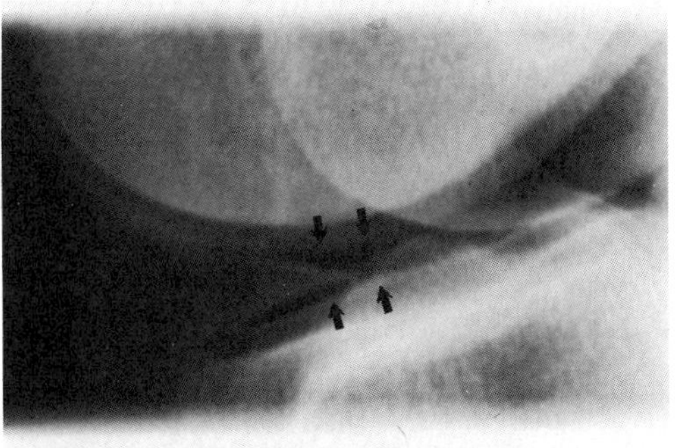

Figure 7.2 Double-contrast knee arthrogram demonstrating surface coating of triangular-shaped medial meniscus. Note also double-contrast display (arrows) of articular cartilage.

often resulted in image artifacts. Moreover, the instilled gas could not readily displace any synovial fluid remaining in meniscal tears, thus rendering their radiographic demonstration inadequate and their diagnosis difficult (Foote GA, 1977).

The initial successes and deficiences of pneumoarthrography prompted the search for a positive contrast agent that would readily mix with the synovial fluid upon its introduction into the joint. The agent would ideally provide adequate radiographic opacification of the fluid space and demonstration of the intraarticular structures for a sufficient period of time to permit completion of the examination, followed by its rapid absorption from the joint and systemic excretion. Of course, the ideal arthrographic contrast medium should also be devoid of physiological effects and observable adverse reactions.

In the early 1920s, positive-contrast arthrography was performed using Lipiodol (iodized poppy seed oil). However, this medium is water insoluble and immiscible with joint fluid, thus requiring joint aspiration prior to contrast injection. It also soon became recognized that the arthrographic use of Lipiodol was associated with the production of severe synovitis (Burman MS, et al, 1932), apparently related to its prolonged retention in the joint combined with its direct irritant effects. Positive-contrast arthrography was therefore not performed extensively until development of the water soluble, iodinated contrast media for urographic and angiographic procedures. Following their injection into the joint, these media mix readily with the synovial fluid and demonstrate rapid systemic absorption and excretion. Moreover, their arthrographic use is associated with relatively low morbidity.

CHEMISTRY

The water-soluble, iodinated contrast media indicated for arthrography procedures are meglumine or combination meglumine-sodium salts of the radiopaque anion, diatrizoate (Table 7.1). Arthrographic use of the ratio-1.5 medium, iothalamate meglumine, and the ratio-3 (low-osmolality) nonionic and ionic-dimeric media has also been reported; however, these agents are not, at the time of this writing, indicated for this purpose. The reader should refer to Chapter 1, Angiographic Contrast Media, for a complete discussion of the chemical properties of these contrast agents.

PHARMACOKINETICS

The water-soluble, iodinated contrast media mix rapidly with the synovial fluid following their introduction into the joint space. Thus the injected medium rapidly comes into direct contact with the highly vascularized synovial membrane responsi-

Table 7.1   **WATER-SOLUBLE, IODINATED CONTRAST MEDIA INDICATED FOR ARTHROGRAPHY PROCEDURES**[a]

GENERIC NAME	CONCENTRATION % W/V	BRAND NAME[b]	MG IODINE/ ML	OSMOLALITY[c] (MOSM/KG)	VISCOSITY (CPS)[c] 25° C/37° C
Diatrizoate meglumine	60	Angiovist-282 (B)	282	1400	6.1/4.1
Diatrizoate meglumine	60	Reno-M-60 (S)	282	1500	4.6/4.0
Diatrizoate meglumine	60	Hypaque-M 60 (W)	282	1415	6.2/4.1
Diatrizoate meglumine (52%)-sodium (8%)	60	Angiovist-292 (B)	292	1500	5.9/4.2
Diatrizoate meglumine (52%)-sodium (8%)	60	Renografin-60 (S)	292	1420	5.9/4.0

[a] U.S. market only
[b] (B) Berlex Imaging
(S) Squibb Diagnostics
(W) Winthrop-Breon Laboratories
[c] Adapted from Fischer HW, Catalog of intravascular contrast media. *Radiology* 1986, 159:561–563

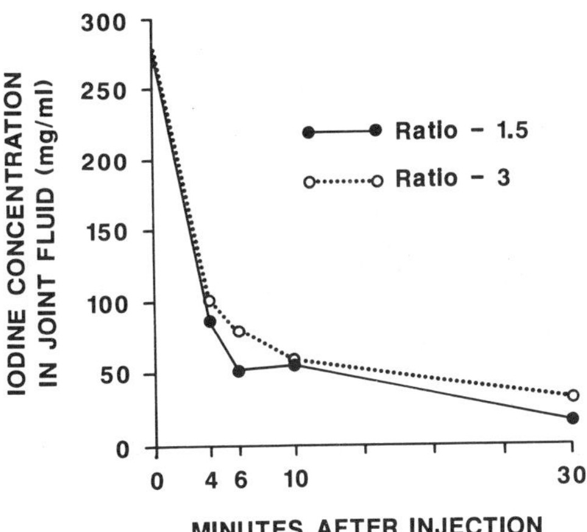

Figure 7.3 Intraarticular iodine concentration as a function of time post injection of a ratio-1.5 ionic (iothalamate meglumine) and ratio-3 nonionic (metrizamide) contrast medium. (Adapted from Katzberg RW, et al, 1976.)

ble for the production and absorption of joint fluid. During the first 5–20 minutes following injection, there is an exponential decrease in the intraarticular contrast medium and, hence, iodine concentration (Figure 7.3). This occurs due to rapid systemic absorption of the medium via the synovial membrane combined with a net flux of extrasynovial fluid into the joint space in an attempt to dilute the hyperosmolar environment created by the injected agent (Katzberg RW, et al, 1976).

The rate at which a contrast medium is absorbed from the joint space appears to be related to its molecular size and, perhaps, viscosity. Large, high-molecular-weight ionic-dimeric (mol. wgt. $\cong$ 1200) media have been shown to have a slower rate of synovial absorption than smaller, lower molecular-weight nonionic (mol. wgt. $\cong$ 800) or ionic-monomeric (mol. wgt. $\cong$ 600) media (Katzberg RW, et al, 1976; Obermann WR and Kieft GJ, 1987). The importance of viscosity as it relates to the rate of contrast absorption from the joint space is unclear. Increased viscosity may delay the rate at which the contrast medium mixes with the joint fluid and comes into contact with the synovial

membrane (Belli A, et al, 1984). It is also known that viscosity increases as a function of the molecular weight of the substance in solution. Therefore the slower rate of contrast-medium absorption with increased viscosity may reflect the previously described effect of increased molecular weight and size. At equivalent % weight/volume (w/v) and iodine concentrations, pure meglumine salts of diatrizoate have greater viscosities than combination meglumine-sodium derivatives (Table 7.1). The ratio-3 nonionic and ionic-dimeric media exhibit respectively greater viscosities than the ratio-1.5, ionic-monomeric media (see Chapter 1, Chemistry).

The degree to which a contrast medium induces hydrarthrosis, increases the intraarticular volume, and promotes self-dilution is directly dependent on its hyperosmolality. At equivalent iodine concentrations, pure meglumine salts of diatrizoate have a lower osmolality than pure sodium salts or combination meglumine sodium derivatives (Table 7.1). The osmolalities of the ratio-3 nonionic and ionic-dimeric media are 50–70% lower than those of the ratio-1.5 media (e. g., diatrizoate meglumine) at equivalent iodine concentrations. The ratio-3 low-osmolality media therefore demonstrate less hydrarthrosis (Figure 7.4) and dilution of intraarticular and iodine concentrations (Figure 7.3) than the ratio-1.5 ionic media (Katzberg RW, et al, 1976).

PHYSIOLOGICAL EFFECTS

Synovial Irritation. The injection of conventional (i. e., ratio-1.5) iodinated contrast media into the joint space commonly produces signs (e. g., pain, swelling) of local synovial irritation. Macroscopic findings include edema and hyperemia of the synovial membrane followed by its contraction and adherence to the joint capsule. Leukocyte and eosinophil infiltration have also been observed in histological evaluations. These effects are usually observed within 2–24 hours post

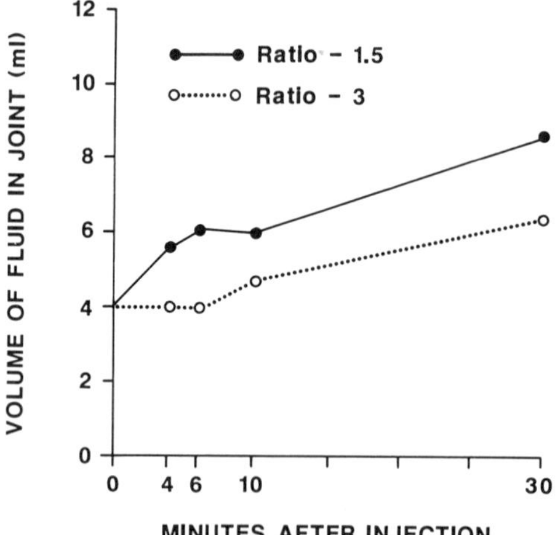

Figure 7.4 Intraarticular volume as a function of time post injection of a ratio-1.5 ionic (iothalamate meglumine) and a ratio-3 nonionic (metrizamide) contrast medium. (Adapted from Katzberg RW, et al, 1976.)

contrast injection, with regression normally occurring within a few days (Johansen JG and Berner A, 1976; Pastershank SP, et al, 1982).

This transient local irritation of the synovium is apparently due to direct molecular toxicity of the injected contrast medium and varies with the chemical nature of the injected agent. Sodium-containing derivatives of the radiopaque anions, diatrizoate and iothalamate, have been shown to produce substantially more leukocyte infiltration than pure meglumine salts. The ratio-3 nonionic media produce minimal direct irritation of the synovium as evidenced by a lack of leukocyte infiltration or alteration in synovial protein concentrations with the intraarticular injection of iohexol and iopamidol (Corbetti F, et al, 1986).

Hydrarthrosis. As previously discussed, the injection of a water-soluble, iodinated contrast medium into the joint space can produce an increase in the intraarticular volume due to a hyperosmolality-induced shift in fluid from the extrasynovial to the intrasynovial space. The resulting hydrarthrosis can produce capsular distension, a worsening of preexisting effusion, and

pain. The degree of hydrarthrosis produced by an intraarticular contrast medium is primarily dependent on its osmolality. At a given iodine concentration, pure meglumine salts of the ratio-1.5 media (i. e., diatrizoate, iothalamate) have a lower osmolality and produce less hydrarthrosis than pure sodium or combination meglumine-sodium salts. The osmolalities of the ratio-3 nonionic and ionic-dimeric media are 50–70% lower than those of equivalent iodine concentrations of the conventional, ratio-1.5 media. Hence, the ratio-3 low-osmolality media produce less hydrarthrosis and potential for capsular distension than the conventional ratio-1.5 agents (Hall FM, et al, 1981). Hydrarthrosis may also be partially related to direct irritative effects of the injected contrast medium on the synovial membrane since it has also been observed, to a milder degree, with the use of isosmotic concentrations of iodinated contrast media (Johansen JG and Berner A, 1976).

CLINICAL CONSIDERATIONS

Procedure Indications. Arthrography is indicated for the diagnosis and evaluation of congenital, post traumatic, or degenerative joint diseases. It is useful for the demonstration of synovial rupture, meniscal tears (Figure 7.1), loose bodies, torn ligaments or communicating bursae, or cysts and soft tissue masses. Arthrography is also utilized to evaluate complications of total joint replacement surgery.

Although controversy exists regarding the relative merits of single-contrast versus double-contrast arthrography (Tegtmeyer CJ, et al, 1979), it is now generally recognized that the double-contrast technique is preferable for the evaluation of subtle articular and meniscal abnormalities (Figure 7.5), especially if combined with computed tomographic techniques (Figure 7.6). If a double-contrast procedure is performed, the use of filtered air versus carbon dioxide represents another area of debate. Carbon dioxide is absorbed rapidly from the joint space (i. e.,

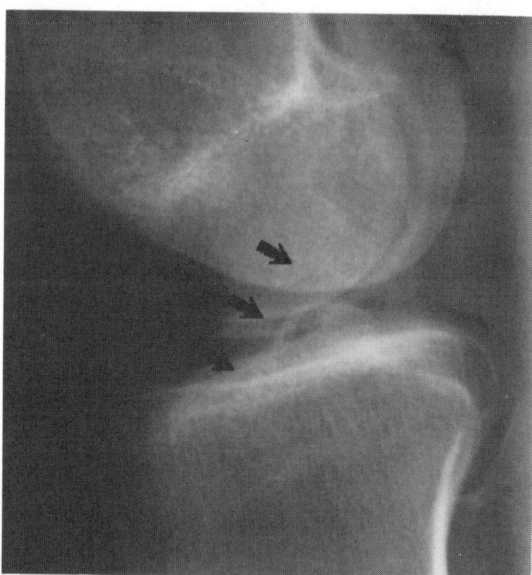

Figure 7.5 Double-contrast knee arthrogram demonstrating (arrows) the configuration of the anterior cruciate ligament.

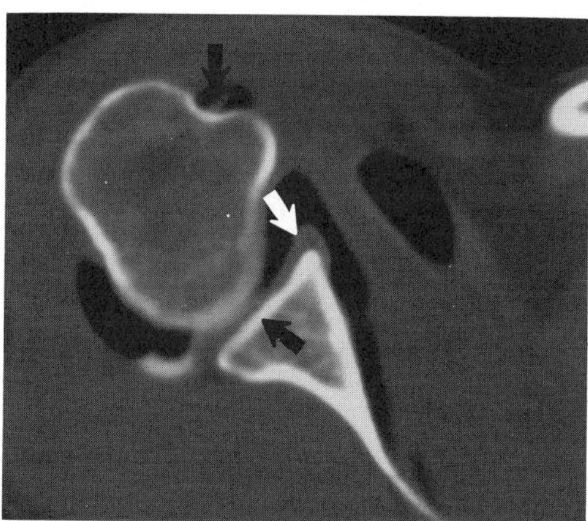

Figure 7.6 Double-contrast computed tomogram of the left shoulder demonstrating the glenoid articular cartilage (closed arrows) and the labrum (open arrow). Note also the bicep tendon (arrowhead) within its respective sheath.

marked reduction in negative contrast at 10–15 minutes post instillation) and therefore does not produce the "gurgling" sensation often noted with the prolonged (i. e., several days) retention of air or oxygen. The use of carbon dioxide for double-contrast arthrography is, however, associated with slightly greater discomfort

immediately following the procedure, and is also more expensive and less convenient than the use of air. Moreover, the rapid synovial absorption of carbon dioxide may not permit the completion of a lengthy examination without a requirement for readministration (Foote GA, 1977; Mink JH and Dickenson R, 1980; Goldberg RP, et al, 1981).

Contrast Medium Considerations. The local discomfort or pain commonly experienced following arthrography is related to soft-tissue trauma induced by the needle used for contrast injection, the direct irritative effects of the intraarticular contrast medium on the synovial membrane, capsular distension produced by the hydrarthrotic effects of the hyperosmolar contrast medium, or a combination of the above (Kaplan P, et al, 1985). Based on respective differences in their irritative and hydrarthrotic effects (see Physiological Effects), pure meglumine salts of the ratio-1.5 ionic media (i. e., diatrizoate, iothalamate) produce less postarthrography discomfort and pain than equivalent iodine concentrations of their combination meglumine-sodium or pure sodium derivatives (Hall FM, et al, 1985). Although the ratio-3 nonionic and ionic-dimeric media have been shown to produce less postarthrography discomfort and a longer duration of intraarticular contrast enhancement than the ratio-1.5 media (Hall FM, et al, 1985; Appel JS, et al, 1985; Katzberg RW, 1984; Kaplan P, et al, 1985), their substantially greater costs (i. e., at the time of this writing) probably warrants limiting their use to patients with severe preexisting joint pain or effusion. As might be expected, the reduced volume of contrast medium required for a double-contrast technique results in less hydrarthrosis and capsular distension, and hence, less postprocedure discomfort than observed with a corresponding single-contrast procedure (Hall FM, et al, 1981).

Patient Preparation. The subcutaneous administration of lidocaine (1% w/v, 1 mL) is usually performed to produce local anesthesia of the skin and subcutaneous tissues prior to intraarticular insertion of the contrast instillation needle. If joint pain is severe, an additional 1–2 mL of lidocaine (1% w/v) may be injected directly into the joint space prior to the arthrography procedure.

Adjunctive Drugs/Techniques.

Epinephrine. As a result of its alpha adrenergic agonistic effects, the intraarticular injection of epinephrine produces constriction of the vasculature of the synovial membrane and thereby decreases both the rate of synovial absorption and the rate of intraarticular dilution of a co-administered contrast medium. The adjunctive administration of epinephrine (1:1000, 0.3 mL) has therefore been shown to improve the sharpness of initial arthrographic films and to prolong the duration that films of acceptable quality can be obtained (Hall FM, 1974). It finds particular use and benefit with the more lengthy procedures such as double-contrast arthrography of the knee.

The adjunctive administration of epinephrine for improved arthrographic quality is, however, associated with an increased incidence and severity of postprocedure discomfort and pain (Hall FM, et al, 1985). By decreasing the rate of absorption and dilution of the intraarticular contrast medium, the epinephrine-enhanced study prolongs exposure of the synovial membrane to the chemotoxic, irritative effects of the injected medium (Corbetti F, et al, 1986). Little is known about the direct irritative effects of epinephrine, itself, on the synovial membrane or its rate of systemic absorption from the joint space. It is, however, recommended that the adjunct arthrographic use of epinephrine be performed with caution in patients with severe cardiac disease (Hall FM, 1974).

Contrast Aspiration. Whether or not aspiration of the injected contrast medium upon completion of the arthrography procedure will reduce the incidence or severity of immediate or delayed pain remains debatable and may depend on the particular joint undergoing examination. For example, it has been shown that postprocedure aspiration of the contrast medium resulted in no alteration of immediate or delayed pain with knee arthrography (Goldberg RP, et al, 1981), but produced substantially less delayed pain with shoulder arthrography (Hall FM, et al, 1985).

Precautions/Contraindications. In addition to postprocedure joint discomfort and pain, the performance of arthrography has also been associated with vasovagal reactions (e. g., sweating, bradycardia, hypotension) and urticaria or hives. The latter pseudo-allergic reactions are related to systemic absorption of the intraarticular contrast medium (see Chapter 8), and may occur up to several hours following the procedure (Newberg AH, et al, 1985).

Contrast Media–Laboratory Test Interaction. Certain (e. g., Reno-M-60®, Renografin-60®, Renografin-76®) of the water-soluble, iodinated contrast media that may be used for arthrography have been shown to exhibit a bacteriocidal or bacteriostatic activity, whereas others (e. g., Conray-60®, Hypaque Sodium-50®) have not (Kim KS and Lachman R, 1982). This contrast inhibition of bacterial growth does not appear to be related to iodine concentration, hyperosmolality, or the nature of the cation or radiopaque anion; but may be related to the nature of sequestrating and buffering agents used in the respective formulations (see Chapter 1, Angiographic Contrast Media). Based on this observation, the removal of joint fluid for bacterial culture should be performed prior to contrast instillation.

DOSAGE

Table 7.2 lists recommended dosages for single- and double-contrast examinations of various joint spaces. Intraarticular injections of contrast media are typically monitored by fluoroscopy to ensure adequate injection technique and opacification while preventing overdistension of the joint space. Faulty injection of an iodinated contrast medium into the soft tissues surrounding the joint can obscure subsequent intraarticular detail and result in increased discomfort, especially with the use of sodium-containing agents (Freiberger RH, et al, 1966; Angell FL, 1971). Injection of iodinated contrast media at excessive iodine concentrations

Table 7.2 RECOMMENDED DOSAGES OF DIATRIZOATE MEGLUMINE (60% w/v, 282 mg iodine/mL) FOR COMMON SINGLE- AND DOUBLE-CONTRAST ARTHROGRAPHY PROCEDURES[a]

ARTHROGRAPHY PROCEDURE	SINGLE-CONTRAST TECHNIQUE DIATRIZOATE DOSE (ML)	DOUBLE-CONTRAST TECHNIQUE DIATRIZOATE DOSE (ML)	AIR DOSE (ML)
Ankle	6–10	1–3	8
Elbow	6–10	0.1–1	6–10
Hip	10–20[b]	—	—
Knee	—	3–5[c]	30–80
Shoulder	20	1–4	10–15
Temporomandibular joint	0.5–0.8	—	—
Wrist	1.5–2.5	—	—

[a] Adult doses

[b] Infant: 1.5–2 mL; adolescent: 5–8 mL

[c] Increase to 8–10 mL with effusion

or volumes into the joint space may also initially obscure intraarticular detail requiring that delayed studies be performed following systemic absorption of the contrast medium and dilution of intraarticular opacification. Capsular distension produced by excessive contrast doses increases the potential for procedure-induced discomfort or pain. Excessive doses and capsular distension may also promote leakage of the contrast medium from sites of injection or previous joint aspiration, rendering the diagnosis of synovial rupture difficult (Foote GA, 1977).

II. Hysterosalpingographic Contrast Media

Dennis P. Swanson
Carol J. Maywood

Hysterosalpingography involves the direct instillation (i. e., using a specialized vacuum cervical adapter cannula or balloon-catheter) of a radiopaque contrast medium into the uterine cavity for the radiographic demonstration of intrauterine abnormalities and the evaluation of fallopian tube patency (Figure 7.7). This procedure previously represented the

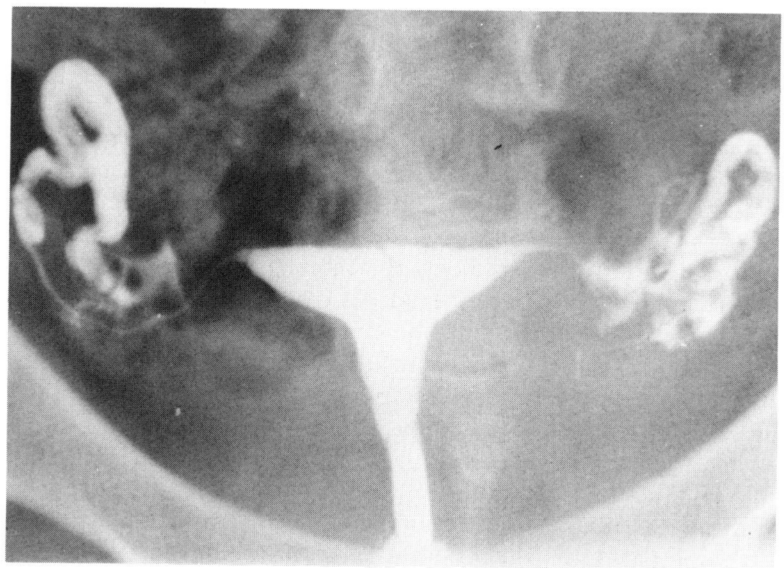

Figure 7.7 Normal hysterosalpingogram demonstrating contrast (Sinografin®) filling of the uterine cavity and both fallopian tubes with spillage into the peritoneal cavity.

primary method for diagnosing uterine and tubal factors responsible for fertility disorders. More recently, hysterosalpingography has been largely replaced by laparoscopy, which provides a more accurate assessment of tubal patency and peritoneal disorders (Rice JP, et al, 1986).

HISTORY

Uterography was first reported in 1910 incorporating the intrauterine administration of a bismuth solution (Rindfleisch, 1910). During the ensuing 10 years several other radiopaque materials were investigated for uterography-hysterosalpingography including thorium nitrate, colloidal silver (Collargol), and sodium iodide and bromide. In general, these agents proved unsatisfactory due to inadequate opacification properties and/or marked peritoneal irritation following their passage through patent fallopian tubes (Yune HY, 1977; Soules MR and Spadoni LR, 1982).

The water-insoluble contrast agent, Lipiodol, was first utilized for hysterosalpingography in the early 1920s (Heuser C, 1925). This agent, comprising glycerin esters of the iodinated fatty acids of poppy seed oil, contained approximately 40% iodine. Its extremely high viscosity and slow rate of clearance from the uterotubal system combined with its iodine content permitted adequate levels of opacification for the required multiple sequential radiographs utilized for hysterosalpingography during this era. It was believed, however, that the viscosity of Lipidol was excessive, resulting in problems associated with a requirement for uterine instillation under high pressure. Lipidol F, an ethyl rather than glyceryl ester of the iodinated fatty acids of poppy-seed oil, provided a less viscous alternative. This agent became eventually known as Ethiodol® (Lipiodol Ultrafluid), an oil-soluble contrast medium currently indicated for hysterosalpingography (Yune HY, 1977; Soules MR and Spadoni LR, 1982).

Although the majority of the Lipiodol instilled into the uterine cavity is discharged into the vagina following completion of the procedure, any of the medium trapped within dilated or obstructed fallopian tubes or spilled into the peritoneal cavity is absorbed very slowly over a period of several months or years. This prolonged retention of Lipiodol combined with its direct irritant effects resulted frequently in the formation of oil granulomas, retention cysts, or adhesions. In addition, intravasation of the water-insoluble Lipiodol via the uterine venous plexus resulted in reported deaths due to pulmonary embolism (Yune HY, 1977).

Lipiodol remained the contrast medium of choice for hysterosalpingography for approximately 30 years. However, the problems related to foreign body reactions and pulmonary embolism led to a search for a water-soluble contrast medium that would be rapidly absorbed from the uterotubal system and peritoneal cavity following completion of the examination, and would subsequently demonstrate rapid systemic excretion. Of course, the ideal medium should also be devoid of local mucosal irritation and systemic side effects.

With the development of the water-soluble, iodinated contrast media for urography and angiography (see Chapter 1) came their investigation as potential hysterosalpingographic agents. It was soon recognized, however, that the relatively low viscosity and rapid systemic absorption of these media often resulted in inadequate levels of uterotubal opacification to permit completion of the radiographic filming sequence. Attempts were made to overcome this problem by adding viscosity extenders, such as polyvinyl pyrolidone, carboxymethylcellulose, and dextran to various water-soluble, iodinated agents (e.g., Slapix®, Visco Rayopake®). However, in general, these additives led to an increased level of mucosal irritation and potential for foreign body reactions (Soules MR and Spadoni LR, 1982). In an alternate approach to increased viscosity, the iodinated dimeric medium, iodipamide meglumine (see Chapter 6, II. Cholangiographic Contrast Media), was combined with the urographic-angiographic medium, diatrizoate meglumine, to form a water-soluble contrast agent indicated specifically for hysterosalpingography: Sinografin®. This agent remains in use today.

With the advent of fluoroscopic radiographic techniques in the latter 1950s, the time required to perform a complete hysterosalpingographic examination was reduced to 20–30 minutes. Therefore, the problems associated with the rapid rate of uterotubal clearance of the low-viscosity, water-soluble media became less important. Hence, certain of the iodinated contrast routinely used for urographic and angiographic procedures were recognized as being safe and effective for routine fluoroscopic examinations of the uterotubal system and are currently indicated for this purpose.

CHEMISTRY

Oil-Soluble Contrast Media. The only oil-soluble contrast medium currently available (i. e., in the United States) and indicated for hysterosalpingography is Ethiodol® (Savage Laboratories). This agent consists of a mixture of ethyl esters of the iodinated fatty acids of poppy-seed oil. It contains 370 mg Iodine/mL, primarily in the form of mono- and diiodoethyl sterates (Figure 7.8).

Ethiodol® is insoluble in water. As an oily liquid, the medium has a relatively high viscosity of 25–30 centipoise at 37° C. The aliphatic carbon-iodine bonds of Ethiodol® are not extremely stable, and therefore it should be protected from prolonged exposure to heat or light. A light amber color is normal, but the medium should not be used if a dark yellow coloration is observed.

Water-Soluble Contrast Media. The water-soluble, iodinated contrast media currently indicated for hysterosalpingography are listed in Table 7.3. As previously described, Sinografin® consists of a mixture of the meglumine salts of the monomeric anion, diatrizoate, and the dimeric anion, iodipamide (Figure 7.9), and is specifically indicated for hysterosalpingography. The remainder of the listed agents are primarily utilized for angiography or excretory urography procedures, but are also indicated for hysterosalpingography. The reader should refer to Chapter 1, Angiographic Contrast Media, for a complete discussion of the chemical properties of the ratio-1.5 ionic-mono mer, diatrizoate, and the ratio-3 ionic-dimer, ioxaglate; and to Chapter 6, II. Cholangiographic Contrast Media, for respective information on iodipamide.

Hysterosalpingographic use of the ratio-1.5 medium, iothalamate meglumine, and the ratio-3 low-osmolality medium, metrizamide have also been reported; however, these intravascular agents (see Chapter 1) are not currently indicated for this purpose.

$$CH_3 - (CH_2)_4 - \overset{I}{CH} - (CH_2)_3 - \overset{I}{CH} - (CH_2)_7 - \overset{O}{\overset{\|}{C}} - O - CH_2 - CH_3$$

Diiodoethylstearate

$$CH_3 - (CH_2)_7 - \overset{I}{CH} - (CH_2)_8 - \overset{O}{\overset{\|}{C}} - O - CH_2 - CH_3$$

Monoiodoethylstearate

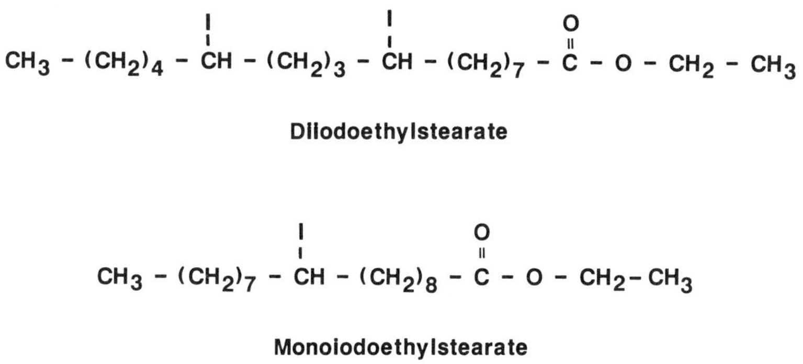

Figure 7.8 Chemical structures of the primary radiopaque components of Ethiodol®, the ethyl esters of diiodo- and monoiodostearic acid.

Table 7.3 WATER-SOLUBLE, IODINATED CONTRAST MEDIA INDICATED FOR HYSTEROSALPINGOGRAPHY[a]

GENERIC NAME	BRAND NAME®[b]	CONCENTRATION (% w/v)	MG IODINE/ ML	VISCOSITY (CPS)[c] 25° C	37° C
Diatrizoate meglumine-Iodipamide meglumine	Sinografin (S)	52.7–26.8	380	27.5[d]	15.9[d]
Diatrizoate meglumine (60%)-sodium (30%)	Hypaque-M 90 (W)	90	462	34.7	19.5
Diatrizoate sodium	Hypaque 50 (W)	50	300	3.4	2.4
Diatrizoate sodium	Urovist Sodium 300 (B)	50	300	3.3	2.4
Ioxaglate meglumine (39.3%)-sodium (19.6%)	Hexabrix (M)	58.9	320	15.7	7.5

[a] U.S. market only
[b] (B) Berlex Imaging
(S) Squibb Diagnostics
(W) Winthrop-Breon Laboratories
(M) Mallinckrodt Inc.
[c] Adapted from Fischer HW, Catalog of intravascular contrast media. *Radiology* 1986, 159: 561–563 (unless otherwise indicated)
[d] Provided by Squibb Diagnostics

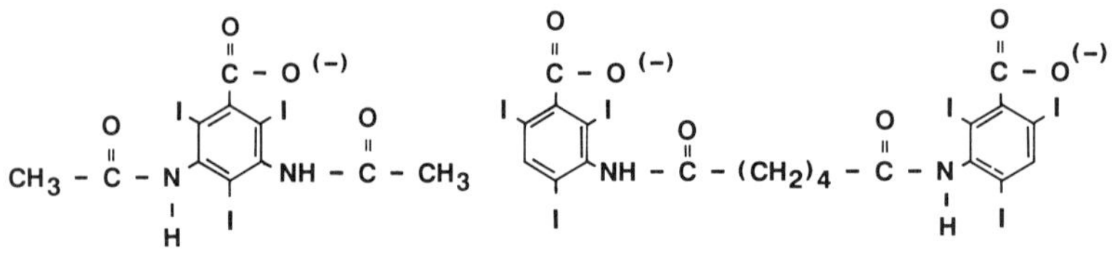

Diatrizoate   Iodipamide

Figure 7.9 Chemical structures of the radiopaque components of Sinografin®.

PHARMACOKINETICS

General. Maximum opacification of the uterus and fallopian tubes occurs immediately following intrauterine instillation of a hysterosalpingographic contrast medium. The majority of the instilled dose drains from the uterotubal system into the vagina following completion of the examination and removal of the instillation device (i. e., vacuum cervical adaptor cannula or balloon catheter). That portion of the contrast medium that passes through patent fallopian tubes into the peritoneal cavity (Figure 7.7) or is trapped within obstructed or dilated fallopian tubes or peritubal adhesions is subject to subsequent systemic absorption.

Ethiodol®. Ethiodol is slowly absorbed from the peritoneal cavity into the blood over a period of several months or longer (Palmer A, 1960). Medium trapped within the fallopian tubes or peritubal adhesions demonstrates even slower systemic absorption, requiring years for complete elimination (Soules MR and Spadoni LR, 1982). With slow absorption, the small amount of water-insoluble Ethiodol® entering the blood is subsequently phagocytized by cells comprising the reticuloendothelial system. It is eventually degraded with the liberation of free iodine and fatty acids.

Water-Soluble Contrast Media. The water-soluble, iodinated contrast media are rapidly absorbed from the peritoneal cavity; their complete elimination usually occurring within one hour (Soules MR and Spadoni LR, 1982; Griffiths HJL, 1969). Medium tapped within the uterus or fallopian tubes is absorbed at a slower rate; however, complete removal still occurs within hours. Systemic diatrizoate and ioxaglate are excreted rapidly via the kidneys (see Chapter 1), whereas systemic iodiapamide undergoes rapid excretion via the hepatobiliary system (see Chapter 6).

PHYSIOLOGICAL EFFECTS

Mucosal Irritation/Pain. Abdominal discomfort and pain are common complaints with hysterosalpingography, with reported incidences as high as 75% (Griffiths HJL, 1969; Winfield AC, et al, 1982a). Pain occuring during the early portions of the procedure is primarily associated with insertion and positioning of the instillation device rather than the instilled contrast medium. However, delayed pain appears to be related to spillage of the contrast medium into the peritoneal cavity and its direct irritant effect on the respective mucosal surfaces (Moore DE, 1982). In an experimental study, water-soluble iodinated contrast media injected directly into the peritoneal cavity were shown to produce an acute inflammatory response with polymorphonuclear infiltration and fibrin deposits (McAlister WH, et al, 1972). This inflammatory response peaked at 48 hours and subsided at 72 hours with no residual scarring or irritation. These observations correlate with the transient pain of hysterosalpingography.

Several comparative studies have addressed the level of pain associated with the use of various contrast media for hysterosalpingography. In general, it has been shown that the oil-soluble contrast media (e. g., Lipiodol, Ethiodol®) produce less pain with spillage into the peritoneal cavity than the water-soluble, iodinated agents (Fullenlove TM, 1969; Moore DE, 1982; Soules MR and Spadoni LR, 1982). This may be related to respective differences in the molecular toxicities and direct irritant effects of the two classes of agents. Another explanation may be related to the fact that the insolubility of the oil-soluble contrast media in the peritoneal fluid results in globule formation. These spherical globules have a limited surface area for direct contact with the mucosal surfaces as compared to the intimate contact of the dissolved water-soluble media.

Based on comparative studies of water-soluble contrast media performed to date, no clear-cut statements can be made regarding the relative efficacy of various contrast medium factors in reducing the mucosal irritation and pain of hysterosalpingography. Unlike their respective effects on the vascular endothelium (see Chapter 1, Angiographic Contrast Media) or synovial membrane (see Chapter 7, I. Arthrographic Contrast Media), meglumine salts of the radiopaque anions do not appear to produce less irritation of the peritoneal mucosal surfaces than do sodium salts (McAlister WH, et al, 1972). Also, no apparent difference appears to exist between the diatrizoate and iothalamate anions. Peritoneal irritation does not seem to be related to the hyperosmolality of the instilled medium since minimal pain differences have been observed in comparative studies of the ratio-1.5 ionic versus ratio-3 low-osmolality media (Davies AC, et al, 1985; Stiris G and Andrew E, 1979; Winfield AC, et al, 1984). This is not particularly surprising since the small volume of a contrast medium passing through the patent fallopian tubes would be rapidly diluted in the large volume space of the peritoneal cavity. In summary, the intensity of hysterosalpingographic pain does vary with the use of different water-soluble contrast media, but no specific responsible factors can be identified. This situation is further compounded by the lack of a well-controlled clinical trial comparing each of the water-soluble contrast media currently indicated for hysterosalpingography.

Pain with hysterosalpingography may be more related to the hydrostatic pressure employed during contrast instillation and the subsequent volume of medium entering the peritoneal cavity than it is to the medium's direct irritant effect on the mucosal surfaces. The intrauterine instillation of physiological solutions has been shown to produce a similar increase in patient discomfort (Stiris G and Andrew E, 1979; Beyth Y, et al, 1985). This response does not appear to be related to pressure-induced tubal spasm since adjunctive administration of the antispasmotic agent, glucagon, had no effect on the level of discomfort (Ansari AH and Shimoura B, 1978).

Foreign Body Reactions. As previously discussed, early hysterosalpingographic use of the oil-soluble contrast medium, Lipiodol, was associated with the frequent production of oil granulomas, retention cysts, and adhesions. The incidence of these foreign-body reactions was increased in the presence of preexisting inflammation of the respective mucosal surfaces and with prolonged retention of the medium in obstructed or dilated fallopian tubes or the peritoneal cavity (Yune HY, 1977).

Although the respective incidences of granuloma formation have not been established, it is clear that the oil-soluble contrast medium, Ethiodol®, has more potential to produce foreign body reactions than the rapidly absorbed water-soluble agents (Soules MR and Spadoni LR, 1982). However, such reactions can also be observed with the water-soluble media if glove talc, lubricant material, glass fragments, and so on are inadvertently administered (Yune HY, 1977). That the incidence of foreign body reactions with the current use of Ethiodol® is undoubtedly less than that reported with the earlier use of Lipiodol may reflect a reduced irritant effect of the former agent or the corresponding recent incorporation of fluoroscopic techniques for more accurate monitoring of dosage and, hence, reduced peritoneal spillage.

Pseudo-allergic Reactions. Pseudo allergic reactions to intravascular iodinated contrast media occur independent of the concentration or dose of the administered agent above a certain threshold level (see Chapter 8). Hence, pseudo-allergic reactions can occur with rapid systemic absorption of the contrast media used for hysterosalpingography. Since previous contrast media reactors are known to be at increased risk for such reactions, their pretreatment with an appropriate steroid-antihistamine-ephedrine regimen (see Chapter 8) should be

considered. All patients should be carefully monitored during and following the hysterosalpingography examination, and appropriate drugs for the treatment of contrast-media reactions should be readily available.

PRECAUTIONS/ CONTRAINDICATIONS

Contrast Medium–Laboratory Test Interactions. Iodinated contrast media (or liberated iodine) absorbed into the systemic circulation can interfere with thyroid function tests based on the measurement of iodine (e. g., radioactive iodine uptake test, serum-protein-bound iodine). Such laboratory tests should be performed prior to contrast administration or alternate tests of thyroid function utilized.

Contrast Intravasation. Intravasation of the contrast media used for hysterosalpingography can occur via the uterine venous plexus or ovarian veins (Figure 7.10). The risk of this procedure-induced complication is greatest in the presence of conditions (e. g., menstrual period, recent surgical manipulations, polyps, fibroids, endometrial disease) that result in a thin or fragile uterine mucosa, with tubal obstruction or disease, and with excessive injection pressures or contrast-medium doses (Yune HY, 1977).

Upon intravasation, the water-soluble iodinated contrast media rapidly disperse in the blood and undergo systemic excretion. However, the intravasation of large volumes of the oil-soluble contrast media can result in the formation of water-insoluble globules that can subsequently embolize the vascular bed of the lungs or other organs. As previously discussed, deaths due to pulmonary embolization were reported with hysterosalpingographic use of the early oil-soluble medium, Lipiodol. Although incidences as high as 13% have been reported for intravasation of the current oil-soluble medium, Ethiodol®, this event does not appear to pose a serious complication

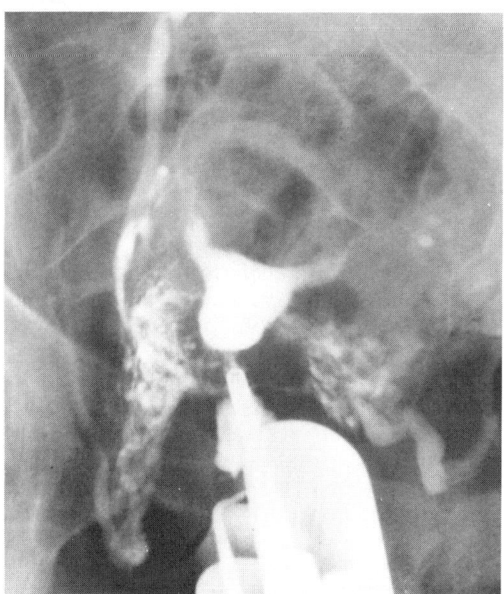

Figure 7.10 Hysterosalpingography performed subsequent to tubal ligation on a patient presenting with unexplained vaginal discharge. The pressure of the injection against the obstructed tubes resulted in the backflow of contrast (Sinografin®) into draining veins and lymphatics.

(Alper MM, et al, 1986). Compared to Lipiodol, the globules formed systemically with intravasation of the less viscous medium, Ethiodol®, may be subject to more rapid fragmentation and cleareance from the pulmonary vascular bed. In addition, the recent incorporation of fluoroscopic techniques into the hysterosalpingographic procedure provides a method to detect the onset of intravasation and to prevent the systemic accumulation of a large amount of the contrast medium.

Pelvic Inflammatory Disease. The reported incidence of serious pelvic inflammatory disease following hysterosalpingography ranges from 0.3–3.0% (Pittaway DE, et al, 1983a; Stumpf PG and March CM, 1980). The risk of this procedure-induced complication increases with a prior history of pelvic inflammatory disease and is especially high with the diagnosis of dilated fallopian tubes, in particular with concomitant spillage of con-

trast medium into the peritoneal cavity. The risk is relatively low with non-dilated tubes or with proximal tubal obstruction or peritubal disease (Pittaway DE, et al, 1983a). Hysterosal pingographic-associated pelvic inflammatory disease is not related to the nature of the contrast medium utilized for the procedure.

Pelvic inflammatory disease post hysterosalpingography is primarily associated with the genital pathogens, chlamydia trachomatis and mycoplasma hominus (Moller BR, et al, 1984). Proper antiseptic preparation of the cervix and endocervix prior to initiation of the examination may help to prevent this complication (Stumpf PG and March CM, 1980). In patients demonstrating tubal dilation, the prophylactic administration of antibiotics should be considered (see Clinical Considerations, Adjunctive Drugs).

CLINICAL CONSIDERATIONS

Procedure Indications. Hysterosalpingography may be useful in evaluating congenital abnormalities of the uterus or in diagnosing intrauterine disorders responsible for habitual abortions, irregular bleeding, or amenorrhea. Although largely replaced by laparoscopy, hysterosalpingography was previously a primary methodology for determining the patency of the fallopian tubes in the evaluation of fertility disorders.

Contrast Media Considerations. Hysterosalpingography may be performed using the oil-soluble contrast medium, Ethiodol®, or one of the water-soluble iodinated contrast media currently indicated for this purpose (Table 7.3). As previously discussed (see Physiological Effects), hysterosalpingographic use of the oil-soluble medium is generally associated with less subjective discomfort or pain than the water-soluble agents. Use of Ethiodol® may also provide slight advantages related to its slow rate of uterotubal migration and the cohesiveness of its radiopaque column, resulting in clearer and sharper radiographic images. However, this slow rate of migration requires that delayed images be obtained at 24 hours to demonstrate the free movement of contrast within the peritoneal cavity and the lack of peritubal adhesions or peritoneal loculations.

Unlike Ethiodol®, the water-soluble, iodinated contrast media are rapidly absorbed from the uterotubal system and peritoneal cavity, thus reducing the potential for foreign-body reactions. Moreover, the water-soluble agents present a negligible risk for pulmonary embolism in the event of contrast intravasation. The rapid flow of the water-soluble media through the utero-tubal system obviates the requirement for delayed images to evaluate contrast distribution in the peritoneal cavity. In addition, the diminished degree of opacification exhibited by the water-soluble media with time may permit better evaluation of the contours of mucosal surfaces such as demonstration of ampullary rugae (Yune HY, 1977; Soules MR and Spadoni LR, 1982).

Within the group of water-soluble, iodinated contrast media indicated for hysterosalpingography, the viscosities of the diatrizoate sodium 50% w/v media are considerably lower than that of ioxaglate-meglumine-sodium, Sinografin®, or the diatrizoate meglumine-sodium 90% w/v preparation (Table 7.3). Although a lower viscosity will facilitate ease of handling and injection of the hysterosalpingographic medium, it will also result in its more rapid kinetics through the uterotubal system. Thus, use of the low-viscosity media requires that the examination incorporate fluoroscopic techniques.

As described, there are certain advantages and disadvantages associated with the use of each of the contrast media currently indicated for hysterosalpingography. It is important that the radiologist be familiar with the pharmacokinetic properties of the medium selected in order to optimize study performance and interpretation. If fluoroscopic techniques are available, the reduced potential for adverse effects probably warrants the use

of a water-soluble iodinated medium over Ethiodol®.

Pregnancy Rates Post Hysterosalpingography. Early clinical studies suggest that the incidence of pregnancy post hysterosalpingography was greater if an oil-soluble versus a water-soluble contrast medium was used for the procedure. These studies were, however, questioned extensively due to their retrospective nature and nonrandomized patient-entry format (Soules MR and Spadoni LR, 1982). Recently, two well-controlled prospective studies have addressed this issue (Alper MM, et al, 1986; Schwabe MG, et al, 1983). Although neither study could demonstrate a significant difference in postprocedure pregnancy rates between the oil-soluble and water-soluble media if the total patient population was considered, it was shown that the subsequent incidence of pregnancy was significantly greater with an oil-soluble medium in a specific group of patients with infertility of unknown origin (i.e., no hysterosalpingographic evidence of tubal dilation or obstruction) (Schwabe MG, et al, 1983).

Several mechanisms were proposed to explain the early observations of an increased post-hysterosalpinography pregnancy rate with oil-soluble versus water-soluble contrast media (Table 7.4). More recently, in vitro studies have demonstrated that Ethiodol® significantly inhibits the phagocytic activity of pelvic peritoneal macrophages, whereas Sinografin® has no effect (Boyer P, et al, 1986). Since high levels of pelvic peritoneal macrophage activity are often found in women with unexplained fertility disorders, the Ethiodol®-induced inhibition of sperm phagocytosis by these macrophages may explain the higher incidence of postprocedure pregnancy observed with this agent. It has also been recently shown that the water-soluble contrast media can inhibit the rate of ciliary transport within the fallopian tubes (Patton DL, et al, 1984). The oil-soluble medium evaluated in this study had no such ef-

Table 7.4 POSSIBLE MECHANISMS TO EXPLAIN AN INCREASED PREGNANCY RATE POST HYSTEROSALPINGOGRAPHIC USE OF AN OIL-SOLUBLE CONTRAST MEDIA[a]

Bacteriostatic effect
Lubricating effect
Chemical stimulation of tubal mucosa
· Increased ciliary transport
· Increased tubal peristalsis
Mechanical stimulation/lavage of fallopian tubes
· Removal of foreign or inspissated material
· Dilation of incompletely obstructed tube
· Release of peritubal adhesions

[a] Adapted from Yune HY, 1977 and Cooper RA, et al, 1983

fect. Since inhibition of tubal ciliary transport may have a negative effect on fertility, these findings may provide yet another explanation for differences in postprocedure pregnancy rates between the two classes of hysterosalpingographic media.

Adjunctive Drugs

Lidocaine. Injection of 3–5 ml of a 1% w/v solution of lidocaine into the lip of the cervix may aid in reducing the discomfort and pain associated with introduction and positioning of the special instillation devices (e. g., cannula with vacuum cervical adaptor, balloon catheter) used for hysterosalpingography. Such use of lidocaine does not, however, affect the incidence or intensity of delayed pain associated with contrast medium spillage into the peritoneal cavity (Birnbaum MD, 1985).

Glucagon. Anxiety, discomfort, or excessive injection pressures associated with performance of the hysterosalpingography procedure can result in spasm of the fallopian tubes. It has been suggested that such an occurrence may represent the primary cause for false-positive studies in the diagnosis of tubal obstruction (Ansari AH and Shimoura H, 1978). Intravenous glucagon (0.5–2 mg) has been shown to be effective in preventing tubal spasm (Gerlock AJ and Hooser CW, 1976; Ansari AH and Shimoura H, 1978; Winfield AC, et al, 1982b). This action of glucagon is probably related to its known relaxant effect on the smooth muscle of the gastrointestinal tract and the fact that segments of the fallopian tubes are composed of the same muscular layers as found in the gastrointestinal mucosa (Gerlock AJ and Hooser CW, 1976). The hypotonic effect of glucagon on the utero tubal system occurs within 1 minute following injection, but may be greatly diminished or absent by 20 minutes (Pittaway DE, 1983b), especially with use of lower dosages.

Side effects following the intravenous injection of glucagon are infrequent and mild. Commonly observed reactions include nausea, vomiting, headache, and flushing. Hypersensitivity reactions can occur, with the possibility of anaphylaxis. Glucagon should be administered with extreme caution to patients with pheochromocytoma or insulinoma due to its potential to release massive amounts of catecholamines or insulin, respectively. Of course, the adjunct use of glucagon may induce hyperglycemic reactions in diabetic patients.

Antibiotics. For patients demonstrating dilated or obstructed fallopian tubes, the prophylactic administration of antibiotics should be considered to prevent the possible occurrence of procedure-induced, pelvic inflammatory disease (see Precautions/Complications). The antibiotic selected should be effective against the genital pathogens (e. g., chlamydia trachomatis, mycoplasma hominus) commonly responsible for this complication. Tetracycline (500 mg twice daily for 10 days) or doxycycline (100 mg twice daily for 5 days) are generally effective agents for initial consideration. In patients allergic to tetracycline, erythromycin (500 mg twice daily for 10 days) represents a possible alternative (Pittaway DE, et al, 1983a; Møller BR, et al, 1984).

Contraindications. The performance of hysterosalpingography is contraindicated in the presence of any condition (e. g., menstruation, intrauterine bleeding, recent surgical procedures) that may increase the risk for uterine perforation. It should also be delayed until 6 months following the termination of pregnancy. Steps should be taken to ensure the absence of an intrauterine pregnancy prior to initiation of the procedure. Hysterosalpingography is also contraindicated in the presence of acute pelvic inflammatory disease or active infections of the genital tract.

DOSAGE

It is recommended that the hysterosalpingographic contrast media be instilled into the uterine cavity under controlled pressure with fluoroscopic monitoring of the dose. Excessive injection pressures (e. g., > 200 mm Hg) or doses increase the potential for discomfort and pain, contrast intravasation, or tubal spasm (Yune HY, 1977). Warming the contrast media to 37° C prior to administration substantially reduces their viscosities (Table 7.3) and the required injection pressure.

Each of the contrast media indicated for hysterosalpingography contains the required iodine concentration of 280 mg/mL or greater (Stiris G and Andrew E, 1979). Under fluoroscopic guidance, a sufficient volume of the medium is initially instilled (via a special vacuum cervical adaptor cannula or balloon catheter) to provide filling of the uterus. Fractional 1–2 mL doses are subsequently injected until fallopian tube patency is demonstrated or intolerable patient discomfort occurs. Tubal patency, peritubal adhesions, and peritoneal loculations are routinely demonstrated at the time of instillation of a water-soluble medium. However, delayed imaging (e. g., at 24 hours) may be required to evaluate the peritoneal distribution of Ethiodol®.

III. Lymphographic Contrast Media

Dennis P. Swanson
P.C. Shetty

Lymphography is defined as a radiographic examination of the lymphatic system. Since the lymph vessels, nodes, and fluid demonstrate the same degree of x-ray absorption as surrounding soft tissues, the introduction of a radiopaque contrast medium into the lymphatic system is required for its adequate visualization using standard radiographic techniques. Nonopacified abnormal lymph nodes can often be demonstrated with computed tomography based on their spatial location relative to surrounding tissues.

Indirect lymphography involves the injection of a radiopaque contrast medium subcutaneously into tissues or into body cavities. The medium is subsequently transported into adjacent lymph vessels and nodes by the lymph fluid formed in these regions. With a direct lymphography technique, the radiopaque contrast medium is injected into a previously isolated and cannulated lymph vessel (i. e., direct lymphangiography) or, rarely, directly into a lymph node (i. e., direct lymphadenography).

HISTORY

The indirect technique represents the most convenient method of performing lymphography. The lymph nodes of living humans were first demonstrated radiographically in the early 1930s following the indirect injection of Lipiodol (iodized poppy seed oil) into the maxillary sinus. However, an injection-to-imaging interval of 1 week was required for adequate lymphatic migration of the contrast medium and nodal opacification (Pfahler GE, 1932). This and subsequent studies confirmed the impracticality of the indirect technique for radiographic evaluation of the lymphatic system. The lymph vessels do not absorb radiopaque contrast media efficiently or rapidly enough to permit their visualization or the visualization of distant lymph nodes. The majority of the subcutaneous or cavitary contrast medium remains at the injection site or enters the vascular system.

In the early 1950s, Kinmonth observed that the indirect, subcutaneous injection of Patent Blue dye produced staining of lymph vessels responsible for drainage of the respective region (Kinmonth JB, 1952). This staining permitted the localization and surgical isolation of lymph vessels for subsequent cannulation and direct injection of a radiopaque contrast medium into the lymphatic system.

The first contrast media evaluated for direct lymphography were the water-soluble, iodinated agents (e. g., acetrizoate, metrizoate, iothalamate) originally developed for urography and angiography procedures (see Chapter 1, Angiographic

Contrast Media). These agents were, however, rapidly absorbed from the lymphatic system. Moreover, their hyperosmolar nature resulted in an increased formation of lymph fluid and rapid dilution of their opacification properties. As a result of these characteristics, lymphographic use of the water-soluble, iodinated contrast media permitted only transient visualization of superficial lymph vessels and regional nodes (Fisher HW, 1959). They were unsatisfactory for radiographic evaluation of the total lymphatic system communicating with the injected vessel.

It was soon recognized that the ideal contrast medium for direct lymphography must be retained within the lymph vessels and nodes for a sufficient period of time and at a suitable level of opacification to permit evaluation of the total lymphatic system. Following completion of the examination, the ideal medium should be rapidly cleared from the lymph vessels and nodes and excreted systemically. Its viscosity (and particle size, if colloidal in nature) must be low enough to permit injection through the small-bore needles used for lymph-vessel cannulation. The medium must also be able to flow readily through the small diameter (0.1–10 mm) lymph vessels and should not alter the normal flow patterns of lymph fluid. Likewise, the ideal medium should not alter the normal filtering and protective activities of the lymph nodes. Of course, it should also be devoid of local or systemic physiological effects or adverse reactions (Svoboda M, 1971).

Based on initial successes with the indirect administration of Lipiodol for lymphography, this oily-contrast medium was evaluated using the direct technique. Although it was retained within the lymph vessels and nodes and provided an acceptable level of opacification, problems were encountered as a result of its extremely high viscosity. Lipiodol-F, an ethyl rather than glyceryl ester of the iodinated fatty acids of poppy seed oil, provided a less viscous alternative. This agent became eventually known as Ethiodol® (Lipiodol Ultrafluid), the oil-soluble contrast medium currently indicated for lymphography (Svoboda M, 1971; Fisher HW, 1977).

CHEMISTRY

The oil-soluble contrast medium, Ethiodol®, is the only agent currently approved and indicated for lymphography in the United States. It consists of a mixture of ethyl esters of the iodinated fatty acids of poppy seed oil, primarily in the form of mono- and diiodoethyl stearates (Figure 8.8), and contains 370 mg iodine/mL.

Ethiodol® is insoluble in water. As an oily liquid the medium has a high viscosity of approximately 55 centipoise at 20° C and 25–30 centipose at 37° C. The aliphatic carbon-iodine bonds of Ethiodol® are not extremely stable; therefore, it should be protected from prolonged exposure to heat or light. A light amber color is normal, but the medium should

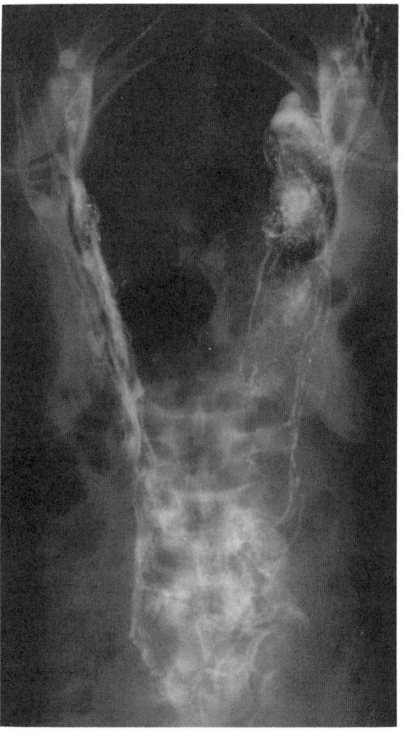

Figure 7.11 Lymphangiogram obtained at 1 hour following the bilateral injection of Ethiodol® into pedal lymphatic vessels.

not be used if a dark yellow coloration is observed (Fischer HW, 1977).

PHARMACOKINETICS

In the absence of obstructing lesions, Ethiodol® will distribute throughout the entire lymphatic system communicating with the lymph vessel at its site of direct injection. Maximum opacification of the lymph vessels occurs during or immediately following administration (Figure 7.11), however contrast will persist in the vessels for several hours. Optimal radiographic differentiation and visualization of the lymph nodes occurs at 24–48 hours following injection (Figures 7.12 and 7.13). Ethiodol® is retained in the lymph nodes for several weeks to months. Its rate of nodal clearance varies considerably, being dependent on several factors including macrophage activity, pathological status, and patient age (Sovak M, 1984).

Following its injection into the lymphatic system, Ethiodol® enters the systemic circulation via lymphatic-venous anastomoses or terminally via the thoracic duct into the left subclavian vein. The amount of contrast medium entering the circulation via the lymphatic-venous anastomoses increases in the presence of obstruction of the lymphatic system, whereas the amount of medium normally exiting the lymphatic system via the thoracic duct increases with increasing doses.

Ethiodol® enters the systemic circulation in the form of water-insoluble globules that are capable of embolizing the first vascular bed they encounter. A medium entering the venous circulation is predominantly trapped within the capillary bed of the lungs. Up to 50–70% of the administered dose of Ethiodol® has been demonstrated in the lungs following direct lymphography (Koehler PR, et al, 1964; Fallat R, 1970). Contrast medium may be detected in the lungs as early as

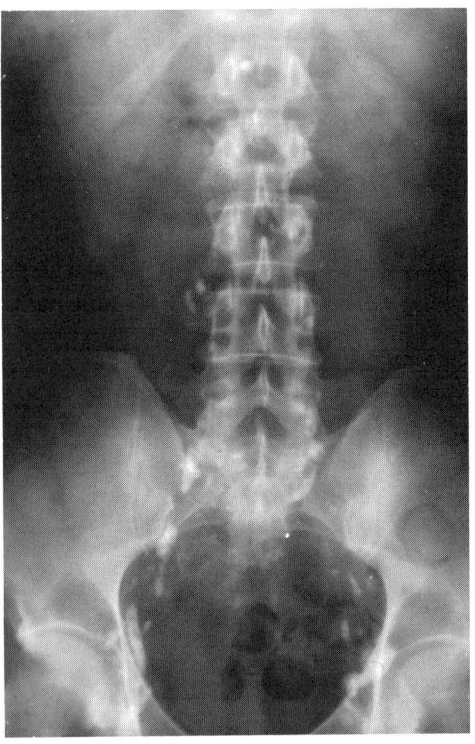 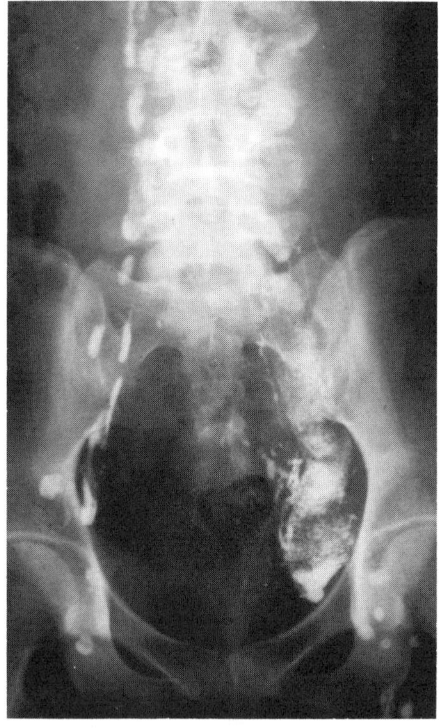

Figure 7.12   Normal lymphogram (anterior and lateral views) obtained at 24 hours following bilateral injection of Ethiodol® into pedal lymphatic vessels.

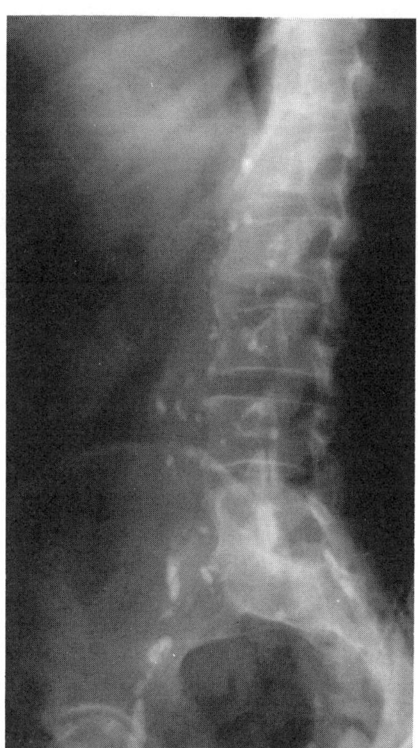

Figure 7.13 Lymphogram (same patient as Figure 8.11) demonstrating a lymphoma involving the left paraaortic and left iliac lymph nodes.

15–20 minutes after lymphatic injection (Deprez-Curely JP, et al, 1962) with maximum localization occurring at 24–48 hours (Fallat R, 1970). Ethiodol® is gradually eliminated (T1/2 of approximately 8 days) (Fallat R, 1970) from the pulmonary vasculature by several processes including its phagocytosis by macrophages within the alveolar space, metabolic degradation to free fatty acids and iodine, or globular fragmentation with subsequent passage through the capillaries (Koehler PR, 1967). Small particulates of Ethiodol® are subsequently phagocytized and degraded by cells comprising the reticulo endothelial system.

The principal route of systemic elimination of iodine following the direct lymphatic administration of Ethiodol® is via the kidney. However, only approximately 10% of the administered iodine dose can be recovered in the urine within a 6-day interval following injection (Deprez-Curely JP, 1962; Koehler PR, et al, 1964).

PHYSIOLOGICAL EFFECTS

Lymph Nodes. With initial Ethiodol® localization, there may be a corresponding increase in the size of the lymph nodes. As the medium clears from the nodes, there is a return to normal configuration. These processes should not be confused with pathological alterations in lymph node anatomy (Svoboda M, 1971).

The localization and retention of Ethiodol® in the lymph nodes also results in a foreign body reaction consisting of an early infiltration of inflammatory cells followed by the appearance of foreign body giant cells that surround the retained oil droplets. This reaction is usually of minimal clinical importance, the abnormal cellular response disappearing after a few months. Some reduction in normal nodal activity may occur during the foreign body reaction phase, especially with excessive doses and nodal localization of the Ethiodol® (Deprez-Curely JP, et al, 1962).

Lung. A primary concern associated with the lymphatic administration of Ethiodol® is the invariable occurrence of oil embolism of the pulmonary microvasculature. Respiratory distress post Ethiodol® lymphography is uncommon (i. e., incidence of approximately 2%) (Dolan PA, 1966), however, subclinical alterations in lung function (e. g., decreases in pulmonary vital capacity and capillary volume) and hypoxemia may be routinely observed at 3–4 hours after injection (Gold WM, et al, 1965). Massive embolism associated with excessive doses can result in hypotension, cyanosis, tachycardia, and electrocardiographic abnormalities. Pulmonary infarct has been reported, and deaths have occurred in patients with preexisting pulmonary disease (Koehler PR, 1967).

Ethiodol®-induced chemical pneumonitis with pulmonary edema and inflammatory changes occurs rarely (e. g., incidence of approximately 0.06%) (Koehler, PR, 1967), but is a common finding in procedure-related fatalities. The edematous effects of Ethiodol® appear to be related to its degradation by esterases of lung tissue or leukocyte origin. The resulting free fatty acids are extremely irritating to the vascular endothelium leading to an increase in pulmonary capillary permeability. In addition, activated leukocytes release proteases, histamine, and other vasoactive substances that produce inflammatory effects that are additive to those of the free-fatty acids. Symptoms (e. g. cough, hempotysis, fever) of chemical pneumonitis may occur shortly after completion of the procedure or after several months, and may persist for several days (Silvestri RC, et al, 1980; Fuchs WA, 1962).

Systemic Embolization. With excessive lymphatic doses of Ethiodol® or in the presence of pulmonary arterio-venous malformations or cardiac right-to-left shunt, the filtering capacity of the lung may be exceeded or bypassed (respectively) resulting in the oil embolism of other vascular beds. For example, cerebral embolism has been reported as a rare complication of Ethiodol® lymphography, resulting in transient or permanent motor dysfunction, paraplegia, blindness, hemiparesis, or psychotic disorders (Fuchs WA, 1962; Nelson B and Rush EA, 1965; Sane DC, et al, 1985). Ethiodol® embolization of the liver vasculature has also been observed, primarily in patients with testicular tumors and multiple metastases, and is apparently associated with the lymphatic-venous passage of oil globules into the portal circulation in the presence of an obstructed common iliac vein and inferior vena cava (Thornbury JR, 1968).

Other Side Effects. Fever is a common occurrence following Ethiodol® lymphography with reported incidences of 10–20% (Dolan PA, 1966; Sovak M, 1984). Other less common side effects include nausea, vomiting, weakness, and fatigue. Symptoms of iodism may also occur with degradation of the administered Ethiodol®

As discussed in detail in Chapter 8, low systemic concentrations of iodinated contrast media can elicit pseudo-allergic reactions ranging from mild urticaria to severe anaphylaxis. Hence, pseudo-allergic reactions can occur with the lymphographic use of Ethiodol®. As a result of its slow lymphatic clearance, the potential for the occurrence of such a reaction can be prolonged. Appropriate drugs for the treatment of potentially serious pseudo-allergic reactions should be readily available during and after the lymphography procedure.

PRECAUTIONS/COMPLICATIONS

Contrast Medium—Laboratory Test Interactions. The lymphatic administration of Ethiodol® has been shown to produce prolonged elevations of total serum iodine and protein-bound iodine (Jacobssen L and Saltzman GF, 1971). Thyroid tests based on the measurement of iodine (e. g., radioactive iodine uptake test, protein-bound iodine) may therefore be altered for several months following a lymphography procedure. Ethiodol® administration may also be associated with transient leukopenia and increased levels of gamma globulin (Tentarelli T, et al, 1965). Return to normal values occurs within 48–60 hours.

Contrast Medium–Diagnostic Procedure Interactions. The embolic localization of Ethiodol® in the microvasculature of the lungs will appear as abnormalities in the lung base on a subsequent computed tomography examination. This should not be confused with lung pathology (Frances RA, et al, 1983).

Ga-67 citrate scintigraphy performed subsequent to lymphography may demonstrate false-positive involvement of the lung associated with Ethiodol®-induced chemical pneumonitis (see Physiological Effects). An abnormal localization of gallium-67 in lymph nodes can also be expected with the respective occurrence of Ethiodol®-induced foreign body reactions (Lentle BC, et al, 1979).

Procedure Complications. Improper aseptic technique in the performance of the surgical cutdown for direct lymphography can result in wound infections, delayed wound healing, and lymphangitis. Excessive pressure during lymphatic injection of the viscous Ethiodol® can result in a rupture of the fragile lymph vessel and extravasation of the contrast medium into the surrounding soft tissues. This event may precipitate localized pain or discomfort, inflammation, or dermatitis (Svoboda M, 1971).

CLINICAL CONSIDERATIONS

Procedure Indications. The historical indications for performing Ethiodol® lymphography are listed in Table 7.5. This procedure has, however, been largely replaced by computed tomography, which permits the demonstration of abnormal lymph nodes without a requirement for the invasive, direct injection of a radiopaque contrast medium into the lymphatic system.

Patient Preparation.

Lymph Vessel Identification. Patent Blue V, the dye used originally to produce staining of the lymphatic vessels to facilitate their subsequent localization for isolation and cannulation (Kinmonth JB, 1952), is not available as an approved drug. Although its tissue-staining characteristics may be less optimal, Methylene Blue Dye is currently available as a sterile, pyrogen-free preparation for parenteral administration. It is recommended that 1 ml of the commercially available product (i. e., 10 mg/mL) be diluted in 10 mL of 1% w/v lidocaine prior to injection. The incorporation of a local anesthetic such as lidocaine reduces the severe pain often associated with subcutaneous administration of the dye and helps to prevent spasm of the lymph vessels when manipulated for cannulation (Fischer HW, 1977). For the identification of adjacent lymph vessels, 1–2 mL total doses of the diluted Methylene Blue are injected subcutaneously at multiple sites (e. g., web spaces between fingers or toes) with gentle massaging of the respective region to promote lymphatic uptake.

Subcutaneous injection of the Methylene Blue Dye will produce discoloration of the skin and urine. Adverse effects associated with dye injection are rare, however, hypersensitivity reactions of a mild to severe nature may occur. With experience, many radiologists can localize the lymphatic vessels without a requirement for dye administration, thus avoiding the objections or potential complications associated with its use.

Local Anesthesia. The subcutaneous administration of a local anesthetic such as lidocaine (1% w/v, 1–2 mL) and antiseptic preparation of the respective site are obvious requirements prior to the surgical cut-down procedure for isolation and cannulation of the lymph vessel. The administration of an appropriate sedative and immobilization of the involved extremity may also be advised.

Contraindications. Ethiodol® lymphography should be performed with extreme caution in patients with preexisting pulmonary dysfunction, emphysema, or congestive heart failure. If required for such patients, only one lymphatic system should be evaluated per setting with a minimum interval of 4 days between examinations (Fisher HW, 1977). Procedures (e. g., anesthesia, surgery) known to affect lung function should also be delayed for several days following Ethiodol® lymphography.

The lymphatic administration of Ethiodol® is contraindicated in patients with known or suspected cardiac right-to-left shunts or pulmonary arteriovenous malformations. It should not be performed subsequent to radiation therapy of the lung since treatment-induced opening of pulmonary arteriovenous shunts may predispose the patient to an increased risk of cerebral (or other organ) embolization (Davidson JW, 1969).

Table 7.5 HISTORICAL INDICATIONS FOR ETHIODOL® LYMPHOGRAPHY

Evaluation of:
- Edema of an extremity of unknown cause
- The nature of intraabdominal masses when biopsy is not available
- Metastatic involvement in patients with intraabdominal nodal disease

Staging of lymphoma, adenopathy

Localization of lymph nodes for subsequent surgical resection or radiation therapy

DOSAGE

Ethiodol® should be prewarmed to 37° C to reduce its viscosity and facilitate its injection through the small-bore needles used for cannulation of the lymph vessel. The medium is injected into the lymph vessel under constant, low pressure at a rate of approximately 0.1–0.2 mL/minute. An excessive injection rate or pressure increases the level of pain and the potential for rupture of the lymph vessel and should therefore be avoided. Ethiodol® administration should be monitored fluorographically and discontinued if an inadvertent intravenous injection, extravasation, or lymphatic-venous shunting is noted. The injection of Ethiodol® should be terminated with the observance of collateral lymph vessels or other signs of lymphatic obstruction, or the appearance of contrast medium in the thoracic duct.

Lower extremity lymphography for the demonstration of inguinal, external iliac, common iliac, para-aortic, and supraclavicular lymph nodes typically involves the administration of 6–8 mL (2–5 mL for children) of Ethiodol® over a 40–60 minute interval. Upper extremity doses of 2–4 mL are used to visualize the axillary and supraclavicular nodes. Radiographs of the lymphatic system are normally obtained immediately following injection and, for optimal nodal visualization, also at 24–48 hours (Fisher HW, 1977).

IV. Bronchographic Contrast Media

Dennis P. Swanson
Rajinder P. Sharma

Bronchography is a radiographic examination of the bronchial tree following the direct instillation of a radiopaque contrast medium. Although useful for identifying endobronchial lesions and abnormal bronchial anatomy, bronchography has been largely replaced for these purposes by bronchoscopy or radiographic tomography techniques.

The ideal contrast medium for bronchography should readily mix with bronchial secretions and provide uniform coating of the bronchial mucosa to the level of the terminal bronchi. An adequate degree of opacification must exist for the required duration of the examination, followed by rapid and complete pulmonary and systemic elimination of the instilled medium. Since contrast medium localized distal to the terminal bronchi will not be readily removed from the lungs by the normal bronchial cleansing processes, the viscosity of the ideal contrast medium must be sufficiently high to prevent excessive filling of the alveoli. Conversely, the viscosity of the medium must be low enough to permit its ease of administration and flow to the small branches of the bronchial tree. Of course, the ideal bronchographic medium should not demonstrate local irritation of the bronchial mucosa, effects on pulmonary physiology, or systemic reactions (House AJS, 1977a; DiGuglielmo L, 1971).

HISTORY

Iodinated Oils. The first contrast medium used extensively for bronchography was Lipiodol. This oily medium, comprising a mixture of the glyceryl esters of iodinated fatty acids of poppy seed oil, produced good coating of the bronchial mucosa and was generally well tolerated. However, due to its relatively low viscosity (i. e., approximately 280 centipoise) a substantial amount of the medium flowed distal to the terminal bronchi and localized in the alveoli. Lipiodol within the alveoli is retained for weeks to months or longer, especially in areas of disease involvement. This prolonged retention was associated with the induction of foreign body granulomatous reactions, fibrosis, and lipoid pneumonia. In addition, Lipiodol expectorated into the gastrointestinal tract during or following the bronchography procedure undergoes rapid degradation with the liberation of iodine. Systemic absorption of this free iodine resulted in side effects (e. g., headache, skin eruptions, weakness, nasal discharge, salivation) of iodism (House AJS, 1977b; DiGuglielmo L, 1971).

In an attempt to reduce its penetration into the alveoli, various powders (e. g., talc, calcined magnesia, sulfanilamide) were added to Lipiodol to increase its viscosity. Although this approach did help to prevent alveolar localization, the potential for foreign body granulomatous reactions still existed, especially with incorporation of the water-insoluble (i. e., talc, calcined magnesium) powders. The inclusion of sulfanilamide powder introduced additional risks of sulfonamide hypersensitivity or toxicity. Based on these considerations, these agents never gained widespread clinical acceptance (House AJS, 1977b).

Water-Soluble, Iodinated Contrast Media. Bronchographic use of the water-soluble, iodinated contrast media originally developed for urographic and angiographic procedures (see Chapter 1, Angiographic Contrast Media) was evaluated in anticipation of their rapid systemic absorption in the event of alveolar localization. As a result of their very low viscosities (i. e., less than 20 centipoise at 25° C) these media flowed rapidly through the bronchial tree with substantial filling of the alveoli, thus permitting only transient and often obscured radiographic visualization of the bronchi. Moreover, these agents are hyperosmolar at the iodine concentrations required for adequate bronchographic opacification and therefore extremely irritating to the bronchial mucosa (House AJS, 1977b; DiGuglielmo L, 1971). Alveolar accumulation of fluid in an attempt to dilute the hyperosmotic environment created by these media could also result in liquid pneumonia.

Viscosity extenders (e. g., dextran, carboxymethyl cellulose, polyvinyl pyrrolidone) were also added to the water-soluble iodinated media in an attempt to limit their rate of flow, alveolar localization, and systemic absorption. However, the addition of these substances did not reduce the degree of hyperosmolarity-

induced mucosal irritation and added further risks of foreign body granulomatous reactions associated with their slow rates (i.e., 10–15 days) of pulmonary elimination (DiGuglielmo L, 1971).

Aqueous Suspensions of Iodinated Contrast Media. In recognition of the fact that suspensions of insoluble particles would not exhibit the colligative properties and, hence, the hyperosmolarity-induced irritative effects of water-soluble agents, attention was directed at the potential use of water-insoluble, iodinated contrast media for bronchographic procedures. Hytrast®, an aqueous suspension of water-insoluble iopydol (46% w/v) and iopydone (30.5% w/v) (Figure 7.14) was used extensively for bronchography during the 1960s. Its carboxymethylcellulose-enhanced viscosity (i.e., 240–280 centipoise at 37° C) and iodine concentration of 500 mg/mL provided excellent mucosal-coating and opacification characteristics. However, medium entering the alveoli was not readily eliminated by the normal bronchial cleansing processes or by degradation, resulting in prolonged alveolar retention, especially in areas of disease involvement. The retained crystals of contrast media (or retained carboxymethylcellulose) were associated with significant inflammatory reactions and subclinical

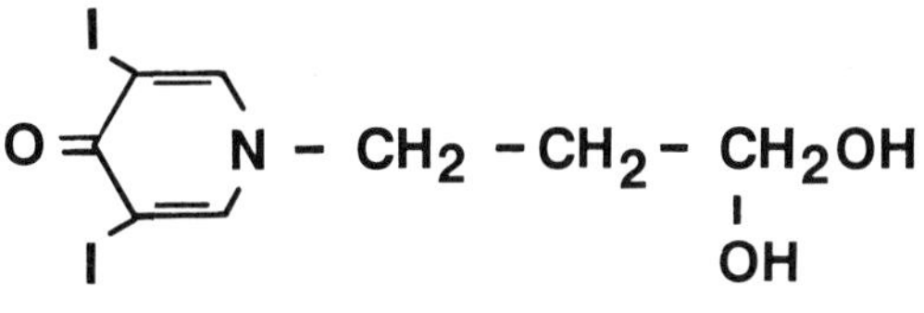

O $=$ N – CH$_2$ – CH$_2$ – CH$_2$OH
         OH

Iopydol

O $=$ NH

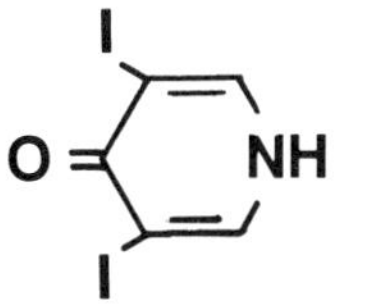

Iopydone

Figure 7.14 Chemical structures of the radiopaque components of Hytrast®.

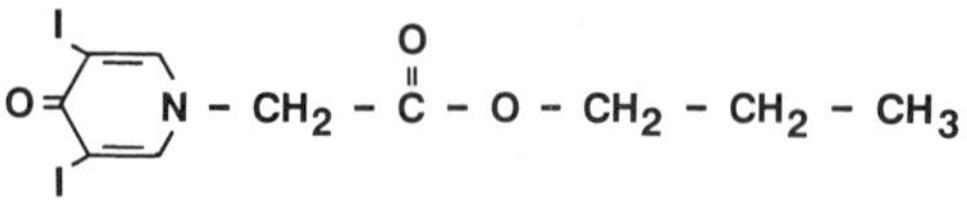

$$O=\!\!\!\overset{I}{\underset{I}{\bigcirc}}\!\!\!\overset{O}{N-CH_2-\overset{\|}{C}-O-CH_2-CH_2-CH_3}$$

Figure 7.15 Chemical structure of propyliodone (Dionosil®).

crystalline pneumonia. These problems led eventually to disuse of this bronchographic medium (House AJS, 1977b).

Dionosil-aqueous®, a 46.8% w/v suspension of insoluble propyliodone (Figure 7.15) in water with carboxymethylcellulose provided advantages related to the fact that any propyliodone localized to the alveoli undergoes enzymatic hydrolysis to water-soluble propyl alcohol and diiodopyridone acetate; by-products that are rapidly eliminated from the lungs and, subsequently, from the systemic circulation. Hence, although the iodine concentration (i. e., 280 mg iodine/mL) of Dionosil-aqueous® resulted in a lower degree of opacification compared to Hytrast®, its use was associated with less bronchial and alveolar irritation. The bronchial mucosal coating and opacification characteristics of Dionosil-aqueous® were generally acceptable for bronchography, thus making this agent preferable over the previously described media (House AJS, 1977b).

In addition to the carboxymethylcellulose-aqueous formulation, this propyliodone contrast agent was also made available as a 56.8% w/v suspension in peanut oil. Compared to the aqueous suspension, Dionosil-oily® demonstrated somewhat poorer mucosal-coating characteristics and perhaps a greater tendency to alveolar filling. It was, however, less irritating to the lungs than Dionosil-aqueous®. Although debatable, the increased level of irritation with Dionosil-aqueous® may have been related to prolonged alveolar retention of the carboxymethylcellulose viscosity-extender and associated inflammatory or foreign body reactions (House AJS, 1977b). This slight difference in irritating effects combined with the higher iodine concentration (i. e., 340 mg iodine/mL) of Dionosil-oily® apparently led to discon-

tinued availability and use of the aqueous formulation.

CHEMISTRY

The only contrast medium currently available in the United States and indicated for bronchography is Dionosil-oily® (Picker International,Inc.). This agent is a 56.8% w/v sterile suspension of propyliodone (Figure 7.15) in peanut oil, containing approximately 340 mg iodine/mL. It appears as a clear oil with an almost white precipitate of propyliodone particles of a diameter of 5–14 microns (Holden WS, and Crone RS, 1953). The viscosity of Dionosil-oily® approaches 1250 centipoise, and it has a specific gravity of 1.26 (House AJS, 1977b).

Dionosil-oily® should be stored in a manner to prevent its prolonged exposure to heat (e. g., great than 30° C) or light. Since the medium is a suspension rather than a colloidal solution, it will settle out with time; thus it requires vigorous shaking prior to use.

PHARMACOKINETICS

Following its introduction into the tracheobronchial system, Dionosil-oily® distributes to the main and lobar bronchi primarily due to gravitational forces as augmented by patient positioning and its relatively high specific gravity. Distribution into the more distal segmental and small bronchi and the bronchioles requires that the patient breathe deeply. This process may be facilitated by mild coughing. Forceful inspirations or coughing can, however, promote filling and obstruction of the terminal bronchioles and the alveoli (Figure 7.16), and should be avoided. At routine dosages (see Dosage), Dionosil-oily® provides uniform coating of the mucosal surfaces of the bronchial tree and a double-contrast effect (Figure 7.17). Adequate levels of bronchographic opacification will persist for the normally required examination time.

Contrast medium localized proximal to or within the segmental bronchi is elim-

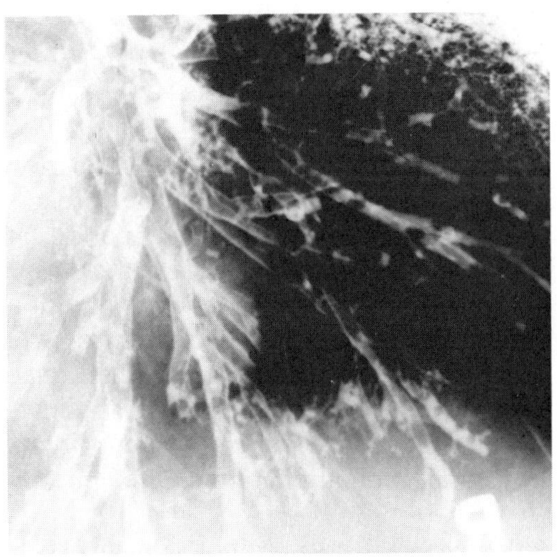

Figure 7.16 Bronchogram demonstrating bronchiectasis of the right lower lobe. Note alveolarization of contrast (Dionosil-oily®) in the right upper lobe.

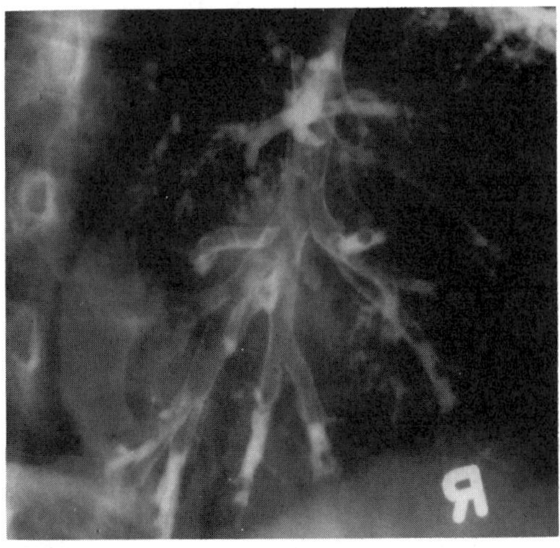

Figure 7.17 Normal bronchogram of the right lower lobe obtained using Dionosil-oily®. Note uniform coating of the mucosal surfaces of the bronchial tree.

inated primarily by expectoration. Removal of the medium from these regions can be enhanced by coughing and the incorporation of postural drainage techniques. Proximal migration and eventual expectoration of medium localized distal to the segmental bronchi is dependent on the normal mucociliary activity of the bron-

chial mucosa and contractions of the bronchial smooth muscle. Mucous in the bronchial tree is produced primarily by mucous glands, which may be found as distal as the small bronchi, and to a lesser extent by the goblet cells of the terminal bronchioles. Hence, due to a loss of mucociliary activity, contrast medium localized distal to the terminal bronchioles is not readily eliminated from the bronchial tree by its normal cleansing processes (Holden WS, 1957).

Propylidone localized to and retained within the alveoli undergoes enzymatic hydrolysis to diodopyridone acetate and propyl alcohol (Tomich EG, et al, 1953; Dunbar JS, et al, 1959). Both of these water-soluble agents are rapidly absorbed from the lung and excreted systemically. Alveolar opacification usually disappears by 2–4 days (Dunbar JS, et al, 1959); however, contrast may persist for several weeks in regions of altered pulmonary ventilation and perfusion (i. e., decreased systemic absorption of enzymatic by-products) or bronchiectasis (i. e., reduced mucociliary activity). Propyliodone expectorated into the gastrointestinal tract undergoes a similar degradation process with systemic absorption and renal excretion of the diiodopyridone acetate by-product. Some deiodination of the parent medium or by-product does occur, as evidenced by the effect of Dionosil-oily® administration on subsequent thyroid function tests (see Precautions).

The peanut oil component of Dionosil-oily® localized to the alveoli does not undergo metabolic degration. It is apparently slowly eliminated from this region via phagocytosis by lung macrophages. The oil-filled macrophages migrate to the bronchial tree where they are eliminated by the normal mucociliary and expectoration processes, or they are absorbed by the regional lymphatics (House AJS, 1977b).

PHYSIOLOGICAL EFFECTS

Pulmonary Function. The bronchographic use of Dionosil-oily® invariably produces a transient alteration of pulmonary function (Richez M, et al, 1980). Immediate reductions of greater than 20% (unilateral study) or 30% (bilateral study) in both vital capacity and maximum breathing capacity may be demonstrated (Christoforidis AJ, et al, 1962); the duration of these functional abnormalities typically ranging from 24–72 hours. Although the contrast-induced functional alterations are usually subclinical, atelectasis with coughing, hemoptysis, dyspnea, and hypoxia can occur with excessive dosages and filling of the terminal bronchioles and alveoli. Acute respiratory failure has been reported in patients with preexisting pulmonary dysfunction (Committee Report, 1967).

Histological studies have demonstrated that Dionosil-oily® produces microatelectasis in close association with retained propylidone crystals and peanut-oil droplets. The medium appears to cause this effect by decreasing the surface activity of lung surfactant, resulting in a collapse of the surface film. Studies involving the administration of peanut oil, alone, indicate that this component of Dionosil-oily® may be primarily responsible for the interaction with surfactant. However, the propyliodone component can also be a factor if the surface density of retained crystals in high (Schürch SF and Roach MR, 1976).

Foreign Body Reactions. Although propyliodine localized to the alveoli underfoes fairly rapid degradation and elimination, the peanut oil component of Dionosil-oily® is retained for a relatively long duration (see Pharmacokinetics). Both components may demonstrate prolonged retention in areas of disease involvement. With this retention, there is a potential for foreign body reactions. Mild to moderate inflammatory reactions with granulomata formation have been observed in animal studies using Dionosil-oily®; however, this does not appear to present a significant clinical problem (Holden WS, et al, 1958; Chaudhry BS, et al, 1983).

Pseudo-allergic Reactions. Pseudo-allergic reactions to intravascular, iodinated contrast media occur independent of their systemic concentration above a certain low threshold value (see Chapter 8). Hence, there is a possibility that a pseudo-allergic reaction may occour with the systemic absorption of the propyliodone by-product. Since this absorption process may occur over an extended period of time, the appearance of a pseudo- allergic reaction may be delayed. Consideration should be given to administering an appropriate pretreatment regimen (see Chapter 8) to bronchography patients who have suffered a previous major reaction to an iodinated contrast medium.

Other Side Effects. Minor side effects including fever, headache, epigastric pain, nausea, and vomiting are frequently observed following bronchography with Dionosil-oily®. The incidence of these transient (i. e., usual duration less than 24–48 hours) reactions can approach 30% (Rayl JE, 1965) and appears to be related to alveolar localization of the contrast medium.

PRECAUTIONS

Contrast Medium–Laboratory Test Interactions. Increased levels of protein-bound iodine have been observed for several weeks following the bronchographic use of Dionosil-oily®. Hence, thyroid tests based on the measurement of iodine (e. g., protein-bound iodine, radioactive iodine uptake test) may be altered for a prolonged period after the procedure. In addition, there is some evidence that propyliodone or its degradation by-product may interfere with the conversion of thyroxin to triiodothyronine (Benker G, et al, 1983).

Contrast Medium–Diagnostic Procedure Interactions. The increase in bronchial secretions associated with bronchoscopy may alter the normal kinetics of Dionosil-oily® if bronchography is performed immediately after the endoscopy procedure (House AJS, 1977a). Contrast-induced embolism of the cerebral circulation resulting in grand mal scizures and transient

Table 7.6 COMMON INDICATIONS FOR THE PERFORMANCE OF BRONCHOGRAPHY

Bronchiectasis
Hemoptysis of unknown cause
Suspected bronchogenic tumor
Pulmonary tuberculosis
Anomalies of the bronchopulmonary segments
Miscellaneous complications post pulmonary resection
Pulmonary parenchymal shadows of unknown nature

neurological deficits has been reported during bronchography performed immediately after bronchoscopy with transbronchial biopsy (Oldendberg FA and Newhouse MT, 1978). Based on these considerations, attention should be given to the elapsed period of time between performance of the respective procedures.

CLINICAL CONSIDERATIONS/ CONTRAINDICATIONS

Procedure Indications. Common indications for the performance of bronchography are listed in Table 7.6. This procedure has, however, been largely replaced by bronchscopy and radiographic tomography techniques.

Patient Preparation. Patients should fast for 4–6 hours prior to bronchography. The pre-procedure administration of an appropriate sedative or analgesic is also recommended.

Since excessive bronchial secretions may interfere with the effectiveness of tracheobronchial anesthesia and the bronchial mucosa-coating properties of Dionosil-oily®, premedication with atropine sulfate (0.4–0.6 mg IM or SQ at 30–60 minutes prior) should be considered. Postural drainage may be required in the presence of profuse secretions.

Adequate anesthesia of the throat and upper tracheobronchial tree is a requirement to suppress the cough reflex associated with insertion of the tracheobronchial catheter and contrast instillation. General anesthesia is normally employed in children. In adults, local anesthesia of the pharyngeal region and larynx can be achieved by the direct application of a topical anesthetic (e.g., 4% w/v lido-

caine, Xylocaine-Duo-Trach®, Astra). With catheter introduction, additional anesthetic may be employed to anesthetize the lower trachea and main bronchi. In addition, suppression of the central cough reflex (and analgesia sedation) can be achieved by administering 30–60 mg of codeine sulfate at 1 hour prior to the study (Paul LW and Juhl JH, 1972).

Contraindications. Bronchography should be performed with extreme caution in patients with preexisting pulmonary dysfunction or obstructive disease. In addition to being concerned about the additive alterations in pulmonary dysfunction normally caused by the administration of Dionosil-oily®, alveolar filling and retention will be further enhanced in these patients due to an impairment of the normal contrast-elimination mechanisms. Tracheobronchial instillation of Dionosil-oily® may also precipitate bronchospasms in highly atopic or asthmatic patients. If required in these patient groups, selective bronchography should be performed unilaterally using the smallest possible dose of contrast medium. Several days should elapse prior to the performance of additional bronchography studies or other procedures known to reduce pulmonary function.

Bronchography is contraindicated in the presence of acute penumonia, upper respiratory tract infections, or pulmonary parenchymal infections. Due to the potential risk of systemic embolization, it should not be performed in the presence of acute or recent substantial hemoptysis. (Minimal hemoptysis is probably not a contraindication.) Patients with severe heart disease may not be able to tolerate the procedure-induced alterations in pulmonary function (Paul LW and Juhl JH, 1972; House AJS, 1977a).

DOSAGE

Prior to administration, the Dionosil-oily® should be throughly agitated to ensure a uniform suspension. It has been suggested that, prior to agitation, 30–50%

of the supernatant peanut oil may be removed to provide a medium of increased viscosity and iodine concentration (Nelson SW and Christoforidis AJ, 1973; Brunner S, 1967). The contrast medium should be administered at room temperature. Excessive warming will substantially reduce its viscosity and increase its potential for alveolar localization. The product information for Dionosil-oily® warns against prolonged contact with plastic syringes that may be used for dose withdrawal and administration.

Dionosil-oily® may be introduced directly into the trachea (bilateral study), the right or left main bronchus (unilateral study), or selectively into the lobar bronchi via a soft catheter. It may also be injected directly into the trachea by percutaneous puncture through the cricothyroid membrane. The increased risk of complications associated with excessive contrast filling of the terminal bronchioles and alveoli can be minimized by incorporating fluoroscopic monitoring to ensure the use of the lowest possible dosage for an adequate study. Commonly used adult dosages of Dionosil-oily® approach 10–20 mL for a unilateral and 20–40 mL for a bilateral examination (Holden WS, et al, 1953). The recommended pediatric dosage is 0.75–1 mL for each year of age. The dosages are administered fractionally, with multiple patient positioning and fluoroscopic monitoring, until adequate visualization of the area under investigation has been obtained.

Upon completion of the examination, the patient should be encouraged to cough lightly to facilitate expectoration of the contrast medium. Postural drainage may also be considered. The patient should be cautioned to avoid anything by mouth until the anesthetic effect on the laryngeal reflex has worn off (Paul LW and Juhl JH, 1972).

References

Alper MM, Garner PR, Spence JEH, et al. Pregnancy rates after hysterosalpingography with oil- and water-soluble contrast media. *Obstet Gynecol* 1986, 68:6–10.

Angell FL. Fluoroscopic technique of double-contrast arthrography of the knee. *Radiol Clin N Am* 1971, 9:81–85.

Ansari AH, Shimoura H. Hypotonic hysterosalpingography with glucagon. *Fertil Steril* 1978, 309:476–477.

Appel JS, Martinez S, Khoury MB, et al. A comparison of Hexabrix and Renografin-60 in knee arthrography. *AJR* 1985, 145:139–142.

Belli A, Renton P, Stroker DJ. Comparative study of iohexol and meglumine iothalamate in double-contrast knee arthrography. *Clin Radiology* 1984, 35:375–377.

Benker G. Vosskuhler A, Hoff HG, et al. Thyroid function after bronchography with propylidone. *Horm Res* 1983, 17:121–127.

Beyth Y, Navot D, Lax E. A simple improvement in the technique of hysterosalpingography achieving optimal imaging and avoiding possible complications. *Fertil Steril* 1985, 44:543–545.

Bjork L, Lodin H. Pulmonary changes following bronchography with Dionosil oily. *Acta Radiol* 1957, 47:177–180.

Birnbaum MD. Reduction of pain following hysterosalpingogram by prior analgesic administration. *Fertil Steril* 1985, 43:947.

Boyer P, Territo MC, deZiegler D, et al. Ethiodol inhibits phagocytosis by pelvic peritoneal macrophages. *Fertil Steril* 1986, 46:715–717.

Brunner S. Bronchography during infancy and childhood. *Dis Chest* 1967, 52:201–204.

Burman MS, Tunick IS, Pomeranz M. The injection of Lipiodol into the knee joint: A warning against its use. *AJR* 1932, 28:787–795.

Chaudhry BS, Gupta NK, Luhadia SK, et al. Comparison of barium sulfate and Dionosil as contrast media for bronchography. *Indian J Chest Diseases and Allied Sciences* 1983, 25:96–100.

Christoforidis AJ, Nelson SW, Tomashefski JF. Effects of bronchography on pulmonary function. *Am Rv Respir Dis* 1962, 663–668.

Cooper RA, Jabamoni R, Pieters CH. Fertility rate after hysterosalpingography with Sinografin. *AJR* 1983, 141:105–106.

Committee Report. Bronchography: A report of the committee on bronchoesophagology. *Dis Chest* 1967, 51:663–668.

Corbetti F, Malatesta V, Composampiero A, et al. Knee arthrography: Effects of various contrast media and epinephrine on synovial fluid. *Radiology* 1986, 161:195–198.

Davidson JW. Lipid embolism to the brain following lymphography: Case report and experimental study. *AJR* 1969, 105:763–771.

Davies AC, Keightley A, Borthwick-Clarke A, et al. The use of a low-osmolality contrast medium in hysterosalpingography: Comparison with a conventional contrast medium. *Clin Radiol* 1985, 36:533–536.

Desprez-Curely JP, Bismuth V, Laugier A, et al. Accidents et incidents de la lymphographie. *Ann Radiol (Paris)* 1962, 5:577–588.

DiGuglielmo L. Radiocontrast agents for bronchography. In *Radiocontrast Agents* (Knoefel PK, section ed.) Intl Encyclopedia of Pharmacology and Therapeutics, Vol. II: New York, Pergamon Press, 1971, pp. 395–411.

Dolan PA. Lymphography: Complications encountered in 522 examinations. *Radiology* 1966, 86:876–880.

Dunbar JS, Skinner GB, Wortzman G, et al. An investigation of the effects of opaque media on the lungs with comparison of barium sulfate, Lipiodol, and Dionosil. *AJR* 1959, 82:902–926.

Fallat R. Pulmonary disposition and clearance of ^{131}I-labeled oil after lymphography in man. Correlation with lung function. *Radiology* 1970, 97:511–520.

Fischer HW. Catalog of intravascular contrast media. *Radiology* 1986, 159:561–563.

Fischer HW. Lymphangiography and lymphadenography with various contrast agents. *Ann NY Acad Sci* 1959, 78:799–808.

Fischer HW. Lymphographic contrast agents. In *Radiographic Contrast Media*, (RE Miller and J Skucas, eds.) Baltimore, University Park Press, 1977, 463–475.

Foote GA. Arthrographic contrast media. In *Radiographic Contrast Agents* (Miller RE, Skucas J, eds.) Baltimore, University Park Press, 1977, 451–462.

Francis RA, Barnes PA, Libshitz HI. Pulmonary oil embolism after lymphangiography. *JCAT* 1983; 7:170–171.

Freiberger RH, Killoran PJ, Cardona G. Arthrography of the knee of double-contrast method. *AJR* 1966, 97:736–747.

Fuchs WA. Complications in lymphography with oily contrast media. *Acta Radiol* 1962, 57:427–432.

Fullenlove TM. Experience with over 2000 uterosalpinographies. *AJR* 1969, 106:463–466.

Gerlock AJ, Hooser CW. Oviduct response to glucagon during hysterosalpingography. *Radiology* 1976, 119:727–728.

Gold WM, Youker J, Anderson S, et al. Pulmonary function abnormalities after lymphangiography. *N Eng J Med* 1965, 273:519–524.

Goldberg RP, Hall FM, Wyshak G. Pain in knee arthrography. Comparison of air versus CO_2 and reaspiration versus no reaspiration. *AJR* 1981, 136:377–379.

Griffiths HJL. A clinical and radiological evaluation comparing the use of two contrast media in hysterosalpingography—Salpix and Urografin. *Br J Radiol* 1969, 42:835–837.

Hall FM. Epinephrine-enhanced knee arthrography. *Radiology* 1974, 111:215–217.

Hall FM, Rosenthal DI, Goldberg RP, et al. Morbidity from shoulder arthrography: Etiology, incidence, and prevention. *AJR* 1981, 136:59–62.

Hall FM, Goldberg RP, Wyshak G, et al. Shoulder arthrography: Comparison of morbidity after use of various contrast media. *Radiology* 1985, 154:339–341.

Heuser C. Lipiodol in the diagnosis of pregnancy. *Lancet* 1925, 2:1111–1112.

Holden WS, Crone RS. Bronchography using Dionosil-oily®. *Br J Radiol* 1953, 26:317–322.

Holden WS. The behaviour of contrast medium in the bronchial tree. *Br J Radiol* 1957, 30:530–536.

Holden WS, Cowdell RH. Late results of bronchography using Dionosil-oily®. *Acta Radiol* 1958, 49:105–112.

House AJS. Introduction to bronchographic agents. In *Radiographic Contrast Agents*, (Miller RE, Skucas J, eds.) Baltimore, University Park Press, 1977a, 379–387.

House AJS. Iodinated bronchographic agents. In *Radiographic Contrast Agents* (Miller RE, Skukus J, eds.) Baltimore, University Park Press, 1977b; 389–401.

Jacobssen L, Saltzman GF. Effect of iodinated roentgenographic contrast media on butanol-extractable, protein-bound, and total iodine in serum. *Acta Radiol* 1971; 75:310–320.

Johansen JG, Berner A. Arthrography with Amipaque (metrizamide) and other contrast media. *Invest Radiol* 1976, 11:534–540.

Kaplan P, Tu H, Ludiatt D, et al. Temporomandibular joint arthrography of normal subjects: Prevalence of pain with ionic versus nonionic contrast agents. *Radiology* 1985, 156:825–827.

Katzberg RW, Burgener FA, Fischer HW. Evaluation of various contrast agents for improved arthrography. *Invest Radiol* 1976, 11:528–533.

Katzberg RW. Preliminary evaluation of Hexabrix for temporomandibular joint arthrography. *Invest Radiol* 1984, 19 (Suppl): S387–S388.

Kim KS, Lachman R. In vitro effects of iodinated contrast media on the growth of staphlococci. *Invest Radiol* 1982, 17:305–309.

Kinmonth JB. Lymphangiography in man: Method of outlining lymphatic trunks at operation. *Clin Sci* 1952, 11:13–20.

Koehler PR, Meyers WA, Shelley JF, et al. Body distribution of Ethiodol following lymphangiography. *Radiology* 1964, 82:866–871.

Koehler PR. Lymphography. Complications and accidents. In *Progress in Lymphology* (A Ruttiman, ed.) Stuttgart, Thieme, 1967, 306–307.

Lentle BC, Scott JR, Nougaim AA, et al. Iatrogenic alterations in radionuclide biodistributions. *Semin Nucl Med* 1979, IX:131–143.

McAlister WH, Shackleford GD, Kissane J. The histologic effects of some iodine containing contrast media on the rat peritoneal cavity. *Radiology* 1972, 105:581–582.

Mink JH, Dickerson R. Air or CO_2 for knee arthrography. *AJR* 1980, 134:991–993.

Møller BR, Allen J, Toft B, et al. Pelvic inflammatory disease after hysterosalpingography associated with chlamydia trachomatis and mycoplasma hominis. *Br J Obstet Gynaecol* 1984, 91:1181–1187.

Moore DE. Pain associated with hysterosalpingography. Ethiodol versus Salpix media. *Fertil Steril* 1982, 38:629–631.

Nelson B, Rush EA, Takasugi M. Lipid embolism to the brain after lymphography. *N Engl J Med* 1965, 273:1132–1134.

Nelson SW, Christoforidis AJ. Bronchography in diseases of the adult chest. *Radiol Clin North Am* 1973, 11:125–152.

Newberg AH, Munn CS, Robbins AH. Complications of arthrography. *Radiology* 1985, 155:605–606.

Obermann WR, Kieft GJ: Knee arthrography: A comparison of iohexol, ioxaglate sodium-meglumine, and metrizoate. *Radiology* 1987, 162:729.

Oldenberg FA, Newhouse MT. Cerebral dye embolism. A complication of selective bronchography following trans-bronchial biopsy. *Chest* 1978, 73:872–873.

Palmer A. Ethiodol hysterosalpingography for the treatment of infertility. *Fertil Steril* 1960, 11:311–315.

Pastershank SP, Resnick D, Niwayama G, et al. The effect of water-soluble contrast media on the synovial membrane. *Radiology* 1982, 143:331–334.

Patton DL, Soules MR, Engel CC, et al. Induced hydrosalpinges in rabbits: Comparison of hysterosalpingographic media and development of an animal model. *Fertil Steril* 1984, 42:466–473.

Pfahler GE. A demonstration of the lymphatic drainage from the maxillary sinuses. *AJR* 1932, 27:352–356.

Paul LW, Juhl JH. *The Essentials of Roentgen Interpretation*, Third Edition, Hagenstown, MD, Harper and Row, 1972, pp 743–747.

Pittaway DE, Winfield AC, Maxson W, et al. Prevention of acute pelvic inflammatory disease after hysterosalpingography: Effect of doxycycline prophylaxis. *Am J Obstet Gynecol* 1983a, 147:623–626.

Pittaway DE. Use of glucagon in hysterosalpingography. *Fertil Steril* 1983b, 39:858.

Rayl JE. Clinical reactions following bronchography. *Ann Otol Rhinol Laryngol* 1965, 74:1121–1132.

Rice JP, London SN, Olive DL. Reevaluation of hysterosalpingography in infertility investigation. *Obstet Gynecol* 1986, 67:718–721.

Rindfleisch W. Darstellung des Cavum uteri. *Berlin Klin Wschr* 1910, 47:780–781.

Richez M, Ravez P, Godart G, et al. Changes in regional and overall lung function after bronchography. *Eur J Nucl Med* 1980, 5:477–480.

Sane DC, Massey EW, Moore J. Lipid cerebral embolism following lymphogram. *Clin Neuropharmacol* 1985, 8:184–188.

Schürch SF, Roach MR. Interference of bronchographic agents with lung surfactant. *Respir Physiol* 1976, 28:99–117.

Schwabe MG, Shapiro SS, Haning RV. Hysterosalpingography with oil contrast media enhances fertility in patients with infertility of unknown origin. *Fertil Steril* 1983, 40: 604–606.

Silvestri RC, Huseby JS, Rughani I, et al. Respiratory distress syndrome from lymphangiography contrast medium. *Am Rev Resp Dis* 1980, 122:543–549.

Soules MR, Spadoni LR: Oil versus aqueous media for hysterosalpingography: A continuing debate based on many opinions and few facts. *Fertil Steril* 1982, 38: 1–11.

Sovak M. Contrast media in lymphography. In *Radiocontrast Agents* (M Sovak, ed.), Springer-Verlag, New York, 1984, 463–477.

Stiris G, Andrew E. Hysterosalpingography with Amipaque. *Radiology* 1979, 130:795–796.

Stumpf PG, March CM. Febrile morbidity following hysterosalpingography: Identification of risk factors and recommendations for prophylaxis. *Fertil Steril* 1980, 33:487–492.

Svoboda M. Radiocontrast agents for lymphography. In *Radiocontrast Agents, Vol. II*, International Encyclopedia of Pharmacology and Therapeutics (PK Knoefel, section ed.), New York, Pergamon Press, 1971, 413–430.

Tegtmeyer CJ, McCue FC, Higgins SM, et al. Arthography of the knee. A comparative study of the accuracy of single- and double-contrast techniques. *Radiology* 1979, 132:37–41.

Tentarelli T, Scattelin F. Nota preliminare sulla variazzioni sierologiche ed ematologiche dopo linfadenografia. *Urologia (Venezia)*, 1965, 32:407–409.

Thornbury JR. Lymphatico-venous anastomoses involving the portal system: Lymphographic changes in man. In *Progress in Lymphology* II, (A Ruttiman, ed.) Stuttgart, Thieme Verlag, 1968, 105.

Tomich EG, Basil B, Davis B. The properties of n-propyl 3:5 di-iodo-4-pyridone-N-acetate (propyliodone) *Br J Pharmacol* 1953, 8:166–170.

Werndorff R, Robinsohn I. Ueber intra articulare und interstitielle sauerstoff insufflation zu radiologisch—diagnostischen and therapeutischen. *Zwecken Verhandl Dtsch Ges Orthop* 1905, 4: 9–11.

Winfield AC, Maxson WS, Harding DR, et al. Hexabrix as a contrast agent for hysterosalpingography. *Radiology* 1984, 152:232–233.

Winfield AC, Henderson-Slayden R, Wentz AC, et al. Hysterosalpingography: Comparison of Conray-60 and Sinografin. *AJR* 1982a, 138:559–560.

Winfield AC, Pittaway D, Maxson W, et al. Apparent cornual occlusion in hysterosalpingography. Reversal by glucagon. *AJR* 1982b, 139:525–527.

Yune HY. Hysterosalpingography. In *Radiographic Contrast Agents* (RE Miller and J Skucas, eds.) Baltimore, University Park Press, 1977, pp. 307–321.

Adverse Reactions to Contrast Media: Etiology, Incidence, Treatment, and Prevention

James H. Thrall

With the advent of new imaging modalities including computed tomography and digital subtraction angiography, the indications for the administration of intravascular contrast media continue to expand. The number of patients undergoing studies involving intravascular contrast is on the order of 10 to 12 million per year in the United States. Adverse reactions to contrast media are a fact of life in radiology departments and, while infrequently fatal, represent collectively the most important day-to-day complications in medical imaging.

The past two decades have seen an increasing number of investigations regarding the incidence of adverse reactions to contrast media and their etiology. Approaches to the treatment of patients experiencing adverse reactions have been developed, although the clinical judgment of the radiologist must still guide the decision to treat and the specific therapy rendered. Categories of patients at predictably increased risk for reactions have been established, and strategies have been developed for their identification and their pretreatment prior to studies requiring intravascular contrast media administration.

CLASSIFICATION AND TERMINOLOGY

Adverse reactions to contrast media can be broadly classified into two major groups (1) predictable reactions that are usually dose dependent and related to the effects of the media on vascular and organ physiology, for example, chemotoxic re-

Table 8.1 CLASSIFICATION OF REACTIONS TO CONTRAST MEDIA

Predictable Reactions
  · Chemotoxic effects
  · Drug/contrast media interactions
Unpredictable Reactions
  · Pseudo-allergy or mediator release effects (effects due to activation of immunologic effector mechanisms)
  · Vagal reactions
Intercurrent Complications
(E. g., complications unrelated to contrast media but temporally related to contrast media administration; myocardial infarction, pulmonary embolism, convulsions, septicemia)

actions, and (2) unpredictable reactions that are generally dose independent beyond a threshold (Table 8.1) (De-Swarte RD, 1984; 1986; Swanson DP, 1986). Both of these types of reaction must also be distinguished from intercurrent complications that are unrelated causally to contrast media but may occur in the immediate time frame following their administration (Baum S, 1965).

The important mediating factors of chemotoxic effects are listed in Table 8.2. These factors have been discussed in previous chapters as they relate to chemotoxicity in the respective organ systems. As noted in those discussions, the number of mediating factors has made it difficult to completely control comparisons of the

Table 8.2 CHEMOTOXIC EFFECTS: MEDIATING FACTORS

Dose/concentration
Site of injection
Rate of injection
Osmolality
Formulation
Viscosity
Molecular toxicity

chemotoxic effects of different contrast agents. For example, in comparing the arm pain experienced following injections of agents with meglumine versus sodium cations, it is generally not possible to completely control iodine versus salt concentration, osmolality, and viscosity, each of which may influence the amount of pain experienced. The reader is referred to the appropriate chapters for in-depth discussions of chemotoxic effects and, in particular, for discussions of the reduced chemotoxicity of the new low-osmolality contrast agents.

Many terms have been used in the radiological literature in referring to "unpredictable" reactions. These terms include "idiosyncratic," "anaphylactoid," "allergic," "pseudo-allergic," "generalized systemic," and "immediate generalized" reactions. The variability in terminology is largely a reflection of incomplete and evolving knowledge of the etiology of the unpredictable reactions.

The term "idiosyncratic" reaction should probably not be used in referring to adverse reactions to contrast media. This term has been reserved in the allergy/immunology literature to refer to drug-induced reactions in susceptible individuals who have genetic enzymatic deficiencies (DeSwarte RD, 1986). For example, patients with erythrocyte glucose-6-phosphate dehydrogenase deficiency develop a hemolytic anemia when they receive primaquine. Susceptible individuals react differently from normals but predictably and characteristically, that is, idiosyncratically. Enzymatic deficiencies or other genetic defects have not been demonstrated in contrast media reactors. The meaning of the term "idiosyncratic" in the context of the literature dealing with contrast media is synonymous with "unpredictable."

The terms, "allergic reaction" or "hypersensitivity reaction," imply that a specific immunologic mechanism (i. e., antigen/antibody reaction) is the cause of the reaction. Current evidence suggests that a reaction between contrast media and contrast media specific antibodies is

probably not the primary etiology of most adverse reactions and these terms should also be limited appropriately in discussing contrast media reactions (Brasch RC, 1980a; 1980b; Carr DH and Walker AC, 1984).

Perhaps the best general qualifying term for the majority of unpredictable reactions to contrast media is "pseudo-allergic." Pseudo-allergic reactions may have entirely similar clinical manifestations as true allergic reactions. The term implies that the initiating event does not involve a reaction with a drug-specific antibody, but can still involve activation of one or more immunologic effector systems by another mechanism. Many other adverse drug reactions fall into this category (DeSwarte RD, 1986). A small percentage of unpredictable reactions are vagal in nature and have distinctly different manifestations as discussed below.

The terms "generalized systemic reaction" or "immediate generalized reaction" have also been used as a way to identify unpredictable adverse reactions but without having to imply a specific mechanism or etiology. These terms are not widely used outside the radiology literature.

The most serious expression of pseudo-allergic unpredictable reactions is the "anaphylactoid" reaction (Table 8.3).

Table 8.3 MANIFESTATIONS OF ANAPHYLACTIC (ANAPHYLACTOID) REACTIONS

Respiratory
- Laryngeal and upper airway edema (epiglottis, hypopharynx, trachea)
- Bronchospasm
- Bronchial secretions and peribronchial congestion

Cardiovascular
- Hypotension
- Cardiac arrhythmias
- Shock
- Cardiac arrest

Gastrointestinal
- Nausea
- Vomiting
- Intestinal cramping
- Diarrhea

Cutaneous
- Pruritis
- Urticaria, hives
- Angioedema

Genitourinary
- Uterine cramps
- Urgency to urinate

This term is used to indicate the same clinical manifestations or clinical syndrome as in anaphylactic reactions but the term "anaphylactoid" implies a non-immunologic etiology (as does the term "pseudo-allergic"). Some authorities now use the terms "anaphylactic" and "anaphylactoid" interchangeably, thereby focusing on the nature of the reaction or clinical syndrome and not the etiology that classically is an IgE-mediated, antigen-induced reaction. The anaphylactic reaction or syndrome is an explosive multiorgan system response to a variety of potent biologically active mediators.

Each of the manifestations of anaphylactic reactions listed in Table 8.3 may be seen alone or in combination up to the full-blown life-threatening response. Because many of these manifestations (e. g., nausea, vomiting, hypotension, cardiac arrhythmias) may also be caused by the chemotoxic effects of contrast media, it is often impossible in individual cases to distinguish which manifestations are due to chemotoxic versus pseudo-allergic effects. Full-blown *anaphylactic* (anaphylactoid) reactions represent only a small fraction of the *unpredictable pseudo-allergic* reactions to contrast media, and the two terms should therefore not be used interchangeably.

ETIOLOGY OF UNPREDICTABLE REACTIONS

Since the first recognition of severe and potentially catastrophic unpredictable reactions to contrast media, the etiology of such reactions has been the subject of intense investigation, particularly in the past two decades. Several hypotheses have now been proposed for the mechanism of these reactions. No single theory or hypothesis has yet been uniformly accepted as the complete explanation for all types of observed reactions, and it may well be that more than one etiology or mechanism is important.

Histamine Release. Radiographic contrast media have been demonstrated to cause the release of histamine, serotonin, and other biologically active mediators from both mast cells and basophils (Brasch RC, et al, 1970; Ring J, et al, 1978; Rockoff SD, et al, 1970; Simon RA, et al, 1979). Histamine was a logical candidate for study due to the overlap of its known effects and the reactions observed following contrast media administration. Both histamine and radiographic contrast media can produce the so-called triple response or wheal and flare response when injected intradermally. Histamine is also a potent vasodilator at the capillary level and can induce alterations of vascular endothelial permeability. The transcapillary passage of plasma proteins and fluid into the extracellular space lead to the formation of edema. Following the administration of histamine, the skin becomes erthematous followed by edema and crops of hives, particularly over the trunk. Histamine is also known to cause bronchoconstriction, and its direct stimulation of nerve endings can produce sensations of burning, itching, and the feeling of warmth. These are also observed following intravascular administration of contrast media.

In in vitro studies, the release of histamine by radiographic contrast media has been shown to be dose dependent (Ring J, et al, 1978). In cells from different subjects, the prosthetic groups on the benzene ring may be specific in determining the degree of response. The presence of iodine on the benzene ring is not necessary for the release of histamine, and no definite receptor has been found on the cells to suggest a consistent structure/function relationship. Methylglucamine salts have a greater releasing effect than sodium salts (Rockoff SD, et al, 1972), and in one investigation, diatrizoate was found to have a greater effect than other derivatives (Ring J, et al, 1978). The new low-osmolality media also cause release of histamine. In in vitro experiments, the degree of release compared to conventional ratio-1.5 ionic media is less (Assem ESK et al, 1983), but the relative in vitro effects remain to be fully investigated.

The contrast-induced in vitro release of histamine is enhanced by serum (Ring J, et al, 1978). The enhancement is reversed when complement is removed from the serum, suggesting more than one mechanism for release. In the absence of serum, the onset of release is delayed (10 minutes) with a slow peak (45 minutes). It has been suggested that the time course of the in vitro release in the absence of serum is akin to that seen with ionophors while the presence of serum and, presumably complement, is necessary for the more immediate release corresponding to the time course of many clinically observed reactions. Release of histamine from basophils of atopic subjects and prior contrast media reactors is greater than in normal subjects (Erffmeyer JE, et al, 1985).

In in vivo studies, contrast-induced histamine release has been demonstrated in both reactors and nonreactors (Brasch RC, et al, 1970). Early studies in vivo were hampered by the insensitivity of chemical methods for measuring histamine. With more sensitive techniques, the release of histamine has been demonstrated in all patients following the intravascular administration of radiographic contrast media (Kaliner M, et al, 1984).

Theories proposed for in vivo release include: (1) a direct cellular effect mediated by a receptor or receptors not yet identified, (2) release secondary to the generation of anaphylatoxins from activation of the complement system and, (3) release due to the hyperosmolarity of the radiographic contrast media, either directly or through indirect hypertonic damage to cell membranes and vascular endothelium. At the biochemical level, an increase in intracellular calcium concentration may set in motion the secretory response of the mast cells and basophils, which is energy dependent. The cellular diuretic effects of hypertonic intravascular contrast media cause an increase in the intracellular calcium concentration.

While histamine is probably an important mediator in contrast reactions, a number of observations suggest that its release is not solely responsible for initiating or mediating severe and fatal adverse reactions to radiographic contrast material. First, in several clinical studies, both reactors and nonreactors demonstrated release of histamine. In a study by Simon and colleagues, 40% of 43 patients had measurable increases in plasma histamine, but there were no statistically significant differences in the rise in plasma histamine between six patients who experienced reactions and 37 who did not (Simon RA, et al, 1979). Likewise, in Brasch's study, no correlation was observed between an increase in plasma histamine concentration and subjective or objective side effects (Brasch RC, et al, 1970). Furthermore, it is now clear that histamine antagonists do not completely suppress or eliminate adverse reactions to radiographic contrast media. The direct administration of histamine alone does not cause anaphylactic reactions. Thus the actions of histamine can only be considered to provide a partial explanation for the spectrum of effects seen in severe and fatal contrast media reactions.

Complement Activation/MultiMediator Release. Subtantial experimental and clinical data has been presented in the last decade that demonstrate activation of the complement system by radiographic contrast media and their analogs (Arroyave CM and Tan EM, 1977; Hasselbacker P and Hahn J, 1980; Gorsette RE and Delmotte P, 1980; Kolb WP, et al, 1978; Lang JH, et al, 1976; Lasser EC, et al, 1981; 1979; 1980; Lasser EC, 1981; Siegle RL, et al, 1980, 1983; Till G, et al, 1978). Activation has been demonstrated both in vitro and in vivo. The new ratio-3 low-osmolality media appear to have less effect on complement activation than conventional ratio-1.5 media.

The complement system consists of at least 15 plasma proteins that interact sequentially. Many of the functions of the complement system support the immune system in host defense and in the inflammatory response. For example, the terminal components (C5–C9) are cytolytic and play a role in host defense against bacterial invasion. Components C3a and C5a are known as "anaphylatoxins" due to their roles as mediators of histamine release. Other important effects of mediators in the complement system that may contribute to adverse reactions to contrast media include release of lysosomal enzymes, increase in vascular permeability, contraction of smooth muscle, and chemotaxis of leukocytes. The complement system is interrelated with the coagulation, fibrinolytic, and kinin systems. Activation of the complement system can therefore result in the release of the mediators associated with these latter systems and vice versa. Contrast media reactors have now been shown to have evidence of activation of these systems as manifested, for example, by the presence of fibrin split products in their serum. Bradykinin may account for the profound hypotension seen as the predominant event in some reactions and activation of the coagulation system may account for the consumptive coagulopathy reported in isolated cases of adverse reactions.

The complement system can be activated in a number of ways. The "classic" pathway is activated immunologically by the interaction of antigens with subclasses of IgG and IgM. The alternative (properidin) pathway is activated by lipopolysaccharides such as bacterial endotoxins or other polysaccharides and immune complexes containing IgA or IgD. It was originally thought that the activation of the complement system by radiographic contrast media was via the alternative pathway. It has now been shown that the activation is not through either the classical or alternative pathways. Rather, the activation is nonsequential and probably mediated by a factor in the plasma. There are simultaneous reductions of CH-50, C3, C4, C1, and factor B. In vivo, the reductions occur rapidly within minutes and may return to baseline within 30 minutes. Lasser has also summarized findings that suggest a primary role for the contact system beginning with activation

of Factor XII by damage to vascular endothelium from hyperosmolar contrast media and proceeding through a cascade of proteins involving prekallikrein and kinins, including bradykinin. Bradykinin is a more potent mediator than histamine and can also play a role in release of mediators and activation of other cascade systems (Lasser EC, 1985).

Interestingly, measured decreases in complement in response to contrast administration have not been shown to correlate with reactions. A much higher percentage of patients demonstrate reduction in complement activity in response to radiocontrast media administration than demonstrate reactions. Rather, the key association may be the presence of a "perturbed" system at the time of contrast injection. Evidence for this comes from the evaluation of $C\bar{1}$ esterase inhibitor concentrations in baseline samples from reactors and nonreactors. In Lasser's work, mean levels for $C\bar{1}$ esterase inhibitor were 20% higher in nonreactors than in reactors (Lasser EC, Lang JH, Lyon SG, et al 1980). Moreover, both baseline and postcontrast injection values for total hemolytic complement activity were significantly different for reactors versus nonreactors. The importance of these observations has been suggested by animal models where depletion of $C\bar{1}$ esterase inhibitor by serial contrast injections led to increased reactivity (Lasser EC, et al, 1979c; Laner EC, Lang JH, lyon SG et al, 1980). Stimulation or protection of $C\bar{1}$ esterase inhibitor levels by administration of steroids was demonstrated to be protective. Thus, it may be hypothesized that clinical and environmental conditions that result in ongoing activation of the complement, coagulation, kinin, or fibrinolysin systems may result in a decrease in the concentration of $C\bar{1}$ esterase inhibitor. When the already compromised balance between activation and inhibition is challenged by injection of radiographic contrast media, it is tipped farther in the direction of activation (Rapoport S, et al, 1982). The reaction can then be self-sustaining and amplified in the presence of a reduced concentration of inhibitor. The resulting release and/or synthesis of multiple mediators from the different "cascade" systems could well explain the wide variety of clinical syndromes seen in adverse reactions. This hypothesis could also explain the increased incidence of reactions in patients with allergies and why prior reactors may or may not react subsequently if it is dependent on the "balance" of their cascade systems.

Antigen/Antibody Reactions. Historically, it was logical to explore the possibility that adverse reactions to contrast media could represent antigen/antibody reactions. The weight of evidence appears to be against this mechanism in the majority of cases, although there is some evidence that antigen/antibody reactions play a role in specific cases.

Brasch has summarized indirect and direct evidence to support an allergic mechanism for adverse reactions to radiographic contrast media (Brasch RC, 1980a). Indirect evidence includes the observation that the manifestations are "allergic" in nature and mimic IgE-mediated hypersensitivity reactions. Important characteristics are the suddenness of onset and the types of manifestations seen, including hypotension, bronchospasm, edema of the airway, and hives. The reactions are not dose related past a critical threshold, which is again characteristic of IgE-mediated allergic reactions. Moreover, patients with allergic histories have a two-to fivefold increased risk of reactions, and there is some increase in risk for atopic patients.

As direct evidence of an allergic etiology, Brasch cites both clinical and experimental observations. There have, in fact, been three documented case reports wherein patients with severe or fatal reactions have had proven antibody activity against radiographic contrast media. Brasch and colleagues have also documented increased binding of the radiographic media with IgG in reactors compared to nonreactors. Brasch has reported the induction of IgG and IgE antibodies in a rabbit model (Brasch RC, 1980b). Analogs of contrast media were bound to proteins and administered with Freund adjuvant for the induction. Last, it has been pointed out that there is often cross-reactivity between antibodies and antigens. This could explain the occurrence of an antibody/antigen reaction in a patient never previously exposed to contrast material. Radiographic contrast media are halogenated benzene rings that are used commonly enough in other applications to provide exposure opportunities to the general public.

The major evidence against an allergic etiology for the majority of contrast reactions comes from the converse of the above observations. The lack of demonstrable antibodies in the vast majority of reacting patients is a major argument against an allergic etiology. Contrast media molecules are small, typically less than 1000 in molecular weight, and have not been generally shown to act as haptens. Carr has pointed out that analogs of contrast media rather than the media per se were used in Brasch's experimental attempts to induce antibodies and that numerous investigators using ideal conditions have not been able to reproduce those observations with actual contrast media (Carr DH and Walker AC, 1984).

In the study evaluating IgG binding noted above, there was considerable overlap in binding levels between reactors and nonreactors and, in essence, with the exception of a very few case reports, specific antibodies have not been found to date, clinically (Carr DH and Walker AC, 1984; Brasch RC, 1980a). The common occurrence of reactions in patients with no prior exposure and the continued unpredictability with repeat exposure are further evidence against an allergic etiology.

The Central Nervous System Hypothesis. A novel alternative hypothesis to explain adverse reactions to contrast media has been suggested by Lalli (Lalli

AF, 1974; 1980; Lalli AF and Greensteet R, 1981). He has proposed a theory attempting to unify the myriad clinical observations in patients adversely reacting to contrast media by invoking a central nervous system mechanism. In this theory, the patient is preconditioned by fear and anxiety. The patient senses the injection of contrast and/or small amounts of contrast cross the blood-brain barrier. The limbic lobe of the cerebrum is stimulated and acts upon and through the hypothalamus to elicit reactions in the respiratory center, the vasomotor center, the vomiting center, and so on. Discharges through the autonomic nervous system could then account for such diverse events as pulmonary edema, ventricular fibrillation, cardiac arrest and urticaria (via the sympathetic system), and bronchospasm and bradycardia (via the parasympathetic system). Lalli notes that an underlying characteristic of contrast media reactions is their suddenness, which he feels is indirect evidence for a CNS mechanism due to the ability of the nervous system to respond rapidly.

Lalli has presented experimental data in mice to support his hypothesis. Diazepam and hexamethonium significantly affected the LD_{50} of radiopaque contrast media and markedly decreased the death rate experimentally. These drugs block autonomic ganglia and conjoint functions of the limbic lobe and hypothalamus.

The CNS hypothesis has not received support in the literature and must be regarded at this time as purely conjectural. Indeed, the number of factors requiring control in order to critically test the hypothesis clinically is daunting. However, there may be specific cases where the CNS hypothesis is operative. Vasovagal reactions are known to be enhanced by fear or anxiety and can be elicited by pain such as experienced from venipuncture. The "activation systems–mediator release" hypothesis and the CNS hypothesis need not be considered mutually exclusive in that the end organs are obviously the same. The potential for interaction and synergism would seem to be present.

Other Possible Etiologies. A number of other mechanisms and mediators have been put forward as possible causes or contributors to contrast media reactions. In cases where patients are taking other drugs, a contrast medium–drug interaction could play a role, as could contrast-induced alterations in calcium metabolism or enzyme inhibition. These effects of contrast media are discussed in greater detail in the previous chapters as they relate to organ-specific chemotoxic effects.

CLINICAL MANIFESTATIONS AND INCIDENCE

Numerous investigators have conducted surveys to determine the incidence and manifestations of adverse reactions to intravascular administration of radiographic contrast media (Ansell G, 1970; Ansell G, 1980; Berg GR, et al, 1973; Davies P, et al, 1975; 1985; Fischer HW and Donst VL, 1971; Gooding CA, et al, 1975; Hartman GW, et al, 1982; Littner MR, et al, 1977; Ochsner SF and Colonje MA, 1971; Ponto PN and Davies P, 1986; Pfister RC, 1983; Schrott KM, et al, 1986; Shehadi WH, 1975; 1982; Shehadi WH and Toniolo G, 1980; Stadalnik RC, et al, 1977; Witten DM, 1975; Witten DM et al, 1973). It is difficult to strictly compare the statistical data provided in different series due to major differences in the design of the respective investigations. Problems in comparing statistical data include the actual definition of what constitutes an "adverse" reaction versus an "expected" side effect, retrospective versus prospective study design, rigorousness and attention to detail in data collection, type and amount of contrast media administered, route of administration, and other aspects of injection including injection rate and contrast media temperature.

As noted by Witten, virtually all patients receiving conventional ionic contrast media experience some mild transient symptoms that can be considered physiologic effects and that are of no clinical significance (Witten DM, 1975). These symptoms include a mild feeling of

Table 8.4 CLASSIFICATION OF REACTION SEVERITY

MINOR	INTERMEDIATE	SEVERE	DEATH
Nausea, retching	Faintness	Syncope, convulsion	
Mild vomiting	Severe vomiting	Pulmonary edema	
Limited number of urticaria or hives	Extensive urticaria	Shock, hypotension	
Sensation of heat or warmth, flushing	Edema of face or larynx	Life-threatening cardiac arrhythmia (ventricular tachycardia)	
	Bronchospasm		
Pruritis	Dyspnea	Cardiac or respiratory arrest	
Mild pallor	Chills		
Diaphoresis	Chest or abdominal pain		
Injection-site pain	Headache		
Transient cardiac arrhythmia (isolated PVCs)			

warmth or a flushing sensation, metallic or brassy taste in the mouth, mild nausea without emesis, local pain at the site of injection, and "peculiar" sensations over the body. These effects are largely chemotoxic and are reduced in patients receiving low-osmolality agents.

Beyond these mild and expected symptoms, most investigators have found it useful for reporting purposes to categorize adverse reactions with respect to severity. Shehadi, reporting for the Committee on Contrast Media of the International Society of Radiology, graded reactions as (1) mild—no therapy needed; (2) moderate—therapy needed; (3) severe—hospitalization needed; and (4) fatal (Shehadi WH, 1975). Ansell noted that any classification of reactions must be arbitrary and used a similar scheme, again with four categories: (1) minor reactions—those which usually required no treatment; (2) intermediate rections—usually required some form of treatment, but there was no undue alarm for the patient's safety, and the response to treatment was usually rapid; (3) severe reac-

tions—there was often fear for the patient's life, and intensive treatment was required in most cases; and (4) death (Ansell G, 1970). Witten and co-workers distinguished between "minor side effects" and "acute reactions," which they subdivided into mild, moderate, and severe (Witten DM, 1975). Table 8.4 lists the clinical manifestations of adverse reactions in a classification scheme similar to that proposed by Ansell.

The overall reported incidence of acute adverse reactions with conventional ratio-1.5 ionic media has ranged from approximately 5–9%, with an incidence of severe or life-threatening reactions encountered in from 1/1,000 (0.1%) to 1/2,000 (0.05%) cases. The reported incidence of fatal reactions has ranged from a low of 1/93,000 to a high of approximately 1/10,000 cases (see Table 8.5) (Shehadi WH, 1975; Fischer HW and Doust VL, 1971; Hartman GW, et al, 1982; Ansell G, 1970; Ansell G, et al, 1980; Hobbs BB, 1981). In a pediatric series reported by Gooding, et al., the overall incidence of adverse reactions was 3.4% (Gooding

Table 8.5 CONVENTIONAL IONIC CONTRAST MEDIA: INCIDENCE OF REACTIONS

	OVERALL INCIDENCE	SEVERE	FATAL
Fischer and Doust (1972)	—	1/1,900	1/52,000
Witten (1973)	6.8%	1/1,000	1/33,000
Shehadi (1975)[a]	4.95%	1/2,900	1/10,000
Shehadi and Toniolo (1980)	4.73%	1/1,400	1/17,000
Ansell (1980)	—	1/4,100	1/41,000
Hobbs (1981)	—	1/2,000	1/93,000

[a] Includes both intravenous and intraarterial studies

CA, et al, 1975). No deaths were encountered in 12,419 urograms and 5 patients, or roughly 1/2,500, had major reactions. The somewhat lower incidence of adverse reactions in children is also supported by data from Shehadi and Ansell.

The incidence of specific individual manifestations and their relative severity as well as the overall reaction rates is of clinical importance. Shehadi has provided the most detailed information (Shehadi WH, 1975). In his 1975 series, the most common individual manifestations were nausea and vomiting, which accounted for approximately 34% and 20% respectively of all reported reactions. In 85%, no treatment was given and no patients required hospitalization. Flushing accounted for 12.5% and urticaria 15.5% of reactions. Three-fourths of the patients with urticaria required some form of treatment and 8 of 1,624 patients were hospitalized. Edema of the face (2.5%) and larynx (.41%) were important reactions that were usually judged to require some form of treatment. The most common reactions requiring hospitalization were related to the cardiovascular system (circulatory collapse, hypotension) followed by respiratory distress. Combined neurologic reactions accounted for less than 0.4% of reactions, with convulsions being the most common manifestation.

Ansell and Witten have provided detailed information on the more serious reactions in their respective series. Ansell reported on 164 patients experiencing intermediate reactions and 43 with severe reactions by his criteria (Ansell G, 1970). Individual manifestations in the intermediate group in descending order of incidence were mucocutaneous (66), hypotension (46), rigors (29), bronchospasm (23), vomiting (20), headache (14), abdominal pain (8), chest pain (7), paresthesias (7), sneezing (4), and convulsions (3). For the severe reactors, the most common manifestations were hypotension (35), myocardial infarction (12), mucocutaneous (7), and bronchospasm (5). Of the 13 deaths in the series, 8 were judged to be primarily cardiac (cardiac arrest),

with 1 each judged due to tracheobronchial edema, vomiting and aspiration, and renal failure; 2 neonates were judged to have died of contrast "overdose," without a more specific mechanism cited (Ansell G, 1970).

Among Witten's 30 "severe" reactors, shock with erythema was noted in 15, followed by angioneurotic edema (5), hives (4), convulsions (3), asthma (1), laryngospasm (1), and cardiac arrest (1). Dermal manifestations accounted for 472 of the 538 other less severe reactions in the series (Witten DM, 1975). The one death in Witten's series was due to cardiac arrest.

Lalli abstracted the primary causes of death in 140 patients experiencing fatal reactions during urography from documentation supplied to the Food and Drug Administration by manufacturers of contrast media. Cardiac manifestations including myocardial infarction (13), ventricular fibrillation (16), and cardiac arrest (14) were collectively the most common etiology being cited in 60 cases. Pulmonary edema (20) and respiratory arrest (11) were the next most common causes of death (Lalli AF, 1980).

Combinations of signs and symptoms become more common as reaction severity increases. In a follow-up to the original survey data on reaction incidence, Shehadi summarized combination patterns. As might be expected, nausea and vomiting was the most common combination of two, followed by urticaria and facial edema. More important, the majority of patients with life-threatening reactions had one or more manifestations in addition to the primary one requiring treatment (Shehadi WH, 1982).

There has been intense interest in the relative rates of adverse reactions for the conventional ratio-1.5 ionic media compared to the more recently introduced ratio-3 low-osmolality nonionic and dimeric preparations. Without question, the low-osmolality media are associated with fewer and less severe effects on vascular and organ physiology than conventional ratio-1.5 media (Bettmann MA, et al, 1984; Grainger RE 1979; 1980). The reasons for this are largely related to the reduced osmolality of the newer agents and have been reviewed in detail in the organ system chapters.

Initial data on the incidence of pseudo-allergic reactions and severe life-threatening reactions for the low-osmolality agents is encouraging but has not yet been collected in a controlled fashion to allow direct comparisons. The early literature has cited historical survey data to make these comparisons rather than double-blind prospective studies, which is obviously not ideal.

In one large series comprising 50,660 patients undergoing urography with the ratio-3 nonionic agent iohexol, the overall incidence of reactions was reported to be 2.1% (Schrott KM, et al, 1986). Using the classification system proposed by Shehadi (Shehadi WH, 1975), there were 570 (1.3%) mild reactions, 467 (0.9%) moderate reactions, 6 (0.01%) severe reactions, and no deaths. Patients identified as being at high risk due to history of allergy or prior reactions to contrast media experienced a reaction rate of 2.7% compared to 1.3% for patients without risk factors. The types of reactions were similar to those reported with conventional media. Although it is impossible to know how the physicians involved in this study compared in their assessments to those involved in prior studies with the ratio-1.5 media, these are lower percentages than those generally reported for the conventional ratio-1.5 agents (see Table 8.5).

Delayed reactions to intravascular contrast media have not been studied to the same extent as the acute reactions decribed above. Depression of 24 hour radioiodine uptake in the thyroid due to flooding of the iodine pool and iodide-induced sialadenitis are well-established, delayed sequelae to intravascular contrast media. Ponto has reported a questionnaire-based study of delayed reactions in 841 patients undergoing nonemergent urography. Seventy percent of the patients reported no adverse reactions. Five percent reported delayed skin rashes, and

13% reported delayed arm pain, typically above the injection site. The incidence of delayed rashes was higher in patients receiving agents containing the meglumine versus sodium cation, and the incidence for sodium iothalamate preparations was the same as that recorded for the ratio-3 nonionic agents (Panto PN and Davies P, 1986).

Impairment of renal function is another well-recognized delayed complication of intravascular contrast media administration (Byrd L and Sherman RL, 1979; Cruz C, et al, 1986; Harvey LA, et al, 1983; Lang EK, et al, 1981; Swanson DP, et al, 1985; Swanson DP, et al, 1986; Swartz RD, et al, 1978). However, the literature is divided on the incidence of renal failure and the importance of risk factors. Frequently cited risk factors include dysproteinemia including multiple myeloma, diabetes mellitis, preexisting renal insufficiency and/or impaired renal blood flow, and age greater than 60 years. These types of risk factors cannot be avoided. Dehydration, concommitant use of nephrotoxic drugs, high doses of contrast media, and repeat studies at close intervals are "avoidable" factors that are also cited as increasing the risk of renal failure (Cruz C, et al, 1986; Byrd L and Sherman RL, 1979).

The incidence of contrast-induced acute renal failure reported in the literature has ranged from 0–13% (Byrd Lard and Sherman RL, 1979). Most series have been retrospective and have not involved attempts to control or correct "avoidable" risk factors, thus making it difficult to assess the true risk due to the unavoidable factors, such as diabetes mellitus or other medical conditions including preexisting degrees of renal insufficiency. Hyperosmolality, dehydration, and acidosis resulting in renal hypoperfusion increase the susceptibility of the kidneys of diabetic patients to damage. In one prospective study where the protocol eliminated these "avoidable" risk factors (and the concomitant use of nephrotoxic drugs), the effect of contrast media on renal function in diabetes was no different than in nondiabetic subjects, and no differences were found in BUN or creatinine values between subjects younger than 40 years of age compared with those over 40 (Cruz C, et al, 1986).

It seems reasonable to conclude from all the available data that there is an increasingly greater likelihood for renal impairment as the number and severity of underlying risk factors increase, but the risks can be minimized by correcting "avoidable" complicating factors prior to examination. The use of mannitol was recommended in the past in cases where the hemodynamics of renal perfusion were in question (Cruz C, et al, 1986; Becker JA, 1980). In current practice, a ratio-3 medium is recommended.

FACTORS AFFECTING THE RISK OF ADVERSE REACTIONS

A number of factors have now been established that are associated with an increased risk of both chemotoxic and unpredictable pseudo-allergic adverse reactions. The organ-specific factors associated with increased chemotoxicity such as impaired renal function or abnormalities in the blood-brain barrier are discussed in the chapters dealing with contrast studies of the respective organ systems. Several other factors are pertinent to all types of studies and to unpredictable reactions.

History of Allergy/Asthma. In Witten's series, a careful prospective history of allergy was obtained in 9,934 patients (Witten DM, 1975). The incidence of minor side effects by his grading system was one and one-half times greater in patients with a history of allergy versus those with no prior history. The difference for mild, moderate, or severe acute reactions was even greater with a two-and-one-half-fold increase in the chance of a significant reaction in patients with a history of allergy. Patients with a specific history of asthma had a fivefold greater chance of significant acute reactions compared to nonallergic patients. These data are supported by other series wherein two to fourfold increases in the risk of severe reactions were encountered overall in patients with a history of allergy and higher risks in patients with histories of asthma (Ansell G, 1970; Shehadi WH, 1975; Kalimo K, et al, 1980). Although iodine is not necessary on the benzene ring for induction of adverse reactions, a history of "iodine allergy" (and seafood) has been among the allergies associated with increased incidence of reaction. The increased risk is on the same order as other allergies.

Previous Reaction to Contrast Media. The most important risk factor reported uniformly is the history of a prior reaction to intravascular contrast media. In patients who have not received any form of premedication or pretreatment and who have a history of significant previous reaction to intravascular contrast media, the incidence of repeat reaction is 15–40% or approximately 3–8 times that expected in all patients (Ansell G, 1970; Shehadi WH, 1975; Witten DM, 1975).

Although the increased risk in known previous reactors is higher than in the general population or patients who have not reacted to a previous contrast study, the unpredictable nature of contrast reactions is well illustrated by numerous reported cases wherein patients have alternately reacted and not reacted during multiple examinations or have had fatal reactions after numerous uncomplicated previous procedures. Thus, a history of prior reaction should alert the radiologist to the increased risk of another reaction but a negative reaction history should not lull the radiologist into a false sense of security.

Quantity of Contrast Medium Administered. Acute adverse reactions including fatal reactions have been noted after intravenous administration of as little as 0.5 ml of contrast material or less, and it is generally accepted that there is no clinically relevant threshold below which reactions will not be encountered. In large series in which the incidence of reactions has been related to the amount of contrast given, there is usually a cluster of reactors who have received small amounts and in whom the injection was terminated. In these cases, the reason for the patient receiving a limited amount of contrast must be understood, as it may look paradoxically in some reports as though there is a greater risk of adverse reaction with small doses! Beyond this observation, the literature is divided on whether the incidence of severe and fatal acute reactions is dose dependent. In Witten's series, no difference was noted between patients receiving 30 ml and 50 ml of a mixture of diatrizoate sodium-meglumine (Renovist®—Squibb) (Witten DM, 1975). In the same series, the incidence of minor side effects was no different in a small number of patients receiving more than 50 ml but the incidence of other acute reactions was somewhat greater. The number of subjects in the above 50-ml category was too small for statistical comparison.

Ansell arbitrarily divided his patients between those receiving 5–19 grams of iodine (equivalent to 17–65 ml of a contrast medium containing 300 mgm Iodine per ml) versus those receiving greater than 20 grams of iodine. In the group receiving the larger dose, there were 2.5 times as many severe and fatal reactions compared to those receiving lesser amounts (Ansell G, 1970).

It is important to note that amounts of contrast media administered for intravenous urography have steadily increased. Between Ansell's reports of 1970 and 1980, the estimated mean dose increased from 12 grams of iodine to 21 grams of iodine (i.e., from 40 to 70 ml of contrast media containing 300 mgm Iodine per ml) (Ansell G, 1970; 1980). It is not unusual for patients to routinely receive 100 ml of a contrast medium containing 400 mgm Iodine per ml or equivalent for intravenous urography, and many radiology departments now routinely administer 150 ml of 282 mgm Iodine per ml contrast media for contrast enhancement in computed tomography studies.

The effect, if any, on the incidence of adverse reactions of these increases in dose over the past decade have not really been prospectively studied in a systematic fashion, but the increases have apparently been reasonably well tolerated. Chemotoxic effects are predictably greater with higher doses and may account for some of the differences found in the series described above.

Route of Administration. Early studies reporting adverse reactions to contrast media administration focused largely on intravenous urography and intravenous cholangiography. In the past two decades, arteriography has become increasingly important, and it is now recognized that there is a significantly lower overall incidence of acute pseudo-allergic adverse reactions with intraarterial compared to intravenous administration of contrast media. This is borne out in the large series reported by Shehadi and Toniolo (Shehadi WH and Toniolo G, 1980). The incidence of reactions in intravenous urography was 4.8% with a mortality of approximately 1/20,000. The overall incidence of reactions in combined intraarterial studies was approximately 2.5%. However, fatal reactions in all types of arteriography were encountered in 1/12,000 cases or roughly twice as frequently as with intravenous urography. The study did not address the effects of intercurrent illness, complications of catheterization, or injections into a particular arterial system as contributors to the mortality for arterial studies. This is a particularly important consideration for coronary arteriography where it may not be possible, in a particular case, to distinguish catheter-induced from contrast-induced complications such as arrhythmias, or between pseudoallergic and chemotoxic effects. The study also did not address the possible effects of premedication, especially sedatives which are commonly given for arteriography but not frequently given for intravenous urography. A combination of these factors could explain the lower overall reaction rate and higher mortality rate.

Bolus Injection Versus Drip Infusion for Intravenous Administration. Single bolus injection in intravenous urography has been reported in two of the largest series to demonstrate a significantly lower incidence of reactions than administration of contrast media by drip infusion. Ansell reported a two-to-threefold increase in the rate of intermediate and severe reactions with infusion versus bolus injections (Ansell G, 1970). Shehadi did not distinguish between the severity of reactions but found overall incidence rates of 5.4% for bolus injection versus 7.06% for drip infusion respectively (Shehadi WH, 1975). Neither series was controlled for patient selection or total contrast administered. More prolonged exposure to the contrast medium could account for the increased overall incidence of reactions with drip infusion.

For the specific case of intravenous cholangiography, the results in both series were reversed with a higher incidence of reaction following single or bolus dose versus drip infusion. Ansell divided patients somewhat arbitrarily into two groups: those receiving the dose for intravenous cholangiography (ioglucamate) in a span of 1–19 minutes and greater than 20 minutes. The latter group had one-third as many minor reactions. The number of patients divided between the two groups was too small to conclude any statistically significant difference for intermediate and severe reactions (Ansell G, 1970). It should be noted that intravenous cholangiography is very seldom used in current practice, having been largely replaced by hepatobiliary scintigraphy and ultrasound imaging, respectively.

Age and Sex. The overall incidence of adverse reactions is lowest in the first two decades of life, peaks in the middle three decades, and declines again in the older age groups. However, the incidence of fatal reactions is greater above the age of 50 than in the younger age groups. This is probably due to the presence of intercurrent disease and, in particular, cardiac disease. Ansell calculated an increase in risk for severe reactions of 4.5 times that expected in normals in patients with a history of cardiac disease and an even greater increased risk of death (Ansell G, 1970). These risk factors were for patients undergoing intravenous urography, and therefore the increased risk cannot be attributed to a procedure-related complication such as catheter-induced arrhythmia or to the increased chemotoxic effects of direct injections in the coronary artery or left ventricle.

No consistent difference in the overall incidence of adverse reactions has been demonstrated between men and women.

Type of Contrast Medium—Conventional Ratio-1.5 Agents. Conventional ratio-1.5 contrast media demonstrate significantly different respective chemotoxities related to their chemical composition, formulation, and a number of other factors ennumerated in Table 8.2. These differences in chemotoxicity have been discussed in detail in previous chapters with respect to their effects on each major organ system. Expression of the chemotoxic effects is most marked for selective arterial injections, and the selection criteria or efficacy criteria for agents used in specific angiography applications are based on a systematic analysis of these effects as described.

With respect to pseudo-allergic reactions following intravenous administration of modern conventional ionic media, the literature does not provide sufficient data to conclude relatively higher or lower risks of severe or fatal reactions between agents of different chemical composition or formulation.

However, before the different ratio-1.5 agents are accepted as of essentially equal risk for significant adverse reactions following intravenous administration, it should be noted that most of the available data are from studies reporting only clinical observations. For example, systematic electrocardiographic monitoring has not been performed in any of the large series cited above that involved thousands of patients. It has now been recognized through a number of investigations that there is a significant incidence of electrocardiographic abnormalities even with intravenous contrast media administration (Berg GR, et al, 1973; Pfister RC, et al, 1983; Stadalnik RC, et al, 1977). These arrhythmias are probably associated with the chemotoxic and related psychogenic effects of pain and subjective discomfort and tend to occur more often in patients with prior electrocardiographic abnormalities, known cardiovascular disease and renal impairment, and in patients older than 50 years. The dependence on clinically observed reactions, combined with the lack of control of the multiple contrast media variables including the total dose and administration rate, the nature of the contrast anion and cation, formulation characteristics (i. e., binding and sequestering agents), and total osmolality, make it difficult to use currently available adverse-reaction data to form conclusions regarding the "optimal" conventional ratio 1.5 agent for intravenous administration.

Viscosity. Decreasing the viscosity of contrast media by warming decreases the pain and subjective discomfort of injection. Part of the effect is flow related due to reduced time of exposure of a given vessel wall segment to the agent and hence less vasodilatation and vascular endothelial effects. However, no correlation has been established between contrast media viscosity and incidence of severe reactions. In a small prospective randomized study, Turner found no statistical difference in anaphylactoid reactions in patients receiving contrast media at room temperature versus body temperature (37° C) (Turner E, et al, 1982).

PREVENTION OF ADVERSE REACTIONS

Pretesting. The concern held by radiologists for adverse contrast media reactions is well illustrated by the history of efforts to develop pretesting regimens to identify at-risk patients. In the early going, radiologists and others thought that adverse reactions were primarily on an allergic basis and developed a number of "sensitivity-testing" procedures analogous to those used by allergists. These included intradermal, subcutaneous, ocular, and intraoral tests. As it became increasingly apparent that these tests were not of value in identifying at-risk patients and that a classical immunological mechanism was not the dominant causative factor, the tests were dropped. However, by the late 1950s and 1960s, it became quite popular among radiologists to use "provocative testing," wherein a test dose, typically 0.5–1.0 ml, was injected intravenously and the patient observed for several minutes (Fischer HW and Doust VL, 1971).

A number of investigators have studied the efficacy of provocation testing using the intravenous method and have concluded that this approach is also of no value in predicting reactions and, in fact, may be overtly misleading. In Fischer's large multiinstitutional survey of 3.8 million patients, no statistically significant difference in death rates or rates of serious reactions was found between institutions where all patients were pretested, some patients were pretested, and pretesting was not used at all (Fischer HW and Doust VL, 1971). In the same series, 59 patients experienced serious reactions and 2 patients died in response to the pretest dose of contrast media. Twenty-three deaths and 714 serious reactions were encountered in patients with negative pretests. Although the percentages are somewhat different, these observations are supported by Witten's experience. All of the 32,964 patients in his series received an intravenous test dose of 0.5 ml. Nine patients reacted to the test dose, of whom two had severe reactions. At the same time, there were 559 reactions recorded in patients with negative pretests. Witten concluded that pretesting in this manner was of no practical value and recommended abandonment since the procedure was not justified on either medical or legal grounds. Many other observers have reached the same conclusion. The practice of routine intravenous provocation pretesting has been increasingly abandoned in the last decade.

Although provocative testing, as it has been used in routine clinical practice, has not been found to be of value, it would still be helpful to have a means of identifying potential reactors, particularly in high-risk groups of patients such as those with a prior history of significant reaction to contrast media. An alternative pretesting method has been described by Yocum wherein serial dilutions of the contrast media to be used in the clinical study are administered at 15-minute intervals (Yocum MW, et al, 1978). The initial dose is 0.1 ml of a 1:10,000 dilution progressing through seven levels to as much as 5 ml of the full-strength material. In a series of 204 patients, this method was successful in separating patients into groups with positive pretests and a subsequent high probability of reaction and negative pretests with a subsequent, statistically significant, lower probability of reaction. An obvious disadvantage of the approach is the time-consuming nature of the sequential tests, which require over 1 1/2 hours. This may be acceptable in selected high-risk patients but makes it impractical as a routine pretesting procedure. This approach has not found clinical acceptance. In clinical practice, it is easier and probably more efficacious to simply pretreat all high-risk patients as described (as follows) than to go through this elaborate process.

The clinical experience with provocative testing strongly suggests that unpredictable pseudo-allergic reactions to contrast material are indeed threshold dependent. The response curve may be very steep over the range of 0–2.0 ml with a variable threshold between subjects. This would explain both the incidence of severe and fatal reactions to small amounts of contrast media and the failure of provocative testing with a single fixed small amount to detect all or even the majority of reactors.

Table 8.6 PRETREATMENT REGIMEN FOR HIGH-RISK PATIENTS

I. Elective Procedures
  Prednisone—50 mgm orally q 6 hr × 3, last dose 1 hr prior to procedure
  Diphenhydramine—50 mgm IM 1 hr prior to procedure
  (Ephedrine—25 mgm orally 1 hr prior to procedure)
II. Emergency Procedures
  Hydrocortisone—200 mg IV as soon as possible and q 4 hr thru the procedure
  Diphenhydramine—50 mgm IM 1 hr prior to procedure

Pretreatment. Another approach to the high-risk patient is the prophylactic administration of one or more premedications. Table 8.6 provides a summary of the pretreatment regimens that evolved for elective and emergency procedures respectively. Table 8.7 summarizes categories of patients at increased risk. Details may differ slightly between authors, but the therapeutic objectives are the same (Greenberger PA, et al, 1985; Kelly JF, et al, 1978). The combination of a corticosteroid and an antihistamine (H_1 blocker) has been uniformly found to reduce the incidence of repeat contrast-media reactions in prior reactors. In untreated subjects, 15–40% will be expected to have a repeat reaction as discussed above. In Greenberger's experience, the combination of prednisone and diphenhydramine hydrochloride pretreatment reduced the incidence of repeat reactions to 10.8% (Greenberger PA, et al, 1985). The addition of ephedrine sulfate further reduced the incidence to 5%. In a series of prior reactors reported by Kelly, prednisone and diphendydramine pretreatment resulted in a reaction rate of 4.95% (Kelly JF, et al, 1978). Thus, premedication appears to significantly reduce but not eliminate adverse reactions in this high-risk group (Madowitz JS and Schweiger MJ,

Table 8.7 CONDITIONS WHERE PREMEDICATION SHOULD BE CONSIDERED

Seizure history
Pheochromocytoma
Dehydration
History of allergies
Asthma
History of prior reactions

1979). Although some authorities have recommended that premedication be considered in other high-risk groups such as patients with histories of asthma and allergy (Table 8.7), data are not available to assess the efficacy of this approach. The relative increased risk in these groups is not as great as in prior reactors and it is, therefore, more difficult to show a beneficial effect.

The potential beneficial protective effects of routine pretreatment with corticosteroids have been studied in a major prospective multiinstitutional trial by Lasser and colleagues (Lasser EC, et al, 1987). They showed that a two-dose regimen of oral methylprednisolone, 32 mgm, given 12 hours and 2 hours prior to intravascular administration of conventional ionic contrast media significantly reduced the incidence of reactions overall ($P < .0001$). More important, severe reactions ($P < 0.05$) and reactions requiring therapy ($P < 0.01$) were significantly reduced. When compared to reported reaction rates with nonionic intravascular contrast media, the results of this series suggest that the overall incidence of reactions requiring therapy following administration of conventional ionic media may be reduced to the same range in both low- and high-risk patients when corticosteroid pretreatment is used (Lasser EC, et al, 1987; Schrott KM, et al, 1986). If this experience can be sustained in routine clinical practice, it will provide a less expensive alternative to the use of nonionic media.

The rationale for using corticosteroids, antihistamines, and sympathomimetics is partly theoretical and partly empirical. Steroids have been shown experimentally to be protective, possibly by their effect of increasing the level of $C\overline{1}$ esterase inhibitor (Lasser EC, et al, 1980; Lasser EC, et al, 1987). This is an attractive theory, but the dominant effect in man is unknown at this time.

The rationale for antihistamines follows from the recognized ability of contrast media to promote the release of histamine and the likelihood that histamine plays an important role in producing many of the manifestations of adverse reactions (Small P, et al, 1982). It should be noted that antihistamines are maximally effective only if given prior to the injection of contrast media. The antihistamines block histamine receptors but do not reverse or antagonize end-organ responses to previously bound histamine. They may also have some beneficial effect due to their weak anticholinergic properties.

Ephedrine is a sympathetic amine that stimulates both alpha and beta receptors. It differs from epinephrine in its longer duration of action and its efficacy after oral administration. Which of its effects are important in reducing the incidence of adverse reactions is unknown. It is used clinically to treat bronchospasm, which is an important adverse reaction to radiographic media. Ephedrine promotes vasoconstriction, which may counteract the formation of edema.

On theoretical grounds, it has been suggested that the addition of a histamine$_2$ receptor antagonist such as cimetedine might also be efficacious in reducing adverse reactions in high-risk patients (Kaliner M, 1984). However, in Greenberger's experience, cimetedine actually increased the observed incidence of reactions (Greenberger PA, et al, 1985). The mechanism for this adverse effect is again unknown, but cimetedine and other histamine$_2$ receptor antagonists are not recommended as part of the pretreatment regimen.

Patients with specific medical problems warrant special pretreatment considerations (Table 8.7). With a history of prior seizures, if the patient is not currently on medication, diazepam 5–10 mg administered intravenously at a rate of no more than 5 mg per minute may be given 10–20 minutes prior to the procedure (Pagani JJ, et al, 1983). Patients with suspected pheochromocytoma will usually already be receiving appropriate medications. Oral phenoxybenzamine is a mainstay of treatment. The dose is started at 10–20 mg per day and titrated for the desired effect. Phentolamine, 2-5 mg intravenously, may be added to block the effects of large amounts of catecholamines that may be released suddenly during a radiographic procedure. Phenoxybenzamine and phentolamine are alpha adrenergic blocking agents.

The problem of dehydration has been discussed in the context of urological procedures. In general, dehydration should be avoided both for its adverse effects on renal toxicity and to reduce the likelihood of hypotension secondary to contrast-induced vasodilation and hypovolemia.

THERAPY OF ADVERSE REACTIONS

Proper therapeutic response to adverse reactions to radiographic contrast media requires recognition that a reaction has occurred, correct identification of the type of reaction, assessment of its severity, and application of specific therapy (Erffmeyer JE, et al, 1985; Goldberg M, 1984; Greenberger PA, 1984; Lieberman P, et al, 1978; Siegle RL and Lieberman P, 1978). Most reactions are mild and require no medication or other therapy beyond reassurance of the patient and continued observation.

In some cases, the radiologist may decide to treat a patient to alleviate discomfort rather than because a life-threatening condition is present. This most commonly occurs with cutaneous manifestations such as urticaria and pruritis, with mild bronchospasm, or with vomiting. These manifestations can be treated by administering 0.2–0.5 mg of aqueous epinephrine subcutaneously (0.2–0.5 ml 1 : 1,000 aqueous epinephrine). The patient may also respond to 50 mgm of diphenhydramine IM or IV.

For more severe reactions where the patient is in obvious acute distress, the radiologist must determine as quickly as possible whether he or she is dealing with a predominantly anaphylactoid reaction, a vasovagal reaction, a reaction secondary to a specific chemotoxicity of contrast media, or to an intercurrent problem such as myocardial infarction or pulmonary embolism (Table 8.8) (Barnhard HJ and

Table 8.8 CAUSES OF CARDIORESPIRATORY ARREST FOLLOWING ADMINISTRATION OF INTRAVASCULAR CONTRAST MEDIA

Pseudoallergic anaphylactoid reaction
Vagal reaction
Chemotoxic sequelae
Intercurrent (incidental) events unrelated to CM (e. g., pulmonary embolism, myocardial infarction)

Barnhard FM, 1968). This differential diagnosis is obviously complex and can only be partially addressed due to the open-endedness of the possibilities.

Sudden collapse without antecedent respiratory or cutaneous signs or symptoms suggests a primary cardiac problem, either due to anaphylaxis or chemotoxicity-induced arrhythmias, and illustrates the importance of continuous direct patient observation. Arrhythmias such as ventricular tachycardia and ventricular fibrillation may be detected clinically but are better diagnosed and followed by ECG monitoring. Most patients are not continuously monitored during intravenous and noncardiac intraarterial procedures, but equipment should be kept readily available. If cardiorespiratory arrest occurs, the differential diagnosis is moot, and the therapy for arrest should be begun.

Myocardial infarction should be suspected if the dominant clinical symptom is chest pain. Pulmonary embolism may also present with sudden chest pain and is very difficult to diagnose clinically. Individual signs and symptoms of pulmonary embolism are nonspecific and may not be clinically distinguishable from those of myocardial infarction. The patient with chest pain but without cardiorespiratory arrest should be treated expectantly while other diagnostic tests are carried out (e. g., ECG, lung scan, serum enzymes, etc.).

Vasovagal reactions are uncommon but well-documented sequelae of contrast media administration. The patient is typically pale and intensely diaphoretic without cyanosis or respiratory difficulty. Severe bradycardia (pulse rate < 40/min) is the hallmark of the vasovagal reaction and the key differential feature. In fatal reactions, the blood pressure falls precipitously, the patient becomes apneic, and shock ensues. In anaphylactic reactions, the patient is flushed due to peripheral vasodilation and is hypotensive and tachycardic due to loss of fluid from the central compartment. Anaphylactic reactions are more common than the other conditions in the differential diagnosis of cardiorespiratory arrest following contrast media administration.

Treatment of Anaphylactic Reactions. The clinical manifestations of anaphylactic reactions are listed in Table 8.3. Several manifestations such as nausea and vomiting are nonspecific, and others such as urticaria and pruritis may be seen in patients who do not go on to develop a life-threatening reaction. Thus, determination of when a set of manifestations is serious enough to warrant the term "anaphylaxis" is arbitrary. For the purposes of this discussion, "anaphylactic reaction" will imply a clinical syndrome considered by the attending physician to be potentially life-threatening and embodying these manifestations.

Even within this broad definition, the presentation of the anaphylactic syndrome may be quite variable between patients. Three distinct reaction patterns cover the majority of cases. Respiratory distress may be the principal feature due either to edema of the larynx or other upper-airway structures or due to bronchospasm. In these presentations, hypotension and cardiac dysrhythmia occur secondary to hypoxemia. Alternatively, the presentation may be a primary vascular collapse without significant respiratory difficulties. Combinations of upper-airway, lower-airway, and cardiovascular manifestations can be seen as well. Although it remains speculative, the different patterns of presentation in the anaphylactic reaction may represent the greater or lesser roles of different mediators. For example, histamine, sero-

tonin, bradykinin, and slow-reacting substance of anaphylaxis each exert different primary effects.

Regardless of which reaction pattern is encountered, the basic therapy for anaphylactoid reactions is the same (Barnhard HJ and Barnhard FM, 1968; Patterson R and Valentine M, 1982). Epinephrine is the principal therapeutic drug. When treating severe anaphylactic reactions, and in the presence of shock, it can be administered slowly by intravenous injection of the *dilute* formulation. Recommended dosages in the literature are somewhat variable, but should be in the range of 0.3–1.0 mg (3–10 cc 1:10,000 aqueous epinephrine). The duration of effect is very short, and epinephrine may be readministered every 5–15 minutes guided by patient response. The same effect can be achieved by a constant intravenous infusion of 0.1–0.4 mg per minute after the initial dose. The reason for specifying an intravenous route of administration rather than a subcutaneous route is the unpredictable absorption from the subcutaneous injection site and the delayed onset of action. The local vasoconstrictive properties of epinephrine contribute to poor and delayed absorption, which may be further accentuated by poor circulation in patients with vascular collapse. In patients with underlying cardiac disease, there may be hesitation to use epinephrine due to its fibrillatory potential. However, a life-threatening anaphylactic reaction must still be treated as the first priority with careful monitoring for signs of myocardial infarction, cardiac arrhythmia, or other serious complications of epinephrine therapy such as cerebral hemorrhage. A slow rate of intravenous injection is emphasized to reduce the potential for electrocardiographic abnormalities.

Epinephrine is not a specific antidote to the mediators responsible for the anaphylactic reaction but, more than any other single drug, it counteracts their effects on multiple organs. Epinephrine stimulates both alpha and beta adrenergic receptors.

Epinephrine is a potent bronchodilator, and since its action is directed at its own receptors, it is more effective than competitive antagonists such as antihistamines in the relief of histamine-induced bronchospasm. It must be remembered, however, that concurrent drug therapy involving alpha- or beta-receptor antagonists can interfere with the respective actions of epinephrine in the treatment of anaphylactic reactions. Moreover, in the presence of a beta blocker, the alpha-receptor activity of epinephrine will predominate and may actually lead to a worsening of the patient's condition. Epinephrine counteracts airway edema through its alpha-receptor action of vasoconstriction. Epinephrine is readily absorbed transtracheally and transbronchially and may be administered as an aerosol if IV access has not been established or in the presence of upper-airway edema.

Epinephrine through its stimulation of beta$_1$ receptors promotes myocardial contraction. Heart rate, cardiac output, and stroke volume are increased, and there is a shift of blood volume to the central compartment. One other possible beneficial effect of epinephrine may be the reduction of histamine release from mast cells and basophils by its action of increasing the concentration of intracellular cyclic-AMP.

If bronchospasm is a dominant feature of the anaphylactoid reaction, it may be appropriate to add a methylxanthine such as aminophylline to the treatment regimen. Effective treatment with aminophylline requires an initial loading dose followed by a maintenance dose. The recommended loading dose is 6 mg per kilogram administered over 20–40 minutes. In otherwise healthy nonsmokers, the maintenance dose is 0.5 mg per kilogram per hour. Smokers and children below the age of 12 require up to 0.9 mg per kilogram per hour for effective therapy. The maintenance infusions should be only continued for 6 hours without measurement of the drug concentration in plasma.

The therapeutic effectiveness of the methylxanthines is partly related to their ability to release and/or interact synergistically with beta-adrenergic agonists. In either case, cardiac arrhythmias may be induced, and as with patients receiving epinephrine, cardiac monitoring is advisable. The use of aminophylline may not be advisable if the patient is hypotensive. Slow injection is again emphasized to decrease the possibility of a hypotensive response or CNS effects.

Antihistamines are frequently included in the treatment of patients experiencing adverse reactions to radiographic contrast media. Diphenhydramine 25–50 mg IM or IV or equivalent is the recommended dosage. The value of antihistamines in the treatment of reactions is limited after histamine has been released; the specific H$_1$ receptors blocked by the histamine receptor antagonists, such as diphenhydramine, are already activated. However, most authors continue to recommend their use, arguing that the antihistamines should be effective in blocking the effects of subsequently released histamine. The weak anticholinergic effects of antihistamines may also beneficially contribute to reduced secretions in the respiratory tree. H$_2$-blocking agents do not have an identified role at this time in the treatment of radiographic contrast media-induced anaphylactic reactions.

Corticosteroids (glucocorticoids) are another class of drug frequently recommended in the treatment of anaphylactic reactions. A review of the literature indicates that the rationale for steroid administration is largely empirical and is not based on a specific mechanism relevant to containing the acute process. The anti-inflammatory effects of steroids that may be valuable in controlling edema, fibrin deposition and capillary dilatation require time to be effective, on the order of 4–6 hours. However, a single dose of a corticosteroid is innocuous, and it is argued that steroids may be beneficial in combating delayed or prolonged effects. If used, steroids should be given intravenously.

Dexamethasone sodium phosphate, 8–20 mg or equivalent, is the recommended dosage. A single dose does not significantly affect subsequent adrenal gland function, and tapering of subsequent doses is not necessary.

In addition to the drug therapy described above, general supportive measures should be instituted. Oxygen is useful and should be administered if hypoxia occurs. Intravenous fluid therapy may be required to replace fluid lost from the intravascular space and is indicated in treating hypotension and shock. The value of fluid replacement in the vascular compartment in treating life-threatening hypotension following contrast administration has been emphasized by VanSonenberg and colleagues (VanSonnenberg E, et al, 1987).

In some patients, cardiorespiratory arrest will have occurred before initial therapeutic steps can be taken. In that event, the protocol for cardiopulmonary resuscitation should be initiated. The administration of epinephrine is appropriate in either case (e. g., anaphylactic reaction with or without actual cardiorespiratory arrest). Moreover, it may be critical in that bronchospasm is not readily diagnosed in an unconscious patient who is not breathing. If not appropriately treated, bronchospasm may obviate other therapeutic measures. Physicians, technologists, and other personnel observing patients following contrast administration should be specifically trained not only to recognize when a reaction is occurring but also to note the signs and symptoms in the mode of presentation and to provide that information to the arrest team.

Treatment of Vagal Reactions. Atropine is the drug of choice for treatment of vagal reactions. Atropine is a muscarinic cholinergic blocking agent that acts principally on autonomic effector cells and to a much lesser extent on ganglionic transmission. The desired effect is to reduce vagal tone on the S–A nodal pacemaker and to increase the heart rate. The dose should be administered intravenously in the amount of 0.4 mgm–0.8 mgm. Intravenous fluids may be required to support the blood pressure: Vagal stimulation can cause reflex peripheral vasodilation with peripheral pooling and decreased venous return to the heart. If the vagal reaction is profound or not promptly recognized and treated, the ensuing hypoxemia may result in myocardial infarction. Electrocardiographic monitoring should be initiated as soon as possible to help assess therapeutic response and to assist in diagnosing other arrythmias or intercurrent infarction (Andrews EJ, 1976; Stanley RJ and Pfister RC, 1976).

Drugs useful in the treatment of contrast media reactions are summarized in Table 8.9. Detailed guidelines for basic and advanced cardiac life support have been published by the American Medical Association (National Conference on Cardiopulmonary Resuscitation (CPR) and Emergency Cardiac Care (ECC), 1986). The reader who is involved with administration of radiographic contrast media is urged to be familiar with these guidelines and to strongly consider acquiring basic and advanced cardiac life support certification. Most hospitals have developed protocols for dealing with "codes" or cardiac arrests. Radiology Department personnel must be trained to both respond to the patient and initiate the code procedure. Emergency carts or trays minimally containing the drugs summarized in Table 8.9 or equivalents should be immediately at hand. Oxygen, intravenous fluids, airways, and defibrillators should also be available. In practice, the radiologist is fortunate in not having to respond frequently to life-threatening reactions but

Table 8.9   DRUGS USEFUL IN TREATING CONTRAST MEDIA REACTIONS

I. Primary
      Epinephrine
      Diphenhydramine
      Atropine
      Oxygen
      IV Fluids
II. Secondary
      Corticosteroids
      Aminophylline

<table>
<tr><td colspan="2">ADVERSE DRUG REACTION REPORT</td><td colspan="2">Henry Ford Hospital
DEPT. OF DIAGNOSTIC RADIOLOGY</td></tr>
<tr><td colspan="4">1. PRODUCT INFORMATION</td></tr>
<tr><td>a. Brand Name</td><td>b. Manufacturer</td><td colspan="2">c. Lot Number</td></tr>
<tr><td colspan="2">d. Generic Name(s)/Concentration(s)</td><td colspan="2">e. Expiration Date
f. Lot Administered to Other Patients
☐ No ☐ Yes</td></tr>
<tr><td colspan="4">2. STUDY INFORMATION</td></tr>
<tr><td>a. Study Performed</td><td>b. Date/Time of Administration</td><td colspan="2">c. Previous Radiology Studies (within 72 hrs.)
☐ No _______ Study
_______ Drug(s) Admin.
☐ Yes _______</td></tr>
<tr><td>d. Total Volume Administered</td><td>e. Route of Administration</td><td colspan="2">f. Time Course (ml./min.) of Admin.</td></tr>
<tr><td colspan="4">3. REACTION INFORMATION</td></tr>
<tr><td colspan="2">a. Date/Time of Reaction Onset

b. Observed Reaction(s) (Time Sequence of Events)</td><td colspan="2">c. Outcome
☐ Recovered, no treatment required
☐ Recovered, required following treatment(s):

☐ Alive, with following sequelae:

☐ Expired (date _______)</td></tr>
<tr><td colspan="4">4. PATIENT INFORMATION</td></tr>
<tr><td>a. Name</td><td>b. H.F.H. Hospital No.</td><td>c. Patient Status
☐ IPD ☐ OPD</td><td>d. Age   e. Sex
☐ M ☐ F</td></tr>
</table>

<table>
<tr><td>f. History of</td><td>No</td><td>Yes</td><td></td><td>No</td><td>Yes</td></tr>
<tr><td>(1) Previous contrast reaction(s)</td><td>☐</td><td>☐</td><td>(7) Renal dysfunction
B.U.N. _______
Serum Creat. _______</td><td>☐</td><td>☐</td></tr>
<tr><td>(2) Allergies (i.e. hay fever, asthma, drug sensitivities)</td><td>☐</td><td>☐</td><td>(8) Heart disease(s)
Specify _______</td><td>☐</td><td>☐</td></tr>
<tr><td>(3) Multiple Myeloma</td><td>☐</td><td>☐</td><td></td><td></td><td></td></tr>
<tr><td>(4) Diabetes mellitus</td><td>☐</td><td>☐</td><td></td><td></td><td></td></tr>
<tr><td>(5) Pheochromocytoma</td><td>☐</td><td>☐</td><td>(9) Other significant diseases
Specify _______</td><td>☐</td><td>☐</td></tr>
<tr><td>(6) Other medications last 6 hours Specify _______</td><td>☐</td><td>☐</td><td></td><td></td><td></td></tr>
<tr><td>g. Pretreatment:</td><td>No</td><td>Yes</td><td></td><td>No</td><td>Yes</td></tr>
<tr><td>(1) Antihistamines</td><td>☐</td><td>☐</td><td>(3) Other:</td><td>☐</td><td>☐</td></tr>
<tr><td>(2) Corticosteroids</td><td>☐</td><td>☐</td><td>Specify _______</td><td></td><td></td></tr>
</table>

<table>
<tr><td colspan="4">5. REPORTED/ADMINISTERED BY:</td></tr>
<tr><td>a. Technologist Name</td><td>b. Physician's Name</td><td>c. Division</td><td>d. Date of Report</td></tr>
<tr><td colspan="4">. SIGNATURE (Person Reporting): _______</td></tr>
<tr><td colspan="4" align="center">QUALITY ASSURANCE DOCUMENT — CONFIDENTIAL
MCLA 333.21513, .21515, .20175 331.531. 533</td></tr>
<tr><td colspan="4">DO NOT DUPLICATE OR CIRCULATE — ROUTE VIA PINK CONFIDENTIAL ENVELOPE</td></tr>
</table>

ORIGINAL TO RADIOLOGICAL PHARMACY (ATTN: D. SWANSON) COPY TO QUALITY ASSURANCE DEPT.

Form 6-67 12/84

Figure 8.1 Form for adverse drug reaction reporting.

must keep his knowledge and skills well honed because of the rapidity with which the reactions can take place and therefore the lack of a temporal margin for uncertainty in response.

Reporting Adverse Reactions. Departments of Radiology should develop policies and guidelines for the reporting and review of adverse reactions to contrast media (and all other drugs used in radiology practice). A useful approach is to include the reporting of adverse reactions to contrast media as a quality-assurance monitor in coordination with the hospital quality-assurance program. Such programs are required by the JCAH to encompass the reporting of all drug reactions. The same forms can be used, and all reactions requiring specific therapy should be reported (see Figure 8.1).

References

Andrews EJ The vagus reaction as a possible cause of severe complications of radiological procedures. *Radiology* 1976, 121:1–4.

Ansell G. Adverse reactions to contrast agents: Scope of problem. *Invest Radiol* 1970, 5:374–390.

Ansell G, Tweedie MCK, West CR, et al. The current status of reactions to intravenous contrast media. *Invest Radiol* 1980, 15 (Suppl):S32–S39.

Arroyave CM, Tan EM. Mechanism of complement activation by radiographic contrast media. *Clin Exp Immunol* 1977, 29:89–94.

Assem ESK, Bray K, Dawson: Release of histamine from human basophils by radiological contrast agents. *Br J Radiol* 1983, 56:647–652.

Barnhard HJ, Barnhard FM: The emergency treatment of reactions to contrast media: Update 1968. *Radiology* 1968, 91:74–84.

Baum S, Stein GN, Kuroda KK. Complications of "no arteriography." *Radiology* 1966, 86:835–838.

Becker JA. Prevention of radiocontrast-induced acute renal failure with mannitol. *Lancet* 1980, 1:1147.

Berg GR, Hatter AM, Pfister RC. Electrocardiographic abnormalities associated with intravenous urography. *N Engl J Med* 1973, 289:87–88.

Bettmann MA, Bourdillon MA, Barry WH, et al. Contrast agents for cardiac angiography: Effects of a nonionic agent versus a standard ionic agent. *Radiology* 1984, 153:583–587.

Brasch RC, Rockoff SD, Kuhn C, et al. Contrast media as histamine liberators. II. Histamine release into venous plasma during intravenous urography in man. *Invest Radiol* 1970, 5:510–513.

Brasch RC. Evidence supporting an antibody mediation of contrast media reactions. *Invest Radiol* 1980a, 15 (Suppl):S29–S31.

Brasch RC. Allergic reactions to contrast media: Accumulated evidence. *AJR* 1980b, 134:797–801.

Byrd L, Sherman RL. Radiocontrast-induced acute renal failure: A clinical and pathophysiological review. *Medicine* 1979, 58:270–279.

Carr DH, Walker AC. Contrast media reactions: Experimental evidence against the allergy theory. *Br J Radiol* 1984, 57:469–473.

Cruz C, Hricak H, Samhouri F, et al. Contrast media for angiography: Effect on renal function. *Radiology* 1986, 158:109–112.

Davies P, Roberts MB, Roylance J. Acute reactions to urographic contrast media. *Br Med J [Clin Res]* 1975, 2:434–437.

Davies P, Panto PN, Buckley J, et al. The old and the new. A study of five contrast media for urography. *Br J Radiol* 1985, 58:593–597.

DeSwarte RD. Drug allergy—Problems and strategies. *J Allergy Clin Immunol* 1984, 74:209–221.

DeSwarte RD, Patterson R. Adverse drug reactions: The clinician's role in reporting. *Arch Intern Med* 1986, 146:649–650.

Erffmeyer JE, Siegle RL, Lieberman P. Anaphylactoid reactions to radiocontrast material. *J Allergy Clin Immunol* 1985, 75:401–410.

Fischer HW, Doust VL. An evaluation of pretesting in the problem of serious and fatal reactions to excretory urography. *Radiology* 1971, 103:497–501.

Fischer HW, Thomson KR. Contrast media in coronary arteriography: A review. *Invest Radiol* 1978, 13:450–459.

Goldberg M. Systemic reactions to intravascular contrast media. *Anesthesiology* 1984, 60:46–56.

Gorsette RE, Delmotte P. In vivo activation of serum complement by contrast media: A clinical study. *Invest Radiol* 1980, 15 (Suppl):S26–S28.

Gooding CA, Bordon WE, Brodear AE, et al. Adverse reactions to intravenous pyelography in children. *AJR* 1975, 123:802–804.

Grainger RE. A clinical trial of a new low-osmolality contrast medium: Sodium and meglumine ioxaglate (Hexabrix) compared with meglumine iothalamate (Conray) for carotid arteriography. *Br J Radiol* 1979, 52:781–786.

Grainger RE. Osmolality of intravascular radiological contrast media. *Br J Radiol* 1980, 53:739–746.

Greenberger PA. Contrast media reactions. *J Allergy Clin Immunol* 1984, 74:600–605.

Greenberger PA, Patterson R, Tapio CM. Prophylaxis against repeated radiocontrast media reactions in 857 cases. *Arch Intern Med* 1985, 145:2197–2200.

Hartman GW, Hattery R, Witten DM, et al. Mortality during excretory urography: Mayo Clinic Experience. *AJR* 1982, 139:919–922.

Harvey LA, Caldicott WJH, Kuruc A. The effect of contrast media on immature renal function. *Radiology* 1983, 148:429–432.

Hasselbacker P, Hahn J. In vitro effects of radiographic contrast media on the complement system. *J Allergy Clin Immunol* 1980, 66:217–222.

Hobbs BB. Adverse reactions to intravenous contrast agents in Ontario, 1975–1979. *J Can Assoc Radiol* 1981, 32:8–10.

Kalimo K, Jansen CT, Kormano M. Allergological risk factors as predictors of radiographic contrast media hypersensitivity. *Ann Allergy* 1980, 45:253–255.

Kaliner M, Dyer J, Merlin S et al: Increased urine histamine and contrast media reactions *Invest Radial* 1984: 19:116–118.

Kelly JF, Patterson R, Lieberman P, et al.

Radiographic contrast media studies in high-risk patients. *J Allergy Clin Immunol* 1978, 62:181–184.

Kolb WP, Lang JH, Lasser EC. Nonimmunologic complement activation in normal human serum induced by radiographic contrast media. *J. Immunol* 1978, 121:1232–1238.

Lalli AF. Urographic contrast media and anxiety. *Radiology* 1974, 112:267–271.

Lalli AF. Contrast media reactions: Data analysis and hypothesis. *Radiology* 1980, 134:1–12.

Lalli AF, Greenstreet R. Reactions to contrast media: Testing the CNS hypothesis. *Radiology* 1981, 138:47–49.

Lang EK, Foreman J, Schlagel JU, et al. The incidence of contrast medium-induced acute tubular necrosis following arteriography. *Radiology* 1981, 138:203–206.

Lang JH, Lasser EC, Kolb WP. Activation of serum complement by contrast media. *Invest Radiol* 1976, 11:303–308.

Lasser EC. Adverse reactions to intravascular administration of contrast media. *Allergy* 1981, 36:369–373.

Lasser EC. Etiology of anaphylactoid responses: The promise of the nonionics. *Invest Radiol* 1985, 20:579–583.

Lasser EC, Lang JH, Lyon SG, et al. Complement and contrast material reactors. *J Allergy Clin Immunol* 1979, 64:105–112.

Lasser EC, Berry CC, Talner LB, et al. Pretreatment with corticosteroids to alleviate reactions to intravascular contrast media. *N Engl J Med* 1987, 317:845–849.

Lasser EC, Lang JH, Hamblin AE, et al. Activation systems in contrast idiosyncrasy. *Invest Radiol* 1980, 15 (Suppl):S2–S5.

Lasser EC, Lang JH, Lyon SG, et al. Changes in complement and coagulation factors in a patient suffering a severe anaphylactoid reaction to injected contrast material: Some considerations of pathogenesis. *Invest Radiol* 1980, 15 (Suppl):S6–S12.

Lasser EC, Lang JH, Lyon SG, et al.

Prekallikrein-kallikrein conversion rate as a predictor of contrast-material catastrophies. *Radiology* 1981, 140:11–15.

Lasser EC, Sliuka J, Lang JH, et al. Complement and coagulation: Causative considerations in contrast catastrophies. *AJR* 1979, 132:171–176.

Lieberman P, Siegle RL, Taylor WW. Anaphylactoid reactions to iodinated contrast material. *J Allergy Clin Immunol* 1978, 62:174–180.

Littner MR, Rosenfield AT, Ulreich S. Evaluation of bronchospasm during excretory urography. *Radiology* 1977, 124:17–21.

Madowitz JS, Schweiger MJ. Severe anaphylactoid reaction to radiographic contrast media: Recurrence despite premedication with diphenhydramine and prednisone. *JAMA* 1979, 241:2813–2815.

National Conference on Cardiopulmonary Resuscitation (CPR) and Emergency Cardiac Care (ECC); Standards and Guidelines for Cardiopulmonary Resuscitation and Emergency Cardiac Care. *JAMA* 1986, 255:2905–2984.

Ochsner SF, Calonje MA. Reactions to intravenous iodides in urography *South Med J* 1971, 64:907–911.

Pagani JJ, Hayman LA, Bigelow RH, et al. Diazepam prophylaxis of contrast media-induced seizures during computed tomography of patients with brain metastases. *AJR* 1983, 140:787–792.

Panto PN, Davies P. Delayed reactions to urographic contrast media. *Br J Radiol* 1986, 59:41–44.

Patterson R, Valentine M. Anaphylaxis and related allergic emergencies including reactions due to insect stings. *JAMA* 1982, 248:2632–2636.

Patterson R, Anderson J Allergic reactions to drugs and biologic agents. *JAMA* 1982, 248:2637–2645.

Pfister RC, Hutter AM, Newhouse JH, et al. Contrast medium-induced electrocardiographic abnormalities. *AJR* 1983, 140:149–153.

Rapoport S, Bookstein JJ, Higgins CB, et al. Experience with metrizamide in patients with previous severe anaphylactoid reactions to ionic contrast agents. *Radiology* 1982, 143:321–325.

Ring J, Arroyave CM, Frizler MJ, et al. In vitro histamine and serotonin release by radiographic contrast media (RCM). *Clin Exp Immunol* 1978, 32:105–118.

Rockoff SD, Brasch R, Kuhn C, et al. Contrast media as histamine liberators. I. Mast-cell histamine release in vitro by sodium salts of contrast media. *Invest Radiol* 1970, 5:503–509.

Rockoff SD, Kuhn C, Chraplyvy M. Contrast media as histamine liberators. V. Comparison of in vitro mast cell histamine release by sodium and methylglucamine salts. *Invest Radiol* 1972, 7:177.

Schrott KM, Behrends B, Clauss W, et al. Iohexol in excretory urography. *Fortschr Med* 1986, 104:153–156.

Shehadi WH. Adverse reactions to intravenously administered contrast media. *AJR* 1975, 124:145–152.

Shehadi WH. Contrast media adverse reactions: Occurrence, recurrence, and distribution patterns. *Radiology* 1982, 143:11–17.

Shehadi WH, Toniolo G. Adverse reactions to contrast media. *Radiology* 1980, 137:299–302.

Siegle RL, Lieberman P. A review of untoward reactions to iodinated contrast material. *J Urol* 1978, 119:581–587.

Siegle RL, Lieberman P, Jennings BR, et al. Iodinated contrast material: Studies relating to complement activation, atopy cellular association and antigenicity. *Invest Radiol* 1980, 15 (Suppl):S13–S17.

Siegle RL, Lieberman P, Rice MC. In vitro complement consumption by contrast materials and analogues: Reactors vs. nonreactors. *Invest Radiol* 1983, 18:387–389.

Simon RA, Schatz M, Stevenson DD, et al. Radiographic contrast media infusions: Measurement of histamine, complement and fibrin split products and correlation with clinical parameters. *J Allergy Clin Immunol* 1979, 63:281–288.

Small P, Satin R, Palayew MJ, et al. Prophylactic antihistamines in the management of radiographic contrast reactions. *Clin Allergy* 1982, 12:289–294.

Stadalnik RC, Vera Z, DaSilva O, et al. Electrocardiographic response to intravenous urography: Prospective evaluation of 275 patients. *AJR* 1977, 129:825–830.

Stanley RJ, Pfister RC. Bradycardia and hypotension following use of intravenous contrast media. *Radiology* 1976, 121:5–7.

Swanson DP, Dick TJ, Simms SM, et al. Product selection criteria for intravascular ionic contrast media. *Clin Pharm* 1985, 14:527–538.

Swanson DP, Thrall JH, Shetty PC. Evaluation of intravascular low-osmolality contrast agents. *Clin Pharm* 1986, 5:8771–891

Swartz RD, Rubin JE, Leeming BW, et al. Renal failure following major angiography. *Am J Med* 1978; 65:31–37.

Till G, Rother U, Gemsa D. Activation of complement by radiographic contrast media: Generation of chemotactic and anaphylatoxin activities. *Int Arch Allergy Appl Immunol* 1978, 56:543–550.

Turner, E, Kentor P, Melamed JL, et al. Frequency of anaphylactoid reactions during intravenous urography with radiographic contrast media at two different temperatures. *Radiology* 1982, 143:327–329.

VanSonnenberg E, Neff CC, Pfister RC. Life-threatening hypotensive reactions to contrast media administration: Comparison of pharmacologic and fluid therapy. *Radiology* 1987, 162:15–19.

Witten DM. Reactions to urographic contrast media. *JAMA* 1975, 231:974–977.

Witten DM, Hirsch FD, Hartman GW. Acute reactions to urographic contrast medium. *AJR* 1973, 119:832–840.

Yocum MW, Heller AM, Abels RI. Efficacy of intravenous pretesting and antihistamine prophylaxis in radiocontrast media-sensitive patients. *J Allergy Clin Immunol* 1978, 62:309–313.

RADIOPHARMACEUTICALS

CHAPTER
9
▼▼▼

Fundamentals of Radiopharmaceuticals

Henry M. Chilton
Richard L. Witcofski

Nuclear medicine is the relatively new field of medical practice that employs unsealed forms of radioactive materials for diagnosis and therapy. These clinical applications of radioactivity center upon two different approaches: *in vivo* studies and *in vitro* techniques.

As the name implies, in vivo studies involve the administration of radioactivity to patients usually by oral or intravenous means. The majority of in vivo applications involve the determination of diagnostic information (such as organ function, shape, or position) from a picture, or image, of the radioactivity distribution within that organ or body part. Certain types of radioactivity are also administered for therapeutic purposes and deliver relatively high doses of radiation to selected tissues.

With in vitro methods, radioactive materials are not administered to the patient, but rather body fluids or tissues are analyzed by radioimmunoassay and other techniques that utilize radioactivity. The radioactive drugs used for all these purposes differ in many ways from traditional pharmaceuticals; hence, specialized knowledge is required of the physicians, pharmacists, and technologists who are responsible for their handling and use.

EARLY USES OF RADIOACTIVITY

By most accounts, the earliest application of radioactivity for diagnostic purposes occurred around 1927 when Blumgart, Yens, and Weiss determined circulation times by injecting Radium C into one antecubital vein and observed its arrival in the other arm using a cloud chamber as the detection device. In 1934, Hevesy, another pioneer in radioactivity, used the principle of isotope dilution to determine the water content of the human body following the administration of deuterated ("heavy") water. For practical purposes, however, the use of radioactive materials as diagnostic and therapeutic drugs began in the United States in 1946 when radionuclides produced at the Oak Ridge, Tennessee, reactor were made available for biological and medicinal applications. Clinical determinations of the suitability and usefulness of radioactive materials in medicine soon followed, and the concept of nuclear medicine was born.

Initially, radioactive materials employed in medicine were called "radiotracers," since the radionuclides were often radioisotopes of biologically relevant elements, such as iodine or calcium, that were used to trace the biological distribution (biodistribution) of these elements (Means JH, 1955; Heaney RP and Whedon GD, 1958). These early "radiotracer" agents were simple chemical forms, such as sodium or chloride salts of radioactive metals, in which the nonradioactive portion of the compound had little effect upon its biological behavior. The biodistribution depended largely upon the elemental properties of the radionuclide (e. g., radioiodine for thyroid function studies).

With time, however, more and more radionuclides were developed that were neither radioisotopes of biologically occurring elements nor their analogs, yet possessed attractive nuclear properties for use in medical imaging.

In many cases, radiochemical techniques were developed to complex these radionuclides onto various chemical components that provided tissue-specificity for the radionuclide, thus allowing the use of an individual radionuclide for a variety of diagnostic or therapeutic applications. Because of these developments, the term "radiotracer" gradually evolved into "radioactive pharmaceutical" and eventually to *radiopharmaceutical*, a term that has endured until today (Briner WH, 1965; 1968).

Although the term *pharmaceutical* implies therapeutic properties, the vast majority of radiopharmaceuticals are used for diagnostic purposes. This diagnostic capability results from the type of radiation (gamma rays) emitted by the agents employed in nuclear medicine, since these radiations become externally accessible for detection and imaging. Alternatively, radionuclides that emit highly ionizing beta radiations that are absorbed locally are chosen for selective therapeutic irradiation of tissues or malignancy. At present, more than 95% of nuclear medicine procedures are diagnostic in nature. Therapeutic applications that account for the remaining studies involve the treatment of hyperthyroidism, thyroid cancer, polycythemia vera, or malignant effusion.

Radiopharmaceuticals differ from traditional pharmaceuticals in several other important ways. First, like most other diagnostic agents that are employed for imaging, radiopharmaceuticals are administered only infrequently, usually as a single dose, to achieve the diagnostic result (similar to x-ray contrast materials). Radiopharmaceuticals are usually administered intravenously so that tissue biodistribution will occur rapidly, and the opportunity will be highest for radiopharmaceutical localization in the tissues of interest (e. g., the "target" tissues). Occasionally, special routes of administration will be required in order to achieve optimal localization within the target tissues. Radioactive gases, for example, that are used to observe lung ventilation function, are necessarily administered by inhalation, whereas studies of cerebrospinal fluid (CSF) kinetics are performed by administering the radiopharmaceutical directly into the spinal cord.

Pictures, or images, of the radiopharmaceutical localized within a given organ or tissue are called *scintiphotos* (Figure 9.1) and are obtained at a period of time post-administration when target-tissue uptake is high and blood and soft tissue levels ("background") are sufficiently low to permit adequate visualization of the organ of interest. Specialized cameras that capture radiation emissions and relate them to their origin within the body are employed to gather and display this type of information. In the majority of cases, the information display is planar, with the imaging plane most often parallel to the camera surface. Computer-assisted reconstruction techniques are available today, however, that permit three-dimensional tomographic projections in almost any orientation.

Unlike most other pharmaceuticals and contrast-enhancement agents, which depend upon relatively large amounts of drug to achieve the desired effect, only very small quantities of radiopharmaceuticals are necessary to perform diagnostic imaging. The radionuclide component of most radiopharmaceuticals provides levels of 10^{-5}–10^{-9} mg/kg body weight, thus enabling the safe use of radioisotopes of even the most toxic elements. It follows that adverse effects associated with the use of radiopharmaceuticals are extremely rare (see Adverse Reactions Involving Radiopharmaceuticals), and those that do occur usually involve hypersensitivity reactions.

PRINCIPLES OF RADIOACTIVITY

The phenomenon of radioactivity was discovered around the turn of this century in naturally occurring elements such as

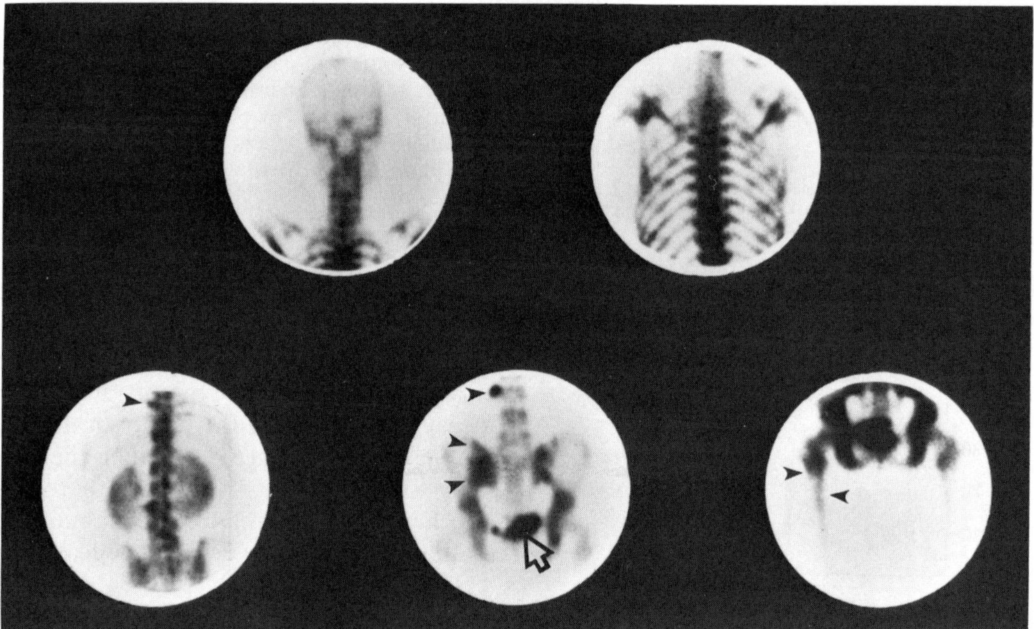

Figure 9.1 Scintillation images of patient injected Tc-99m medronate (MDP), a radiopharmaceutical that localizes in bone with relatively higher uptake in boney lesions (arrows) and areas of skeletal trauma. The relatively large amount of activity noted in the anterior pelvic views (arrow head) is within the bladder. Approximately one-half the administered dosage of these radiopharmaceuticals is excreted by the kidneys via glomerular filtration.

radium, polonium, and thorium. Radioactivity was explained by Rutherford and Soddy in 1910 as a process that transforms atoms of an unstable element into a stable element through the emission of energy. Why some atoms of an element are stable and others are unstable and radioactive is not fully understood but apparently involves the number of protons and neutrons in the atom. In stable atoms that are small and less complex, protons and neutrons are essentially equal in number. As atoms become larger, however, relatively more neutrons must be present for stability.

When the ratio of protons to neutrons is outside the range of stability (Figure 9.2), the unstable atoms seek stability by changing to a more favorable proton-to-neutron balance. This process, which is accompanied by the emission of energy (radiation), is known as radioactive transformation or "decay" and involves a decrease in the number of radioactive atoms with time. The time necessary for the decay of radioactive atoms to one-half their original number is known as the physical half-life and is specific for any given radionuclide.

TYPES OF RADIATION

Alpha Radiation. Alpha particles are emitted from the nuclei of the very heavy naturally occurring elements. Because of their mass and charge (they are composed of two protons and two neutrons), alpha particles are the least penetrating form of radiation and are usually absorbed or stopped within a few centimeters of air. Alpha particles do not penetrate tissues and currently have no applications in diagnostic nuclear medicine. It has been suggested, however, that notwithstanding the difficulties encountered in their use and safe handling, radionuclides that decay by alpha emission may prove useful for therapeutic applications.

Beta Radiation. Beta radiation also originates in the nucleus and may be either negatively (B^-) or positively (B^+) charged. The B^- particle is emitted during a nuclear transformation in which a neutron is converted into a proton; the B^+ particle is formed when a

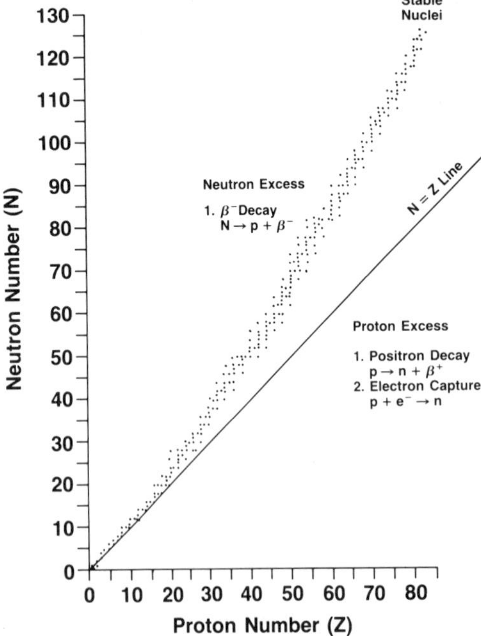

Figure 9.2 Proton-neutron plot of stable nuclei (represented by dots). Note that stable nuclei tend to have a neutron excess (i.e., lie above the nuetron = proton, N = Z, line). Increasing the neutron imbalance, however, creates unstable nuclei that favor decay by B⁻ emission. Unstable nuclei created by too few neutrons favor decay by either positron (B⁺) emission or electron capture.

proton is converted into a neutron. In air, beta particles travel several meters; in tissues, up to a few millimeters. In nuclear medicine, B⁻ radiation is employed primarily for therapeutic applications. B⁺ emissions are utilized in a special form of diagnostic imaging called positron emission tomography (PET).

Gamma Rays. Unlike the particulate emissions of alpha and beta radiations, gamma rays are a form of electromagnetic radiation that are highly penetrating and travel at the speed of light. Gamma rays originate within the nucleus as a result of transitions between energy levels and therefore have one or a few discrete energies. Gamma ray emission is of primary importance in radionuclides that are utilized to prepare radiopharmaceuticals for diagnostic purposes.

Characteristic X-rays. Characteristic x-rays are also a form of electromagnetic radiation; however, the essential difference between gamma rays and characteristic x-rays is in their origin and their energy spectrum. X-rays are generated by energy transitions occurring within the electron shells of an atom. For example, some radioactive decay processes result in the loss of an inner orbital electron from an atom. When outer electrons fill these inner vacancies, x-rays whose energies are characteristic of that particular atom are produced.

TYPES OF RADIOACTIVE DECAY

In general, radionuclides may decay by any one of five different decay processes or a combination of these processes. With any radionuclide, the type of radioactive decay depends upon the nature of the unstable nucleus, that is, whether there is only excess energy or whether there are too many protons relative to the number of neutrons, or vice versa. The decay processes, as outlined in this section, result in the emission of particles or energy as the radioactive atom seeks to become stable. After decay has occurred, the transformed nucleus (daughter radionuclide) may be either stable or radioactive.

Alpha Decay. During alpha decay, the atomic number (Z) and atomic mass number (A) decrease by 2 and 4, respectively (Figure 9.2). Radionuclides that decay by alpha emission are not important at present in nuclear medicine, but alpha particles might have future therapeutic applications.

Beta Minus. Radioactive nuclei that contain too many neutrons emit negatively charged beta particles as a neutron changes to a proton. While the mass number of the nucleus remains the same, its atomic number increases by 1. A gamma ray may or may not accompany the emission of the B⁻ particle. Several radiopharmaceuticals are composed of radionuclides that decay by B⁻ emission (Table 9.1).

B⁺ (positron) Decay. Positron decay occurs in the nuclei with excessive numbers of protons and sufficient energy to convert a proton into a neutron. The B⁺ particle (a positive electron or positron) loses energy over a very short distance and then interacts with a negative electron in a nearby atom. At the moment of this interaction (called "annihilation"), two gamma rays are emitted in opposite directions, each with an energy of 511 keV. These gamma rays are suitable for obtaining tomographic images using special radiation detectors that detect these "paired" gamma rays in "coincidence," thus eliminating other extraneous radiations. These imaging devices and the

Table 9.1   SELECTED RADIONUCLIDES USED IN NUCLEAR MEDICINE

RADIONUCLIDE	PHYSICAL HALF-LIFE	DECAY MODE	PRIMARY MODE OF PRODUCTION	
			Reactor	*Accelerator*
Tc-99m	6.0 hrs	I.T.	√	
I-131	8.0 days	B⁻	√	
T1-201	73.1 hrs	E.C.		√
Ga-67	78.1 hrs	E.C.		√
Xe-127	36.4 days	E.C.		√
Xe-133	5.27 days	B⁻	√	
I-123	13.0 hrs	E.C.		√
In-111	2.81 days	E.C.		√
C-11	20.3 min	B⁺		√
N-13	10 min	B⁺		√
O-15	2.0 min	B⁺		√
F-18	110 min	B⁺		√

technique of tomographic reconstruction using positron-emitting radionuclides (PET), can be employed to image a variety of short-lived positron-emitting radionuclides (Table 9.1).

Gamma Decay (Isomerism). Unlike alpha and beta decay, during gamma decay, the nucleus changes only in its energy status, from high to low, by the emission of a gamma ray. Therefore, during gamma decay, both the mass number and the atomic number of the decaying radionuclide and the daughter remain the same, and the nuclide pair are known as isomers. In most cases, the radioactive half-life of the parent or energetic nucleus is very short (less than 10^{-10} seconds) but may be as long as several minutes or hours. Whenever this prolonged transitional state occurs, the decaying radionuclide is called metastable (indicated by adding an "m" to the mass number). In nuclear medicine, the metastable radionuclide Tc-99m is the most commonly utilized radionuclide.

Electron Capture. Radioactive nuclei that contain relatively larger amounts of protons tend to decay by electron capture whereby the nucleus "captures" an inner orbital electron and converts a proton into a neutron. As outer shell electrons move inward to fill the vacancy created by the electron capture, characteristic x-rays are emitted.

Units of Radioactivity. Traditional pharmaceuticals are prescribed in well-known units of weight (grams or molar-equivalents) or volume, whereas radiopharmaceuticals are dispensed in amounts of activity that are expressions of the decay rate of the contained radionuclide. The development of the traditional unit of radioactivity, called curie, was based upon the presumed rate of decay of one gram of radium-226 (3.7×10^{10} disintegrating atoms per second). Because the curie is so large, the millicurie and the microcurie are more commonly used as expressions of radioactivity.

$$
\begin{aligned}
1 \text{ curie (Ci)} &= 3.7 \times 10^{10} \text{ dps} \\
&= 2.2 \times 10^{12} \text{ dpm} \\
1 \text{ millicurie (mCi)} &= 3.7 \times 10^{7} \text{ dps} \\
&= 2.2 \times 10^{9} \text{ dpm} \\
1 \text{ microcurie } (\mu\text{Ci}) &= 3.7 \times 10^{4} \text{ dps} \\
&= 2.2 \times 10^{6} \text{ dpm}
\end{aligned}
$$

Recently, the becquerel, which is a measurement unit of the Systeme Internationale (SI), has been proposed as a replacement for the curie [1 becquerel (Bq) = 1 disintegration/second].

$$
\begin{aligned}
1 \text{ becquerel (Bq)} &= 1 \text{ dps} \\
&= 2.703 \times 10^{-11} \text{ Ci} \\
1 \text{ kilobecquerel (kBq)} &= 10^{3} \text{ dps} \\
&= 2.703 \times 10^{-8} \text{ Ci} \\
1 \text{ megabecquerel (MBq)} &= 10^{6} \text{ dps} \\
&= 2.703 \times 10^{-5} \text{ Ci} \\
1 \text{ gigabecquerel (GBq)} &= 10^{9} \text{ dps} \\
&= 2.703 \times 10^{-2} \text{ Ci} \\
1 \text{ terabecquerel (TBq)} &= 10^{12} \text{ dps} \\
&= 27.03 \text{ Ci}
\end{aligned}
$$

The two units of radioactivity are related as follows:

$$
\begin{aligned}
1 \text{ microcurie} &= 37 \text{ kilobecquerels} \\
&\quad (0.037 \text{ megabecquerels}) \\
1 \text{ millicurie} &= 37 \text{ megabecquerels} \\
1 \text{ curie} &= 37 \text{ gigabecquerels}
\end{aligned}
$$

PRODUCTION OF RADIOACTIVITY

Several radionuclides occur in nature as members of chains, or series, of radioactive elements, beginning with thorium-232, actinium-235, and uranium-238, and decay to stable isotopes of lead. These radionuclides constitute "natural" radioactivity and, with few exceptions, have no usefulness in medicine today. All radionuclides currently used in medicine are artificially produced.

Man-made radionuclides are produced by bombarding nuclei of stable elements with subatomic particles (such as neutrons or protons) in order to create unstable proton/neutron ratios. That radioactivity could be made by man was first demonstrated during the 1930s by Joliot and Curie when they produced radioactivity by bombarding light elements with natural alpha particles and by Fermi and others who used radium combined with beryllium to form a neutron source that was used to create a variety of radionuclides.

Today, this process of preparing radionuclides (known as nuclear reaction, or activation) occurs primarily in either a nuclear reactor (neutron activation) or a particle accelerator, such as a cyclotron (proton bombardment).

PRODUCTS OF NUCLEAR REACTORS

Neutron Activation. Nuclear reactors serve as sources of low-energy neutrons that can be used to bombard nuclei of stable atoms to produce unstable (radioactive) nuclei. In the process, the stable nucleus (or target) "captures" a neutron to produce an unstable nucleus that is neutron rich. Radionuclides prepared in this manner decay by β^- emission, often with accompanying gamma emissions that may be useful for diagnostic imaging purposes. The product of neutron activation is a radiosotope of the target nucleus, since both are of the same proton number (no change in proton number occurs).

$$X \,(n, \gamma)\, X^*$$

where,

$$X \;=\; \text{stable target}$$
$$X^* \;=\; \text{radioactive product}$$

NOTE: both X and X^* are "isotopes" of each other, since they possess the same number of protons. X^*, however, is a "radioisotope" of X, since it is radioactive.

Since most of the stable atoms are not activated during the neutron bombardment process, they are carried over into the final product (the target and product nuclei share the same proton number and hence have the same chemical nature). In radiochemistry, these stable atoms are known as *carrier* atoms because they were once purposefully employed to "carry" the much smaller number of radioactive atoms during certain types of chemical syntheses and prevent their plating onto glassware. Carrier atoms are undesirable because their presence may affect radiopharmaceutical biodistribution or toxicity. Most radiopharmaceutical products today are described as either *carrier-free* or *no-carrier-added* (Wolf AP, 1981).

Fission Products. Neutron bombardment of fissionable materials results in the immediate formation of a highly unstable nucleus that promptly breaks into two smaller radioactive fragments (fission products). In practice, the most widely used fission material is uranium-235. Since in nature nonfissionable U-238 is the principal isotope of uranium (99.3% vs. 0.7% natural abundance for U-235), the concentration of U-235 to U-238 is sometimes increased or "enriched." When an atom of U-235 captures a neutron, the resulting nucleus exists for only a fraction of a second before it splits into fission fragments and more neutrons. In the fission reaction in a reactor, the emission of neutrons is maintained at a level that will sustain a nuclear chain reaction so that the energy emitted through fission may be used to generate power. Fission products of these reactions are generally from atomic mass numbers of about 70 to

170 but are most often split in a 40:60 ratio, with peaks at mass numbers of 90 and 140. Many of the by-products of this fission reaction are radionuclides that are useful for incorporation into radiopharmaceuticals, including radioisotopes of xenon, iodine, and molybdenum.

Proton Bombardment

In proton bombardment, positively charged protons are accelerated to energies sufficient to overcome repulsion by the positively charged nuclei. As a result, a proton can enter the nucleus to produce changes in the atomic number with accompanying nuclear instability. This nuclear rearrangement leaves the nucleus in an excited state that is described as being proton-rich (or neutron-deficient). Radionuclides prepared in this manner regain stability by undergoing electron capture (EC), with accompanying characteristic x-ray production, or by positron (B^+) emission.

Radionuclide Generators

Radiopharmaceuticals composed of radionuclides that have short half-lives are most desirable for use in medicine for several reasons. First, the rapid decay of short-lived radionuclides results in lower radiation dose to the patient. Second, short-lived radionuclides yield high intensities of gamma ray photons, thereby providing the count rates that are necessary for high-resolution images. In summary, short-lived radionuclides can be administered in relatively large amounts and yield significantly greater numbers of photons than radionuclides that decay at much slower rates.

Very short-lived radionuclides, however, often present special problems in availability. Supplying these radionuclides to sites great distances from their reactor or accelerator-production facilities often necessitates rapid daily shipments. The problems and expense associated with air freight shipments, however, can be overcome with the use of radionuclide *generators*. These devices, which contain a rel-atively longer-lived parent radionuclide that decays to a shorter-lived daughter radionuclide, make possible the convenient supply of these highly desirable radionuclides.

Radionuclide generators make use of the existing relationship between two radionuclides in which a relatively longer-lived radionuclide (the parent) continually decays to form a short-lived radionuclide (the daughter) (Richards P, 1966). The parent radionuclide, prepared in either a nuclear reactor or an accelerator, is chemically bound or adsorbed onto some type of anion exchange column (such as aluminum oxide). The column containing the parent radionuclide is housed within a glass sleeve that is prepared in a sterile and apyrogenic manner. Because the daughter radionuclide is chemically different from the parent, it binds loosely to the anion exchange material, allowing separation and collection in some type of solvent system that serves as a vehicle for efficient removal without removing the parent radionuclide. Physiologic solutions (such as normal saline) are preferred because they facilitate patient administration without the need for extensive chemical manipulation that would otherwise be required to render the radionuclide suitable for use in humans.

The separation of the daughter radionuclide from the parent is known as elution (or more commonly, "milking"), and the radionuclide generator is usually called a "cow." Because the parent radionuclide is continually decaying to form a new daughter radionuclide, the process of daughter elution can be repeated several times until decay of the parent results in such a low level of activity that only a minimal amount of daughter activity is formed. The entire process of elution is conveniently accomplished in a closed system in order to maintain sterility.

In nuclear medicine, the Tc-99m daughter radionuclide supplied by the Mo-99/Tc-99m generator is employed in more than 90% of the in vivo studies performed today. The relatively convenient means of operation of the Mo-99/Tc-99m generator and its high degree of reliability, coupled with the extremely desirable imaging properties of Tc-99m, have made it the cornerstone of nuclear medicine practice. The Mo-99/Tc-99m radionuclide generator was developed in 1966 by Powell Richards at the Brookhaven National Laboratory. The characteristics of operation of this generator remain much the same as its original design. The ion exchange material is alumimun trioxide, and a vacuum-assisted process is employed for the removal and collection of the daughter radionuclide, Tc-99m. In the milking process, normal saline is "pulled" over the column containing the parent-daughter radionuclide pair by placing a sterile, pyrogen-free evacuated vial at the end opposite the saline source. Various quality-control procedures on the generator product are desirable to ensure that the material obtained is of the highest purity and does not contain appreciable amounts of either the longer-lived parent (Mo-99, physical half-life 67 hours) or the alumimun trioxide employed to prepare the ion exchange column. In the former case, the presence of Mo-99 in generator eluate administered to patients could result in significantly larger radiation exposures than necessary. In the latter case, altered biodistribution of some Tc-99m radiopharmaceuticals has been associated with the presence of aluminum ions contained in the generator eluate used to prepare these radiopharmaceuticals.

In the case of the Mo-99/Tc-99m generator, the daughter radionuclide, Tc-99m sodium pertechnetate, can be administered directly to patients because its biodistribution closely mimics that of iodide. It can also be used to radiolabel a variety of other tissue-specific radiopharmaceuticals, such as those employed for bone, liver, lung, and renal imaging. The 6.0-hour physical half-life of Tc-99m, coupled with its isomeric decay mode and 140 keV principal photon, is nearly ideal for use in diagnostic imaging.

Limitations to the use of Tc-99m are principally related to its chemical char-acteristics. In practice, complex formation with technetium occurs primarily with compounds possessing hydrophilic groups, such as hydroxyl, carboxylic acid or phosphate moieties; compounds composed largely of lipophilic groups do not bind technetium (Richards P and Steigman J, 1975). Because chemical techniques for labeling with Tc-99m involve acidic media, only compounds stable under these conditions are suitable for Tc-99m labeling. Unfortunately, many biological compounds and a significant number of drug products are predominantly lipid soluble or unstable at acid pH and cannot be successfully labeled with Tc-99m.

Even though a particular compound can be radiolabeled with Tc-99m, this radionuclide may not be the most desirable radiolabel especially for those materials that possess lengthy blood clearance or slow target uptake and thereby undergo considerable decay before sufficient amounts of the materials are taken up by the desired tissues (i.e., high target: nontarget ratios are achieved). For these compounds and biological agents, as well as those that cannot be labeled with Tc-99m other means for radiolabeling and different radionuclides are required (see Other Radionuclides).

Radioisotopes of Iodine. Radioisotopes of iodine were among the earliest radionuclides employed in medicine, and their use continues today. Radioiodine can be used in its salt form (simple sodium iodide) or it can be employed for radioiodination of certain compounds or biological materials. The process of radioiodination is largely governed by the oxidation state of iodine (the I_2 state is required). All radioiodination methods, then, use potent oxidizing substances that can damage the compound to be labeled. In radioiodination, iodide binds firmly to aromatic compounds with the primary binding site on proteins occurring at the tyrosyl group; the next important binding site is the imidazole ring of histidine (Francis GE, et al, 1951, Hughes WL and Straessle R, 1950).

Among the 24 known radioisotopes of

iodine, only three (I-123, I-125, and I-131 have properties suitable for use in medicine (Myers WG, 1966).

Other Radionuclides. Indium-111, a cyclotron product, is useful for the preparation of several radiopharmaceuticals (Thakur M and Gottschalk A, 1980). In the free ionic state, In-111 behaves much like iron and will bind many of the same serum proteins, including transferrin. Although its behavior is not identical to that of iron (it is not involved in erythropoiesis), its distribution in bone marrow closely parallels that of iron, so that it is useful in the evaluation of bone marrow function related to hematopoiesis.

As In-111 oxine, this radionuclide can be employed for the radiolabeling of cellular blood products, including leukocytes and platelets. It can also be bound to larger chelate structures (such as DTPA, or pentetate) and employed for the study of cerebrospinal fluid (CSF) kinetics. Chromium-51 sodium chromate is often used in nuclear medicine to label red blood cells and certain types of proteins, such as human serum albumin. A variety of other radionuclides are used in nuclear medicine, including radioisotopes of xenon (Xe-133 and Xe-127), phosphorous-32, gallium-67, thallium-201.

PRINCIPLES OF RADIATION DETECTION

In nuclear medicine, several different types of radiation-detection systems are required to accurately measure radiation exposure rates and amounts of radioactivity, to identify types of radioactivity, and to accurately depict the biodistribution of radioactivity or to measure its concentration in tissue samples (i. e., blood and urine). Images of radioactivity localized within body organs and vascular spaces are obtained with electronic systems that depict relative concentrations of activity.

Radiation detection is based upon the ability of radiation to ionize molecules. Ionizing radiation dissipates energy into matter with the subsequent transformation of energy into a measurable signal. This signal can be employed to generate either electrical pulses (counts) as in a Geiger-Mueller counter, or steady electrical current that permits the detection and measurement of radioactivity. The interaction of radiation within a radiation detector, such as the gamma scintillation camera, provides the basis of the nuclear medicine image, the type of specialized pictures that portray the positional distribution of radioactivity within the body.

THE SCINTILLATION DETECTOR

In nuclear medicine, the most commonly utilized piece of equipment is the scintillation camera (Figure 9.3), which is also known as the gamma camera, or Anger camera. The basic scintillation detector is a crystal composed of a substance that becomes fluorescent whenever energy, such as ionizing radiation, is absorbed (most other clinical instruments that measure radioactivity, but do not always express its presence as an image, also utilize scintillation-detector crystals). In the detector, the energy transformation from interaction with a gamma ray culminates in a photoelectric effect and the formation of a flash of light (i. e., scintillation). The amount of energy that is deposited within the crystal by the gamma ray, which depends upon the energy of the gamma ray, is proportional to the brightness of the flash of light.

The fluorescent material that makes up scintillation detectors is sodium iodide that has been "spiked" with small amounts of impurity atoms, known as "activators," that are added in order to produce usable scintillations. Because the activators in the sodium iodide detector system employed in nuclear medicine are thallium (Tl) atoms, the detectors are described as NaI(Tl) crystals.

In a simple scintillation detector, the crystal interfaces directly to a photomultiplier tube (PMT) (Figure 9.4), a device that converts light to an amplified electrical pulse. The pulse is then transmitted

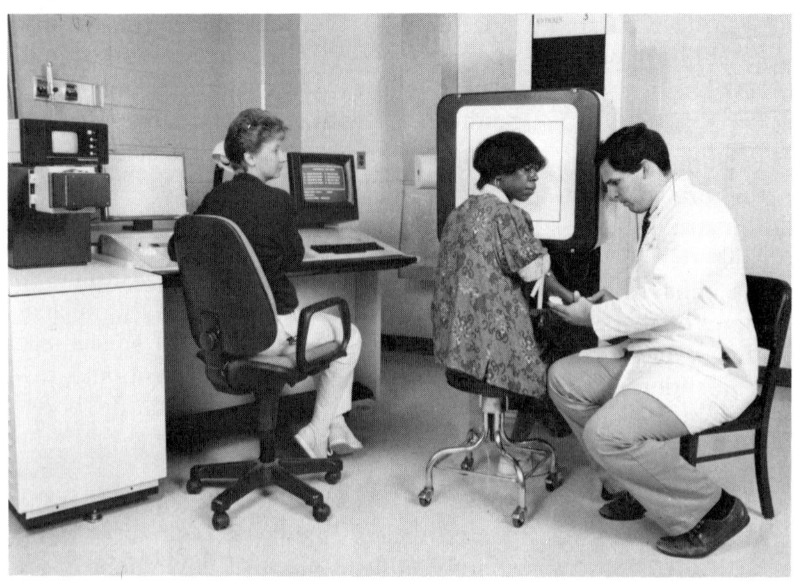

Figure 9.3 Gamma scintillation camera with patient shown undergoing brain imaging. The patient is positioned in the desired orientation to permit visualization of a known lesion during perfusion imaging (see also Figure 9.4).

through a preamplifier to the main electronics for additional amplification. Within the PMT, the electronic pulses are multiplied to form a voltage output pulse that is directly proportional to gamma ray energy. After the pulses are linearly increased in size by an amplifier, they are sorted, according to size, by a spectrometer.

The spectrometer discriminates various gamma ray energies by the use of energy-dependent "windows" that may be used to select the energies to be counted. This type of information can be displayed either in a cathode-ray-tube format, where energies are shown across an energy continuum of a selected range, or it may be displayed as counts within a region that is derived manually by progressively advancing a window along an energy scale. Such displays are called "pulse height spectra" (Figure 9.5) (Rollo FD, 1977).

Scintillation Cameras. The clinical images employed in nuclear medicine are usually produced by a scintillation camera. The image of the distribution of radioactivity in the patient is formed by a grid of PMTs that are arranged to view overlapping regions of a large scintillation crystal so that the scintillation created in the crystal by any radiation interaction is detected by several adjacent PMT tubes. With computer assistance, the relative brightness of each scintillation as seen by all the PMTs is used to identify the point of origin of the gamma rays. This is reproduced on an oscilloscope in the same X-Y coordinates. The image that is derived in this manner can be stored for computer-assisted processing or reproduced directly onto film. Images obtained in either manner are known as scintiphotos (Figure 9.6).

Scintillation Scanners. In the early days of nuclear medicine, before the introduction of the stationary scintillation camera system, the scintillation scanner was employed to obtain images of radioactivity distribution. This device, which employed the scintillation detector system mounted onto a rigid, motor-driven beam that moves the detector back and forth, actually mapped out the radioactivity biodistribution within its viewing area. The information is displayed as scan lines along

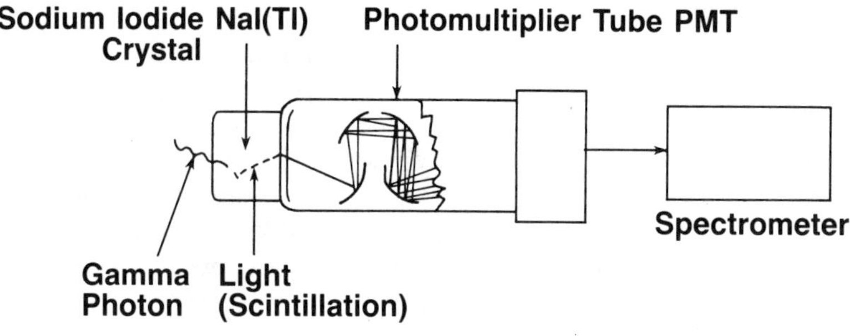

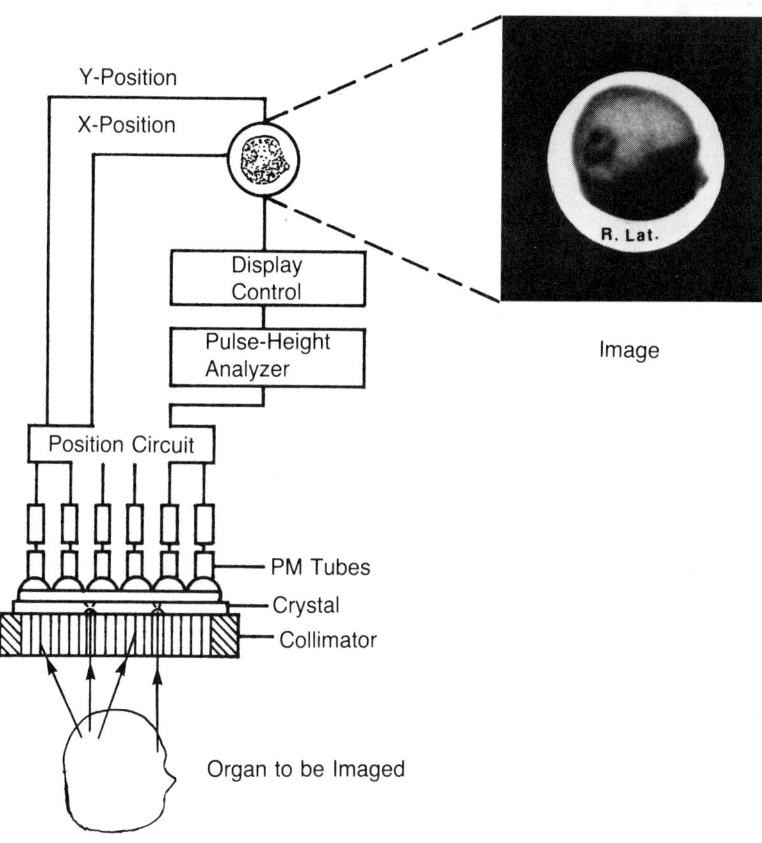

Figure 9.4 A. Diagram of scintillation detector consisting of sodium iodide [NaI(Tl)] detector, photomultiplier tube (PMT). Gamma rays strike the detector crystal wherein the electromagnetic energy is converted to light (a "scintillation"). Within the photomultiplier tube, light is converted to electrons that are multiplied in number to create a pulse that is proportional to the light source. The output pulse signal is further amplified, then sorted according to size. B. Schematic of the components of the gamma scintillation camera employed to form a scintiphoto.

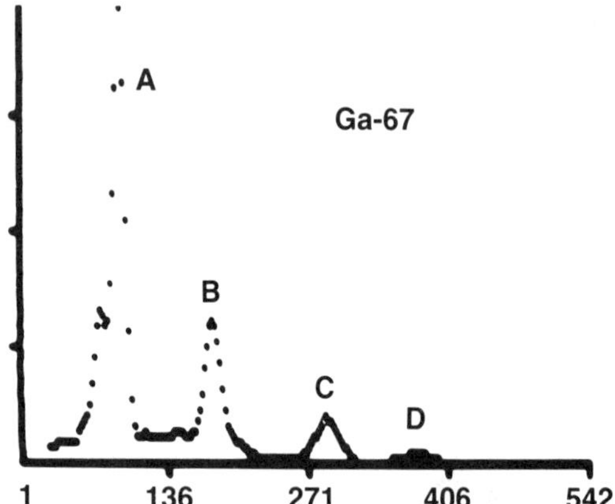

Figure 9.5 Pulse height spectrum of Ga-67 showing the multiple photon emissions of this radionuclide. Note the relative differences in heights of the photon emissions A (94 keV), B (184 keV), C (300 keV) and D (397 keV). Photons are not formed in the same abundances (number per disintegrating atoms).

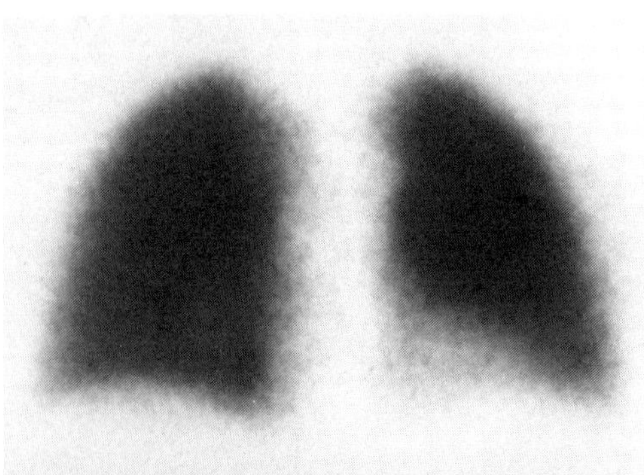

Figure 9.6 Scintillation images showing the appearance of the pulmonary perfusion agent, Tc-99m macroaggregated albumin (MAA), in a patient with apparently healthy lungs. The radiopharmaceutical distributes in the lung in relation to regional pulmonary perfusion, localizing by capillary blockade. Radioactivity appears in this image as dark areas.

the viewing path as successive accumulations of "dots." The so-called scans (a name that persists today even for the images obtained with the stationary scintillation camera) could be displayed as either life size or miniaturized depictions of body organs or tissues.

For the most part, scintillation scanner devices have been replaced by the scintillation camera systems. The major advantage of camera systems over scanners is their speed of image production, which permits visualization of dynamic processes, such as organ blood flow, through serial images over very short periods of time.

Collimation. Radioactivity is focused onto the crystal of a detector system by permitting radiations to pass through the holes of a lead collimator. The holes are arranged so as to permit a limited area beneath each hole to be focused onto the crystal and to prevent radiation from outside the field of view from appearing in that region. Only gamma rays that originate directly below a hole in the collimator will interact with the crystal above this region.

Several different types of collimators are in use today in nuclear medicine. They differ primarily in the size, shape, and arrangement of holes within the lead collimator (Figure 9.7).

The design and configuration of a lead collimator affect the relationship between *sensitivity* and *resolution*, two very important concepts in medical imaging. The sensitivity and resolution of a specific imaging system are a function of the design characteristics of the lead collimator employed for imaging. Sensitivity increases as more gamma rays are counted; it is inversely related to imaging time. Resolution is the ability of the imaging device to accurately reproduce the distribution of radioactivity as it exists in the field of imaging. As a general rule for any given radionuclide, collimation designed to achieve high sensitivity (high count rate, or short imaging time) utilizes relatively large holes in lead; collimation designed to provide high resolution will have lower count rates because smaller holes in the lead collimator are required. As a result, any gain in count rate (sensitivity) during imaging is attained by a decrease in image quality (or image resolution).

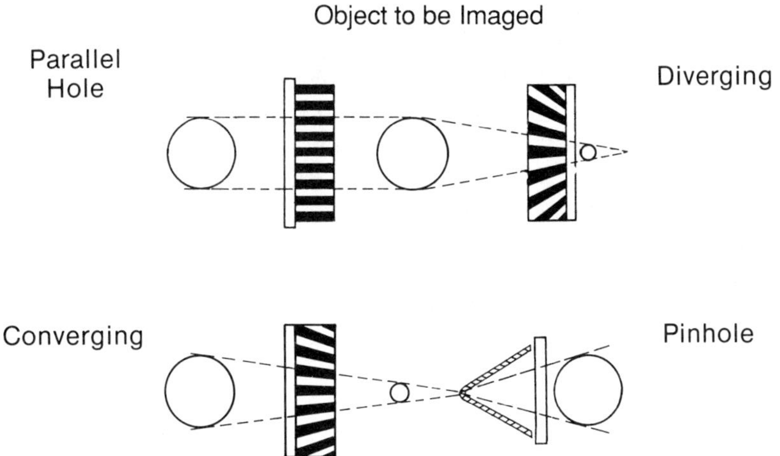

Figure 9.7 Types of collimators used with the scintillation camera and the effect they have upon the image-gathering process in nuclear medicine. Object to be imaged is shown in center column. Effect of various collimators upon the image that is produced is shown in outer columns.

RADIATION DOSIMETRY

Although traditional pharmaceuticals and radiological contrast agents may be associated with some measured toxic pharmacologic manifestations, toxicity from the use of radiopharmaceuticals is essentially nonexistent. The primary concern associated with the medical use of radioactivity is the exposure of the patient and personnel to ionizing radiation and its associated risk. Although the radiation dose associated with diagnostic nuclear medicine procedures has not been shown to cause a significant increase in cancer in patients, the number of nuclear medicine and radiologic procedures performed each year cause concern in both physicians and patients. However, only a small portion of the population's total radiation exposure is from medical radiation, and most of that is from x-ray procedures.

Radiation Dosimetry Units

Measurements of radiation *exposure* describe primarily the quantity of ionizations caused by ionizing radiation. The amount of energy absorbed in air or tissues is called the *absorbed dose*, and is measured in rads. The measure of delete-rious effect, for both radiation workers and the general public, is called the *dose equivalent* and is measured in rem.

Roentgen. The roentgen is a unit of exposure. During decay, the emitted radiation ionizes molecules in air and produces a charge (i. e., ion pairs) that corresponds to the quantity of radiation. The roentgen (R) expresses the quantity of x-rays or gamma rays that produces one electrostatic unit of either positive or negative charge in 1 cc of air at a specified temperature and pressure. Because the roentgen is a measure of radiation quantity, rather than intensity, it measures total radiation exposure without regard to time relationships. The roentgen does not measure exposure from nonelectromagnetic (alpha or beta) emissions.

Rad (Radiation Absorbed Dose). The rad is a measure of the amount of energy imparted to a medium such as tissue by any form of ionizing radiation. One rad is equal to 100 ergs of absorbed energy per gram of tissue. It has been proposed that the rad be replaced by the new SI unit of absorbed dose, the gray (Gy). One gray is equivalent to 100 rads.

Rem: (Roentgen Equivalent Man). The rem was developed as a unit of radiation absorbed dose that adjusts for the apparent differences in biologic damage that may be created by the same total absorbed energy (the same rad dose). Highly ionizing radiation, such as alpha particles or neutrons, produces significantly greater degrees of tissue damage than less densely ionizing radiations such as x-rays, gamma rays, or beta particles because the intensity of ionization is greater for the former. The new SI unit for radiation dose equivalent, the sievert (Sv), is equivalent to 100 rem.

Regarding radioactivity and radiation exposure, the following nomenclature has become standard. The amount of radioactivity administered to a patient is known as the *dosage*. For example, lung scans are often performed with a *dosage* of 5 millicuries of Tc-99m MAA. The amount of radiation one would receive from this dosage, however, is known as the radiation *dose*. A lung scan performed in an adult with a *dosage* of 5 millicuries, for example, would provide a radiation *dose* of approximately 1 rad to the patient's lungs.

FACTORS AFFECTING RADIATION DOSIMETRY

The radiation dose (the amount of radiation received) is a surrogate measure of the relative risk associated with any procedure that involves radioactivity (as with radiopharmaceuticals) or radiation (as with x-rays or radiation therapy). While radiation dose calculations for radiopharmaceuticals are based upon several readily definable parameters (such as the types and quantities of radioactivity employed), they are only estimates of risk because many variables affect the exact radiation dose received in a given patient. Among these factors are the presence of disease states, the patient's physiology, and the patient's age (ICRP, 1988). For any given radionuclide, other variables include the chemical and physical state of the radionuclide, and redistribution and clearance patterns of the radiolabeled complex.

Types of Radiation. The majority of diagnostic nuclear medicine procedures employ radionuclides that emit gamma photons, since these emissions can be detected externally. Ideally, these radionuclides should decay by the emission of a single gamma photon, but other forms of radiation accompany the release of a gamma photon. Most gamma-emitting radionuclides that are used in medicine also emit particulate radiation (such as β^- particles or conversion electrons) or low-energy x-rays that contribute the greater fraction of the radiation dose without any clinical benefit. Radiopharmaceuticals such as I-131 or P-32 are usually employed for therapeutic applications because of their highly ionizing beta emissions.

Amount of Radioactivity Administered. It can be logically assumed that the larger the amount of radioactivity administered, the larger the radiation dose received. In nuclear medicine, the diagnostic value of the information obtained from an examination involving radioactivity will vary with the amount of administered activity. In general, there is a threshold of administered activity below which no useful information will be generated (Figure 9.8). Dilution of the relatively small amounts of activity administered can result in insufficient count density for diagnostic utility. Diagnostic quality can be improved, however, by increasing the amount of administered activity. With the acquisition of an acceptable image, though, one reaches a point at which any larger amount of activity administered serves only to increase patient radiation exposure without any appreciable improvement in image quality. Therefore, there is an optimal amount of radioactivity to be administered for each type of diagnostic nuclear medicine examination.

Radionuclides that decay by the emission of highly ionizing β^- radiation, and also emit gamma rays, may be administered for either diagnostic or therapeutic purposes depending upon the amount of radioactivity administered. For example,

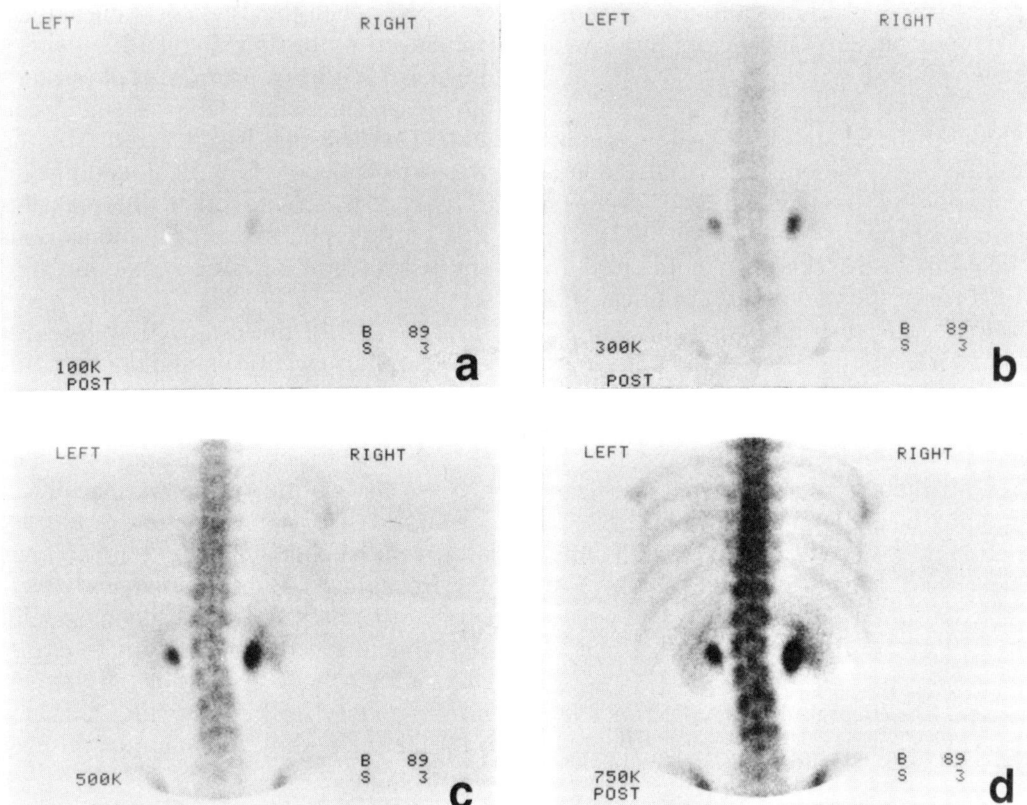

Figure 9.8 Scintillation images (*scintiphotos*) taken of a patient who has been administered the bone-seeking radiopharmaceutical, Tc-99m medronate (MDP). Scintiphoto A was obtained with 100,000 counts, scintiphoto B with 300,000 counts, scintiphoto C with 500,000 counts, and scintiphoto D with 750,000 counts. Note that increasing numbers of photons produce greater image detail.

I-131, a gamma-emitting radionuclide that also undergoes β^- decay, can be safely administered in relatively small doses (10–20 microcurie amounts) for diagnostic evaluation of thyroid function (e. g., radioactive iodine uptake test) or in much larger quantities to deliver therapeutic amounts of radiation to a hyperplastic or cancerous thyroid gland. Thus, with any nuclear medicine procedure, the goal of the clinician is to employ sufficient amounts of radioactivity to be able to obtain the needed diagnostic information while using no amounts larger than are absolutely necessary.

Physical Half-Life. The ability of nuclear medicine instrumentation to provide high-quality images depends upon the availability of large numbers of gamma photons that can be externally detected. For any given radionuclide, larger amounts of radioactivity provide higher "count" rates—that is, more gamma photons. This translates into images of higher resolution. A concern with the use of larger amounts of radioactivity, however, is that the radiation dose must be kept within acceptable limits. It is possible, however, to balance the desire for high count rates with acceptable radiation exposures by the use of radionuclides that have short physical half-lives (they decay soon after administration). However, the half-life cannot be so short that there is insufficient time for the radiopharmaceuticals to localize within target tissues before appreciable decay losses occur. With some radiopharmaceuticals, lengthy blood-clearance rates or slow uptake by target tissues precludes the use of short-lived radionuclides and favors those with longer physical half-lives.

Physicochemical States. Since the biodistribution of a radionuclide is determined primarily by its physical and chemical (physicochemical) state (Table 9.2), the radiation dose is likewise influenced by the form of the radiopharmaceutical. For example, the distribution of Tc-99m sodium pertechnetate, one of the more commonly employed radiopharmaceuticals, involves uptake by the gastric mucosa and the thyroid gland (they receive the highest radiation dose) with significant amounts cleared by the kidneys by glomerular filtration (Beasley TM and Palmer HE, 1966; Hayes MT and Green FA, 1977; Lathrop KA and Harper PV, 1972).

Table 9.2 MECHANISMS OF LOCALIZATION FOR RADIOPHARMACEUTICALS CLASSIFIED ACCORDING TO PHYSIOCHEMICAL PROPERTIES[a]

SUBSTRATE SPECIFIC

Isotopically substituted biochemical
  [C-11] palmatic acid
  [C-11] glucose
Metabolic trapping
  2-deoxy-2-[F-18] fluoro-D-glucose
Enzyme inhibitor or enzyme substrate
  6-β[I-131]-iodomethyl-19-norcholesterol (NP-59)?
  I-123, I-131-sodium iodide for thyroid imaging
Receptor-binding biochemical or drug
  radiolabeled steroids
  meta-iodo [I-131] benzylguanidine (mIBG)
  cholinergic blocking agents
Antibodies against tumor-associated or pathology-derived
  antigens
  CEA antibody
  Anti-fibrin antibody
  Anti-melanoma antibody
  Anti-myosin antibody
Miscellaneous
  Tc-99m IDA-analogs for hepatobiliary imaging

SUBSTRATE NONSPECIFIC

Diffusion
  Tc-99m for brain imaging
  Xe-133, Xe-127, Kr-81m for lung ventilation imaging
Compartmental space
  Tc-99m-penetate for ECF measurements
  Tc-99m-labeled RBCs for blood volumes, cardiac function
  In-111-penetetate for CSF kinetics
Capillary blockade
  Tc-99m-macroaggregated albumin for regional pulmonary perfusion
Cell sequestration
  Tc-99m-RBCs (heat damaged) for splenic sequestration studies
Phagocytosis
  Tc-99m-sulfur colloid for RES imaging

[a] Modified from Eckelman WC and Reba RC, 1979

However, when the physicochemical form is changed by complexing Tc-99m with a molecule that has a prominent physical or biological character, such as sulfur colloid, a particle that is sequestered by the phagocyte cells of the reticuloendothelial (RE) system, an altogether different pattern of radiopharmaceutical biodistribution results with differing radiation exposure.

Ideally, all of the radioactivity present in radiopharmaceuticals should be composed of the desired radionuclide in the preferred physicochemical state. However, trace impurities of other radionuclides may occur within radiopharmaceutical preparations, or some fraction of the desired radionuclide may exist in another physicochemical form. In the above example, the presence of Tc-99m sodium pertechnetate within a preparation of Tc-99m sulfur colloid would not only diminish the quality of the liver study but also bring about a shift in radiation dose to other organs.

Radiopharmaceutical Elimination. The rate of radiopharmaceutical disappearance is a composite of radioactive decay, known as the physical half-life ($T_{1/2_{phy}}$), and normal metabolic excretion, known as the biologic half-life ($T_{1/2_{biol}}$). The net effect of both these half-lives is to decrease the amount of radioactivity within the body. They can be combined to form a new half-life, called the effective half-life ($T_{1/2_{eff}}$) that takes into account clearance by both radioactive decay and biological elimination. In all cases the $T_{1/2_{eff}}$ is shorter than either the physical or the biological half-life. The $T_{1/2_{eff}}$ is calculated as the *product* of the physical and biological half-lives *divided* by their sum.

$$T_{1/2_{eff}} = \frac{T_{1/2_{biol}} \times T_{1/2_{phy}}}{T_{1/2_{biol}} + T_{1/2_{phy}}}$$

Patient Age and Size. While few product monographs specify their use in pediatrics, many radiopharmaceuticals are routinely administered to infants and children in activity levels that are "in proportion" to those of adults (Shore RM and

Hendee WR, 1986). Reduction of activity according to body weight still results in greater radiation doses to infants and children than to adults, since significant physiologic differences exist between children and adults. For example, young children have profoundly different rates of renal blood flow and glomerular filtration that can affect the clearance of radiopharmaceuticals and, consequently, radiation dose. Compared to adults, children also demonstrate a greater uptake of bone-seeking radiopharmaceuticals and have a poorly developed blood-brain barrier, an incomplete enzyme complement (Coffey JL, et al, 1987), and a pulmonary vasculature that is not fully developed at birth (Rhurlbeck W, 1976). (The number of pulmonary arteries develops rapidly during the first year of life, usually reaching the number found in an adult by 8 years of age (Davies G and Reid L, 1970).) For calculation of pediatric dosages a variety of methods have been developed that take into account age, weight, body surface area, or combinations of these factors. Table 9.3 provides one method for determining pediatric dosages that utilizes body surface area.

While for infants and children the concern is for a reduction in the amount of radioactivity administered, in large adults it may be necessary to administer more than the routine dosage in order to perform an adequate study. For example, a very large patient undergoing a bone study may require a proportionally larger dosage of the bone-seeking radiopharmaceutical to compensate for the relatively larger number of photons that are absorbed by the patient due to soft tissue attenuation. Dosages of radiopharmaceuticals for patients of all sizes should be carefully determined in order that the least amount of radioactivity is utilized that will result in a quality study.

Presence of Disease.   In nuclear medicine imaging, alteration of radiopharmaceutical distribution, which permits disease diagnosis, can have a profound effect on radiation dosimetry. For example, during bone imaging, a significant fraction of the radiopharmaceutical not taken up by the bone is cleared from blood by renal excretion. Any reduction in renal function can result in prolonged blood clearance of the radiopharmaceutical with a correspondingly higher whole-body radiation dose.

Similarly, in patients with severe liver disease, radiopharmaceuticals that are normally removed from blood by the Kupffer's cells of the liver will be taken up by the other cells of the reticuloendothelial system, principally the spleen and bone marrow (Figure 9.9), with correspondingly higher radiation to those organs (MIRD, 1975).

Use of Radioactive Materials during Pregnancy and Breast feeding.   In women of childbearing age, the possibility of pregnancy should always be considered, and the patient should be carefully interviewed to assess the likelihood of pregnancy. Irradiation of the fetus results from the placental transfer and distribution of the radiopharmaceutical into the fetal tissues, or from external irradiation resulting from radioactivity localized within various organs of the mother, such as the bladder. Some radiopharmaceuticals are known to undergo placental transfer and localize in fetal tissues, whereas others do not. Radioisotopes of iodine, for example, readily cross the placenta and are concentrated within the fetal

Table 9.3   BODY SURFACE AREA METHOD FOR THE CALCULATION OF RADIOPHARMACEUTICAL DOSAGES FOR PEDIATRIC PATIENTS[a]

| PATIENT WEIGHT | | BODY SURFACE | FRACTION OF |
lb	*kg*	AREA (M^2)	ADULT DOSE
4.4	2	0.15	0.09[b]
8.8	4	0.25	0.14
13.2	6	0.33	0.19
17.6	8	0.40	0.23
22.0	10	0.46	0.27
33.0	15	0.63	0.36
44.0	20	0.83	0.48
55.0	25	0.95	0.55
66.0	30	1.08	0.62
77.0	35	1.20	0.69
88.0	40	1.30	0.75
99.0	45	1.40	0.81
110.0	50	1.51	0.87
121.0	55	1.58	0.91

[a] Based upon average adult body surface area of $1.7\,M^2$ adapted from Modell W, 1958.

[b] Minimal amounts of activity should be established for each study that are necessary to provide adequate image quality.

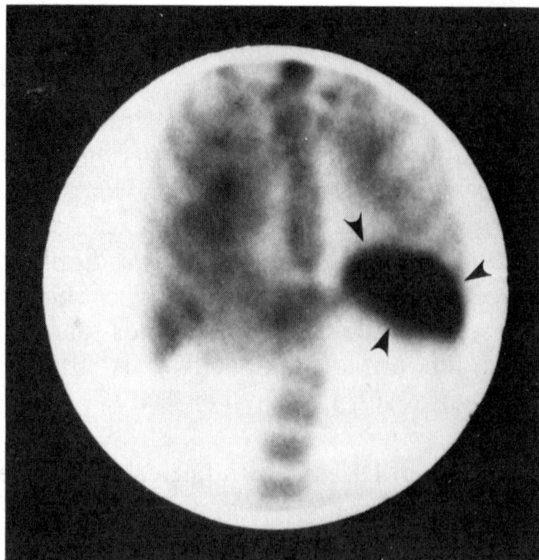

Figure 9.9 Scintiphoto of patient (anterior projection) who has been administered Tc-99m sulfur colloid, a radiopharmaceutical that localizes in the cells of the reticuloendothelial system. As a result of the patient's severe liver disease, significant amounts of the radiopharmaceutical are shifted to the spleen (arrows) and bone marrow. The liver is only faintly visualized in this patient.

thyroid after the first 10 weeks of pregnancy (Hibbard B and Herbert R, 1960). Radiopharmaceuticals that fail to cross the placenta act only as external sources of irradiation to the fetus, and their contribution to the radiation dose to the fetus depends upon the amount of activity administered and the distribution in the mother's organs and tissues. In the case of radiopharmaceuticals that do not cross the placenta but are rapidly eliminated by the kidneys, the urinary bladder, acting as a reservoir, can become a major source of radiation exposure to the fetus.

Whenever a nuclear medicine examination is proposed for a woman known to be pregnant, the benefits should clearly outweigh any risks. Exposure of the patient who is unaware of her pregnancy can later lead to considerable concern and apprehension about the possible effects on the embryo. As a general rule, the amount of conceptus irradiation that occurs from a diagnostic procedure is small and rarely justifies termination of pregnancy. When such inadvertent radiation exposure occurs, a qualified individual should prepare an estimate of the absorbed dose to the fetus and a description of the associated risks.

Since many radiopharmaceuticals are secreted in milk (Mountford PJ and Coakley AJ, 1988), it is advisable to assume that, unless evidence exists to the contrary, some radioactive component may be found in the milk whenever a radiopharmaceutical is administered to a lactating female. The International Commission on Radiological Protection (ICRP) Task Group on the Protection of the Patient in Nuclear Medicine (1988) suggests that, whenever radiopharmaceuticals are considered for use in a nursing female, the risk to the breast-fed child should be considered. Postponing the procedure is one possibility. However, if the anticipated benefit of performing the procedure is thought to be substantial, the child should be removed from breast-feeding until the levels of secreted radiopharmaceutical fall to acceptable levels. The ICRP recommends that the following actions be taken for various radiopharmaceuticals.

Group I: Stop nursing for at least 3 weeks.
- All I-131 and I-125 radiopharmaceuticals, except radioiodinehippuran (OIHA)
- Ga-67 citrate, T1-201 chloride

Group II: Stop nursing for at least 12 hours.
- OIHA labeled with I-131, I-125, or I-123
- All Tc-99m radiopharmaceuticals, except RBCs, phosphonates, and pentetate (DTPA)

Group III: Stop nursing for at least 4 hours.
- Tc-99m RBCs, phosphonates, and pentetate (DTPA)

Group IV: No necessity to stop breast-feeding.
- Cr-51 EDTA

ADVERSE REACTIONS INVOLVING
RADIOPHARMACEUTICALS

In the United States, information relating to adverse reactions involving radiopharmaceuticals has been compiled largely through the efforts of the Society of Nuclear Medicine (SNM) and a reporting system that originated in 1967.

For the most part, the greater volume of information currently known about adverse reactions in the United States comes from data that has been acquired since 1976 in a cooperative effort of the SNM, the United States Pharmacopeial Convention, and the Food and Drug Administration (Cordova MA and Rhodes BA, 1980; Cordova MA, et al, 1982; Cordova MA, et al, 1984).

Reported reactions involving radiopharmaceuticals most commonly involve small numbers of pyrogenic or allergic manifestations (rash, flushing, chills, tachycardia, etc.) that occur soon after radiopharmaceutical administration. The notable exceptions appear to be late-onset rashes and itching associated infrequently with the use of the skeletal imaging radiopharmaceutical, Tc-99m medronate (MDP).

For the most part, reported reactions have more commonly occurred with radiopharmaceuticals that contain known immunogens, such as radiolabeled human serum albumin and aggregates of human serum that are used for blood-pool imaging and pulmonary perfusion imaging, respectively. A number of adverse reactions is also associated with the use of Tc-99m sulfur colloid, a radiopharmaceutical that is routinely employed for liver and spleen imaging. Commercial formulations of this radiopharmaceutical contain gelatin, an animal protein, as a particle-size stabilizer.

Still, the number of adverse reactions that occur with radiopharmaceuticals is very low. From 1976 through 1984, the total number of adverse reactions reported to the SNM Adverse Reactions Registry was less than 400; based upon these figures, the overall incidence is estimated at less than 40 per 100,000 radiopharmaceutical administrations (Cordova MA, et al, 1987).

REGULATORY CONSIDERATIONS INVOLVING THE USE OF RADIOPHARMACEUTICALS

The regulation of radiopharmaceuticals was for many years the sole jurisdiction of the Atomic Energy Commission (which later became the Nuclear Regulatory Commission [NRC]). The Food and Drug Administration initially determined that the interests of nuclear medicine and the regulation of these radioactive drugs could be best served by the Atomic Energy Commission because radioactivity was the central property of these agents, and the FDA had no expertise in this area. During the early 1970s, however, the FDA recognized that, excepting the distinction of radioactivity, the many similarities that existed between radiopharmaceuticals and traditional pharmaceuticals required careful scrutiny in order to determine the safety and efficacy of these drug products.

THE NUCLEAR REGULATORY
COMMISSION (NRC)

The Atomic Energy Commission (AEC) was created in 1954 to promote and regulate the use of atomic energy. This responsibility includes the regulation of the possession, use, and transfer of certain types of radioactive materials, specifically, reactor by-product materials (anything produced in a reactor), and other types of source and special nuclear materials that generally involve weapons-grade research or reactor operations. Naturally occurring or accelerator-produced radionuclides and radiation from machines (such as x-ray units) were not included in its jurisdiction.

A 1959 amendment to the Atomic Energy Act of 1954, provided that individual states, by agreement with the AEC, could accept the responsibility for regulating radioactive materials, so long

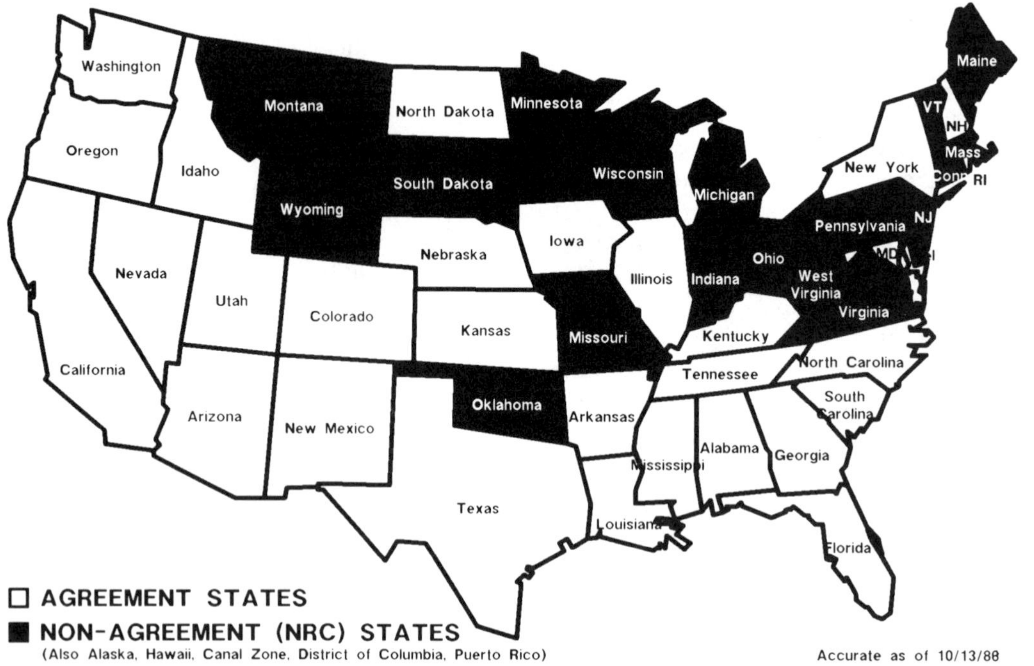

Figure 9.10   Jurisdiction of Nuclear Regulatory Commission (NRC) and Agreement States.

as these states (so-called Agreement States, Figure 9.10) developed a regulatory program that was compatible with that of the AEC. Agreement states, unlike the AEC, are not limited to the regulation of reactor by-product materials only and can adopt regulations for all forms of radioactive materials, including those radionuclides produced in an accelerator, as well as radiation-producing machines. It is important to note that Agreement States enjoy some degree of latitude in their regulations, which may be more, or less, stringent than those of the commission.

In 1974, the Energy Reorganization Act abolished the AEC and created the Nuclear Regulatory Commission (NRC) to regulate for public health and safety, and the Energy Research and Development Administration for promotional activities. The regulatory endeavors of the NRC (like those of the AEC) continued to be limited to regulation of reactor by-product materials. (However, for compliance, the NRC includes radiation dose from by-product materials and other sources of radiation, regardless of its ori-

gin.) The NRC's regulations affected the practice of medicine by requiring licensed users of radioactive materials to use radiopharmaceuticals only for those indications listed in the package insert. A 1979 policy statement noted that regulatory authority over the medical use of radioisotopes provides for the radiation safety of workers and the general public, including patients. The NRC further stated its intention to avoid any exercise of authority in areas where there exists "adequate regulations by other federal and state agencies or well-administered professional standards."

Also in 1979, the NRC announced that although the FDA regulates the manufacture, interstate distribution, investigation, and research use of drugs (including radiopharmaceuticals), the NRC is the only agency authorized to regulate the routine use of radiopharmaceuticals (an interpretation that is derived from their chartered objectives to provide for the radiation safety of the public). In 1979, the NRC also announced that licensees could use by-product radioactive materials for clinical procedures other than those specified in the product package insert so long as the user complied with the product labeling regarding the radiopharmaceutical's chemical and physical form, route of administration, and dosage range. Still left unanswered, however, were questions involving the NRC's restriction of the practice of medicine, since a number of often new and unapproved indications for approved radiopharmaceuticals involve a variance in the route of administration as recorded on the product package insert. In these situations, the product could not be used, except in violation of NRC guidelines.

This question was answered, at least in part, however, when the NRC decided to review requests for such uses and to authorize those which are in their opinion within the reasonable practice of medicine. The first such exemption to the "route of administration" restriction was issued in a 1983 NRC rule permitting the use of Tc-99m pentetate as an aerosol for pulmonary imaging. Previouslly, this radiopharmaceutical had been approved for intravenous administration only.

Overview of Medical Licensing Information. The NRC (and Agreement State agencies) grant two types of licenses for the use of radioactive materials: (1) general licenses for in vitro use, and (2) specific licenses for in vivo use. The general licenses for in vitro use are issued either to individuals (physicians, veterinarians) or to institutions and specify possession limits for certain radionuclides that are used for in vitro applications. Specific licenses are of either limited scope (either for physicians in private practice or institutions) or broad scope (large institutions with active radioactive materials programs only). Medical institutions and physicians who use by-product materials often need more by-product material than can be permitted under the general license program. A specific license that authorizes a larger inventory of by-product material and a wider variety of uses may be issued for different types of medical use (Table 9.4). The types of use comprise diagnostic or therapeutic procedures

Table 9.4 TYPES OF MEDICAL USE OF REACTOR BY-PRODUCT MATERIALS (ACCORDING TO NRC[a]) MADE ON THE BASIS OF USER'S TRAINING AND EXPERIENCE, FACILITIES AND EQUIPMENT NEEDED, AND RADIATION SAFETY REQUIREMENTS

10 CFR 35.100 "Use of radiopharmaceuticals for uptake, dilution, and excretion studies."
Diagnostic use of prepared radiopharmaceuticals for measurement of uptake, dilution, and excretion studies. A prepared radiopharmaceutical is one that has been manufactured in the form to be administered to the patient and that has been labeled, packaged, and distributed in accordance with the manufacturer's radioactive materials license.

10 CFR 35.200 "Use of radiopharmaceuticals, generators, and reagent kits for imaging and localization studies."
Diagnostic use of prepared radiopharmaceuticals for imaging and tumor localization, and diagnostic use of radionuclide generators and kits for preparation and use of radiopharmaceuticals.

10 CFR 35.300 "Use of radiopharmaceuticals for therapy."
Use of prepared radiopharmaceuticals for therapy that may or may not require hospitalization for radiation safety purposes.[b] Licenses that authorize the therapeutic use of prepared radiopharmaceuticals that do not require patient hospitalization for radiation safety purposes will be issued to private practitioners.

10 CFR 35.400 "Use of sources for brachytherapy."
The use of sealed or encased sources for implant therapy.

10 CFR 35.500 "Use of sealed sources for diagnosis."
The use of sealed sources in diagnostic devices such as portable imaging devices or bone mineral analyzers.

10 CFR 35.600 "Use of sealed sources in a teletherapy unit."
The use of cobalt-60 or cesium-137 in a teletherapy unit, usually for cancer treatment.

[a] See Title 10 of the Code of Federal Regulations, Part 35, Medical use of By-product Material. Note that Agreement States may use a different taxonomy for classification of medical use.
[b] Patients administered 30 mCi or more for therapy must be hospitalized until the body burden diminishes to less than this amount of activity.

that require similar physician training and experience and radiation safety procedures.

Broad-scope licenses are issued only to medical centers that are engaged in significant amounts of research that would make frequent amendments to their licenses impractical. These institutions are staffed with full-time radiation safety personnel who, in concert with a Radiation Safety Committee, oversee the research and medical use of radioactivity according to NRC guidelines. In this regard, broad-scope licensees assume much of the responsibility for the management of the radiation safety program.

Applications for a radioactive materials license are generally made along NRC guidelines. They include the names of the persons who will be authorized to use radioactive materials, a description of available facilities and equipment (including radiation detection instruments), quality control and instrument calibration procedures, radiation protection measures (including procedures for ordering and handling radioactive materials, and rules for their safe use, storage, and disposal), and the types of radioactive materials for which the application requests authorization.

Applicants request the use of one or more of the different classes of radiopharmaceuticals that are necessary in their clinical practices. Physicians who wish to use radioactive materials must have proper training and experience in basic radionuclide handling techniques and in the clinical application of the materials being requested. Different types and amounts of training and experience are required according to the types of materials requested and their intended use. An NRC license is valid for 5 years.

It is worthwhile to note that Agreement States have a degree of flexibility in their regulatory programs. Requirements and authorizations may be different. Also, the NRC does not have regulatory authority over accelerator-produced radioactive material such as thallium-201, gallium-67, xenon-127, or cobalt-57. The appropriate state authority should be consulted for requirements involved in the possession, use, transfer, and disposal of such radionuclides.

THE FOOD AND DRUG ADMINISTRATION (FDA)

During the early years of nuclear medicine, the FDA opted to allow radiopharmaceuticals prepared from by-product materials to be distributed primarily under the regulatory supervision of the Atomic Energy Commission. In 1962, the FDA formalized a temporary exemption for radioactive pharmaceuticals and biolo-

gics from investigational new drug (IND) requirements, provided that reactor by-product materials were shipped in compliance with AEC regulations (the FDA exemption did not include accelerator-produced radionuclides). In 1971, however, the FDA determined that the 1962 exemption of the radiopharmaceuticals should be revoked. A final order to this effect, issued on July 25, 1975, required radiopharmaceuticals in commercial distribution to possess an approved new-drug application (NDA), biologic product license, or exemption as an investigational new drug (IND). Investigational new drug (IND) studies for radiopharmaceuticals, like traditional pharmaceuticals, are intended to demonstrate a drug's safety and efficacy for a given clinical situation prior to its release into interstate commerce (Table 9.5) (Swanson DP and Lieto RP, 1984). As a general rule, the average time for approval of radiopharmaceutical NDAs since 1974 has been slightly more than 2 years (Siegel BA, 1983).

The FDA has traditionally recognized that the prerogative to utilize an approved drug in a way that is not contained in the approved product labeling is the responsibility of the physician and that such a decision does not constitute a violation of FDA guidelines. In fact, the FDA provided support in this area by stating that "labeling for a marketed drug does not always contain all of the current informa-

Table 9.5 INVESTIGATIONAL NEW DRUG STUDIES INCLUDE PRECLINICAL AND CLINICAL EVALUATIONS OF A DRUG'S SAFETY AND EFFICACY. CLINICAL STUDIES IN HUMANS MAY BE CLASSIFIED INTO THREE DISTINCT PHASES

Phase I—	Initial carefully controlled studies in a limited number of individuals to determine basic pharmacokinetic information (absorption, distribution, metabolism, and excretion) as well as toxicity, dosage range, and routes of administration.
Phase II—	Studies are conducted on a limited number of subjects for a specific disease in order to provide further evidence of safety and initial evidence of diagnostic or therapeutic efficacy.
Phase III—	Larger clinical trials intended to assess the safety and efficacy of the drug in a given diagnostic or therapeutic condition. Specific (optimum) dosages are determined. Studies are usually performed independently by several investigators.

tion available to physicians relating to the proper use of the drug, in good medical practice," and further, that the physician "has the responsibility to be well-informed about the drug and to base such use on firm scientific rationale or sound medical evidence" (Federal Register, Vol. 43, March 17, 1978, p. 11211) (Siegel BA, 1983). While it may be argued that FDA policy permits the use of radiopharmaceuticals for almost any indication and in any manner, NRC policies are not so lenient. The NRC does permit specific licensees to use diagnostic radiopharmaceuticals for unapproved purposes. Use of therapeutic radiopharmaceuticals is limited to indications and methods of administration identified in the product package insert (10 CFR 35.200 and 35.300).

The Radioactive Drug Research Committee (RDRC). The RDRC was established by the FDA to obviate the need for submission of an investigational new drug (IND) application whenever research trials are necessary to determine basic pharmacokinetic information and biodistribution data on new drugs. RDRC studies, however, are intended only as a means for obtaining basic knowledge of new drugs and are not intended as a substitute for the IND mechanism to determine the safety and efficacy of a new drug.

Radioactive Drug Research Committees are individually chartered by the FDA and are empowered by the FDA to authorize basic research studies in a small number of patients with a radioactive drug that has been shown to provide radiation doses less than prescribed maximums and that will not cause any clinically detectable pharmacological effect. The protocol, which must be approved by the institutional Investigational Review Board (IRB), should not be intended for immediate therapeutic, diagnostic, or similar purposes, or to determine the safety and effectiveness of the drug in humans. While the results of certain basic research studies may have eventual therapeutic or diagnostic implications, the ini-

tial RDRC studies are considered to be basic research only (21 CFR Part 361.6). An annual report of all RDRC activities is submitted to the FDA for approval.

Misadministration of Radiopharmaceuticals. NRC defines a misadministration of a radiopharmaceutical as being the administration of

1. A radiopharmaceutical other than the one intended; or
2. A radiopharmaceutical to the wrong patient; or
3. A radiopharmaceutical by a route of administration other than that intended by the prescribing physician; or
4. A diagnostic dose of a radiopharmaceutical differing from prescribed dosage by more than 50%; or
5. A therapy dosage of a radiopharmaceutical differing from prescribed dosage by more than 10%.

It is not always necessary to file a report of the misadministration with the NRC (or the appropriate Agreement States agency). For example, the NRC requires that a report be filed only if the misadministration involved a by-product material not intended for medical use, or if the administered dosage differed fivefold from the intended dosage, or if administration of by-product material made it likely that the patient would receive an organ dose greater than 2 rem or a whole-body dose greater than 500 mrem. Otherwise when a misadministration involves a diagnostic procedure, the institutional Radiation Safety Officer shall promptly investigate its cause, make a record for NRC review, and retain the record for a period of 10 years. Such a record must contain the names of all individuals involved in the event (physician, nuclear medicine technologist, pharmacist, patient, and patient's referring physician), the patient's social security number or hospital identification number, a brief description of the event, the effect upon the patient, and the action taken, if any, to prevent a recurrence.

Whenever a misadministration involves a therapeutic procedure, the licensee must notify by telephone the appropriate regional NRC office, as well as the patient's referring physician and the patient (or a responsible family member or guardian), unless the referring physician agrees to inform the patient or believes, based upon medical judgement, that informing the patient (or the patient's family or guardian) would be harmful to one or the other. These actions must be taken within 24 hours after the licensee discovers the misadministration. If the licensee cannot reach the above-mentioned individuals within 24 hours, it is the responsibility of the licensee to notify them as soon as practical.

Within 15 days after an initial therapy misadministration, the licensee shall report in writing to the regional NRC office and to the referring physician, and furnish a copy of the report to the patient (or the patient's family or responsible guardian) if either was previously notified. The written report involving a therapeutic misadministration must include the following: the licensee's name, referring physician's name, a brief description of the event, the effect upon the patient (if any), the action taken to prevent recurrence, whether the licensee informed the patient (or family or guardian), and if not, why. The patient's confidentiality should be protected by the information contained in the report. Reports of misadministration must be kept for 10 years.

The reporting rule (as outlined) applies to NRC states only. However, the Nuclear Regulatory Commission directed Agreement States to develop similar reporting programs by April 1990. At the time of this writing, the NRC was in the early stages of reviewing this reporting rule and another rule on quality assurance in the medical use of radionuclides.

Department of Transportation. In the early 1950s, the Interstate Commerce Commission (ICC) first established regulations that were intended to provide protection against excessive exposure to radiation during transportation of radioactive materials. The ICC regulations were designed to protect radiation-sensitive cargo, such as film, from radiation by establishing limits on radiation levels that emanate from these packages.

Jurisdiction over the safe transportation of materials was transferred to the Department of Transportation (DOT) in 1966 by virtue of the Department of Transportation Act. The DOT now has regulatory responsibility for safety in the transportation of all hazardous materials, including radioactive materials, in shipments by all modes of transportation (rail, highway, air, water) in interstate or foreign commerce, and by all means except postal shipments (postal shipments come under the jurisdiction of the U.S. Postal Service).

The NRC (and equivalent state agencies) have uniform requirements for licensees who turn over radioactive materials to carriers for transport. The NRC also provides assistance to the DOT in developing regulatory guidelines and inspects licensees for compliance with DOT regulations (Guide for the Preparation of Applications for Medical Use Programs, 1987).

For purposes of transportation, radioactive materials are defined as those materials that spontaneously emit ionizing radiation and have a specific activity in excess of 0.002 microcuries per gram of material. All materials are to some degree radioactive. The demarcation of 0.002 microcuries per gram allows a distinction between materials not normally considered radioactive and those that are regulated as radioactive in transportation. Materials with a specific activity lower than 0.002 microcuries per gram are not regulated by the DOT (but may be subject to regulation by the NRC).

DOT regulations for the transportation of radioactive materials place certain requirements on the packaging of these materials based upon the form, type, and quantity of the radionuclide being shipped. Packages must be labeled accordingly. Occasionally, the vehicles that transport these materials on public highways or rail must bear appropriate warnings. Radioactive materials can be transported on passenger-carrying aircraft; however, the transportation of radioactive materials by passenger-carrying buses is not permitted.

References

A review of the Department of Transportation (DOT) regulations of transport of radioactive materials: US DOT, Washington, DC, 1983.

Beasley TM, Palmer HE, Nelp WB. Distribution and excretion of technetium in humans. *Health Phys* 1966, 12:1425–1435.

Blumgart HL, Weiss S. Studies on the velocity of blood flow in normal resting individuals, and a critique of the method used. *J Clin Invest* 1927, 4:15–28.

Blumgart HL, Yens OC. Studies on the velocity of blood flow. I. The method utilized. *J Clin Invest* 1927, 4:1–14.

Briner WH. New dimensions for pharmacy. *Hosp Top* 1965, 43:79–90.

Briner WH. Radiopharmacy: The emerging young speciality. *Drug Intell Clin Pharm* 1968, 2:8–13.

Cloutier RJ, Coffey JL, Snyder WS, et al. *Radiopharmaceutical dosimetry symposium*. Washington, DC, DHEW Publication, FDA 76-8044, 1976, pp. 293–304.

Coffey JL, Watson EE, Hubner KF, et al. Radiopharmaceutical absorbed dose considerations. In *Essentials of nuclear medicine science*. Hladik WB III, Saha G, Study KT (eds). Baltimore, Williams and Wilkins, 1987, pp. 51–74.

Cordova MA, Hladik WB III, Rhodes BA, et al. Adverse reactions associated with radiopharmaceuticals. In *Essentials of nuclear medicine science*. Hladik WB III, Saha G, Study KT (eds), Baltimore, Williams and Wilkins, 1987, pp. 303–320.

Cordova MA, Hladik WB III, Rhodes BA. Validation and characterization of adverse reactions to radiopharmaceuticals. *Noninvasive Med Imag* 1984, 1:17–24.

Cordova MA Rhodes BA. Adverse reactions to radiopharmaceuticals: Incidence in 1978, and associated symptoms. Report of the adverse reactions subcommittee of the Society of Nuclear Medicine. *J Nucl Med* 1980, 21:1107–1110.

Cordova MA, Rhodes BA, Atkins HL, et al. Adverse reactions to radiopharmaceuticals. *J Nucl Med* 1982, 23:550–551.

Davis G, Reid L. Growth of the alveoli and pulmonary arteries in children. *Thorax* 1970, 25:669–681.

Eckelman WC, Reba RC. The classification of radiotracers. *J Nucl Med* 1978, 19:1179–1181.

Fermi E. Radioactivity induced by neutron bombardment. *Nature* 1934, 133:757–765.

Francis GE, Mulligan W, Wormall A. Labeling of proteins with iodine-131, sulfur-35, and phosphorous-32. *Nature (London)* 1951, 167:748–755.

Guide for the preparation of application for medical use programs: Regulatory Guide 10.8, Revision 2, US NRC, Washington, DC, August 1987.

Hayes MT, Green FA. In vitro studies of pertechnetate-99m binding by human serum and tissues. *J Nucl Med* 1977, 14:149–158.

Heaney RP, Whedon GD. Radiocalcium studies of bone formation rate in human metabolic bone disease. *J Clin Endocrinol Metab* 1958, 18:1246–1267.

Hevesy G. *Adventures in radioisotope research*. London, Pergamon, 1962.

Hibbard B, Herbert R. Foetal radiation dose following administration of radioiodinated albumin. *Clin Sci* 1960, 19:337–344.

Hughes WL, Straessle, R. Preparation and properties of serum and plasma proteins. XXIV. Iodination of human serum albumin. *J Am Chem Soc* 1950, 72:452–459.

ICRP Publication 52, *Protection of the patient in nuclear medicine*. Oxford, Pergamon, 1988.

Joliot F, Curie I. Artificial production of a new kind of radioelement. *Nature (London)* 1934, 133:201–202.

Lathrop KA, Harper PV. Biologic behavior of Tc-99m from Tc-99m pertechnetate ion. *Prog Nucl Med* 1972, 1:145–149.

Means JH. Historical background of the use of radioactive iodine in medicine. *N Engl J Med* 1955, 252:936–940.

MIRD—Medical Internal Radiation Dose Committee: Summary of current radiation dose estimates to humans with various liver conditions from Tc-99m sulfur colloid. MIRD dose estimate report 3. *J Nucl Med* 1975, 16:108A–108B.

Modell W. Principles of the choice of drugs. In *Drugs of choice*, Modell W (ed.), St. Louis, C.V. Mosby, 1958.

Mountford PJ, Coakley AJ. A review of the secretion of radioactivity in human breast milk: data, quantitative analysis and recommendations. *Nuclear Medicine Communications* 1989, 10:15–27.

Myers WG. Radioisotopes of iodine. In *Radioactive pharmaceuticals*, Andrews GA, Kniseley RM, Wagner HN Jr (eds), USAEC symposium series 6, Springfield, Va, National Bureau of Standards, Report CONF-651111, 1966, pp. 217–243.

Rhurlbeck W. Postnatal growth and development of the lung. In *Lung disease-state of the art* (1974–1975), Murray J (ed). New York, American Lung Association, 1976, pp. 33–74.

Richards P. Nuclide generators. In *Radioactive pharmaceuticals*, Andrews GA, Kniseley RM, Wagner HN Jr (eds), USAEC symposium series 6, Report CONF-651111, Springfield, Va, National Bureau of Standards, 1966, pp. 155–163.

Richards P, Steigman J. Chemistry of technetium as applied to radiopharmaceuticals. In *Radiopharmaceuticals*, Subramanian G, Rhodes BA, Cooper JF, Sodd VJ (eds), New York, Society of Nuclear Medicine, 1975, pp. 23–35.

Rollo FD. *Nuclear medicine physics, instrumentation and agents*. St. Louis, C.V. Mosby, 1977.

Siegel BA. Radiopharmaceuticals and FDA: A clinician's perspective. *J Nucl Med Technol* 1983, 11:177–186.

Shore RM, Hendee WR. Radiopharmaceutical dosage selection for pediatric nuclear medicine. *J Nucl Med* 1986, 27:287–298.

Swanson DP, Lieto RP. The submission of IND applications for radiopharmaceutical research: When and why. *J Nucl Med*, 1984, 25:714–717.

Thakur M, Gottschalk A (eds) *Indium-111 labeled neutrophils, platelets, and lymphocytes*. New York, Trivirum, 1980.

Wolf AP: Terminology concerning specific activity of radiopharmaceuticals. Author's reply. *J Nucl Med* 1981, 22:392–393.

Radiopharmaceuticals for Central Nervous System Imaging: Blood-Brain Barrier, Function, Receptor-Binding, Cerebral Spinal Fluid Kinetics

Henry M. Chilton
James H. Thrall

THE BLOOD-BRAIN BARRIER

Unlike other organs, the brain is protected from severe changes or fluctuations in levels of nutrients and other essential substances in blood by a complex anatomic and physiologic mechanism known as the blood-brain barrier (BBB). Functionally, the BBB limits the free exchange of substances between the normal brain and blood (Lajtha A and Toth J, 1963) and acts to exclude from the brain a variety of toxins, drugs (including most water-soluble radiopharmaceuticals) and other undesirable substances.

The histologic site of the BBB appears to involve the cerebral capillary endothelium, which is structurally different from capillaries generally found elsewhere in the body (Crone C, 1965). Specifically, the endothelial cells form a continuous layer of adjacent cells joined together at the periphery, causing the endothelium to appear fused when observed on electron microscopy. Physically open clefts between general capillary cells permit the passage of small polar molecules, but the tight-junctioned nature of the brain capillary cells prohibits passage of lipophobic molecules (Areskog NH, et al, 1964). Passive entry can occur, however, with substances that are sufficiently lipid soluble to cross the intact cellular membrane (Oldendorf WH, 1974a).

Studies have also shown the BBB to be almost completely impermeable to macro-molecules (Sisson WB and Oldendorf WH, 1971); this property is probably related to the virtual absence of pinocytic vesicles associated with the brain capillary-cell cytoplasm (Reese TS and Kornovsky MJ, 1967). Pinocytic vesicles are a prominent feature of general capillary-cell cytoplasm and may account for the slight permeability of general capillaries to macromolecules (Renkin EM, 1964). These two structural features of the healthy CNS capillaries, tight cell junctions and the absence of pinocytosis, seem to explain the impermeability of these cells to most hydrophilic substances.

The BBB is not a completely impermeable barrier, but rather a selectively permeable barrier that regulates the concentration of metabolic substrates and nutrients in the brain, permitting the exchange of these substances between the brain and the general extracellular fluid. As a result, molecules that are not protein bound and have a high degree of lipid solubility and low ionization at blood pH readily diffuse across the lipid membrane of the cerebral capillary cell. On the other hand, substances that are either hydrophilic or protein bound will *not* cross the intact BBB (Oldendorf WH, 1974b). Radiopharmaceuticals that are used for brain imaging can be classified accordingly, with the agents utilized for conventional brain imaging best fitting the latter category. These radiopharmaceuticals are discussed first.

I. Radiopharmaceuticals for Conventional Brain Imaging

In cerebral neoplasm and other pathologies, the integrity of the BBB is altered to allow substances that are normally confined to the cerebral vasculature to diffuse into the involved cerebral tissues (Raimondi AJ, 1966). Since radiopharmaceuticals used for conventional brain imaging are water-soluble agents that cannot permeate the intact BBB (Figure 10.1), accumulation occurs only in areas where the BBB has been damaged (Figures 10.2 and 10.3) (Oldendorf WH, 1981). However, because, alterations in the permeability of the BBB are not limited to tumor, brain imaging by conventional nuclear medicine has also proven valuable in the diagnosis of a variety of additional cerebral pathologies (Table 10.1). On the other hand, the large number of pathologies that cause similar alterations in the permeability of the BBB has limited the specificity of conventional brain scintigraphy studies. Additionally, the development of other diagnostic modalities, such as computerized axial tomography (CAT) and magnetic resonance (MR) imaging, has further contributed to the decrease in the number of conventional brain imaging studies performed. However, nuclear medicine brain imaging continues to be valuable in several clinical situations, most notably the determination of clinical brain death (Figure 10.4).

BACKGROUND/HISTORY

A common property of the water-soluble radiopharmaceuticals employed for conventional brain imaging is their exclusion from healthy brain tissues by the intact BBB. In principle, then, any radiopharmaceutical can be used for this purpose so long as it remains in blood and is prevented from crossing the BBB because of its molecular size, hydrophilicity, or protein-binding characteristics.

Among the earliest radiopharmaceuticals used for imaging of cerebral tumors were P-32 sodium phosphate (Erickson TC, et al, 1949) and radioiodinated (I-131)

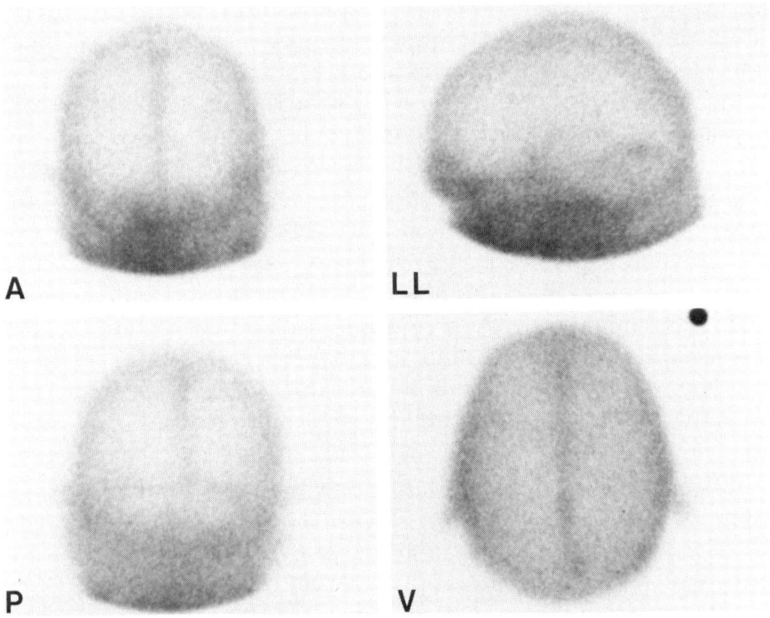

Figure 10.1 Static brain scintigrams obtained 2 hours after the injection of Tc-99m pentetate demonstrate normal activity in the scalp, dural sinus, and facial areas with no lesions in the brain. A = anterior view, LL = left lateral view, P = posterior view, V = vertex view.

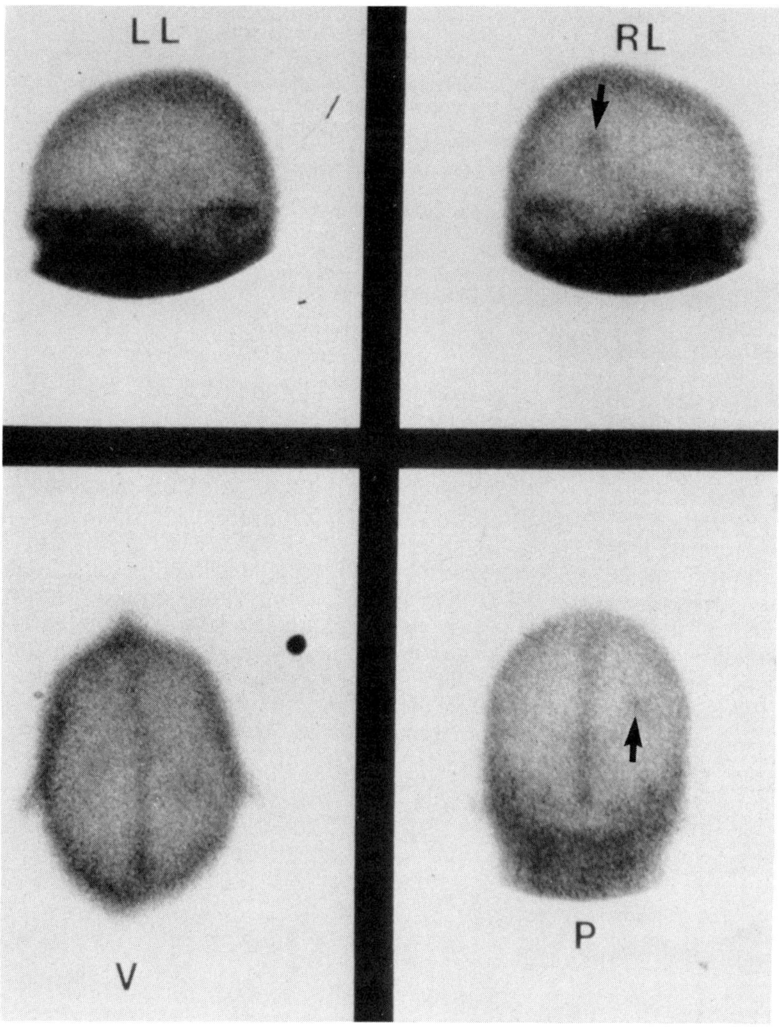

Figure 10.2 Static brain scintigrams obtained 2 hours after the injection of Tc-99m pentetate reveal (arrows) a right parietal glioma. LL = left lateral view, RL = right lateral view, V = vertex view, P = posterior view.

diiodofluorescein (Moore GE, 1948), a derivative of fluorescein. Surgical exposure of tumor was required for detection of P-32 sodium phosphate because of its exclusive Beta decay mode (Selverstone B, et al, 1949), whereas external detection devices such as Geiger–Mueller detectors were used for tumor detection and localization of the gamma-emitting I-131 diiodofluorescein. Radioiodinated (I-131) human serum albumin was also evaluated for brain imaging, using external detection devices.

Conventional nuclear medicine brain imaging developed rather slowly, however, prior to availability of radionuclides that decayed purely by the highly desirable gamma emission modes. Notable advances in this area came with the development of the Mo-99/Tc-99m radionuclide generator, which made possible widespread availability of the short-lived (6.0-hour physical half-life) radionuclide Tc-99m (Richards P, 1966). Initially, Tc-99m sodium pertechnetate from this generator was extensively used for conventional brain imaging (McAfee JG, et al, 1964). This radiopharmaceutical, which is

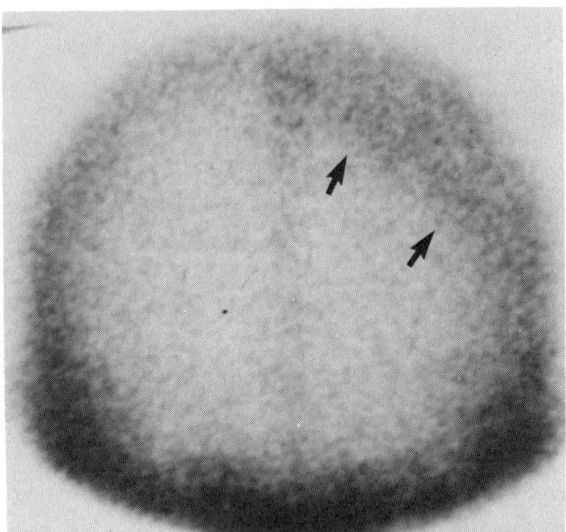

Figure 10.3 Static brain scintigram (anterior view) obtained 2 hours after the injection of Tc-99m gluceptate in a patient who had sustained head trauma. The study reveals (arrows) an abnormal crescent of activity on the left corresponding to a subdural hematoma.

Table 10.1 CLINICAL INDICATIONS FOR CONVENTIONAL BRAIN IMAGING

1. Screening for the presence of primary tumors, both benign and malignant
2. Detecting cerebral metastases
3. Evaluating patients with cerebrovascular disease
4. Detection of intracranial injury due to trauma, such as subdural hematoma, intracerebral hemorrhage
5. Localization of intracranial abscesses
6. Localization of arteriovenous malformations
7. Evaluation of patients with intracranial diseases, such as meningitis, encephalitis
8. Determination of legally defined "brain death"

conveniently obtained directly from the Mo-99/Tc-99m generator in a sterile, apyrogenic, ready-to-use form, could be administered to patients soon after generator elution with only minimal manipulation.

Although the radionuclidic properties of Tc-99m are, in general, nearly optimal for nuclear medicine studies, the biodistribution properties of the generator product, Tc-99m sodium pertechnetate, are less than ideal for brain imaging. For example, the pertechnetate anion closely resembles that of iodide

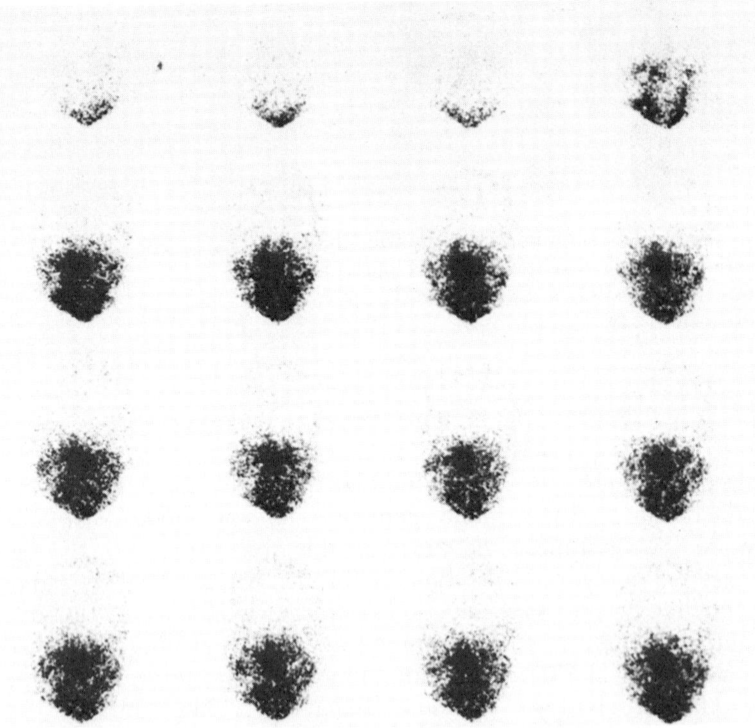

Figure 10.4 Radionuclide cerebral angiogram obtained with Tc-99m gluceptate in a brain-dead patient. There is absence of blood flow in the cerebral circulation with intense activity in the facial and nasopharynx (i. e., "hot nose"-sign) areas.

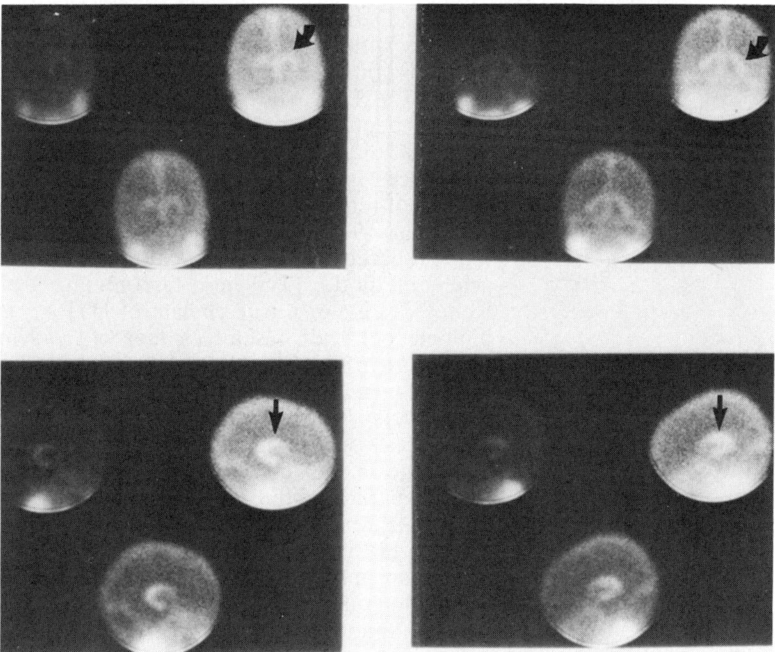

Figure 10.5   Static brain scintigrams obtained 4 hours after the injection of Tc-99m sodium pertechnetate. Note (arrows) intense choroid plexus activity in this otherwise normal subject who had not been pretreated with potassium perchlorate.

(McAfee JG, et al, 1979) both having a net −1 charge and an ionic radius of approximately the same value. Therefore, pertechnetate biodistribution resembles that of iodide, with localization occurring in the gastrointestinal mucosa, salivary and thyroid glands, and the choroid plexus (Figure 10.5). Because pertechnetate is taken up by the choroid plexus, patients should be pretreated with a blocking agent, such as potassium perchlorate (200–400 mg administered orally 30 minutes prior to radiopharmaceutical injection), in order to prevent the appearance of pertechnetate in this structure during brain imaging (Witcofski RL, et al, 1967). Also, because of the relatively long blood-pool clearance of Tc-99m sodium pertechnetrate, static brain imaging must be delayed as long as 3 or 4 hours after its intravenous administration for adequate visualization of tumor against levels of the radiopharmaceutical in blood and soft tissues (Ramsey RG and Quinn JL, 1972).

The beneficial imaging properties of Tc-99m can be utilized for conventional brain imaging, however, by preparing water-soluble complexes of Tc-99m with superior biodistribution properties, i. e., more rapid blood-pool clearance rates and less soft-tissue uptake than with Tc-99m sodium pertechnetate (Hauser W, et al, 1970; Waxman AD, et al, 1976). Among the current radiopharmaceuticals employed for conventional brain imaging studies are Tc-99m pentetate and Tc-99m gluceptate. An additional advantage to the use of either of these agents for brain imaging is that neither normally localizes in the choroid plexus or thyroid gland (Haynie TP, et al, 1970; Waxman AD, et al, 1976). Patient pretreatment with a blocking agent, such as potassium perchlorate, is therefore not required with the use of Tc-99m pentetate or Tc-99m gluceptate for brain imaging.

CHEMISTRY

Technetium in a +7 valence state (VII), obtained as Tc-99m sodium pertechnetate directly from the Mo-99/Tc-99m radionuclide generator, is chemically inert; however, other oxidation states of technetium can be formed and subsequently incorporated into a variety of chelates of differing biodistribution and tissue affinities

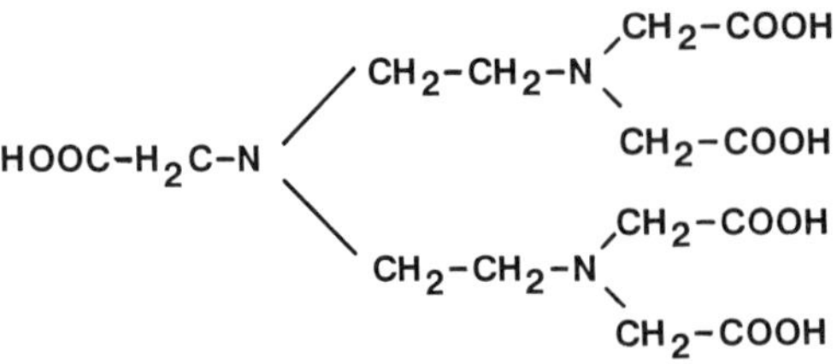

Figure 10.6 Chemical structure of the pentetate (DTPA) chelating agent.

(Benjamin PR, et al, 1970). Generally, when Tc-99m is bound to chelating substances, the reduced Tc (IV) state predominates, although the Tc (III) and Tc (V) states are also noted in several Tc-99m products. Reduced states of technetium can be achieved by treatment of generator-produced Tc-99m sodium pertechnetate with any one of several different reducing substances (Fritzberg AR, et al, 1977).

Tc-99m Pentetate (DTPA). Tc-99m pentetate is a complex of technetium and the chelate diethylenetriaminepentaacetic acid (DTPA) (Figure 10.6). The formation of Tc-99m pentetate requires the use of a suitable reducing agent in order to reduce the technetium (VII) to a chemically reactive oxidation state. Initially, a variety of reducing substances were employed, including ferrous sulfate, ferric chloride with ascorbic acid, electrolysis, and stannous ions (Eckelman WC and Levenson SM, 1977). However, among the products of Tc-99m pentetate prepared by these various methods, different biologic behavior (notably differences in blood-clearance rates and the pattern of renal excretion) were noted (Atkins HL, et al, 1971). For example, Tc-99m pentetate prepared by the ferric chloride/ascorbic acid method (Tc-99m ferpentetate or Renotec®) is not a true chelate of DTPA; its biologic behavior resembles that of Tc-99m ferrous-ascorbic acid (Atkins HL, et al, 1971). Whereas a significant fraction of the radiolabeled product prepared by the ferric chloride/ascorbic acid method concentrates over time in the renal cortex, Tc-99m pentetate prepared by the stannous ion reduction method is rapidly excreted by the kidneys with no long-term retention. Additionally, W. C. Eckelman and colleagues (1972) have shown that technetium in Tc-99m pentetate prepared by the stannous ion reduction method is in the +4 oxidation state, whereas in the Tc-99m pentetate products prepared by alternate methods appreciable amounts of the +5 oxidation state of technetium also exist.

Today, the stannous ion reduction method is routinely used for the preparation of Tc-99m pentetate. Commercially available kit-type formulations of these products and their components are listed in Table 10.2. Although both the calcium trisodium and pentasodium salts of pentetate are available, there appear

Table 10.2 FORMULATION INFORMATION AND NAMES OF COMMERCIALLY AVAILABLE PENTETATE PRODUCTS

MANUFACTURER	NAME	EACH VIAL CONTAINS:
E.R. Squibb & Sons	Techneplex®	10 mg pentetate calcium trisodium 0.5 mg stannous chloride pH adjusted with HCl (lyophilized mixture stored under nitrogen)
Syncor International	AN-DTPA®	20.6 mg pentetate calcium trisodium 0.15–0.3 mg stannous chloride pH adjusted 3.9–4.1 with HCl/NaOH (lyophilized mixture stored under nitrogen)
Medi-Physics	MPI DTPA Kit (Multidose)	5 mg pentetate pentasodium 0.17 mg (minimum) stannous chloride pH adjusted with HCl/NaOH (lyophilized mixture stored under nitrogen)
	Tc-99m DTPA Unit Dose (Single dose)	3.0 mg pentetate calcium trisodium 0.15 mg stannous chloride pH adjusted with HCl (lyophilized mixture stored under nitrogen)
Dupont-NEN	DTPA	10 mg pentetate calcium trisodium 0.5 mg $SnCl_2 \cdot 2H_2O$ pH adjusted with HCl (lyophilized mixture stored under nitrogen)

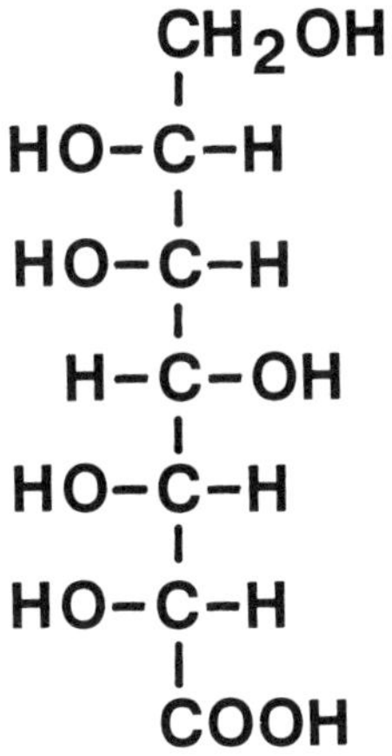

$$CH_2OH$$
$$HO-C-H$$
$$HO-C-H$$
$$H-C-OH$$
$$HO-C-H$$
$$HO-C-H$$
$$COOH$$

Figure 10.7 Chemical structure of the gluceptate (glucoheptonate) chelating agent.

to be no significant differences between the radiolabeled salts in regard to their biodistribution as brain imaging radiopharmaceuticals.

Tc-99m Gluceptate. Although official nomenclature for this radiopharmaceutical is Tc-99m gluceptate, in past years it was known as Tc-99m glucoheptonate, which identifies its seven-carbon, sugar-like structure (Figure 10.7). Like pentetate, the gluceptate chelate also requires reduction of pertechnetate to a more chemically reactive species in order for radiolabeling to occur. Although electrolytic-assisted reduction and complexation of Tc-99m to gluceptate can result in a preparation that is at least equal to the radiochemical quality of Tc-99m gluceptate prepared by stannous ion method (Shiow-Ling C, et al, 1978; Steigman J, et al, 1979), the stannous method is preferred for its relative ease and convenience (Table 10.3).

Both the +4 and +5 oxidation states of technetium have been reported for Tc-99m gluceptate. W. C. Eckelman and S. M. Levenson (1977) determined (based on studies involving a similar technetium compound, Tc-99m gluconate) that technetium in Tc-99m gluceptate most likely exists as the +4 oxidation state, whereas W. de Kieviet (1981) used stannous ion titration to show an oxidation state of +5 for Tc-99m gluceptate. The molecular configuration of Tc-99m gluceptate was determined by de Kieviet (1981) as a central technetium atom surrounded by two gluceptate ligands. The chelate is a carbohydrate-type in which the oxygens from hydroxide units act as donor ligands providing the necessary electrons to form the coordination complex. Analysis by nuclear magnetic resonance demonstrates two five-membered gluceptate rings, bidentate bound to technetium by the oxygens of the end carboxyl group and the adjacent hydroxyl group. Experiments with the reducing agent sodium borohydride in preparing Tc-99m gluceptate demonstrated the absence of tin in the formed complex and that the biologic behavior was independent of the reducing agent employed.

Package/Storage. All currently available commercial "kit" formulations of both pentetate and gluceptate are lyophilized. An earlier report had demonstrated difficulty with aqueous (nonlyophilized) formulations leading to deterioration of these products particularly when stored at room temperature. The observed effect, which involved slower than normal plasma clearance and urinary excretion, was not attributable to the presence of free pertechnetate (Hosain F, 1974). Suggested packaging and storage data for these radiopharmaceuticals are shown in Table 10.4.

PHARMACOKINETICS

Tc-99m Pentetate. Uptake of Tc-99m pentetate in brain lesions occurs as a result of the localized disruption of the BBB. With time, falling levels of the

Table 10.3 FORMULATION INFORMATION AND NAMES OF COMMERCIALLY AVAILABLE GLUCEPTATE PRODUCTS

MANUFACTURER	NAME	EACH VIAL CONTAINS:
Dupont-NEN	Glucoscan®	200 mg gluceptate sodium 0.06 (minimum) stannous chloride (lyophilized mixture stored under nitrogen)
Mallinckrodt	TechneScan Gluceptate®	50 mg gluceptate calcium 0.7–1.1 mg stannous chloride (lyophilized mixture stored under nitrogen)

TABLE 10.4 COMPENDIAL (USP XXI) RECOMMENDATIONS FOR PACKAGING AND STORAGE OF Tc-99m PENTETATE AND GLUCEPTATE

	Tc-99m PENTETATE	Tc-99m GLUCEPTATE
Packaging/storage:	Preserve in single dose or multidose containers at temperature of 2–8° C.[a] Protect from freezing	
pH:	3.8–7.5	4.0–8.0
Radiochemical purity:	Should not be less than 90%	
Stability:	Should be injected within 6 hours of preparation	

[a] Note, however, that package inserts for several of these commercial products specifically state that storage before and after preparation be at room temperature.

radiopharmaceutical in blood permit visualization of radioactivity in the lesion as a result of increasing target to non-target ratios.

Following intravenous injection, Tc-99m pentetate rapidly distributes throughout the extracellular fluid space. Plasma clearance is multiexponential with biological half-lives of 3.8 minutes (58%), 16 minutes (24%), 2.0 hours (16%), and 14 hours (2%) (McAfee JG, et al, 1979). The extremely fast component represents diffusion into the extravascular extracellular fluid space whereas the slowest component probably represents plasma protein binding. The fraction of the administrated dose remaining in the plasma is approximately 15–20% after 1 hour, 10–12% after 2 hours, and 4% after 6 hours. Plasma clearance may be delayed in patients with renal disease. Less than 5% of the injected dose is bound to plasma proteins (Russell CD, et al, 1986). There is negligible binding of Tc-99m pentetate of red blood cells.

Tc-99m pentetate is rapidly eliminated from the body by glomerular filtration. Whole-body clearance is biexponential with biological half-lives of 1.0 hour (58%) and 9.2 hours (42%). Approximately 90% of the injected dose is eliminated in the urine within the first 12 hours following intravenous administration.

Tc-99m Gluceptate. Whether Tc-99m gluceptate might localize in brain tumor via mechanisms other than increased permeability of the BBB is not clear. Tumors extract relatively large amounts of glucose as an energy-producing substrate. It has therefore been postulated that gluceptate's sugarlike chemical structure might result in tumor tissues recognizing Tc-99m gluceptate as a metabolic substrate (Léveillé J, et al, 1977), thus accounting for some measure of its uptake in cerebral tumors.

Following intravenous injection, Tc-99m gluceptate is rapidly cleared from the blood. The blood-pool clearance is triexponential with biological half-lives of 5 minutes (84%), 1 hour (10%), and 24 hours (6%) (Arnold RW, et al, 1975). After 1 hour, 2–15% of the injected dose remains in the blood pool. The rate of blood clearance may be delayed in patients with renal disease. Virtually all the blood-pool activity is in the plasma, with little or no diffusion into the red blood cells. Protein binding increases from 47% initially after injection to 55% at 1 hour and 87% at 24 hours (Arnold RW, et al, 1975).

Tc-99m gluceptate is rapidly eliminated from the body by both glomerular filtration and renal tubular secretion. Whole-body clearance is also triexponential with biological half-lives of 20 minutes (35%), 2.4 hours (30%), and 89 hours (35%). Urinary excretion accounts for the elimination of approximately 40% of the administered dose within the first hour, with 70% appearing in the urine by 24 hours (Arnold RW, et al, 1975). The hepatobiliary system represents a normal alternate route of excretion for a small fraction of Tc-99m gluceptate (Prince JR, et al, 1978; Tyler JL and Powers TA, 1982).

PRECAUTIONS

Drug Interactions. Corticosteroid therapy to reduce cerebral edema in space-occupying diseases of the brain may also reduce the cerebral tumor uptake of conventional radiopharmaceuticals (Marty R and Cain ML, 1973) by decreasing peritumor edema. Though steroid interference with the brain uptake of Tc-99m pentetate or gluceptate may not be as great a problem as that earlier reported with Tc-99m sodium pertechnetate, it is generally advised that steroid therapy should be discontinued for at least 2 days prior to brain imaging, if at all possible, in order to decrease any likelihood of a false-negative study.

Cancer chemotherapy drugs may also interfere with brain imaging based on the observation of patchy, increased radiopharmaceutical uptake in brain in patients who exhibit chemotherapy neurotoxicity (Sherkow LH, 1979). Similarly, ventricular localization of brain-imaging radiopharmaceuticals has been shown in patients with ventriculitis caused by intrathecal methotrexate therapy (Makler PT, Jr, et al, 1978).

Interference of Tc-99m sodium pertechnetate brain imaging may be caused by the prior administration of stannous ion-containing drugs (Ancri D, et al, 1977; Chandler WM and Shuck LD, 1975) and certain antimicrobials (Castronovo JJ, et al, 1985). It has been shown that Tc-99m pertechnetate radiolabeling of red blood cells occurs in the presence of stannous ions and sulfonamides (Chervu LR, et al, 1981). For stannous ions the mechanism involves reduction of the Tc-99m pertechnetate ion intracellularly with subsequent binding to hemoglobin (Callahan RJ, et al, 1981; Dewanjee MK, 1974). The mechanism for the sulfonamide-induced erythrocyte labeling is unclear. Both drug-induced interferences result in a failure of the Tc-99m pertechnetate to leave the vascular space with resultant increased activity noted in the superior sagittal and transverse sinuses and decreased lesion-to-background ratios. The significance of this interference has been lessened since pertechnetate is no longer preferred for routine brain imaging. This interaction has not been reported with either Tc-99m pentetate or gluceptate.

Side Effects/Adverse Reactions. At present, there are no known side effects associated with the use of diagnostic doses of either Tc-99m pentetate or gluceptate.

Use During Pregnancy/Breastfeeding. It is generally advisable that radiopharmaceuticals not be utilized during pregnancy because of the risk of fetal radiation exposure. As with most radiopharmaceuticals, studies in either animals or humans have not been performed to determine teratogenic effects of these radio brain imaging agents; therefore, risk benefit should be considered. Also, it is suggested that breastfeeding should be discontinued for approximately 24 hours following the administration of either Tc-99m pentetate or gluceptate since the excretion of either radiopharmaceutical or their breakdown products in breast milk can cause radiation exposure to the feeding infant (Mountford PJ and Coakley AJ, 1985).

CLINICAL CONSIDERATIONS

Several clinical studies have been performed to compare the Tc-99m radiopharmaceuticals for brain imaging including evaluations of the overall sensitivities of both early and delayed static imaging. Although it is generally agreed that static imaging delayed for 1–3 hours post injection improves the diagnostic accuracy for all conventional Tc-99m brain imaging radiopharmaceuticals, it is not entirely clear which is the optimum agent for static brain imaging.

In the early 1970s, clinical comparisons of radiopharmaceuticals for brain imaging utilized the two commonly available Tc-99m agents, Tc-99m pentetate and Tc-99m sodium pertechnetate. These studies, in general, found that superior static imaging was obtained with Tc-99m pentetate. The availability of Tc-99m gluceptate during the mid-1970s and its subsequent application for brain imaging caused others to include this new radiopharmaceutical in clinical comparisons. In 1977, J. Léveillé and colleagues reported improved detectability of primary and metastatic brain lesions with Tc-99m gluceptate compared to pertechnetate. No difference was noted in the detection of either infarcts or ischemic lesions even on delayed images. F. D. Rollo and colleagues (1977) found Tc-99m gluceptate superior to pertechnetate and DTPA for the detection of strokes and neoplasms. Soon afterwards, however, T. W. Ryerson and colleagues (1978) compared these same radiopharmaceuticals in patients with proven brain lesions and found no significant difference between Tc-99m gluceptate and Tc-99m pentetate in the numbers of lesions detected or in lesion-to-background ratios. M. R. Tetalman and colleagues (1978) also compared Tc-99m pentetate with gluceptate yet found greater lesion detection with Tc-99m pentetate. J. E. Seabold and colleagues (1983) found Tc-99m pentetate superior to Tc-99m gluceptate for the detection of CVAs and infarcts, noting that 17% of patients with CVAs (N = 24) were not detected with Tc-99m gluceptate although all were studied within 1–2 days of a positive Tc-99m pentetate study. In that same study, Tc-99m pentetate was either superior to (43%) or equivalent to (43%) Tc-99m gluceptate in the detection of metastatic brain lesions. Tc-99m gluceptate was reported superior to pentetate in only 17% of the respective cases. J. I. Banzo and coworkers (1982) reported no difference in the sensitivity of either Tc-99m pentetate or Tc-99m gluceptate for detecting brain lesions (both 96%) although they noted that lesion-to-background ratios were higher with Tc-99m pentetate in 38% of their cases as opposed to 18% with Tc-99m gluceptate.

Why clinical experiences differ with these agents is not clear. It is possible that earlier reports comparing Tc-99m pentetate and Tc-99m gluceptate may have utilized the ferric chloride/ascorbic acid DTPA formulation (ferpentetate) rather than the currently available stannous ion (pentetate) formulation. Neither Rollo nor Ryerson described the specific formulation of Tc-99m pentetate that they utilized. Others who found Tc-99m pentetate superior clearly described the use of the stannous ion formulation. Since different renal excretory rates have been described for the two formulations, it is likely that different lesion-to-background ratios could be obtained with these products, which may result in lower lesion detectability with the more slowly clearing product. Tc-99m ferpentetate has been shown to clear much more slowly from blood than Tc-99m pentetate (Atkins HL, et al, 1971).

Although it is debatable whether Tc-99m gluceptate or Tc-99m pentetate is the superior radiopharmaceutical for routine static imaging, it appears that no significant difference exists in the diagnostic quality of radionuclide angiograms performed with either Tc-99m sodium pertechnetate, Tc-99m pentetate, or Tc-99m gluceptate (Rollo FD, et al, 1977). As a result of the greater convenience of generator-produced Tc-99m sodium pertechnetate and its lesser expense (compared to Tc-99m gluceptate and Tc-99m pentetate), Tc-99m sodium pertechnetate is often utilized whenever only flow-type diagnostic information is desired (e. g., as in the determination of brain death). It should be pointed out, however, that Tc-99m pentetate is the preferred radiopharmaceutical for flow-type imaging because of its lower patient radiation dosimetry (Table 10.5).

DOSAGE/DOSIMETRY

With both Tc-99m pentetate and gluceptate, adults receive 15–20 millicuries intravenously for brain imaging. The recommended dose of Tc-99m sodium pertechnetate for dynamic imaging in adults is 20–25 mCi. Pediatric dosages should be individualized according to established methods utilizing either body surface (preferred), weight, or age.

The patient radiation dosimetry for

Table 10.5   ESTIMATED ABSORBED RADIATION DOSES IN ADULT PATIENTS FROM INTRAVENOUSLY ADMINISTERED Tc-99m PERTECHNETATE, PENTETATE AND GLUCEPTATE[a]

ORGAN	RADS/20 MILLICURIES		
	Tc-99m Sodium Pertechnetate[b]	*Tc-99m Pentetate*	*Tc-99m Gluceptate*
Kidneys		0.44	3.4
(renal cortices)			4.8[c]
Total body	0.27	0.15	0.2
Bladder wall	1.10		
· 2.4-hour void		2.8[c]	2.4[c]
· 4.8-hour void		5.6[c]	5.6[c]
Testes	0.27	0.20	0.2
Ovaries	0.28	0.32	0.4
Liver	0.30	0.30	0.24
Thyroid	2.60		
G.I. tract			
· Stomach wall	5.0[c]		

[a] From respective product information

[b] Values are for resting population and patients *not* pretreated with blocking agents, such as potassium perchlorate.

[c] Critical organ(s).

Tc-99m pertechnetate, pentetate, and gluceptate are shown in Table 10.5 (Arnold RW, et al, 1975; Thomas SR, et al, 1984). Radiation exposure to the bladder from these radiopharmaceuticals can be minimized by increasing the intake of fluids and encouraging frequent voiding during the first 4–6 hours after radiopharmaceutical administration.

IMAGING TECHNIQUE

With either Tc-99m pentetate or Tc-99m gluceptate, the conventional nuclear medicine brain imaging study consists of two phases: the radionuclide angiogram (or "dynamic") portion and the delayed (or "static") images.

"Dynamic" Phase.   The initial portion of the conventional brain image study requires that the radiopharmaceutical is injected intravenously via a large arm vein in order to facilitate bolus delivery of the radiopharmaceutical to the brain. Immediately following intravenous administration, images are obtained serially every few seconds. These dynamic images record the appearance of the radiopharmaceutical during the arterial, capillary, and venous phases of cerebral circulation (Figure 10.8) and reflect relative blood flow to areas in the head.

Dynamic images are usually taken with the patient in the anterior position, although the posterior or vertex view may occasionally be preferred for visualization of the suspected blood-flow abnormality. Generally, lateral views are not routinely employed in dynamic imaging of the brain since comparison of symmetry during the various phases of cerebral blood flow assists in image interpretation. Computer-assisted analysis techniques may be desirable during the dynamic phase in order to derive comparative blood-flow information among various areas of the brain.

The initial dynamic imaging portion is of particular diagnostic value in evaluating (1) arteriovenous malformations that are often visible as perfusion abnormalities, (2) cerebral infarctions, (3) subdural and epidural hematomas, and (4) brain death where cerebral blood flow is absent (Figure 10.4).

Delayed or "Static" Images.   Static images of the brain are obtained 1–3 hours following intravenous administration of the radiopharmaceutical when levels of the radiopharmaceutical in blood have fallen sufficiently to permit visualization of the uptake in cerebral lesions (Wolfstein RS, et al, 1974; Fink-Bennett D, et al, 1982). Images are usually obtained in at least four projections, lateral views from each side and anterior and posterior views (Figures 10.1 and 10.2).

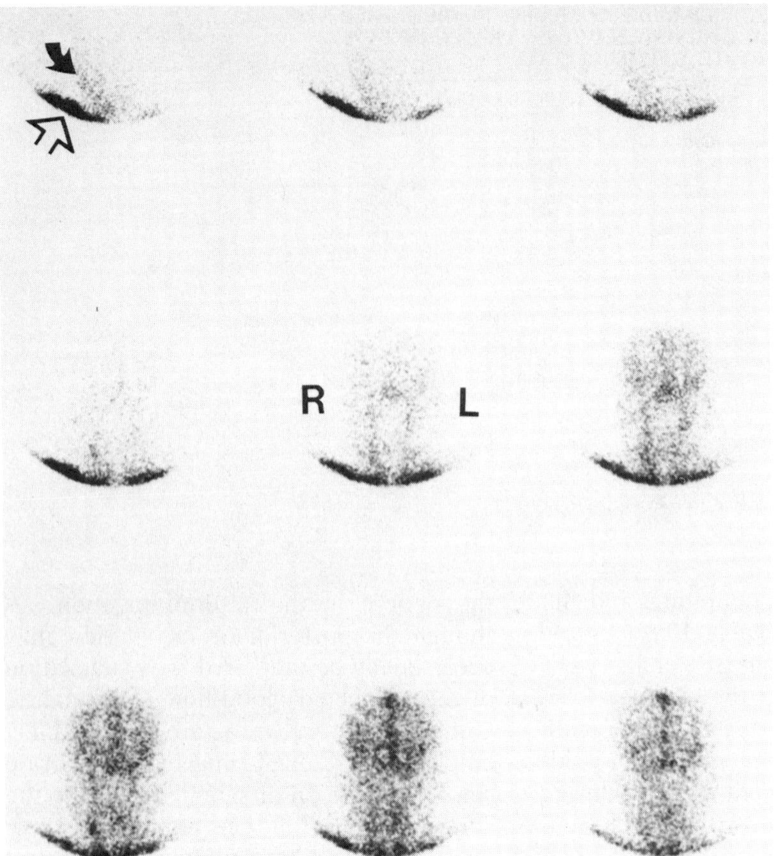

Figure 10.8 Tc-99m pentetate cerebral angiogram in a normal subject (same patient as Figure 10.1). Early frames (top row) demonstrate "pseudo-activity on the right side (solid arrow) resulting from scatter of radiation off the face and neck as the radioactive bolus passes through the subclavian vein (open arrow). Flow of activity through the carotid arteries (middle row) is symmetrical, as is cerebral perfusion. Late frames (bottom row) demonstrate activity in the superior sagittal sinus.

Though static brain imaging has a reported sensitivity as high as 70–90% for many types of cerebrovascular disease and head tumors, the radionuclide angiogram, when performed in conjunction with static imaging, is reported to increase diagnostic sensitivity for some diseases by as much as 10–15% (Cowan RJ, et al, 1973; Maynard CD and Cowan RJ, 1974).

II. Radiopharmaceuticals for Measuring Cerebral Function

Although conventional nuclear medicine brain imaging permits observation of tumor or diseases that affect the integrity of the blood-brain barrier (BBB), a variety of central nervous diseases affect brain tissue without involving the BBB and cannot be demonstrated using conventional brain-imaging radiopharmaceuticals. To evaluate these diseases, it is necessary to employ radiopharmaceuticals that are capable of measuring functional parameters involved in cerebral physiology, including cerebral perfusion, glucose metabolism, and oxygen utilization. To evaluate these processes, radiopharmaceutical uptake in brain must involve passage through the intact BBB utilizing nonpathological mechanisms. Two general processes have been identified in the BBB for the transport of substances into brain. They involve (1) carrier-mediated transport utilizing specific binding mechanisms involving membrane carriers and (2) passive diffusion as a result of substrate lipophilicity.

CARRIER-MEDIATED TRANSPORT OF RADIOPHARMACEUTICALS IN THE BRAIN

Carrier-mediated transport of ions and metabolic substances across cellular membranes is initiated by the attachment of these materials onto a carrier protein. Carrier-transport proteins have markedly high affinities for substances to be transported, and, once binding has occurred, the complex is many orders of magnitude more lipid soluble than the substance itself, thus facilitating its transport across the capillary membrane (Crone C, 1965). The movement of substances into brain via carrier-mediated transport is essentially independent of plasma concentration. However, with significantly elevated plasma concentrations, carrier sites may be saturated, and the transfer rates will then be limited by the dissociation constants of the carrier and the substance. As a result, increases in the plasma concentration of the ion or metabolic substrate may have no effect on its concentration in the brain (Holman BL, et al, 1983).

At least nine carrier transport proteins for the BBB have been identified (Table 10.6), each with high affinities for specific precursors of cellular metabolism (Oldendorf WH, 1983). Because most of the metabolic substances transported into brain via these proteins are chemically composed solely of carbon, hydrogen, oxygen, and nitrogen, radioisotopes of these

Table 10.6 SUBSTANCES FOR WHICH CARRIER-TRANSPORT PROTEINS ARE KNOWN TO EXIST IN THE BLOOD-BRAIN BARRIER

Hexoses (glucose and its analogues)
Short chained monocarboxylic acids
Amino acids (neutral, basic, and acidic)
Choline
Purine
Nucleic acid precursors
Thyroxine
Triiodothyronine

elements or their analogues have been necessarily used in preparing radiolabeled metabolic tracers as radiopharmaceuticals for functional brain imaging.

Substances that have been radiolabeled and used to study cerebral metabolism include glucose (and its analogues), amino acids, and radioisotopes of oxygen. Fluorine-18 fluorodeoxyglucose is currently the most prevalently used radiopharmaceutical for the evaluation of cerebral metabolism.

CEREBRAL METABOLISM: F-18 FLUORODEOXYGLUCOSE

Background/History. Though glucose is the major energy source for the brain, brain cells have no mechanism for its storage and must be continually supplied glucose from blood by transport through cell membranes. In brain, glucose uptake is proportional to metabolic activity, and in diseases affecting the central nervous system, changes occur in rates of regional brain glucose utilization.

Although the transport mechanism for glucose across the BBB has been extensively studied, efforts directed at developing nonhexose analogues that enter brain by this pathway have been unsuccessful, since the carrier transport is stereospecific for glucose. Fortunately, the specificity of this carrier-transport protein for individual hexose analogues is less than that of enzyme systems that are required for subsequent glucose metabolism. For example, even though the transport of glucose shows marked stereospecificity (i. e., D-glucose but not L-glucose enters brain), the carrier-mediated transport system accepts more hexose analogues than does hexokinase, the first enzyme in the glycolytic pathway (Lund-Anderson H, 1979).

Radiolabeled glucose and a variety of radiolabeled glucose analogues can be synthesized and utilized to measure regional glucose metabolism. Among these, glucose labeled with Carbon-11 (C-11) and glucose analogues labeled with C-11 and Fluorine-18 (F-18) have been most successful.

Chemistry. Early methods used to prepare C-11 glucose were mostly impractical since the lengthy times of the respective syntheses (patterned after those used to prepare glucose radiolabeled with relatively long-lived Carbon-14) were inconsistent with the short half-life (i. e., 20 minutes) of the C-11 radionuclide. Subsequently, rapid synthetic techniques were developed that are suitable for preparing C-11 glucose either by photosynthesis from C-11 dioxide (Lifton JF and Welch MJ, 1971), or by chemical synthesis, using various C-11 precursors.

By substituting a hydroxyl group for a hydrogen atom on the second carbon of D-glucose, a glucose analogue is formed that has all the characteristics of glucose, including its transport and utilization, except that it fails to undergo intracellular enzymatic glycolysis beyond initial phosphorylation (Sols A and Crane RK, 1954; Diamond I and Fishman RA, 1973). This glucose analogue, 2-deoxyglucose, appears to inhibit all subsequent enzymatic steps of intracellular glycolysis that follows the hexokinase reaction. Thus, 2-deoxyglucose becomes metabolically trapped within brain cells (i. e., as 2-deoxyglucose-6-phosphate) as a function of respective metabolic requirements.

Provided there is negligible loss of 2-deoxyglucose-6-phosphate from the intracellular site of phosphorylation during its measurement and a suitable radiolabel can be found, this type of radiopharmaceutical can permit the noninvasive measurement of regional glucose utilization in man using emission tomography (Raichle ME, et al, 1975; Raichle ME, et al, 1979). In animals, the use of 2-deoxy-D-[C-14] glucose and autoradiography to determine regional brain glucose metabolism is a widely accepted technique (Kennedy C, et al, 1975). Carbon-11 labeled 2-deoxyglucose can be synthesized by a variety of methods including nuc-displacement of 2,3:4,5-di-o-isopropyl-leophilic displacement of 2,3:4,5-di-o-isopropylidene-1-o-trifluoromethyl sul-fonyl-D-arabinitol with C-11 cyanide followed by reduction and hydrolysis (Shiue CY, et al, 1979) or by enzymatic synthesis (Bessell EM and Thomas P, 1973).

Fluorine can substitute for a hydroxyl group in several biological substrates to create analogues with approximately the same biological activity as the natural metabolite (Goldman P, 1969). Of the several fluorine-labeled glucose analogues that have been developed, 2-fluorodeoxyglucose (2FDG) possesses biochemical properties that most closely resemble that of D-glucose. Fluorinated deoxyglucose is stable in vivo, is transported intracellularly via the hexose carrier protein, and is a suitable substrate for hexokinase (Bessell EM, et al, 1971). Like 2-deoxyglucose, 2FDG also fails to undergo subsequent metabolic steps following intracellular phosphorylation (Figure 10.9) (Bessell EM and Thomas P, 1973).

Fluorine-18 (Table 10.7) is the most commonly employed radioisotope of fluorine used in the preparation of 2FDG. Several synthetic reactions have been used to prepare F-18 fluorodeoxyglucose (F-18 FDG) (Barrio JR, et al, 1981). Positron emission tomography (PET) is used to image the cerebral biodistribution of the C-11 and F-18 radiolabeled glucose analogues. PET imaging of both C-11 and F-18-labeled 2-deoxyglucose is useful for evaluating regional glucose metabolism (Figure 10.10).

Pharmacokinetics. Following intravenous administration, distribution of F-18 FDG is relatively uniform throughout the body (Gallagher BM, et al, 1977). Localization in the brain occurs with an uptake half-time of approximately 8 minutes; by 35 minutes after injection, 95% of the peak uptake is achieved. Brain uptake in human subjects averages approximately 4% of the administered dose. The F-18 FDG is freely filtered by the glomerulus but is partially reabsorbed by the tubules. Urinary elimination is variable, ranging from 8% to 42% (average 21%) of the injected dose in the first 2 hours.

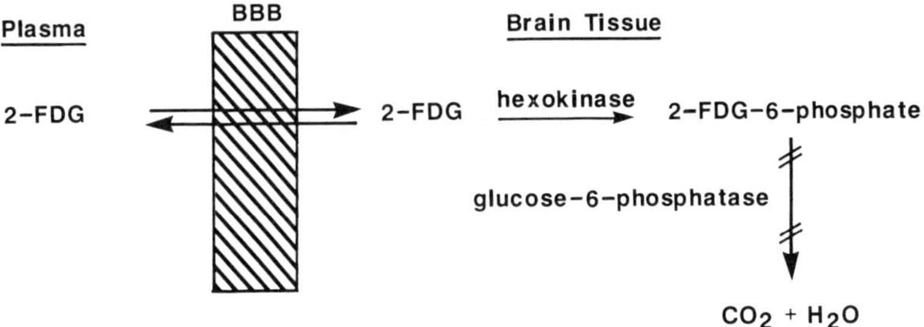

Figure 10.9 Steps involved in the cerebral location of 2-fluorodeoxyglucose (2-FDG). The 2-FDG freely enters brain tissue via the stereospecific carrier transport system responsible for glucose uptake. Although the 2-FDG is a suitable substrate for the initial hexokinase phosphorylation reaction, it is unable to undergo further enzymatic glucolysis and thus becomes trapped in brain cells as a function respective of metabolic activity.

Table 10.7 NUCLEAR AND PHYSICAL PROPERTIES OF FLUORINE-18 (F-18)

Physical $T_{1/2}$:	110 minutes
Decay mode:	$Beta^+$ (97%), EC (3%)
Principal emission:	Positron
Energy/Yield:	511 keV/194%

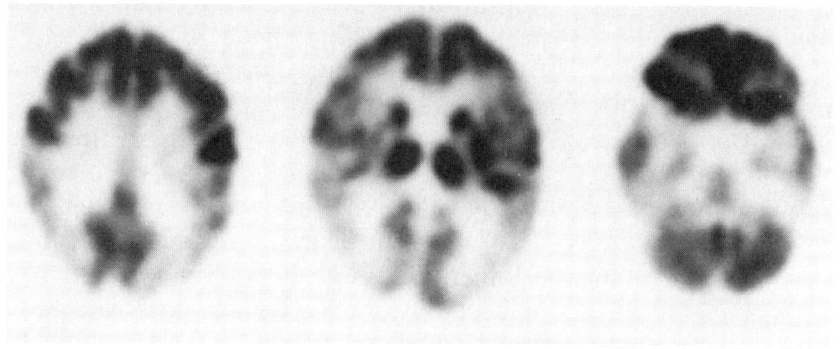

Figure 10.10 Positron emission tomography study in a patient with Alzheimer's disease obtained following the intravenous administration of F-18 2-fluorodeoxyglucose. Glucose utilization is especially impaired in the parietal cortex but is normal in the deep gray-matter structures and in the cerebellum. (Courtesy of David E, Kuhl, M.D., University of Michigan Medical Center, Ann Arbor, MI).

Table 10.8 PATIENT
RADIATION DOSIMETRY
ESTIMATES TO SELECTED
ORGANS FROM [F-18]
FLUORO-2-DEOXY-D-
GLUCOSE[a]

ORGAN	RADS/mCi
Kidneys	0.071
Lungs	0.063
Liver	0.059
Spleen	0.14
Urinary bladder	0.41
Whole body	0.04

[a] Dose estimates from Radiopharmaceutical Dosimetry Center, Oak Ridge Associated Universities, Oak Ridge, TN, and are based upon distribution data from B.M. Gallagher and colleagues (1977), assuming a $T_{1/2}$ eff of 1.83 hours (except urinary bladder, for which the assumptions are taken from S.C. Jones and colleagues (1982). All values for 2-hour voiding of urinary bladder.

Precautions. There are no known contraindications to the use of F-18 FDG. Because of the relatively short physical half-life of F-18 (110 minutes), breastfeeding may be resumed 24 hours after radiopharmaceutical administration.

Dosage/Dosimetry. Radiation dosimetry for F-18 FDG is shown in Table 10.8.

CEREBRAL PERFUSION: LIPOPHILIC RADIOPHARMACEUTICALS

Background/History. For nonionic substances without a specific transport mechanism, the penetration rate from blood into brain is directly related to lipid solubility. A substance with sufficient lipid solubility will diffuse from blood into the lipid of the vascular endothelial cell membrane and eventually into the cell cytoplasm. Once it crosses the outer membrane of the capillary endothelium, the substance enters the extracellular fluid of the brain (Oldendorf WH, 1983).

A variety of substances and drugs are sufficiently lipophilic to cross the intact BBB, including oxygen, carbon dioxide, inert gases (e.g., xenon), and several drugs such as barbituates, ethanol, amphetamines, and phenothiazines. Blood-brain barrier permeability can be predicted by measuring the lipid/water solubility of substances (Oldendorf WH, 1974a). The ratio between the solubility of the radiopharmaceutical in lipid and in water is called the *partition coefficient*. When, for example, the olive oil/water partition coefficient of a substance is greater than 0.04, the material penetrates substantially into the brain during a single microcirculatory passage (Oldendorf WH, et al, 1972; Oldendorf WH, 1981). Substances with lower partition coefficient values will also penetrate the BBB, but at a slower rate.

In principle, radiopharmaceuticals intended for the evaluation of cerebral perfusion should possess partition coefficients that allow them to be nearly completely cleared by brain during a single passage and be sufficiently retained within the brain in order to provide flow-dependent images. In this situation, activity in brain is proportional to regional cerebral blood flow. In addition to being completely cleared from blood during a single passage through the brain, radiolabeled substances for imaging cerebral perfusion should also be (1) metabolized to a polar configuration or bound to neuroreceptor sites in order to avoid significant washout from the brain during the period of imaging, and (2) ideally, not trapped in the lungs during the initial passage, since subsequent lung clearance would result in prolonged delivery time to the brain and the need for a prolonged steady state in blood flow in order to accurately measure cerebral perfusion (Holman BL, et al, 1983). Such radiopharmaceuticals must also be nontoxic and pharmacologically inert in order to avoid undesirable alterations in brain perfusion induced by the radiopharmaceutical during the imaging procedure. It is also known that brain uptake of lipophilic substances can be affected by factors such as the retention of the drug at the injection site, plasma protein binding, the rate of metabolic degradation, accumulation of the agent by the liver and other tissues,

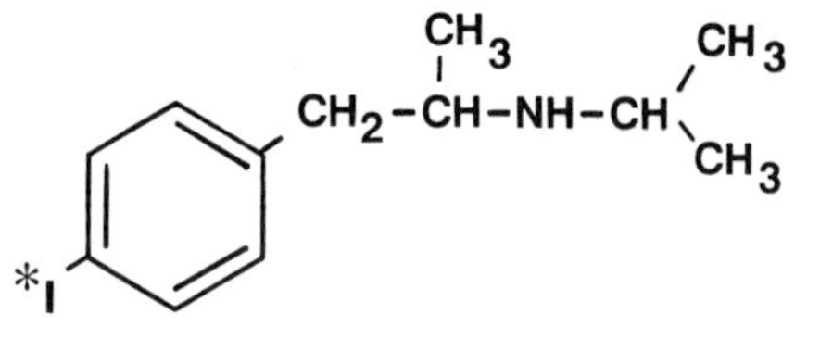

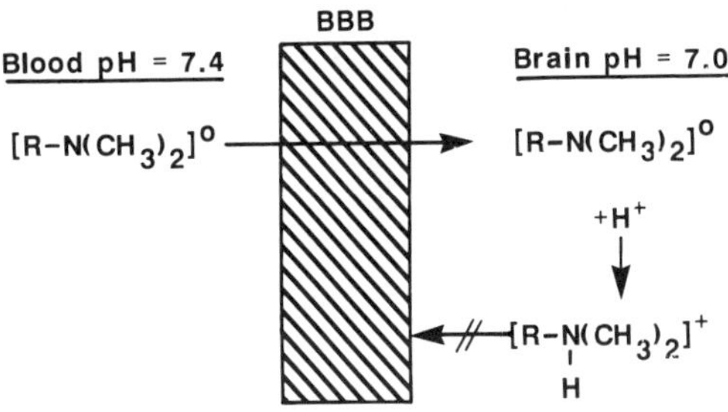

IMP

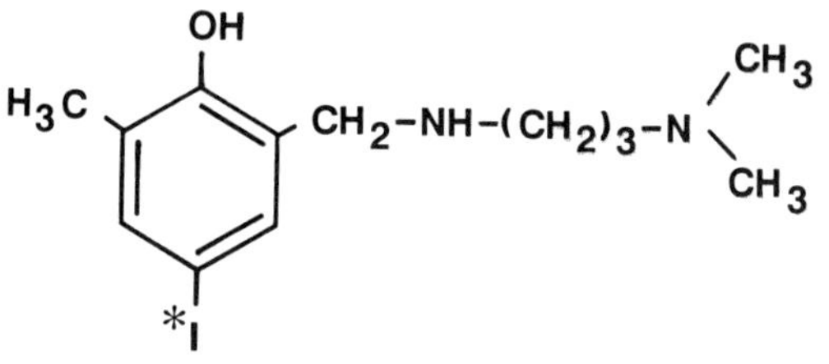

HIPDM

Figure 10.11   Chemical structures of N-isopropyl-p-iodoamphetamine (IMP) and N,N,N'-trimethyl-N'-[2-hydroxy-3-methyl-5-iodobenzyl]-1,3-propanediamine (HIPDM).

and the degree of brain tissue binding (Oldendorf WH, 1974b).

In nuclear medicine, several lipophilic compounds have been developed that exhibit brain uptake and potential usefulness for cerebral perfusion imaging. These agents have included I-123 4-iodoantipyrine (Uzler JM, et al, 1975), C-11 alpha-p-iodoanilinophenylacetonitrile (Winstead MB, et al, 1979) and 2,5-dimethoxyphenylisopropylamine, a catecholamine analogue that has been radio-labeled with both Br-77 (Sargent T, III, et al, 1975) and I-123 (Sargent T, III et al, 1978). Although these radiolabeled substances represented the initial phase of development of radiopharmaceuticals for cerebral perfusion imaging, none were ideal.

Radiolabeled Amines and Diamines.   A number of radioiodinated (I-123) compounds have been shown to possess clinical usefulness in delineating cerebral blood flow (LaFrance ND, et al, 1981; Holman BL, et al, 1983). H. S. Winchell and colleagues (1980a) investigated a large group of radioiodinated monoamines and found

that N-isopropyl-p-[I-123] iodoamphetamine (I-123 IMP, or Spectamine®) (Figure 10.11) provided the highest blood-brain barrier permeability and retention in the brain parenchyma. Although the mechanism of brain uptake of I-123 IMP is dependent upon its lipid solubility, it has been suggested that its brain retention is a result of "non-specific, high-capacity" binding to receptor sites in CNS tissue (Winchell HS, et al, 1980b; Kuhl DE, et al, 1982).

Radiolabeled diamines are another group of compounds that have been evaluated for cerebral perfusion imaging. The development of radiolabeled diamines occurred through research on a series of selenium-75 (Se-75) piperidine (PIPSE) and morpholine (MOSE) derivatives, frequently referred to as "pH shift agents." The pH shift mechanism of cerebral perfusion imaging (Figure 10.12) centers on the pH gradient that exists between blood (pH 7.4) and brain (pH 7.0). At the higher pH of blood, the pH shift agents are neutral and lipid soluble and can readily diffuse into brain parenchyma. Upon encountering the lower pH of the brain, these agents become ionized and, as such, are incapable of reverse diffusion (Kung HF and Blau M, 1980a). Hence, the pH shift agents become trapped in the brain as a function of their initial delivery (i. e., cerebral perfusion).

Figure 10.12   Illustration of "pH shift mechanism." At the pH of blood, the agent is neutral and lipid soluble and therefore capable of rapidly penetrating the intact blood-brain barrier (BBB). Upon encountering the more acidic pH of brain tissue, the agent acquires a charge and in the ionic state is incapable of reverse diffusion.

The Se-75 diamines displayed high brain uptake and retention after intravenous administration in animals and humans (Kung HF and Blau M, 1980b); however, the suboptimal radionuclidic characteristics of Se-75 limited the clinical usefulness of these agents, thereby prompting the search for radioiodinated diamines. Of the radioiodinated diamines evaluated, I-123 labeled N,N,N^1-trimethyl-N^1-[2-hydroxy-3-methyl-5-iodobenzyl]-1, 3-propanediamine (HIPDM) (Figure 10.11) appears most promising for clinical cerebral perfusion imaging applications. Moreover, I-123 HIPDM can be prepared on-site using a "kit" reagent approach, similar to that used in the preparation of Tc-99m radiopharmaceuticals (Kung HF, et al, 1983). I-123 HIPDM, however, is not approved for use in the U.S.; I-123 IMP (Spectamine®) has been approved for use in the evaluation of stroke.

Pharmacokinetics. After intravenous injection, I-123 IMP is rapidly cleared from the plasma with uptake in the brain, lungs, and liver. While I-123 HIPDM also accumulates initially in the lungs, the clearance from the lungs is faster with IMP than with HIPDM. By 60 minutes after injection, the lung activity is 30% of maximum for IMP and 50% for HIPDM (Holman BL, et al, 1984a). With I-123 IMP, liver and lung activity progressively increases over the first 5 hours, the percentages in these organs at 1 and 5 hours being 4.1 and 2.1; and 14.1 and 5.1, respectively. By 22 hours, liver and lungs contain 10.1 and 6.1 percent of the injected dose respectively (Spectamine® product literature, 1987). At 1 hour after injection, thyroid uptake is approximately 1%, probably reflecting the presence of free iodide in the I-123 IMP preparation. Cumulated urinary excretion averages 23% during the first 24 hours and 40% at 48 hours (Bischof-Delaloye A, et al, 1984).

Following injection in humans, I-123 IMP is metabolized to a number of compounds including p-iodoamphetamine, p-iodophenylacetone, p-iodobenzoic acid, p-iodohippuric acid, free iodide, and un-identified compounds. The two major metabolites are p-iodoamphetamine and p-iodobenzoic acid, which is a further breakdown product of p-iodoamphetamine. Plasma metabolites are negligible until 30 minutes after injection, increasing to almost 1% of the injected dose at 24 hours (Holman BL, et al, 1983). Plasma p-iodoamphetamine levels initially increase up to 8 to 10 hours post-dosing and then decrease with a terminal half-life of approximately 48 hours. p-iodobenzoic acid is noted to continually accumulate in the plasma up to 44 hours after dosing (Spectamine® product literature, 1987).

Brain uptake of I-123 IMP is observed within 30 seconds following injection and is greater than 80% of peak activity by 10 minutes (Hill TC, et al, 1982). Brain activity appears constant from 20–60 minutes after injection with approximately 5.6–7.5% of the injected dose respectively deposited (Holman BL, et al, 1983; Bischof-Delaloye A, et al, 1984). Studies by Kuhl and colleagues (1982) have shown that I-123 IMP undergoes back diffusion from brain into blood. The half-time for this occurrence is approximately 60 minutes. Despite this brain clearance, the net brain uptake is reasonably constant over the period of 20–60 minutes after injection because of the continued influx of I-123 IMP from the lung to brain during this period.

Kuhl and colleagues (1982) found in dogs that the measurement of cerebral blood flow using I-123 IMP and labeled microspheres correlated closely whenever blood flow was 75–200% of normal. Single-pass brain extraction, however, appears to be either flow or pH dependent, since the percent extraction decreased from 92% at normal blood flow (pH 7.35) to 74% at one-half normal blood flow (pH 7.10). In normal humans, the measurement of mean cerebral blood flow with I-123 IMP was calculated at 47 ml/min per 100 g; in close agreement with the accepted value of 50 ml/min/100 g.

Though early biodistribution studies had shown I-123 IMP to concentrate in the eyes of animals (Holman BL, et al,

1984b), later studies in humans showed no routine eye accumulation above background levels. In animals, the eye uptake of I-123 IMP appears to be related to active melanin synthesis and probably does not occur in the human eye, wherein melanin synthesis ceases at the embryonic stage (Holman BL, et al, 1983).

Following intravenous injection, I-123 HIPDM is rapidly cleared from the blood. Initial uptake by the lungs is high (approximately 50–60% of administered dose) with a biexponential clearance of 2.9 hours ($\cong$20%), and 49 hours ($\cong$60%). Liver uptake is variable but averages approximately 20% of the injected dose with prolonged retention. Occasionally uptake in the pancreas is noted (1–2% injected dose). Cumulative urinary excretion of the administered activity is approximately 20% at 24 hours and 30% at 48 hours, principally in the form of free radioiodide (Kung HF, et al, 1983).

Brain uptake of I-123 HIPDM is prompt, reaching about 4.6–8.5% of the injected dose at 15 minutes post injection. Compared to I-123 IMP, the peak brain uptake of I-123 HIPDM is 30–40% lower; however, its rate of uptake is faster. At 2 minutes post injection, 75% of the maximum brain uptake is achieved for I-123 HIPDM compared to only 45% for I-123 IMP. At 30–60 minutes post injection, the brain activity of each of these agents is relatively constant, and images obtained during this period are similar in appearance (Holman BL, et al, 1984a).

Clinical Considerations. Both I-123 IMP and HIPDM have blood-brain extraction fractions of 90% (Kung HF, et al, 1983; Kuhl DE, et al, 1982); however, as previously discussed, the brain activity of I-123 IMP is greater than that of I-123 HIPDM during the time at which imaging would normally be performed (i. e., at 20–60 minutes after injection). As a result, I-123 IMP offers some advantage over I-123 HIPDM for cerebral perfusion imaging, particularly with imaging procedures, such as SPECT, which require high count rates. On the other hand, I-123

HIPDM demonstrates a rapid accumulation in the brain soon after administration and for this reason, the steady state for cerebral blood flow need not be as long for I-123 HPDM as I-123 IMP. Iodine-123 HIPDM may, therefore, be preferable to use for quantitative studies of cerebral blood flow or for studies involving rapid changes in cerebral blood flow. For example, in patients with active epileptic seizures, I-123 HIPDM can be injected during the ictus with imaging of respective cerebral perfusion patterns performed later when the seizure has been brought under control. Assuming that cerebral blood flow changes associated with the seizure last only a short time, rapid uptake of the radiopharmaceutical used to map these changes is a requirement (Holman BL, et al, 1984a).

Unlike I-123 HIPDM, the cerebral distribution of I-123 IMP appears to change over time. In one report, there was a 42% decrease in cerebellum activity, an 18% decrease in cortex activity, and a 21% increase in cerebral infarct activity from early (i. e., 15–45 minutes post injection) to late (210–240 minutes post injection) I-123 IMP images (Creutzig H, et al, 1986). Similarly, Buell and colleagues (1985) demonstrated that I-123 IMP distribution at 13–27 minutes post injection correlated well with regional cerebral blood flow (measured with Xe-133), whereas the I-123 IMP distributions at 33–47 minutes and 5.5 hours post injection were significantly different. Based on these observations, regional cerebral perfusion studies using I-123 IMP (Figure 10.13) should be performed within 30 minutes post injection.

Dosage/Dosimetry. Patient radiation dosimetry estimates for I-123 IMP and HIPDM are presented in Table 10.9.

Tc-99m Propyleneamineoxime (PAO) Derivatives. The development of lipophilic complexes of technetium-99m for cerebral perfusion imaging would provide substantial advantages associated with its "ideal" radionuclide properties. The development

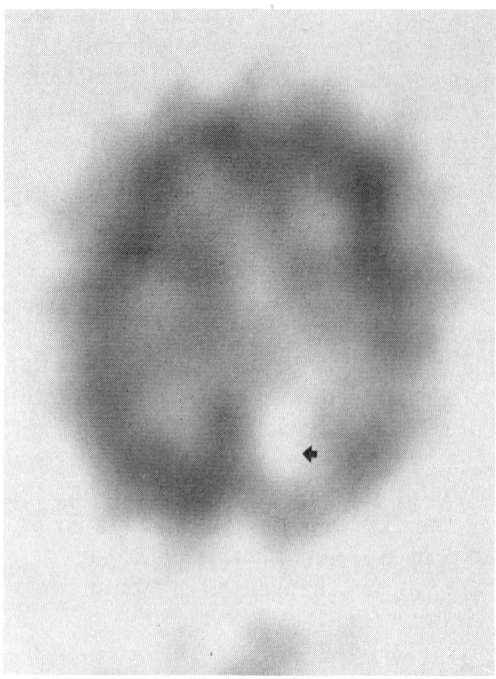

Figure 10.13 Single photon emission tomography evaluation of cerebral perfusion using I-123 IMP. Note (arrow) area of hypoperfusion corresponding to a cystic brain tumor.

Table 10.9 PATIENT RADIATION DOSIMETRY ESTIMATES FOR I-123 HIPDM AND I-123 IMP[a]

	RAD/5 mCi	
ORGAN	I-123 IMP[b]	I-123 HIPDM
Brain	0.5	0.70
Retina	3.7	—
Lung	1.1	2.9
Liver	1.1	1.85
Bladder	—	0.5
Total body	0.4	0.2

[a] From Spectamine® product literature (1988), and R. Wicks and colleagues (1983).
[b] At time of calibration.

of such an agent, however, has been hindered by basic problems with incorporating Tc-99m into an organic complex with sufficient lipophilicity to cross the intact blood-brain barrier and be retained by the brain. D. E. Troutner and coworkers (1983; 1984) prepared a neutral, lipophilic complex, propyleneamine oxine (PAO), that demonstrated, in animals, brain localization as a function of cerebral blood flow and had a first-

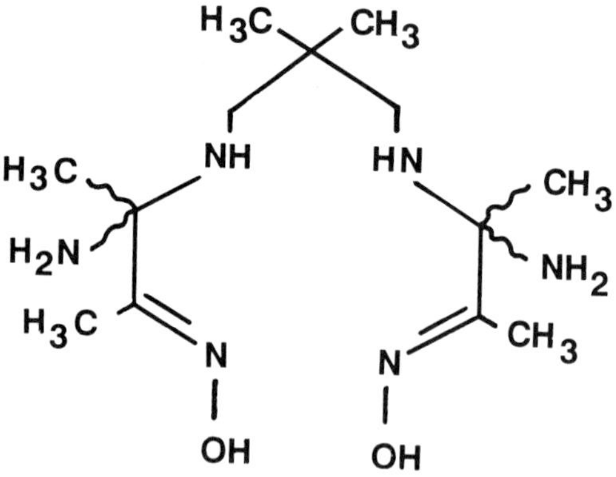

Figure 10.14 Chemical structures of hexamethylpropyleneamineoxime (HM-PAO).

pass extraction efficiency of 80% (Volkert WA, et al, 1984). Although this compound rapidly localized into the brain, it was not retained by the brain, and it passively diffused back into blood when its plasma concentration fell below its cerebral concentration.

HM-PAO. The hexamethyl derivative of PAO (HM-PAO, Figure 10.14) developed by Neirinckx and colleagues (1987) demonstrates prolonged retention in the brain (Nowotnik DP, et al, 1985) and appreciable extraction across the blood-brain barrier (Lassen NA, et al, 1987) (Figure 10.15). Of the d,l and $meso$stereoisomers of HM-PAO, the d,l mixture has been shown to have a higher brain retention than the $meso$isomer with 70–80% of the d,l complex that reaches the brain crossing the blood-brain barrier (Sharp PF, et al, 1986). Tc-99m-d,l-HM-PAO (hereafter $exametazime$, also known as Ceretec®, Amersham Corp., Arlington Heights, IL) has been shown to contain equimolar amounts of the d and l isomers. Each single-dose vial contains a lyophilized mixture of 0.5 mg exametazime (d,l,-4,8-diazo-3,6,6,9-tetramethylundecane-2,10-dione bisoxime), 7.5 μg stannous chloride dihydrate (minimum stannous tin 0.6 μg; maximum total stannous and stannic tin 4.0 μg/vial) and 4.5 mg sodium chloride. The vial is sealed in a nitrogen atmosphere and contains no bacteriostatic agent or preservative.

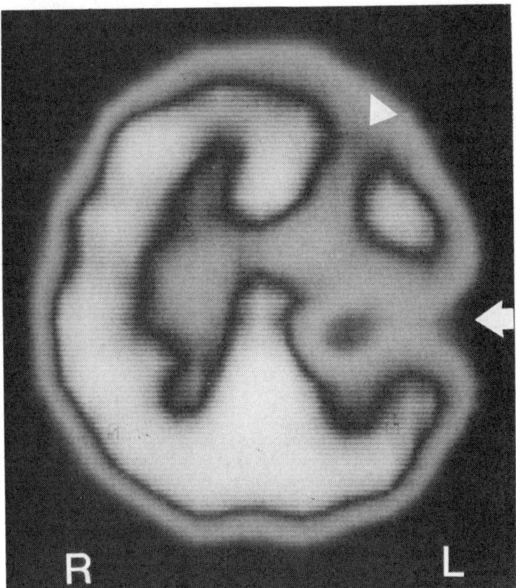

Figure 10.15 Transverse section of a Tc-99m HM-PAO SPECT study demonstrating decreased cerebral blood flow to the mid-left parietal cortex (arrow) and the left-frontal parietal (arrowhead) regions. Images compliments of James M. Mountz, M.D., University of Michigan Medical Center, Ann Arbor, MI.

In normal humans, Tc-99m exametazime is rapidly cleared from the blood after intravenous administration reaching a peak value within seconds, then declining exponentially after about 10 minutes to a steady-state level that represents about 40–50% of the peak activity (Lassen NA, et al, 1988). Tc-99m exametazime has an extraction efficiency across the blood-brain barrier of about 0.75 (Andersen AR, et al, 1988a) with the initially rapid accumulation of Tc-99m exametazime due to its lipophilicity. The mechanism of cerebral localization appears to involve conversion of Tc-99m exametazime into a polar metabolite that is no longer capable of permeating the blood-brain barrier. Since not all Tc-99m exametazime is converted and trapped immediately upon crossing the blood-brain barrier, however, diffusion of the radiopharmaceutical from brain tissues to blood occurs that accounts for the failure of Tc-99m exametazime to behave as a

perfect "microsphere-type" agent for the evaluation of cerebral blood flow (Andersen AR, et al, 1988b).

The conversion of Tc-99m exametazime to a hydrophilic species has been shown to occur in aqueous solutions at a rate much too slow to account for the in vivo retentions. Neirinckx and coworkers (1988) presented evidence that the in vivo conversion to nondiffusible forms may be dominated by an intracellular reaction with glutathionine. Glutathionine is present in relatively high concentrations intracellularly while only relatively small amounts exist in plasma. They have shown that conversion to hydrophilic species corresponds to levels of glutathionine in brain whereby buffered aqueous solutions of glutathionine rapidly converted HM-PAO to hydrophilic forms having the same chromatographic characteristics as found in the homogenates of rat brains (Neirinckx RD, et al, 1988). In support of this hypothesis, H. Matsuda and colleagues (1988) have shown that Tc-99m exametazime concentrates similarly in both gray and white matter, tissues known to have nearly equal concentrations of glutathionine.

Approximately 30% of the injected dose distributes into the GI tract immediately after injection, and about one-half of this activity is excreted over 48 hours. Another 40% of the injected dose is excreted through the urine over the 48 hours following injection (Ceretec® Product Literature, 1988).

Precautions. Because of the significant chemistry involved, special consideration must be given to the manner of preparation and the use of this radiopharmaceutical. Minimal amounts of stannous ions (as the reductant) are contained in the product, therefore, only freshly eluted Tc-99m sodium pertechnetate should be used to prepare the Tc-99m exametazime. Generator eluate more than 2 hours old should not be used, nor should eluate be used from a generator that was not eluted within the previous 24 hours. The lyophilized vial should not be reconstituted with more than 10–30 mCi or 5 ml total volume. Tc-99m exametazime may be stored at room temperature. Because Tc-99m exametazime undergoes in vitro conversion with time to secondary hydrophilic species, the radiopharmaceutical preparation should not be used after 30 minutes from the time of reconstitution. It is suggested that radiochemical purity be established prior to administration in order to determine and quantify the presence of the three principal radiochemical impurities (a secondary Tc-99m exametazime complex, free unbound pertechnetate, and hydrolyzed, reduced Tc-99m). The manufacturer specifies a 3-phase system to isolate the impurities (ITLC/SG and methylethyl ketone; ITLC/SG and normal saline; and Whatman No. 1 and 50% aqueous acetonitrile). Alternatively, W.A. Volkert (personal communication, 1989) suggests a single phase system, using solvent separation pads (Gelman Sciences, Inc., Ann Arbor, MI) and ethyl acetate, that resolves the primary lipophilic complex from all other radiochemical impurities. Radiochemical purity should be not less than 80%.

Adverse Reactions. Rash with generalized erythema, facial edema, and fever has been reported with the use of Tc-99m exametazime. A transient increase in blood pressure has been noted in up to 8% of patients (Ceretec® product literature, 1988).

Dosage/Dosimetry. Adults should be intravenously administered 15–20 mCi of Tc-99m exametazime that has been prepared within 30 minutes of the time of administration. Dynamic brain imaging may be performed immediately upon injection; static imaging, from 15 minutes up to 6 hours post injection.

Radiation dosimetry is shown in Table 10.10.

Tc-99m exametazime has also been shown useful for demonstrating a variety of pathologic and physiologic changes in brain, including epilepsy, extrapyramidal disorders, dementias, and psychiatric disorders (Podreka I, et al, 1987; Leonard JP, et al, 1986).

Table 10.10 PATIENT RADIATION DOSIMETRY ESTIMATES FOR Tc-99m EXAMETAZIME (HM-PAO)[a]

ORGAN	RADS/20 mCi
Lachrymal glands	5.2
Liver	1.1
Gallbladder wall	3.8
Small intestine wall	0.88
Upper large intestine wall	1.60
Lower large intestine wall	1.10
Kidneys	2.60
Urinary bladder wall	1.0
Ovaries	0.46
Testes	0.14
Brain	0.52
Whole body	0.26

[a] Personal communication from Radiopharmaceutical Dosimetry Center, Oak Ridge Associated Universities, Oak Ridge, TN

Labeling of white blood cells (WBCs). White blood cells that have been labeled in vitro with Tc-99m exametazime have been employed to obtain images that are diagnostically equivalent to those obtained with In-111 labeled white blood cells (Mock BH, et al, 1988; Roddie ME, et al, 1987). Unlike labeling with In-111 oxine, Tc-99m exametazime labeling of white blood cells is accomplished in plasma and is not adversely affected by the presence of transferrin. Typical white blood cell labeling efficiencies with Tc-99m exametazime range from 50–65%. Whether Tc-99m exametazime will prove as popular as In-111 oxine for labeling white blood cells for imaging inflammatory lesions is not assured. Though the greater convenience and widespread availability of Tc-99m is a significant advantage, the relatively shorter physical half-life of Tc-99m (6 hours) may limit the usefulness of this label for imaging at 24 hours when abscess-to-background ratios are typically highest.

Other New Tc-99m Agents for Brain Imaging. In addition to Tc-99m exametazime, work has proceeded on several other new Tc-99m radiopharmaceuticals that have demonstrated effectiveness for brain imaging, including Tc-99m DADT (diamine dithiol) and the ester-derivative dimer Tc-99m ECD (L,L-ethyl cysteinate dimer) (Lever SZ, et al, 1985; Cheesman

EH, et al, 1988). Presently, Tc-99m ECD has been shown in clinical trials to yield rapid brain uptake with good retention. At 2 minutes post injection, 4.6–6.8% of the injected dose localizes in brain, with a half-life of 17–20 hours (Walovitch RC, et al, 1988; Demonceau G, et al, 1988). Compared to Tc-99m exametazime, Tc-99m ECD shows more rapid brain clearance, higher brain-to-soft tissue ratios and more rapid urinary excretion (Demonceau G, et al, 1988). The mechanism of brain uptake appears to involve a rapid de-esterization of ECD. Presently, Tc-99m ECD (also known as Neurolite®, Dupont, N. Billerica, MA) is classified as an investigational new drug with availability limited to clinical trials only.

II. Receptor-Specific Radiopharmaceuticals

William C. Eckelman, Ph.D.

In nuclear medicine studies of the brain, several radiopharmaceuticals are available for measuring changes in blood-brain barrier permeability or cerebral blood flow (*vide supra*). Relatively fewer agents are available, however, that measure biochemical processes. Of the classes of radiotracers that are useful in studying biochemical processes, receptor-binding radiotracers are especially interesting since they have the potential to measure changes in receptor concentrations that occur in certain disease states (Melnechuk T, 1978; Blecher M and Bar RS, 1981; Gibson RE, 1982; Wagner, HN, Jr, 1982).

CHARACTERIZATION OF RECEPTORS AND RECEPTOR-SPECIFIC SUBSTANCES

Provided that receptor systems can be determined that are primarily affected by disease, receptor-binding radiopharmaceuticals could prove useful in respective disease detection or screening. Few receptors, however, have been isolated for structural determination. As a result, the definition of a receptor is operational and largely based upon certain properties observed in vitro. The usual criteria are high ligand affinity, specificity, saturability, and distribution in relation to physiologic response. The determination of those properties has been made possible by development of high specific activity radiotracers. For example, E. V. Jensen and H. I. Jacobson (1962) used radiolabeled estradiol to identify the cytosolic estradiol receptor in the early 1960s. In general, receptor protein is present in limited concentration, about 10^{-7} to 10^{-10} M in homogenized tissue. Therefore, the receptor is easily saturated by the appropriate ligand. Specificity and high ligand affinity are closely related because, by nature of the high affinity between the re ceptor and the ligand, specificity results. Often, ligands at high concentration can cause physiologic effects at numerous receptors but are specific for only one receptor at low concentration.

One of the most important properties of receptors is stereoselectivity. When stereoisomers exist for receptor-specific substances, one is typically far more potent than the other in binding affinity and physiologic response. For in vivo studies, this property will allow proof of receptor binding because it can be tested using the high specific activity, nonphysiologically active radioisomer.

In vivo tests for saturability would require the injection of a physiologically active amount of the biochemical or drug. The final criterion for the existence of a receptor is that the binding of ligand to the receptor sites can be related to the biological effect of the ligand. This can be determined experimentally by comparing the affinity of various ligands with their in vivo biological effect. If a correlation is obtained, then the receptor is defined.

In the radiotracer context, the distribution of the receptor is determined in vivo or from in vitro assays of various organs and tissues. In general, receptor-binding radiotracers offer an area of research that will allow the noninvasive monitoring of the change in receptor as a function of disease. The development of receptor-binding radiotracers is, however, a two-part problem: (1) the development of a radioligand that has a high receptor-to-nonreceptor binding and thus fulfills the operational definition and (2) the development of an analytical technique that shows a high sensitivity between the radioactivity in the target organ and the receptor concentration. Many radioligands have been shown to localize in receptor-containing tissue and have fulfilled the operational definition for a receptor-binding radiotracer (Eckelman WC, 1986).

Background/History. It is difficult to trace the history of the development of gamma-emitting, receptor-binding radiotracers. J.A. Katzenellenbogen, et al (1982), in their review of the history of steroid receptor-binding radiotracers quote Albert and colleagues' 1949 work as the earliest study. The interest in radiolabeling steroid receptor ligands is reflected in the large number of compounds that soon appeared in the literature (Katzenellenbogen JA, 1982; Counsell RE and Klausmeier WH, 1979). Most were evaluated by in vivo distribution studies in small animals. The identification of cytosolic estradiol receptors in 1960 led to the systematic study of the requirements for receptor binding by those in the drug industry and those developing radiotracers (Jensen EV and Jacobson HI, 1962). The major focus of gamma-emitting receptor-binding radiotracers has been on the steroid hormones (Eckelman WC, 1986). One of the first iodinated estrogens with a high affinity constant and high specific activity was 16-alpha estradiol reported in 1979 (Hochberg RB, 1979). Of the iodinated steroids, 11-beta methoxy-17-alpha iodovinylestradiol appears to be optimal in consideration of its ease of synthesis, attainable effective and chemical specific activity, affinity constant, and nonspecific binding.

Ready availability of a radionuclide was often the guiding force for the selection of a radiolabel in the early studies. In this regard, I-131 and I-125 are today the most often used radionuclides for radiolabeling receptor-specific ligands, along with Br-77. Because the x-ray emissions of I-125 are of relatively low energy and cannot be detected easily by external imaging, this radionuclide is used primarily for in vitro or small-animal work, whereas I-123, a cyclotron product, is used along with I-131 for in vivo imaging studies (Myers WB, 1966).

The first receptor system having the distinction of being studied using the highly desirable radionuclide, Tc-99m, is hepatic-binding protein (HBP) (Vera DR, et al, 1984a; 1984b; Vera DR, et al, 1985). The radiolabeled ligand, Tc-99m galactosylneoglycoalbumin (Tc-99m NGA), binds to HBP, a receptor that is located at the plasma membrane of the hepatocytes. HBP normally recognizes and binds galactose-terminated glycoproteins that are transported to hepatic lysosomes where the ligand complex is catabolized and the receptor is subsequently recycled to the cell surface. Tc-99m NGA is formed by combining albumin with galactose in various molar ratios with subsequent Tc-99m radiolabeling occurring via electrolysis. Because of its relatively low toxicity, this compound can be used in large enough concentrations so that the interaction between the ligand and the receptor is on the linear portion of the second-order binding curve. This produces a second-order response that is sensitive to the binding affinity, the ligand concentration, and the receptor concentration.

Stadalnik and colleagues (1985) studied Tc-99m NGA in patients and found HBP concentration directly related to the clinical biochemical manifestations of reduced functional hepatocyte mass in liver disease such as hepatoma, cirrhosis, and liver metastases.

Brain Receptor-Specific Radiopharmaceuticals. The neuroleptic receptor binding systems have received tremendous interest recently because of their importance in neurological disease and their potential for diagnosis. A.M. Friedman and colleagues, (1982; 1984) studied Br-77 bromospiroperidol in various species and concluded that this compound reached steady state rapidly compared to spiperone itself. They suggested that an equilibrium model could be used to account for specific binding and for competition of endogenous dopamine for the same D-2 receptors. It was also found that Br-77 bromospiperone was readily extracted and that its fraction of specific binding was high. While reasonably good images could be obtained using a pinhole collimator, the lack of availability and poor imaging characteristics of Br-77 prevented extensive clinical studies with these agents. Bromine-77 bromo-benperidol is another substrate for D-2 receptors that achieves a relatively high specific-to-nonspecific ratio in primates (Moerlein SM and Stöklin GL, 1984; 1985). Even though this radiotracer binds to the receptor according to the operational definition of a receptor, the target-to-nontarget ratio was not as high as spiperone itself, perhaps due to its relatively high lipophilicity.

The muscarinic acetylcholine receptor (mAChR) system has also been studied extensively (Eckelman WC, 1982; Gibson RE, et al, 1984). The radioiodinated analogue of 3-quinuclidinyl benzilate (QNB) has been shown to bind to the mAChR by testing saturability and stereoselectivity in the corpus striatium, cerebellum, and the heart of rats. 3-quinuclidinyl-4-iodobenzilate (4-IQNB) receptor binding can be inhibited by co-injection of small amounts of nonradioactive mAChR ligands as well as displaced by the same materials after the 4-IQNB has bound to the receptor binding. The in vivo experiments involve a complicated set of variables including the total receptor concentration, the dissociation rate, transport of the displacing ligands, and the input function (i.e., IQNB still available for uptake from the blood). Nevertheless, the combined evidence along with the regional distribution indicates a receptor mediated localization. Another important proof is obtained by using two stereomers of IQNB differing in the chirality of the quinuclidinyl carbon. In those organs containing mAChR, the difference in distribution between the pharmacologically active form, the 3-R-quinuclidinyl-4-iodobenzilate, and the pharmacologically inactive form, the 3-S-quinuclidinyl-4-iodobenzilate, is striking. Only limited human studies with 4-IQNB in disease states have been undertaken (Holman BL, et al, 1985).

Many receptor systems have been studied, and the necessary experiments by which to validate in vivo receptor binding are in place. From the validation of a gamma-emitting, receptor-binding radiotracer to its use to determine the change in receptor concentration is, however, a major advance. Many gamma-emitting radiotracers have been validated, but few have been used clinically. One of the most often studied in man is the positron-emitting derivative C-11 N-methylspiperone (C-11 MS).

In clinical studies by D.F. Wong and colleagues (1984), the dopamine D2 and the serotonin S2 receptors were imaged with C-11 MS and measured in human volunteers. The relative receptor concentration was derived from tissue-ratio data using the corpus striatum, which contains D2 receptors, and the cerebellum, which does not. Assuming that the change in tissue ratio is related to a change in receptor concentration, the D2 and S2 receptor concentration decreased as a function of age. Recently, the same group studied eleven normal volunteers—ten drug-naive and five previously treated schizophrenic patients (Wong DF, et al, 1985). Although the tissue ratio using no carrier added C-11 MS did not show a difference in relative receptor concentration because of the effect of blood-flow differences, the use of the high and a low specific activity preparation resulted in the differentiation of receptor number in normal and drug-naive schizophrenics. The drug-naive schizophrenics showed increased receptor concentration.

Many receptor-binding radiotracers targeted for neurological receptors have been developed (Eckelman WC, 1986;

Welch MJ, et al, 1986). Two major tasks remain before these radiopharmaceuticals become clinically useful. The determination of the receptor number and the sensitivity to change in receptor concentration must be validated. Then, using a radioligand deemed to be sensitive to receptor change, clinical studies must be carried out verifying their clinical sensitivity and selectivity. This is the challenge for both single-photon and positron-emitting, receptor-binding radiotracers in the coming years.

III. Imaging of Cerebrospinal Fluid Dynamics

Henry M. Chilton
Robert J. Cowan

Nuclear medicine studies evaluating cerebrospinal fluid (CSF) dynamics have been primarily used (1) to detect and distinguish between two types of hydrocephalus—communicating hydrocephalus and hydrocephalus resulting from cerebral atrophy—and (2) to determine the presence of CSF leaks (CSF rhinorrhea, otorrhea, etc.). In CSF imaging, the radiopharmaceutical is usually administered intrathecally but may also be rarely administered intracisternally. Normally, the radiopharmaceutical introduced into the spinal subarachnoid space ascends, enters the basal cisterns, and proceeds supratentorially through the subarachnoid space over the cerebral hemispheres, draining eventually via the Pacchnionian granules into the superior sagittal sinus. It has been shown (Bering EA, Jr and Sato O, 1963) that CSF fluid produced within the choroid plexus sets up a current that flows out of the ventricular system. It is generally accepted that radiopharmaceuticals administered intrathecally ascend and move by bulk transport into the extraventricular fluid. Whether this is true for substances of all molecular weights appears unlikely in that computed tomography (CT) has shown the route of exit of water-soluble contrast material from the CSF to be dependent upon the specific gravity of the contrast molecules. Most of the radiopharmaceuticals employed for CSF imaging, however, have relatively small molecular weights (usually less than 700) or are radiolabeled substances that are normal constituents of the CSF (e. g., albumin).

While in the past CSF imaging has been employed widely for evaluation of communicating hydrocephalus, its use has decreased substantially since CT and magnetic resonance imaging provides improved resolution of the ventricles and subarachnoid spaces. Still, CSF imaging is a useful diagnostic aid in the evaluation of the patency of surgical ventricular shunts and for the localization of CSF leaks.

Background/History. The use of radiopharmaceuticals to evaluate CSF dynamics can be traced to the work of R.E. Rieselbach and colleagues (1962) who evaluated the subarachnoid spaces of monkeys and several patients with colloidal Gold-198. Later, G. DiChiro and colleagues (1964) investigated the intrathecal and intraventricular injection of radioiodinated [I-131] human serum albumin (RISA) in patients with brain tumor, internal hydrocephalus, or CSF rhinorrhea. Other radiopharmaceuticals have been investigated for use in CSF imaging, including the lipid-insoluble, high molecular weight polysaccharide, Tc-99m inulin (Bell EG, et al, 1970). Although inulin is a nontoxic, nonirritating, nonantigenic substance that has been used extensively by physiologists to research the CSF, Tc-99m inulin achieved only limited popularity with clinicians because its relatively short physical half-life (6.0 hours) prevented CSF imaging at 24 hours when radiopharmaceutical ascent to the parasagittal region normally occurs. Similarly, Tc-99m labeled human serum albumin was found unsuitable for routine CSF imaging (DiChiro G, et al, 1968). This latter agent has, however, retained some favor with clinicians for imaging CSF leaks since detection of leakage can often be accomplished on the day of administration, usually within a few hours of intrathecal injection of the radiopharmaceutical.

In-111 transferrin was originally recommended by P. Matin and D.A. Goodwin (1971) for CSF imaging. This radiopharmaceutical, which was prepared on-site by radiolabeling the patient's serum transferrin, distributed nearly identically to I-131 HSA. Like I-131 RISA and Tc-99m inulin, In-111 transferrin is believed to be absorbed unchanged at the Pacchionian granulations. A principal drawback to the use of In-111 transferrin was that the patient's own serum could not be used as a source of transferrin whenever septicemia or bacteremia were suspected. Although the nuclear properties of I-131 are less than ideal, I-131 RISA endured for many years as the agent of choice for CSF imaging, primarily as a result of (1) its widespread availability, (2) acceptable radiation dosimetry, and (3) the fact that albumin is a normal constituent of the CSF (Brocklehurst G, 1968).

During the late 1960s, cases of aseptic meningitis associated with the use of I-131 RISA (Detmer DE and Blacker HM, 1965; Nicol CF, 1967; Oldham RK and Staab EV, 1970) caused investigators to seriously consider the development of other radiopharmaceuticals for CSF imaging. The use of very high specific activity RISA had already been attempted to decrease the incidence of this reaction, but it did not eliminate it entirely. J.F. Cooper and J.C. Harbert (1973) suspected that a pyrogenic chemical contaminant rather than the albumin concentration was the cause of the aseptic meningitis frequently seen with the use of I-131 RISA. Using the Limulus Amebocyte Lysate (LAL) test that was purported to be specific for bacterial endotoxin (Cooper JF, et al, 1971; Yin ET, et al, 1972), they detected the presence of endotoxin in drug lots of I-131 RISA that had been previously given patients who had developed aseptic meningitis. Since these lots had earlier tested negative for pyrogens with the U.S.P. pyrogen test, Cooper and Harbert concluded that the LAL pyrogen test was inadequate as the sole test for radiopharmaceuticals intended for intrathecal injection and that it should be supplemented by the Limulus Amebocyte Lysate test, which is considerably more sensitive for the detection of gram negative endotoxins.

Yb-169 AND In-111 PENTETATE (DTPA)

Although radioiodinated HSA was the original agent used by G. DiChiro and colleagues (1964), the first radiolabeled chelate suggested for CSF imaging was Ytterbium-169 (Yb-169) pentetate, previously known as diethylenetriaminepentaacetic acid, or DTPA (Wagner HN, Jr et al, 1970). Despite having a molecular weight of only approximately 600 (considerably less than the 70,000 molecular weight of albumin), this chelate demonstrated a pattern of movement in the CSF similar to that of albumin and appeared to be absorbed principally through the Pacchionian granules. The Yb-169 radionuclide had the disadvantageous properties of a relatively long physical half-life (32 days) and multiple gamma emissions ranging in energy from 63 to 308 keV, in addition to being only moderately abundant (less than 45%). The radiation-absorbed dose to the spinal cord surface following intrathecal administration of 500 microcuries of Yb-169 pentetate was approximately 8 rads and could be considerably higher in the presence of an obstructing lesion that prevents normal ascent of the radiopharmaceutical. Following absorption from the CSF, Yb-169 pentetate is cleared from blood by renal excretion (primarily glomerular filtration). Patients with impaired renal function require careful evaluation before this radiopharmaceutical is employed because significant increases in radiation dose occurred with prolonged blood clearance. As a result of these concerns and the approval of In-111 pentetate for cisternography, Yb-169 pentetate realized limited clinical use and was recently withdrawn from the market.

In-111 pentetate was introduced for CSF imaging in the early 1970s (Hosain F and Som P, 1972; Goodwin DA, et al, 1973). With its 2.8 day physical half-life, In-111 pentetate is well suited for imaging CSF kinetics at 24–48 hours post injection while providing low patient radiation exposures. The two principal gamma emissions of 173 and 247 keV are formed in relatively high abundance (89 and 94%, respectively) and are acceptable for use with the scintillation camera. In-111 pentetate meets the characteristics for an ideal agent for CSF imaging as summarized by F.H. DeLand and colleagues (1971): high photon yield for images of good resolution, adequate effective half-life for extended imaging beyond 24 hours, acceptable radiaiton dose, biological safety, photon emission of an appropriate energy for available instrumentation, and acceptable availability and cost.

Chemistry. In-111 pentetate is available as a sterile, pyrogen-free, isotonic aqueous solution. At the time of calibration each milliliter contains 1.0 millicurie of In-111, 20–50 micrograms of pentetic acid, and sodium bicarbonate for pH adjustment (i. e., 7–8). Principal radionuclidic impurities are In-114m (<0.1%) and Zn-65 (<0.1%). The currently available formulation in the United States (Medi-Physics Inc. Emeryville, CA) contains no antimicrobials or preservatives and is intended to be discarded after single use.

Pharmacokinetics. Following intrathecal administration, In-111 pentetate is primarily absorbed from the subarachnoid space at the arachnoid villi. Some portion of the administered activity is absorbed across both the cerebral and spinal leptomeninges. A smaller fraction may also be absorbed across the ventricular ependyma. Whenever major routes of CSF flow are pathologically impaired, alternate routes of CSF absorption may assume primary importance.

In normal individuals, radiopharmaceutical migration usually reaches the cisterna magna within 3–4 hours of administration. From there, the radiopharmaceutical passes forward along the base of the brain and ascends symmetrically in front of and along the sides of both cerebral hemispheres to reach the parasagittal region by 24 hours (Figure 10.16).

The biological half-life of In-111 pentetate is CSF is 12 hours (Goodwin DA, et al, 1973). Compared to RISA, In-111 pentetate appears to have a significantly higher rate of egress through the lining of the subarachnoid space. The effective half-life of In-111 pentetate is 10 hours, which approaches the optimum effective half-life of 17 hours for an imaging procedure performed at 24 hours (Wagner HN, Jr and Emmons H, 1966). Cumulative activity in the urine approaches 66% of the administered dose at 1 day post injection, 82% by 2 days and 90% by the third day. Once In-111 pentetate reaches blood, it has biexponential clearance with 80% having a whole-body half-life of 0.5 hours, and the remaining 20% having an 8-hour half-life.

PRECAUTIONS

Breastfeeding/Pregnancy. It is not known whether In-111 pentetate can cause fetal harm when administered during pregnancy. Likewise, it is not known whether this radiopharmaceutical is excreted in human breast milk. Therefore, In-111 pentetate should be given during pregnancy only if clearly needed, and caution should be exercised regarding the administration of this radiopharmaceutical to a nursing mother.

Adverse Reactions. One death has been reported to have occurred within 20 minutes following the administration of In-111 pentetate and appears to have been drug related. Two cases of aseptic meningitis have also been reported to have occurred at one institution (Alderson PO and Siegel BA, 1973). Clinically, these cases resemble reactions that occurred in association with I-131 RISA. Documentation of pyrogenic contaminants in the offending lot by the limulus lysate test was not made against the manufacturer's negative U.S.P. pyrogen test since the vials of In-111 pentetate had been discarded following patient administration. The incidence of aseptic meningitis and pyrogen reactions associated with the use of In-111 pentetate is reported to be less than 0.4%. Due to the highly sensitive

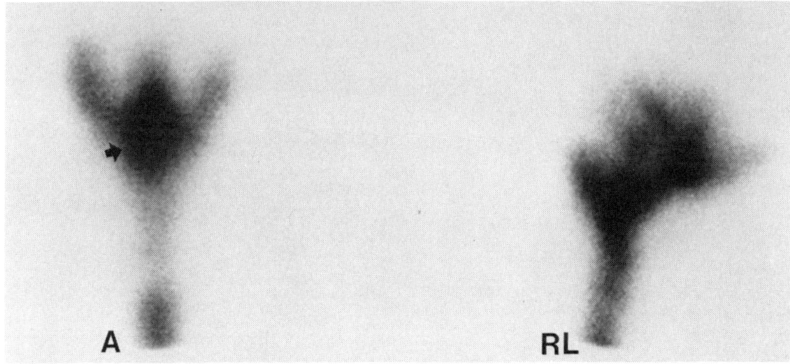

Figure 10.16A   Anterior (A) and right lateral (RL) cisternograms obtained in a normal subject at 2 hours following the intrathecal injection of In-111 pentetate. Note (arrow) the concentration of the radiotracer in the basal cisterns.

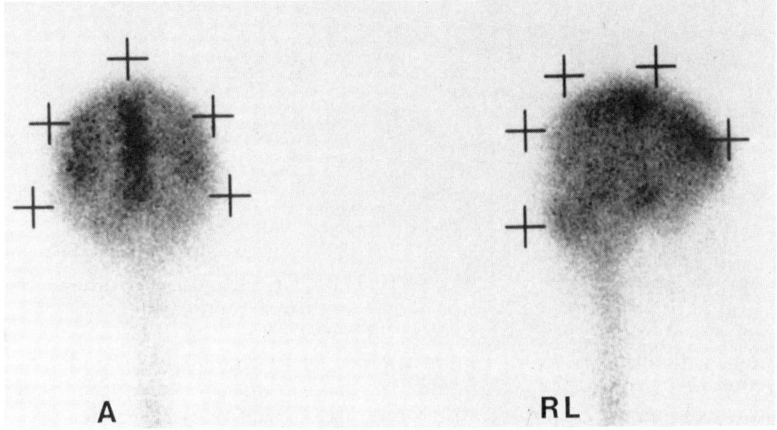

Figure 10.16B   Anterior (A) and right lateral (RL) cisternograms obtained in the same patient at 24 hours after injection. Note normal cephalad migration of the radiotracer over the complexities of the cerebrum and the lack of ventricular penetration.

nature of the meningeal lining to pyrogens (Barnes B and Fish M, 1972), extreme care should be exercised in the dose preparation and intrathecal injection of In-111 pentetate to assure aseptic conditions.

CLINICAL CONSIDERATIONS

Compared to air encephalography and iodinated contrast ventriculography, CSF radionuclide imaging has several advantages for the evaluation of CSF flow and the investigation of subarachnoid space. Specifically, nuclear medicine CSF imaging is of low morbidity and utilizes diagnostic agents that are near physiologic in nature and that distribute in a pattern characteristic of CSF flow. Unlike air, radiopharmaceuticals do not normally enter the cerebral ventricles. Alterations in the normal intracranial flow pattern of the CSF caused by obliteration of the subarachnoid space can lead to fluid and In-111 pentetate diffusion into the ventricles provided the communicating foramen are patent (Figure 10.17).

DOSAGE/DOSIMETRY

Patients for CSF imaging with In-111 pentetate normally receive up to 500

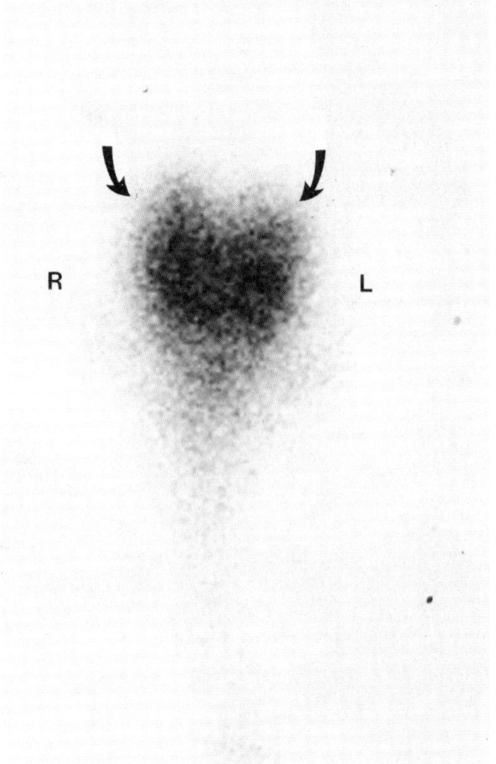

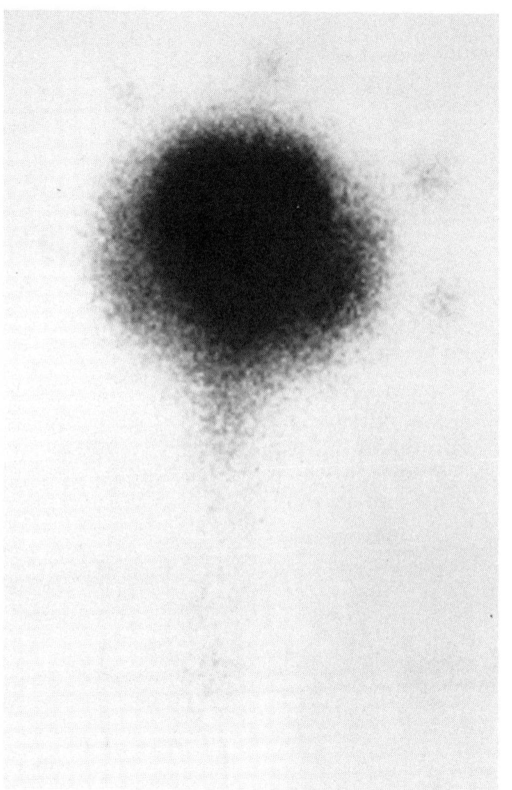

Figure 10.17A Cisternogram (anterior view) obtained 4 hours following the intrathecal injection of Yb-169 pentetate in a patient with normal pressure hydrocephalus. Note (arrows) abnormal radiotracer penetration into the ventricular system of the brain.

Figure 10.17B Cisternogram (anterior view) obtained in the same patient at 24 hours after injection. Note more intense ventricular activity and failure of the radiotracer to demonstrate migration over the convexities of the cerebrum. Radioactive markers outline the cranium.

microcuries by intrathecal injection into the lumbar subarachnoid space. Reduced dosages should be considered in patients with renal dysfunction since prolonged blood retention results in increased radiation dosimetry. Aseptic techniques should be carefully maintained throughout the preparation and injection of the radiopharmaceutical. Following the administration of In-111 pentetate, patients should remain supine for at least 1 hour. Imaging is usually begun 4 hours after radiopharmaceutical injection and may be repeated 24, 48, and 72 hours later.

Images of 50,000–100,000 counts/projection, including posterior, lateral, and vertex views, may be helpful. In the presence of communicating hydrocephalus (normal pressure hydrocephalus), there is characteristically abnormal ventricular penetration of the radiopharmeceutical and marked delay or lack of ascent over the cerebral hemisphere (Figure 10.17).

Since CSF flow may be increased in the presence of a subarachnoid leak, images of the suspected area may be desirably obtained as early as 1–4 hours post injection. The use of nasal pledgets inserted after radiopharmaceutical injection and subsequently assayed for radioactivity in a well-counter are often helpful in confirming the presence and location of CSF leakage. Essentially no radioactivity should appear on the pledgets within this time in the absence of leakage.

Since early imaging may be sufficient for the detection of CSF rhinorrhea, Tc-99m pentetate ($T_{1/2}$ 6.0 hours) may be

Table 10.11 PATIENT RADIATION ABSORBED DOSIMETRY ESTIMATES FOR IN-111 PENTETATE (DTPA)[a]

ORGAN	RADS/500 uCi
Total body	0.041
Kidneys	0.22
Spinal cord	
· Surface	5.0
· Average	1.5
Brain	
· Surface	4.1
· Average	0.4
Bladder	
· 2-hour void	0.21
· 48-hour void	0.5
· Testes	
· 2-hour void	0.04
· 4.8-hour void	0.05
Ovaries	
· 2-hour void	0.06
· 4.8-hour void	0.06

[a] From respective product-insert information, Medi-Physics, Inc., Paramus, NJ.

acceptable for this use. It is conveniently prepared from materials commonly available in most nuclear medicine departments. Whenever Tc-99m pentetate is employed for detection of CSF rhinorrhea, it is often advisable to perform the in-house Limulus Amebocyte Lysate (LAL) test for pyrogens on the final product to ensure apyrogenicity prior to injection (Cooper JF, 1985).

Radiation dosimetry values for In-111 pentetate are shown in Table 10.11.

References

Albert S, Heard RDH, LeBlond CP, et al. Distribution and metabolism of iodo-alpha-estradiol labeled with radioactive iodine. *J Biol Chem* 1949, 177: 247–258.

Alderson PO, Siegel BA. Adverse reactions following ^{111}In-DTPA cisternography. *J Nucl Med* 1973, 14:609–611.

Ancri D, Lonchampt MF, Basset JY. The effect of tin on the tissue distribution of ^{99m}Tc-sodium pertechnetate. *Radiology* 1977, 124:445–450.

Andersen AR, Friberg H, Lassen NA, et al. Assessment of the arterial input curve for [^{99m}Tc]-*d,l*-HM-PAO by rapid octanol extraction. *J Cereb Blood Flow Metab* 1988a, 8(Suppl 1):S23–S30.

Andersen AR, Friberg HH, Schmidt JF, et al. Quantitative Measurements of cerebral blood flow using SPECT and [^{99m}Tc]-*d,l*-HM-PAO compared to xenon-133. *J Cereb Blood Flow and Metab* 1988b, 8(Suppl 1):S69–S81.

Areskog NH, Arturson G, Grotte G, et al. Studies on heart lymph. II. Capillary permeability of the dog's heart, using dextran as a test substance. *Acta Physiol Scand* 1964, 62:218–223.

Arnold RW, Subramanian G, McAfee JG, et al: Comparison of ^{99m}Tc complexes for renal imaging. *J Nucl Med* 1975, 16:357–367.

Atkins HL, Cardinale KG, Eckelman WC, et al. ^{99m}Tc-DTPA prepared by three different methods. *Radiology* 1971, 98:674–677.

Banzo JI, Banzo J, Abós MD, et al. ^{99m}Tc-DTPA and ^{99m}Tc-GH cerebral imaging: A comparative analysis. *Nucl Med Commun* 1982, 3:304–308.

Barnes B, Fish M. Chemical meningitis as a complication of isotope cisternography. *Neurology* 1972, 22:83–91.

Barrio JR, MacDonald NS, Robinson GD. Remote, semi-automated production of F-18 labeled 2-deoxy-2 fluoro-D-glucose. *J Nucl Med* 1981, 22:372–375.

Bell EG, Subramanian G, McAfee JG, et al. Gamma cisternography with ^{99m}Tc-labeled inulin. *J Nucl Med* 1970, 11:(Abst) 299.

Benjamin PP, Rejali A, Friedell H. Electrolytic complexation of ^{99m}Tc at constant current: Its applications in nuclear medicine. *J Nucl Med* 1970, 11:147–153.

Bering EA, Jr, Sato O. Hydrocephalus: Changes in formation and absorption of cerebrospinal fluid within the cerebral ventricles. *J Neurosurg* 1963, 20:1050–1063.

Bessell EM, Foster AB, Westwood JH. The use of deoxy-fluoro-D-glucopyranoses and related compounds in a study of yeast hexokinase specificity. *Biochem J* 1971, 128:199–204.

Bessel EM, Thomas P. The effect of substitution at C-2 of D-glucose 6-phosphate on the rate of dehydrogenation by glucose 6-phosphate dehydrogenase (from yeast and from rat liver). *Biochem J* 1973, 131:83–89.

Bischof-Delaloye A, Hungerbühler JP, Regli F, et al. Biodistribution of I-123-iodo-amphetamine in man. *J Nucl Med* 1984, 25:(Abst)P108.

Blecher M, Bar RS. *Receptors and Human Disease*. Baltimore, Williams and Wilkins, 1981.

Brocklehurst G. Use of radio-iodinated serum albumin in the study of cerebrospinal fluid flow. *J Neurol Neurosurg Psychiatry* 1968, 31:162–168.

Buell U, Krappel W, Schmiedek P, et al. I-123 amphetamine vs. Xe-133 SPECT. A comparative study in patients with unilateral cerebrovascular disease. *J Nucl Med* 1985, 27:25.

Callahan RJ, Froelich JW, McKusick KA, et al. Studies on red blood cell (RBC) labeling: Rate of binding of Tc-99m to hemoglobin (Hgb) in the intact cell and Hgb solution. *J Nucl Med* 1981, 22:70.

Castronovo JJ, Chervu LR, Milstein DM. Altered distribution of technetium-99m sodium pertechnetate associated with antimicrobial therapy. *Clin Nucl Med* 1985, 10:868–871.

Chandler WM, Shuck LD. Abnormal technetium-99m pertechnetate imaging following stannous pyrophosphate bone imaging. *J Nucl Med* 1975, 16:518–519.

Ceretec® Product Literature, Amersham Corporation, Arlington Heights, IL, 1989.

Cheesman EH, Blanchette MA, Ganey MV, et al. Technetium-99m ECD: Ester-derivatized diamine-dithiol Tc complexes for imaging brain perfusion. *Abst J Nucl Med* 1988, 29:788.

Chervu LR, Castronovo JJ, Huq SS, et al. Alterations in red cell tagging with sulfonamides. *J. Nucl Med* 1981, 22:70.

Cooper JF. Pyrogen testing: Practical considerations. In *Quality Assurance of Radiopharmaceuticals Manufactured in the Hospital*. (Warbick–Cerone AL, Johnston LF, eds.) Pergamon Press, Dublin, 1985, 123–132.

Cooper JF, Harbert JC. Bacterial endotoxin as a cause of aseptic meningitis following radionuclide cisternography. *J Nucl Med* 1973, 14:(Abst)387.

Cooper JF, Levin J, Wagner HN, Jr. Quantitative comparison of in vitro and in vivo methods for the detection of endotoxin. *J Lab Clin Med* 1971, 78:138–148.

Counsell RE, Klausmeier WH. Radiotracer interaction with sex steroid hormone receptor proteins (receptor mapping). In *Principles of Radiopharmacology*. Vol. II (Colombetti L, ed.) Boca Raton, FL, CRC Press, 1979, 59–91.

Cowan RJ, Maynard CD, Meschan I, et al. Value of the routine use of the cerebral dynamic radioisotope study. *Radiology* 1973, 107:111–116.

Creutzig H, Schober D, Gielow P, et al. Cerebral dynamics of N-isopropyl (^{123}I) p-iodoamphetamine. *J Nucl Med* 1986, 27:178–183.

Crone C: Facilitated transfer of glucose from blood into brain tissue. *J Physiol (Lond.)* 1965, 181:103–113.

de Kieviet W: Technetium radiopharmaceuticals: Chemical characterization and tissue distribution of Tc-glucoheptonate using Tc-99m and carrier Tc-99. *J Nucl Med* 1981, 22:703–709.

DeLand FH, James AE Jr, Wagner HN, Jr, et al. Cisternography with ^{169}Yb-DTPA. *J Nucl Med* 1971, 12:683–689.

Demonceau G, Leveille J, De Roo M, et al: Comparison of Tc-99m ECD and Tc-99m HMPAO: First human results. *J Nucl Med* 1988, 29:747 (abstract).

Detmer DE, Blacker HM. A case of aseptic meningitis secondary to intrathecal injection of ^{131}I human serum albumin. *Neurology* 1965, 15:642–643.

Dewanjee MK. Binding of ^{99m}Tc ion to hemoglobin. *J Nucl Med* 1974, 15:703–706.

Diamond I, Fishman RA. High affinity transport and phosphorylation of 2-deoxy-D-glucose in synaptosomes. *J Neurochem* 1973, 20:1533–1542.

DiChiro G, Ashburn WL, Briner WH. Technetium (Tc-99m) serum albumin for cisternography. *Arch Neurol* 1968, 19:218–227.

DiChiro G, Reames PM, Matthews WB, Jr. RISA-ventriculography and RISA cisternography. *Neurology* (Minneap.) 1964, 14:185–191.

Eckelman WC. Clinical potential of receptor-based radiopharmaceuticals. In *Radiopharmaceuticals: Progress and Clinical Perspectives* (Fritzberg A, ed.) Vol. II, Boca Raton, FL, CRC Press, 1986, 89–113.

Eckelman WC. Receptor-specific radiopharmaceuticals. In *Computed Emission Tomography* (Ell PJ and Holman BL, eds.) Oxford, Engl., Oxford University Press, 1982, 263–284.

Eckelman WC, Meinken G, Richards P. The chemical state of ^{99m}Tc in biomedical products. II. The chelation of reduced technetium with DTPA. *J Nucl Med* 1972, 13:577–581.

Eckelman WC, Levenson SM. Radiopharmaceuticals labeled with technetium. *Int J Appl Radiat Isot* 1977, 28:67–82.

Ell PJ. A new lipophilic brain scanning agent: Experience with Tc-99m hexamethyl-PAO. Presented at the 32nd Annual Meeting of the Society of Nuclear Medicine, Houston, 1985.

Erickson TC, Larson F, Gordon ES. Uptake of radioactive phosphorus by malignant brain tumors. *J Lab Clin Med* 1949, 34:587–591.

Fink-Bennett D, Uppal TK, Wesolowski DP. Tc-99m glucoheptonate brain scintigraphy: A clinical comparison between one- and two-hour delayed images. Concise communication. *J Nucl Med* 1982, 23:17–19.

Friedman AM, DeJesus OT, Revenaugh J, et al. Measurements in vivo of parameters of the dopamine system. *Ann Neurol* 1984, 15:S66–S76.

Friedman AM, Huang CC, Kulmala HA, et al. The use of radiobrominated p-bromospiroperidol for x-ray imaging of dopamine receptors. *Int J Nucl Med Biol* 1982, 9:57–61.

Fritzberg AR, Lyster DM, Dolphin DH. Evaluation of formamidine sulfinic acid and other reducing agents for use in the preparation of Tc-99m-labeled radiopharmaceuticals. *J Nucl Med* 1977, 18:553–557.

Gallagher BM, Ansari A, Atkins H, et al. Radiopharmaceuticals XXVII. ^{18}F-labeled 2-deoxy-2-fluoro-D-glucose as a radiopharmaceutical for measuring regional myocardial glucose metabolism in vivo: Tissue distribution and imaging studies in animals. *J Nucl Med* 1977, 18:990–996.

Gibson RE. Quantitative changes in receptor concentrations as a function of disease. In *Receptor-Binding Radiotracers.* (Eckelman WC, ed.), Vol. II. CRC Series in Radiotracers in Biology and Medicine (Colombetti LG, ed.), Boca Raton, FL, CRC Press, 1982, 185–212.

Gibson RE, Rzeszotarski WJ, Jagoda EM, et al: [^{125}I] 3-quinuclidinyl-4-iodobenzilate: A high-affinity, high-specific activity radioligand for the M_1 and M_2- acetycholine receptors. *Life Sci* 1984, 34:2287–2296.

Goldman P. The carbon-fluorine bond in compounds of biological interest. *Science* 1969, 164:1123–1130.

Goodwin DA, Song CH, Finston R, et al. Preparation, physiology and dosimetry of ^{111}In-labeled radiopharmaceuticals for cisternography. *Radiology* 1973, 108:91–98.

Hauser W, Atkins HL, Nelson KG, et al. Technetium-99m DTPA: A new radiopharmaceutical for brain and kidney scanning. *Radiology* 1970, 94:679–684.

Haynie TP, Konikowski T, Jhingran SG, et al. Brain scintigrams with ^{99m}Tc-iron DTPA complex in experimental and metastatic neoplasms: Comparison with radioactive chloromerodrin and pertechnetate. *J Nucl Med* 1970, 11:(Abst) 324–325.

Hill TC, Holman BL, Lovett B, et al. Initial experience with SPECT (single-photon computerized tomography) of the brain using N-isopropyl I-123 p-iodoamphetamine: Concise communication. *J Nucl Med* 1982, 23:191–195.

Hochberg RB. Iodine-125 labeled estradiol: A gamma-emitting analog of estradiol that binds to the estrogen receptor. *Science* 1979, 205:1138–1140.

Holman BL, Hill TC, Lee RGL, et al. Brain imaging with radiolabeled amines. In *Nuclear Medicine Annual 1983*, (Freeman LM, Weissman HS, eds.), New York, Raven Press, 1983.

Holman BL, Lee RGL, Hill TC, et al. A comparison of two cerebral perfusion tracers, N-isopropyl I-123 p-iodoamphetamine and I-123 HIPDM, in the human. *J Nucl Med* 1984a, 25:25–30.

Holman BL, Wick MM, Kaplan ML, et al. The relationship of the eye uptake of N-isopropyl-p-[^{123}I]iodoamphetamine to melanin production. *J Nucl Med* 1984b, 25:315–319.

Holman BL, Gibson RE, Hill TC, et al. Muscarinic acetylcholine receptors in Alzheimer's disease. In vivo imaging with iodine 123-labeled 3-quinuclidinyl-4-iodobenzilate and emission tomography. *JAMA* 1985, 254:3063–3066.

Hosain F. Quality control of ^{99m}Tc-DTPA by double-tracer clearance technique. *J Nucl Med* 1974, 15:442–445.

Hosain F, Som P. Chelated ^{111}In: An ideal radiopharmaceutical for cisternography. *Br J Radiol* 1972, 45:677–679.

Jensen EV, Jacobson HI. Basic guides to the mechanism of estrogen action. *Recent Prog Horm Res* 1962, 18:387–414.

Jones SC, Alavi A, Christman D, et al. The radiation dosimetry of 2-[F-18] fluoro-2-deoxy-D-glucose in man. *J Nucl Med* 1982, 23:613–617.

Katzenellenbogen JA, Heiman DF, Carlson KE, et al. In vivo and in vitro steroid receptor assays in the design of estrogen radiopharmaceuticals. In *Receptor-Binding Radiotracers* (Eckelman WC, ed.), Vol. I, CRC Series in Radiotracers in Biology and Medicine (Colombetti LG, ed.), Boca Raton, FL, CRC Press, 1982, 93.

Kennedy C, DesRosiers MH, Jehle JW, et al. Mapping of functional neural pathways by autoradiographic survey of local metabolic rate with [^{14}C] deoxyglucose. *Science* 1975, 187:850–853.

Kuhl DE, Barrio JR, Huang SC, et al. Quantifying local cerebral blood flow by N-isopropyl-p-[^{123}I] iodoamphetamine (IMP) tomography. *J Nucl Med* 1982, 23:196–203.

Kung HF, Blau M. Regional intracellular pH shift: A proposed new mechanism for radiopharmaceutical uptake in brain and other tissue. *J Nucl Med* 1980a, 21:147–152.

Kung HF, Blau M. Synthesis of selenium-75 labeled tertiary diamines: New brain imaging agents. *J Med Chem* 1980b, 23:1127–1130.

Kung HF, Tramposch KM, Blau M. A new brain perfusion imaging agent: [I-123] HIPDM:N,N,N'-trimethyl-N'-[2-hydroxy-3-methyl-5-iodobenzyl]-1,3-propanediamine. *J Nucl Med* 1983, 24:66–72.

LaFrance ND, Wagner HN Jr, Whitehouse P, et al. Decreased accumulation of isopropyl-iodoamphetamine (I-123) in brain tumors. *J Nucl Med* 1981, 22:1081–1083.

Lajtha A, Toth J. The brain barrier system. V. Stereospecificity of amino acid uptake, exchange and efflux. *J Neurochem* 1963, 10:909–920.

Lassen NA, Andersen AR, Friberg H, et al. The retention of [^{99m}Tc]-*d,l*-HM-PAO in the human brain after intracarotid bolus injection: A kinetic analysis *J Cereb Metab Blood Flow* 1988, 8 (Suppl 1):S13–S22.

Lassen NA, Andersen AR, Friberg H, et al. Technetium-99m-HMPAO as a tracer of cerebral blood flow distribution: A kinetic analysis. *J Cereb Blood Flow Metab* 1987, 7(Suppl 1):S535.

Leonard JP, Nowotnik DP, Neirinckx RD: Technetium-99m-*d,l*-HM-PAO: A new radiopharmaceutical for imaging regional brain perfusion using SPECT. A comparison with Iodine-123 HIPDM. *J Nucl Med* 1986, 27:1819–1823.

Léveillé J, Pison C, Karakand Y, et al. Technetium-99m glucoheptonate in brain-tumor detection: An important advance in radiotracer techniques. *J Nucl Med* 1977, 18:957–961.

Lever SZ Burns HD, Kervitsky TM, et al.

Design, preparation and biodistribution of a technetium-99m triaminedithiol complex to assess regional cerebral blood flow. *J Nucl Med* 1985, 26:1287–1294.

Lifton JF, Welch MJ. Preparation of glucose labeled with 20-minute half-lived carbon-11. *Radiat Res* 1971, 45:35–40.

Lund-Anderson H. Transport of glucose from blood to brain. *Physiol Rev* 1979, 59:305–359.

Makler PT, Jr, Gutowicz MF, Kuhl DE. Methotrexate-induced ventriculitis: Appearance on routine radionuclide scan and emission computed tomography. *Clin Nucl Med* 1978, 3:22–23.

Marty R, Cain ML. Effects of corticosteroid (dexamethasone) administration on the brain scan. *Radiology* 1973, 107:117–121.

Matin P, Goodwin DA. Cerebrospinal fluid scanning with ^{111}In. *J Nucl Med* 1971, 12:668–672.

Matsuda H, Oba H, Seki H, et al. Determination of flow and rate constants in a kinetic model of [^{99m}Tc]-Hexamethyl-propylene amine oxime in the human brain. *J Cereb Blood Flow and Metab* 1988, 8(Suppl 1):S61–S68.

Maynard CD, Cowan RJ. Static dynamic imaging of the brain. *CRC Critical Reviews in Clinical Radiology and Nuclear Medicine*. 1974, 5:447–477.

McAfee JG, Fueger CF, Stern HS, et al. ^{99m}Tc-pertechnetate for brain scanning. *J Nucl Med* 1964, 5:811–827.

McAfee JG, Gagne G, Atkins JL, et al. Biological distribution and excretion of DTPA labeled with Tc-99m and In-111. *J Nucl Med* 1979, 20:1273–1278.

Melnechuk T. *Cell Receptor Disorders*. LaJolla, CA, Western Behavioral Sciences Institute, 1978.

Mock BH, Schauwecker DS, English D, et al: In vivo kinetics of canine leukocytes labeled with technetium-99m HM-PAO and indium-111 tropolonate. *J Nucl Med* 1988, 29:1246–1251.

Moerlein SM, Stöklin GL. Specific in vivo binding of ^{77}Br-brombenperidol in rat brain. *Life Sci* 1984, 35:1357–1363.

Moerlein SM, Stöklin GL. Synthesis of high specific activity [^{75}Br]- and [^{77}Br]-bromoperidol and tissue distribution studies in the rat. *J Med Chem* 1985, 28:1319–1324.

Moore GE. Use of radioactive diiodofluorescein in the diagnosis and localization of brain tumors. *Science* 1948, 107:569–571.

Mountford PJ, Coakley AJ. Radiopharmaceuticals in breast milk. In 4th International Radiopharmaceutical Symposium CONF.851113. Schlafke-Stelson AT and Watson EE (eds), Oak Ridge, TN, Oak Ridge Associated Universities, 1986, 167–180.

MPI Indium DTPA In-111 product literature, Med-Physics, Paramus, NJ.

Myers WB. Radioisotopes of iodine. In *Radioactive Pharmaceuticals* (Andrews GA, Kniseley RM, Wagner, HN, Jr, eds.), USAEC, NTIS, 1966, 217–243.

Neirinckx RD, Canning LK, Piper IM, et al. Tc-99m *d,l*-HM-PAO: A new radiopharmaceutical for SPECT imaging of regional cerebral blood perfusion. *J Nucl Med* 1987, 28:191–202.

Neirinckx RD, Burke JF, Harrison RC, et al: The retention mechanism of technetium-99m-HM-PAO: Intracellular reaction with glutathione. *J Cereb Blood Flow Metab* 1988, 8:S4–12.

Nicol CF. A second case of aseptic meningitis following isotope cisternography using ^{131}I human serum albumin. *Neurology* 1967, 17:199–200.

Nowotnik DP, Canning LR, Cumming SA, et al. Development of a Tc-99m-labelled radiopharmaceutical for cerebral blood flow imaging. *Nucl Med Commun* 1985, 6:499–506.

Oldendorf WH. Lipid solubility and drug penetration of the blood-brain barrier. *Proc Soc Exp Biol Med* 1974a, 147:813–816.

Oldendorf WH. Blood-brain barrier permeability to drugs. *Annu Rev Pharmacol Toxicol* 1974b, 14:239–248.

Oldendorf WH. Clearance of radiolabeled substances by brain after arterial injection using a diffusable internal standard. In *Research Methods in Neurochemistry* (Marks N, Rodnight R, eds.).

Vol. 5, New York, Plenum Press, 1981; 91–112.

Oldendorf WH. The blood-brain barrier and its relevance to modern nuclear medicine. In *Functional Radionuclide Imaging of the Brain* (Magistretti PL, ed.). Serono Symposia Publications from Raven Press. Vol. 5, New York, Raven Press, 1983, 1–10.

Oldendorf WH. Hyman W, Braun L, et al. Blood-brain barrier: Penetration of morphine, codeine, heroin, and methadone after narcotic injection. *Science* 1972, 178:984–986.

Oldham RK, Staab EV. Aseptic meningitis following the intrathecal injection of radioiodinated serum albumin. *Radiology* 1970, 97:317–321.

Podreka I, Suess E, Goldenberg G, et al: Initial experience with technetium-99m HM-PAO brain SPECT. *J Nucl Med* 1987, 28:1657–1666.

Prince JR, Dukstein WG, White WE. Gallbladder visualization with the renal imaging agent glucoheptonate. *Clin Nucl Med* 1978, 3:68.

Raichle ME, Larson KB, Higgins CS, et al. Three dimensional in vivo mapping of brain metabolism and acid base status. In *Cerebral Function, Metabolism and Circulation* (Ingvar DH and Lassen NA, eds.). *Acta Neurol Scand* [Suppl], 1979, 56 (Suppl 64): 188–189.

Raichle ME, Larson KB, Phelps ME, et al. In vivo measurement of brain glucose transport and metabolism employing glucose-^{11}C. *Am J Physiol* 1975, 228:1936–1948.

Raimondi AJ. Ultrastructure and the biology of human brain tumors. *Prog Neurol Surg* 1966, 1:1–63.

Ramsey RG, Quinn JL, III. Comparison of accuracy between initial and delayed ^{99m}Tc-pertechnetate brain scans. *J Nucl Med* 1972, 13:131–134.

Reese TS, Karnovsky MJ. Fine structural localization of a blood-brain barrier to exogenous peroxidase. *J Cell Biol* 1967, 34:207–217.

Renkin EM. Transport of large molecules across capillary walls. *Physiologist* 1964, 7:13–28.

Richards P. The technetium-99m generator. In *Radioactive Pharmaceuticals* (Andrews GA, Knisely RM, and Wagner HN, eds.). USAEC Symposium Series, No. 6. CONF-651111, Springfield, VA, National Bureau of Standards, 1966, 335–357.

Rieselbach RE, DiChiro G, Freireich EJ, et al. Subarachnoid distribution of drugs after lumbar injection. *N Engl J Med* 1962, 267:1273–1278.

Roddie ME, Peters AM, George P, et al: Comparison of white cells labeled with Tc-99m-HM-PAO and In-111 for imaging inflammation. *J Nucl Med* 1987, 28:574 (abstract).

Rollo FD, Cavalieri RR, Born M, et al. Comparative evaluation of ^{99m}Tc-GH, ^{99m}TcO$_4$ and ^{99m}Tc-DTPA as brain imaging agents. *Radiology* 1977, 123:379–383.

Russell CD, Rowell K, Scott JW. Quality control of technetium-99m DTPA: Correlations of analytic tests with in vivo protein binding in man. *J Nucl Med* 1986, 27:560–562.

Ryerson TW, Spies SM, Singh NB, et al. A quantitative clinical comparison of three ^{99m}technetium labeled brain imaging radiopharmaceuticals. *Radiology* 1978, 127:429–432.

Sargent T, III, Budinger TF, Braun G, et al. An iodinated catecholamine congener for brain imaging and metabolic studies. *J Nucl Med* 1978, 19:71–76.

Sargent T, III, Kalbhen DA, Shulgin AT, et al. A potential new brain-scanning agent: 4-^{77}Br-2, 5-dimethoxyphenyl-isopropylamine (4-Br-DPIA). *J Nucl Med* 1975, 16:243–245.

Seabold JE, Boyd CM, Saha GB, et al. A clinical comparison of Tc-99m DTPA and Tc-99m glucoheptonate as brain imaging radiopharmaceuticals. *Nucl Med Commun* 1983, 4:78–87.

Selverstone B, Solomon AK, Sweet WH. Location of brain tumors by means of radioactive phosphorus. *JAMA* 1949, 140:277–278.

Sharp PF, Smith FW, Gemmell HG, et al: Tc-99m HM-PAO stereoisomers for imaging regional cerebral blood flow. *J Nucl Med* 1986, 27:171–177.

Sherkow LH. Chemotherapeutic neurotoxicity on brain scintigraphy. *Clin Nucl Med* 1979, 4:439–440.

Shiow-Ling C, Hoag SG, Yanchick VA. Electrolytic complexing of glucoheptonate and technetium-99m. *J Nucl Med* 1978, 19:520–524.

Shiue CY, MacGregor RR, Lade RE, et al. A new synthesis of 2-deoxy-D-*arabino*-hexose. *Carbohydr Res* 1979, 74:323–326.

Sisson WB, Oldendorf WH. Brain distribution spaces of mannitol-^{3}H, inulin-^{14}C, and dextran-^{14}C in the rat. *Am J Physiol* 1971, 221:214–217.

Sols A, Crane RK. Substrate specificity of brain hexokinase. *J Biol Chem* 1954, 210:581–595.

Spectamine® product literature, Medi-Physics, Paramus, NJ, 1987.

Stadalnik RC, Vera DR, Woodle ES, et al. Technetium-99m NGA functional hepatic imaging: Preliminary clinical experience. *J Nucl Med* 1985, 26:1233–1242.

Steigman J, Chin EV, Solomon NA. Scintiphotos in rabbits made with Tc-99m preparations reduced by electrolysis and by $SnCl_2$: Concise communication. *J Nucl Med* 1979, 20:766–770.

Tetalman MR, Deutchman AJ, Scheu J, et al. The optimal pharmaceutical for brain imaging. *J Nucl Med* 1978, 19:(Abst)673.

Thomas SR, Atkins HL, McAfee JG, et al. Radiation absorbed dose from Tc-99m diethylenetriaminepentaacetic acid (DTPA). *J Nucl Med* 1984, 25:503–505.

Troutner DE, Volkert WA, Hoffman TJ, et al. A tetradentate amine oxime complex of Tc-99m. *J Nucl Med* 1983, 24:10.

Troutner DE, Volkert WA, Hoffman TJ, et al. A neutral lipophilic complex of ^{99m}Tc with a multidentate amine oxime. *Int J Appl Radiat Isot* 1984, 35:467–470.

Tyler JL, Powers TA. Gallbladder visualization with technetium-99m gluco-heptonate: Concise communication. *J Nucl Med* 1982, 23:870–871.

Uzler JM, Bennett LR, Mena I, et al. Human CNS perfusion scanning with ^{123}I-iodoantipyrine. *Radiology* 1975, 115:197–200.

Vera DR, Krohn KA, Stadalnik RC, et al. Tc-99m galactosyl-neoglyco-albumin: In vivo characterization of receptor-mediated binding to hepatocytes. *Radiology* 1984a, 151:191–196.

Vera DR, Krohn KA, Stadalnik RC, et al. Tc-99m galactosyl-neoglyco-albumin: In vivo characterization of receptor-mediated binding. *J Nucl Med* 1984b, 25:779–787.

Vera DR, Stadalnik RC, Krohn KA. Technetium-99m galactosyl-neoglyco-albumin: Preparation and preclinical studies. *J Nucl Med* 1985, 26:1157–1167.

Volkert WA. Personal communication, 1989.

Volkert WA, Hoffman TJ, Seger RM, et al. ^{99m}Tc-propylene amine oxime (^{99m}Tc-PnAO); a potential brain radiopharmaceutical. *Eur J Nucl Med* 1984, 9:511–516.

Wagner HN, Jr. Introduction: The role of receptors in disease. In *Receptor-Binding Radiotracers* (Eckelman WC, ed.), Vol. II. CRC Series in Radiotracers in Biology and Medicine (Colombetti LG, ed.), Boca Raton, FL, CRC Press, 1982, 177–183.

Wagner HN, Jr, Emmons H. Characteristics of an ideal pharmaceutical. In *Radioactive Pharmaceuticals* (Andrews GA, Kniseley RM, Wagner HN, Jr (eds.). AEC Symposium Series No. 6, CONF-651111, Springfield, VA, National Bureau of Standards, 1966, p1–32.

Wagner HN, Jr, Hosain F, DeLand FH, et al. A new radiopharmaceutical for cisternography; chelated ytterbium 169. *Radiology* 1970, 95:121–124.

Walovitch RC, Makuch J, Knapik G, et al: Brain metabolism of Tc-99m ECD is related to in vivo metabolism. *J Nucl Med* 1988, 29:747 (abstract).

Waxman AD, Tanacescu D, Siemsen JK,

et al. Technetium-99m-glucoheptonate as a brain-scanning agent: Critical comparison with pertechnetate. *J Nucl Med* 1976, 17:345–348.

Welch MJ, Chi DY, Mathias CJ, et al. Biodistribution of N-alkyl and N-fluoroalkyl derivatives of spiroperidol: Radiopharmaceuticals for PET studies of dopamine receptors. *Int J Rad Appl Instrum* [B], 1986, 13:523–526.

Wicks R, Billings J, Kung HF, et al. Biodistribution in humans and radiation dose calculations for the brain perfusion imaging agent I-123 HIPDM. *J Nucl Med* 1983, 24:95–96.

Winchell HS, Baldwin RM, Lin TH. Development of I-123 labeled amines for brain studies: Localization of I-123 labeled amines for brain studies: Localization of I-123 iodophenylalkylamines in rat brain. *J Nucl Med* 1980a, 21:940–946.

Winchell HS, Horst WD, Braun L, et al. N-isopropyl-[^{123}I]-p-iodoamphetamine: Single-pass brain uptake and washout; binding to brain synaptosomes; and localization in dog and monkey brain. *J Nucl Med* 1980b, 21:947–952.

Winstead MB, Dischino DD, Winchell HS. Concentration of activity in brain following administration of ^{11}C-labeled α-p-iodoanilinophenylacetonitrile. *Int J Appl Radiat Isot* 1979, 30:293–295.

Witcofski RL, Janeway R, Maynard CD, et al. Visualization of the choroid plexus on the technetium-99m brain scan. Clinical significance and blocking by potassium perchlorate. *Arch Neurol* 1967, 16:286–291.

Wolfstein RS, Tanacescu D, Sakimura IT, et al. Brain imaging with ^{99m}Tc-DTPA: A clinical comparison of early and delayed studies. *J Nucl Med* 1974, 15:1135–1137.

Wong DF, Wagner HN, Jr, Dannals RF, et al. Effects of age on dopamine and serotonin receptors measured by positron tomography in the living human brain. *Science* 1984, 226:1393–1396.

Wong DF, Wagner HN, Jr, Pearlson G, et al. Dopamine receptor binding of C-11-3-N-methylspiperone in the caudate in schizophrenia and bipolar disorder: A preliminary report. *Psychoparmacol Bull* 1985, 21:595–598.

Yin ET, Galanos C, Kinsky S, et al. Picogram-sensitive assay for endotoxin: Gelation of Limulus polyphemus blood cell lystate induced by purified lypopolysaccharides and lipid A from Gram-negative bacteria. *Biochem Biophys Acta* 1972, 261:284–289.

Radiopharmaceuticals for Endocrine Imaging

I. Thyroid Imaging

James H. Thrall

Radiotracer studies of the thyroid gland were the first clinically important procedures in nuclear medicine and provided a fundamental stimulus to the creation and early development of the entire field. Radioiodine first became available from cyclotron production in the late 1930s on a limited basis. With the development of the atomic reactor in the 1940s, availability was significantly improved, and the United States Atomic Energy Commission began providing I-131 for widespread clinical use shortly after the end of World War II (Beierwaltes WH, 1979).

The central role of iodine in thyroid metabolism provides a situation in which a radiotracer is almost uniquely matched to its purpose; the thyroid cannot discriminate between different isotopes of iodine, radioactive or stable. (The "isotope effect" in biological systems is most marked with tritium and is not observed with elements heavier than sulfur or phosphorus.) In many respects, the ideal match of radioiodine to studies of the thyroid gland has not been duplicated for other organ-specific nuclear medicine studies, but continues to serve as a prototype for the development of radiotracers (Gross, et al, 1984).

CHEMISTRY/PHYSICS

Radioiodines. All isotopes of iodine have 53 protons in the nucleus and 53 orbital electrons. I-127 is the only stable or nonradioactive isotope of iodine and has 74 neutrons in the nucleus. In addition to I-127, there are 24 radioactive isotopes of iodine. Approximately ten of these have been used in biomedical applications.

Those radioisotopes with a greater number of neutrons than stable I-127 undergo beta-minus decay with the exception of I-128, which also decays by electron capture 6.4% of the time. The beta particles (electrons ejected from the atomic nucleus) are emitted with a continuous spectrum of kinetic energies up to a maximum value characteristic of that particular radioisotope. The maximum beta energy is an important parameter. It defines the distance or range in soft tissue over which the energy from the beta particles will be deposited. Radioisotopes of iodine with fewer neutrons in the nucleus than I-127 undergo decay primarily by electron capture or by positron emission. The absence of particulate emissions in the former of these two processes significantly reduces the radiation absorbed dose resulting from the use of respective isotopes.

I-131

Iodine-131 is the "classic" radioisotope of iodine from the standpoint of its medical use. Its sodium salt was used almost exclusively for two decades for percent thyroid uptake measurements and imaging applications. Its current use has been somewhat restricted due to the relatively high radiation dose to the thyroid gland. The beta particles from I-131 have a maximum energy of 0.606 MeV and deposit the majority of their energy within 2.2 millimeters of their site of origin (Table 11.1). The most abundant photon emission from I-131 has an energy of 364 keV and occurs in approximately 85% of decays. This energy is higher than optimal

Table 11.1   RADIOISOTOPES USED TO IMAGE THE THYROID

	RADIONUCLIDE		
	I-123	*I-131*	*Tc-99m*
Mode of decay	Electron capture	Beta minus	Isometric transition
Physical half-life	13 hr	8.06 days	6.03 hr
Decay constant	$0.0533\ hr^{-1}$	$0.0860\ days^{-1}$	$0.1149\ h^{-1}$
Average effective life	18.8 hr	11.63 days	8.7 hr
Photon energy (meV)	0.028 (0.867)	0.030 (0.046)	0.0186 (0.077)
(Mean number per disintegration)	0.159 (0.836)	0.080 (0.026)	0.1405 (0.879)
	0.529 (0.011)	0.284 (0.058)	
		0.364 (0.820)	
		0.637 (0.065)	
		0.723 (0.017)	
Relative cost	High	Low	Low

for the gamma-scintillation camera or available collimation due to relatively low crystal efficiency and high septal penetration, respectively. The half-life of I-131 is 8.06, days which is substantially longer than necessary for most studies of the thyroid gland and contributes to the high radiation dose. Iodine-131 continues to be valuable for selected studies of the thyroid. Specifically, delayed imaging at 24, 48, and 72 hours is frequently useful in evaluating extrathyroidal spread of differentiated thyroid cancer (Keyes JW, et al, 1978). In this application, the longer half-life is advantageous. The combination of a relatively high-energy beta particle and a detectable photon make I-131 the agent of choice for most therapeutic applications in patients with hyperthyroidism and thyroid carcinoma. (Therapeutic applications are discussed in Chapter 18.)

I-125

The alternative use of I-125 for thyroid studies was extensively explored in the 1960s. It was felt at one time that the low-photon energies of I-125 (27.5–35.4 keV) afforded better resolution for cold nodules (Charkes ND, 1971). However, low-energy photons arising from posterior aspects of the thyroid are highly attenuated, negating any advantage for superficial structures. The half-life of I-125 is 60 days, and even though it decays 100% of the time by electron capture with no particu-

late emissions, the radiation dose is similar to I-131, variably estimated at approximately 0.4–1.0 rads per microcurie administered in patients with normal percent uptakes (Tables 11.1 and 11.3). The long half-life of I-125 has an advantage in economy and availability. In current practice, I-125 remains extremely valuable as a radiolabel for in vitro laboratory procedures due to its long half-life and low-energy emissions. It is not used for clinical imaging or uptake studies.

I-123

Many investigators have concluded that I-123 may represent the "ideal" radionuclide of iodine for most thyroid-imaging applications and for uptake studies (Wellman and Anger, 1971; Atkins HL, et al, 1973; Nishiyama H, et al, 1974; Arnold and Pinsky, 1976; Keyes JW, et al, 1978). The half-life of I-123 is 13.3 hours, which is satisfactory for routine clinical imaging, and with the appropriate adjustment in administered dose, can be satisfactory for studies up to 24 or even 48 hours (Table 11.1). I-123 has a useful principal gamma photon of 159 keV that occurs in 84% of decays. This gamma energy is readily collimated and efficiently detected by modern gamma cameras. There is also a lower energy photon of 27.5 keV, occurring in 92% of decays, which is not useful for gamma camera studies. Iodine-123 decays 100% of the time by electron capture, resulting in no particulate emissions and favorable radiation dosimetry.

In spite of its many useful properties, I-123 has some disadvantages that have retarded its clinical utilization. The theoretical advantage in low-radiation dose is offset in some commercial preparations by the presence of contaminants that reduce the usable shelf-life of I-123, increase the actual absorbed dose, and cause a degradation of image quality due to high-energy gamma photons (Keyes JW, et al, 1978; Baker GA, et al, 1976). The presence of I-124 in early commercial preparations of I-123 resulted in increased radiation dose to the patient and contamination with high-energy photons of 602 keV and 722 keV, leading to degraded images due to collimator septal penetration and scattering. The relative contamination from I-124 increases with time due to the longer half-life of I-124 (4.1 days) compared to I-123 (13.3 hours). Current production methods have reduced the contamination problems. The $(p, 5n)$ reaction on I-127 and the $(p, 2n)$ reaction on Xenon-124 are the preferred production methods that have fewer energetic impurities consisting of I-125 for the former reaction and tellurium-121 m for the latter (Ziessman HA, et al, 1986). The short physical half-life and hence shelf-life of I-123 creates logistical problems in maintaining a reliable supply and is partly responsible for the substantially greater cost of I-123 compared to I-131.

OTHER RADIOIODINES

The first radioisotope of iodine used for experimental studies was I-128; however, this radionuclide never became clinically important. Radioiodine-132 enjoyed a brief vogue and was used more extensively in Europe than the United States (Goolden and Mallard, 1958). I-132 has a half-life of 2.3 hours resulting in a substantially lower radiation dose per microcurie administered than I-131. At one time, it was recommended for tests in children or pregnant women or in situations requiring repeat testing at short intervals. The short half-life of I-132 made it unsuitable for longer tests such as 24-hour radioiodine uptake measurements. Iodine-129 and I-130 have been used in highly specialized applications. Iodine-129 has a half-life of 1.6×10^7 years, making it suitable for experimental studies requiring isotopic equilibrium. Iodine-130 is produced by neutron activation of I-129 providing a mechanism for increasing the sensitivity of measuring compounds containing I-129. Iodine-130 itself has a short 12.5-hour half-life and is not optimal for primary use from either the standpoint of radiation dose or photon energy.

RADIOIODINE FORMULATIONS

Iodine-131 and I-123 are available for thyroid studies as their sodium salts either in liquid or capsule form. Historically, only liquid preparations were available, which required pipetting of aliquots for the preparation of uptake and scanning doses as well as therapy doses. The volatility of iodine represents a health physics hazard with liquid formulations, resulting in airborn I-131 activity that can exceed maximum permissible concentrations. Measurable amounts of radioiodine can be found frequently in personnel handling unsealed quantities of liquid formulations of sodium iodide. Internal contamination is minimized by handling the I-131 preparations in properly designed fume hoods. The exposure to personnel handling radioiodine is a particular problem for therapeutic amounts. Volatilization is enhanced by oxidation of the iodide ion to iodine by dissolved oxygen in acidic solutions. Maintaining an alkaline pH through the use of buffers results in a decrease in iodine volatility. Current formulations use distilled water, antioxidants, and chelating agents to reduce the problem of oxidation and volatility.

More recently, I-131 and I-123 have become available in capsule form, which is more convenient for handling and storage. Early in the experience with capsules, some preparations did not completely dissolve in the gut, resulting in spuriously low 24-hour uptake values (Halpern S, et al, 1973; Robertson JS, et al, 1974; Green JP, et al, 1976). This problem has been largely solved but remains a theoretical cause of falsely low uptake measurements. In new radioiodine capsule formulations, polyethylene glycol base is used for suspending radioiodine rather than gelatin. This has prevented spurious radioiodination of gelatin and retention of iodine in the gut. Polyethylene glycol base rapidly dissolves in gastric fluid allowing bioavailability of radioiodine in a time course similar to that of oral solutions. The capsule formulations are less flexible from the standpoint of dose administration, but this is outweighed by the health physics considerations associated with a reduction in the chance for facility contamination and exposures to clinical personnel from I-131 in the air. When using I-131 capsules, it is possible to allow higher activity capsules to decay to lower levels when a lesser amount of radioactivity is desired for a clinical study. However, Ziessman and co-workers have pointed out that a similar strategy should not be followed with I-123 capsules that contain long-lived contaminants such as I-125 and I-124. (Ziessman HA, et al, 1986). The time from calibration to administration of I-123 is the major determinant of overall radiation dose to the thyroid gland and I-123 should never be decayed down in order to obtain a recommended pediatric-administered activity. Rather, if a smaller dose of I-123 is clinically indicated for a young child or for an uptake versus an imaging study, the correct amount should be ordered and administered as promptly as possible on the day of delivery.

Technetium-99m Pertechnetate. The limitations of the available radioisotopes of iodine for thyroid imaging and function studies led to a search for noniodine radionuclides that would localize in thyroid tissue (Atkins and Richards, 1968;

Atkins HL, et al, 1973; dosRemedios LV et al, 1971; Keyes JW, et al, 1978; Gross MD, et al, 1984). Technetium-99m pertechnetate is trapped by the thyroid but not further organified. The Tc-99m radionuclide has a half-life of 6 hours and a principal photon energy of 140 keV. This energy is ideally suited to modern gamma scintillation cameras, which have in fact been optimized for Tc-99m. Technetium-99m pertechnetate delivers the lowest radiation dose to the thyroid gland of all clinically used agents and is readily available as the daughter product of molybdenum-99 in molybdenum-99/technetium-99m generator systems. The half-life of the parent compound is just over 3 days. With appropriate initial activity, the generator system can provide a continuous supply of Tc-99m activity with replacement on a weekly basis.

Technetium-99m pertechnetate is obtained as a sodium salt from the molybdenum-99 generator system by elution with 0.9% Sodium Chloride for Injection, U.S.P. After appropriate dose calibration, the Tc-99m pertechnetate in normal saline is used for thyroid imaging without further modification.

Miscellaneous Agents. In addition to radionuclides that specifically localize in functioning thyroid tissue, a number of other radiotracers have been evaluated for a variety of clinical applications. Selenium-75 selenomethionine, wherein radioactive selenium is substituted for the sulfur of methionine, accumulates in areas of rapid protein synthesis (Weinstein MO, et al, 1971). The rationale for this tracer was the hypothesis that thyroid cancers should demonstrate active protein synthesis resulting in a positive uptake of tracer. Selenomethionine is, however, avidly incorporated in normal thyroid tissue and, hence, the sensitivity and specificity for differentiating benign from malignant lesions is low. Selenomethionine is not currently used for this application.

Gallium-67 citrate has been suggested for a number of thyroid-imaging applications (Erjavec M, et al, 1974; Heidendal GAU, et al, 1975; Kaplan WO, et al, 1974; Koutras OA, et al, 1976; Higashi T, et al, 1981; Higashi T, et al, 1982; Grove RB, et al, 1973). The sensitivity of gallium uptake in differentiated thyroid carcinomas has not been sufficient to warrant routine clinical application. Gallium-67 citrate has been shown to demonstrate increased uptake in areas of subacute thyroiditis as a marker of inflammatory disease. However, this diagnosis is usually made on the basis of history, physical exam, and selected other laboratory evaluations and does not require gallium-67 citrate imaging. In selected cases where the diagnosis is in doubt, gallium may be helpful.

Thallium-201 chloride has been suggested for a number of applications in evaluating thyroid disease (Keyes JW, et al, 1978; Tonami N, et al, 1978; Hisada K, et al, 1978; Fukuchi M, et al, 1979; Tonami and Hisada, 1980; Hoefnagel CA et al, 1986). Although thallium-201 chloride has found greatest application in myocardial perfusion imaging, it also localizes in skeletal muscle and many other well-perfused, highly cellular tissues, including the thyroid. The combination of diminished radioiodine uptake and increased thallium-201 accumulation suggests a metabolically active thyroid lession (Figure 11.1), although the pattern is not specific for thyroid cancer. Some studies have suggested the utility of thallium-201 for detecting metastases from thyroid cancer. A potential advantage is the ability to image metastatic deposits without having to discontinue thyroid replacement therapy.

Another radiopharmaceutical proposed for specific thyroid imaging applications is modified technetium-99m dimercaptosuccinic acid (Tc-99m DMSA). In usual Tc-99m DMSA preparations, technetium is in a plus-3 valence state and the preparations do not demonstrate tumor affinity. In preparations where the technetium is in a plus-5 valence state, tumor affinity has been reported, and modified Tc-99m

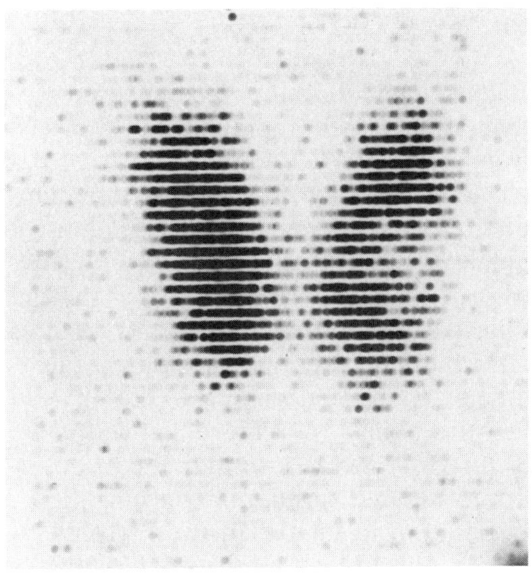

Figure 11.1A Radioiodine-131 scan demonstrates a cold nodule in the lateral aspect of the mid-portion of the left lobe.

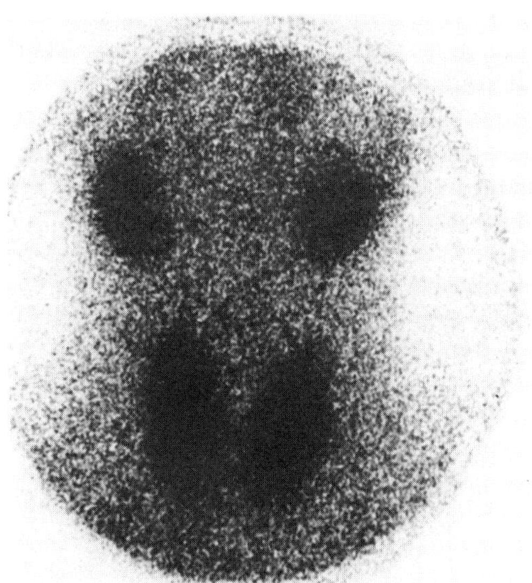

Figure 11.1B Corresponding Thallium-201 scan demonstrates uptake in the radioiodine cold nodule. Surgery revealed a papillary-follicular thyroid cancer.

DMSA has been proposed as an agent for imaging medullary thyroid cancer (Ohta H, et al, 1984; Ohta H, et al, 1985). Sufficient information is not currently available to assess the efficacy of this agent.

PHARMACOKINETICS

Radioiodines. Orally administered iodine is absorbed rapidly from the gastrointestinal tract. Radioiodine can be detected in the thyroid gland within minutes. Oxidation and organic binding of iodine also occur rapidly, and radioactivity can be demonstrated in the thyroid follicular lumen within 20 to 30 minutes after parenteral administration of radioiodine. In normal subjects, the thyroid has the ability to achieve a twenty-five to fortyfold increase in iodine concentration compared to plasma concentrations. In addition to uptake in the thyroid, iodine is concentrated in the salivary glands and gastric mucosa. Between 50–75% of the tracer amounts of radioactive iodine are excreted in the urine of euthyroid subjects with normal renal function within 48 hours. The percentage is correspondingly lower for thyrotoxic subjects and higher for patients with diminished thyroid function. A small fraction of administered activity is excreted via the colon. After its uptake in the thyroid gland, radioactive iodine is incorporated into thyroid hormones and their metabolites. These radioactive molecules are secreted by the thyroid, and radioactivity is redistributed through the body with appreciable uptake in the liver.

The specific pharmacokinetics of radioiodine uptake in the thyroid correlate with the functional status of the thyroid. Radioiodine uptake studies have therefore been used as clinical means of assessing thyroid function. The factors affecting the measured percent uptake include the size of the iodide pool from which the fractional clearance into the thyroid is occurring, the functional status of the gland, and the time post administration.

The importance of the iodide pool is illustrated by differences in percent uptakes regionally and over time in the United States. As recently as the early and mid 1960s, the normal range for the 24-hour I-131 uptake in many laboratories was given as 20–45%. In most parts of the United States, this range has fallen to a low end of 7–10% and an upper end of 25–30% (Pittman JA, et al, 1969; Bernard JO, et al, 1970). The explanation for this is the use of periodate additives in food and hence a generally much higher dietary intake of iodine in the United States than historically. The expanded iodine pool results in a lower fractional clearance of administered radioiodine into the normal thyroid gland. In parts of the world with low amounts of iodide in the diet, normal uptakes may be as high as 50% or greater.

The specific activity of radioiodine preparations is high enough so that carrier iodine does not have an effect on tracer pharmacokinetics. It should be noted that as little as 1 milligram of stable iodine can substantially reduce the 24-hour radioiodine uptake by expanding the pool. Ten milligrams or more of stable iodide is essentially a blocking dose that can reduce the 24-hour radioiodine uptake by 98%. The ability of stable iodine to block radioiodine uptake is the rationale for its use in subjects exposed to fallout from nuclear accidents, which typically involve the release of I-131. The recommended thyroid-blocking dose of potassium iodide is 130 mgm per day, which provides approximately 100 mgm of iodine. The same amount of iodine is available in 0.8 ml of Lugol's solution or 0.13 ml SSKI.

In patients with renal failure, the net clearance of iodine through the kidneys is diminished, resulting in an expanded iodine pool. The predictable effect of decreased thyroid radioiodine uptake is offset by a longer exposure of the gland to circulating tracer, since it is not cleared by the kidney. In clinical practice, renal failure may result in apparent decrease or increase in thyroid radioiodine uptake depending on how these opposing factors balance each other.

The measurement of percent uptake of iodine in the thyroid gland at 24 hours has been adopted as a standard and provides good separation of euthyroid from hypothyroid individuals. It also provides a good separation between euthyroid and hyperthyroid subjects in most cases. One exception is the floridly hyperthyroid patient in whom the percent uptake may peak as early as 5 hours after radiotracer administration, and the 24-hour uptake may actually be less than the earlier measurement (Figure 11.2).

Technetium-99m   Pertechnetate. As noted previously, Tc-99m pertechnetate is trapped by the thyroid but not further organified or incorporated into thyroid hormones. The trapping process is rapid following parenteral administration, with the majority of subjects demonstrating peak uptake within 20–30 minutes, thus forming the basis for selecting this time frame for clinical imaging and uptake studies. In normal euthyroid subjects, 0.5–3.75% of an intravenously administered dose of Tc-99m pertechnetate is taken up in the gland. The 20–30-minute percent uptake of Tc-99m pertechnetate has been shown to correlate well with clinical and laboratory assessments of thyroid function (Atkins and Richards, 1968).

PRECAUTIONS

Drug–Radiopharmaceutical Interactions. A history of previous administration of iodine-containing radiographic contrast materials or other drugs or foods containing large amounts of iodine should be addressed for patients undergoing radioiodine percent uptake determinations and thyroid scanning. The percent uptake can be spuriously depressed if the iodine pool is flooded. For water-soluble contrast media, the effect is typically gone by 1–2 weeks. For lipid soluble media, such as Pantopaque® or Ethiodol®, the effect may be observed for months or even years until the iodine reservoir is depleted. Table 11.2 summarizes various agents that can affect thyroid percent uptake and provides an estimate of the duration of the interaction. The unpredictable effect of impaired renal function has been previously noted and the percent uptake determination is of limited value diagnostically in patients with renal failure. It may still be

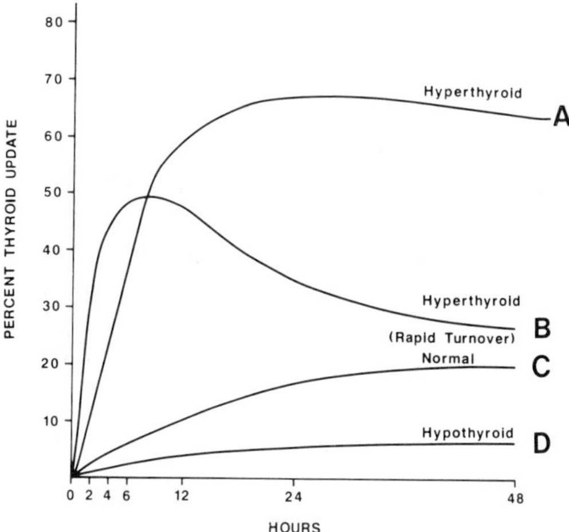

Figure 11.2 Graphical representation of radioiodine uptake kinetics in a normal subject and patients with hypo- and hyperthyroidism. In some cases of hyperthyroidism, the 24-hour measurement can be misleading because of rapid turnover (e. g., curve B).

Table 11.2 **NONTHYROIDAL FACTORS INFLUENCING THYROID UPTAKE OF IODINE**

DECREASED UPTAKE	DURATION OF EFFECT
Excess Iodine (expanded iodine pool)	
· Lugol's solutions, SSKI	2–4 wk
· Tincture of Iodine	2–4 wk
· Kelp	2–4 wk
· Some mineral supplements, cough medicines, and vitamin preparations	2–4 wk
· Iodinated drugs and skin ointments, iodochlorhydroxyquin	2–4 wk
Radiographic Contrast Media	
· Water-soluble intravascular contrast media	2–4 wk
· Oral cholecystographic agents	4 wk–indef
· Fat-soluble brochographic, lymphographic, and myelographic agents	4 wk–Yrs
Thyroid Hormones	
· Thyroxine	4–6 wk
· Triiodothyronine	2–3 wk
Noniodine-Containing Drugs	Variable
· ACTH, adrenal steroids	
· Antithyroid drugs	
· Monovalent anions (perchlorate)	
· Penicillin	
· Antithyroid drugs (propylthiouracil, methimazole)	
Goitrogenic Foods	Variable
· Genus brassicae (cabbage, turnips)	

INCREASED UPTAKE
Iodine deficiency
Pregnancy
Rebound phase after discontinuance of thyroid hormones and antithyroid drugs and recovery from subacute thyroiditis
Choriocarcinoma
Hydatid-form mole
Renal failure

valuable as an adjunct to calculating therapy doses for hyperthyroidism.

Pregnancy. The problem of exposure to the fetus is a common one in all radiological imaging and has special aspects for thyroid radiotracers. Radioiodine and Tc-99m pertechnetate both cross the placental membranes (Book and Goldman, 1975; Herbert RJT, et al, 1969). Therefore, the fetus is potentially exposed from both circulating radioactivity in the maternal tissues and from radioactivity crossing the placenta. Prior to the twelfth week of gestation, the fetal thyroid does not concentrate radioiodine. During this period, the absorbed dose to the fetal thyroid is only 1 millirad per microcurie of I-131 administered to the mother. After the fetal thyroid attains the ability to trap radioiodine, the dose increases. By 13 weeks, the dose is estimated at 0.7 rads per microcurie increasing to 6.0 rads per microcurie by 22 weeks. At term, the estimated absorbed dose is 8 rads per microcurie of I-131 administered (Table 11.3).

Table 11.3   ABSORBED RADIATION DOSES TO THE THYROID FROM RADIOIODINE AND TECHNETIUM-99m IMAGING AGENTS

| | ABSORBED DOSE (RADS/mCi) OF ADMINISTERED RADIOPHARMACEUTICAL | |
Radiopharmaceutical	*Adult[a]*	*Newborn[b]*
I-131 sodium iodide	800.0	16,000.0
I-125 sodium iodide	450.0	11,100.0
I-123 sodium iodide (100% radionuclide purity)	7.5	160.0
I-123 sodium iodide (with radionuclide impurities)	21.0	233.0
Tc-99m sodium pertechnetate	0.13	3.4

[a] Assuming a maximum thyroid uptake of 15% (13.8% 24-hr uptake) and a 19.6 gm thyroid gland.

[b] Assuming that dose to newborn is approximately 10–20 times that of adult.

Breastfeeding. Radioiodine and Tc-99m pertechnetate are both excreted in the breast milk of lactating women (Figure 11.3) (Romney BM, et al 1986; Ahlgren L, et al, 1985). Any activity secondarily ingested by the nursing infant may concentrate in the thyroid gland. The question frequently arises in clinical practice

A

B

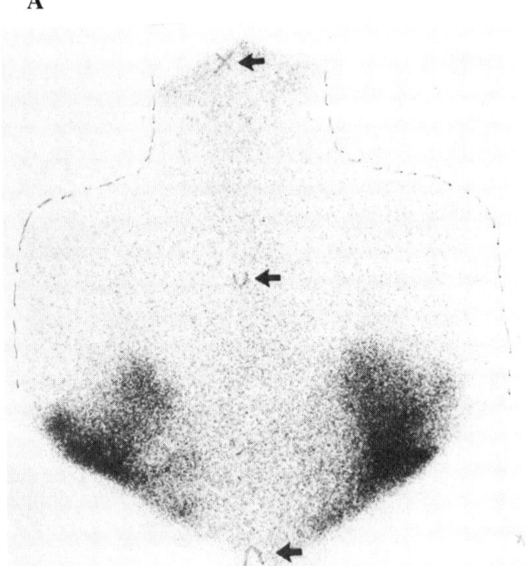
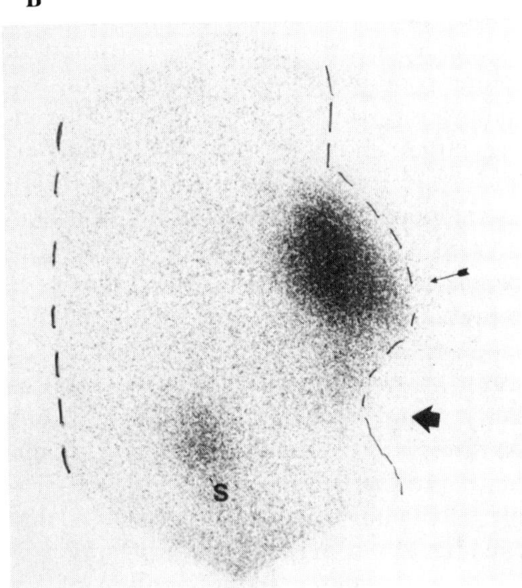

Figure 11.3 Anterior (A) and lateral (B) scintiphotos obtained with I-131 reveal significant breast uptake in a patient undergoing a thyroid cancer follow-up evaluation 6 weeks postpartum. Uptake on anterior view could be mistaken with lung uptake without proper history or lateral view. (Anterior view arrows are at the level of the chin, sternal notch, and xiphoid; lateral view arrows indicate breast and xiphoid. "S" indicates radioactivity in the stomach.)

Table 11.4   GUIDELINES FOR SAFE RESUMPTION OF NURSING AFTER RADIONUCLIDE ADMINISTRATION[a]

RADIONUCLIDE	BREAST MILK ACTIVITY AT WHICH NURSING CONSIDERED SAFE	MAXIMUM DELAY REQUIRED BEFORE RESUMING NURSING
Tc-99m	$8.2 \times 10^{-2}\,\mu$Ci/ml (30.34×10^{-4}MBq/ml)	24 hr after 20 mCi (740 MBq)
Ga-67 citrate	$2.1 \times 10^{-3}\,\mu$Ci/ml (7.77×10^{-5}MBq/ml)	4 wk after 3 mCi (111 MBq)
I-131 orthoiodohippurate	$1.65 \times 10^{-5}\,\mu$Ci/ml (6.10×10^{-7}MBq/ml)	4.5 days after 200 μCi (7.4 MBq)
NaI-131	$4.1 \times 10^{-7}\,\mu$Ci/ml (15.17×10^{-9}MBq/ml)	8 wk after 5 μCi (0.185 MBq)
NaI-123	$1.2 \times 10^{-4}\,\mu$Ci/ml (4.44×10^{-6}MBq/ml)	2–3 days after 10–30 μCi (0.37–1.11 MBq)

[a] From Romney, et al, *Radiology*, 1986; 160: 549–554; with permission.

concerning the advisability of resuming breastfeeding after a diagnostic study with an agent known to be excreted in breast milk. This is obviously dependent on the specific tracer employed, the amount administered, and the guidelines for maximum permissible doses established by the NCRP or ICRP. Most authors have conservatively taken 1/10 or 1/15 of the maximum permissible dose guidelines in calculating recommendations for safe resumption of nursing. Table 11.4 provides calculations for maximum breast milk activity at which nursing is considered safe and the maximum delay required before resuming nursing.

CLINICAL CONSIDERATIONS

Clinical Indications.   The radioiodine uptake test is indicated for evaluation of thyroid gland function (Table 11.5). Hypothyroid subjects have diminished percent uptakes compared to the normal range, and patients with primary and secondary hyperthyrodism have increased percent uptakes. The radioiodine uptake test is probably not as sensitive as newer infusion tests for making these distinctions but retains an important role in patients being considered for radioiodine therapy of hyperthyroidism. In particular, the radioactive iodine uptake test will be decreased in patients who are hyperthyroid secondary to subacute thyroiditis and in patients with factitious hyperthyroidism due to ingestion of thyroid hormone. Historically, the percent uptake value has been used in many laboratories to help

Table 11.5   INDICATIONS FOR RADIONUCLIDE STUDIES OF THE THYROID

RADIOIODINE UPTAKE

Assessment of thyroid gland function
· Hypothyroidism
· Hyperthyroidism
· (Differential diagnosis of primary hyperthyroidism versus subacute thyroiditis and factitious hyperthyroidism)
Radioiodine treatment planning
Assessment of thyroid functional reserve
Evaluation of thyroid gland autonomy

RADIONUCLIDE SCINTIGRAPHY

Assessment of thyroid gland position, size, and morphology
Detection of accessory or ectopic thyroid tissue
Assessment of the functional status of thyroid nodules
Evaluation of upper mediastinal masses
Detection of metastatic thyroid cancer and response to therapy
Evaluation of acute thyroid pain

determine or calculate the amount of radioiodine administered for therapy. It is now well established that hyperplastic thyroid tissue is more sensitive to radiation damage than normal tissue. Successful treatment requires between 5000 and 10,000 rads for patients with diffuse toxic goiter (Graves' disease). This amount of radiation is delivered to the thyroid when 80–100 microcuries are retained in the gland per gram of tissue. Table 11.6 illustrates a typical calculation of an individualized treatment dose based on estimated thyroid gland weight and measurement of the 24-hour radioiodine percent uptake.

Response of the radioiodine uptake to adjunctive maneuvers such as TSH stimulation and T3 suppression are described

Table 11.6   CALCULATION OF I-131 THERAPY DOSE FOR HYPERTHYROIDISM

INPUT DATA

Thyroid gland weight	45 gm
Radioiodine uptake (24 hours)	70%
Desired retained dose[a]	100 μCi/gm

CALCULATIONS

$$\text{Required dose } (\mu\text{Ci}) = \frac{45 \text{ gm} \times 100 \text{ } \mu\text{Ci/gm}}{0.70} = 6420 \text{ } \mu\text{Ci}$$

$$\text{Dose in mCi} = \frac{6,429}{1,000} = 6.4 \text{ mCi}$$

[a] Selected to deliver 8,000–10,000 rads to the thyroid.

below. Evaluation of the autonomy of individual thyroid nodules often requires imaging rather than global estimates of radioiodine uptake.

The thyroid scan is most frequently employed in the evaluation of patients with palpable abnormalities of the gland especially when the clinical findings are equivocal and confusing (Table 11.5). The finding that a palpable nodule demonstrates radioiodine uptake significantly reduces the likelihood of malignancy although it does not eliminate the possibility of cancer completely. The demonstration of Tc-99m pertechnetate uptake in a nodule is a less certain indicator of a benign process and may require reimaging with radioiodine. Some thyroidologists now advocate fine needle biopsy rather than imaging in the initial evaluation of thyroid nodules. This approach is however, by no means universally accepted, and the scan remains valuable in demonstrating overall thyroid gland morphology and in detecting clinically occult nodules (Arnold and Pinsky, 1976).

The thyroid scan is indicated in the

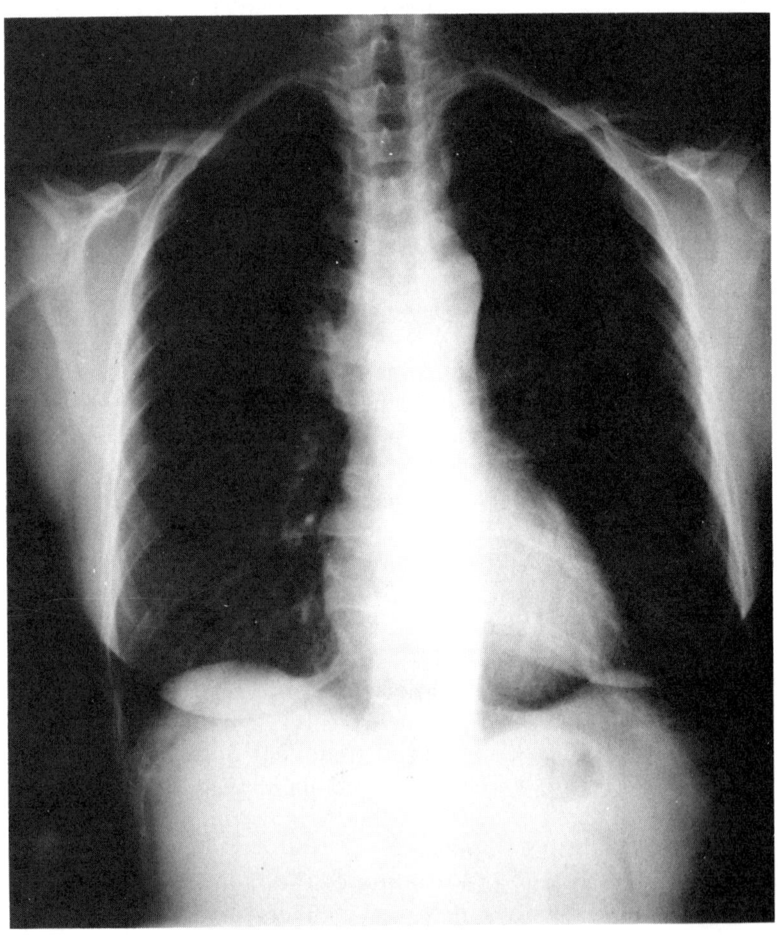

Figure 11.4A   Anterior chest film reveals large mediastinal mass.

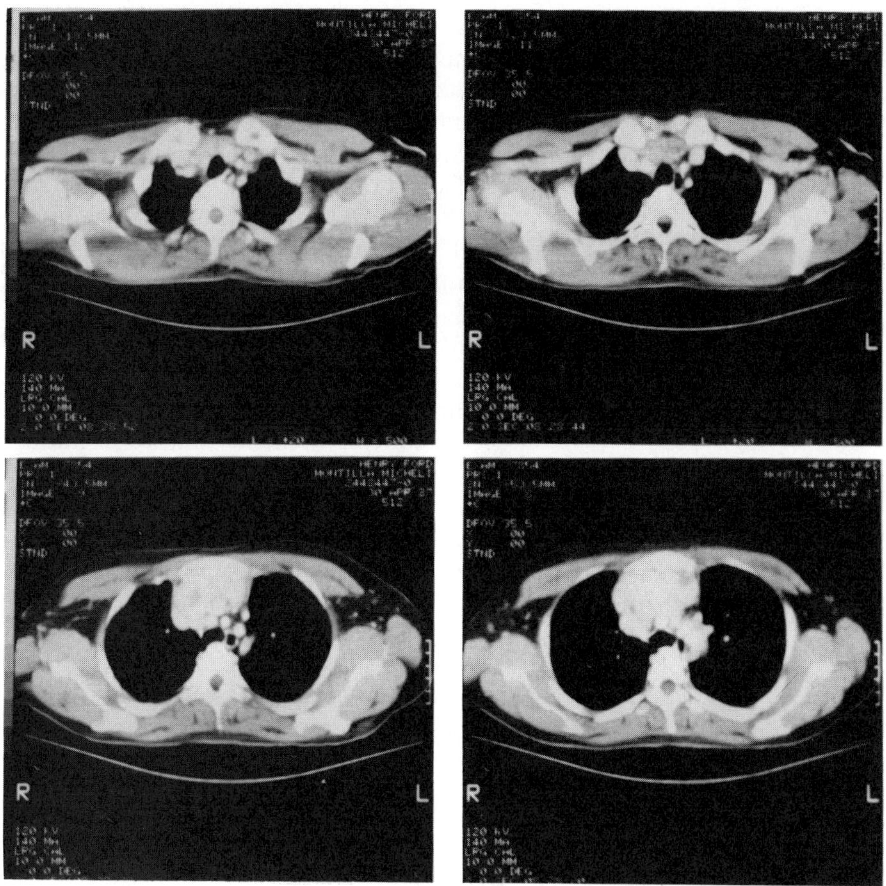

Figure 11.4B   Selected levels from computed tomogram demonstrate the mass to be in the mediastinum with extension superiorly.

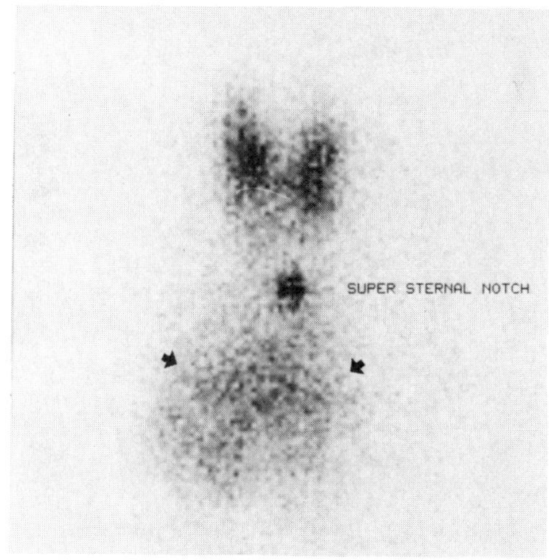

Figure 11.4C   Radioiodine (I-131) neck and chest scintigram reveals (arrows) a functioning goiter with radiotracer uptake corresponding to the mass seen by chest x-ray and computed tomography.

differential diagnosis of neck masses arising adjacent to the thyroid bed or in known ectopic locations such as the base of the tongue or superior mediastinum (Figures 11.4A, 11.4B). Demonstration of functioning thyroid tissue establishes the diagnosis (Figure 11.4C). For these applications, radioiodine is preferred to permit delayed imaging (Figure 11.5A). Blood pool activity in the great vessels makes evaluation of substernal goiter difficult with Tc-99m pertechnetate (Figure 11.5B).

An infrequent but useful indication for thyroid scintigraphy is the evaluation of patients with acute thyroid pain. The most common etiologies are subacute thyroiditis and hemorrhage. The latter condition is seen more commonly in hyperplastic glands and during pregnancy. Both abnormalities present as areas of reduced

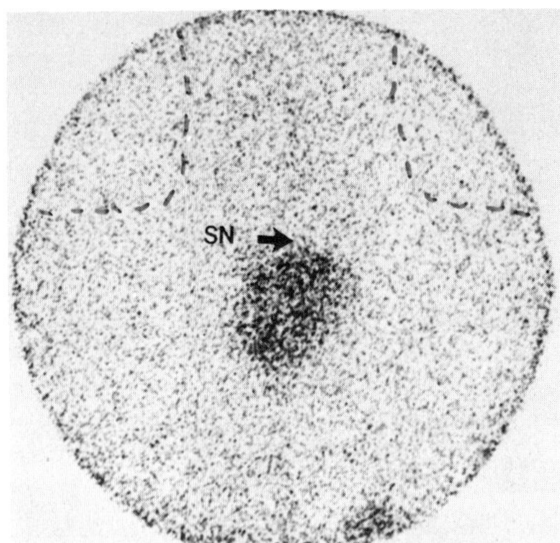

Figure 11.5A Pinhole view of the neck and chest reveals radioiodine uptake in the superior mediastinum below the level of the sternal notch. (Outline of the neck [dotted line] and level of sternal notch [SN and arrow] provided for reference.)

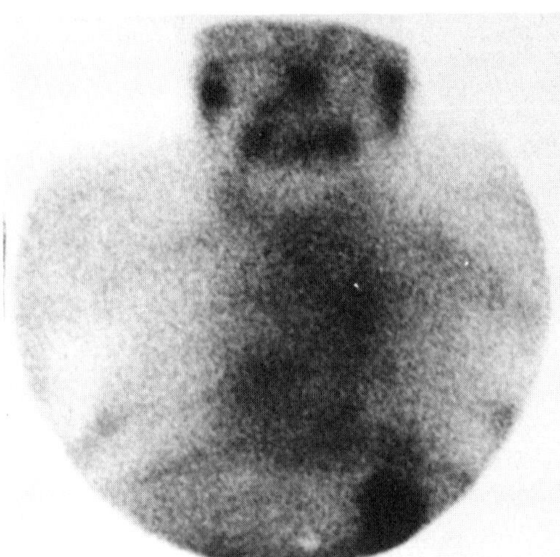

Figure 11.5B Same patient as in Figure 11.5A imaged with Tc-99m pertechnetate at 30 minutes post injection. Substernal thyroid is obscured in general soft tissue and vascular background activity.

may be mistakenly diagnosed as having Graves' disease. Radioiodine uptake and/or imaging studies readily differentiate subacute thyroiditis from primary and secondary hyperthyroidism.

Detection of metastases from differentiated thyroid cancer is an important clinical indication for radioiodine thyroid scanning (Figure 11.6). As a minimum, the neck and chest should be imaged. With modern extended field imaging systems, a complete evaluation includes the entire body. The rationale for detecting metastatic disease is that even though differentiated thyroid cancer does not demonstrate the same degree of function as normal thyroid tissue, it can frequently demonstrate sufficient function to be seen above soft tissue background activity in the absence of normal thyroid tissue. With the normal thyroid gland removed and in the absence of exogenous hormone therapy, the pituitary produces TSH and

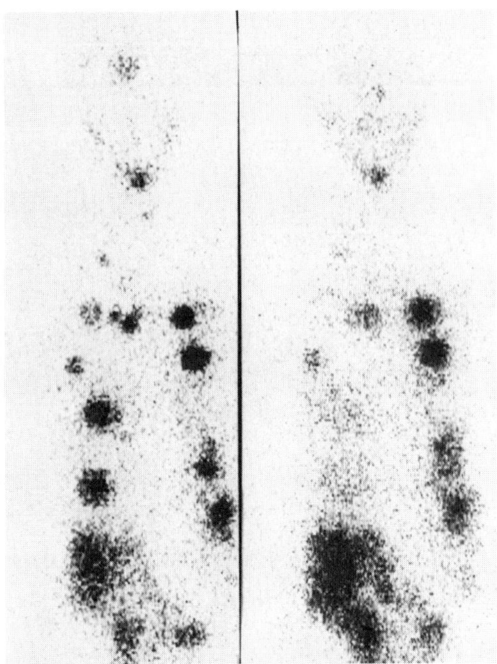

Figure 11.6 Anterior (left) and posterior (right) whole body scintigram obtained with I-131 in a patient with widely metastasized thyroid cancer. Some normal activity is expected in the colon, bladder, and salivary glands. Other regions of focal uptake correspond to metastases.

radionuclide concentration. The release of stored thyroid hormone in patients with subacute thyroiditis can result in clinical hyperthyroidism. In some patients, subacute thyroiditis is not associated with pain (silent thyroiditis), and the patient

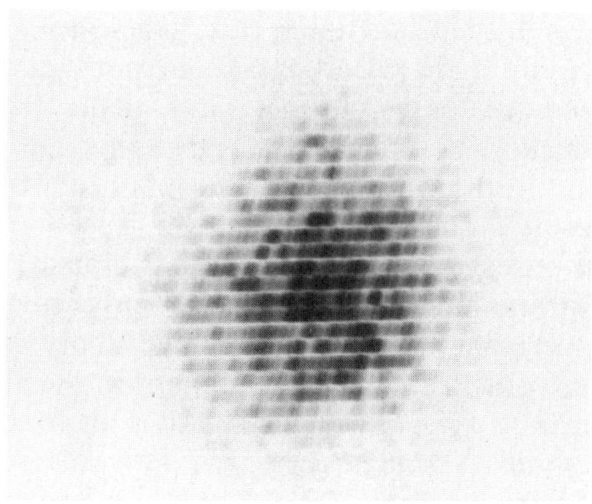

Figure 11.7A Tc-99m pertechnetate scan reveals large "hot" nodule in left lobe of thyroid. Virtually no activity is seen in the right lobe.

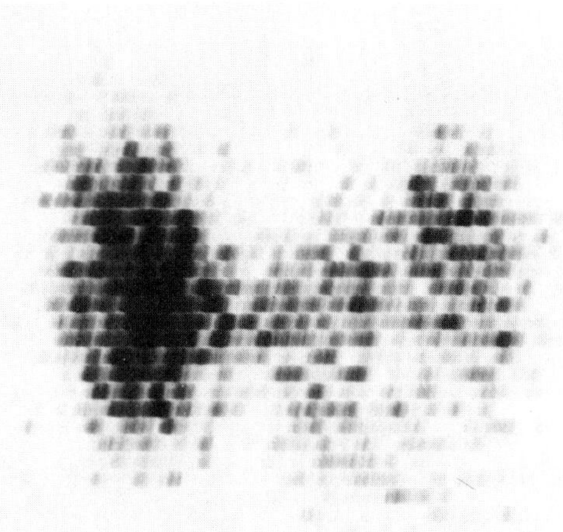

Figure 11.7B Corresponding I-131 scan reveals diminished uptake in area of nodule illustrating the problem of discordant findings on Tc-99m pertechnetate and radioiodine scintigrams.

stimulates radioiodine uptake in metastatic deposits.

Radiopharmaceutical Considerations. As noted above, Tc-99m pertechnetate has found widespread clinical use for thyroid imaging due to its low cost, ready availability, and favorable imaging characteristics. However, Tc-99m pertechnetate is only trapped in the thyroid and not organified. The demonstration of a "hot" or functioning nodule by Tc-99m pertechnetate imaging may or may not correspond to a "hot" nodule by radioiodine imaging (Figure 11.7), and it has now been reported by multiple authors that a small percentage of such cases can involve malignancy. Out of 188 "hot" (i. e., Tc-99m pertechnetate) nodules summarized from the literature by H. L. Atkins, 2.1% harbored cancer (1984). Among 727 "warm" nodules, 4% were histologically malignant. One approach to addressing the problem of discordance between Tc-99m pertechnetate and radioiodine studies is to routinely re-image technetium "hot" nodules with radioiodine when there is concern about thyroid cancer.

Radioactivity in the esophagus is another important artifact or variant encountered in thyroid imaging when Tc-99m pertechnetate is used. Tc-99m pertechnetate is secreted by the salivary glands into the oral cavity and then swallowed with the potential for "staining" of the esophagus above or below the thyroid. The activity is usually slightly off the midline due to the displacement of the esophagus by the trachea when the neck is hyperextended during the imaging procedure (Figure 11.8). When the activity occurs above the thyroid, it can be confused with a pyramidal lobe. This potentially confusing activity is readily cleared by having the patient take several swallows of water. Although iodine is also secreted by the salivary glands, the problem of esophageal activity is not encountered due to the more delayed imaging time and early clearance of iodine from the salivary structures.

Radioiodine may be preferred to Tc-99m pertechnetate in a number of nonmalignant conditions. Delayed imaging at 24 or even 48 hours with radioiodine may be preferable to early imaging in highly vascular areas and in looking for ectopic thyroid tissue at the base of the tongue or in the mediastinum or when looking for struma-ovarii. These, however, are not frequent clinical problems.

Patient Preparation. For the vast majority of indications, no special patient preparation is required. In patients undergoing metastatic evaluations, thyroid

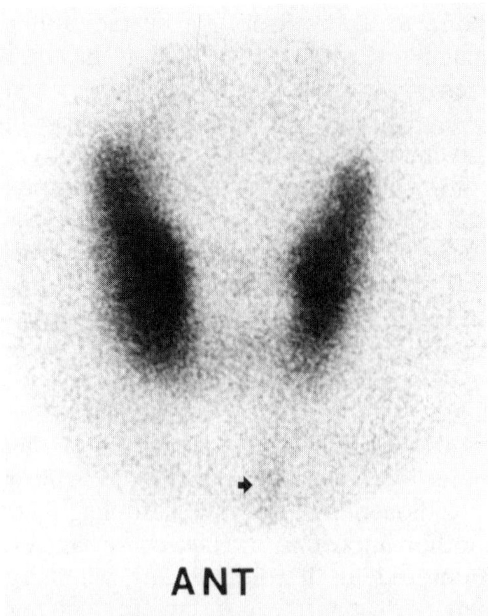

Figure 11.8 Tc-99m pertechnetate scintigram reveals (arrow) esophageal activity below the thyroid slightly to the left of midline.

medication should be discontinued for 6 weeks. This results in an elevation of thyroid stimulating hormone (TSH) and a correspondingly greater sensitivity for detection of metastatic deposits. Measurements of TSH can be used to monitor the patient's response to discontinuation of thyroid hormone. A number of alternative schemes have been described to prepare patients for whole-body imaging in order to reduce the symptoms of hypothyroidism experienced by these thyroidectomized subjects. One alternative approach is to substitute T3 for T4 for a number of weeks and then to image after the patient has been off T3 for 2 weeks. The rationale for this is the shorter biological half-life of T3 compared to T4 (Table 11.3). No controlled series are available to assess the true difference, if any, in sensitivity between these approaches.

Adjunctive Techniques. Historically, hormonal manipulations of the thyroid-pituitary axis were frequently used in evaluating the thyroid gland. Thyroid stimulating hormone (TSH) was used to assess thyroid functional reserve and to stimulate radiotracer uptake in nonvisualized or suppressed tissues in patients with functioning nodules. No value is currently placed clinically on the concept of thyroid reserve, and it is rarely, if ever, necessary to assess the distribution of suppressed extranodular tissue. These indications have essentially been eliminated from clinical practice. The one remaining use of TSH is the occasional patient with functioning thyroid cancer who may not be able to undergo the 6-week wait for an imaging evaluation following discontinuation of thyroid hormone. When this approach is indicated, 10 units of thyrotropin are given daily for 3 or 4 days. Some caution must be exercised in using exogenous TSH. The available commercial preparations contain bovine thyrotropin. As a foreign protein, these preparations may cause anaphylactic reactions and usually induce neutralizing antibodies after a number of injections. The endogenous stimulation approach with discontinuation of thyroid hormone for 6 weeks has been shown to provide greater radioiodine uptake in thyroid carcinoma than injections of TSH and represents a safer approach.

Suppression of thyroid function by administering exogenous thyroid hormone is another historically important adjunctive technique. After a baseline 24-hour radioiodine uptake test, 50–100 micrograms of T3 is administered daily for 7 to 10 days. Failure of a repeat radioiodine uptake to suppress by more than 50% of the baseline value is considered evidence of thyroid autonomy. This is a characteristic feature of active Graves' disease, and the test is occasionally useful in establishing this diagnosis in patients with questionable or borderline increased function studies. It may also be useful in the evaluation of euthyroid subjects with suspected Graves' eye disease. In current practice, the T3 suppression test has been replaced by nonimaging techniques. Thyrotropin-releasing hormone (TRH) is infused with measurement of the TSH response. In patients with

Graves' disease, the response of TSH is diminished.

The T3 suppression test has also found utility when combined with imaging to determine the autonomy of individual functioning nodules of the thyroid. The test must be employed with caution for patients with coronary artery disease. If thyroid function is indeed nonsuppressible, the exogenous hormone is additive, and cardiotoxicity may result with tachyarrhythmias and angina.

The third interventional modification of the radioiodine uptake procedure is the perchlorate discharge test, which provides a measure of the degree of dissociation between trapping and organification of iodine in the thyroid gland. The test is performed by administering a tracer dose of radioiodine followed by a determination of baseline uptake at 1 to 2 hours. After the initial measurement, 1 gram of potassium perchlorate is given orally and sequential hourly uptake measurements obtained. In normal subjects, there should be a fall of less than 10% in thyroid uptake over a 2-hour period following perchlorate administration. In patients with congenital metabolic defects in organification and patients with Hashimoto's thyroiditis, a discharge of trapped but unbound radioiodine occurs. More than a 15% discharge is considered abnormal. The phenomenon is also seen in patients on adequate antithyroid drug therapy.

DOSAGE/DOSIMETRY

Dosage. Table 11.7 provides a summary of typical dosages for uptake and imaging procedures of the thyroid. For Tc-99m pertechnetate, 3–10 millicuries are typically administered intravenously. Maximum uptake occurs relatively soon (i.e., 15–40 minutes) after administration, and imaging is typically begun following a 20–30-minute delay. When Tc-99m pertechnetate is used for uptake studies, the measurement is made at 20–30 minutes with 0.50–3.75% of the administered dose expected in normals.

For I-131 sodium iodide, the administered dose varies significantly depending on the application. Follow-up whole-body scans on patients with differentiated thyroid cancer are now accomplished with a dose of at least 1 millicurie, and in some laboratories, up to 5–10 millicuries are administered. If only a percent uptake determination is required, as little as 2–6 microcuries of I-131 are given. In selected situations (i.e., patients without known cancer) involving uptake and imaging studies, 30 microcuries may be given. In all applications, the dose is administered orally in liquid or capsule form.

For I-123 sodium iodide, the recommended dose is 100–500 microcuries. The dose is administered orally. Imaging is begun at 4 to 6 hours although imaging is also feasible at 24 hours. Uptake studies

Table 11.7 RADIOPHARMACEUTICALS FOR THYROID IMAGING—CLINICAL STUDY PARAMETERS AND DOSIMETRY

RADIOPHARMACEUTICAL	DOSE	ROUTE OF ADMINISTRATION	TIME TO IMAGING	ABSORBED DOSE (RAD/MCI) *Whole Body*	*Gonads*
Technetium 99m (Sodium Pertechnetate)	3–10 mCi	Intravenous	20–40 min	0.01	0.01–0.04
I-123 (Sodium Iodide)	100–500 μCi (scan)	Oral	4–24 hr	0.02–0.04	0.01–0.03
	10–20 μCi (uptake)		4–24 hr		
I-131 (Sodium Iodide)	30–50 μCi (Routine scan)	Oral	24 hr	0.50–4.00	0.08–0.18
	1–5mCi (Whole-body scan—cancer follow-up)		24–72 hr		
	2–6 μCi (uptake)		4–24 hr		

with I-123 may give false values if the uptake probe system cannot handle the count rate, resulting in counting errors due to dead-time losses.

Dosimetry. Estimates of absorbed radiation dose in thyroid imaging are summarized in Tables 11.3 and 11.7. Technetium-99m pertechnetate delivers the lowest dose per millicurie administered among clinically important radiopharmaceuticals, followed in order by I-123, I-125, and I-131. Doses of Tc-99m pertechnetate used in clinical practice are substantially greater than the other agents and the dose per millicurie somewhat overestimates the differences actually observed in clinical studies (Task Force on short-lived radionuclides of the Bureau of Radiologic Health of the Food and Drug Administration, Washington, DC, June 1976). The recommended administered activities for imaging and uptake studies are provided in Table 11.7. Using the recommended activity for Tc-99m pertechnetate of 3–10 millicuries results in an estimated absorbed dose to the thyroid of 0.39–1.3 rads. With an upper limit dose of 10 millicuries, Tc-99m pertechnetate delivers approximately one-third the radiation exposure from I-123 and one-eighteenth that from I-131 when the latter agents are also used in the recommended amounts.

As noted above, preparations of I-123 commonly have radionuclidic impurities including I-124, I-125, I-126, I-130, and I-131. All except I-130 have longer half-lives than I-123 and therefore become relatively more abundant with increasing time after production (Ziessman HA, et al, 1986). The increasing relative abundance of impurities increases both radiation exposure to the patient and degrades scintigraphic images due to high-energy photons from the contaminants. For these reasons, I-123 should not be administered beyond the day for which the dose was calibrated.

Radiation dosimetry is of special importance in children and pregnant or breastfeeding women. For children, the radiation absorbed doses per millicurie of administered activity are higher than for adults. This is because the percentage of radioactivity localizing in the thyroid gland is roughly the same for children and adults, but the weight of the gland and therefore the volume of distribution of radioactivity increases with age (Table 11.3). For subjects with normal thyroid function, the dose to the thyroid of a newborn is estimated at 11 times that to the adult per millicurie administered. The use of I-123 or Tc-99m pertechnetate in children is emphasized for these reasons.

FLUORESCENT THYROID SCANNING

Fluorescent thyroid scanning is a nuclear imaging procedure that does not require administration of a radiotracer to the patient but provides a qualitative and quantitative map of the distribution of stable iodine within the thyroid gland (Hoffer PB, 1969). In brief, an external radiation beam is directed at the thyroid gland. The energy of the beam is chosen to be higher than the binding energy of the K-shell electrons of stable I-127, which is 33.5 keV. Americium-241 with a principal photon energy of 59.5 keV has been used as well as x-ray beams. The x-ray or gamma-ray photons from the external beam interact with K-shell electrons and displace them from the iodine atom (photoelectric effect) resulting in a vacancy in the K-shell that is filled immediately by an outer orbit electron. In 85% of these events, an L-shell electron fills the vacancy, and in making this transition, the L-shell electron gives up energy in the form of a characteristic x-ray (stimulated x-ray fluorescence). This x-ray with energy of 27.5 keV is characteristic for the transition from the L-shell to the K-shell of I-127 and can be detected externally. By systematically scanning the thyroid with a fluorescent imaging system consisting of the stimulating external photon beam and a detector optimized for the low-energy iodine characteristic x-rays, the distribution of stable iodine can be mapped. Iodine can actually be quantitated with appropriate calibration and standardization of the imaging technique (Patton JA, et al, 1976; Gillin MT, et al, 1977; Thrall JH, et al, 1978).

In addition to the ability to quantitate stable iodine in the gland, fluorescent thyroid imaging affords the potential for imaging the gland in clinical settings where radiotracer uptake is suppressed, such as subacute thyroiditis or flooded iodine pools, and in the extranodular tissues of patients with autonomous nodules. Fluorescent thyroid scanning has not become clinically important but has provided valuable insight into thyroid iodine content in different clinical conditions affecting the thyroid gland.

II. Parathyroid Scintigraphy

James H. Thrall

The diagnosis of hyperparathyroidism is accomplished clinically through radioimmunoassays for parathyroid hormone and its metabolites. However, the localization of parathyroid adenomas, particularly after initial surgery or when they are multiple, remains a clinical problem that has led to an ongoing search for radiopharmaceuticals demonstrating specific localization in parathyroid tissues.

One of the first agents studied for this purpose was Selenium-75 selenomethionine (DiGuilio and Beierwaltes, 1964; Weinstein MB, et al, 1971). This radiolabeled amino acid is rapidly incorporated into polypeptides in areas of hormone and protein synthesis and has been shown to be incorporated in vivo within the peptide segments of the parathyroid hormone (PTH) molecule. Superimposition of selenomethionine uptake in the thyroid and the small size of the parathyroids and many parathyroid adenomas have, however, contributed to a lack of success in the general clinical application of this agent. Thyroid suppression with T3 to reduce Se-75 selenomethionine uptake in the thyroid gland has been of limited value.

An alternative approach to imaging

parathyroid adenomas has been described using Tl-201 thallous chloride. As noted previously, Tl-201 localizes in metabolically active tissues and is rapidly concentrated in parathyroid adenomas. However, Tl-201 is also taken up in the thyroid, requiring the utilization of a dual tracer subtraction technique to permit visualization of parathyroid adenomas (Gimlette TMD, et al, 1986). The patient is initially injected with Tl-201 thallous chloride with imaging in multiple views (Figure 11.9A). The view that is felt to provide the most positive indication of possible abnormality is selected and the patient is subsequently injected with Tc-99m pertechnetate (Figure 11.9B). Imaging is accomplished without moving

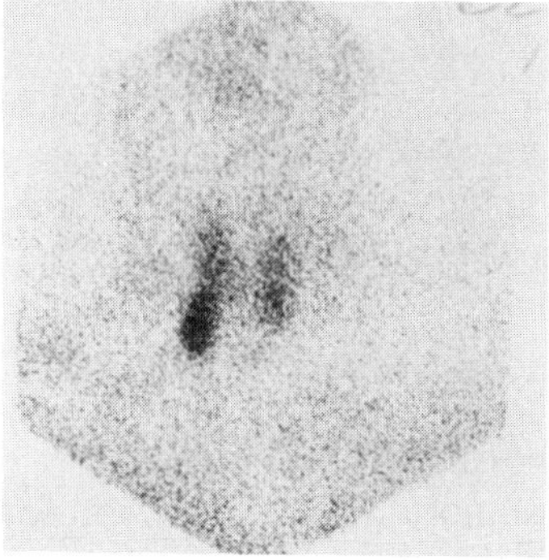

Figure 11.9A Anterior view obtained with T1-201 in a patient with hyperparathyroidism and suspected adenoma. Note asymmetry between right and left lobes.

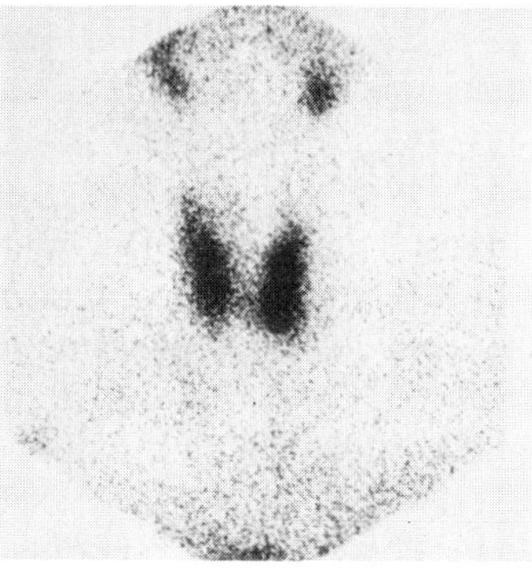

Figure 11.9B Tc-99m pertechnetate scan with patient in same position as Figure 11.9A.

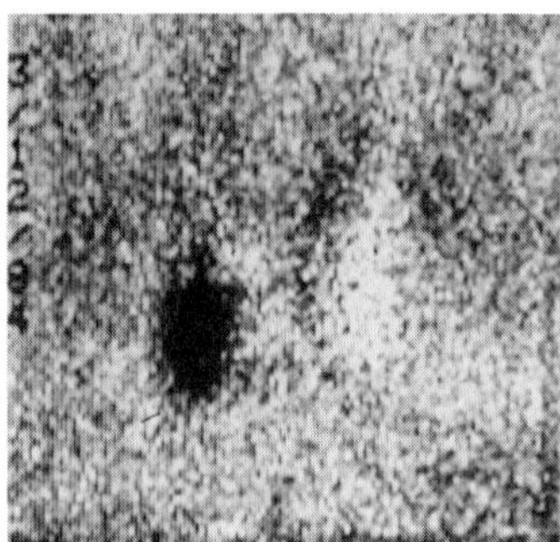

Figure 11.9C Subtraction scan reveals positive differential accumulation of T1-201 in a parathyroid adenoma adjacent to the lower pole of the right lobe.

the patient. A nuclear medicine computer system is then used to subtract the thyroidal component of Tl-201 localization, thereby theoretically unmasking thallium uptake due solely to localization in parathyroid adenomas (Figure 11.9C). This technique assumes an identical distribution of Tc-99m pertechnetate and Thallium-201 in the thyroid so that the activity levels can be normalized for the subtraction step. This may or may not be a good assumption in patients with goiters. In patients with normal thyroid glands, it is a reasonable assumption, and the subtraction imaging technique has found modest clinical utility. A recent study reported correct localization of 96% of parathyroid adenomas over 1.0 gm in size and 0% below 0.3 gm using the Tl-201–Tc-99m pertechnetate subtraction technique (Gimlette TMD, et al, 1986).

III. Adrenocortical Imaging

Dennis P. Swanson

Circulating plasma cholesterol is avidly taken up by and concentrated within adrenal cortical cells, and is eventually utilized for respective biosynthesis of a number of steroid hormones (Samuels and Uchikawer, 1967). It is therefore not surprising that the development of radiopharmaceuticals for imaging the adrenal cortex centered originally on radiolabeled derivatives of the cholesterol nucleus.

CHEMISTRY

History. The first attempt to synthesize a radiolabeled cholesterol suitable for external imaging involved direct iodination (I-131) of the 5-6 double bond using a chloramine-T method (Nagai T, et al, 1968). The resulting agent, most likely a diiodocholesterol, demonstrated insufficient target-to-background radioactivity ratios for further investigation. Radioiodine was subsequently introduced into the neopentyl C-19 position of cholesterol to produce an agent, I-131 19-iodocholesterol (Figure 11.10), that exhibited canine adrenal: liver and adrenal: kidney radioactivity ratios in the range of 150:1 and 250:1, respectively, at 6 days following its intravenous injection (Counsell RE, et al, 1970). Further investigation of this radiopharmaceutical eventually led to successful scintigraphic imaging of the human adrenals and its use in the evaluation of adrenal cortical diseases (Beierwaltes WH, et al, 1971; Lieberman LM, et al, 1971).

In the early syntheses of I-131 19-iodocholesterol a radiochemical impurity was consistently observed at varying levels depending on the nature of the solvent used as the refluxing medium (Kojima M, et al, 1975; Basmadjian GP, et al, 1975). This radiochemical impurity, which did not correspond to free radioiodide, was isolated and identified as 6β-iodomethyl-19-norcholesterol (Figure 11.10), a homallylic isomer of 19-iodocholesterol (Maeda, and Kojima 1975). Subsequent tissue distribution studies revealed that the 6β-derivative concentrated substantially greater (i. e., by a factor of 5–50) in

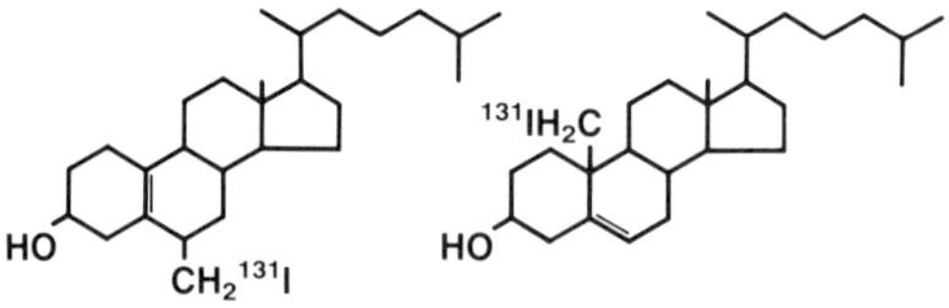

Figure 11.10 Chemical structures of 19-iodocholesterol and 6β-iodomethyl-19-norcholesterol (NP-59).

the adrenal cortex than 19-iodocholesterol (Kojima M, et al, 1975; Sarkar SD, et al, 1975; Couch and Williams, 1977) and was also more stable in vivo (Scott KN, et al, 1977). Although the target-to-background radioactivity ratios achieved with 6β-iodomethyl-19-norcholesterol were essentially equivalent to 19-iodocholesterol, its increased adrenocortical localization and stability permitted earlier and improved scintigraphy of the human adrenals (Sarker SD, et al, 1975). Hence, I-131 6β-iodomethyl-19-norcholesterol rapidly replaced I-131 19-iodocholesterol as the imaging agent of choice for the nuclear medicine evaluation of adrenocortical disease.

Although numerous derivatives of cholesterol and several radiolabeled inhibitors of adrenal cortical enzymes have been synthesized and evaluated in an attempt to improve upon the imaging characteristics of I-131 6β-iodomethyl-19-norcholesterol (Beierwaltes WH, et al, 1978; 1981), this agent is currently the only radiopharmaceutical available in the United States for adrenocortical scintigraphy. Extensive, developmental research in this area has, in general, been restricted as a result of the relatively low prevalence of adrenocortical disease and the respective limited role of scintigraphy compared to other routinely available diagnostic modalities (i. e., laboratory testing, computed tomography).

NP-59. 6β-iodomethyl-19-norcholesterol (Figure 11.10) is insoluble in water and slightly soluble in ethyl alochol. It is therefore commercially available in the form of a sterile, pyrogen-free surfactant solution consisting of absolute ethanol (7.3% v/v) and Tween-80 (1.8% v/v) in Bacteriostatic Sodium Chloride Injection, U.S.P. (Product Information, NP-59, Nuclear Pharmacy, University of Michigan, Ann Arbor). This formulation of I-131 6β-iodomethyl-19-norcholesterol (NP-59) is clear to slightly turbid and colorless to pale yellow with a pH approximately 6.0. Strongly yellow preparations indicate product degradation with the lib-

eration of free iodine/radioiodine, and should therefore be discarded.

The manufacturer of NP-59 specifies (Product Information, NP-59, Nuclear Pharmacy, University of Michigan, Ann Arbor) a radiochemical purity in excess of 90%, a radionuclidic purity of greater than 99%, and a specific activity of 1.3–1.8 mCi/mg at the time of shipment. When stored at freezer temperatures (2–5° C), the I-131 6β-iodomethyl-19-norcholesterol is stable to deiodination for the indicated expiration dating of 14 days post synthesis (Beierwaltes WH et al, 1978). Storage at elevated temperatures will, however, result in a more rapid rate of product degradation (Scott KN, et al, 1977).

The I-131 radiolabel decays by β^- particle emission with a physical half-life of 8 days. External imaging is performed utilizing the 364 keV gamma radiation that accompanies this decay process.

PHARMACOKINETICS

Adrenal cortical cells obtain cholesterol for steroid hormone biosynthesis primarily from the plasma cholesterol pool (Samuels and Uchikawer, 1967). In plasma, insoluble cholesterol is transported in the form of a low-density lipoprotein complex. Uptake of this bound cholesterol by the adrenocortical cells occurs via a specialized transport system which involves a specific low-density lipoprotein (LDL) recepter (Brown and Goldstein, 1976; Faust JR, et al, 1977). Studies indicate that the number and affinity of these LDL-receptors are controlled by the amount of intracellular and extracellular cholesterol (Brown and Goldstein, 1975), and by plasma adrenocorticotropic hormone (ACTH) and prostaglandin levels (Gwynne JT et al, 1976). The localization of I-131 6β-iodomethyl-19-norcholesterol in the adrenal cortex appears to occur by this same LDL-receptor mechanism. The radiocholesterol is apparently circulated in plasma bound to LDL (Fikuski K, 1978), and its adrenal uptake is affected by factors known to alter

LDL-receptor activity. For example, decreased or increased amounts of circulating cholesterol have been shown to stimulate or suppress, respectively, the adrenocortical localization of I-131 6β-iodomethyl-19-norcholesterol (Gordon L, et al, 1980). Also, increased plasma levels of ACTH result in an expected enhancement of radiocholesterol uptake by the adrenal cortex (Blair RJ, et al, 1971; Fukuchi K, et al, 1976). Unlike native cholesterol, however, the I-131 6β-iodomethyl-19-norcholesterol does not appear to participate in the metabolic processes involved in steroid hormone biosynthesis, but is simply stored within the lipid pools of adrenocortical cells for a prolonged period of time (Sarkar SD, et al, 1975).

Following intravenous injection, I-131 6β-iodomethyl-19-norcholesterol demonstrates progressive accumulation in the adrenal cortex. In rats, a peak localization of 2.6% of the injected dose/organ was observed at 7 days following administration (Couch and Williams, 1977). Distribution to the rat adrenal cortex at 1 and 3 days post injection were 1.0% and 2.2% of the dose/organ, respectively. As mentioned previously, I-131 6β-iodomethyl-19-norcholesterol demonstrates prolonged retention in adrenocortical cells, with a biological half-life of approximately 30 days (rat data) (Ice RD, et al, 1976). The biological half-life of respective radioactivity in potential background organs such as the liver (i.e., 10.5 days, rat data) and kidney (i.e., 8.6 days, rat data) is substantially less, resulting in progressively increasing target-to-background radioactivity ratios with time. In fact, low adrenal-to-liver radioactivity ratios preclude adequate scintigraphic visualization of the normal adrenal cortices (Figure 11.11) until two–three days following the administration of NP-59 (Thrall JH, et al, 1978; Gross MD, et al, 1980).

The localization of I-131 6β-iodomethyl-19-norcholesterol in the human adrenal cortex appears to be significantly less than that observed in rats. A mean uptake per normal human gland of 0.16% of the administered dose (range of 0.073–

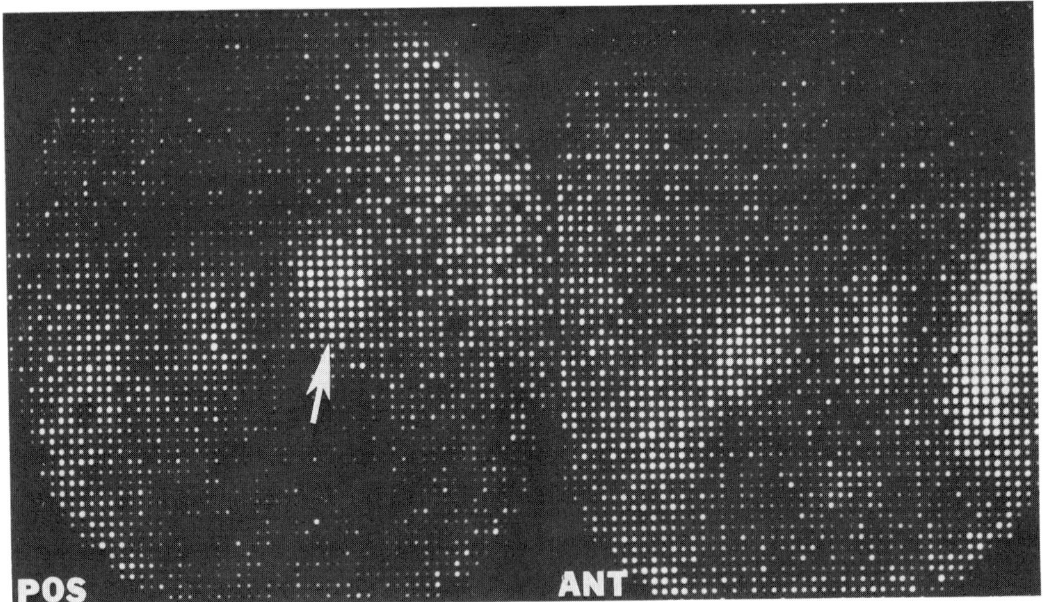

Figure 11.11 Normal adrenal scintigram obtained using I-131 6β-iodomethyl-19-norcholesterol. Note (arrow) the more intense appearance of the right versus left adrenal on the posterior view (POS) due to the more proximal location of the right gland relative to the gamma camera. The anterior view (ANT) shows a reversal in the degree of intensity of the right versus left adrenal. (See Freitas, et al, 1978.)

0.26%) has been determined using external counting techniques (Carey JE, et al, 1979). Tissue sampling at 20 hours post injection has revealed a testicular uptake of 0.07% of the administered dose and an ovarian uptake of 0.08% of the administered dose (Ice RD, et al, 1976). The human whole-body clearance of I-131 6β-iodomethyl-19-norcholesterol is triexponential with biological half-lives of approximately 1.5 days (40% of administered dose), 4.5 days (35%) and 400 days (25%) (Ice RD, et al 1976). Elimination occurs almost equally between the kidney and liver.

PRECAUTIONS

Formulation Incompatibilities. I-131 6β-iodomethyl-19-norcholesterol is insoluble in aqueous solutions, thus requiring the use of a surfactant (i. e., Tween-80) in its formulation for intravenous injection. To avoid precipitation of the radiocholesterol, dilution, if required, should be performed using this same surfactant solution (see Chemistry).

Adverse Reactions. Adverse reactions including immediate shortness of breath, tightness in the chest, palpitations, hypotension, and nausea or dizziness have been reported with the intravenous injection of NP-59 (Product Information, NP-59, Nuclear Pharmacy, University of Michigan, Ann Arbor). These reactions, which occur with an overall incidence of approximately 0.1%, are transient in duration, normally persisting for 5–20 minutes post injection. Although not proven, it is currently felt that the Tween-80 component of the NP-59 formulation may be the precipitating factor for these reactions. Polyoxyethylene sorbitan fatty acid esters (i. e., Tweens) have been shown to cause the release of histamine from various internal cellular sources following their intravenous administration (Marks and Kolmen, 1971; Burnell and Maxwell, 1974). The type and duration of adverse reactions observed with the ad-

ministration of NP-59 appear to be consistent with the expected effects of released histamine on pulmonary and cardiac physiology.

In an attempt to avoid these adverse effects of NP-59, it is recommended that patient dosages be administered as soon as possible following receipt of the agent in order to minimize the injected volume. The dosage should be administered slowly over a 1–2 minute interval with constant patient monitoring. Finally, pretreatment with an antihistamine should be considered in patients with a significant atopic history (Product Information, NP-59, Nuclear Pharmacy, University of Michigan, Ann Arbor).

Pregnancy/Breastfeeding. It is currently not known whether I-131 6β-iodomethyl-19-norcholesterol will cross the placenta to directly expose and/ or cause harmful effects on the fetus. However, the normal localization and retention of this agent in the maternal liver, spleen, kidneys, and ovaries will result in substantial fetal radiation exposure. The I-131 6β-iodomethyl-19-norcholesterol does undergo some in vivo deiodination with the liberation of free radioiodine, which can cross the placenta and is also excreted in breast milk during lactation (Committee on Drugs, 1983). Based on these considerations, the administration of NP-59 to pregnant or possibly pregnant women should be avoided unless the potential benefits to be gained from the study clearly outweigh the aforementioned risks. Formula-feeding should be substituted for breastfeeding if applicable.

Drug–Radiopharmaceutical Interactions. Several drugs can potentially alter the normal uptake of I-131 6β-iodomethyl-19-norcholesterol by the adrenal cortex via their direct or indirect action on adrenocortical activity. Table 11.8 summarizes the known or expected effects of various drugs on NP-59 scintigraphy and the mechanism(s) responsible for the respective drug–radiopharmaceutical interaction.

Table 11.8   DRUGS KNOWN OR EXPECTED TO CAUSE AN ALTERATION IN THE NORMAL UPTAKE OF I-131 6β-IODOMETHYL-19-NORCHOLESTEROL BY THE ADRENAL CORTEX

DRUG	EFFECT ON RADIO-PHARMACEUTICAL UPTAKE BY ADRENAL CORTEX	MECHANISM RESPONSIBLE FOR DRUG—RADIOPHARMACEUTICAL INTERACTION	REFERENCE(S)
ACTH (exogenous)	Increase	General stimulation of adrenocortical activity	Blair, et al, 1971; Gross, et al, 1981
Glucocorticords (exogenous)	Decrease	Suppression of ACTH release from the pituitary	Gross, et al, 1981
Adrenal Enzyme Inhibitors (e. g. mitotane, metyrapone, aminoglutethimide)	Increase	Reduction in synthesis and release of steroid hormones stimulates ACTH release from the pituitary	Gross, et al, 1980; 1981
Diuretics (general)	Increase	Hypovolemic stimulation of reninangiotensin system results in increased zona glomerulosa activity (i. e., aldosterone synthesis and release)	Gross, et al, 1980; 1981; Fischer, et al, 1982
Spironolactone (long-term therapy)	Decrease	Inhibition of aldosterone biosynthesis by zona glomerulosa	Gross, et al, 1981
Oral contraceptives	Increase	Stimulation of renin-angiotensin system results in increased zona glomerulosa activity	Gross, et al, 1980; 1981
Beta-blockers	Decrease	Suppression of renin-angiotensin system results in decreased zona glomerulosa activity	Gross, et al, 1981
Indomethacin	Decrease	Suppression of renin-angiotensin system results in decreased zona glomerulosa activity	Gross, et al, 1981
Cholestyramine resin	Increase	Reduction in serum cholesterol levels results in an increase in the number and af'nity of LDL receptors	Gross, et al, 1981

CLINICAL CONSIDERATIONS

Patient Preparation. The I-131 6β-iodomethyl-19-norcholesterol does exhibit some in vivo degradation resulting in the release of free radioiodine. To block thyroidal uptake of this released radioiodine and radioiodine that may be present as a radiochemical impurity in the injected radiopharmaceutical, it is recommended that patients be pretreated with oral Lugol's Iodine, 3 drops twice daily, commencing 24 hours prior to NP-59 administration and continued for 14 days (Thrall JH, et al, 1978; Gross MD, et al, 1980). Other oral thyroid-blocking agents such as Saturated Solution of Potassium Iodide (S.S.K.I.), 1 drop three times daily, or potassium perchlorate, 200 mg four times daily, may be used alternatively for the same dosage duration. (See also Appendix B.)

The normal renal and hepatic elimination of radioactivity following the administration of I-131 6β-iodomethyl-19-norcholesterol can result in kidney, gallbladder, and intestinal activity that may interfere with interpretation of the adrenal scintigrams. Adequate patient hydration and a bowel cleansing regimen administered the day prior to imaging will help to avoid this problem (Thrall JH, et al, 1978; Gross MO, et al, 1980).

Adjunctive Techniques. The adrenal cortex is anatomically and functionally divided into three histological zones; the zona glomerulosa, zona fasciculata, and the zona reticularis (Liddle and Melmon, 1974). To facilitate scintigraphic evaluation of the zona glomerulosa or the zona reticularis in the face of hyperaldosteronism or hyperandrogenism, respectively, it is recommended that the adjunct administration of dexamethasone be incorporated to suppress the release of ACTH from the pituitary and thus reduce substantially the activity of the zona fasciculata (Thrall JH, et al, 1978; Gross MD, et al, 1980). Using a dexamethasone suppression regimen of 4 mg daily, in divided doses, commencing 7 days prior to the scheduled injection of NP-59 and continued throughout the imaging sequence, the normal adrenal cortices should not visualize until at least 5 days following radiopharmaceutical administration (Gross MD, et al,

1979). Breakthrough visualization of the adrenals prior to this 5-day interval is an indication of hyperactivity or tumor involvement of the adrenocortical zone under investigation (see Clinical Indications).

Clinical Indications. The three histologic zones of the adrenal cortex synthesize and secrete distinct steroid hormones with differing biological functions. In this regard, the principal hormones produced by the zona glomerulosa, zona fasciculata, and zona reticularis are aldosterone, cortisol, and angrogens, respectively (Liddle and Melmon, 1974). Adrenocortical scintigraphy following the intravenous injection of NP-59 can be used to evaluate abnormalities of each of these zones. However, the scintigraphic patterns observed will have relevance only if combined with a knowledge of the specific hormonal imbalance in question (Thrall JH, et al, 1978; Gross MD, et al, 1980). In general, adrenocortical scintigraphy is useful in determining whether the hormonal imbalance is due to bilateral hyperactivity or tumor involvement of the respective zone, and in the latter case, which adrenal is involved for subsequent surgical removal.

The scintigraphic patterns that may be observed in the presence of various hormonal imbalances are discussed in the following subsection (Thrall JH, et al, 1978; Gross MD, et al, 1980). Included are the probable clinical diagnoses based on these patterns and a knowledge of hormonal abnormality.

HYPERCORTISOLISM (CUSHING'S SYNDROME)

The excess production and secretion of cortisol associated with an abnormality of the zona fasciculata will exert negative feedback on the pituitary to suppress the release of ACTH. In the absence of this adrenocortical-stimulating hormone, normal adrenal tissue should demonstrate negligible uptake of I-131 6β-iodomethyl-19-norcholesterol and therefore should not visualize scintigraphically.

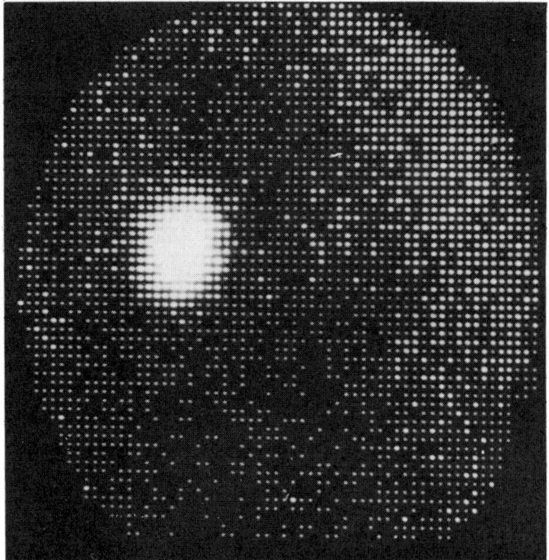

Figure 11.12 I-131 6β-iodomethyl-19-norcholesterol scintigraphy on a patient with Cushing's syndrome demonstrates unilateral (left) adrenal activity consistent with a Cushing's adenoma involving the left gland.

1. Unilateral adrenal visualization (Figure 11.12): A scintigraphic pattern of intense activity in one, possibly enlarged adrenal with no uptake in the contralateral normal adrenal is consistent with a Cushing's adenoma.
2. Bilateral adrenal visualization (Figure 11.13): Scintigraphic visualization of both adrenals in a patient with confirmed hypercortisolism is indicative of hyperplasia of the zona fasciculata of both adrenals. A small degree of asymmetry in the observed intensity of adrenal activity may be noted as a result of the more posterior location of the right versus left gland (Figure 11.11). Reversed or marked asymmetry suggests the coexistence of Cushing's adenoma with hyperplasia (Gross MO, et al, 1979).
3. Bilateral nonvisualization (Figure 11.14): A failure to scintigraphically display either adrenal in the presence of confirmed hypercortisolism is commonly associated with an adrenocortical carcinoma. Carcinomas function poorly per gram of tissue and may therefore demonstrate minimal uptake

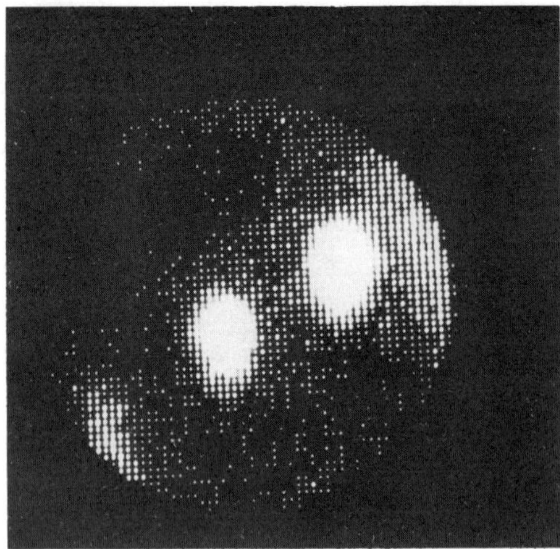

Figure 11.13 I-131 6β-iodomethyl-19-norcholesterol scintigraphy on a patient with Cushing's syndrome demonstrates symmetrical, intense adrenal activity consistent with bilateral hyperplasia.

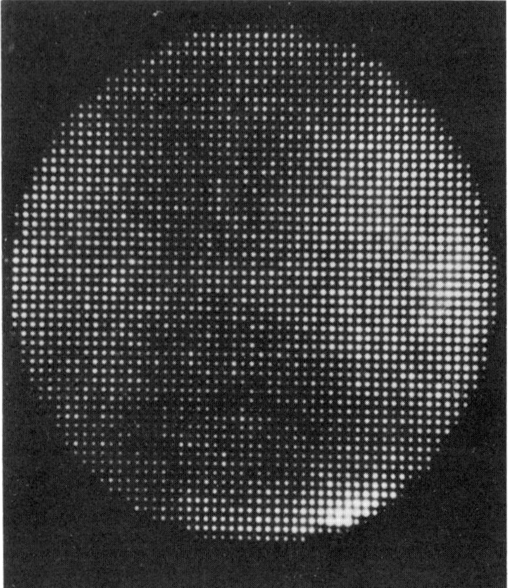

Figure 11.14 I-131 6β-iodomethyl-19-norcholesterol scintigraphy on patient with Cushing's syndrome demonstrates bilateral nonvisualization of the adrenals consistent with an adrenocortical carcinoma.

of the I-131 6β-iodomethyl-19-norcholesterol. However, large adrenocortical carcinomas may secrete a sufficient amount of cortisol to produce Cushingnoid symptoms and to also suppress

radiopharmaceutical uptake in the contralateral, normal gland. Technical problems, such as extravasation of the injected dose or the exogenous administration of glucocorticords, should be examined as other potential causes of adrenal nonvisualization when this pattern is observed.

HYPERALDOSTERONISM

The excess production and secretion of aldosterone associated with abnormalities of the zona glomerulosa does not result in feedback inhibition of the release of ACTH by the pituitary. Normal adrenal tissue will therefore continue to localize I-131 6β-iodomethyl-19-norcholesterol in the presence of hyperplasia or tumor involvement of the zona glomerulosa, thus rendering the respective diagnosis difficult. The adjunct administration of the glucocorticoid, dexamethasone (see Adjunctive Techniques), will suppress ACTH release and the uptake of I-131 6β-iodomethyl-19-norcholesterol by normal adrenal tissue for up to 5 days post radiopharmaceutical injection. Hence, in patients with confirmed hyperaldosteronism, this pharmacological intervention facilitates the scintigraphic differentiation of bilateral hyperplasia versus aldosteronoma as the causative disease process and permits lateralization of the tumor in the latter event (Thrall JH, et al, 1978; Gross MD, et al, 1980).

1. Unilateral adrenal visualization (with dexamethasone suppression) (Figure 11.15): Distinct scintigraphic visualization of a single adrenal occurring prior to 5 days following the injection of I-131 6β-iodomethyl-19-norcholesterol is highly specific for an aldosteronoma. Scintigraphic visualization of the contralateral, normal gland is suppressed via the action of the exogenous dexamethasone.

2. Bilateral adrenal visualization (with dexamethasone suppression) (Figure 11.16): Scintigraphic visualization of both adrenal glands occurring prior to

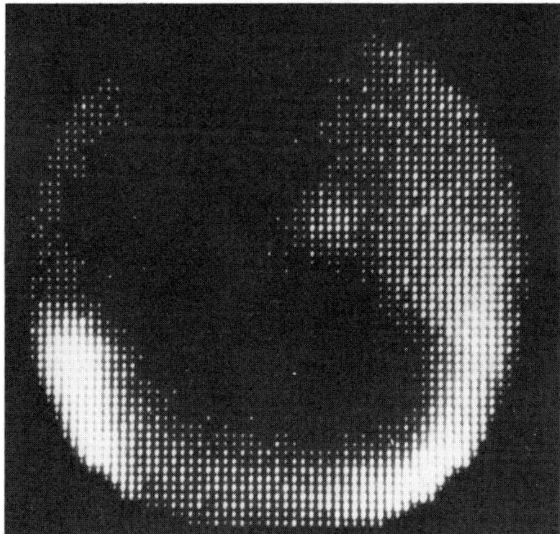

Figure 11.15 I-131 6β-iodomethyl-19-norcholesterol scintigraphy (with dexamethasone suppression) on a patient with hyperaldosteronism [hyperandrogenism] demonstrates distinct unilateral visualization of the right adrenal at 3 days post radiopharmaceutical injection. Such an imaging pattern in the presence of the respective hormonal imbalance is indicative of a right adrenal aldosteronoma [androgenoma].

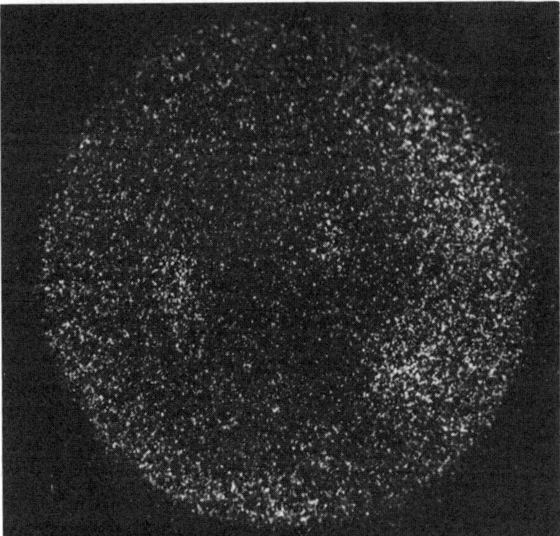

Figure 11.16 I-131 6β-iodomethyl-19-norcholesterol scintigraphy (with dexamethasone suppression) on a patient with hyperaldosteronism [hyperandrogenism] demonstrates distinct visualization of both adrenals at 3 days post radiopharmaceutical injection. Such an imaging pattern in the presence of the respective hormonal imbalance is indicative of bilateral hyperplasia of the zona glomerulosa [zona reticularis].

5 days following the injection of I-131 6β-iodomethyl-19-norcholesterol is indicative of hyperplasia of the zona glomerulosa of both adrenals.

HYPERANDROGENISM

The source of excess androgens in women with virilism may be of adrenal or ovarian origin, or may result from the peripheral conversion of precursor hormones. Adrenocortical scintigraphy can be used to evaluate whether an abnormality of the zona reticularis is responsible for the hormonal imbalance (Thrall JH, et al, 1978; Gross MD, et al, 1980). As with hyperaldosteronism, an excess of circulating androgens does not result in feedback inhibition of the release of ACTH by the pituitary. Hence, the adjunct administration of dexamethasone is required to accurately diagnose and differentiate bilateral hyperplasia or tumor involvement of the zona reticularis. With hyperandrogenism, the scintigraphic

patterns and interpretation criteria are the same as those described for hyperaldosteronism (Figures 11.15 and 11.16). If no scintigraphic abnormalities of the adrenals are observed, the aforementioned alternate sources of excess androgen should be considered.

ADRENAL HYPOFUNCTION

Hypofunctioning or nonfunctioning adrenal tissue will demonstrate minimal or no uptake of I-131 6β-iodomethyl-19-norcholesterol. The exogenous administration of ACTH combined with repeat adrenal scintigraphy can be used to differentiate hypofunctioning adrenocortical tissue from an absence or infarct of the adrenal (Thrall JH, et al, 1978). Distinct regions of nonfunctioning adrenal tissue (e. g., adrenal cyst) or adrenal medullary diseases (e. g., pheochromocytoma, hyperplasia) will frequently yield a scintigraphic pattern (Figure 11.17) of photopenic defects within the visualized adrenal

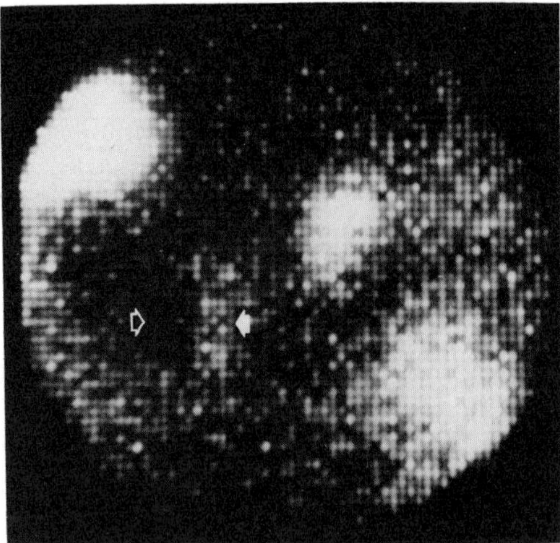

Figure 11.17 I-131 6β-iodomethyl-19-norcholesterol scintigraphy on a patient with a pheochromocytoma. Note the diffuse appearance of the adrenal cortex (closed arrow) and the photopenic area (open arrow).

(Thrall JH, et al, 1978; Gross MD, et al, 1980).

DOSAGE/DOSIMETRY

Dosage. The recommended dosage of NP-59 for adrenocortical scintigraphy is 1-2 mCi/1.7 m^2 (Thrall JH, et al, 1978; Gross MD, et al, 1980). This dosage should be administered slowly (i. e., over 1–2 minutes) by the intravenous route (Product Information, NP-59, Nuclear Pharmacy, University of Michigan, Ann Arbor).

Table 11.9 ESTIMATED RADIATION DOSIMETRY FOR I-131 6β-IODOMETHYL-19-NORCHOLESTEROL[a]

ORGAN	RADS/mCi
Adrenals	26[b]
Thyroid (unblocked)	42–161[c]
Liver	0.6–2.1[c]
Kidneys	1.3–2.1[c]
Spleen	2.0–2.5[c]
Ovaries	8.0[b]
Testes	2.3[b]
Total body	1.2[b]

[a] (Adapted from Ice et al, 1976; Carey et al, 1979; Brookeman, 1978.)
[b] Based on human distribution data.
[c] Based on rat distribution data extrapolated to humans.

Adrenocortical imaging is normally delayed until 2 days post radiopharmaceutical administration to permit adequate clearance of liver background activity. The patient is then imaged daily for another 3–5 days or until sufficient information is obtained to make an accurate diagnosis (Thrall JH et al, 1978; Gross MD, et al, 1980).

Dosimetry. Radiation-absorbed dose estimates for I-131 6β-iodomethyl-19-norcholesterol are summarized in Table 11.9.

IV. Adrenomedullary Imaging

Neil A. Petry
Brahm Shapiro

INTRODUCTION/HISTORY

The adrenal gland consists of two embryologically and functionally distinct regions, the cortex and the medulla. The first scintigraphic images of human adrenal cortex were obtained in 1970 utilizing I-131 19-iodocholesterol, an adrenocortical imaging agent (see Adrenocortical Imaging); however, the introduction of I-131 meta-iodobenzylguanidine (MIBG) as an adrenomedullary imaging radiopharmaceutical was delayed by a decade. The development of I-131 MIBG has been previously described by several authors (Wieland and Beierwaltes, 1981a; Gross MO, et al, 1982; 1984; McEwan AJ, et al, 1985). A review of these works reveals that research efforts have focused on the synthesis of radiolabeled catecholamines, enzyme inhibitors, and neuronal blocking agents.

Initial efforts to develop adrenomedullary imaging agents were based upon the central role of the adrenal medulla in the synthesis and storage of catecholamines. In 1967, J.O. Morales and co-workers reported the results of C-14-labeled catecholamine adrenomedullary uptake studies in the dog. Study results demonstrated that of the labeled catecholamines investigated, C-14 dopamine provided the highest tissue–plasma ratio. In 1969, L.M. Lieberman and co-workers demonstrated that C-14 dopamine concentrated selectively in human neuroblastoma and that uptake was considerably greater than that found in the normal adrenal medulla. Four years later, labeled dopamine was shown to concentrate in human pheochromocytoma (Fowler JS, et al, 1973; Anderson BC, et al, 1973). During 1975 and 1976 developmental efforts focused on the synthesis of 6-iodopamine labeled with I-131 or I-123. The adrenomedullary uptake of labeled 6-iododopamine was found to be similar to that of C-14 dopamine; however, uptake was inadequate for satisfactory imaging (Fowler JS, et al, 1976; Ice RD, et al, 1975).

An alternative approach to the direct radioiodination of the catechol ring (Larsen AA, et al, 1967) led to an evaluation of radiolabeled sulfanilide analogues of dopamine (Ice RD, et al, 1975). Uptake studies demonstrated that only one of these analogues exhibited adrenomedullary localization similar to that of C-14 dopamine, thus indicating that these sulfanilide analogues would prove inadequate for adrenomedullary imaging. Alternative catecholamine analogues bearing a substituted sulfonyl or sulfonalkyl group in the meta position have been suggested (Uloth RH, et al, 1966; Kaiser C, et al, 1975). These catecholamine analogues do not act as substrates for catechol-O-methyltransferase (COMT), and their enhanced metabolic stability suggested that peak adrenal uptake may occur at longer time intervals than those observed with labeled catecholamines. Some of these analogues may be susceptible to radiolabeling with gamma-emitting radionuclides; however, these compounds have not been adequately evaluated as potential radiopharmaceuticals for adrenal medulla or neuroendocrine tumor imaging.

Successful adrenocortical imaging with radiolabeled enzyme inhibitors of adrenocortical enzymes (Beierwaltes WH, et al, 1979) identified a second potential approach to the development of adrenomedullary radiopharmaceuticals. Efforts to utilize this approach focused on two of the four well-characterized enzymes responsible for the biotransformation of tyrosine to epinephrine. Tyrosine hydroxylase, the rate-limiting enzyme for catecholamine synthesis, was initially targeted, as it is present in high concentration in adrenal medulla. A radioiodinated analogue of the tyrosine hydroxylase inhibitor alpha-methyl-paratyrosine, I-125 3-iodo-alpha-methyltyrosine, demonstrated no adrenal uptake presumably due to rapid invivo deiodination (Beierwaltes WH et al, 1978). The adrenal uptake of 26 radioiodinated tyrosine derivatives were investigated and a number were found to concentrate selectively in the mouse adrenal (Kloss and Leven, 1979). However, most of these agents did not concentrate significantly in the canine adrenal medulla, which has proven to be the animal model of greatest predictive value in the evaluation of potential adrenomedullary imaging agents. Subsequently, phenylethanolamine-n-methyl transferase (PNMT) was targeted, as it is found almost exclusively within the adrenal medulla with small amounts in the brain. R. G. Pendleton and co-workers (1979) identified 7,8-dichloro-1,2,3,4-tetrahydroisoquinoline hydrochloride (SKF-64139) as a potentially useful, selective inhibitor of PNMT. T. Yu and associates (1979) subsequently reported that SKF-64139 and other tetrahydroisoquinoline analogues were capable of being radioiodinated and therefore may be of interest as potential imaging agents. Specific adrenal gland uptake was demonstrated with four of the radiolabeled tetrahydroisoquinoline analogues studied; however, low absolute uptake and rapid washout was observed (Yu T, et al, 1979).

A conceptual breakthrough in the development of adrenomedullary imaging agents occurred when research efforts turned to the investigation of a class of antihypertensive drugs called adrenergic neuron blocking agents. In 1977, N. Korn and co-workers reported the first evaluation of radiolabeled neuronal blocking agents, radioiodinated bretylium analogues (RIBA, Figure 11.18), which showed selective concentration invivo in

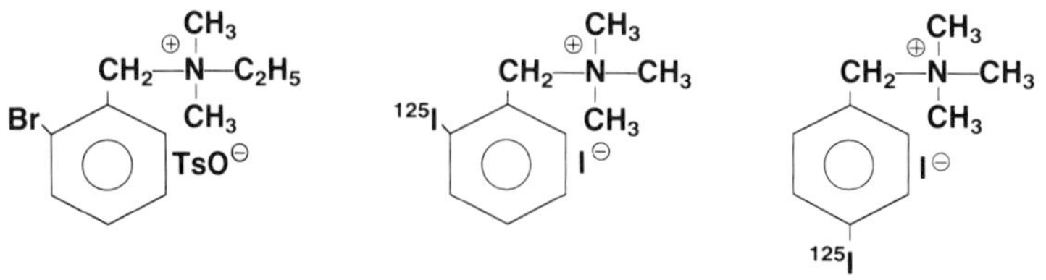

Figure 11.18 Modifications of the chemical structure of bretylium tosylate (I) result in I-125 ortho-RIBA and I-125 para-RIBA (III). (From Korn, et al, 1977, with permission.)

the canine adrenal medulla. Biodistribution studies in the dog showed that the ortho isomer localized in myocardium and that the para isomer concentrated maximally in the adrenal medulla. In 1979, D. M. Wieland and associates confirmed that these radiolabeled bretylium analogues concentrated in canine adrenal medulla. However, they observed that the ortho isomer (Figure 11.19) of the ethylhydroxy derivative gave maximal organ concentration and kinetics, which enabled the canine adrenal medulla to be visualized 3 and 4 days after intravenous injection (Wieland DM, et al, 1979). A clinical trial with this I-131 labeled bretylium analogue was undertaken in three patients with suspected pheochromocytoma; however, the agent failed to provide useful images of the adrenal medulla (Beierwaltes WH, et al, 1978). In retrospect, none of the studied patients in fact had pheochromocytomas, so although it failed to visualize the normal adrenal medulla, it is an open question whether this radiopharmaceutical may in fact visualize pheochromocytomas. Subsequent efforts focused on the examination of the adrenergic neuronal blocking agent guanethi-

dine, which is believed to have pharmacologic properties similar to bretylium.

Guanethidine is a potent neuron blocking agent that depletes peripheral tissues of their catecholamine stores by direct action on adrenergic nerves (Chang CC, et al, 1967; Giachetti and Hollenbeck, 1976). This drug is not readily iodinated; however, the combination of the benzyl portion of bretylium (Figure 11.18) with the guanidine group of guanethidine (Figure 11.20) yields a series of aromatic arakylguanidines (Figure 11.20) that are well suited for radioiodination. Many of these aromatic aralkylguanidines have also been shown to be potent neuronal blocking agents (Short and Darby, 1967). During 1979 and 1980, Wieland and associates reported (Wieland DM, et al, 1979; 1980; Wu JL, et al, 1979) the radioiodination (I-125) and avid concentration of the ortho, para, and meta isomers of iodobenzylguanidine in the canine adrenal medulla. Scintigraphic visualization of the canine adrenal medulla was demonstrated with I-131 labeled para-iodobenzylguanidine (PIBG) and metaiodobenzylguanidine (MIBG). The I-131 PIBG permitted adrenomedullary visualization 72

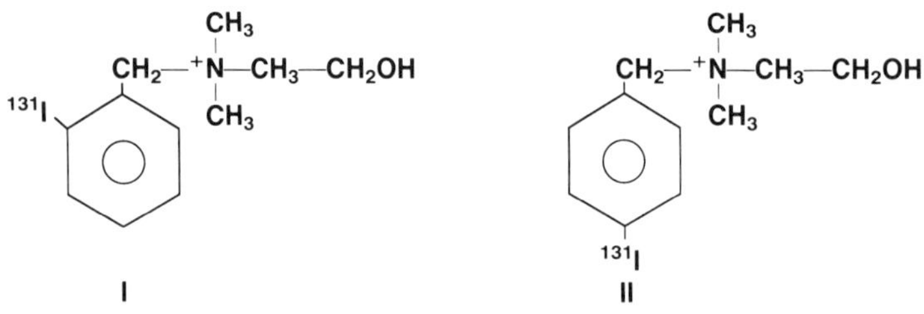

Figure 11.19 Ortho (I) and para (II) isomers of I-131 iodobenzyldimethyl-2-hydroxyethyl ammonium.

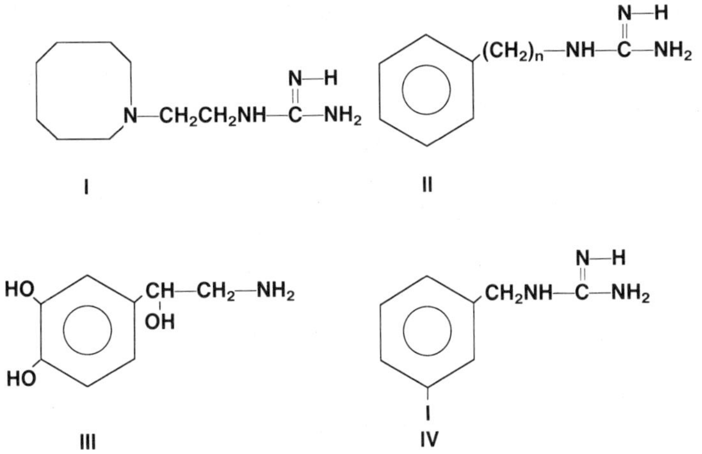

Figure 11.20 Chemical structures of gaunethidine (I), aralkylguanidines (II), norepinephrine (III), and meta-iodobenzylguanidine (IV).

hours post injection; however, better visualization with the I-131 MIBG was achieved at 24 and 48 hours due to lower background activity and tenfold less in-vivo deiodination (Wieland DM, et al, 1980; Wieland and Beierwaltes, 1981a). Significant heart uptake, reflecting the rich sympathetic innervation of the organ, was observed for all three isomers. This observation provided the impetus to evaluate I-123 MIBG as a potential myocardial agent (Wieland DM, et al, 1981b; 1981c; Kline RC, et al, 1981).

In 1981, Wieland and co-workers (1981c) reported the first successful scintigraphic imaging of primate adrenal medulla utilizing I-123 and I-131 labeled iodobenzylguanidine. The imaging superiority of MIBG over PIBG was again documented in the monkey. Liver uptake was lower, and thyroid uptake was significantly reduced for the MIBG, implying that it was more stable invivo with consequently reduced free iodine concentrations. In the same year, J. C. Sisson and co-workers (1981) reported the scintigraphic localization of human pheochromocytomas utilizing I-131 MIBG. This study of eight patients with known tumors demonstrated that a broad spectrum of pheochromocytomas could be localized with high sensitivity; however, normal adrenal medulla was not visualized with I-131 MIBG. When a larger series of patients was examined, M. Nakajo and associates (1983a) demonstrated that the normal adrenal medulla was in fact visualized in a minority of patients ($< 20\%$). Subsequently, M. D. Lynn and associates (1984; 1985) demonstrated that the normal adrenal medulla could be regularly visualized and pheochromocytomas could be better visualized with I-123 MIBG primarily due to the superior physical characteristics of the I-123 label.

In 1985, B. Shapiro and co-workers reported an overall sensitivity of 87.4%, and an overall specificity was 98.9% in the first 400 patients (441 studies) investigated for suspected pheochromocytoma. This experience led the authors to conclude that I-131 MIBG scintigraphy is a safe, noninvasive, and efficacious technique for localization of pheochromocytoma. In the same year, J. C. Sisson and associates (1984a; 1984b) reported the results of treating pheochromocytoma with therapeutic I-131 MIBG. Currently, clinical trials to evaluate the efficacy of this agent in the diagnosis and treatment of other neuroendocrine tumors are in progress.

CHEMISTRY

I-131 Meta-Iodobenzylguanidine sulfate (I-131 MIBG) is a radioiodinated aralkylguanidine that is a physiological analogue of norepinephrine and of guanethidine (Figure 11.20). This diagnostic radioactive agent was first synthesized by D. M. Wieland and associates (1980) utilizing heat exchange radioiodination of m-iodobenzylguanidine sulfate with sodium iodide I-131. The m-iodobenzylguanidine sulfate occurs as colorless crystals that are soluble in water and sparingly soluble in ethanol. The I-131 radiolabel decays by beta (negatron) particle emission to Xenon-131 (stable) with a physical half-life of 8.06 days. External imaging is performed utilizing the 364 keV gamma radiation (81.2% abundant) that accompanies this decay process. The I-123 radiolabel decays by electron capture to Tellurium-123 (half-life 1×10^3 years) with a physical half-life of 13.1 hours. The 159 keV gamma radiation (83.4% abundant) that accompanies this decay process is utilized for external imaging.

The current supplier of I-131 MIBG (Nuclear Pharmacy, University of Michigan, Ann Arbor) prepares this agent as described by T. J. Mangner and co-workers (1983). It is packaged in multiple dose vials as a sterile, nonpyrogenic, aqueous solution for intravenous injection with a radiochemical purity of greater than 90%, a radionuclidic purity of greater than 99% and a specific activity of 2.9–3.6 mCi/mg (0.94–1.17 Ci/mmol) at the time of calibration. At calibration time each milliliter of the solution contains 2.0–2.4 mCi of I-131 MIBG; 0.67–0.70 mg of m-iodobenzylguanidine sulfate; 0.53 ml of 0.0135 M sodium acetate buffer (containing 0.22 mg sodium acetate and 0.27 mg of glacial acetic acid); 0.47 ml Bacteriostatic Sodium Chloride Injection, 0.9%, U.S.P., and 0.01 ml benzyl alcohol. Benzyl alcohol is utilized in this radiopharmaceutical preparation as a free radical scavenger to protect against autoradiolysis. The I-131 MIBG for injection is a clear, colorless solution with a pH of 4.5–7.0. It has an expiration date (shelf-life) of 8 days following the date of calibration. Strongly yellow preparations of radiolabeled MIBG indicate the liberation of free iodine/radioiodine and should be discarded.

The I-131 MIBG for injection is very stable to the invitro liberation of free radioiodine. Stability studies indicate that diagnostic I-131 MIBG is optimally stored at freezer temperature ($^-$20–$^-$10°C); however, refrigerator temperature (2–8°C) may also be utilzied with caution. At expiration, vials stored at freezer temperature will typically show 2% or less free radioiodine from invitro deiodination whereas those stored at refrigerator temperature will typically show 10% or less free radioiodine. Storage at controlled room temperature (15–30°C) is not recommended, as greater than 10% free radioiodine is typically observed at expiration under these storage conditions. The product is shipped at ambient temperature, consequently investigators are advised to incorporate a chromatographic test of radiochemical purity prior to patient administration.

PHARMACOKINETICS

Biodistribution. The normal and abnormal invivo distribution of I-131 MIBG in man, as revealed by scintigraphic imaging techniques, was first described in detail by Nakajo and co-workers (1983a). Following intravenous injection, the normal distribution of I-131 MIBG includes uptake in the salivary glands, liver, spleen, and urinary bladder, organs which are clearly portrayed in all cases with scintigraphy (Figure 11.21). The heart is scintigraphically demonstrated in patients with normal catecholamine levels but not in those patients with elevated catecholamines (Nakajo M, et al, 1983b). The mechanism associated with this observation remains obscure but may involve competition between MIBG and catecholamines for cellular uptake or a down-regulation of such uptake. The middle and lower lung zones and colon are less frequently or less clearly seen whereas the upper lung zones and kidneys are rarely seen. The normal adrenal glands are visualized with I-131 MIBG in 2% of injected patients at 24 hours post injection and 16% at 48 hours; however, the organs are seen in almost all cases when studied with I-123 MIBG

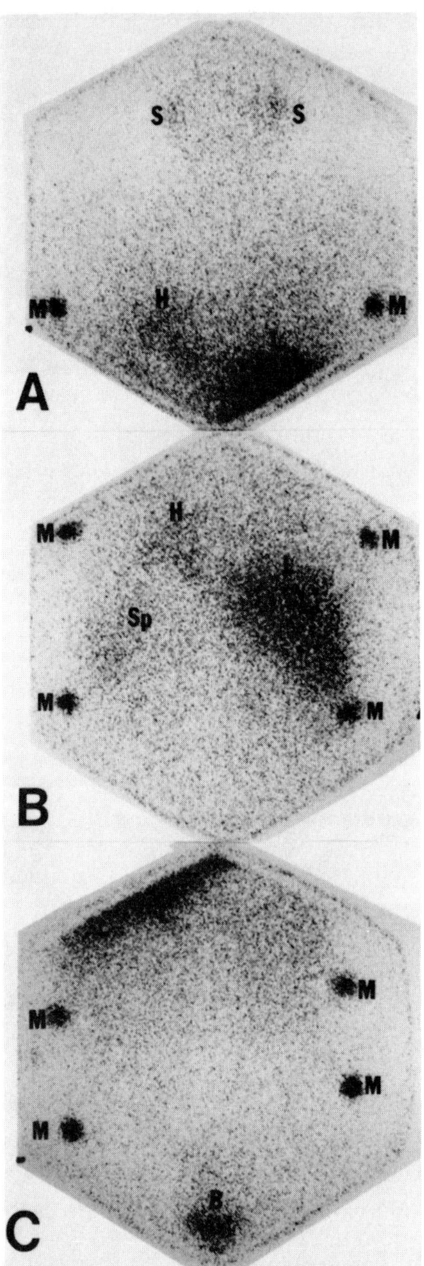

Figure 11.21 Overlapping I-131 MIBG images obtained in a normal patient at 48 hours after injection. A. Posterior head and chest; B. posterior mid-abdomen; and C. anterior lower abdomen. Note accumulation of I-131 MIBG in the salivary glands (S), heart (H), Liver (L), spleen (SP), and urinary bladder (B). Radioactive markers (M). (From Nakajo, et al, 1983a; with permission.)

(Nakajo M, et al, 1983a; Lynn MD, et al, 1984; 1985). The adrenal medulla is also frequently visualized following large ther-apeutic doses of I-131 MIBG. Adrenal medulla visualization is probably a function of the small size of the organs and their depth, which when combined with the limited photon flux from a tracer dose of I-131 MIBG makes them seldom visible. The accumulation of I-131 MIBG at sites other than those described above must be considered abnormal and may indicate the presence of pheochromo-cytoma (Figures 11.22 and 11.23), especially if intense uptake is observed in the region of the adrenals. The 159 keV gamma and high photon flux associated with I-123 MIBG permits a more precise scintigraphic portrayal of the normal and abnormal distributions of MIBG (Figure 11.24) and provides greater sensitivity in the detection and localization of pheo-chromocytomas (Lynn MD, et al, 1984; 1985). Unfortunately, the relatively short half-life, limited availability, and cost of I-123 have limited the utilization of I-123 MIBG.

Excretion and Metabolism. The excre-tion and metabolism of I-131 MIBG in nine patients with metastic pheochro-mocytoma, given both diagnostic and therapeutic doses, has been studied in de-tail by Mangner and co-workers (1986). In the patient population studied, 40–55% of the injected radioactivity from diagnos-tic doses appeared in the urine within 24 hours and 70–90% was recovered within 4 days. Fecal excretion was not determined, as a previous unpublished study of a sepa-rate patient population indicated that less than 1% of the injected diagnostic dose was found in fecal collections obtained over 4 days post I-131 MIBG injection. In other studies, fecal excretion ranged from 1–4% of the administered dose, whereas only minute amounts of radioactivity were detected in the saliva, sweat, and exhaled breath (Nakajo M, et al, 1983a; 1984; Sipila LN, et al, 1985). Fecal excretion of radioactivity results in occasional ($\cong 20\%$) visualization of the colon, espe-cially in the descending colon. If there is doubt as to the location of probable co-lonic activity, imaging should be repeated after laxatives and/or enemas.

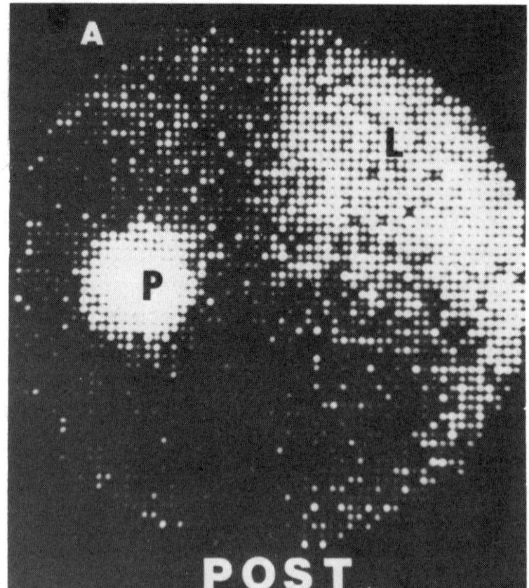

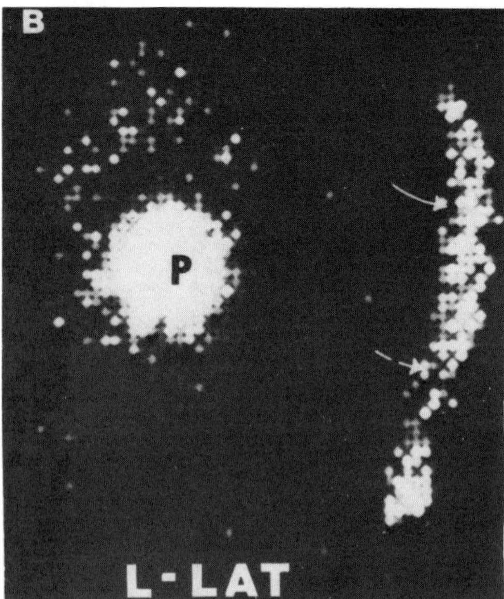

Figure 11.22   Scintigrams obtained at 24 hours after the injection of I-131 MIBG in a patient with a 24-gram tumor involving the left adrenal. The pheochromocytoma (P) is readily identified in both the posterior (A) and left lateral (B) images. The liver (L) is also seen in the posterior view (A). The arrows on left lateral image (B) point to a radioactive marker positioned on the patient's back. (From Sisson, et al, 1981; with permission.)

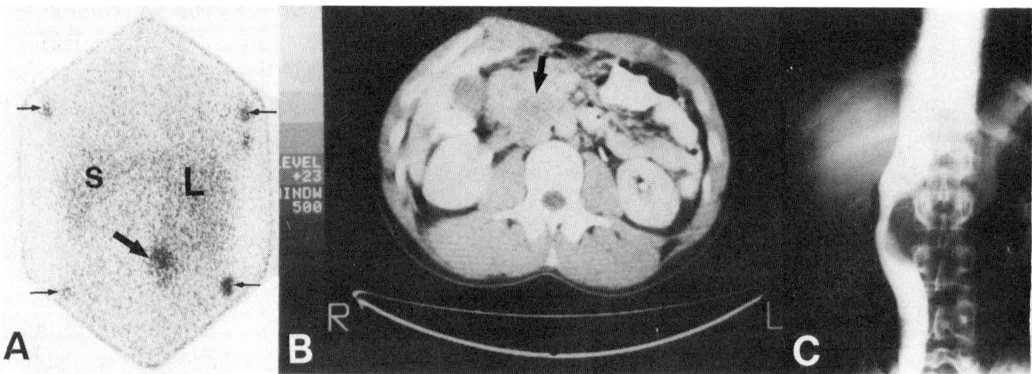

Figure 11.23   A. Anterior abdominal scintigram obtained following the administration of I-131 MIBG shows (large arrow) a right, para-renal (extra-adrenal) pheochromocytoma and normal uptake in the liver (L) and spleen (S). Small arrows designate surface markers. B. Abdominal computed tomography shows (arrow) the tumor arising from the right renal hilar region. C. Inferior venacavogram reveals indentation of the inferior vena cava at the level of the kidney. (From Glowniak, et al, 1985; with permission.)

The rate of urinary excretion was similar in six of nine patients and closely paralleled that reported for normal volunteers (Mangner TJ, et al, 1986; Swanson DP, et al, 1981), indicating that the presence of tumors that concentrate the agent have little effect on the rate, amount or route of elimination. Three patients with moderately elevated blood urea nitrogen and serum creatinine levels were observed to have lower urinary excretion rates. This observation was attributed to differences in kidney function as lower rates of urinary excretion were observed

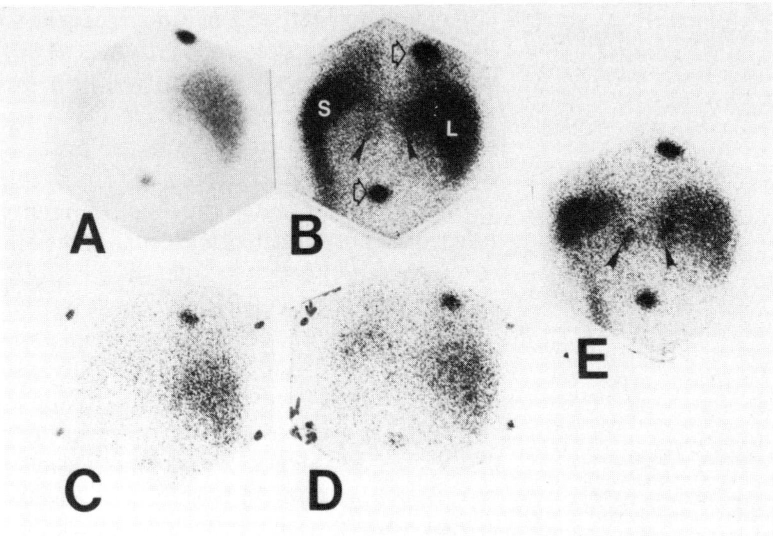

Figure 11.24 Posterior abdominal scintigrams obtained on a patient with malignant, metastatic pheochromocytoma: A. 10 mCi I-123 MIBG imaged at 24 hours post injection (484 K counts, 3.5 min.); B. 10 mCi I-131 MIBG imaged at 48 hours post injection (404 K counts, 15 min.); C. 0.5 mCi I-131 MIBG imaged at 48 hours post injection (100 K counts, 12 min.); D. 0.5 mCi I-131 MIBG imaged at 48 hours post injection (100 K counts, 20 min.); E. 179 mCi I-131 MIBG imaged at 6 days post injection (200 K counts, 1.5 min.). Arrowheads indicate adrenal glands, open arrows indicate metastatic lesions. L = liver, S = spleen. (From Lynn, et al, 1984; with permission.)

on repeat studies, and there were no significant differences in agent specific activity or the dosage of radioactivity administered. Subsequent studies of these patients following therapeutic doses of I-131 MIBG indicated that urinary excretion rates were similar to those observed with diagnostic doses. This indicates that the kinetics of elimination are relatively constant with loading doses of I-131 MIBG ranging from approximately 0.15 mg (typical diagnostic dose) to approximately 5 mg (typical therapeutic dose) and relatively independent of activity and specific activity of the administered dose (Mangner TJ, et al, 1986).

The chemical structure of I-131 MIBG is similar to that of the endogenous catecholamine norephinephrine (Figure 11.20); however, it is not a catecholamine and thus would not be expected to be a substrate for monoamine oxidase (Kuntzman and Jacobson, 1963) or catechol-O-

methyltransferase (Brochardt RT, 1980). The agent is also structurally similar to guanidines such as the antihypertensive drugs bethanidine, guanoxan, and debrisoquin, which are metabolized to varying degrees in man with the major metabolite generally being a ring-hydroxylated product (Turnbull LB, et al, 1976; Jack DB, et al, 1971; Allen JG, et al, 1975; Maxwell and Wastila, 1977). Metabolic studies in the canine model indicate that I-131 MIBG is not extensively deiodinated (Wieland DM, et al, 1980). In 1983, M. Inbasekaran and co-workers showed that a polar derivative of MIBG, 4-hydroxy-3-iodobenzylguanidine (HIBG), accumulated in the dog adrenal medulla. This observation suggested that a minor metabolite of I-131 MIBG might contribute to or be responsible for the accumulation of activity in the adrenal medulla, thus prompting Mangner and co-workers to undertake a detailed study of the invivo

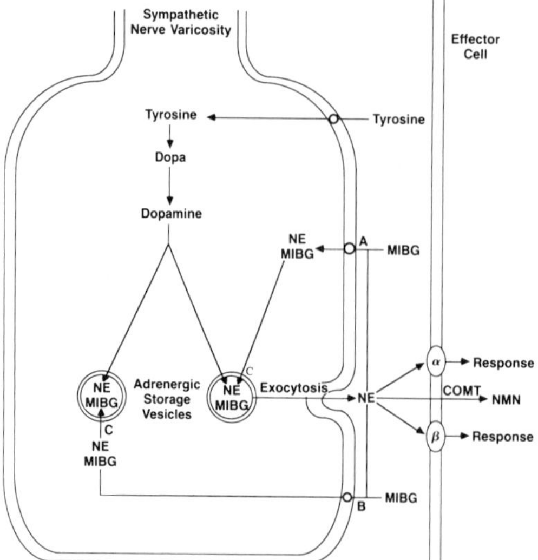

Figure 11.25 Proposed mechanism and site of localization of meta-iodobenzyl-guanidine in adrenergic neuronal tissues. A. Type I, sodium-dependent uptake; B. Type II, sodium-independent uptake; C. Vesicle uptake and storage.

metabolism of I-131 MIBG (Mangner TJ et al, 1983). In this study reverse-phase high-performance liquid chromatography was utilized detecting six radioactive metabolites of I-131 MIBG. However, study results indicated that I-131 MIBG is not metabolized appreciably, and is excreted by the kidneys primarily as the unaltered parent compound.

Mechanism of Localization. A model of a sympathetic neuroeffector junction (Figure 11.25) can be utilized to describe the proposed mechanisms associated with the invivo localization of radiolabeled MIBG in adrenergic tissues and neuroendocrine tumors. The radiopharmaceutical is a physiological analogue of the endogenous neurotransmitter-hormone norepinephrine (NE) which is the transmitter of most sympathetic postganglionic fibers and of certain tracts of the central nervous system. Norepinephrine is synthesized de novo from the amino acid tyrosine, which is actively transported into the axoplasm of adrenergic neurons and adrenal medullary cells. Tyrosine is then

converted to DOPA and subsequently to dopamine by cytoplasmic enzymes. Ultimately, dopamine is transported into the vesicles of the varicosity where it is converted to NE and stored. Via the process of exocytosis, NE is released from the storage vesicles into the neuroeffector junction where it activates alpha and beta receptors in the membrane of the postsynaptic effector cell. Released NE that does not bind to receptors is rapidly inactivated by catechol-O-methyltransferase (COMT) or monoamine oxidase (MAO). However, the active re-uptake of the NE into nerve and storage vesicles represents the most important mechanism for the termination of the physiologic action of this neurotransmitter. Current evidence indicates that this active re-uptake mechanism is involved in the accumulation of MIBG in both normal and tumorous adrenergic tissues.

The specific localization mechanisms associated with I-131 MIBG uptake have been studied utilizing a variety of models, most important of them the normal adrenal medulla of intact animals (Wieland DM, et al, 1981c; VonMoll L, et al, 1987; Shapiro B, et al, 1984a). Animal studies of the pharmacologic effects of reserpine, desmethylimipramine, cocaine, insulin hypoglycemia, and 6-hydroxydopamine on invivo I-131 MIBG distribution strongly suggest that this radiopharmaceutical enters adrenergic tissue and is stored in the granules of the adrenal medulla by mechanisms very similar to those described above for the re-uptake of NE (Jacques S, et al, 1984).

Invitro localization studies in primary cultures of bovine adrenomedullary cells have contributed additional knowledge. S. Jacques, Jr., and co-workers (1984) observed the uptake of NE and MIBG to be affected by two uptake systems as characterized by their respective sodium-dependency, ouabain sensitivity and energy dependency. The Type I sodium-dependent uptake system, which is specific for catecholamines, was characterized to be ouabain sensitive, energy and temperature dependent, of high affinity-low capacity, and saturable. Type I uptake has been shown to predominate at the less than 1 μ molar I-131 MIBG concentrations typically achieved in patients following the intravenous administration of diagnostic doses (VonMoll L, et al, 1987; Jaques S, et al, 1984; Tobes MC, et al, 1985). The sodium-independent uptake system, designated Type II uptake, is diffusional in nature and is characterized to be ouabain insensitive, energy independent, temperature dependent, and non-saturable out to 5 μ molar. Type II uptake has been found to predominate at higher concentrations of MIBG (VonMoll L, et al, 1987; Jaques S, et al, 1984; Tobes MC, et al, 1985). The results of these invitro experiments suggest that both the sodium-dependent (Type I) uptake and the sodium-independent (Type II) uptake systems are important for I-131 MIBG and I-123 MIBG scintigraphy of the adrenal medulla and its tumors. Once within the cytoplasm, MIBG and catecholamines are concentrated into the adrenergic storage vesicles by another energy-dependent system similar to, but distinct from, the Type I-uptake mechanism.

PRECAUTIONS

Adverse Reactions. In the limited clinical experience, to date, adverse reactions to diagnostic dosages of I-131 MIBG have been extremely rare. However, as with any drug, the possibility of an adverse reaction or side effect in certain individuals cannot be completely discounted.

Following therapeutic I-131 MIBG significant but reversible falls in white blood cell and platelet counts have been observed. This myelosuppression may last for 6–8 weeks or longer and appears to be related to the whole-body radiation dose (Sisson JC, et al, 1987). Hypothyroidism has been observed in one patient following four treatments ($\cong$ 200 mCi) with I-131 MIBG. No incidence of significant hepatic, renal, or sympathetic nervous system dysfunction has been observed following therapy with this radiopharmaceutical.

Pregnancy/Breastfeeding. Ideally, examinations using I-131 labeled radiopharmaceuticals in women of childbearing potential should be performed during the first 10 days following the onset of menses and/or appropriate testing performed to rule out pregnancy. It is not known if I-131 MIBG can cause fetal harm if administered to pregnant women; therefore, this radiopharmaceutical should be used in pregnancy only if the potential benefits to be gained clearly outweigh the potential risk. Under such circumstances, consideration should be given to the use of I-123 MIBG rather than the I-131 labeled material.

Radioiodinated MIBG may undergo both invitro and invivo degradation resulting in the liberation of free radioiodine. Free radioiodine is excreted in human breast milk during lactation; thus breastfeeding is generally contraindicated for an appropriate period of time as best determined by assaying the specific concentration of the collected breastmilk.

Drug–Radiopharmaceutical Interactions. Drug-MIBG interactions have been documented in rats, mice, and dogs (Wieland DM, et al, 1981c; Shapiro B, et al, 1984a; Sherman DS, et al, 1985; Guilloteau D, et al, 1984; Wieland DM, et al, 1981d), and in case reports (Shapiro B, et al, 1984a) and clinical studies in man (Sisson, JC, et al, 1981). These interactions may be of clinical significance in that scintigraphy may be adversely affected by the presence of drugs that inhibit uptake of the radiotracer in adrenergic tumors. Patients receiving these interfering drugs are typically excluded from the examination; thus, additional studies are necessary to determine the true significance of potential interactions. Tables 11.10–11.15 list several drugs known to inhibit the reuptake of norepinephrine into presynaptic adrenergic neurons and may therefore inhibit the localization of I-131 MIBG in neuroendocrine tumors. These lists of medications include a variety of tricyclic antidepressants (Table 11.10) that should not be taken for 6 weeks prior to the

Table 11.10 POTENTIAL DRUG-MIBG INTERACTION: TRICYCLIC ANTIDEPRESSANTS AND RELATED DRUGS (GENERIC NAMES)

Amitriptyline HCl
Amoxapine
Desipramine HCl
Doxepine HCl
Imipramine HCl, pamoate
Maprotaline HCl
Nortriptyline HCl
Protriptyline HCl
Trimipramine maleate
Trazodone HCl

Table 11.11 POTENTIAL DRUG-MIBG INTERACTION: PHENOTHIAZINE DERIVATIVES (GENERIC NAMES)

Acetophenazine maleate
Chlorpromazine HCl
Fluphenazine decanoate, enanthate, HCl
Mesoridazine besylate
Perphenazine
Prochlorperazine
Prochlorperazine edisylate, maleate
Promazine HCl
Thioridazine HCl
Trifluoperazine HCl
Triflupromazine HCl

Table 11.12 POTENTIAL DRUG-MIBG INTERACTION: AMPHETAMINES (GENERIC NAMES)

Amphetamine sulfate
Benzphetamine HCl
Dextroamphetamine sulfate
Diethylpropion HCl
Flenfluramine HCl
Mazindol
Methamphetamine HCl
Methylphenidate HCl
Phendimetrazine tartrate
Phenmetrazine HCl
Phenteramine HCl

Table 11.13 POTENTIAL DRUG-MIBG INTERACTION: "OVER-THE-COUNTER" NASAL DECONGESTANTS AND SYMPATHOMIMETICS

GENERIC DRUG	COMMON BRAND NAMES®
Pseudo-ephedrine HCl	Halofed, Sudafed, Sudrin, Cenafed, Neofed, Dorcol Pediatric Formula, Neo-Synephrinol Day Relief, Decofed Syrup, Novafed, Peedee Dose Decongestant
Pseudo-ephedrine Sulfate	Afrinal Repetabs
Phenylpropanolamine HCl	Propagest, Sucrets Cold Decongestant Formula, Rhinedecon
Phenylephrine HCl	Neo-Synephrine, Alconefrin, Rhinall, Allerest Nasal, Doktros Nose Drops, Nostril, Coricidin Nasal Mist, Sinex, Sinophen, Sinarest Nasal, Duration Mild

Table 11.14 POTENTIAL DRUG-MIBG INTERACTION: "OVER-THE-COUNTER" DIET-CONTROL AGENTS

Phenylpropanolamine HCl	Diadex, Resolution II Half-Strength, Prolamine, Control, Dex-A-Diet, Dexatrim, Unitrol, Acutrim, Appedrine, Grapefruit Diet Plan with Diadex

Table 11.15 POTENTIAL DRUG-MIBG INTERACTIONS: OTHER DRUG CATEGORIES

GENERIC DRUG	COMMON BRAND NAMES®
Labetalol HCl	Normodyne, Trandate
Bretylium tosylate	Bretylol
Guanethidine monosulfate	Ismelin
Reserpine	Serpasil, Sandril
Haloperidol lactate	Haldol
Thiothixene HCl	Navane

administration of MIBG. Medications such as phenothiazines (Table 11.11), amphetamines (Table 11.12), nasal decongestants containing sympathomimetics (Table 11.13), "diet-control" pills (Table 11.14), and other categories of drugs (Table 11.15) should not be taken for at least 2 weeks prior to radiopharmaceutical administration.

CLINICAL CONSIDERATIONS

Clinical Considerations. Diagnostic I-131 MIBG is an investigational radiopharmaceutical currently undergoing clinical evaluation as a diagnostic adjunct in patients with pheochromocytoma, a typically benign tumor originating from the adrenal medulla or sympathetic paraganglia. The incidence of pheochromocytoma in the adult population has been reported as being between 0.01% and 0.001% (McEwan AJ, et al, 1985). The incidence of the tumor is approximately 0.1% in patients with hypertension (Mayer and Gifford, 1982). It has been reported that 10% occur in children, 10% are malignant, 10% are extra-adrenal, 10% are

Table 11.16 COMPARISON OF RESULTS OF I-131 MIBG SCINTIGRAPHY FOR THE DIAGNOSIS OF SUSPECTED PHEOCHROMOCYTOMA

STUDY SITE	PATIENTS	SENSITIVITY (%)	SPECIFICITY (%)	−PDA[a] (%)	+PDA[b] (%)	REFERENCE
U. Michigan, U.S.A.	475	87	99	95	97	Shapiro, et al, 1985
U. Michigan, U.S.A. (Recent summary)	600	88	99	95	98	
Combined German	191	88	99	94	98	German, anonymous, 1983
Combined French[c]	99	91	96	95	92	Chatal and Carbonnel, 1985
Southampton, England	46	88	95	88	95	Ackery, et al, 1984
Mayo Clinic, U.S.A.	42	79	96	85	94	Swensen, et al, 1985
Tours, France	27	89	94	94	89	Baulieu, et al, 1984

[a] Negative predictive accuracy.
[b] Positive predictive accuracy.
[c] Equivocal negative added to true negative and equivocal positive added to true positive.

familial, and they are often associated with the Multiple Endocrine Neoplasia (MEN 2) Syndrome, von Hippel-Lindau disease, and neurofibromatosis (Schonebe, 1969). No convincing sex predominance has been reported, and the tumor is most common in the fourth and fifth decade of life (McEwan AJ, et al, 1985). Clinical trials with this agent have demonstrated that pheochromocytomas of all types, including sporadic adrenal and extra-adrenal lesions (Shapiro B, et al, 1985; 1984b), metastatic deposits (Shapiro B, et al, 1984c), familial pheochromocytomas (Valk TW, et al, 1981; Glowniak JV, et al, 1985), and medullary hyperplasia (Valk TW, et al, 1981) can be visualized with greater than 85% sensitivity and greater than 95% specificity (Table 11.16). I-131 MIBG is *not* a screening tool for pheochromocytoma or other tumors. However, it may be utilized as a diagnostic adjunct for the localization of possible tumors when the history, clinical examination, and biochemistry indicate a reasonable probability that such a tumor may be present and other radiological imaging procedures do not confirm tumor presence.

More recently, it has been demonstrated that I-131 MIBG can be used effectively to visualize neuroblastoma (Treuner J, et al, 1984; Geatti O, et al, 1985), a highly malignant tumor derived from the adrenergic nervous system, which is the fourth most common cause of death from cancer in children under age 15 years (Miller RW, 1969). The sensitivity and specificity for neuroblastoma (Table 11.17) appear to be similar to those observed in pheochromocytoma (Table 11.16), although the number of patients studied is smaller. The potential clinical utility of I-131 MIBG scintigraphy in

Table 11.17 COMPARISON OF RESULTS OF I-131 MIBG SCITIGRAPHY FOR THE DIAGNOSIS OF SUSPECTED NEUROBLASTOMA

STUDY SITE	PATIENTS	SENSITIVITY (%)	SPECIFICITY (%)	−PDA[b] (%)	+PDA[b] (%)	REFERENCE
U. Michigan, U.S.A.	10	90	—	—	100	Geatti, et al, 1985
U. Michigan, U.S.A. (Recent summary)	45	80	100	39	100	
Amsterdam, Holland	26	95	100	80	100	Hoefnagel, et al, 1985
Villejuif, France[c]	24	70	100	40	100	Lumbroso, et al, 1985
Philadelphia, U.S.A.	19[d]	57[e]	60[e]	60[e]	80[e]	Heyman and Evans, 1986
Copenhagen, Denmark	16	75	—	—	100	Munker, 1985
Tubingen, West Germany	5	100	100	100	100	Feine, et al, 1984

[a] Negative predictive accuracy.
[b] Positive predictive accuracy.
[c] Majority of studies performed using I-123 MIBG.
[d] Nineteen sites of disease in thirteen patients.
[e] In four cases, tumor was present but had matured to ganglioneuroma or ganglioneuroblastoma (i. e., four false negative studies).

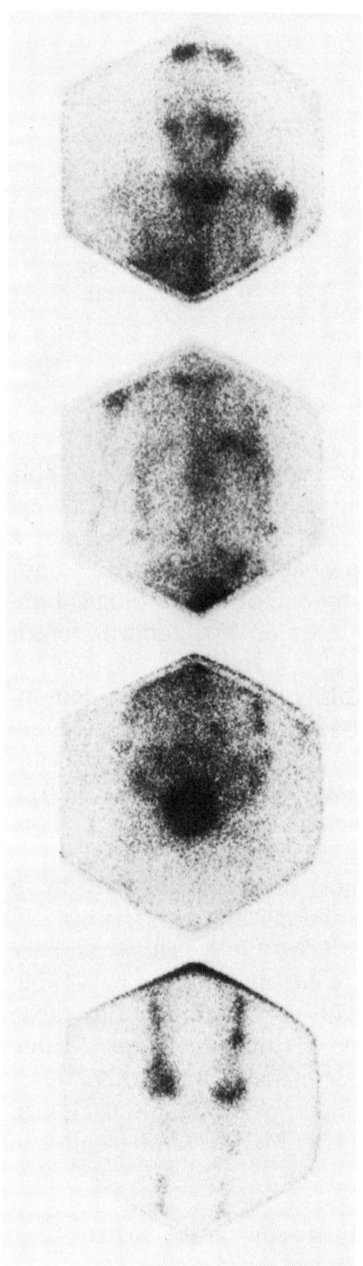

Figure 11.26 I-131 MIBG scintigraphy reveals extensive skeletal and bone marrow metastases in a patient with neuroblastoma. (From Geatti, et al, 1985; with permission.)

neuroblastoma is demonstrated in Figure 11.26. Neuroendocrine tumors derived from the amine precursor uptake and decarboxylation (APUD) system, including carcinoids (VonMoll L, et al, 1987; Fischer M, et al, 1984), medullary carcinoma of

the thyroid (Sone T, et al, 1985), and other tumors, have demonstrated an affinity for I-131 MIBG, thus making scintigraphic characterization of these tumors possible. The localization of I-131 MIBG in a primary pulmonary carcinoid is demonstrated in Figure 11.27. Diagnostic I-123 MIBG may also be utilized as an adjunct in the scintigraphic portrayal of neuroendocrine tumors.

The successful scintigraphic characterization of these tumors has led to the treatment of pheochromocytoma (Sisson JC, et al, 1984a; 1984b) neuroblastoma, (Fischer M, et al, 1983), and carcinoids (Hoefnagel CA, et al, 1986) with large doses of therapeutic I-131 MIBG. However, treatment experience is exremely limited, and further clinical trials are required to adequately assess the efficacy of therapeutic I-131 MIBG. Even though I-125 MIBG has been utilized primarily for biodistribution studies in animals and for invitro studies of cellular uptake mechanisms, there are theoretical reasons to believe that this agent may hold promise as a therapeutic agent (Shapiro and Gross, 1987). The physical decay of I-125 produces highly abundant low-energy Auger electrons that may be ideal for the delivery of therapeutic doses of radiation to isolated cells and cell clusters of neuroblastoma found in the bone marrow. The nonpenetrating nature of the Auger electrons would permit irradiation of the nucleus and organelles of tumor cells that specifically concentrate I-125 MIBG without the excessive irradiation of surrounding normal bone marrow elements. Even though there is reason to believe that this approach to therapy may offer advantages, there have been no reported treatments to date.

Patient Preparation.

Catecholamine Measurements. Biochemical studies of plasma and urinary catecholamines are performed in conjunction with imaging in patients suspected of having pheochromocytoma. Samples for the determination of plasma epinephrine and norepinephrine levels are obtained following an overnight fast and after the patient has been recumbent for at least

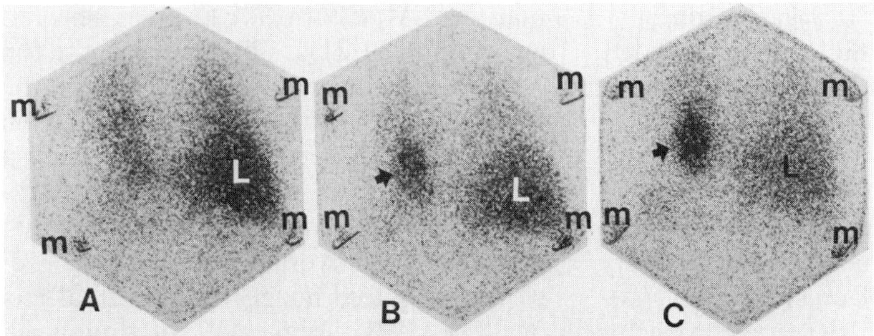

Figure 11.27 Posterior images of the chest obtained following the injection of 0.5 mCi of I-131 MIBG. Primary pulmonary carcinoid is not demonstrated at 24 hours post injection (A), but becomes increasingly obvious (arrows) on the 48 hour (B) and 72-hour (C) images. L = liver, M = surface markers. (Adapted from Von Moll, et al, 1987; with permission.)

one-half hour with an indwelling venous cannula in situ (Shapiro B, et al, 1985). The urinary excretion rates of catecholamines and catecholamine metabolites are typically determined on 12-hour, overnight urine samples. Attention should be paid to the host of potential dietary and pharmacologic interactions and interferences that may occur with the various assays for catecholamines and catecholamine metabolites (DeQuatro and Campase, 1979). Urinary catecholamines may be increased with severe physical or mental stress after myocardial infarction, after surgery, or after infusion of isoproterenol and epinephrine or norepinephrine. False-positive urinary catecholamines will also be observed during therapy with tetracycline drugs, quinine, dopa, and alpha-methyldopa. Food and beverages high in vanillin (e. g., bananas, coffee, nuts, and other fruits) may cause up to 10–15% false positives when testing for catecholamine metabolites such as vanillymandelic acid.

Thyroid Blockade. As in the use of any radioiodine-containing radiopharmaceutical, it is advantageous to suppress thyroidal uptake and encourage excretion of unbound radioiodide by pharmacologic intervention. Thyroidal uptake of radioiodide associated with the administration of I-131 MIBG can be suppressed by the oral administration of Lugol's solution or SSKI in a dose equivalent to 30–130 mg of potassium iodide per day given prior to radiopharmaceutical administration, and continued for at least 7 days following injection. The administration of potassium iodide also encourages excretion of radioiodide and thus decreases background activity and reduces the radiation dose to the patient. With proper thyroid blockade, Shapiro and co-workers (1985) found that thyroidal uptake

of free I-131 was seldom visible (<5% of cases) on the image obtained of the posterior head, neck, and upper thorax. Faint thyroid uptake could, however, be discerned in 70% in which an anterior neck view was obtained. Alternative blocking agents for those patients who are allergic to iodide include anions such as perchlorate or thiocyanate that act as competitive inhibitors of the thyroid gland's anion transport mechanism. (See also Appendix B.)

DOSAGE/DOSIMETRY

Currently diagnostic and therapeutic I-131 MIBG and to a lesser extent I-123 MIBG are commercially available for routine clinical use in many European countries and throughout the world from several radiopharmaceutical manufacturers. However, these radiopharmaceuticals have not been approved by the United States Food and Drug Administration (FDA) largely because New Drug Applications (NDA) have not been submitted by a commercial sponsor. Diagnostic I-131 MIBG, which has been identified as an orphan drug by the FDA, is currently available on a limited basis in the United States from the Nuclear Pharmacy, University of Michigan, Ann Arbor. It is made available only to those physician-sponsors who possess a FDA-approved Notice of Claimed Investigational Exemption for a New Drug (IND) and therefore is limited to investigational use only.

I-131 MIB (Diagnostic Dosage/Imaging.
The recommended adult dosage of I-131 MIBG injection for diagnostic imaging studies is 0.5 mCi/1.7 m^2 administered intravenously over a 15–30 second interval. Slow intravenous injection is desirable as MIBG is a norepinephrine analogue and thus there is a theoretical possibility that MIBG may displace endogenous norepinephrine from its storage vesicles and precipitate a hypertensive crisis. A 1 mCi dose may be considered for patients who have had surgery for pheochromocytoma, ganglioneuroma, or adrenal medullary hyperplasia where postoperative confirmation of adequacy of resection is required. Additionally, this higher dosage may also be considered when equivocal foci of abnormal uptake are seen or when recurrence of new tumor is suspected. For patients under 18 years of age, it is suggested that the dosage be adjusted on the basis of body weight according to the formula of Modell (Modell, 1958). The minimum diagnostic dose required for a clinically acceptable study is approximately 0.135 mCi. This minimum dosage is obtained utilizing Modell's formula and the assumption that patients will be 1 year of age or greater and have a minimum body weight of 10 Kg.

Patients who receive diagnostic I-131 MIBG are typically imaged at 24, 48, and 72 hours post injection utilizing a wide-field-of-view Anger camera with a high-energy parallel-hole collimator and computer. Twenty-four hour images are frequently positive in patients having pheochromocytomas even though background activity tends to be high. Imaging at 72 hours, when background activity is low, may prove useful especially in those cases where the 48-hour images are weakly positive or equivocal. Patients are imaged from the base of the skull to the urinary bladder utilizing multiple overlapping images. The anterior pelvis-lower abdominal image (Figure 11.21) is obtained with the emptied urinary bladder located near the bottom of the field and radioactive markers placed on the lateral iliac crests and lateral lower rib margins. A posterior head and chest image (Figure 11.21) is obtained with the top of the skull located near the top of the field with radioactive markers placed on the axillae. The posterior abdomen-chest image (Figure 11.21), with axillary markers, is then obtained in a manner that provides clear overlap with the two previously acquired images. If abnormal foci of I-131 MIBG uptake are noted they can be more accurately located with scintigraphic images of adjacent organs (e. g., kidneys with Tc-99m pentetate, liver with Tc-99m sulfur colloid, bone with Tc-99m medrenate, cardiac blood pool with Tc-99m labeled red blood cells, and myocardium using Tl-201 thallous chloride [Figure 11.28]). In malignant pheochromocytomas (Figure 11.29), a whole-body bone scan should be obtained, and all areas of abnormal bone uptake should be imaged during the I-131 MIBG imaging study.

Scintigrams obtained with radiolabeled MIBG should be interpreted in the light of the medical history, physical findings, laboratory studies, and all other available radiologic imaging procedures. Prior external radiation therapy, chemotherapy, and patient medications may cause decreased visualization or nonvisualization of tumors. Special attention should be given to observed plasma and urinary catecholamine and urinary catecholamine metabolite (i. e., normetanephrines and VMA) levels. I-131 MIBG directed computed tomography (CT) and magnetic resonance imaging (MRI) procedures have been utilized in selected patients and may prove useful in further confirming and/or defining the exact anatomical relationships of the disease (Francis, et al, 1983). All images should be checked carefully for foci of abnormal MIBG uptake as pheochromocytomas may be multiple and/or metastatic in nature.

I-123 MIBG (Diagnostic Dosage/Imaging).
Clinical experience has demonstrated that I-123 MIBG is clearly superior to I-131 MIBG when utilized in imaging the normal adrenal medulla, pheochromo-

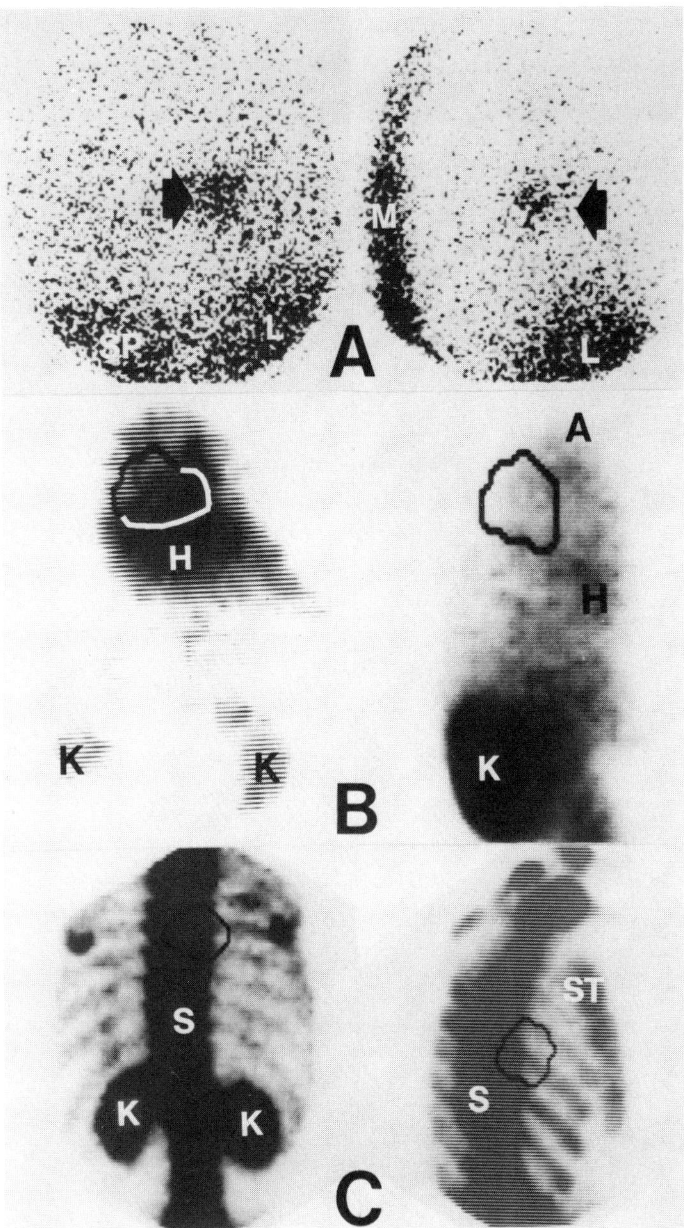

Figure 11.28   Scintigraphic studies in a patient with a left atrial, extra-adrenal pheochromocytoma. A I-131 MIBG images: Left panel = posterior view of chest, right panel = right lateral view of chest, arrow = pheochromocytoma, M = external marker along spine, L = liver, SP = spleen. B. Tc-99m RBC blood-pool images with abnormal focus of I-131 MIBG uptake superimposed: Left panel = anterior view of chest, right panel = right lateral view of chest, K = kidney, H = cardiac blood pool, A = aortic arch. C. Tc-99m medronate bone scan with abnormal focus of I-131 MIBG uptake superimposed: Left panel = posterior view of chest, right panel = right posterior oblique view of chest, K = kidney, S = spine, ST = sternum. (From Shapiro, et al, 1984b; with permission.)

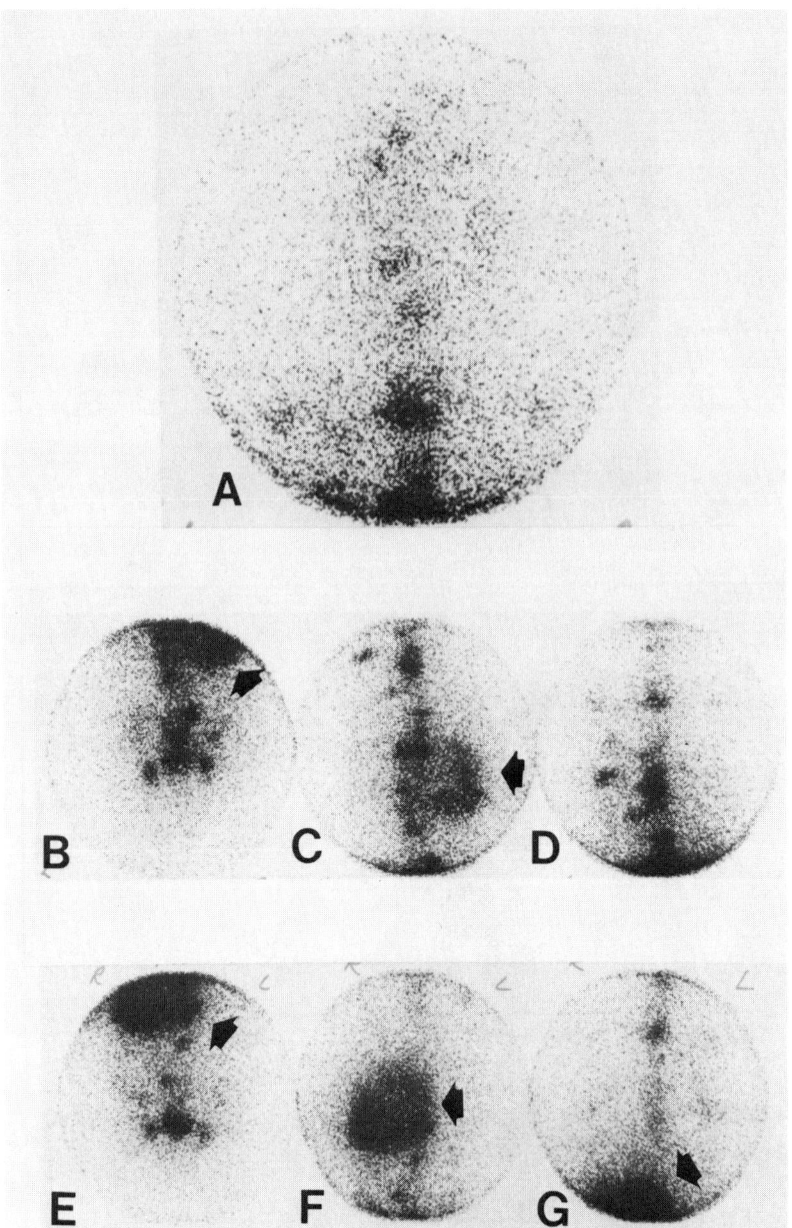

Figure 11.29 Extensive skeletal metastases demonstrated by I-131 MIBG scintigraphy. A. Anterior head and neck; B. posterior pelvis; C. posterior abdomen; D. posterior chest; E. anterior pelvis; F. anterior abdomen; and G, anterior chest. Solid arrow indicates large right adrenal primary with necrotic center manifesting as a "halo" sign. (From Shapiro, et al, 1984c; with permission.)

cytoma, and other neuroendocrine tumors. However, I-123 MIBG has not been made widely available largely due to its high costs of production and distribution. Consequently, only a limited number of clinical studies have been initiated at institutions with the resources to produce the radiopharmaceutical onsite. A diagnostic dose of 10 mCi of I-123 MIBG can be administered with radiation dosimetry nearly equivalent to a 0.5 mCi diagnostic dose of I-131 MIBG (Lynn MD,

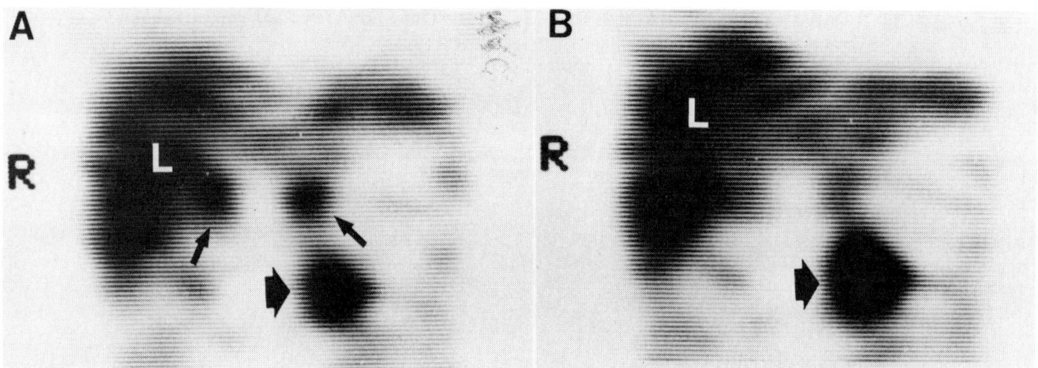

Figure 11.30 Pheochromocytoma (large arrow) localized to the left renal hilum as demonstrated by I-123 MIBG and SPECT imaging. A. coronal section; B. sagittal section. The normal adrenal medullae (small arrows) and liver (L) are clearly visualized.

et al, 1984; Swanson DP, et al, 1981). Therefore, the recommended maximum adult diagnostic dosage of I-123 MIBG injection for scintigraphic imaging studies is 10 mCi/1.7 m² administered intravenously over a 15–30-second interval. The recommended dosage for patients under 18 years of age can be calculated as described above.

Initial images of patients given I-123 MIBG are obtained 2 to 3 hours post injection utilizing a wide-field-of-view Anger camera with a low-energy, parallel-hole collimator and computer. Patients may also be imaged at 18–24 hours and even as late as 48 hours post injection, as the photon flux at this latter time is similar to that at 48 hours post injection of 0.5 mCi of I-131 MIBG. Images from the base of the skull to the pelvis are acquired as described above for I-131 MIBG imaging. Single photon emission tomographic (SPECT) imaging techniques (Figure 11.30) can also be utilized in an attempt to more clearly locate foci of abnormal radiopharmaceutical uptake. SPECT imaging is performed utilizing a rotating gamma camera with data collection over 64 projections in 360° at 15–20 seconds per projection (Lynn MD, et al, 1985). Acquired images are reconstructed to yield transaxial, sagittal, and coronal sections, whereas dynamic rotating displays of the sixty-four projections are helpful in fully appreciating tumor location.

I-131 MIBG (Therapeutic Dosage). Clinical experience in treating neuroendocrine tumors with therapeutic I-131 MIBG is extremely limited. The therapeutic dose is determined in part by invivo determination of tumor concentration/retention and whole-body elimination kinetics utilizing diagnostic doses of I-131 MIBG and/or I-123 MIBG. CT images may also be utilized to estimate tumor volumes. A dose sufficient to deliver greater than 2,000 rads to primary tumors typically requires the administration of 100–200 mCi of I-131 MIBG. High specific activity I-131 MIBG is utilized to limit the dosage of MIBG sulfate to approximately 5 mg and to minimize the theoretical possibility of adverse pharmacologic effects due to induced catecholamine release. Therapy doses are administered intravenously over approximately 90 minutes with an infusion pump. The dosage of therapeutic I-131 MIBG for patients under 18 years of age must be determined on a case-by-case basis as described above.

Dosimetry. Comparative radiation dose estimates (Table 11.18) for I-123 and I-131 MIBG in patients of various ages have been calculated. The radiation dose estimates are based upon the distribution data of Swanson and associates (1981). The dose to the adrenals is the average organ dose and the adrenal medulla dose for the adult is 35.9 Rads/mCi for I-131

Table 11.18 COMPARATIVE RADIATION DOSIMETRY ESTIMATES FOR I-131 AND I-123 MIBG[a]

| | ESTIMATED RADIATION DOSE (RADS/MCI) | | | | | | | |
| | 1-YEAR OLD | | 5-YEAR OLD | | 10-YEAR OLD | | ADULT | |
ORGAN	*I-131*	*I-123*[b]	*I-131*	*I-123*[b]	*I-131*	*I-123*[b]	I-131	*I-123*[b]
Adrenals	20.0	0.59	13.0	0.37	9.6	0.27	4.8	0.14
Bladder wall	5.6	0.41	4.4	0.33	2.8	0.22	2.8	0.24
Liver	2.4	0.23	1.3	0.12	0.89	0.09	0.44	0.04
Ovaries	15.2	0.67	6.7	0.31	3.7	0.19	1.18	0.07
Red marrow	4.4	0.29	2.3	0.16	1.4	0.10	0.74	0.06
Spleen	10.0	0.63	5.6	0.35	3.5	0.23	1.6	0.11
Testes	4.1	0.20	2.2	0.11	1.3	0.07	0.70	0.04
Thyroid	370.0	21.1	230.0	11.1	88.8	5.2	34.0	2.1
Total body	4.4	0.22	2.2	0.12	1.4	0.08	0.70	0.04

[a] Calculations based on distribution data from Swanson, et al. 1981.

[b] Assumes "pure" I-123; no I-124 or I-125 radiocontaminants.

MIBG and 1.1 Rads/mCi for I-123 MIBG. Bladder voiding intervals are 1.0 hour for newborns and 1 year olds, 2.0 hours for 5-, 10-, and 15-year olds, and 4.8 hours for adults. Liberal fluid intake and frequent (e.g., every 2 hours) voiding should be encouraged. The listed thyroid doses are for unblocked thyroid; with thyroid blockade, the thyroid dose is approximately the same as the total body dose.

References

Ackery DM, Tippett P, Condon B, et al. New approach to the localization of pheochromocytoma: Imaging with ^{131}I-MIBG. *Brit Med J* 1984, 288:1587–1591.

Ahlgren L, Ivarsson S, Johnsson L, et al. Excretion of radionuclides in human breast milk after administration of radionuclides, *J Nucl Med* 1985, 26:1085–1090.

Allen JG, East PB, Francis RJ, et al. Metabolism of debrisquine sulfate: Identification of some urinary metabolites in rat and man. *Drug Metab Dispos* 1975, 3:332-337.

Anderson BG, Beierwaltes WH, Harrison TS, et al. Labeled dopamine concentration in pheochromocytomas. *J Nucl Med* 1973, 14:781–784.

Arnold JE, Pinsky S. Comparison of Tc-99m and I-123 for thyroid imaging. *J Nucl Med* 1976, 17:261–267.

Atkins HL: The thyroid. In *Freeman and Johnson's Clinical Radionuclide Imaging* (LM Freeman, ed.), New York, Grune and Stratton, 1984, pp 1275–1317.

Atkins HL, Klopper SF, Lambrecht RM, et al. A comparison of Technetium-99m and Iodine-123 for thyroidal imaging. *AJR* 1973, 117:195–201.

Atkins HL, Richards P. Assessment of thyroid function and anatomy with technetium 99m as pertechnetate. *J Nucl Med* 1968, 9:7–15.

Baker GA, Lum DJ, Smith EM, et al. Significance of radiocontaminants in I-123 for dosimetry and scintillation camera imaging. *J Nucl Med* 1976, 17:740–743.

Basmadjian GP, Hetzel KR, Ice RD, et al. Synthesis of a new adrenal cortex scanning agent, 6β-I-131-iodomethyl-19-norcholest-5(10)-en-3β-ol (NP-59). *J Lab Comp* 1975, 11:427 (Abstr).

Baulieu JL, Guilloteau C, Chambon C, et al. Metaiodobenzylguanidine (MIBG) scintigraphy: One-year experience. *J Nucl Med* (Abstr) 1984, 25:111.

Beierwaltes WH. The history of the use of radioactive iodine. *Semin Nucl Med* 1979, 9:151–155.

Beierwaltes WH, Lieberman LM, Ansari AN, et al. Visualization of human adrenal glands in-vivo by scintillation scanning. *JAMA 1971, 216:215–217.*

Beierwaltes WH, Wieland DM, Swanson DP. Radiolabeled enzyme inhibitors for imaging. In *Principles of Radiopharmacology*, Vol. 1 (Colombetti LG, ed.), Boca Raton, CRC Press, 1979, pp 41–57.

Beierwaltes WH, Wieland DM, Swanson DP. Adrenocortical compounds. In *Radio-pharmaceuticals: Structure Activity Relationships* (Spencer RP, ed.), Orlando, FL, Grune and Stratton, Inc., 1981; pp 395–412.

Beierwaltes WH, Wieland DM, Yu T, et al. Adrenal Imaging agents: Rationale, Synthesis, formulation and metabolism. *Semi Nucl Med* 1978, 8:5–21.

Bernard JD, McDonald RA, Nesmith JA. New normal ranges for radioiodine uptake study. *J Nucl Med* 1970, 11:449–451.

Blair RJ, Beierwaltes WH, Lieberman LM, et al. Radiolabeled cholesterol as an adrenal scanning agent. *J Nucl Med* 1971, 12:176–182.

Book SA, Goldman M. Thyroidal radioiodine exposure of the fetus. *Health Phys* 1975, 29:874.

Brochardt RT. N-methylation and O-methylation. In *Enzymatic Basis of Detoxication*, Vol. 2 (Jakoby WB, ed.), New York, Academic Press, 1980, pp 43–62.

Brookeman VA. Radiation dosimetry of adrenal imaging agents, 19-iodocholesterol and 6-iodomethylnorcholesterol. *Int J Appl Radiat Isot* 1978, 29:277–279.

Brown MS, Goldstein JL. Regulation of the activity of the low-density lipoprotein receptor in human fibroblasts. *Cell* 1975, 6:305–316.

Brown MS, Goldstein JL. Receptor-mediated control of cholesterol metabolism. *Science* 1976, 91:150–154.

Burnell RC, Maxwell GM. General and coronary hemodynamic effects of Tween-20. *Aust J Exp Biol Med Sci* 1974, 52:151–155.

Carey JE, Thrall JH, Freitas JE, et al. Absorbed dose to the human adrenals from iodomethyl-norcholesterol (I-131) "NP-59." *J Nucl Med* 1979, 20:60–61.

Charkes ND. Scintigraphic evaluation of nodular goiter. *Semin Nucl Med* 1971, 1:316–333.

Chatal JF, Charbonnel B. Comparison of iodobenzylguanidine imaging with computed tomography in locating pheochromocytomal. *J Clin Endocrinol Metab* 1985, 61:769–776.

Committee on Drugs. The transfer of drugs and other chemicals into human breast milk. *Pediatrics* 1983, 72:375–383.

Couch MW, Williams CM. Comparison of 19-iodocholesterol and 6-iodomethylnorcholesterol as adrenal scanning agents. *J Nucl Med* 1977, 18:724–727.

Counsell RE, Ranade VV, Blair RJ, et al. Tumor localizing agents. IX. Radioiodinated cholesterol. *Steroids* 1970, 16:317–328.

DeQuattro V, Campese VM. Pheochromocytoma: Diagnosis and therapy. In *Endocrincology*, Vol. 2 (DeGroot LJ, Cahill GF, et al, eds.), New York, Grune and Stratton, 1979; pp 1279–1288.

DiGuilio W, Beierwaltes WH. Parathyroid scanning with Selenium-75 labeled methionine. *J Nucl Med* 1964, 5:417–427.

dosRemedios LV, Weber PM, Jasko IA. Thyroid scintigraphy in 1000 patients. Rational use of Tc-99m and I-131 compounds. *J Nucl Med* 1971, 12:673–677.

Erjavec M, Auesperg M, Golouh R, et al. Computer-assisted scanning in evaluation of 67-Ga citrate uptake in thyroid disease. *J Nucl Med* 1974, 15:810–813.

Faust JR, Goldstein JL, Brown MS. Receptor-mediated uptake of low-density lipoproteins and utilization of its cholesterol for steroid synthesis in cultured mouse adrenal cells. *J Biol Chem* 1977, 252:4862–4871.

Feine U, Treuner J, Niethammer D, et al. Erste utenshungen zur scintigraphischen darstellung von neuroblastomen mit 131-J-meta-benzylguanidin. *Nuc Compact* 1984, 15:23–26.

Fikuski K. Adrenal affinity and plasma lipoprotein binding of radiohalogenated derivatives of cholesterol. In *Second International Symposium on Radiopharmaceutical Chemistry*, Oxford, Engl, 1978, Abstract 23.

Fischer M, Kamanabroo D, Sonderkamb H, et al. Scintigraphic imaging of carcinoid tumors with 131-I-metaiodobenzylguanidine. *Lancet* 1984, 2:165.

Fischer M, Winterberg B, Muller-Rensing R, et al. Nuklear medizinische therapid dis phaochromocytoms. *Nucl Compact* 1983, 14:172–178.

Fischer M, Vetter W, Winterg B, et al. Adrenal scintigraphy in primary aldosteronism: Spironolactone as a cause of incorrect classification between adenoma and hyperplasia. *Eur J Nucl Med* 1982; 7:222–224.

Fowler JS, Ansari AN, Atkins HL, et al. Synthesis and preliminary evaluation in animals of carrier-free 11C-L-dopamine hydrochloride. *J Nucl Med* 1973, 14:867–869.

Fowler JS, MacGregor RR, Wolf, AP. Radiopharmaceuticals. 16. Halogenated dopamine analogs. Synthesis and radiolabeling of 6-iododopamine and tissue distribution studies in animals. *J Med Chem* 1976, 19:356–360.

Francis IR, Glazer G, Shapiro B, et al. Complementary roles of CT scanning and 131-I-MIBG scintigraphy in the diagnosis of pheochromocytoma. *AJR* 1983, 141:719–725.

Freitas JE, Thrall JH, Swanson DP, et al: Normal adrenal assymetry: Explanation and interpretation. *J Nucl Med ed* 1978; 19:149–153.

Fukuchi M, Hyodo K, Tachibana K, et al. Uptake of Thallium-201 in enlarged thyroid glands: Concise communication. *J Nucl Med* 1979, 20:827–832.

Fukuchi S, Nakajima K, Muira T, et al. Comparative study of adrenal scanning agents, 6β-[I-131]-iodomethyl-19-norcholest-5(10)-en-3β-ol-^{131}I(NCL-6-^{131}I) and ^{131}I-19-cholesterol (Cl-19-^{131}I). *Jpn J Nucl Med* 1976, 13:775–779.

Geatti O, Shapiro B, Sisson JC, et al. 131-I-metaiodobenzylguanidine (131-I-MIBG) scintigraphy for the location of neuroblastoma: Preliminary experience in 10 cases. *J Nucl Med* 1985, 26:736–742.

German—Anonymous. Clinical value of adrenomedullary scintigraphy with ^{131}I-MIBG. *Nuc Compact* (Editorial) 1983, 14:318.

Giachetti A, Hollenbeck RA. Extravesicular binding of noradrenaline and guanethidine in the adrenergic neurons of the rat heart: A proposed site of action of adrenergic neuron blocking agents. *Br J Pharmacol* 1976, 58:497–504.

Gillin MT, Thrall JH, Corcoran RJ, et al. Evaluation of a thyroid fluorescent scanning system of the concentric source—detector design. *J Nucl Med* 1977, 18:163–167.

Gimlette TMD, Brownless SM, Taylor WH, et al. Limits to parathyroid imaging with Thallium-201 confirmed by tissue uptake and phantom studies. *J Nucl Med* 1986, 27:1262–1265.

Glowniak JV, Shapiro B, Sisson JC, et al. Familial extra-adrenal pheochromocytoma: A new syndrome. *Arch Intern Med* 1985, 145:257–261.

Goolden AWG, Mallard JR. The use of Iodine-132 in studies of thyroid function. *Br J Radiol* 1958, 31:589–595.

Green JP, Wilcox JR, Marriott JD, et al. Thyroid uptake of I-131: Further comparisons of capsules and liquid preparations. *J Nucl Med* 1976, 17:310–312.

Gross MD, Freitas JE, Swanson DP, et al. The normal dexamethasone suppression and adrenal scintiscan. *J Nucl Med* 1979, 20:1131–1135.

Gross MD, Shapiro B, Thrall JH, et al. The scintigraphic imaging of endocrine organs. *Endocr Rev* 1984, 5:221–281.

Gross MD, Swanson DP, Wieland DM, et al. The mechanisms of localization, specificity, and metabolism of adrenal gland imaging agents. In *Studies of Cellular Function Using Radiotracers* (Billinghurst MW and Colombetti LG, eds.), Boca Raton, CRC Press, 1982, pp. 189–223.

Gross MD, Thrall JH, Beierwaltes WH. The adrenal scan: A current status report on radiotracers, dosimetry, and clinical utility. In *Nuclear Medicine Annual 1980* (Freeman LM, Weissman HS, eds.), New York, Raven Press, 1980, pp. 127–175.

Gross MD, Valk TW, Swanson DP, et al. The role of pharmacologic manipulation in adrenal cortical scintigraphy. *Semin Nucl Med* 1981, 11 : 128–148.

Grove RB, Pinsky SM, Brown TL, et al. Uptake of Ga-67 citrate in subacute thyroiditis. *J Nucl Med* 1973, 14 : 403 (Abstr).

Guilloteau D, Baulieu JL, Huguet F, et al. Meta-iodobenzylguanidine adrenal medulla localization; Autoradiographic and pharmacologic studies. *Eur J Nucl Med* 1984, 9 : 278–281.

Gwynne JT, Mahattee D, Brewer AB, et al. Adrenal cholesterol uptake from plasma lipoproteins: Regulation by corticotrophin. *Proc Natl Acad Sci USA*, 1976, 73 : 4329–4333.

Halpern S, Alazraki N, Wittenberg R, et al: I-131 thyroid uptakes: Capsule versus liquid. *J Nucl Med* 1973, 14 : 507–510.

Heidendal GAK, Roos P, Thijs JG, et al. Evaluation of cold areas on the thyroid scan with ^{67}Ga-citrate. *J Nucl Med* 1975, 16 : 793–794.

Herbert RJT, Hibbard BM, Sheppard MA. Metabolic behavior and radiation dosimetry of Tc-99m albumin in pregnancy, *J Nucl Med* 1969, 10 : 224–232.

Heyman S, Evans AE. I-131-metaiodobenzylguanidine (I-131-MIBG) in the diagnosis of neuroblastoma. *J Nucl Med* (Abstract) 1986, 27 : 931.

Higashi T, Watanabe Y, Yamaguchi M, et al. The relationship between the Ga-67 uptake and nuclear DNA Feulgen content in thyroid tumors. *J Nucl Med* 1982, 23 : 988–992.

Higashi T, Ito K, Mimura T, et al. Clinical evaluation of Ca-67 scanning in the diagnosis of anaplastic carcinoma and malignant lymphoma of the thyroid. *Radiology* 1981, 141 : 491–497.

Hisada K, Tonami N, Miyamae T, et al. Clinical evaluation of tumor imaging with Tl-201 chloride. *Radiology* 1978, 129 : 497–500.

Hoefnagel CA, DeKraker J, Marcuse HR, et al. Detection and treatment of neural crest tumors using I-131-meta-benzylguanidine. *Euro J Nucl Med* (Abstr) 1985, 11 : 17.

Hoefnagel CA, Delprat CC, Marcase HR, et al. Role of Thallium-201 total body scintigraphy in follow-up of thyroid carcinoma. *J Nucl Med* 1986, 27 : 1854–1857.

Hoefnagel CA, Den Haartog Jager FCA, Van Gennip AM, et al: Diagnosis and treatment of a carcinoid tumor using iodine-131 metaiodobenzylguanidine. *Clin Nucl Med* 1986, 3 : 150–152.

Hoffer PB. Fluorescent thyroid scanning. *AJR* 1969, 105 : 721–727.

Ice RD, Kircos LT, Coffey JL, et al. Radiation dosimetry of 6β-^{131}I-iodomethyl-19-norcholesterol, NP-59. In *Radiopharmaceutical Dosimetry Symposium* (Cloutier RJ, Coffey JL, et al, eds.), HEW Publication (FDA) 76–8044, Superintendent of Documents, U.S. Government Printing Office, Washington, DC, 1976, pp 246–254.

Ice RD, Wieland DM, Beierwaltes WH, et al. Concentration of dopamine analogs in the adrenal medulla. *J Nucl Med* 1975, 16 : 1147–1151.

Inbasekaran M, Sherman PS, Brown LE, et al. Development of kit-form analogs of meta-iodobenzylguanidine. *J Nucl Med* (Abstr) 1983, 24 : 118.

Jack DB, Stenlake JB, Templeton R. Metabolism and excretion of guanoxan in man. *J Pharm Pharmacol* 1971, 23 : 2225–2235.

Jaques S, Jr, Tobes MC, Sisson JC, et al. Mechanisms of uptake and retention of metaiodobenzylguanidine (MIBG) in the adrenal medulla. *Mol Pharmacol* 1984, 26 : 539–546.

Kaiser C, Schwartz MS, Colla DF, et al. Adrenergic agents. III. Synthesis and adrenergic activity of some catecholamine analogs bearing a substituted sulfonyl or sulfonaylakyl group in the meta position. *J Med Chem* 1975, 18 : 674–683.

Kaplan WD, Holman BL, Selekow HA, et al. ^{67}Ga-citrate and the nonfunctioning thyroid nodule. *J Nucl Med* 1974, 15 : 424–427.

Keyes JW, Thrall JH, Carey JE. Technical considerations in in-vivo thyroid studies. *Semin Nucl Med* 1978, 8 : 43–58.

Khafagi FA, Shapiro B, Mallette S, et al. Reduction of [I-131]-metaiodobenzylguanidine uptake by labetalol. (In preparation.)

Kline RC, Swanson DP, Wieland DM, et al. Myocardial imaging in man with ^{123}I-meta-iodobenzylguanidine. *J Nucl Med* 1981, 22:129–132.

Kloss G, Leven M. Accumulation of radioiodinated tyrosine derivatives in the adrenal medulla and in melanomas. *Eur J Nucl Med* 1979, 4:179–186.

Kojima M, Maeda M, Ogawa H, et al. New adrenal scanning agent. *J Nucl Med* (Abstr) 1975, 16:666.

Korn N, Buswink A, Yu T, et al. A radioiodinated bretylium analog as a potential agent for scanning the adrenal medulla. *J Nucl Med* 1977, 18:87–89.

Koutras DA, Pandos PG, Sfontouris, J, et al. Thyroid scanning with gallium-67 and cesium-131. *J Nucl Med* 1976, 17:268–271.

Kuntzman R, Jacobson MM. Monoamine oxidase inhibition by a series of compounds structurally related to bretylium and guanethidine. *J Pharmacol Exp Ther* 1963, 141:166–172.

Larsen AA, Gould WA, Roth HR, et al. Sulfonanilides. II. Analogs of catecholamines. *J Med Chem* 1967, 10:462–472.

Liddle GW, Melmon KL. The adrenals. In *Textbook of Endocrinology* (Williams RH, ed.), Philadelphia, WB Saunders Co., 1974, p 235.

Lieberman LM, Beierwaltes WH, Conn JW, et al. Diagnosis of adrenal disease by visualization of human adrenal glands with I-131-19-idodocholesterol *N Engl J Med* 1971, 285:1387–1389.

Lieberman LM, Beierwaltes WH, Varma WM, et al. Labeled dopamine concentration in human adrenal medulla and neuroblastoma. *J Nucl Med* 1969, 10:93–97.

Lumbroso J, Hartman O, Lemerle J, et al. Scintigraphic detection of neuroblastoma using 131-I and 123-1 labeled metaiodobenzylguanidine. *Euro J Nucl Med* (Abstr) 1985, 11:16.

Lynn MD, Shapiro B, Sisson JC, et al. Portrayal of pheochromocytoma and normal adrenal medulla by m-^{123}I]Iodobenzylguanidine: Concise communication. *J Nucl Med* 1984, 25:436–440.

Lynn MD, Shapiro B, Sisson JC, et al. Pheochromocytoma and the normal adrenal medulla: Improved visualization with I-123 MIBG scintigraphy. *Radiology* 1985, 156:789–792.

Maeda M, Kojima M. Homallylic rearrangement of 19-iodocholest-5en-3β-ol: New adrenal scanning agent. *Steroids* 1975, 26:241.

Mangner TJ, Anderson-Davis H, Wieland DM, et al. Synthesis of I-131 and I-123-meta-iodobenzylguanidine for diagnosis and treatment of pheochromocytoma. *J Nucl Med* (Abstr) 1983, 24:118.

Mangner TJ, Tobes MC, Wieland DM, et al. Metabolism of iodine-131 metaiodobenzylguanidine in patients with metastatic pheochromocytoma. *J Nucl Med* 1986, 27:44.

Marks LS, Kolmen SN. Tween 20 shock in dogs and related fibrinogen changes. *Am J Physiol* 1971, 220:218–223.

Maxwell RA, Wastila WB. Adrenergic neuron blocking drugs. In *Handbook of Experimental Pharmacology*, Vol. 39. New York, Springer-Verlag, 1977; pp 161–261.

Mayer WM, Gifford RW. Hypertension secondary to pheochromocytoma. *Bull NY Acad Med* 1982; 58:139–158.

McEwan AJ, Shapiro B, Sisson JC, et al. Radio-iodobenzylguanidine for the scintigraphic location and therapy of adrenergic tumors. *Semin Nucl Med* 1985, 15:132–153.

Miller RW. Fifty-two forms of childhood cancer: United States mortality experience, 1960–1966. *J Pediatr* 1969, 75:685–689.

Modell W. *Drugs of Choice*. St. Louis, CV Mosby, 1958–59; pp 53.

Morales JO, Beierwaltes WH, Counsell RE, et al. The concentration of radioactivity from labeled epinephrine and its precursors in the dog medulla. *J Nucl Med* 1967, 8:800–809.

Munker T. [11]I-metaiodobenzylguanidine

scintigraphy of neuroblastomas. *Semin Nucl Med* 1985, 15:154–160.

Nagai T, Solis BA, Koh CS. An approach to developing adrenal gland scanning. *J Nucl Med* 1968, 9:576–580.

Nakajo M, Shapiro B, Copp BJ, et al. The normal and abnormal distribution of the adrenomedullary imaging agent m-[I-131]-iodobenzylguanidine (I-131 MIBG) in man: Evaluation by scintigraphy. *J Nucl Med* 1983a, 24:672–682.

Nakajo M, Shapiro B, Glowniak JV, et al. Inverse relationship between cardiac accumulation of meta-(131-I)-iodobenzylguanidine (I-131 MIBG) and circulating catecholamines: Observations in patients suspected of pheochromocytoma, *J Nucl Med* 1983b, 24:1127–1134.

Nakajo M, Shapiro B, Sisson JC, et al. Salivary gland accumulation of meta-131-I-iodobenzylguanidine. *J Nucl Med* 1984, 25:2–6.

Nishiyama H, Sodd VJ, Berke RA, et al. Evaluation of clinical value of I-123 and I-131 in thyroid disease. *J Nucl Med* 1974, 15:261–265.

Ohta H, Ishii M, Yoshizami M, et al. A comparison of the tumor seeking agent Tc-99m dimercaptosuccinic acid and the renal imaging agent Tc-99m dimercaptosuccinic acid in humans. *Clin Nucl Med* 1985, 10:167–170.

Ohta H, Yamamoto K, Endo K, et al. A new imaging agent for medullary carcinoma of the thyroid. *J Nucl Med* 1984, 25:323–325.

Patton JA, Hollifield JW, Brill AB, et al. Differentiation between malignant and benign solitary thyroid nodules by fluorescent thyroid scanning. *J. Nucl Med* 1976, 17:17–21.

Pendleton RG, Kaiser C, Gessner G. Studies of adrenal phenylethanolamine-N-methyl-transferase (PNMT) with SKF-64139, a selective inhibitor. *J. Pharmacol Exp Ther* 1979, 197:623–632.

Pittman JA, Daily GE, Beschi RJ. Changing normal values for thyroid radioiodine uptake. *N Engl J Med* 1969, 280:1431–1434.

Robertson JS, Verhosselt M, Wahner HW. Use of I-123 for thyroid uptake measurements and depression of I-131 thyroid uptakes by incomplete dissolution of capsule filler. *J Nucl Med* 1974, 15:770–774.

Romney BM, Nickoloff EL, Esser PD, et al. Radionuclide administration to nursing mothers: Mathematically derived guidelines. *Radiology* 1986, 160:549–554.

Samuels LT, Uchikawer T. Biosynthesis of adrenal steroids. In *The Adrenal Cortex* (Eisenstein AB, ed.), Boston, Little, 1967, pp 61–102.

Sarkar SD, Beierwaltes WH, Ice RD, et al. A new and superior adrenal scanning agent, NP-59, *J Nucl Med* 1975, 16:1038–1042.

Schonebe CK. Malignant pheochromocytoma. *Scand J Uro Nephrol* 1969, 3:64–68.

Scott KN, Mareci TH, Couch MW, et al. Chemical and radiochemical stability of adrenal scanning agents, 6β-[I-131]-iodomethyl-19-norcholest-5(10)en-3β-ol and 19-iodocholest-5-en-3β-ol. *Steroids* 1977, 30:511–519.

Shapiro B, Wieland DM, Brown L, et al. I-131-metaiodobenzylguanidine (MIBG) adrenal medullary scintigraphy: Interventional studies. In *Interventional Nuclear Medicine* (Spencer RP, ed.), New York, Grune and Stratton, 1984a, pp 451–481.

Shapiro B, Sisson JC, Kalff V, et al. The location of middle mediastinal pheochromocytoma. *J Thorac Cardiovasc Surg* 1984b, 87:814–820.

Shapiro B, Sisson JC, Lloyd R, et al. Malignant pheochromocytoma: Clinical, biochemical and scintigraphic characterization. *Clin Endocrinol* 1984c, 20:189–203.

Shapiro B, Copp JE, Sisson JC, et al. Iodine-131 metaiodobenzylguanidine for the location of suspected pheochromocytoma: Experience in 400 cases. *J Nucl Med* 1985, 26:576–585.

Shapiro B, Gross MD. Radiochemistry, biochemistry and kinetics of ^{131}I-metaiodobenzylguanidine (MIBG) and ^{123}I-MIBG: Clinical implications of the use of ^{123}I-MIBG. *Med Pediatr Oncol* 1987, 15:170–177.

Sherman PS, Fisher SJ, Wieland DM, et al. Over the counter drugs block heart accumulation of MIBG. *J Nucl Med* (Abstr) 1985, 26:35.

Short JH, Darby TD. Sympathetic nervous system blocking agents. III. Derivatives of benzylguanidine. *J Med Chem* 1967, 10:833–840.

Sipila LN, Carey JE, Shapiro B, et al. Health physics aspects of I-131-metaiodobenzylguanidine therapies—A prototype for I-131 radiolabeled anti-body therapies, *Med Phys* 1985, 12:520.

Sisson JC, Frager MS, Valk TW, et al. Scintigraphic localization of pheochromocytoma. *N Engl J Med* 1981, 305:12–17.

Sisson JC, Shapiro B, Beierwaltes WH, et al. Radiopharmaceutical treatment of malignant pheochromocytoma. *J Nucl Med* 1984a, 24:197–206.

Sisson JC, Shapiro B, Beirwaltes WH, et al. 131-I-metaiodobenzylguanidine treatment of malignant pheochromocytomas. *J Nucl Med* (Abstr) 1984b, 25:72.

Sisson JC, Hutchinson J, Johnson J, et al. Acute toxicity of therapeutic 131-I-MIBG relates more to whole body than to blood radiation dosimetry. *J Nucl Med* (Abstr) 1987, 28:618.

Sone T, Fukunaga M, Otsuka N, et al. Metastatic medullary thyroid cancer: Localization with iodine-131-metaiodobenzylguanidine. *J Nucl Med* 1985, 26:604–608.

Swanson DP, Carey JE, Brown LE, et al. Human absorbed dose calculations for iodine-131 and iodine-123 labeled metaiodobenzylguanidine (MIBG): A potential myocardial and adrenal medulla imaging agent. In *Proceedings of the Third International Symposium of Radiopharmaceutical Dosimetry*. Oak Ridge, TN, Oak Ridge Associated Universities, 1981, pp 213–224.

Swenson SJ, Brown MI, Sheps SG, et al. Use of 131-I-MIGB scintigraphy in the evolution of suspected pheochromocytoma. *Mayo Clin Proc* 1985, 60:299–304.

Task Force on Short-Lived Radionuclides of the Bureau of Radiological Health and the Food and Drug Administration, Washington, DC, June, 1976.

Thrall JH, Gillin MT, Johnson MC, et al. Quantitative thyroid fluorescent scanning: Technical and clinical experience. *AJR* 1978, 130:517–522.

Thrall JH, Freitas JE, Beierwaltes WH. Adrenal scintigraphy. *Semin Nucl Med* 1978, 8:23–41.

Tobes MC, Jaques S, Wieland DM, et al. Effect of uptake-one inhibitors on the uptake of norepinephrine and metaiodobenzylguanidine. *J Nucl Med* 1985, 26:897–907.

Tonami N, Bunko H, Mishigishi T. Clinical application of T1-201 scintigraphy in patients with cold thyroid nodules. *Clin Nucl Med* 1978, 3:217–221.

Treuner J, Feine U, Niethammer D, et al. Scintigraphic imaging of neuroblastoma with [131-I]-iodobenzylguanidine. *Lancet* 1984, 1:333–334.

Turnbull LB, Teng L, Newman J, et al. Disposition of bethanidine, N-benzyl-N', N''-dimethylguanidine, in the rat, dog and man. *Drug Metab Dispos* 1976, 17:269–275.

Uloth RH, Kirk JR, Gould WA, et al. Sulfonanilides. I. Monoalkyl- and arylsulfonamidophenethanolamines. *J Med Chem* 1966, 9:88–96.

Valk TW, Frager MS, Gross MD, et al. Spectrum of pheochromocytoma in multiple endocrine neoplasia. *Ann Intern Med* 1981, 94:762–767.

Von Moll L, McEwan AJ, Shapiro B, et al. 131-I-MIBG scintigraphy of neuroendocrine tumors other than pheochromocytoma and neuroblastoma. *J Nucl Med* 1987, 28:979–988.

Weinstein MB, Ashkar FS, Caron CD. Selenomethionine-75 as a scanning agent for the differential diagnosis of the cold thyroid nodule. *Semin Nucl Med* 1971, 1:390–396.

Wellman HN, Anger RT. Radioiodine dosimetry and the use of radionuclides other than I-131 in thyroid diagnosis. *Semin Nucl Med* 1971, 1:356–378.

Wieland DM, Swanson DP, Brown LE, et al. Imaging the adrenal medulla with a I-131 labeled antiadrenergic agent. *J Nucl Med* 1979, 20 : 155–158.

Wieland DM, Wu J, Brown LE, et al. Radiolabeled adrenergic neuro-blocking agents: Adrenomedullary imaging with [^{131}I]iodobenzylguanidine. *J Nucl Med* 1980, 21 : 349–353.

Wieland DM, Beierwaltes WH. A structure-distribution relationship study of adrenomedullary radiopharmaceuticals. In *Radiopharmaceuticals: Structure-Activity Relationships* (Spencer RP, ed.), New York, Grune and Stratton, 1981a.

Wieland DM, Brown LE, Rogers WH, et al. Myocardial imaging with a radio-iodinated norepinephrine storage analog. *J Nucl Med* 1981b, 22:22–31.

Wieland DM, Brown LE, Tobes MC, et al. Imaging the primate adrenal medulla with (^{123}I) and (^{131}I) iodoben-zylguanidine: Concise Communication. *J Nucl Med* 1981c, 22 : 358–364.

Wieland DM, Brown LE, Marsh DD, et al. The mechanism of MIBG locations: Drug intervention studies. *J Nucl Med* (Abstr) 1981d, 22 : 20.

Wu JL, Wieland DM, Brown LE, et al. Adrenal imaging with I-131-p-iodobenzylguanidine. *J Nucl Med* (Abstr) 1979, 20 : 681.

Yu T, Wieland DM, Brown LE, et al. Synthesis of radiolabeled inhibitors of phenylethanolamine-N-methyl-transferase. *J Labeled Comp* 1979, ,16 : 173–176.

Ziessman HA, Fahey FH, Gochoo JM. Impact of radiocontaminants in commercially available Iodine-123: Dosimetric evaluation. *J Nucl Med* 1986, 27 : 428–432.

Radiopharmaceuticals for Lung Imaging

Henry M. Chilton
James D. Ball

Well-developed scintigraphic methods are available to evaluate both pulmonary ventilation (V) and pulmonary perfusion (Q). These techniques have been applied to diagnose many clinical conditions, but the most important indication for combined pulmonary V/Q imaging is suspected pulmonary embolism. Pulmonary V/Q scintigraphy is considerably less invasive and less expensive than pulmonary angiography and in many patients provides sufficient diagnostic certainty for clinical decision making.

I. Regional Pulmonary Perfusion Imaging

RADIOPHARMACEUTICALS

Following intravenous administration, radiolabeled particles larger than red blood cells become trapped by capillary blockade within the first capillary bed encountered. Localization of such properly sized particles that are injected into an arm vein (for instance, basiliac) occurs in the pulmonary capillaries. Scintillation images of their appearance in the lungs yields diagnostic information about regional pulmonary arterial blood flow provided radiolabeled particles are (1) of the proper size, (2) mixed homogenously in blood in the right side of the heart, and (3) extracted almost entirely in the lungs during their first passage.

The primary indication for pulmonary perfusion imaging is to screen for the presence of pulmonary emboli. Changes in pulmonary perfusion, however, are not limited to pulmonary emboli and can occur with other types of lung diseases, such as emphysema, asthma, pneumonia, and bronchogenic carcinoma.

BACKGROUND/HISTORY.

Experiments in dogs using properly sized ceramic microspheres labeled with Ag-111 and Hg-203 demonstrated that regional pulmonary perfusion could be easily measured using external imaging devices. Radioiodinated (I-131) macroaggregated albumin (MAA) was first developed for this purpose by G. V. Taplin and associates (1963; 1964a,b) and later utilized by H. N. Wagner Jr. and associates (1964) and J. L. Quinn III, et al (1964) to obtain scans of lung perfusion in humans. Compared to the early use of the insoluble ceramic microspheres, I-131 MAA could be safely administerd to humans because the albumin aggregates are metabolized and soon cleared from the lungs. When H. N. Wagner, Jr. and associates initially evaluated radioiodinated MAA, they used 20–50 micron aggregates in dogs and found that the doses presented no hemodynamic, immunologic, or radiation hazard and could effectively localize experimental emboli. In humans, H. N. Wagner, Jr. and colleagues (1969) noted that lung distribution of MAA was proportional to regional pulmonary arterial blood flow.

Initially, macroaggregated human serum albumin was radiolabeled with Iodine-131 and, to a much lesser extent, Chromium-51. Later, I-131 was replaced by other radionuclides with superior imaging properties.

Iron hydroxide (Fe-OH) particles were employed to study lung perfusion and were first labeled with Indium-113m (Stern HS, et al, 1966) and later with Tc-99m (Boyd RE and Ackerman SA, 1969; Yano Y, et al, 1969). Although In-113m Fe-OH represented a slight improvement over radioiodinated MAA, its use was limited because of (1) the relatively high energy (394 keV) principal photon of In-113m, (2) an associated incidence of a moderately benign side effect known as flushing," and (3) the fact that the required Sn-113/In-113m generator was not widely available. Nonbiodegradable iron hydroxide particles (both ferrous and ferric) were also labeled with Tc-99m (Yano Y, et al, 1969; Boyd RE, et al, 1969; Bruno RE, et al, 1970); however, Tc-99m labeled microspheres of biodegradable denatured human serum albumin (HAM) being developed about the same time eventually replaced all other lung perfusion radiopharmaceuticals (Rhodes BA, et al, 1969; Burdine JA, et al, 1970).

The original kit-type formulation of Tc-99m labeled HAM was far from ideal because the labeling procedure was time consuming and required careful manipulation in order to ensure proper labeling. Ultrasonification was necessary during radiolabeling in order to prevent aggregation of particles, and repeat washings were desirable to remove "free" Tc-99m and thus assure reasonably high tagging efficiencies in the final product. Additionally, as microspheres prepared by this formulation had a tendency to aggregate during the labeling procedure or upon standing for several hours afterwards, careful visual examination of the product was imperative, and, occasionally, reultrasonification was required prior to administration to break up any large aggregates that had formed.

To alleviate many of these problems, an "instant" labeling kit that required only the addition of generator-produced Tc-99m sodium pertechnetate was developed for the preparation of Tc-99m HAM. Later, a similar "instant" kit was also developed for Tc-99m macroaggregated albumin (MAA). Both of these products were used extensively for pulmonary perfusion imaging until recently when a decision was made by the manufacturer to remove the product from the marketplace. For historical and comparative purposes, however, a discussion of Tc-99m HAM will be included in the following presentation of radiopharmaceuticals for imaging regional pulmonary perfusion.

Chemistry

Human Albumin Microspheres (HAM). The preparation of HAM particles (Rhodes BA and Bolles TF, 1975) involved a three-step process: (1) emulsification or formation of a suspension of albumin droplets in cottonseed oil, (2) gelatinization or solidification of the albumin droplets into rigid microspheres by heating, and (3) separation and sizing of the microspheres.

Particle-size distribution of albumin microspheres depended primarily upon physical conditions involved in the preparation of the suspension. Because controlling these parameters to provide a reproducible, uniform size distribution proved difficult, particle-size separation incorporated mechanical sieving (Zolle I, et al, 1970; Pasqualini R, et al, 1969).

The original method for radiolabeling HAM particles with Tc-99m involved treatment of HAM particles with thiosulfate (a variation of the method used to prepare Tc-99m sulfur colloid, the radiopharmaceutical commonly employed for imaging the reticuloendothelial system). The stannous ion-assisted reduction and radiolabeling method for preparing Tc-99m HAM proved more convenient and reliable. The stannous ion technique simply required the addition of Tc-99m sodium pertechnetate to a vial containing the stannous ion pretreated microspheres. Ultrasonification remained a requirement during preparation to ensure the dispersion of Pluronic F-68, a detergent that served as a surface active agent to decrease the likelihood of HAM aggregation.

Preparations of microspheres of human serum albumin were extremely uniform in their particle size range. In recent formulations approximately 5% of the microspheres were in the 10 to 18 micron range, more than 90% were between 18 and 40 microns, and less than 2% of the particles were larger than 40 microns.

Macroaggregated Albumin (MAA). Whereas HAM particles were produced by heating albumin in an oil bath, macroaggregated albumin particles are prepared by the heat denaturation of albumin in an aqueous solution. Initially, macroaggregated albumin suspensions were prepared by heating 0.1% radioiodinated (I-131) albumin solutions at pH 5.5 for 20 minutes at 79 degrees centigrade. In this method, the resultant particle size ranged from a few microns to 100 microns, with 60–80% of the aggregates in the 10 to 20 micron range. Subsequent reheating of the I-131 MAA preparation for 5 minutes at 100 degrees centigrade produced a suspension with fewer small particles and only a slight increase in size for the larger aggregates (Taplin GV, et al, 1967). Later, microwave heating and ultrasound agitation were added to this technique to produce a narrower particle-size distribution and to convert large macroaggregates to a smaller and more uniform suspension (Taplin GV, et al, 1967).

A variety of methods have been utilized for radiolabeling macroaggregated albumin (MAA) with Tc-99m; however, none approaches the simplicity and demonstrated effectiveness of the stannous method. Near instantaneous radiolabeling of MAA occurs when generator-produced Tc-99m sodium pertechnetate is added to MAA previously treated with stannous ions (usually stannous chloride). No special manipulation or treatment (e. g., ultrasonification) is required for radiolabeling or to ensure product integrity. Technetium-99m MAA is usually ready for use within a few minutes following the addition of Tc-99m sodium pertechnetate. Certain commercial formulations, however, suggest a brief incubation period (5–10 minutes) to ensure that optimal radiolabeling has occurred.

All commercially available MAA products utilize the stannous ion radiolabeling method (Table 12.1). For MAA, the majority of particles are between 10 and

Table 12.1 COMMERCIALLY AVAILABLE MACROAGGREGATED ALBUMIN KITS FOR TECHNETIUM-99m RADIOLABELING[a]

NAME®	MANUFACTURER	VIAL SIZE	NUMBER OF PARTICLES/VIAL	KIT COMPONENTS
MAA—Multidose	Medi-Physics, Inc.	10 ml	4–8×10^6	Aggregated albumin (0.34 mg), stannous tartrate (0.27 mg), isotonic saline (0.6 ml)
MAA—Unit dose	Medi-Physics, Inc.	5 ml	0.5–1.0×10^6	Aggregated albumin (0.11 mg), stannous tartrate (0.09 mg), isotonic saline (0.3 ml)
Macrotec	Squibb Diagnostics	5 ml	1.0–8.0×10^{6b}	Aggregated albumin (1.5 mg), albumin (10 mg), stannous chloride (0.07–0.19 mg), sodium chloride (1.8 mg), acetic acid/sodium acetate/hydrochloric acid (trace)
Pulmolite	DuPont-New England Nuclear	10 ml	3.6–6.5×10^{6b}	Aggregated albumin (1.0 mg), albumin (10 mg), tin (0.12 mg total), stannous chloride (0.02 mg minimum), sodium chloride (10 mg)
TechneScan MAA	Mallinckrodt, Inc.	10 ml	$8(\pm 4) \times 10^6$	Aggregated albumin (2.0 mg), albumin (0.5 mg), stannous chloride (0.12 mg), lactose (80 mg), succinic acid (24 mg), sodium acetate (1.4 mg)

[a] United States market only.
[b] Average number of particles/vial specified on per batch basis.

40 microns. Macroaggregates over 50 microns are seldom encountered in current product formulations.

PHARMACOKINETICS

Following intravenous administration, Tc-99m MAA (and Tc-99m HAM) particles are rapidly cleared from blood into the lungs by the mechanism of capillary blockade. The level of localization within the lungs depends significantly upon particle size since progressively larger particles occlude pulmonary vessels at a higher vascular level than the capillary beds (mean diameter-8 microns).

Particle Clearance from Lungs. A primary difference exists between lung clearance mechanisms and rates of clearance of Tc-99m MAA and Tc-99m HAM. Macroaggregates are cleared from the lungs primarily by aggregate breakup, and the smaller particles ultimately undergo phagocytosis by the cells of the reticuloendothelial system. With human albumin microspheres, however, clearance from the lungs occurs only by dissolution of the albumin particles.

The size of the MAA or HAM particles also affects clearance rate from the lungs. For example, larger particles clear much more slowly than do smaller particles. The slower lung-clearance rate is due to the continual breakup or dissolution of larger particles into smaller ones before they are eventually cleared from the lungs. A particle 40 microns in diameter, for instance, could break into smaller particles sufficiently large to block yet other smaller vessels in the lungs before eventually being cleared.

For MAA and HAM particles of nearly the same size, HAM demonstrated a longer biological clearance from the lungs than MAA (i.e., for 20 to 30 micron particles, HAM had a biological half-life of 4 to 6 hours vs. 2 to 3 hours for the MAA). This observed difference in clearance rates is related at least in part to particle shape. For example, because HAM particles were spherical and equivalent in all three dimensions, a microsphere only slightly larger than the diameter of a capillary segment completely blocks that vessel. On the other hand, since MAA particles are seldom spherical, it is possible that an aggregate larger than the diameter of the capillary bed could pass through the lung vasculature, provided it is properly oriented.

The method of preparation of MAA and HAM also affects the rate of biologic clearance from lung. It has been shown that in HAM preparation, the length of heating and the temperature can have a profound effect upon biodegradability. Among preparations of HAM and MAA of nearly identical particle size, significant differences were noted in lung clearance rates (Davis MA, 1975).

PRECAUTIONS

The relative safety associated with the use of radiolabeled particles to study pulmonary perfusion is due to several factors. First, the normal physiologic and anatomic properties of the lung permit the safe occlusion of a relatively large number of pulmonary vessels before appreciable changes in pulmonary arterial pressure will occur (Mishkin FS and Brashear RE, 1971). Detailed studies of the human lung by E. R. Weibel (1963) have shown approximately 280 billion capillary segments and no less than 300 million precapillary arterioles (Table 12.2). Since pulmonary perfusion imaging is generally accomplished by the administration of a relatively small number of radiolabeled particles, the percentage of pulmonary vessels normally occluded during a lung perfusion study is rather low. In general, less than 0.5% of pulmonary vessels are occluded in the lungs of healthy persons administered routine doses (i. e., less than 1–2 million particles) of Tc-99m MAA (or HAM). An additional safety factor is the highly anastomotic nature of the pulmonary vessels, a condition that results in extensive degrees of blood shunting during hemodynamic crises. As a result, the risk of altering pulmonary hemodynamics

Table 12.2　THE PULMONARY VASCULATURE[a]

VESSEL	APPROXIMATE NUMBER IN ADULT LUNG	APPROXIMATE DIAMETER (MICRONS)
Distribution artery connectors	0.25×10^6	100–150
Distribution arteries	4×10^6	60–100
Precapillary arterioles	300×10^6	17–59
Terminal capillary units	289×10^9	8–16

[a] From Weibel, 1963.

Table 12.3　COMPENDIAL (*UNITED STATES PHARMACOEPIA XXI*) REQUIREMENTS FOR AGGREGATED ALBUMIN (INCLUDING MACROAGGREGATED ALBUMIN AND HUMAN ALBUMIN MICROSPHERES)

Packaging/Storage:	Single or multiple dose containers; 2–8°C
Labeling:	In addition to time and date of calibration and amount of radioactivity, labeling should state that the product should not be used if clumping of the product occurs
Particle size:	Not less than 90% should have a diameter between 10–90 microns with none greater than 150 microns
pH:	Between 3.8–8.0
Radiochemical purity:	Not less than 90% (no more than 10% total radiochemical purity

through the use of biodegradable albumin aggregates in most patients is extremely low (Harding LK, 1973).

During the mid-to-late 1960s, when most nuclear medicine imaging was performed with rectilinear scanning devices, adequate images of lung perfusion were thought to be obtainable with as few as 60,000 particles (Heck LL and Duley JW, 1974). The greater resolution of modern-day scintillation cameras, however, requires that slightly more particles be injected to assure that the scintillation image of lungs will not result in a "patchy" appearance resulting from the random distribution in lung of too few particles (Dworkin HJ, et al, 1977). Today, it is generally advised that the minimum number of particles to be administered for pulmonary perfusion imaging is around 125,000 particles. No more than 2 million particles should be given, because any larger number would unnecessarily occlude many more pulmonary capillaries with no great increase in diagnostic information.

In addition to the number of particles injected, particle size is also an important factor that can affect image quality and patient safety. For example, the injection of particles larger than the diameters of the precapillary arterioles may prove harmful because the larger particles occlude pulmonary blood flow at a much higher vascular level. Conversely, particles much smaller than the terminal capillary units pass through the lungs and eventually appear in the liver as they are subsequently removed from the blood by the cells of the reticuloendothelial system (McLean JR, et al, 1977; 1979). To optimize lung image quality and prevent any likelihood of altered lung hemodynamics from the injection of particles of the improper size, U.S.P. XXI specifies optimal particle-size characteristics of these preparations (Table 12.3).

Side Effects/Adverse Reactions. Reported adverse reactions associated with the use of Tc-99m MAA (or HAM) have included flushing, respiratory and cardiac distress, hives, itching, and redness. Death has been reported in at least four patients (limited to United States data) injected with Tc-99m lung-perfusion radiopharmaceuticals. Anaphylactoid reactions, attributed to the albumin nature of these products, have also occurred. In the United States in 1978, the number of reported adverse reactions for MAA and HAM were 2 and 16 respectively, which gave an incidence (number of reactions/100,000 administrations) of 0.3 for MAA and 4.34 for HAM. In 1981, one adverse reaction was reported for MAA whereas three reports were made involving HAM (Rhodes BA and Cordova MA, 1979, Cordova MA, et al, 1982).

Use During Pregnancy/Breastfeeding. The beneficial use of radiopharmaceuticals during pregnancy, particularly the first trimester, should be carefully weighed against potential risk. It has been reported that radioactivity is excreted in breast milk following the use of Tc-99m MAA (Cranage R and Palmer M, 1985). Therefore, it is advised that breastfeeding should be discontinued for 24 hours after the administration of Tc-99m MAA (Romney BM, et al, 1986).

Toxicity. The first signs of toxicity associated with the use of Tc-99m MAA or Tc-99m HAM are an increase in pulmonary artery pressure and a concommitant decrease in femoral artery pressure (Allen DR, et al, 1974). In normal individuals, 60–70% of the pulmonary circulation must be occluded before changes in lung hemodynamics are observed. These symptoms occur in direct relationship to the particular size distribution and number of particles administered. With the recommended doses (i. e., particle number and size) of these radiopharmaceuticals no adverse hemodynamic effects have been documented. In animals, it has been shown that the first observable signs of distress occur at doses that are at least several hundred times the average lung dose and that a safety factor of greater than 1,000 exists for the mean lethal dose (MLD).

Because death associated with the use of these products has been reported in patients with severe pulmonary vascular disease (Vincent WR, et al, 1968), it is recommended that such patients receive no more than the suggested *minimum* (i. e., 125,000) number of particles. Additionally, patients with right-to-left intrapulmonary or cardiac shunt have exhibited transient ischemic episodes when given these radiopharmaceuticals. Therefore, the use of these agents in these types of patients should also be carefully monitored to ensure that injections contain no more than the minimum number of particles necessary for adequate imaging of pulmonary perfusion.

Use in Pediatrics. As pediatric patients are routinely given proportionally lesser amounts of radioactivity than are adults, the number of particles administered to children must be similarly reduced because the pulmonary vasculature is not fully developed at birth or for several years thereafter (Davies G and Reid L, 1970). If 500,000 particles are considered safe for adults, it has been estimated that newborns should not receive more than 50,000 particles, and 1 year-olds should be given fewer than 165,000 particles (Heyman S, 1979; Levine G, 1980).

CLINICAL CONSIDERATIONS/ CONTRAINDICATIONS

Radionuclide pulmonary perfusion imaging is a sensitive means of evaluating pulmonary arterial blood flow (Figure 12.1). However, several pathophysiological processes (e. g., chronic obstructive lung disease, asthma, pulmonary embolus, etc.) will result in abnormal perfusion of the pulmonary arterial tree. Therefore, while the sensitivity of this study is high, its specificity is less than ideal.

The most frequent reason for performing a pulmonary perfusion study is to evaluate a patient for possible pulmonary emboli. Classically, pulmonary emboli result in multiple bilateral segmental perfusion defects most numerous at the lung bases (Figure 12.2). Often, the chest radiograph is relatively unremarkable. Unfortunately, from a diagnostic point of view, the classic pattern of pulmonary emboli appears all too infrequently. It is apparent that perfusion may be altered by any disease process that directly affects pulmonary arterial blood flow (e. g., pulmonary emboli). Less obvious is the fact that many disease processes indirectly affect pulmonary perfusion by causing blood to be shunted away from regions of lung that are abnormally ventilated. Therefore, diseases that primarily affect the pulmonary parenchyma—pneumonia, for instance—also alter pulmonary arterial blood flow. As a result, pulmonary perfusion defects (Figure 12.3) may be due to chronic obstructive pulmonary disease (COPD), pneumonia, pleural effusion, tumor, foreign bodies, and asthma, to name a few causes. Increased diagnostic specificity of an abnormal perfusion study is accomplished by the addition of a ventilation study. (The utility of ventilation imaging is presented later in this chapter.)

Split pulmonary perfusion imaging is helpful in predicting whether or not a patient may undergo a pneumonectomy without becoming a respiratory cripple. Relative perfusion of each lung is expressed as a percentage of total lung activity. The FEVI (forced expiratory

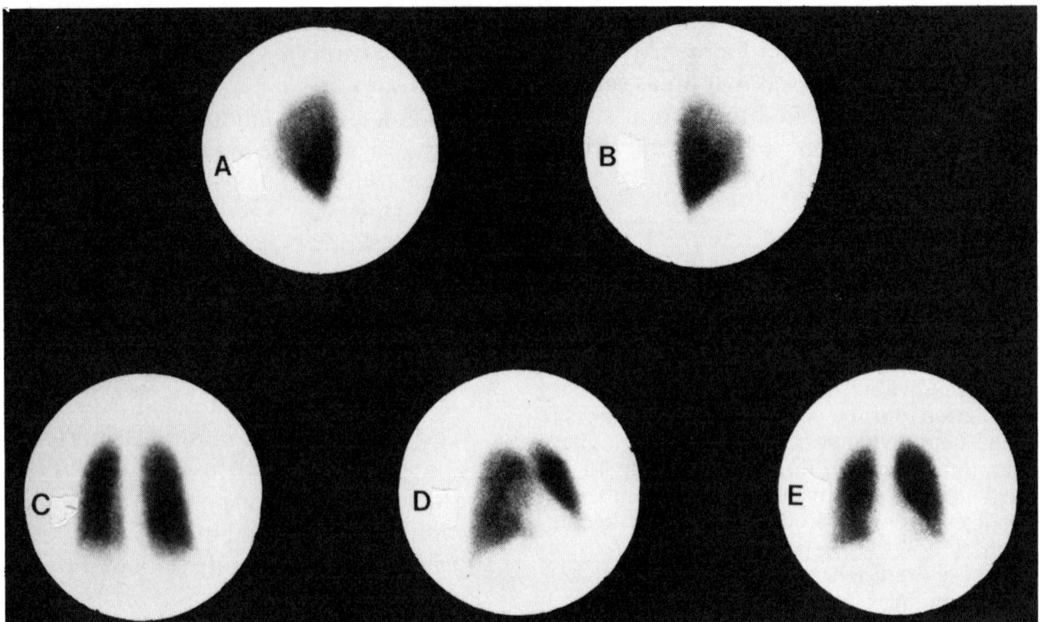

Figure 12.1 Lung perfusion image performed with Tc-99m macroaggregated albumin (MAA) in patient with no evidence of perfusion abnormality. Images shown are (A) left lateral, (B) right lateral, (C) posterior, (D) right anterior oblique, and (E) anterior views. Note the attenuation of activity that is normally seen in anterior view that corresponds to mediastinum.

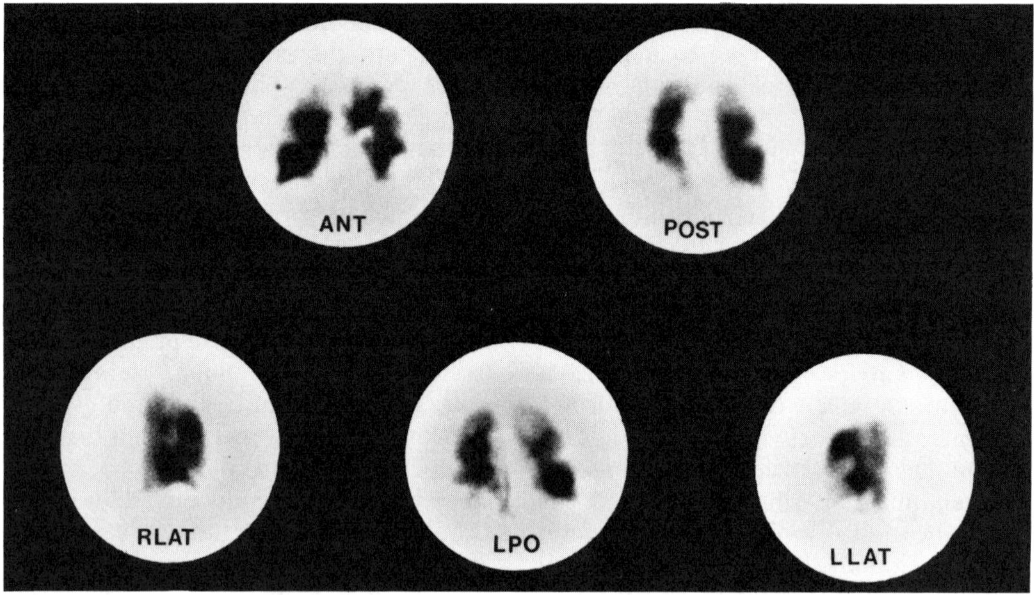

Figure 12.2 Pulmonary perfusion images performed with 3 millicuries Tc-99m MAA demonstrating multiple bilateral segmental perfusion abnormalities that appear to be due to emboli. Perfusion abnormalities are noted throughout the lungs but more prominent at the bases.

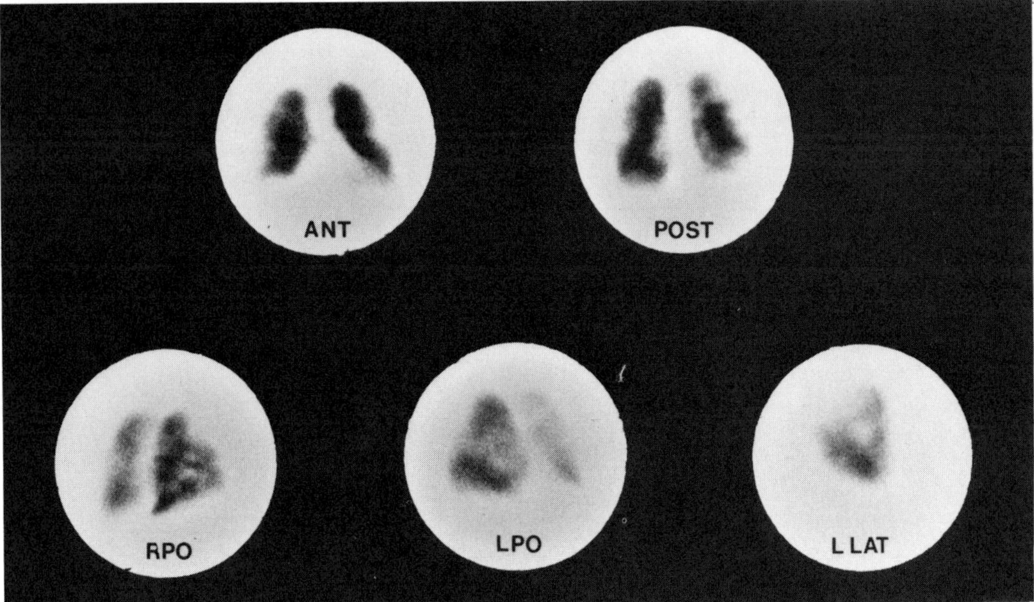

Figure 12.3 Lung images depicting multiple small nonsegmental perfusion defects that appear throughout the lungs. This pattern would suggest a nonembolic parenchymal process such as COPD.

volume in 1 second) obtained from a pulmonary function test is multiplied by the percentage perfusion of the lung remaining after surgery. This procedure accurately predicts the postoperative FEVI.

Contraindications. Technetium-99m MAA (or Tc-99m HAM) should not be administered to patients with severe pulmonary hypertension. The use of these radiopharmaceuticals is also contraindicated in persons with a history of hypersensitivity to human serum albumin and albumin-containing products. The presence of right-to-left cardiac shunts may represent a relative contraindication to the intravenous injection of Tc-99m MAA (or Tc-99m HAM), however, in practice, pulmonary perfusion radiopharmaceuticals are often used to detect right-to-left shunts (Figure 12.4).

Dosage/Dosimetry

Method. In adults, between 3 and 6 millicuries of Tc-99m MAA are administered intravenously via a peripheral vein with the patient supine. The supine posi-

tion is desired during injection of this radiopharmaceutical because in patients injected while upright, gravitational effects produce an uneven distribution of radiolabeled particles in the lungs, with greater numbers appearing at the bases. Provided no right-to-left intrapulmonary or cardiac shunt exists, near-complete localization of the radiolabeled particles occurs during their first passage through the pulmonary arteriocapillary bed.

Injection of Tc-99m MAA should be made over a period of 15 to 30 seconds to permit adequate mixing of the radiolabeled particles in blood and thereby ensure their uniform distribution in the lungs. During the injection of this radiopharmaceutical, the syringe contents should not be allowed to mix with blood for longer than a few seconds because clots that may form in the syringe can incorporate the radiopharmaceutical to produce "hot" spots in the perfusion lung images (Davis MA, 1975). During injection, the patient should be encouraged to breathe freely and deeply because capillaries in the dependent regions of the lung are less likely to be collapsed at high

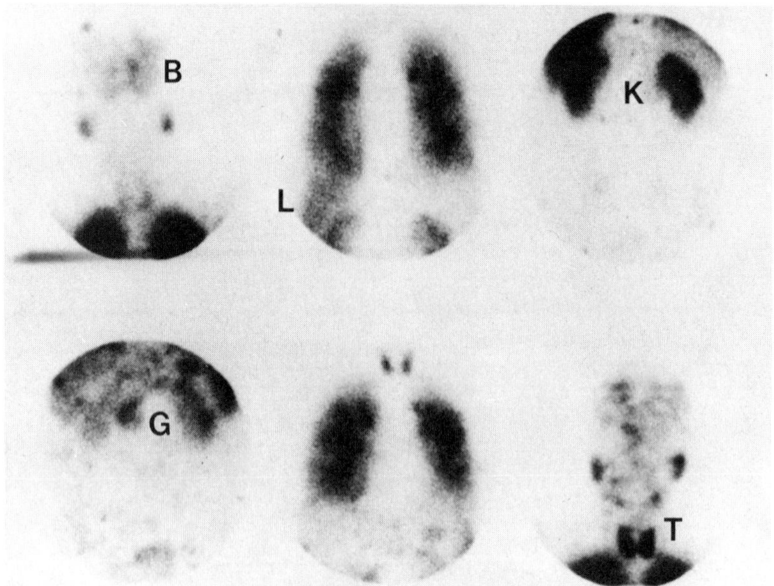

Figure 12.4 Selected views of the head, lungs, and abdomen following the injection of Tc-99m MAA in a patient with right-to-left cardiac shunt. Notice radiopharmaceutical uptake in the brain (B), thyroid (T), liver (L), kidney (K), and gut (G). The extensive brain uptake proves that the abnormal biodistribution is due to shunting and not to the presence of the radiochemical impurity, Tc-99m pertechnetate. (Reproduced with permission from Bank ER, et al. Radionuclide demonstration of intrapulmonary shunting in cirrhosis *AJR* 1983, 140:967–969.)

levels of lung inflation. Imaging with multiple views, can commence immediately following radiopharmaceutical administration.

Dosimetry. Estimated absorbed radiation dosimetry for Tc-99m MAA (and Tc-99m HAM) is shown in Table 12.4.

Table 12.4 ESTIMATED ABSORBED RADIATION DOSE IN ADULTS FOR Tc-99m MAA AND HAM (ADMINISTERED INTRAVENOUSLY)

| | RADS/4 MILLICURIES | |
ORGAN	*Tc-99m MAA*[a]	*Tc-99m HAM*[b]
Lung	0.8	0.9
Kidney	0.4	0.6
Stomach	—	0.3
Bladder wall	0.2	0.12
Ovaries	0.036	0.05
Testes	0.02	0.02

[a] Personal communication, Radiopharmaceutical Internal Dosimetry Information Center, Oak Ridge Associated Universities, Oak Ridge, TN.

[b] Product formerly available from 3M Company, St. Paul, MN.

II. Ventilation Imaging

RADIOAEROSOLS AND RADIOACTIVE GASES

Although pulmonary perfusion imaging is a very sensitive indicator of alterations in lung blood flow, it frequently lacks the specificity necessary to distinguish pulmonary emboli from nonembolic types of lung disease that also produce perfusion defects. To increase the specificity of the study for pulmonary emboli, some measure of regional ventilation is desired. By combining ventilation imaging with pulmonary perfusion imaging, it is possible to obtain in excess of a 90% true-negative diagnosis of pulmonary embolism and to substantially reduce the high false-positive rate that can occur on the basis of pulmonary perfusion imaging only.

BACKGROUND/HISTORY

The use of radioactive gases for the assessment of lung function can be traced to the mid-1950s when H.W. Knipping and colleagues employed Xenon-133 in the early diagnosis of bronchial carcinoma. Gases composed of Oxygen-15, Carbon-11, and Nitrogen-13 were also used with external scintillation detectors to determine the relative distribution of gas ventilation to different regions of the lung. External detectors were later used to obtain profile analysis of radioactivity in the lungs of patients with known pulmonary disease. Scintillation images of the distribution of radiogases in lung were not, however, obtained until the mid-1960s, when gamma-scintillation cameras became available.

Today, ventilation imaging is a routine diagnostic procedure in most nuclear medicine departments and is usually performed with radioisotopes of xenon (e. g., Xenon-133 and Xenon-127), although Krypton-81m, another radiogas, and radioaerosols of short-lived Tc-99m radiopharmaceuticals, such as pentetate (DTPA), are being utilized more frequently.

CHEMISTRY

Radiopharmaceuticals utilized in the evaluation of ventilation can be classified as either radiogases or radioaerosols.

Radiogases of Xenon and Krypton.

Among the radiogases employed for ventilation imaging are the radioisotopes of xenon (Xenon-127 and Xenon-133) and Krypton-81m. A description of the physical and nuclear properties of these agents is found in Table 12.5.

Xenon-133 and Xenon-127 are available from commercial suppliers either as unit-dose products (both Xe-133 and Xe-127) or larger multiple-dose containers (Xe-133 only). With the unit-dose containers, the gas is delivered by the use of a hand-held device that provides positive pressure to the vial in order to displace the vial contents into a shielded, closed-circuit breathing apparatus. With the multiple-dose containers, the gas is initially contained in a larger vessel that serves as a reservoir for dispensing smaller, unit-dose-type preparations on an as-needed basis.

Krypton-81m ($T_{1/2}$ phy = 13 seconds) is a generator-supplied radionuclide produced by the decay of parent rubidium (Rb-81). Since the decay of parent to daughter occurs so rapidly, Kr-81m may be eluted continuously from the generator using as the eluant a stream of humidified oxygen across the generator column. Krypton-81m is administered by inhalation directly from the generator. Rubidium-81/Krypton-81m generators usually contain 2–10 millicuries at the time of calibration. At parent-daughter equilibrium, each millicurie of Rb-81 produces approximately 0.96 millicuries of Kr-81m. Generators are preferably used within 12 hours of generator

Table 12.5 PHYSICAL AND NUCLEAR PROPERTIES OF THE RADIOACTIVE GASES AND RADIOAEROSOLS USED FOR LUNG VENTILATION IMAGING

	PHYSICAL HALF-LIFE	DECAY MODE	PRINCIPAL PHOTON ENERGY (ABUNDANCE)	MEANS OF PRODUCTION
Radiogases				
Xenon-133	5.27 days	β minus	81 keV (35%)	U-235 fission by-product
Xenon-127	36.4 days	E.C.[a]	172 keV (25%)	Accelerator product:
			203 keV (68%)	Cs-133(p, 2p5n)Xe-127
			375 keV (17%)	
Krypton-81m	13 secs	E.C.[a]	190 keV (65%)	Generator product from decay of Rubidium-81 (T-1/2 Phy. = 4.6 hr)
Radioaerosols				
Tc-99m Pentetate	6 hrs	I.T.[b]	140 keV (88%)	Radioaerosol of Tc-99m pentetate via commercial nebulizer

[a] E.C. = electron capture.
[b] I.T. = isomeric transition.

calibration because of the relatively short $T_{1/2}$ of the rubidium parent (4.7 hours). The generator is stored at room temperature.

Radioaerosols. For several years, radioaerosols have been suggested as an alternative to radioactive gases for ventilation imaging. Various radioaerosols have been investigated, and several have been found useful in the investigation of ventilation. Compared to radiogas ventilation imaging, radioaerosol lung imaging has some advantages. For example, since radioaerosols are retained transiently in the lung as a function of inhalation, images of ventilation from different projections can be obtained during a single study. Also, difficulties associated with the use of radioactive gases, including their shielded containment and disposal, can be minimized with the use of radioaerosols.

Despite their availability in nuclear medicine for over two decades, radioaerosols have not been generally accepted because of technical difficulties associated with their use. In the past, devices used to generate radioaerosols produced droplets of a wide particle-size range that distributed nonuniformly in the lung, usually with excessive central lung deposition and relatively poor penetration into the lung periphery. Nebulizer devices capable of producing radioaerosols of the desired size for uniform lung distribution have only recently been made available. Previous techniques for the production of radioaerosols included ultrasonic nebulizers, delivery systems that utilized a heating chamber to reduce the size of "wet" aerosols by evaporation, baffles for removing large particles by impaction, and a large reservoir bag in the delivery line to remove larger particles by preferential settling; none of these were entirely successful. The use of ultrasonic nebulizers should be avoided since they have been shown to produce unacceptably high levels of free unbound Tc-99m pertechnetate in radioaerosol preparations of Tc-99m pentetate (Waldman DL, et al, 1987).

The standard aerosol device employed

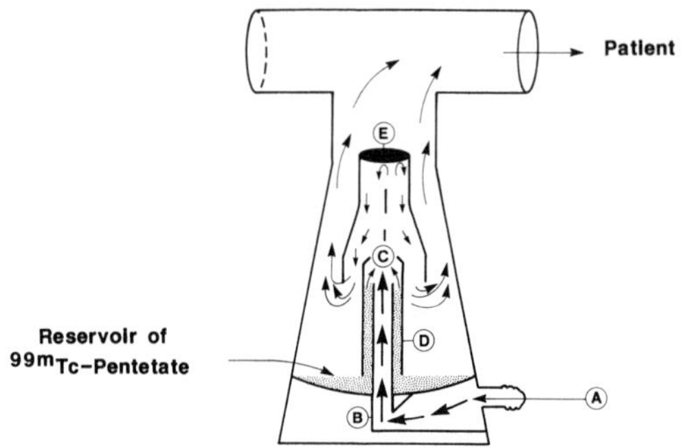

Figure 12.5 Diagram of nebulizer device used to generate radioaerosols for pulmonary imaging. Oxygen flows into the gas inlet (A) and through the Venturi tube (B). At the aerosol formation zone (C), the oxygen flow creates a slightly lower pressure that acts to "pull" the liquid through the Venturi tube sleeve. As the liquid meets the oxygen flow, the liquid is subject to gas shearing with aerosol formation. Large aerosol particles strike the baffle (E) to form small particles that clear the nebulizer and enter the breathing pathway to the patient.

today consists of a reservoir (nebulizer) and a yoke fitted with a mouthpiece through which the aerosol is breathed (Figure 12.5). The return side of the yoke is fitted with a filter through which expired air passes and radioaerosol is trapped. The system's nebulizer if fitted with a Venturi tube that creates the aerosol when a column of liquid is sheared by a jet of compressed air (e. g., oxygen).

Based upon the several studies on the lung deposition of radioaerosols of varying sizes, it appears that the ideal size for aerosol droplets in order to achieve uniformity of distribution in the lungs during deep tidal-volume breathing is 0.1–0.5 microns (Hayes M and Taplin GV, 1980; Brain JD and Valberg PA, 1979) or less. With a preparation of this size, no "settling out" of large particles occurs in the airways or bronchi (Figure 12.6) and, as a result, a high percentage of the inhaled radioaerosol reaches the peripheral air spaces of the lungs. On the other hand, particles greater than 3 microns deposit in

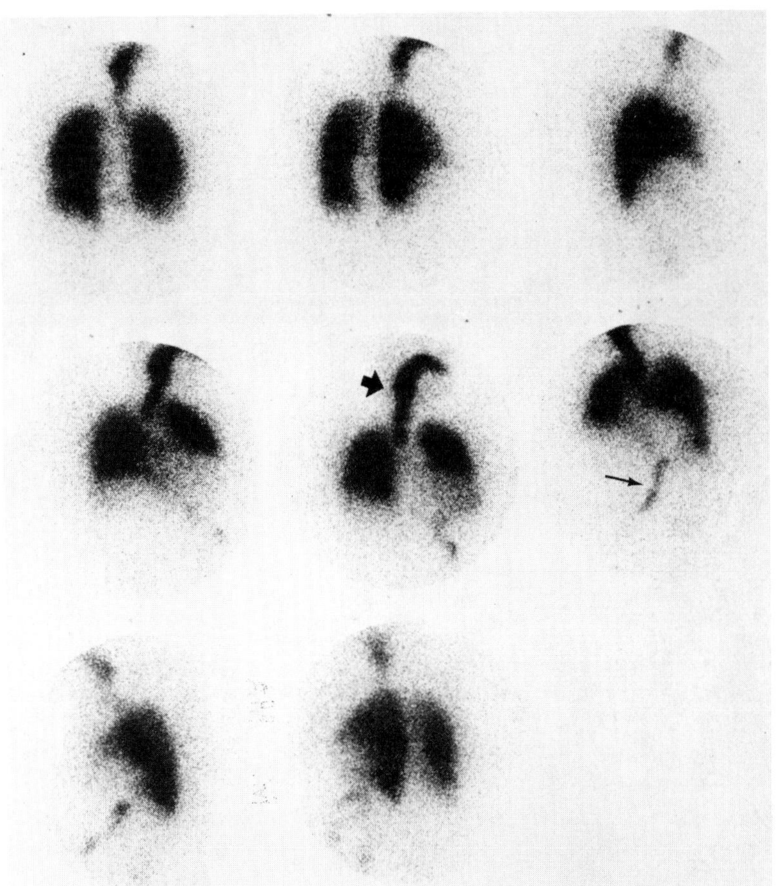

Figure 12.6 Otherwise normal Tc-99m pentetate (DTPA) aerosol study demonstrating substantial tracheal activity (large arrow) with swallowed activity in the stomach (small arrow). (Courtesy of J.W. Keyes, Jr. Georgetown University Hospital, Washington, DC.)

the large airways, failing to penetrate the lung periphery. The mass median average diameter (MMAD) of the aerosol particles prepared by the nebulizer (already described) is estimated at 0.25 millimicrons (Sirr SA, et al, 1985). Because of their submicronic and fairly homogenous particle size, aerosols prepared by this method penetrate the pulmonary parenchyma with minimal deposition in the large airways (Figures 12.7 and 12.8).

The most common radioaerosol is prepared from Tc-99m pentetate (DTPA), although other Tc-99m radiopharmaceuticals, such as sulfur colloid and pyrophosphate, have been used. Technetium-99m pentetate is preferred for radioaerosol imaging because of its ready availability, its relatively rapid clearance from the lung, and its subsequent rapid excretion via the kidneys.

A "pseudo-gas" of Tc-99m has been prepared and utilized for ventilation imaging that has biological behavior much like an aerosol, but is produced as an ultra-fine dry dispersion of Tc-99m labeled carbon (0.005μm) (Fawdry R, et al, 1988; Rimkus DS and Ashburn WL, 1988). The ultra-fine aerosol diffuses like a gas (hence, its name) and is administered in much the same manner as a radioaerosol (Burch WM, et al, 1984). The pseudo-gas is prepared directly from generator eluate using a high-heat oven. It is currently available outside the United States.

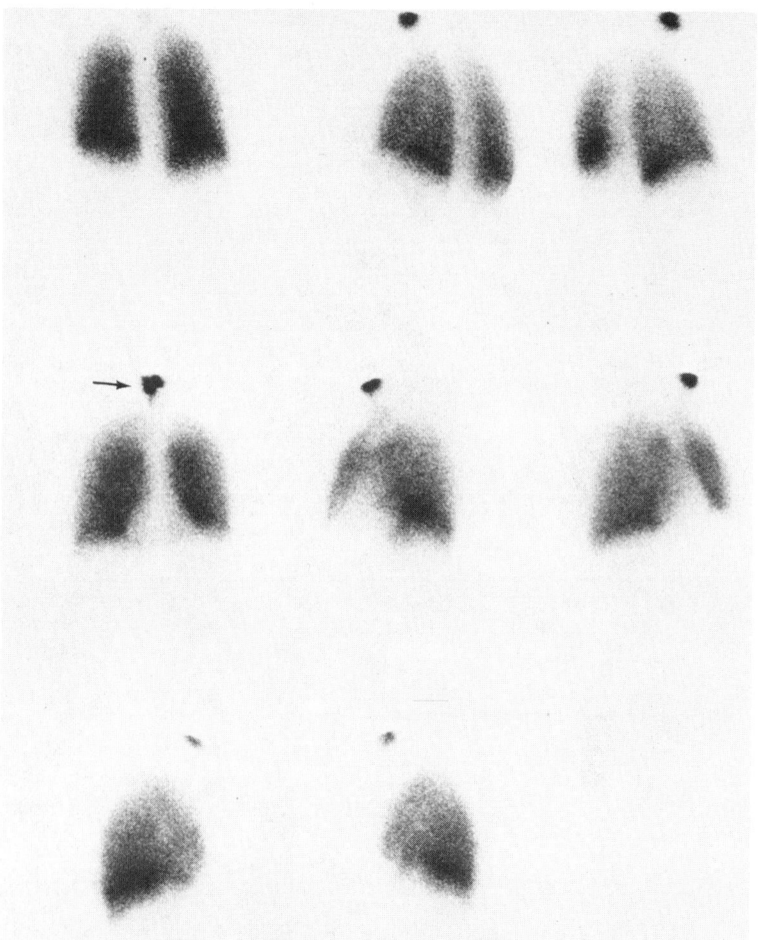

Figure 12.7 Normal Tc-99m pentetate (DTPA) aerosol study. The radiopharmaceutical is well distributed to the lung parenchyma. Some activity is seen (arrow) in the region of the oropharynx. (Study courtesy of J.W. Keys, Jr., Georgetown University Hospital, Washington, DC.)

It is generally accepted that most radioaerosol systems usually deliver to the lungs less than 5% of the total radioactivity placed into the nebulizer system. Associated technical difficulties in the delivery and migration of the aerosol in the necessarily closed system contribute to this relatively low amount of the radioaerosol that reaches the patient's lungs. S. A. Sirr and associates (1985) examined the effect of adding ethanol (10% by volume) to the Tc-99m pentetate and found a significant increase (almost a factor of 2) in the number of aerosol droplets produced per unit of time with no effect upon droplet size. The addition of ethanol did not affect clearance half-times of Tc-99m pentetate from the lungs of healthy patients.

PHARMACOKINETICS

Krypton-81m, Xenon-133, and Xenon-127. Though Krypton-81m and the radioisotopes of xenon are readily diffusible gases that pass freely through cell membranes and exchange between blood and tissues (Yeh SY and Peterson RE, 1963), they are physiologically and biologically inert by virtue of their noble gas properties. As a result of their lipophilic nature, however, xenon concentrates more

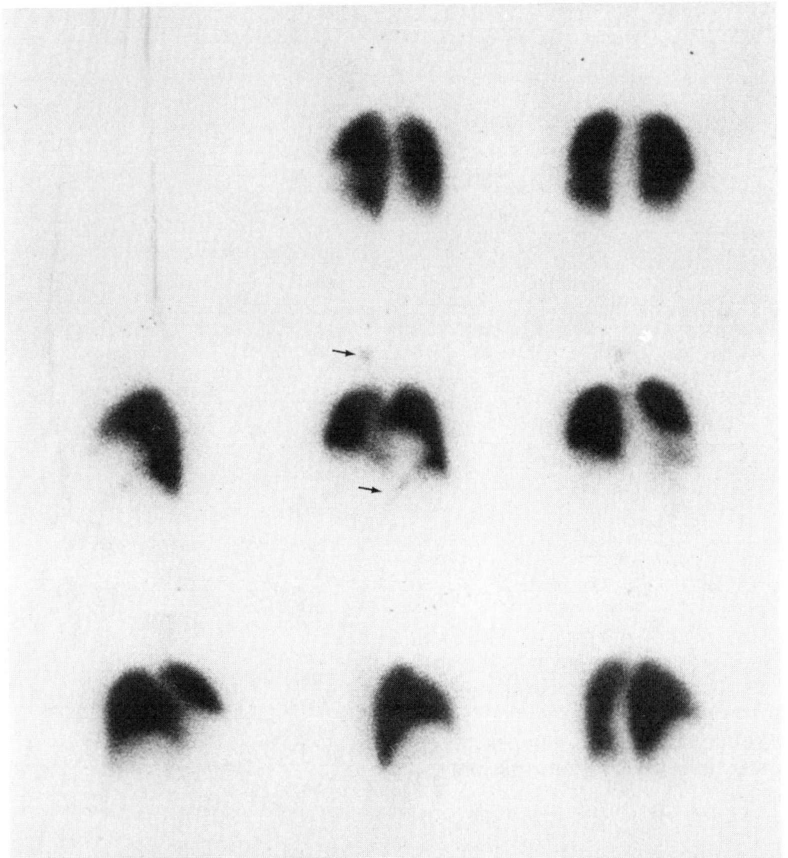

Figure 12.8 Essentially normal Tc-99m pentetate (DTPA) aerosol study. Note evidence of minimal tracheal and gastric activity (arrows). (Courtesy of J.W. Keyes, Jr. Georgetown University Hospital, Washington, DC.)

in body fat than in blood, plasma, water, and protein solutions. Although inhaled krypton and xenon enter the alveolar wall and the pulmonary venous circulation, most of the blood-borne radioactivity is returned to the lungs and exhaled after a single pass through the circulation.

Upon inspiration, the radioxenon gases initially distribute within the lungs as a function of ventilation with eventual diffusion of the gases occurring into nonventilated areas. During rebreathing with room air, the radiogases are rapidly expired from regions of normal ventilation (Figure 12.9). (Following a single inhalation of radioxenon, a biological half-life of less than 2 minutes is observed in normal lungs.) In patients with chronic obstructive pulmonary diseases, trapping of the radioactive xenon gas in the involved areas is observed during this expiratory or "washout" phase of the ventilation study.

The short physical half-life (13 seconds) of Krypton-81m precludes imaging of gas trapping in abnormally ventilated regions of the lung during the washout phase of ventilation imaging. The clinical case of Krypton-81m for demonstrating altered areas of ventilation is based on the fact that its ultra-short physical half-life results in the rapid decay of inhaled Kr-81m and allows visualization of only those areas that ventilate. Equilibration-type images are not obtained; therefore, regions of lung that do not ventilate appear as "cold" defects during continuous breathing of this radioactive gas.

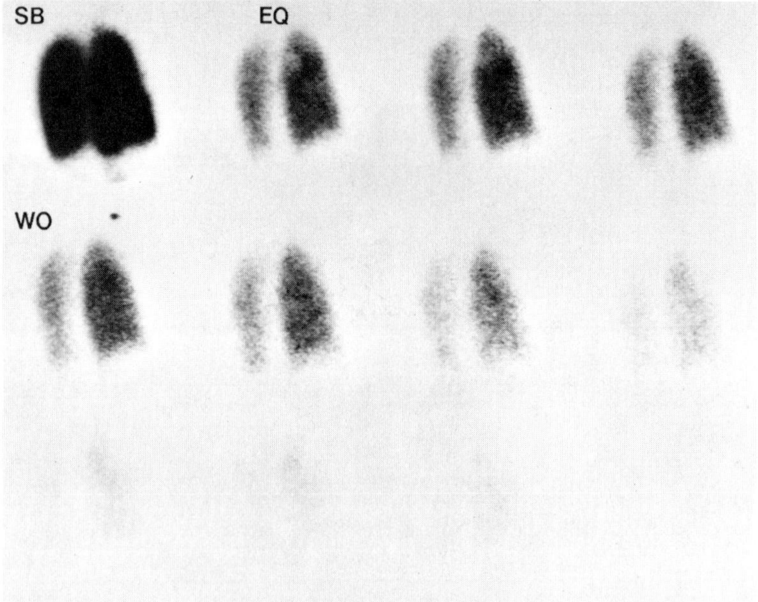

Figure 12.9   Lung ventilation study performed with 5 millicuries of Xenon-127. Patient is imaged in the right posterior oblique orientation and demonstrates uniform ventilation with no appreciable areas of gas trapping. Study consists of single breath image (SB), with subsequent 30-second images taken of gas equilibration (EQ) and washout (WO) from the lungs.

Radioaerosols. Radioaerosols of appropriately small particle size (see Chemistry) distribute within the lungs as a function of ventilation. Agents commonly used as radioaerosols (i. e., Tc-99m pentetate) are highly water soluble and therefore, do not diffuse with time into nonventilated areas of the lungs. Hence, regions of altered ventilation appear as nonradioactive areas (i. e., "cold" defects) on radioaerosol images.

Clearance of Tc-99m pentetate from the lungs appears to depend primarily on diffusion through the alveolar-capillary barrier rather than mucociliary transport or regional blood flow. It is possible, however, that ciliary action may play some role in the clearance of Tc-99m pentetate deposited in the proximal airways. The measurement of the clearance times of Tc-99m pentetate from the lungs of normal controls has been found by several investigators to be slightly less than 1 hour (range: 53–59 minutes). Cigarette smoke and other noxious materials that produce alterations in the epithelial morphology of the lungs may be responsible for an increase in the permeability of this barrier (Mason GR, et al, 1983). J. G.

Jones and associates (1980) and B. D. Minty and associates (1981) reported that the clearance of Tc-99m pentetate is accelerated among smokers and that this abnormality rapidly returns to normal with cessation of smoking. Following absorption, Tc-99m pentetate is rapidly cleared from blood via renal excretion (GFR).

A. T. Isitman and associates (1988) compared radioaerosols of Tc-99m pentetate and Tc-99m pyrophosphate in smokers and nonsmokers and found significantly longer retention of Tc-99m pyrophosphate (clearance $T_{1/2}$ of 1.2 hrs vs 0.6 hrs for Tc-99m pentetate). They obtained superior images with Tc-99m pyrophosphate and suggest the slower alveolar clearance makes it better suited for SPECT and post-perfusion planar imaging.

PRECAUTIONS

Radioisotopes of Xenon. Clinical facilities using radioactive xenon are required by the Nuclear Regulatory Commission (NRC) and most state regulatory agencies to use some type of gas-trapping device to contain and store exhaled xenon for decay. In the past, direct atmospheric release of xenon was a common practice. Atmospheric release is undesirable, however, as xenon released in this fashion may reenter the building through ventilation intakes or open windows. Charcoal trapping of xenon is an effective alternative to direct atmospheric release because the xenon gas is captured and safely contained as radioactive waste for decay. In the trapping procedure, expired breath containing xenon is pumped through an activated charcoal cartridge that binds xenon by adsorption (Bolmsjo MS and Persson BRR, 1982). However, because xenon atoms are only weakly bound to charcoal (by van der Waal's forces), the adsorption of xenon is followed by its desorption with each repeated use of the trap. Movement of xenon through the trap is continually subjected to this adsorptive/desorptive process, so that transit of xenon through the trap is prolonged. Eventually, any xenon remaining after decay clears the effluent side of the trap; however, the amount of xenon activity discharged is low because considerable decay occurs from the time xenon is initially placed onto the trap until it is released.

The discharge of xenon from the trap can be minimized by a trap design that optimizes the relationship between the time xenon is adsorbed and its physical decay. Physical factors affecting xenon hold-up in the trap include charcoal mass, size, and quality; airflow rates through the trap; and the operating temperature of the trap. Since carbon dioxide and moisture decrease gas-trapping efficiency, gas-drying prefilters and carbon dioxide trapping devices are integral to the trap performance and its usable lifetime. Still, with frequent and repeated use, gas saturation of the charcoal cartridge may occur, eventually necessitating its replacement.

Concern for environmental contamination with Krypton-81m is unrealistic because its ultra-short physical half-life of 13 seconds prohibits its presence in the immediate environment in measurable quantities beyond very short periods of time (i. e., less than a minute).

Use During Pregnancy/Breastfeeding. Although both krypton and xenon are physiologically inert, their use during pregnancy should be carefully considered in relation to potential risk. It is not known whether xenon and krypton are excreted in breast milk.

It is not known whether Tc-99m pentetate crosses the placenta; however, Tc-99m pertechnetate, an impurity that exists in varying amounts in Tc-99m pentetate, crosses the placenta. Any decision to use Tc-99m pentetate during pregnancy, therefore, must be carefully weighed against risks that might be reasonably expected to occur. P.J. Mountford and associates (1984) detected levels of radioactivity in breast milk following a Tc-99m pentetate aerosol study and suggested that breastfeeding need not be interrupted for more than 4 hours after the aerosol study.

Side Effects/Adverse Reactions. No adverse reactions have been reported with the use of these ventilatory radiopharmaceuticals.

Causes of Altered Biodistribution/Drug Interference. Case reports have detailed that xenon accumulates in the liver in the presence of excess fat (Susskind H, et al, 1977; Carey JE, et al, 1974). Liver uptake of xenon has been noted in patients with conditions that predispose them to fatty liver, namely, diabetes mellitus, obesity, alcoholic fatty infiltration, hypercholesterolemia, and coronary artery disease.

Radioaerosol Imaging. Upon completion of radioaerosol inhalation, patients should rinse their mouths and expectorate into a disposable container to prevent any activity from appearing in the esophagus and interfering with the interpretation of pulmonary ventilation.

CLINICAL CONSIDERATIONS

Clinical Indications. Pulmonary perfusion imaging is a relatively low-risk procedure that is highly useful in the diagnosis of pulmonary embolism. It is well known that a negative perfusion study virtually excludes the presence of significant pulmonary emboli, and a ventilation study performed in this situation provides no additional diagnostic information. Perfusion abnormalities, however, are too nonspecific to indicate only the presence of pulmonary embolism (Poulose K, et al, 1968). If perfusion defects are similar to or less marked than abnormalities present on a current chest radiograph (less than 24 hours old), the study may be regarded as predictably positive. Ventilation imaging is not indicated because any abnormalities noted on the chest x-ray would also ventilate abnormally. If the chest radiograph is normal or less markedly abnormal than corresponding areas on the perfusion study, an accompanying ventilation study (either radiogas or radioaerosol) would significantly increase diagnostic specificity (McNeil BJ, et al, 1974).

Areas that perfuse *abnormally* but ventilate *normally* (perfusion-ventilation mismatch) favor the diagnosis of pulmonary emboli (Figure 12.10). The probability of pulmonary emboli is directly related to both the number and the size of the perfusion-ventilation mismatches. On the other hand, areas that both perfuse and ventilate abnormally (perfusion-ventilation match) (Figure 12.11) are highly indicative of a primary pulmonary parenchymal disorder such as chronic obstructive pulmonary disease (COPD).

Ventilation studies are also useful in the evaluation of inhalation injuries. Inhalation of noxious agents typically results in areas of air trapping identified on the washout portion of a xenon ventilation study.

Radiopharmaceutical Considerations. Radioisotopes of xenon are used in over half of the ventilation studies performed in the United States, and Xe-133 is employed in the majority of these ventilation studies. The primary advantage of xenon ventilation imaging is its ability to offer physiologic evaluation of the lung in the three phases of ventilation (*single breath, equilibration, and washout*). Xenon is also economical and readily available. Unfortu-

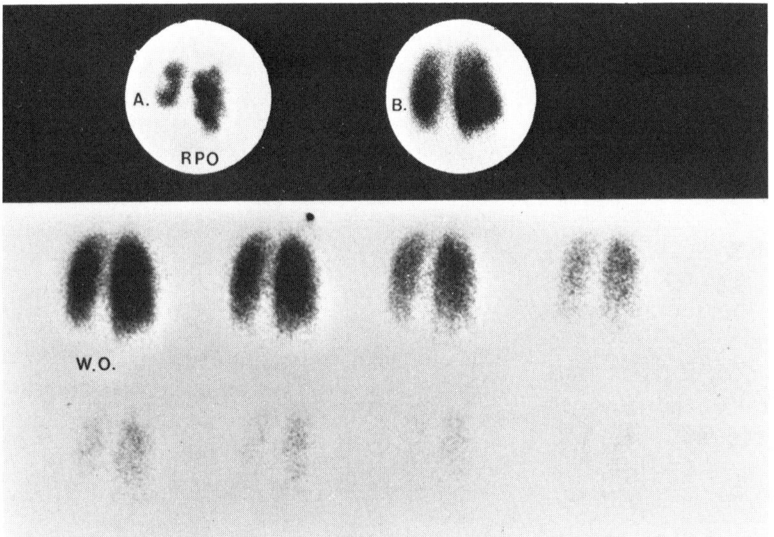

Figure 12.10 Mutiple lung perfusion abnormalities in the lungs of this individual are best observed in the right posterior oblique projection (Image A). The single breath Xenon-127 ventilation image (Image B) shows no ventilation abnormalities and an otherwise normal appearance of the radioactive gas is noted during the washout (W.O.) portion of the ventilation study. The classic "mismatch" of abnormal perfusion with normal ventilation is indicative of pulmonary emboli.

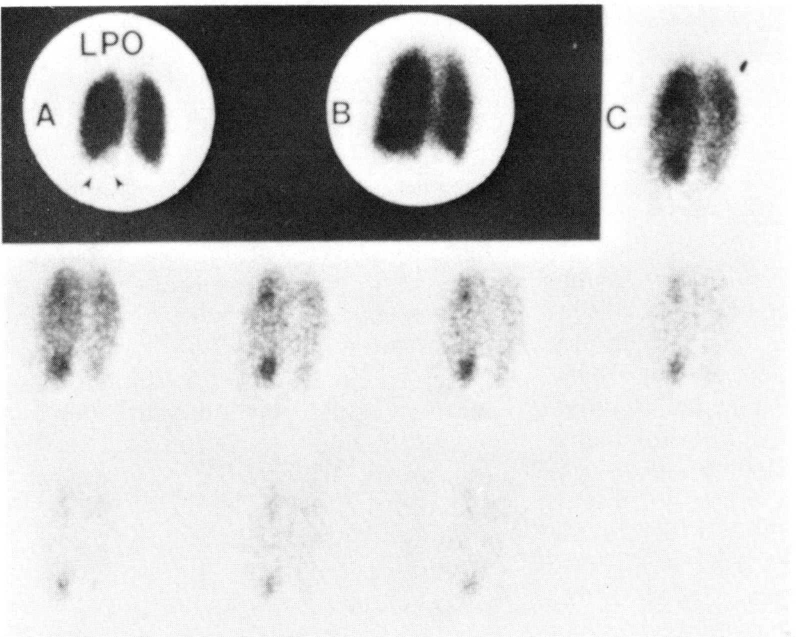

Figure 12.11 Lung perfusion image performed with 5 millicuries of Tc-99m MAA that demonstrates a large perfusion defect best noted at base of left lung in left posterior oblique image (LPO) (Image A). Single breath Xenon-127 ventilation image (B) is essentially normal; however, the area of the previously noted perfusion defect appears as a prominent region of gastrapping during washout imaging (Image C). The "matched" nature of the observed perfusion and the ventilation abnormalities are usually indicative of chronic obstructive lung disease.

nately, the primary 81 keV photon emission of Xe-133 is less than that of Tc-99m (140 keV) so that ventilation imaging with Xe-133 is ideally performed either before the perfusion study or on the following day, after decay and clearance of the Tc-99m lung agent. Alternatively, Xe-133 ventilation imaging can be performed immediately following the Tc-99m perfusion study if computer subtraction techniques are applied (i.e., subtraction of the residual Tc-99m activity that falls within the Xe-133 window).

The implications of performing the ventilation study prior to perfusion imaging are obvious. First, the patient may be unnecessarily ventilated if no perfusion abnormalities are noted on the subsequent perfusion study. Second, the ventilation study may be performed in a projection that does not permit optimal visualization of any yet-to-be-observed perfusion abnormality. Other disadvantageous properties of Xe-133 include the decreased energy resolution of the relatively low energy 81 keV photons and their low photon abundance (i.e., < 35 photons are formed per 100 disintegrating atoms), decay by β^- emission, and the inability to obtain more than one view during a single ventilation study.

Another radioisotope of xenon, Xe-127, is available for use in pulmonary ventilation imaging. The higher-energy, principal photons of Xe-127 (173 and 203 keV) permit ventilation imaging to be performed immediately following a Tc-99m perfusion study without image degradation (Atkins HL, et al, 1977; Coates G and Nahmias C, 1977). Since Xe-127 can be imaged in the presence of Tc-99m, the patient may be placed in the position that allows optimal visualization of the previously noted perfusion defect. Other advantageous properties of Xe-127 include the increased energy resolution associated with the higher energy photons, high proton yields (i.e., approximately 93 usable photons per 100 disintegrating atoms), and decay by electron capture with no particulate emissions. Additionally, its relatively long physical half-life (36.4 days) allows on-site storage for significant periods of time until its use is indicated. The relatively long half-life presents no significant radiation burden to the patient, however, since xenon is physiologically inert and rapidly eliminated from the lungs and blood. Disadvantages of Xe-127 are limited to the inability to obtain more than one view during the ventilation study, restricted availability because few sites are capable of producing Xe-127, and the regulatory requirement to trap and contain expired Xe-127 for decay. This last consideration may require additional lead shielding for existing Xe-133 trapping devices because Xe-127 has principal photon emissions that are more energetic than those of Xe-133. Also, the longer half-life of Xe-127 may require some modifications in trap design (i.e., longer charcoal length) in order to lessen a likelihood of Xe-127 release before substantial decay has occurred.

Krypton-81m, like Xe-127, has a principal photon energy (i.e., 190 keV) higher than that of Tc-99m, thus enabling ventilation imaging to be selectively performed following Tc-99m perfusion imaging (Fazio F, 1975; Goris ML, et al, 1977). Krypton-81m also decays by electron capture and provides relatively minimal radiation exposure to the patient. Another advantage of Kr-81m is that multiple views of ventilation can be obtained, because a patient can continuously breathe the relatively short-lived radiopharmaceutical. However, this extremely short half-life does not permit the buildup of Kr-81m in diseased regions of the lung, and the subsequent visualization of these areas during the gas washout phase (see Pharmacokinetics). A major disadvantage to Kr-81m is that its parent, Rb-81, has a 4.7 hour physical half-life, which necessitates daily air freight shipments and limits generator usefulness to the day of delivery only. As a result, Kr-81m may not be available for use after hours and on weekends when emergency, on-call lung studies are often performed. The 13-second physical half-life of Kr-81m is advantageous for disposal, however, and expired Kr-81m is usually exhausted directly into the room with no need for a gas-trapping device or specialized disposal method.

Radioaerosol imaging (Tc-99m pentetate) has been revitalized recently with the development of reliable nebulizers that produce radioaerosols of the desired, submicronic size necessary for uniform lung distribution. Because radioaerosol particles are temporarily distributed in the airways, multiple views of ventilation are permitted. Radioaerosol imaging can be performed following Tc-99m perfusion imaging; however, because both the perfusion and the radioaerosol radiopharmaceuticals utilize Tc-99m, adjustments are required in the amount of activities administered in order to avoid interpretation problems. When perfusion imaging precedes the radioaerosol study, the amount of Tc-99m MAA agent administered must be adjusted downward (i.e., usually less than 2 mCi) to optimize visualization of the subsequently administered radioaerosol in the presence of the previously administered Tc-99m agent. Furthermore, with radioaerosol imaging it is not possible to evaluate washout phases of ventilation wherein areas of ventilatory disease are often best demonstrated as regions of gas trapping.

Because each ventilation method has advantages and disadvantages that influence its desirability in given clinical settings, which method is superior has been the subject of considerable debate. Clinical comparisons have been made for radioaerosols, Kr-81m, and the radioxenons in different types of lung disease. P.O. Alderson and associates (1984) found diagnostic equivalence for pulmonary emboli. Compared to the radioaerosols and Kr-81m, however, xenon trapping during the washout imaging phase (which is not observed on radioaerosol imaging or Kr-81m imaging) appears to be a more sensitive indicator of obstructive pulmonary disease (Alderson PO, et al, 1974; 1979). Although L. Ramanna and associates (1986) noted this discordance

Table 12.6 DOSAGE AND RADIATION DOSIMETRY INFORMATION RELATING TO THE USE OF Kr-81m, Xe-127, AND Xe-133

	KRYPTON-81M[a]	XENON-127[b]	XENON-133[b]
Activity to administer:	1–10 mCi	5–10 mCi	10–20 mCi
Radiation dosimetry:	*mrads/mCi—min*	*mrads/mCi*	*mrads/mCi*
Lungs	2.5	6.0	8.0
Total body	0.055	1.7	1.1
Ovaries	<0.001	2.0	1.0
Testes	<0.001	0.8	1.0
Bladder	<0.001	1.4	1.4
Kidneys	0.06	1.4	1.4

[a] Administered as a continuous inhalation. (From MPI Krypton Kr-81m gas generator, 1979.)

[b] Administered either as a single inhalation or as a homogeneous mixture of xenon and air. Volume of air in closed-circuit breathing apparatus assumed to be 7.5 L. (From Atkins HL, et al. 1980.)

between xenon and aerosol imaging, they concluded that gas trapping defects noted with xenon were the result of unimpressive perfusion defects that did not change the scintigraphic probability for pulmonary embolism in any patient they studied. Among the currently available radioisotopes of xenon, Xe-127 is superior for ventilation imaging.

Dosage/Dosimetry

Dosage and dosimetry information relating to the use of Kr-81m, Xe-127, and Xe-133 are listed in Table 12.6. Radiation dosimetry for Tc-99m pentetate administered as a radioaerosol is listed in Table 12.7.

Table 12.7 ABSORBED RADIATION DOSIMETRY FOR Tc-99m PENTETATE (DTPA)[a] ADMINISTERED AS A RADIOAEROSOL

ORGAN	^{99m}TC-PENTETATE (AEROSOL) RADS/MCI[b]
Lungs	0.097
Bladder	0.35
Kidneys	0.029
Red marrow	0.022
Ovaries	0.031
Testes	0.017
Total body	0.017

[a] Personal communication, Radiopharmaceutical Internal Dosimetry Information Center, Oak Ridge Associated Universities (ORAU), TN.

[b] Assumptions: (1) Radioaerosol completely absorbed from lungs with corresponding biological half-life in lungs of 1 hour; (2) lung deposition fraction and kinetic model from ICRP-30; and (3) aerosol is approximately 0.25 μ MMAD (Mass Median Aerodynamic Diameter).

Method: Xenon Ventilation Imaging. In xenon ventilation imaging, the patient inhales a small quantity of xenon while images of gas distribution in the lungs are obtained during various phases of breathing (e. g., breathhold, rebreathing, and gas washout from lungs). The prevalent method incorporates a closed-circuit breathing apparatus to safely contain the xenon. The patient inhales the radioactive xenon from this device either as a bolus or as a mixture of xenon in air. As the patient breathes xenon from the closed-circuit breathing apparatus, images of xenon distribution in the lungs are obtained serially, usually requiring approximately 10–30 seconds/image. When the gas concentrations in the patient's lungs

and the breathing device are essentially equal (the "equilibrium" image), the system is opened to allow the patient to breathe room air only. The expired xenon is trapped or contained within the breathing device for subsequent disposal in accordance with applicable regulatory guidelines. Imaging is performed during this later phase to obtain the washout images. An often-performed variation of this procedure is that in which patients are asked at the beginning of the study to hold their breath while an image (the "wash in" image) records the distribution of gas in the lungs during the initial tidal inspiration.

Method: Krypton-81m Ventilation Imaging. Because of the very short physical half-life of Kr-81m, the patient can breathe the gas directly from its generator source without a special gas-containment device or gas-administration system. The procedure requires the use of a full-face mask or a mouthpiece and nose clamp connected in line with the Rb-81/Kr-81m generator (Ruth TJ, et al, 1980). Images of the Kr-81m distribution in the lungs are obtained as the patient breathes Kr-81m directly from the generator. The patient can exhale Kr-81m directly into the room because, as a result of its ultra-short physical half-life, no significant buildup of radioactivity occurs in the room.

Method: Radioaerosol Imaging. Essential elements of any radioaerosol delivery system include an oxygen source (with airflow regulator), a nebulizer, disposable tubing, a bacterial filter (necessary to trap exhaled radioaerosol and prevent environmental contamination), and shielding, as required. For most procedures the radioaerosol is administered to patients seated in an upright position. Although this position is more convenient for administering the radioaerosol, an associated increase in basal deposition of radioactivity can result. A more even distribution of radioaerosol may be obtained by having the patient breathe the radioaerosol while in a supine position. A mouthpiece is utilized for the inhalation of the radioaerosol, and a noseclamp is fitted on the patient to prevent inadvertent exhalation of the radioaerosol into the room.

Between 30 and 75 millicuries of Tc-99m pentetate in a volume of 2–3 milliliters is added to the nebulizer after the patient has been allowed to acclimate to the delivery system. With the patient breathing normally, an oxygen flow rate of 8–10 L/min is maintained for approximately 2–4 minutes in order to deliver the radioaerosol to the patient's lungs. Depending upon the activity added to the nebulizer, the efficiency of the delivery system, and the patient's ability to cooperate during the inhalation procedure, sufficient radioaerosol is usually inhaled over this time period to produce a count rate of 150,000–250,000 per 1–2 minute image. Additionally, it is not a requirement of this procedure that the radio-

aerosol inhalation be performed in the camera room. In fact, since pulmonary distribution of the radioaerosol is transiently retained after administration and does not constitute a source of environmental contamination, any room can be used for the radioaerosol administration. Also for this reason, multiple images of radiopharmaceutical distribution in the lungs can be obtained.

The radiopharmaceuticals employed for both the pulmonary perfusion and the radioaerosol imaging studies utilize Tc-99m. Perfusion imaging can be performed as a follow-up to radioaerosol imaging, provided the amount of the Tc-99m perfusion radiopharmaceutical administration is increased substantially. A disadvantage to this imaging sequence is that radioaerosol studies may be performed unnecessarily whenever the subsequent perfusion study turns out to be normal. If the perfusion study is performed first, the follow-up radioaerosol study may be interpreted with difficulty in the presence of the residual activity of the perfusion radiopharmaceutical. Radioaerosol imaging following lung perfusion imaging can be accomplished by (1) decreasing the amount of Tc-99m perfusion agent to 1–2 mCi, and (2) utilizing longer inhalation times (perhaps as long as 10 minutes) during radioaerosol administration. Though this technique allows for lung studies to be performed in the ideal sequence (i.e., performing selective ventilation imaging only when appropriate), routine perfusion studies take proportionally longer to perform because of the lower administered dose.

Other Clinical Applications (Xenon).

Blood-Flow Measurements. The relatively inert nature of xenon permits its use as a freely diffusible tracer for the measurement of skin and cerebral blood flow (Daly MJ and Henry RC, 1980; Obrist WD, et al, 1975) and to estimate the level of amputation (Malone JM, et al, 1981). For skin blood-flow measurements, xenon is dissolved in saline and injected intradermally, and the clearance (washout) of radioactivity from that site is monitored. For cerebral blood-flow measurements xenon is most often administered by inhalation, and the activity washout is determined by the use of probe-type detectors placed about the head.

References

Alderson PO, Biello DR, Gottschalk A. Tc-99m DTPA aerosol and radioactive gases compared as adjuncts to perfusion scintigraphy in patients with suspected pulmonary embolism. *Radiology* 1984, 153:515–521.

Alderson PO, Lee H, Summer WR, et al. Comparison of Xe-133 washout and single-breath imaging for the detection of ventilation abnormalities. *J Nucl Med* 1979, 20:917–922.

Alderson PO, Secker-Walker BH, Forrest JV. Detection of obstructive pulmonary disease: Relative sensitivity of ventilation-perfusion studies and chest radiography. *Radiology* 1974, 112:643–648.

Allen DR, Nelp WB, Cheney F, et al. Studies of acute cardiopulmonary toxicity of Sn-macroaggregated albumin in the dog. *J Nucl Med* 1974, 15:567–571.

Atkins HL, Robertson JS, Croft BY, et al. Estimates of radiation absorbed doses from radioxenons in lung imaging. *J Nucl Med* 1980, 21:459–465.

Atkins HL, Susskind H, Klopper JF, et al. A clinical comparison of Xe-127 and Xe-133 for ventilation studies. *J Nucl Med* 1977, 18:653–658.

Bolmsjo MS, Persson BRR. Factors affecting the trapping performance of xenon hold-up filters in nuclear medicine applications. *Med Phys* 1982, 9:96–105.

Boyd RE, Ackerman, SA. Lung scanning using ^{99m}Tc-labeled macroaggregated ferrous hydroxide (Tc-MAFH) as the perfusion agent. *J Nucl Med* 1969, 10:737–739.

Brain JD, Valberg PA. Deposition of aerosol in the respiratory tract. *Am Rev Respir Dis* 1979, 120:1325–1373.

Bruno RE, Brookeman VA, Arborelius M, et al. ^{99m}Tc-iron hydroxide aggregates for lung scanning. *J Nucl Med* 1970, 11:134–137.

Burch WM, Tetley, IJ, Gras JL. Technetium-99m "pseudo-gas" for diagnostic studies of the lung. *Clin Phys Physiol Meas* 1984, 5:79–85.

Burdine JA, Sonnemaker RE, Ryder LA, et al. Perfusion studies with technetium-99m human albumin microspheres (HAM). *Radiology* 1970, 95:101–107.

Carey JE, Purdy JM, Moses DC. Localization of xenon-133 in liver during ventilation studies. *J Nucl Med* 1974, 15:1179–1181.

Coates G, Nahmias C. Xenon-127, a comparison with xenon-133 in liver during ventilation studies. *J Nucl Med* 1977, 18:221–225.

Cordova MA, Rhodes BA, Atkins HL, et al. Adverse reactions to radiopharmaceuticals. *J Nucl Med* 1982, 23:550–551.

Cranage R, Palmer M. Breast-milk radioactivity after ^{99m}Tc-MAA lung studies. *Eur J Nucl Med* 1985, 11:257–259.

Daly MJ, Henry RC. Quatitative measurement of skin perfusion with Xenon-133. *J Nucl Med* 1980, 21:156–160.

Davies G, Reid L. Growth of the alveoli and pulmonary arteries in children. *Thorax* 1970, 25:669–681.

Davis MA. Particulate radiopharmaceuticals for pulmonary studies. In *Radiopharmaceuticals* (Subramanian G, Rhodes BA, et al, eds.). New York, Society of Nuclear Medicine, 1975, pp. 267–280.

Dworkin HJ, Gutkowski RF, Porter W, et al. Effect of particle number on lung perfusion images: Concise communication. *J Nucl Med* 1977, 18:260–262.

Fawdry R, Bush V, King T, et al. Initial experience with technegas—a new ventilation agent (Abst). *J Nucl Med* 1988, 29:765.

Fazio F. Assessment of regional lung ventilation by continuous inhalation of radioactive krypton-81m *Br Med J* [*Clin Res*] 1975, 3:673–676.

Finn JP, Myers MJ, Nair KM, et al. Clinical comparison of a new Tc-99m DTPA delivery system with Kr-81m. *J Nucl Med* 1984, 25:P68.

George DL. Permissible concentration in

air of xenon-127: Concise communication. *J Nucl Med* 1978, 19:105–106.

Goris ML, Daspit SG, Walter JP, et al. Applications of ventilation lung imaging with [81m]krypton. *Radiology* 1977, 122:399–403.

Harding LK, Horsfield K, Singhal SS, et al. The proportion of lung vessels blocked by albumin microspheres. *J Nucl Med* 1973, 14:579–581.

Hayes M, Taplin GV. Lung imaging with radioaerosols for the assessment of airway disease. *Semin Nucl Med* 1980, 10:243–251.

Haynie TP, Calhoon JH, Nasjletti CE, et al. Visualization of pulmonary artery occlusion by photoscanning. *JAMA* 1963, 185(4):306–308.

Heck LL, Duley JW. Statistical considerations in lung imaging with ^{99m}Tc albumin particles. *Radiology* 1974, 113:675–679.

Heyman S. Toxicity and safety factors associated with lung perfusion studies with radiolabeled particles (Letter). *J Nucl Med* 1979, 10:1098–1099.

Hoffer PB, Harper PV, Beck RN, et al. Improved xenon images with [127]Xe. *J Nucl Med* 1973, 14:172–174.

Isitman AT, Palmer WT, Hoffman RE, et al. Comparison of Tc-99m DTPA and PYP aerosols in smokers and non-smokers (Abst). Proceedings of 74th Scientific assembly and annual meeting. *Radiology* 1988, 169(P):201.

Jones JG, Minty BD, Lawler P. Increased alveolar permeability in cigarette smokers. *Lancet* 1980, 1:66–68.

Knipping HW, Bolt W, and Valentin H. Regionale funktionsanalyse in der kreislauf- and lungenklinik mit hilfe der isotopenthorakographie und der selektiven angiographie der lungengefasse. *Munch Med Wochenschr* 1957, 99:46–47.

LeBlanc AD, Johnson PC. The handling of Xe-133 in clinical studies. *Phys Med Biol* 1961, 16:105–109.

Levine G. A model for administering the desired number of particles for pulmonary perfusion studies. *J Nucl Med Technol* 1980, 8:33–36.

Lippman M, Yeates DB, Albert RE. Deposition, retention, and clearance of inhaled particles. *Br J Ind Med* 1980, 37:337–362.

Liuzzi A, Keany J, Freedman G. Use of activated charcoal and containment of ^{133}Xe exhaled during pulmonary studies. *J Nucl Med* 1972, 13:673–676.

Malone JM, Leal JM, Moore WS, et al. The "gold standard" for amputation level selection: Xenon-133 clearance. *J Surg Res* 1981, 30:449–456.

Mantel J, Cook KJ, Corrigan KE. Radioactive krypton and xenon trapping by cryogenic technics. *Radiology* 1968, 90:590–591.

Mason GR, Uszler JM, Effros RM, et al. Rapidly reversible alterations of pulmonary epithelial permeability induced by smoking. *Chest* 1983, 83:6–11.

McLean JR, Welch WJ, Rockwell LJ. Quality control procedures for ^{99m}Tc-MAA. *Int J Nucl Med Biol* 1979, 6:142–143.

McLean JR, Wise P. Impurities in a ^{99m}Tc lung imaging kit. *J Nucl Med Technol* 1977, 5:28–31.

McNeil BJ, Holman BL, and Adelstein SJ. The scintigraphic definition of pulmonary embolism. *J Am Med Assoc* 1974, 227:753–756.

Minty BD, Jordan C, Jones JG. Rapid improvement in pulmonary epithelial permeability after stopping cigarettes. *Br Med J* 1981, 282:1183–1186.

Mishkin FS, Brashear, RE. Pulmonary and systemic blood pressure responses to large doses of albumin microspheres. *J Nucl Med* 1971, 12:251–252.

MPI Krypton Kr-81m gas generator, Medi-Physics, Inc, Emeryville, CA, 1979.

Mountford PJ, Hall FM, Wells CP, et al. Breast-milk radioactivity after a Tc-99m DTPA aerosol/Tc-99m MAA lung study. *J Nucl Med* 1984, 25:1108–1110.

Muehlbaecher CA, DeBon FL, Featherstone RM. Further studies on the solubilities of xenon and cyclopropane in blood and protein solutions. *Mol Pharmacol* 1966, 2:86–89.

Obrist WD, Thompson HK, Jr, Wang

HS, et al. Regional cerebral blood flow estimated by Xe-133 inhalation. *Stroke* 1975, 6:245–256.

Pasqualini R, Plassio G, Sosi S. The preparation of albumin microspheres. *J Nucl Med Biol* 1969, 13:80–84.

Ponto RA, Kush GS, Loken MK. Considerations of problems in handling and radiation dosimetry of ^{133}Xe. *J Nucl Med* 1970, 11:352.

Poulose K, Reba RC, Wagner HN, Jr. Characteristics of the shape and location of perfusion defects in certain pulmonary diseases. *N Engl J Med* 1968, 279:1020–1025.

Quinn JL, III, Whitley JE, Hudspeth AS, et al. Early clinical application of lung scintiscanning. *Radiology* 1964, 82:315–318.

Ramanna L, Alderson PO, Waxman AD, et al. Regional comparison of technetium-99m DTPA aerosol and radioactive gas ventilation (xenon and krypton) studies in patients with suspected pulmonary embolism. *J Nucl Med* 1986, 27:1391–1396.

Rhodes BA, Zolle I, Buchanan JW, et al. Radioactive albumin microspheres for studies of the pulmonary circulation. *Radiology* 1969, 92:1453–1460.

Rhodes BA, Bolles TF. Albumin microspheres: Current methods of preparation and use. In *Radiopharmaceuticals* (Subramanian G, Rhodes BA, et al, eds.). New York, Society of Nuclear Medicine, 1975, pp. 282–291.

Rhodes BA, Cordova MA. Adverse reactions to radiopharmaceuticals: Incidence in 1978, and associated symptoms. Report of the Adverse Reactions Subcommittee of the Society of Nuclear Medicine. *J Nucl Med* 1979, 21:1107–1110.

Rimkus DS, Ashburn WL. Lung ventilation scanning with technetium-99m labeled carbon particles ("Technegas") *J Nucl Med* 1988, 29:765.

Romney BM, Nickoloff EL, Esser PD, et al. Radionuclide administration to nursing mothers: Mathematically derived guidelines. *Radiology* 1986, 160:549–554.

Ruth TJ, Lambrecht RM, Wolf AP, et al. Cyclotron isotopes and radiopharmaceuticals—XXX. Aspects of production, elution, and automation of ^{81}Rb–^{81m}Kr generators. *Int J Appl Radiat Isot* 1980, 31:51–59.

Sirr SA, Juenemann PJ, Tom H, et al. Effect of ethanol on droplet size, efficiency of delivery, and clearance characteristics of technetium-99m DTPA aerosol. *J Nucl Med* 1985, 26:643–646.

Stern HS, Goodwin DA, Wagner HN, Jr, et al. ^{113m}In—A short-lived isotope for lung scanning. *Nucleonics* 1966, 24(10):57–59.

Susskind H, Atkins HL, Cohn SH, et al. Whole-body retention of radioxenon. *J Nucl Med* 1977, 18:462–471.

Taplin GV, Dore EK, Johnson DE, et al. Colloidal radioalbumin aggregates for organ scanning. In 10th Annual Meeting of the Society of Nuclear Medicine, Montreal, Can., June, 1963.

Taplin GV, Dore EK, Kennady JC, et al. Aggregated albumin labeled with various radioisotopes. In *Radioactive Pharmaceuticals* (Andrews GA, Knisely RM, Wagner HN, Jr, eds.). U.S. Atomic Energy Commission, Division of Technical Information, Oak Ridge, TN, 1966, pp. 525–552.

Taplin GV, Griswold ML, Hurwit J, et al. Radioalbumin suspensions of higher specific activity and more uniform size. *J Nucl Med* 1967, 8:303.

Taplin GV, Johnson DE, Dore EK, et al. Lung photoscans with macroaggregates of human serum radioalbumin. Experimental basis and initial clinical trials. *Health Phys* 1964a, 10, 1219–1227.

Taplin GV, Johnson DE, Dore EK, et al. Organ visualization by photoscanning using micro- and macroaggregates of radioalbumin. In *Medical Radioisotope Scanning*, Vol. 2, International Atomic Energy Agency, Vienna, Austria, 1964b, pp. 3–31.

Vincent WR, Goldberg SJ, Desilets D. Fatality immediately following rapid infusion of macroaggregates of ^{99m}Tc albumin (MAA) for lung scan. *Radiology* 1968, 91:1181–1184.

Wagner HN, Jr, Rhodes BA, Sasaki Y, et al. Studies of the circulation with radioactive microspheres. *Invest Radiol* 1969, 4:374–386.

Wagner HN, Jr, Sabiston DC, Jr, McAfee JG, et al. Diagnosis of massive pulmonary embolism in man by radioisotope scanning. *N Engl J Med* 1964, 271:377–384.

Waldman DL, Weber DA, Oberdorster G, et al. Chemical breakdown of radio-aerosols during nebulization. *J Nucl Med* 1987, 28:378–382.

Weibel ER. *Morphometry of the Human Lung*. Berlin Springer-Verlag, and New York, Academic Press, 1963.

Yano Y, McRae J, Honbo DS, et al. ^{99m}Tc-ferric hydroxide macroaggregates for pulmonary scintiphotography. *J Nucl Med* 1969, 10:683–686.

Yeh SY, Peterson RE. Solubility of carbon monoxide, krypton, and xenon in lipids. *J Pharm Sci* 1963, 52:453–458.

Zolle I, Rhodes BA, Wagner HN, Jr. Preparation of metabolizable radioactive human serum albumin microsphere for studies of the circulation. *Int J Appl Radiat Isot* 1970, 21:155–167.

Radiopharmaceuticals for Cardiac Imaging: Myocardial Infarction, Perfusion, Metabolism, and Ventricular Function (Blood Pool)

Henry M. Chilton
Ronald J. Callahan
James H. Thrall

Nuclear medicine studies of the heart represent one of the fastest growing areas of research and clinical interest. Only a few years ago, nuclear medicine cardiac studies were limited to evaluations of myocardial infarction by means of "hot spot" Tc-99m pyrophosphate imaging or radionuclide angiographic studies. Recent developments in radiopharmaceutical chemistry and advances in nuclear medicine instrumentation, including computer analysis techniques, however, have made possible widespread advances in cardiovascular nuclear medicine. Techniques and radiopharmaceuticals now exist for the imaging of viable myocardium and the determination of myocardial tissue metabolism. Whereas radionuclide angiography initially produced serial images that were similar to x-ray angiography, it is now possible to obtain quantitative information regarding radiopharmaceutical distribution along time-activity curves that can be used to calculate cardiac output, mean transit times, cardiac volumes, and ejection fractions.

For most purposes, nuclear medicine studies of the heart can be divided into two categories that are based largely upon the clinical information sought: direct imaging of the myocardium (either perfused, healthy, or infarcted tissues), and determination of quantitative cardiac function. In addition, these two categories can be further broken into groups based on specific differences in the diagnostic properties of the radiopharmaceuticals that are currently available and employed for these purposes (Table 13.1).

I. Imaging Myocardial Infarction

Tc-99m PYROPHOSPHATE

The ability to detect the presence, location, and size of necrotic myocardial tissue has long been a goal of nuclear

Table 13.1   CLASSIFICATION OF CARDIOVASCULAR NUCLEAR MEDICINE STUDIES ACCORDING TO TYPE OF DIAGNOSTIC INFORMATION OBTAINED AND RADIOPHARMACEUTICALS EMPLOYED

IMAGING CATEGORY	DIAGNOSTIC CLASSIFICATION	RADIOPHARMACEUTICALS
A. Imaging of myocardium	I. Avid infarct	Tc-99m pyrophosphate (PPi)
		In-111 antimyosin antibody
	II. Myocardial perfusion	T1-201 thallous chloride
		Rb-82 rubidium
	III. Metabolic activity	Radiolabeled modified fatty acids
		Radiolabeled glucose analogues
B. Quantitative measurement of ventricular function (the Radionuclide Ventriculogram	I. First-pass imaging	Tc-99m sodium pertechnetate
		Short-lived generator products
	II. Equilibrium gated blood pool imaging	Tc-99m red blood cells (RBCs)
		Tc-99m human serum albumin (HSA)

medicine. To this end, the accurate differentiation of necrotic tissue from salvageable myocardium has great importance in the evaluation of patients for coronary artery bypass and in the selection of candidates for the newer reperfusion therapies. At present, two radiopharmaceuticals Tc-99m pyrophosphate and In-111 antimyosin are available for the detection of myocardial necrosis (infarct-avid agents).

Infarct-avid imaging ("hot spot") with Tc-99m pyrophosphate, a radiopharmaceutical that adsorbs onto hydroxyapatite tissue of bone, was introduced in 1974 by R. W. Parkey and coworkers, and F. J. Bonte and colleagues when they reported the successful use of this radiopharmaceutical for the localization of acute myocardial infarction. This application of Tc-99m pyrophosphate as a means for localizing infarction supported previous observations by A. N. D'Agostino and M. Chiga (1970) that calcium influx during irreversible myocardial injury resulted in the formation of a crystalline hydroxapatitelike substance that closely resembled the crystalline material of bone.

CHEMISTRY

Over the years, a variety of compounds, the majority of which have been totally unrelated (Table 13.2), have been explored for visualization of infarction. As early as 1963, P. Malek and colleagues utilized fluorescence to show the accumulation of tetracycline within the infarcted myocardium. Attempts at developing a radioiodinated form of tetracycline (I-131) were unsuccessful, and further radiolabeling attempts using additional radionuclides were not pursued, thus ending for that time period any further investigation of this agent for avid infarct imaging. During the mid-1960s, work with chloromerodrin (Carr EA, et al, 1963) and hydroxy mercury derivatives of fluorescein labeled with radioisotopes of mercury showed some degree of success. These compounds appeared to bind directly to protein in damaged myocardial cells (Gorten RJ, et al, 1966; Malek P, et al, 1967). Detailed clinical studies, however, were never performed.

Following the introduction of the Mo-99/Tc-99m radionuclide generator, M. K. Dewanjee and colleagues (1972) prepared Tc-99m labeled tetracycline using the stannous-ion-assisted method for the reduction of technetium. B. L. Holman and colleagues (1973) evaluated Tc-99m tetracycline and found significant localization in the liver and blood clearance so slow that imaging could not be performed until 24 hours after radiopharmaceutical administration, thus limiting its clinical utility. The relatively short physical half-life of Tc-99m (6.0 hrs) diminished the amount of radiopharmaceutical remaining the following day for imaging purposes. Another Tc-99m radiopharmaceutical, gluceptate, was shown in animals to be infarct avid; however, clinical trials with this radiopharmaceutical produced disappointingly low target-to-background ratios with a corresponding low detection rate for acute infarcts (Rossman DJ, et al, 1975).

During the late 1970s, the development of several new and superior Tc-99m bone-seeking phosphate and diphosphonate radiopharmaceuticals inspired many studies searching for superior materials for avid infarct imaging. Comparative clinical studies, however, failed to demonstrate any degree of superiority for the newer bone-seeking Tc-99m radiopharmaceuticals (Kelly RJ, et al, 1979; Wakat MA, et al, 1980). Therefore, Tc-99m pyrophosphate remains the radiopharmaceutical of choice for avid infarct imaging.

Table 13.2 SELECTED RADIOPHARMACEUTICALS THAT HAVE BEEN EVALUATED FOR AVID INFARCT IMAGING

I-131 rose bengal
Hg-203 chlormerodrin
Hg-203 mercuric nitrate
Tc-99m tetracycline
Tc-99m gluceptate
Tc-99m medronate (MDP)
Tc-99m oxidronate (HDP)
Tc-99m oxytetracycline
Tc-99m mercaptoisobutyric acid
Tc-99m succimer (DMSA)

Table 13.3 KIT-TYPE FORMULATIONS FOR PREPARATION OF Tc-99m PYROPHOSPHATE CURRENTLY AVAILABLE IN THE UNITED STATES

| | | COMPOSITION | | STORAGE CONDITIONS | |
NAME®	MANUFACTURER	*Substance*	*Amount*	*Unlabeled*	*Labeled*
TechneScan PYP	Mallinckrodt, Inc.	Sodium pyrophosphate Stannous chloride dihydrate pH adjusted with HCl to 4.5–7.5	11.9 mg 3.2–4.4 mg (min–max).	2–8° C	15–30° C
Pyrolite	DuPont-NEN	Product is lyophilized and packaged under nitrogen atmosphere Sodium pyrophosphate Sodium trimetaphosphate Stannous chloride dihydrate pH adjusted with HCl/NaOH to 4.5–5.5	 10 mg 30 mg 0.95–1.8 mg (min–max)	 15–30° C	 15–30° C
Phosphotec	Squibb Diagnostics	Product is lyophilized and packaged under nitrogen atmosphere Sodium pyrophosphate Stannous fluoride pH adjusted with HCl/NaOH Product is lyophilized and packaged under nitrogen atmosphere	 23.9 mg 0.4–0.9 mg (min–max)	 15–30° C	 15–30° C

Information on the several pyrophosphate formulations that are commercially available is shown in Table 13.3. Only one commercial formulation combines significant amounts of sodium trimetaphosphate with sodium pyrophosphate. The benefit of including trimetaphosphate is not entirely clear, although one report (Nelson MF, et al, 1975) has stated that the skeletal uptake of Tc-99m trimetaphosphate is comparable to that of Tc-99m pyrophosphate. Clinical evaluations of Tc-99m trimetaphosphate alone as an avid infarct agent have not been reported.

PHARMACOKINETICS

Biodistribution. Tc-99m pyrophosphate clears rapidly from blood, with less than 8% remaining in blood 3 hours after intravenous administration. Blood clearance appears to be triphasic; the first component (74% of the injected dose) has a half-life of 0.03 hour, the second component (18.3%) 0.64 hour, and the third component (7.4%) 53.7 hours. From 10 to 30% of the remaining blood activity is contained in the red cell fraction between 1 and 3 hours, increasing to 65% of whole-blood activity at 24 hours. Between 40 and 50% of plasma activity is protein bound within the first hour and 55–60% by 3 hours and beyond. Of the total activity administered, 40–50% is deposited in bone. Cumulative urinary excretion for up to 24 hours accounts for approximately 60% of the administered activity (Subramanian G, et al, 1975).

Mechanisms of Localization. Pyrophosphate is known to occur as an endogenous product of cell metabolism normally present in the plasma (0.16–3.4 N mole/liter) and is sometimes present in abnormally high concentrations in pseudogout, osteoarthritis, and acromegaly, and in low concentrations in osteogenesis imperfecta (Subramanian G, et al, 1975). Whether endogenous pyrophosphate plays some role in the healing process of infarction is not known.

It has been postulated that localization of Tc-99m pyrophosphate within an acute myocardial infarction occurs in response to the calcium influx that accompanies cell death, although the precise uptake mechanism within the damaged myocardium is not completely understood. Calcium deposition that occurs during irreversible tissue injury results in the formation of various calcium phosphate complexes that act as sites of uptake for Tc-99m

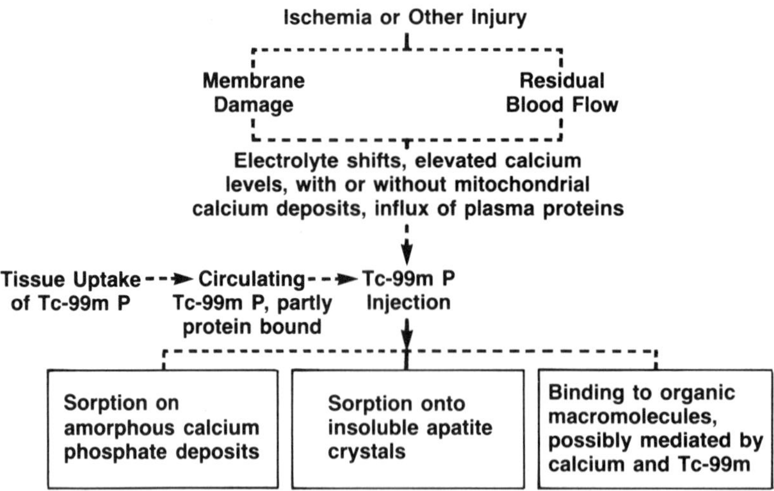

Figure 13.1 Proposed pathophysiologic basis for the scintigraphic detection of myocardial tissue damage with Tc-99m pyrophosphate (Tc-99m-P). (From Buja LM, et al, 1977.)

bone-seeking radiopharmaceuticals (Figure 13.1). In addition to tissue calcification, uptake also depends upon local blood flow and the degree of tissue damage. Residual blood flow is required for the delivery of the radiopharmaceutical to the injury site. Following infarction, the highest concentration ratios of Tc-99m pyrophosphate between damaged and normal myocardium occur when local blood flow is 20–40% of normal. With further reductions in blood flow, localization diminishes, and in regions of minimal blood flow (approximately 5%), uptake may appear normal (Zaret BL, et al, 1976). Where there is no blood flow (for instance, in the central infarct zone), localization fails to occurs. Because uptake of Tc-99m pyrophosphate is not proportional to myocardial damage, infarct imaging cannot be used for quantification of infarcted tissues. The area of radiopharmaceutical uptake does, however, correspond to infarct size (Wahner HK and Dewanjee MK, 1981).

PRECAUTIONS

The course of the relationship between the development of infarction and an abnormal Tc-99m pyrophosphate scintilla-tion study has been examined in animal models. Tc-99m pyrophosphate studies of experimental canine infarcts have shown that abnormal images are obtained within the first 12 to 24 hours following a fixed coronary occlusion and become progressively more abnormal during the initial 24 to 72 hours (Buja LM, et al, 1975; 1976). Images remain positive up to 6 days after infarction and begin to fade thereafter, usually becoming normal by the fourteenth day after experimental canine coronary artery ligation. J. T. Willerson and colleagues (1980) have found the myocardial localization begins approximately 10 to 12 hours after the onset of symptoms with increasingly positive uptake demonstrated during the initial 24 to 72 hours after acute myocardial infarction.

Adverse Reactions. Generalized hypersensitivity reactions have been associated with the use of pyrophosphate. These reported reactions include bronchospasm, hypotension, rash, pruritis, hives, and wheezing (Cordova MA, et al, 1987). From 1976 to 1984, a total of 16 adverse reactions associated with the use of pyrophosphate (both Tc-99m labeled and unlabeled) were reported in the United States (Cordova MA, et al, 1987).

Use During Pregnancy/Breastfeeding.   It is not known whether Tc-99m pyrophosphate can cause harm to the fetus when administered during pregnancy. Use during pregnancy is advised only if the benefits to be received clearly outweigh any risks that might be expected to occur. It is not known whether Tc-99m pyrophosphate is secreted in breast milk. It is advised, however, that lactating patients who receive this radiopharmaceutical suspend breastfeeding for 12 hours afterwards (ICRP, 1988), presumably because preparations often contain in varying amounts, Tc-99m pertechnetate, a radiochemical impurity that is known to be secreted in breast milk.

Alterations in Radiopharmaceutical Biodistribution.   Patients who have received large doses of doxorubicin demonstrate diffuse uptake of Tc-99m pyrophosphate within the myocardium (Chacko AK, et al, 1977). The mechanism appears to involve drug-induced cardiac toxicity, usually manifested as diffuse microscopic damage to the myocardium. L. M. Buja and colleagues (1981) have shown that diphosphonate therapy may decrease uptake of Tc-99m pyrophosphate in infarcted myocardium and increase its uptake in normal myocardial tissues. The mechanism may be due to saturation of Tc-99m pyrophosphate binding sites within the infarcted myocardial tissues and dilution of the radiopharmaceutical in the circulating diphosphonate pool at the time of Tc-99m pyrophosphate administration (Hladik WB III, et al, 1987).

Increased liver uptake of Tc-99m pyrophosphate has also been reported. This increase is often due to pathophysiological changes (Hansen S and Stadalnik RC, 1982) but may also be related to drug-induced alterations or technical problems associated with the radiopharmaceutical preparation. Excessive Al^{+3} levels in the Tc-99m eluate used to prepare Tc-99m pyrophosphate and in the patient's serum (hyperaluminemia secondary to antacid therapy) can result in the localization of

the radiopharmaceutical within the liver (Chaudhuri TK, 1976).

METHOD/DOSIMETRY

Method.   Adult patients usually receive 15–20 millicuries of Tc-99m pyrophosphate via intravenous administration. No special patient preparation is necessary except that patients should be well hydrated, when possible, in order to facilitate the renal excretion of the radiopharmaceutical and reduce the blood background activity. Scintillation images are obtained 90 minutes later in the anterior, 45° left anterior oblique (LAO), and left lateral positions (Figure 13.2). Regions of acute myocardial infarction are reliably positive when performed as early as 12–18 hours following the acute episode or within 14 days of the event (Figure 13.3). Maximum localization in infarcts is limited, however, to a much shorter time span, usually 2–3 days after infarction.

Radiation Dosimetry.   The radiation dosimetry for Tc-99m pyrophosphate to selected organs is shown in Table 13.4.

Table 13.4   ADULT RADIATION DOSE FROM Tc-99m PYROPHOSPHATE

TISSUE		RADS/20 mCi
Bone marrow		0.79
Kidneys		0.56
Total body		0.17
Bladder	2.0 hr void	1.94
	4.8 hr void	4.6
Testes	2.0 hr void	0.2
	4.8 hr void	0.3
Ovaries	2.0 hr void	0.18
	4.8 hr void	0.31

From Radiopharmaceutical Dosimetry Center, Oak Ridge Associated Universities, Oak Ridge, TN.

CLINICAL CONSIDERATIONS

Tc-99m pyrophosphate imaging is sometimes the only indicator of acute myocardial necrosis because the electrocardiogram may be only nonspecifically abnormal, and cardiac enzymes may be

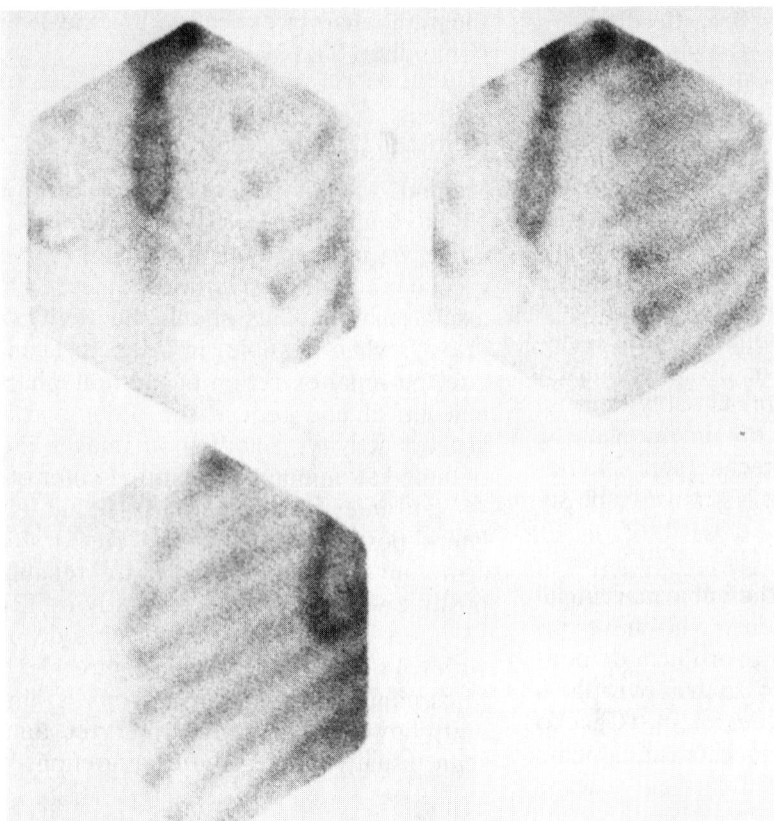

Figure 13.2 Tc-99m pyrophosphate study performed in anterior (A) 45° left anterior oblique (B) and 70° left lateral (C) orientations showing normal distribution with no evidence of myocardial infarction.

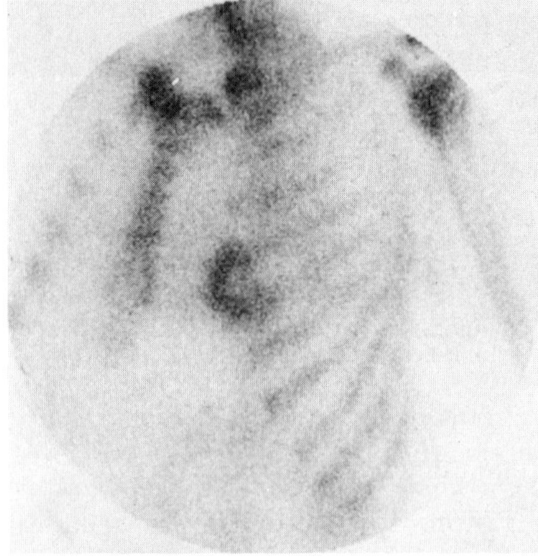

Figure 13.3 Tc-99m pyrophosphate study showing relatively large and intense radiopharmaceutical localization in apical and septal regions in left anterior oblique view.

either normal because of temporal restrictions on their usefulness or elevated because of injury to an organ other than the heart (Willerson JT, et al, 1980). Although the sensitivity of this procedure is quite high, the specificity is not especially high. Several conditions may cause Tc-99m pyrophosphate localization by the mycocardium; including angina, ventricular aneurysm, pericarditis, cardiomyopathy, myocardial trauma, and radiation therapy (Lyons KP, et al, 1980) (Figure 13.4). Other limitations apply, including the fact that the normal uptake of Tc-99m pyrophosphate by bone may limit its utility for estimation of infarct size (Willerson JT, et al, 1980).

Tc-99m pyrophosphate imaging is further limited in that the false-negative rate is relatively high during the initial

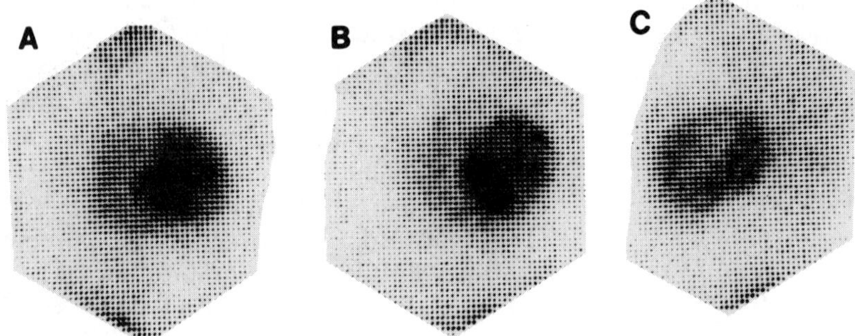

Figure 13.4 False positive Tc-99m pyrophosphate study in a patient with cardiac amyloidosis. Note the extensive uptake in both the left and right ventricles. (A = anterior, B = 45° LAO, C = 70° LAO)

12–18 hours following infarction when a diagnosis is often critical.

Interpretation of radiopharmaceutical uptake by the myocardium is based on a five-level grading system comparing activity in the myocardium to activity in adjacent, normal bone (Table 13.5). There is general agreement that 3+ and 4+ activity is consistent with myocardial infarction, and 2+ activity, while at times the result of acute myocardial infarction, is often seen in coronary artery disease and other forms of myocardial damage in the absence of acute myocardial infarction (Lyons KP, et al, 1980).

A variety of new Tc-99m bone seeking radiopharmaceuticals developed since the introduction of Tc-99m pyrophosphate demonstrate superior skeletal uptake and more rapid clearance from blood. Because all these agents localize in skeletal tissues, it has been postulated that they would also be useful for the detection of myocardial infarction. Several reports have suggested that the newer Tc-99m bone-seeking radiopharmaceuticals, medronate (MDP) (Singh A and Usher M, 1977) and oxidronate (HDP), are comparable to Tc-99m pyrophosphate for myocardial infarct imaging. Comparative clinical analyses, however, support the superiority of Tc-99m pyrophosphate over all other Tc-99m bone-seeking radiopharmaceuticals for the detection of acute myocardial infarction (Kelly RJ, et al, 1979; Wakat MA, et al, 1980; Makler PT, et al, 1979; Singh A and Usher M, 1977).

Adjunctive drug therapy has been mentioned as a means of increasing target-to-background rations by decreasing the amount of Tc-99m pyrophosphate that localizes in bone. E.A. Carr and colleagues (1981) demonstrated that uptake of Tc-99m pyrophosphate can be enhanced in the necrotic myocardium, uptake by bone can be reduced, and the lesion-to-blood ratios can be altered favorably when vitamin D_3 or desoxycorticosterone acetate (DOCA) is administered in pharmacological doses before injection of Tc-99m pyrophosphate. Although enhanced diagnosis of myocardial infarction would be facilitated by the improved imaging quality resulting from higher myocardium-to-background (and bone) ratios, the possibility of a drug-associated adverse effect upon myocardium healing is a serious concern (Wahner HK and Dewanjee MK, 1981)

Table 13.5 GRADING SCALE FOR Tc-99m PYROPHOSPHATE LOCALIZATION IN SUSPECTED MYOCARDIAL INFARCTION[a]

GRADING RANK	RADIOPHARMACEUTICAL APPEARANCE IN MYOCARDIUM
0	No discernable activity
1+	Questionable activity; probably blood pool
2+	Activity less than adjacent bone
3+	Activity equal to adjacent bone
4+	Activity greater than adjacent bone

[a] Berman DS, et al, 1977

that has not been fully examined. To date, drug-induced modulation of Tc-99m pyrophosphate tissue distribution has not been further investigated.

INDIUM-111 ANTIMYOSIN

Since the first use of antibodies in cardiology to treat digitalis toxicity (Smith TW, et al, 1976), the high degree of specificity of these proteins has been of increasing interest in the field of cardiology. The first diagnostic imaging application of radiolabeled antibodies in cardiac nuclear medicine was developed by B.A. Khaw and colleagues (1979) using cardiac myosin as the target molecule.

The cardiac myosin/anticardiac myosin antibody system was chosen for in vivo visualization of myocardial infarction for several reasons. Cardiac myosin is an intracellular contractile protein that exists in large concentrations. It is readily isolated and purified, is immunogenic, and is not exposed to the extracellular environment in normal viable myocytes. The rationale for use of a radiolabeled antimyosin antibody is that following myocyte necrosis from myocardial infarct or any other cause, the intracellular myosin is exposed to the extracellular components. A radiolabeled antibody could therefore penetrate disrupted cell membranes and bind to cardiac myosin, thereby permitting its visualization by scintillation imaging.

CHEMISTRY

Initial studies with the antimyosin antibody began with polyclonal affinity purified antibodies to cardiac myosin that were labeled with radioisotopes of iodine (Khaw BA, et al, 1976; 1978a;b). Since then, optimization of this system has involved both the antibody molecule and the radionuclide.

With the advent of the technology to prepare monoclonal antibodies (Kohler G and Milstein C, 1975), methods to prepare large quantities of purified murine antihuman-cardiac myosin soon followed. Further studies indicated that antibody fragments, namely (Fab')$_2$ and Fab could be prepared. The faster blood clearance rate of the Fab fragment was most suitable for imaging studies.

Although the initial experience with radiolabeled antimyosin was obtained with radioisotopes of iodine, the undesirable physical properties of I-131 and I-125, and the lack of ready availability of high purity I-123, resulted in the development of other labeling strategies using Tc-99m and In-111. Currently, most radiolabeled antibodies utilize multivalent cations, such as In-111, Ga-68, and Tc-99m, through a bifunctional chelating agent that is covalently bonded to the antibody.

In currently available preparations of antimyosin, the Fab fragment of antimyosin is covalently linked to diethylenetriaminepentaacetic acid (DTPA), as described by G.E. Krejcarek and K.L. Tucker (1977) and used by B.A. Khaw and colleagues (1980; 1982; 1984a;b). In any manipulation of an antibody molecule, the effect of such derivitization on immunoreactivity must be considered. For example, with the antimyosin system, increasing the Fab antibody solution concentration from 5 mg/ml to 10 mg/ml results in an increase from 4 to 7 moles DTPA per mole Fab without significant loss of antibody activity. However, increasing the molar ratios of anhydride by increasing the concentration of isobutylchloroformate causes drastic loss of antibody activity.

DTPA-coupled antimyosin Fab has been labeled with Tc-99m by the dithionate reduction system (Khaw BA, et al, 1982, 1986). This method involves the reduction of technetium-99m pertechnetate by a huge excess of sodium dithionate, which is then added to the DTPA-antimyosin. Purification by gel filtration column chromatography is required. This method resulted in quite variable labeling efficiencies, with the major drawback being formation of colloidal technetium and subsequent localization in the reticu-

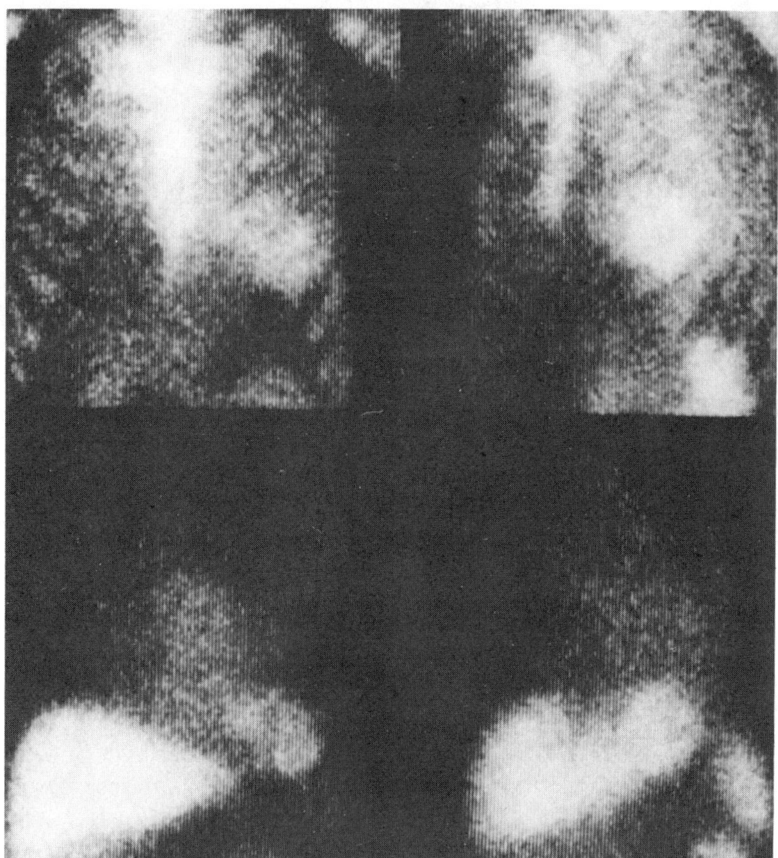

Figure 13.5 Acute myocardial infarction shown in patient with both Tc-99m pyrophosphate images (top row, anterior and 45° left anterior oblique projections) and corresponding In-111 antimyosin images. Note relatively intense uptake of In-111 antimyosin by liver and spleen. (Courtesy of Tsunehiro Yasuda, Massachusetts General Hospital, Boston, MA.)

loendothelial system. Although this agent has been used clinically to detect areas of myocardial infarction, the high level of liver activity resulting from the presence of colloidal impurities severely limited its usefulness, especially in inferior myocardial infarctions (Khaw BA, et al, 1986). To minimize the interference from liver activity and increase time available for imaging, a method was developed for labeling DTPA-antimyosin Fab with In-111 from the weak chelator sodium citrate (0.3 M) at pH 5.5.

Currently, a commercially available kit for the labeling of DTPA-antimyosin Fab with In-111 via this method is undergoing clinical trials in this country and abroad.

Pharmacokinetics

Localization of antimyosin fragments in acute experimental myocardial infarcts results from specific antibody–antigen interaction (Figure 13.5). This localization has an inverse exponential relationship to late regional myocardial blood flow determined by microsphere studies in dogs (Khaw BA, et al, 1976; 1978a; 1978b). Tc-99m monoclonal antimyosin Fab localizes in experimental myocardial infarct within 2 hours of intravenous administration. In clinical studies, antimyosin labeled with Tc-99m by the dithionate reduction method has been used to visualize regions of acute myocardial infarction as early as 12 hours after intravenous injection.

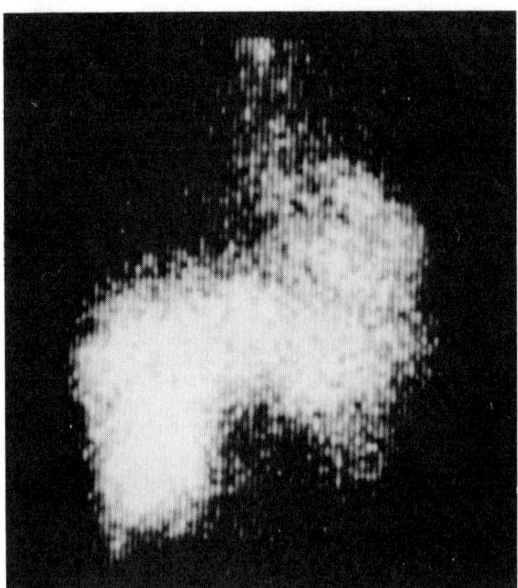

Figure 13.6 In-111 antimyosin study in patient with myocarditis. Activity is noted throughout the myocardium. (Courtesy of Tsunehiro Yasuda, Massachusetts General Hospital, Boston, MA.)

Areas of infarct may be clearly visible even in the presence of significant bone marrow visualization because of colloidal Tc-99m contamination.

With In-111 labeled antimyosin, experimental infarcts have been visualized 5 hours after intravenous injection. However, because of the 2.8-day half-life of In-111, imaging studies can be carried out as long as 72 hours after administration. In clinical studies with In-111 DTPA antimyosin Fab, areas of infarcted myocardium are clearly visible at 20–24 hours post injection. In the diagnosis of acute myocarditis with In-111 antimyosin (Figure 13.6), the optimal interval between injection and imaging is 48 hours.

The utility of In-111 antimyosin must be compared to that of other myocardial imaging techniques such as Tc-99m pyrophosphate and Thallium-201 chloride. These techniques may not be sufficiently specific for assessment of irreversibly damaged myocardial tissue. Tc-99m pyrophosphate may be sequestered by reversibly injured myocardium (Gerber KH and Higgins CB, 1983), resulting in overestimation of the extent of irreversibly damaged tissue.

PRECAUTIONS

Any use of antibodies in clinical applications raises the possibility of eliciting an acute allergic reaction or late serum sickness. In clinical practice at the Massachusetts General Hospital, skin testing is done prior to administration of In-111 antimyosin. To date, no positive skin test and no untoward reactions have been experienced in approximately 350 administrations.

Since these antibodies are of murine origin, the possibility of the production of human antimouse (HAMA) antibody must be considered. In some cases, such as the diagnosis of myocarditis with In-111 labeled antimyosin Fab, multiple injections of the antibody are required for serial imaging. In one study (Nicol PD, et al, 1988) of 28 patients who received 2–3 injections of the antibody, all sera tested indicated an absence of HAMA. This finding supports J.M. Brown and colleagues (1988), who found no detectable HAMA levels in their large-scale study of sera from 1832 patients.

METHOD/DOSIMETRY

The recommended administered dose of In-111 antimyosin is 1.5–2.0 mCi. The estimated radiation-absorbed dose from this administered dose is calculated from total body imaging at 1, 24, and 48 hours after intravenous injection (Table 13.6).

Table 13.6 RADIATION ABSORBED DOSE ESTIMATES FOR IN-III ANTIMOYSIN[a]

	Rem/1.8mCi
Whole body	0.918
Kidneys	7.92
Liver	1.46
Spleen	2.16
Bone marrow	0.90
Gonads (male)	0.918
Gonads (female)	1.06

[a] Myo-scint®, Centocor Corp., Malvern, PA.

CLINICAL CONSIDERATIONS

Radiolabeled Fab of monoclonal antimyosin antibodies binds to cells that have lost the integrity of their plasma membranes, thereby exposing intracellular myosin to extracellular fluid. Imaging with In-111 antimyosin has been used to localize and quantify regions of myocardial necrosis in myocardial infarction (Khaw BA, et al, 1986).

Because myocardial necrosis is an obligatory component of myocarditis (Aretz HT, et al, 1986), In-111 antimyosin has been evaluated in the diagnosis of acute myocarditis (Yasuda T, et al, 1987). This group has found that antimyosin antibody imaging is a reliable screening method for evaluating patients thought to have myocarditis, and that a positive antimyosin scan indicates the need for right ventricular biopsy to establish the histologic diagnosis.

II. Imaging Myocardial Perfusion

TI-201 THALLOUS CHLORIDE

Radiopharmaceuticals that localize in myocardium and are capable of distinguishing ischemia from infarction must distribute into the myocardium in proportion to blood flow and in relation to capillary membrane permeability and cellular functional integrity.

For many years, nuclear medicine techniques have been evaluated for the assessment of regional coronary blood flow. Research has involved the intracoronary injection of both diffusable and nondiffusable tracers, including radioisotopes of the physiologically inert gases, xenon and krypton, and radiolabeled microspheres and aggregates of human serum albumin. Although radioactive xenon and krypton have been used for cardiac flow studies, difficulties associated with the handling and administration of solutions of these poorly soluble substances have limited the appeal of this procedure for routine use. Studies using radiolabeled particulates have not advanced beyond animal studies because of the hazards associated with administering particulates for arterial blockade.

Noninvasive nuclear medicine methods for the evaluation of myocardial perfusion have centered primarily upon various radioisotopes of potassium and its analogues. As a result of the high degree of muscle contractility, normally perfused myocardial cells have a high demand for intracellular potassium. Though other muscles, tissues, and organs also utilize potassium, the myocardium has the highest concentration of this element per gram of tissue. The uptake of these substances by the myocardium occurs at a rate that is related to the coronary blood flow and the rate of exchange of the radioisotope within the circulating blood and viable myocardium. Intracellular localization of these monovalent substances depends upon functional integrity, primarily the intact cellular energy transport mechanism involving the Na-K-ATPase pump.

Potassium is the major intracellular cation, and its concentration within the cell is maintained by the active energy-dependent process. Analogues of potassium (i. e., monovalent alkaline metals) behave similarly, although it has been demonstrated that the efficiency of the Na-K-ATPase mechanism for these ions appears to bear an inverse relationship to the size of the ion, with evidence that larger ions are removed more slowly from blood (Love WD, et al, 1968). Reasonably, the evaluation of myocardial perfusion with a radioisotope of potassium or a suitable analogue would seem most logical, and several have been used successfully to image the normal myocardium (Matthews CME, et al, 1969). However, none of the several that are known to exist possess suitable nuclear properties. Most have suboptimal photon emissions or deliver unacceptably high radiation doses.

Although thallium is not a true analogue of potassium (it is a member of the IIIA series of the periodic group), it distributes in organs and tissue in a manner that is identical to that of potassium (Gehring PJ and Hammond PB, 1967;

Mullins LJ and Moore RD, 1960). M. Kawana and colleagues (1970) suggested the use of radioisotopes of thallium as potassium analogues for imaging. Thallium-199 was initially proposed for medical use; however, its relatively short physical half-life (7.4 hours) presented considerable logistical problems in its supply and delivery. In 1975, E. Lebowitz and colleagues introduced Tl-201 ($T_{1/2_{phy}}$ 73.1 hours) for medical use.

Though the imaging properties of Tl-201 are not ideal—it possesses a lower energy spectrum with x-ray emissions occurring at 65–83 keV—it has become the radiopharmaceutical of choice for the evaluation of myocardial perfusion. However, radiolabeled complexes have been developed (and approved for clinical use) that have biodistribution properties and clinical applications closely approximating those of the thallous ion. Clinical trials of these compounds are currently underway.

CHEMISTRY

Thallium-201 is a cationic monovalent metal ion that results from the decay of Pb-201, a radionuclide produced by the proton bombardment of stable Tl-203.

$$\text{Tl-203 (p, 3n) Pb-201} \xrightarrow{9.4\ \text{hrs}} \text{Tl-201}$$

Following decay of Pb-201, Tl-201 is isolated by ion-exchange chromatography dissolved in HCl (to form the thallous chloride) and evaporated to dryness. Thallous chloride is then dissolved in NaOH, and the pH is adjusted to 4.5–7.0. The United States Pharmacopeia (XXI) specifies radiochemical purity of no less than 95%, and says that the principal radionuclidic impurities Tl-200 ($T_{1/2_{phy}}$ 26.1 hrs) and Tl-202 ($T_{1/2_{phy}}$ 12.0 days) should be less than 2% and 2.7% of total radioactivity, respectively, at the time of calibration. Pb-203 should be less than 0.5%. In practice, radionuclidic purity of most commercially available formulations of Tl-201 thallous chloride at the time of calibration is typically 98% or greater. Significant amounts of these high-energy

Table 13.7   FORMULATION OF CURRENTLY AVAILABLE (U.S.) PREPARATIONS OF THALLOUS CHLORIDE T1-201

MANUFACTURER	pH	COMPONENTS
Mallinckrodt, Inc.	4.5–7.0	Sodium chloride 9.0 mg/ml Benzyl alcohol 0.9% v/v (as preservative)
Medi-Physics, Inc.	4.5–7.5	Isotonic, contains no bacteriostat
DuPont-NEN	5.0–7.0	Isotonic, contains benzyl alcohol 0.9%

impurities may contribute substantially to image degradation.

Activity concentrations at the time of calibration are usually 1 or 2 mCi/ml with most products being utilized 24–48 hours before calibration. Commercial formulations generally contain 0.9% sodium chloride for isotonicity and 0.9% benzylalcohol as a preservative, although one manufacturer lists no preservative in its formulation (Table 13.7). U.S.P. XXI does not require the presence of a stabilizer or preservative. Various radioactivity sizes of Tl-201 thallous chloride are available from commercial manufacturers in the United States. Over the last 2 years, the trend is to make available significantly larger sizes of radioactivity to meet the increasingly larger patient doses.

PHARMACOKINETICS

After intravenous administration, Tl-201 clears rapidly from the blood with maximal concentration in the myocardium achieved at 10 minutes, at which time about 5% of the administered dose localizes within this organ. Five minutes after intravenous administration, only 5–8% of the injected dose remains in blood. Tl-201 clerance from blood follows a biexponential disappearance curve, with 92% of the blood-borne activity clearing with a half-life of about 5 minutes and the remainder clearing with a half-life of about 40 hours. Most of the latter activity is in the red blood cells. Plasma fraction appears to be constant with time but varies from 28–50% of the total blood pool activity (Atkins HL, et al, 1977). About 15% of Tl-201 is taken up by the liver and 3.5% by the kidneys. Biological half-life in these organs is approximately 36 hours (U.S.P. DI, 1988).

Urinary excretion accounts for 4–8% of activity in the first 24 hours after intravenous administration, and fecal excretion is insignificant.

Whole-body counting indicates a mean disappearance time of approximately 10 days. About 0.15% of the injected dose is found in the testes of patients. Animal studies show the total amount of Tl-201 in ovaries and uterus to be 0.2%. Tl-201 uptake occurs in the thyroid but appears to account for less than 0.2% (Atkins HL, et al, 1977).

Thallium localization within the myocardium occurs intracellularly in proportion to regional blood flow, and approximately 85% of Tl-201 that passes through the coronary circulation is extracted during each pass. A close correlation exists between early Tl-201 distribution and microsphere-determined regional blood flow in canine coronary occlusion models has been reported (Hamilton GW, et al, 1978; Mueller TM, et al, 1976; Pohost GM, et al, 1978). The increase in Tl-201 deposition in heart occurred to a lesser extent, however, than microsphere-determined blood flow during reactive hypermia (Strauss HW, et al, 1975) or in response to dipyridamole therapy (Hamilton GW, et al, 1978). In the normal and mildly reduced flow ranges. Tl-201 distribution closely approximately blood flow, whereas in the low-flow range (less than 10% of flow in the nonischemic zone), thallium concentration is usually found in excess of microsphere-determined regional blood flow.

The potassium-like distribution of thallium is due to the similarities that exist between these two elements: Both possess monovalent cationic charges, have similarly sized hydrated ionic radii, and participate in the membrane Na-K-ATPase pump (Ritchie JL and Hamilton GW, 1978). P. J. Gehring and P. B. Hammond (1964) have shown that the thallous ion activates the Na-K-ATPase system and that intracellular binding of the thallous ion appears to be greater than that of potassium. It was also demonstrated (Gehring PJ and Hammond PB, 1967) that thallous ion uptake could be blocked by ouabain and sodium fluoride, agents that are known to block the sodium-potassium ATPase system.

Thallium is also known to bind more firmly to Na-K-ATPase than potassium with an affinity approximately 10 times greater than that of potassium for the potassium-activating site (Britten J and Blank M, 1968).

Within the myocardium, thallium distribution closely follows that of myocardial blood flow to viable tissues where adequate tissue oxygenation occurs to support metabolic activity (Figure 13.7). Whereas viable myocardium accumulates Tl-201 and appears as a region of relatively high activity, Tl-201 uptake does not occur in infarcted tissues or in regions of ischemia brought about by some form of stress induced by either exercise or pharmacologic intervention at the time of radiopharmaceutical administration. After an interval of rest, however, ischemic regions subsequently revert to areas of Tl-201 localization (Figure 13.8), whereas infarcted zones do not localize Tl-201.

Following intravenous administration, approximately 8–10% of the administered dose is initially deposited within the lungs. In patients with increased left arterial pressure, a greater quantity of Tl-201 is deposited in the lungs on the initial transit. Though the activity usually clears by the time of the redistribution image, it has been reported that significant correlation exists between increased lung uptake and various types of coronary artery disease or myocardial injury, particularly with exercise (Kushner FG, et al, 1981). C. A. Boucher and colleagues (1980) have reported that Tl-201 lung uptake correlates closely with the extent of pulmonary artery disease, the number of myocardial segmental thallium perfusion defects, and the prevalence of prior myocardial infarction.

Tl-201 is distributed and extracted by the myocardium, with the major portion

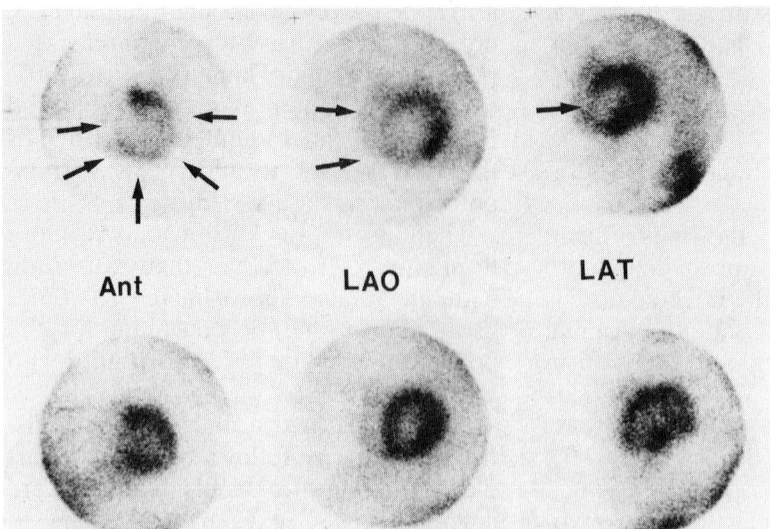

Figure 13.7 Transient ischemia demonstrated by Tl-201 thallous chloride scintigraphy shown as defect in immediate post stress (top row, arrows) images that fills during delayed images performed 3 hours later. "Normalization" during imaging is almost complete.

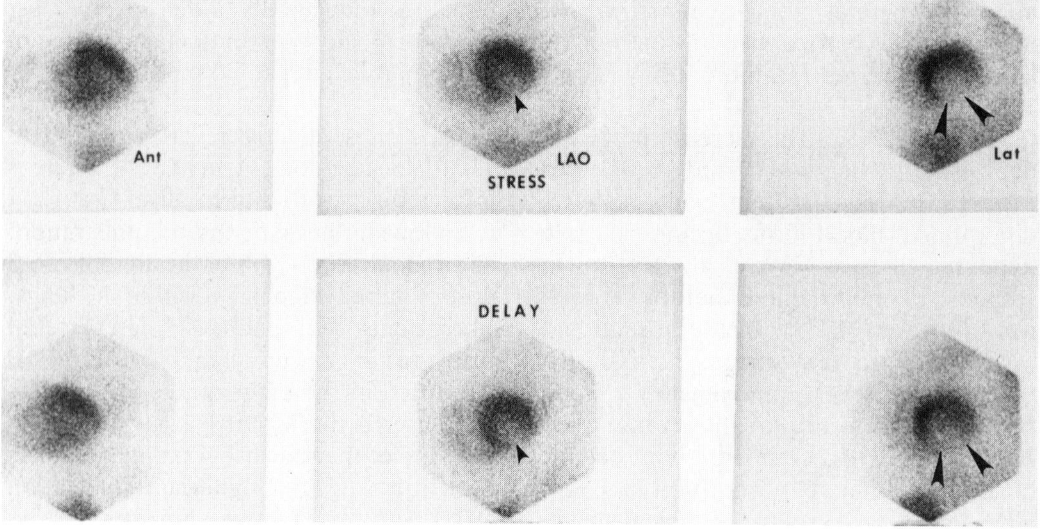

Figure 13.8 Tl-201 thallous chloride scintigraphy demonstrating significant perfusion defect during stress imaging (arrows) that fails to normalize Tl-201 during 3-hour delayed imaging.

of Tl-201 activity within the chest appearing in the left ventricular myocardium because of its relatively larger mass and higher blood flow. Activity is occasionally noted in the right ventricular myocardium; however, atria are rarely visualized due to the limited muscle cell mass. First-pass extraction efficiency by the myocardium typically approaches 90%.

PRECAUTIONS

Though blood glucose, insulin, and pH are known to affect the transport of potassium, it has not yet been shown whether any of these parameters affect Tl-201 uptake by the myocardium.

Drug-related alterations in the distribution of Tl-201 have been reported to include the beta-adrenergic blockers and nitrates (Hockings B, et al, 1983; Henkin RE, et al, 1982; Pohost GM, et al, 1980; Albro PC, et al, 1978; Osbakken MD, et al, 1981; Wolf R, et al, 1979). Both classes of drugs tend to decrease both the number and the size of exercise-induced perfusion defects, creating the likelihood of false-negative exercise scans. For the beta blockers, the effects may stem from drug-induced changes in the exercise performance of patients, whereby the normally associated rise in heart rate and systolic blood pressure that occurs in exercise are significantly lessened. Further, beta blockers may increase myocardial oxygen extraction and augment stroke volume despite a tendency for cardiac output to decrease. For nitrates, it is conceivable that a beneficial redistribution of coronary blood flow occurs resulting in decreased myocardial ischemia (Becker L, 1978). In any event, it is recommended that beta blocker therapy be discontinued 48 hours prior to performance of the study (by the appropriate tapering of dosage) and that nitrate therapy should also be discontinued prior to the Tl-201 study (Hladik WB III, et al, 1987). Phenytoin has been shown in rats to reduce thallium uptake by the myocardium (Schachner ER, et al, 1980); however, no similar effect has been reported in clinical studies.

Use During Pregnancy/Breastfeeding. It is not known whether Tl-201 crosses the placenta or whether it causes harm to the fetus when administered during pregnancy. Reasonably, Tl-201 should be administered to pregnant patients only when benefits clearly outweigh any potential risks.

Tl-201 has been shown to be excreted in breast milk (Stabin M, 1988). Therefore, patients who are breastfeeding should stop nursing for at least 3 weeks (in practical terms, discontinue) following the administration of Tl-201 thallous chloride (ICRP, 1988).

DOSAGE/DOSIMETRY

Method. The method of serial imaging following the administration of a single dose of Tl-201 thallous chloride (Pohost GM, et al, 1977) is almost universally employed to differentiate normal, reversible ischemia from infarcted, or scarred, myocardium during exercise or at rest.

Patients who undergo Tl-201 imaging should be fasting for at least 4 hours to minimize splanchnic localization of this radiopharmaceutical. The patient exercises to the maximal end point (80% of the predicted maximum heart rate) using either treadmill exercise, upright and supine bicycle stress, or handgrips, and the radiopharmaceutical is administered intravenously through an indwelling line. The patient continues to exercise during radiopharmaceutical administration and for 60–90 seconds afterward in order to maintain the desired state of myocardial perfusion during the initial distribution and clearance phase of Tl-201. The exercise stress image should be started immediately and completed within 20 minutes. Beyond this period, significant Tl-201 washout from healthy myocardium occurs with the appearance of the radiopharmaceutical in the transiently ischemic tissues. Rest images (images of Tl-201 redistribution) are usually obtained 2–4 hours following radiopharmaceutical administration. Between the initial and delayed Tl-201, patients should be asked to forego eating because it has been shown that patients who have eaten a high-carbohydrate meal have a significantly lower incidence of transient or persistent myocardial defects in the delayed images (Wilson RA, et al, 1986).

During both exercise-stress and rest, images are usually obtained in the anterior and 45 degree, and 70 degree left anterior oblique (LAO) projections. A left lateral view may be substituted for the 70 degree LAO image.

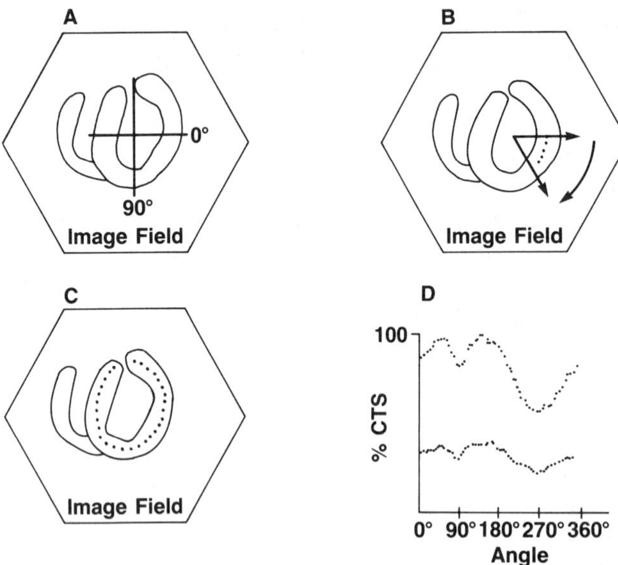

Figure 13.9   The quantitative method of analysis that was applied to both tomographic and planar scintigrams. The polar coordinate reference axis is shown in (A). The image pixels for circumferential profile analysis are found by performing a radial search for maximum value of 6-degree intervals (B) until covering 360 degrees (C). The maximal values shown as black dots in (B) and (C) are then replotted in (D) for each angle as a percent of the maximum value of the circumferential profile. The top curve in (D) represents the circumferential profile from the stress thallium-201 image and the bottom from the 4-hour delayed image. (From Berman DS, et al, 1984.)

Computerization is playing an increasingly significant role in the acquisition, processing, and display of Tl-201 images. Image enhancement has been successfully performed using computer-assisted processing that involves some type of background subtraction or image filtering. Quantitative analysis techniques are becoming more useful in the interpretation of Tl-201 images. The computer approaches that have been investigated express Tl-201 myocardial distribution as a function of space and time (Garcia E, et al, 1981; Berger BC, et al, 1979; Meade RC, et al, 1978; Burow RD, et al, 1979). Generally, these quantitative methods of analysis (Figure 13.9) obtain counts from a circumferential profile, then quantitate the segmental activity as an annular function referenced from the center of the left ventricular cavity (Berman DS, et al, 1984). These circumferential profiles are then plotted as a function of time in order

that Tl-201 distribution may be compared to other areas of the myocardium over time.

Tomographic imaging techniques are often preferable for Tl-201 imaging due to the consequential superimposition of one portion of the myocardium over another that occurs with planar imaging. The types of tomographic imaging employed with Tl-201 involve primarily the use of a seven-pinhole collimator (whereby seven simultaneous images of the heart, at different angles, are projected onto the camera detector) or single photon emission computed tomography (SPECT) imaging. SPECT is performed with single-/or dual-head rotating cameras that separate the myocardium into multiple layers and different axes. Most clinicians who perform SPECT imaging of the heart utilize between 3.5–5.0 millicuries of Tl-201 thallous chloride in order to obtain the high count rates that are necessary for good definition of myocardial structures in the tomographic images.

Pharmacological-Assisted Stress Testing. Occasionally, the accuracy of clinical exercise testing is limited by patient's ability to achieve and maintain adequate levels of exercise. Although the sensitivity and specificity of exercise Tl-201 imaging appears to be somewhat less dependent upon the accuracy of exercise than does ECG (Berman DS, et al, 1984), failure to exercise, or to exercise to the proper level of intensity, can result in a significant decrease in the diagnostic sensitivity of this technique (McLaughlin PR, et al, 1979). B. Massie and colleagues (1982) noted shower rates and Tl-201 washout in patients with submaximal exercise and concluded that the rate of washout depends upon the exercise level rather than the duration of exercise. In patients for whom exercise Tl-201 scintigraphy is not possible, the adjunctive use of dipyridamole, a potent coronary arteriolar vasodilator, can create a desirable stresslike condition.

Outside nuclear medicine, dipyridamole has primary clinical usefulness (often in conjunction with aspirin therapy) in the inhibition of platelet aggregation to prevent postoperative thromboembolic complications as well as for prevention of attacks. The platelet-aggregation inhibitor activity is due to the inhibitor of the enzymes adenosine deaminase and phosphodiesterase, which results in the increased accumulation of adenosine, adenine nucleotides, and cyclic AMP (U.S.P. DI, 1988). In nuclear medicine, the coronary-artery-dilating properties of dipyridamole are a means of increasing coronary blood flow analogous to physiological stress. K. L. Gould and co-workers (1978a; b; Albro PC, et al, 1978) reported that dipyridamole given intravenously could lead to coronary vasodilation in normal vessels, whereas fixed coronary artery stenosis prevents or attenuates this response. In the resting myocardium, dipyridamole has been shown to bring about an increase in myocardium-to-background ratios that are the result of the absolute increase in Tl-201 uptake. Because stenosed vessels are already at maximal vasodilation due to autoregulatory response, dipyridamole brings about no further increase in blood flow (Rabinovitch MA, 1985). The validation of dipyridamole-assisted Tl-201 imaging as a highly sensitive and specific test for coronary artery disease has been determined in several reports (Leppo J, et al, 1982, Francisco DA, et al, 1982). M. A. Josephson and colleagues (1982) reported that the overall sensitivity and specificity of exercise-Tl-201 imaging and dipyridamole-assisted imaging were not significantly different in their study of 33 patients, although dipyridamole-assisted method appeared more sensitive, however, in detecting coronary stenoses in the 40–60% range.

A primary distinction between exercise and dipyridamole is that dipyridamole causes only a minor augmentation in myocardial oxygen demands (Francisco DA, et al, 1982). As a result, myocardial ischemia occurs less frequently with dipyridamole than with exercise. While myocardial ischemia can occur with dipyridamole, it is due primarily to the coronary "steal" phenomenon (Leppo J, et al, 1982).

As a result, relative differences in Tl-201 uptake between areas of the myocardium that are supplied by stenosed and normal coronary arteries are enhanced by dipyridamole.

Dipyridamole-Adjunctive Method. In the method of K. L. Gould and co-workers (1978b), the patient is supine when intravenously injected dipyridamole at a rate of 0.142 mg/kg/min for 4 minutes. Immediately afterwards, the patient is brought to a standing position and allowed to walk in place for approximately 3 minutes, after which time the Tl-201 thallous chloride is administered, and the patient continues to walk in place for 4 additional minutes. Imaging is begun immediately afterwards, with redistribution images performed 2–4 hours later. Heart rate, blood pressure, and EKG should be monitored every minute for the first 15 minutes of the test. The test should not be performed in patients who have rest angina (Rabinovitch M, 1985).

Side effects reported with the use of dipyridamole include headache, chest pain (incidence, approximately 20% in CAD patients), dizziness, nausea, and EKG changes (minor ST-segment depression and T-wave changes) (Leppo J, et al, 1982; Francisco DA, et al, 1982). If necessary, the dipyridamole-antagonist, aminophilline, may be administered to reverse the vasodilator effects (Alfonso S, 1970). To those patients who experience more severe or prolonged chest pain during dipyridamole administration, D. A. Francisco and co-workers (1982) have given nitroglycerine, which is known to reduce myocardial oxygen demands, followed by aminophylline. In such situations, the vasodilator effect may be sustained for the relatively short periods of time to ensure Tl-201 distribution under stress-like conditions prior to the reversal of dipyridamole.

CLINICAL CONSIDERATIONS

Noncardiac Applications. Tl-201 thallous chloride has been evaluated for diagnostic usefulness in other applications, including imaging of the thyroid gland and the kidneys. As a renal imaging agent, it has been shown to concentrate preferentially in the renal medulla (approximately 3.5 times the level that is taken up by the renal cortex) (Bradley-Moore PR, et al, 1975; Raynaud C, et al, 1972).

Parathyroid Imaging. Tl-201 thallous chloride also concentrates in hyperplastic parathyroid tissues in sufficient quantities to permit scintillation imaging. Unfortunately, Tl-201 uptake by the thyroid gland requires some form of thyroid subtraction for adequate visualization of the parathyroid tissues. Most clinicians utilize computer-assisted subtraction techniques and Tc-99m pertechnetate with the thyroid-pertechnetate image performed initially, then stored for subsequent subtraction. Tl-201 parathyroid scintigraphy appears to be limited to the detection of tissues greater than 5 mm in diameter (Ferlin G, et al, 1983) and may not show all hyperplastic tissues in patients with secondary hyperparathyroidism (Young AE, et al, 1983).

BLOOD FLOW MEASUREMENTS WITH POSITON-EMITTING RADIONUCLIDES

Three positron-emitting radionuclides—Nitrogen-13, Oxygen-15, and Rubidium-82—are used for determination of myocardial blood flow in conjunction with position-emitting tomography (PET).

Nitrogen-13. This radionuclide (as ammonia) has been used to image myocardial blood flow at rest and during pharmacological or physical-stress imaging (Gould KL, et al, 1979, Schelbert HR et al, 1982, Tamaki N, et al, 1985). Nitrogen-13 ammonia rapidly diffuses into the myocyte, probably because of the ability of the nonionic, lipophilic species to readily cross the capillary and sacrolemmal membranes (Schelbert HR, et al, 1981). Once intracellular, it converts again to the charged species, but subsequent utilization of N-13 by the glutamate-glutamine reaction slows the exit of N-13 from the myocyte. Retention times of 60–120 minutes are reported following intravenous administration (Bergmann SR, et al, 1980).

A property of all diffusable tracers is a decrease in extraction efficiencies at higher blood flow. Regional N-13 concentrations also relate to blood flow in a nonlinear fashion, with flows greater than 3 ml/min/gm myocardium producing only small increases in N-13 myocardial blood flow. Between 0.5 and 2.5 ml/min/gm, however, an almost linear relationship exists with N-13 myocardial uptake (Shah A, et al, 1985).

Oxygen-15. Oxygen-15 water is employed for blood-flow measurements of the myocardium, as well as the quantification of cerebral blood flow and the measurement of oxygen metabolism (Mazziotta JC and Phelps M, 1986). Extraction of Oxygen-15 water by the myocardium is essentially independent of metabolic variation because this material is metabolically inert. As a result, its uptake is independent of variations that may affect the reliabilities of other metabolic tracers as measurement tools for evaluating blood flow. First-pass capillary transit extraction efficiencies for Oxygen-15 labeled water in myocardium are less affected by blood flow, with measurements approaching 95% (Bergmann SR, et al, 1984; 1985). Because O-15 activity is relatively high in the vascular compartment (inlcuding heart chambers) and the lungs, subtraction techniques must be performed with a suitable blood pool marker, such as O-15 carbon monoxide, which binds to red blood cells.

Rubidium-82. Whereas the relatively short physical half-lives of N-13 and O-15 require on-site accelerators to produce adequate supplies of these positron-emitting radionuclides, Rubidium-82 is an attractive alternative. It is a positron-emitting radionuclide, yet it can be supplied through the convenient decay of a longer lived parent (strontium-82, physical $T_{1/2}$ 25 days) (Horlock P, et al, 1981; Neirinckx RD, et al, 1982). This generator-produced radionuclide is an analogue of potassium and possesses similar biologic distribution (increased myocardial localization and low blood levels) that permits its use as a perfusion agent. Because the generator supply mode obviates the need for a cyclotron and, because the generator may be eluted frequently for use (daughter buildup occurs rapidly), myocardial blood-flow imaging with Rubidium-82 can be performed repeatedly over short-time intervals. Blood flow and Rubidium-82 uptake appear to be in close agreement, as evidenced by radiolabeled microsphere blood flow. Single capillary transit extraction fractions average about 74% at control flows of 1 ml/min/gm

of myocardium but fall with higher flows (Grover M, et al, 1984). It is not yet established whether low extraction fractions at high flow rates will limit delineation of small perfusion abnormalities and lessen the value of Rb-82 perfusion imaging. As a result of its widespread availability through its generator system, Rb-82 imaging is receiving considerable interest.

COMPLEXES OF TC-99M EMPLOYED FOR MYOCARDIAL PERFUSION

Although the development of a suitable Tc-99m complex that distributes in myocardial tissues in a manner analogous to Tl-201 has long been a goal of nuclear medicine, investigators have only recently identified a number of compounds that are taken up by the myocardium in relation to blood flow. E. Deutsch and associates (1981), with Tc-99m DMPE (dichloro(1,2-dimethylphosphino(ethane))), obtained the first high-quality images of myocardial perfusion with a Tc-99m radiopharmaceutical in a dog model (Nishiyama H, et al, 1982). Subsequent clinical trials with this radiopharmaceutical, however, demonstrated the effect of species variability (Ketring AR, et al, 1983), noting low myocardial and high lung uptake in human subjects (Dudczak R, et al, 1983). Other Tc-99m complexes were developed and investigated, including Tc-99m t-butyl isonitrile (TBI), Tc-99m methoxy isobutyl isonitrile (MIBI) (also known as RP-30A), Tc-99m carboxymethoxy isopropyl isonitrile (CPI) and Tc-99m 2-methoxy-2-methylpropyl-isonitrile (MPIN). Various comparisons of these radiopharmaceuticals have been made in clinical trials and animal models.

B. L. Holman and associates (1984) utilized Tc-99m TBI and performed imaging at 1–4 hours in humans to demonstrate high-quality myocardial images. The radiopharmaceutical initially produced high lung and liver uptake that subsided sufficiently at 40–60 minutes to permit optimal visualization of the myocardium. Though the myocardial residence time was relatively long, the lengthy retention by the heart was disadvantageous because it prohibited repeating studies on the same day. A primary distinction between the Tc-99m agents and Tl-201 is that no Tc-99m agent yet developed undergoes myocardial redistribution. (In delayed imaging with these agents, some increase in activity has appeared in transiently ischemic areas. Such occurrence may be attributed to radiopharmaceutical efflux into blood from the activity that is initially deposited in the liver and lungs. The subsequent release of activity by these organs into blood permits uptake by the areas previously noted as ischemic during stress at the time of injection. K. A. McKusick and associates (1986b) called this "defect-normalization"). Therefore, diagnostic evaluation of the myocardium at rest and immediately after stress requires two separate injections of these Tc-99m radiopharmaceuticals.

Comparison of Tl-201 and Tc-99m TBI in patients thought to have coronary artery disease (McKusick KA, et al, 1986b) found high liver uptake that obscured inferior segments of the left ventricle. Liver-to-heart ratios with Tc-99m TBI were 3:4 at 60 minutes.

P. Gerundini and co-workers (1986) evaluated in normal human volunteers three potential Tc-99m agents—trimethylphosphite (TMP), 1,2-bis(dimethyoxyphosphino)ethane, and t-butylisonitrile (TBI)—and found none suitable for clinical use. Detracting biologic properties included lengthy blood clearance (TMP and 1,2-bis(dimethyoxyphosphino)ethane) and high initial lung uptake followed by undesirable activity in the liver and spleen (TBI only).

Others found that Tc-99m CPI produced images of excellent quality with less initial liver and lung uptake and relatively high myocardial-to-background ratios obtained 10 minutes after injection (Sporn V, et al, 1986). Still lower lung and liver levels were noted with Tc-99m MIBI by K. A. McKusick (1986a). McKusick and coworkers (1986b) compared Tc-99m TBI, CPI, and MIBI and found that MIBI yielded the least distracting lung and liver uptake. Myocardium-to-background ratios for TBI, CPI, and MIBI averaged 1.2, 1.9, and 2.5, respectively, at 30 minutes, and 1.3, 2.4, and 2.8, respectively, at 60 minutes. In a recent clinical comparison of MIBI and MPIN, C. Dudczak and colleagues (1988) found MIBI superior to MPIN with higher heart-to-background ratios for MIBI. Respective ratios for MIBI and MPIN were 2.9 and 1.9 (at rest) and 3.1 and 2.3 (after dipyridamole administration). Heart-to-liver ratios were approximately the same. MPIN demonstrated slightly faster myocardial washout than did MIBI (half-life 273 minutes vs. 514 minutes).

Evidence is lacking for a Tc-99m complex that achieves an extraction efficiency as high as that of Tl-201 or that localizes by the same cationic exchange mechanism. Studies in isolated perfused rat hearts have shown Tc-99m MIBI to have a single capillary extraction efficiency of 0.44 at flows of 0.8 ml/min/g myocardium (compared to 0.82 for Tl-201) (Leppo JA, et al, 1986). The earliest Tc-99m myocardial perfusion complex, DMPE, is not transported by the Na^+K^+ ATPase mechanism by either human erythrocytes (Sands H, et al, 1986) or neonatal rat myocytes (Delano ML, et al, 1985). It has been suggested that the localization of Tc-99m TBI differs from that of DMPE and may be related its lipophilicity. Excretion of these agents appears to involve both renal and hepatobiliary mechanisms. Within 1 hour, renal excretion of Tc-99m MIBI accounts for 16% of the administered dose whereas excretion via the biliary pathway is about 8% at the same time (Schelbert HR, 1987).

The difficult nature of the lengthy myocardial retention of the isonitriles may be considered a detriment because same-day imaging requires the administration of a much larger second dose of the radiopharmaceutical to determine infarction from stress-induced ischemia.

BATO (Substituted Oxime) Complexes of Tc-99m. Attempts to develop a Tc-99m labeled complex that undergoes more rapid myocardial clearance have been made by A. D. Nunn and colleagues (1986) with another new class of Tc-99m agents called BATO derivatives (derived from *boronic adducts* of *technetium oxime*). These neutral, seven-coordinate technetium complexes, have shown rapid myocardial clearance and relatively low, rapidly clearing, liver and lung uptake. Good images of the myocardium have been obtained with Tc-99m chloro(methylboron(1-)-tris[1,2-cyclohexane dionedioxime]) (SQ 30217) (Coleman RE, et al, 1986). Newer Tc-99m labeled derivatives of this class, neutral tris oxime and chloro-hydroxy substituted oximes, have also shown excellent myocardial uptake with somewhat longer myocardial washout than the prototype agent (120 minutes vs. 70 minutes) (Narra RK, et al, 1987; Hirth W, et al, 1988; Linder KE, et al, 1988). Imaging with these types of agents may be initiated as early as 2–3 minutes after injection but must be completed within 15–20 minutes because of the rapid clearance.

III. Imaging Myocardial Metabolic Activity

Several agents, collectively called metabolic heart agents, have been studied in animals and man in an attempt to identify severely ischemic but viable myocardium in patients with coronary artery disease. The promise of these agents is to provide definitive evidence that myocardial tissue, shown to be hypokinetic or akinetic by gated cardiac blood pool imaging and/or hypo perfused by Thallium-201 imaging remains viable.

This information is of increasing importance in light of newer reperfusion therapies (Kloner RA, et al, 1983). Therefore, a rapid technique for determining the metabolic function on a regional basis becomes important.

Under aerobic conditions, the primary metabolic substrates of cardiac metabolism are fatty acids. The remainder of myocardial energy requirements are met by catabolism of lactate and glucose. Long-chain fatty acids of between 14 and 18 carbons account for 90% of myocardial energy requirements under aerobic conditions. However, when oxygen delivery is compromised (Opie L, 1984; Marshall RC, et al, 1983), the major substrate is glucose (Liedtke JA, 1981).

Therefore, the design of metabolic agents has followed two paths: first, the use of glucose analogues, which would be expected to show increased uptake in ischemic but viable tissue and, second, the use of long-chain fatty acids, which would be expected to show a discordant distribution pattern with myocardial perfusion agents, for example, Tl-201. By this methodology, areas that are underperfused yet viable could be identified. Currently, the most promising of these agents are the positron-emitting F-18 fluoro-deoxy-glucose and the branched-chain modified fatty acids labeled with I-123.

Since metabolic substrates are in many cases rapidly catabolized with rapid tissue clearance of by-products, metabolic substrate radiopharmaceuticals are usually modified analogues that enter metabolic pathways, undergo at least one step in the metabolic pathway, and then become "trapped" intracellularly for a period of time sufficient to allow external imaging. The modification of the glucose and fatty acid analogues will be discussed below.

ANALOGUES OF GLUCOSE

Regional myocardial uptake of glucose can be measured by the use of the radiolabeled glucose analogues that trace the initial steps of glucose uptake and metabolism. The radiopharmaceutical of choice is 2-fluoro(F-18)-2-deoxyglucose (FDG). This glucose analogue can be suitably labeled with F-18, a short-lived ($T_{1/2_{phy}} = 110$ min), positron-emitting radionuclide that requres a nearby cyclotron for production. FDG exchanges across capillary and cellular membranes in proportion to glucose metabolism and competes with glucose for phosphorylation by hexokinase to FDG-6-phosphate.

At this step, however, this analogue of glucose is no longer competitive with glucose, because FDG-6-phosphate is not a substrate for glycolysis nor can it be synthesized to glycogen. Deoxyglucose-6-phosphate and 2-FDG-6-phosphate are then trapped in the tissue and released very slowly (Phelps ME, et al, 1979; Huang SC, et al, 1980). Kinetic models that substantiate the fact that accurate positron emission tomographic (PET) images reflect glucose metabolism have been studied extensively (Phelps ME, 1977; 1978; 1979; Huang SC, et al, 1980; Kuhl DE, et al, 1976; Budinger TF, et al, 1977).

CHEMISTRY

The synthesis of F-18 labeled 2-deoxy-2 fluoro-d-glucose was first accomplished by T. Ido and associates (1977; 1978) at the Brookhaven National Laboratory. FDG Injection is readily prepared either by the electrophilic reaction of ^{18}F-enriched fluorine gas with 3,4,6-tri-O-acetyl-D-glucal or by the nucleophilic reaction of ^{18}F-labeled acetylhypofluorite with a suitably protected D-mannopyranose. The fluorinated product is hydrolyzed with acid to give a mixture of 2-fluoro-2-deoxy-D-glucose (FDG) and 2-fluro-2-deoxy-D-mannose (FDM). It is purified by column chromatography and dissolved in an appropriate solvent, most commonly 0.9% saline. Increased demand for this product resulted in modifications of the original method to include remote, semi-automated procedures (Barreo JR, et al, 1981; Fowler JS, et al, 1981).

In fact, much of the promise of PET imaging is based on the completely automated synthesis modules ("Black Box" approach) to the production of F-18 FDG in a clinical setting. Many manufacturers of cyclotrons are including this type of technology in their PET facilities packages. Whether these automated synthesis modules will be able to produce products on a routine clinical basis and in a high-quality reproducible form that can be readily processed for human use remains to be seen.

MODIFIED FATTY ACIDS

Currently, fatty acid radiopharmaceuticals that show promise for clinical use include the intrinsically labeled C-11 palmitate (Schon H, et al, 1984; Geltman EM, et al, 1982) and modified fatty acids labeled with either I-123 or C-11 (Freundlieb C, et al, 1980, Livini E, et al, 1982; 1985).

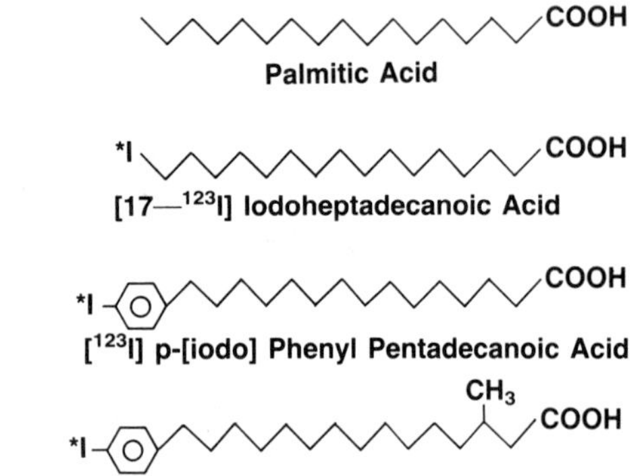

Figure 13.10 Structures of native and selected modified radiolabeled fatty acid molecules that have been used as cardiac metabolic agents.

Chemical modification of fatty acids has as its primary goal the alteration of structure enough to inhibit at least one step in the metabolic pathway thereby increasing myocardial residence time sufficiently to allow scintillation imaging (Dudczak R, et al, 1982; 1983). This goal has been accomplished by the addition of a terminal phenyl group to inhibit terminal beta oxidation and by the synthesis of branched-chain fatty acids, primarily by methylation at the 3 position (Livini E, et al, 1982) (Figure 13.10). A molecule with a phenyl group in the omega position has the added property of providing a moiety that can be iodinated easily and with good in vivo stability.

The net results of these modifications has been an increase in residence time in the heart of up to 5 hours (Miller DD, et al, 1985a;b), allowing sufficient time for imaging (Figure 13.11). The extraction fraction for fatty acids is in the 50–60% range, and serum half-times are less than 2 minutes (Miller DD and Strauss HW, 1988).

Although more centers for positron emission omography are being developed, the number of clinical centers that are capable of utilizing the positron labeled analogues of glucose and the modified fatty acids is still limited. On the other hand, I-123 labeled modified fatty acids can be manufactured commercially

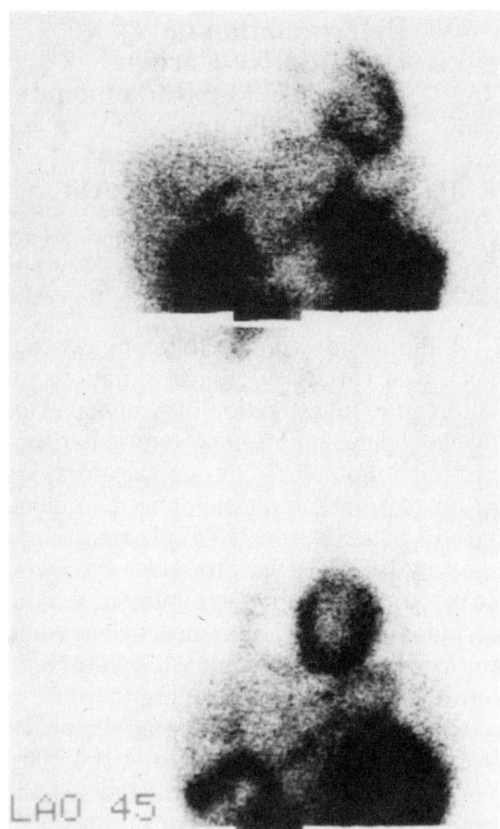

Figure 13.11 I-123 labeled fatty acid images of the heart in a normal volunteer demonstrate excellent uptake in the left ventricular myocardiac. The right ventricle is also demonstrated and well visualized on the 45° LAO view.

and distributed nationwide for use with single photon emission computed tomography (Jansen D, et al, 1984). At this time, one I-123 modified fatty acid preparation is undergoing limited clinical trials in the United States.

PRECAUTIONS

The use of metabolic radiopharmaceuticals requires attention to the metabolic status of the patient. For example, the metabolism of glucose in the aerobic heart depends upon the plasma concentration of glucose and insulin, availability of alternative substrates, especially fatty acids, mechanical work, and the rate of oxidative respiration (Neely JR and

Morgan HE, 1974; Opie LH, et al, 1973; Rovetto MJ, et al, 1975; Hillis LD and Braunwald E 1977; Wildenthal K, et al, 1976; Braunwald E, 1976). Therefore, dietary history becomes an important factor in evaluating images with metabolic agents, as the uptake of F-18 FDG and radiolabeled fatty acids are influenced by insulin and by glucose, and free fatty acid levels, respectively.

The quantitative measurement of myocardial metabolism with these agents is very complex. Detailed mathematical models have been proposed, yet much work remains to be done. Currently, comparison of the distribution pattern of these tracers to perfusion agents such as Tl-201 seems to be the preferred method of interpretation.

Radiation Dosimetry of Metabolic Cardiac Agents. A detailed review of the radiation absorbed dose from potential myocardial imaging agents has been published by the Radiopharmaceutical Internal Dose Information Center at Oak Ridge National Laboratories (Watson EE, et al, 1985). This report is based on human and animal studies that have appeared in the literature. Dosimetry of

Table 13.8 RADIATION DOSE ESTIMATES FOR I-123 BMIP[a]

| | ESTIMATED RADIATION ABSORBED DOSE | |
ORGAN	*2.0 hours[b]* Rad/mCi	*4.8 hours[b]* Rad/mCi
Bladder	0.19	0.38
Stomach	0.050	0.050
Small intestine	0.19	0.19
Upper large intestine	0.42	0.42
Lower large intestine	0.61	0.61
Heart wall	0.094	0.094
Kidneys	0.069	0.069
Liver	0.076	0.076
Lungs	0.058	0.058
Ovaries	0.12	0.13
Red marrow	0.068	0.069
Testes	0.045	0.049
Thyroid	0.28	0.28
Total body[c]	0.053	0.055

[a] 5% I-124 contamination assumed; 0.48% free iodide assumed; treated as in MIRD Dose Estimate Report No. 5 (25% uptake).
[b] Bladder voiding interval.
[c] Dose to the "total body" is dose to the whole body from all source organs plus any activity uniformly distributed in the remainder of the body.

Table 13.9   RADIATION DOSE ESTIMATES FOR F-18 FDG

| ORGAN | ESTIMATED RADIATION ABSORBED DOSE | |
	2.0 hour[a] Rad/mCi	4.8 hour[a] Rad/mCi
Bladder	0.86	1.7
Brain	0.064	0.064
Heart wall	0.23	0.23
Kidneys	0.076	0.077
Liver	0.062	0.064
Lungs	0.067	0.068
Ovaries	0.062	0.082
Pancreas	0.094	0.095
Red marrow	0.054	0.058
Spleen	0.14	0.14
Testes	0.068	0.084
Total Body[b]	0.054	0.060

[a] Bladder voiding interval.

[b] Dose to the "total body" is dose to the whole body from all source organs plus any activity uniformly distributed in the remainder of the body.

the various I-123 labeled modified fatty acids appears similar; however, it is important to consider the presence of the radionuclide impurity, I-124, whenever dosimetric evaluation for I-123 radiopharmaceuticals is made.

The radiation absorbed doses from the typical modified fatty acid, I-123 Beta Methyl Iodophenyl Pentadecanaic Acid and F-18-2-fluoro-2-deoxyglucose, are listed in Tables 13.8 and 13.9, respectively. The critical organ for F-18 FDG is the bladder, whereas for I-123-BMIPP it is the lower large intestine. By way of comparison, the effective whole-body dose equivalent for these two agents is approximately the same as that for Tl-201 thallous chloride.

The ultimate role of cardiac metabolic radiopharmaceuticals in clinical cardiology is yet to be determined. These agents are of research interest in several centers around the world. The availability of a commercially produced, I-123 labeled modified fatty acid would accelerate the process of determining the role of this class of agents. At this time, several years may pass before this occurs.

For the increasing number of centers with positron emission tomography capabilities, the availability of automated synthetic procedures, the so-called Black Box for the preparation of F-18 FDG, will also increase the application of this compound in evaluating cardiac metabolism.

IV. Determination of Quantitative Cardiac Function: The Radionuclide Ventriculogram

RADIOPHARMACEUTICALS FOR FIRST-PASS IMAGING AND EQUILIBRIUM GATED BLOOD POOL IMAGING

Radionuclide ventriculography is beneficial in a variety of clinical situations including the investigation of ischemic heart disease, determination of ventricular-wall motion abnomalities, prognostic grouping of myocardial infarct patients, the follow-up of patients receiving pharmacologic therapy for heart failure and arrythmias. It is also of primary usefulness in the determination of valvular insufficiency and in the assessment of ventricular reserve in aortic and mitral valve regurgitation.

Radionuclide ventriculography can be accomplished by two different techniques: (1) the first-pass technique, and (2) the equilibrium gated blood pool study.

In first-pass imaging radiopharmaceuticals are injected as a bolus and depict blood flow during the immediate flow through the chambers and great vessels. Equilibrium gated blood pool imaging utilizes radiopharmaceuticals that are largely confined to the vascular blood pool. Images are recorded during computer-selected portions of the cardiac cycle using a gating mechanism that usually involves EKG triggering (Figure 13.12).

With the first-pass technique, the radiopharmaceutical is injected as a bolus and its immediate passage through the heart depicts blood flow via scintillation imaging and computer acquistion techniques. The radiopharmaceutical needs to reside within the intravascular system only long enough to transverse the chambers. In order to acquire adequate count rates to yield high-quality images during the short time of radipharmaceutical transit through the heart, however, radiopharmaceuticals utilized for first-pass imaging must provide a high photon flux (which is usually accomplished with materials with

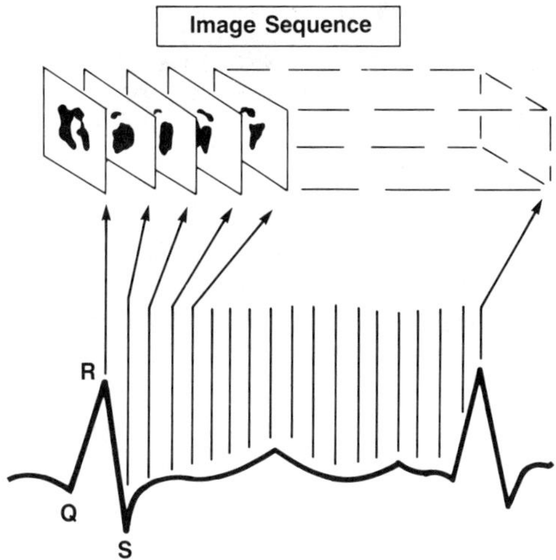

Figure 13.12 Computer imaging sequence for EKG gated blood pool ventriculography. The sequence is normally triggered by the R wave, with the cardiac cycle divided into discrete components. Counts arriving during any division are placed in the computer matrix relevant to that division. After several hundred cardiac cycles, there is sufficient information on each frame to form a useful image. (From Metler FA, Jr. and Guiberteau MJ, 1985.)

short physical half-lives). In this manner, relatively large amounts of radioactivity may be safely administered in order to achieve the desirably high count rates.

In equilibrium gated blood pool imaging (also known as multi-gated acquistion imaging), the radiopharmaceutical must reside within the vascular compartment sufficiently long and at constant levels to permit the computer-assisted acquistion of counts for image formation. Ideally, the attachment of a short-lived gamma-emitting radionuclide, such as Tc-99m, onto either a macromolecule (e. g., human serum albumin, or red blood cells) results in a radiopharmaceutical that demonstrates prolonged intravascular retention.

Both techniques have clinical strengths and weaknesses. Both have the ability to display the image sequence in cinematic format. The first-pass technique is often useful whenever it is desirable to acquire data in the shortest period of time. The

equilibrium gated blood pool technique yields a higher resolution image and data of a higher degree of statistical certainty because of the greater number of counts recorded over longer periods of image acquisition. Equilibrium imaging, because of the persistence of radiopharmaceutical within the blood pool, permits data to be obtained before, during, and after various interventions such as exercise. Exercise radionuclide ventriculography is an important measure of ventricular function.

First-pass imaging requires no specific localization properties of the radiopharmaceutical except that it presents itself within the intravascular compartment suficiently to permit its observations during passage through the heart and great vessels. With the exception of Tc-99m macroaggregated albumin (a radiopharmaceutical that localizes within the pulmonary capilary bed during its first pass through the lungs), almost any other Tc-99m radiopharmaceutical will suffice. Tc-99m pertechnetate is usually the preferred radiopharmaceutical for first-pass imaging. Very short-lived radionuclides have also been utilized for first-pass imaging. These generator-produced radionuclides, W-178/Ta-178, Os-191/Ir-191, and Hg-195/Au-195, which have physical half-lifes of several minutes or less, produce the very high flux of usable photons that are required for high-resolution first-pass imaging (Cheng C, et al, 1980; Brihaye C, et al, 1986; Dymond DS, et al, 1983). Presently, none of these short-lived generator radionuclides is commercially available in the United States.

Occasionally, first-pass imaging is performed in conjuction with equilibrium blood pool imaging by employing for the first-pass imaging a radiopharmaceutical that will be suitably retained by the blood pool. Initial images of flow through the heart depict first-pass information, whereas later images demonstrate blood pool distribution. For this reason, and because information on the several radiopharmaceuticals that are used specifically for first-pass imaging is detailed elsewhere in this text, the remainder of this section is devoted to information on the agents utilized for equilibrium blood pool imaging.

CHEMISTRY

Technetium-99m Human Serum Albumin. Technetium-99m will efficiently label human serum albumin (HSA) by a variety of methods, including electrolysis and stannous ion-assisted. Commercially available formulations at present utilize stannous ions for the reduction of Tc-99m pertechnetate so that complexation with albumin will occur (HSA, Medi-Physics, Inc., Richmond, CA) (Nusynowitz ML, et al, 1978). These kit-type formulations contain a lyophilized mixture of human serum albumin, stannous ions (usually as stannous tartrate), and appropriate buffering substances. Following reconstitution of these kits with Tc-99m pertechnetate, labeling is relatively fast with radiolabeling yields routinely in the 90–99% range (Nusynowitz ML, et al, 1978; Thrall JH, et al, 1978).

Technetium-99m Radiolabeled Red Blood Cells. The most commonly used radiopharmaceutical for equilibrium blood pool imaging is Tc-99m labeled autologus red blood cells. The ability of Tc-99m to label red blood cells was discovered accidentally during Tc-99m pertechnetate brain scans that were performed several days after Tc-99m pyrophosphate bone scans. These scans demonstrated high levels of blood background activity resulting from an unusually high level of Tc-99m activity in the red blood cells. Subsequently, it was determined that the activity within the red blood cells was caused by high levels of unreacted stannous ions that were contained in the previously administered bone-scanning agent, Tc-99m pyrophosphate. Others also noted that Tc-99m red cell labeling occurred only when Tc-99m pertechnetate brain scans followed Tc-99m pyrophosphate bone scans; brain scans performed with Tc-99m pentetate (or other chelates of Tc-99m) failed to demonstrate Tc-99m red blood cell labeling.

Table 13.10 GENERAL STEPS IN THE RADIOLABELING OF RED BLOOD CELLS WITH Tc-99m USING THE STANNOUS ION-ASSISTED TECHNIQUE

1. Treatment of cells with stannous ion
2. Removal of extracellular stannous ion
3. Addition of Tc-99m sodium pertechnetate

Red blood cells can be labeled with Tc-99m by a variety of techniques that all utilize the stannous ion-assisted radiolabeling methodology (Pavel D, et al, 1977; Smith TD and Richards P, 1976; Callahan RJ, et al, 1982a) (Table 13.10). With any of the commonly performed techniques, reasonably high labeling efficiencies can be achieved (Table 13.11). However, because some of the variations employed for Tc-99m red blood cells produce more effective labeling than others, it may be desirable to utilize a single method for certain clinical applications. For example, whenever Tc-99m red blood cell imaging is utilized for detection of gastrointestinal hemorrhage, the Tc-99m radiolabeled red blood cells should have the highest tagging efficiency, because any amounts of unreacted Tc-99m pertechnetate would localize in gastric mucosa and potentially complicate an accurate diagnosis of active gastric bleeding.

Treatment of Red Blood Cells with Stannous Ion. Although it is technetium in the +7 (pertechnetate) oxidation state that crosses the intact erythrocyte membrane (Rabito CA, et al, 1986), only technetium that has been reduced to a lower oxidation state will firmly bind hemoglobulin (Dewanjee M, 1974; Rehani MN and Sharma SK, 1980). Stannous ions are most commonly employed for reduction of technetium and the stannous chloride (as a stannous pyrophosphate complex) is preferred. At physiologic pH, stannous ions are subject to hydrolysis and precipitation that causes their rapid clearance from blood by the RE system. When complexed with pyrophosphate (or other soluble chelates), however, stannous ions are sufficiently soluble to be resistant to these effects, yet are not so strongly bound to pyrophosphate as to prevent their dissociation and attachment to red blood cells. In the in vivo (Pavel D, et al, 1977) and modified in vivo (Callahan RJ, et al, 1982a) methods, treatment with stannous ion is accomplished by the direct intravenous adminis-

Table 13.11   METHODS FOR Tc-99m RADIOLABELING OF RED BLOOD CELLS AND VARIOUS STEPS INVOLVED

A. THE MODIFIED BROOKHAVEN METHOD (IN VITRO)

1. Add 1–6 ml heparinized* whole blood to reagent vial (containing 50 μg Sn^{+2}, 3.67 mg Na citrate, 5.5 mg dextrose, 1.4 mg NaCl)
2. Incubate at room temperature for 5 minutes
3. Add 0.6 ml 0.1% sodium hypochlorite, 1.0 ml 4.4% EDTA solution, mix gently
4. Add 0.5–3.0 ml Tc-99m sodium pertechnetate
5. Incubate for 15 minutes at room temperature

B. THE IN VIVO METHOD

1. Inject stannous pyrophosphate
2. Wait 10–20 minutes
3. Inject Tc-99m sodium pertechnetate

C. MODIFIED IN VIVO METHOD

1. Inject stannous pyrophosphate
2. Wait 10–20 minutes
3. Withdraw 5–8 ml whole blood into shielded syringe containing Tc-99m sodium pertechnetate
4. Gently mix syringe contents for 10 minutes at room temperature

D. ORIGINAL BOOKHAVEN METHOD (IN VITRO)

1. Add 4 ml heparinized[a] whole blood to reagent vial (containing 2.0 mg Sn^{+2}, 3.67 mg Na citrate, 5.5 mg dextrose, 0.11 mg NaCl)
2. Incubate at room temperature for 5 minutes
3. Add 1.0 ml 4.4% EDTA
4. Centrifuge tube for 5 minutes at 1300 G
5. Withdraw 1.25 ml of packed red cells, transfer to sterile vial containing 1–3 ml Tc-99m sodium pertechnetate
6. Incubate at room temperature for 10 minutes

[a] Use only dilute heparin solutions; fewer than 100 units.

tration of stannous pyrophosphate. Other chelates of stannous ions can also be used (such as pentetate, medronate, etc.) and would yield radiolabeled red blood cells in varying degrees of efficiencies (Jones AG, et al, 1977). Pyrophosphate seems nearly ideal, however, because it maintains the solubility of stannous ions in serum until they come into contact with the high-affinity red blood cells.

How much stannous ion is required for RBC labeling has been confusing because reports have described the amounts of tin to be given in terms of either stannous ions, stannous chloride, or stannous pyrophosphate. D. Pavel and associates (1977) used a dose of 0.2 mg/kg stannous pyrophosphate equivalent to 30 μg stannous ions/kg. In animal studies, A.G. Jones and co-workers (1977) observed changes in blood disappearance of Tc-99m pertechnetate at stannous ion doses of 1 μg/kg and a plateau of 10 μg Sn^{+2}/kg. R.G. Hamilton and P.O. Alderson (1977) also found 10 μg Sn^{+2}/kg to be the minimum dose to achieve satisfactory red blood cell labeling and noted no decrease in labeling efficiency at doses up to 40 μg Sn^{+2}/kg. However, A. Khentigan and co-workers (1976) reported a threshold dose of 20 μg Sn^{+2}/kg before any alteration in pertechnetate biodistribution is noted. For Tc-99m red blood cell labeling using either the in vivo or the modified in vivo technique, most clinicians utilize 10–20 μg Sn^{+2}/kg. Depending upon the commercial formulation chosen, it may be necessary to inject one-third to one half the contents of a vial of stannous pyrophosphate or an entire vial to provide this number of stannous ions (Table 13.12). When the in vivo method of radiolabeling is employed, a much smaller number of stannous ions are employed, usually 1–15 micrograms (Smith TD and Richards P, 1976; Srivastava SC, et al, 1983).

Removal of Extracellular Stannous Ions. The presence of stannous ion in the serum can result in the undesirable reduction of Tc-99m pertechnetate prior to its entry into the red blood cell. Such an occurrence is unfortunate because only

Table 13.12   NOMINAL STANNOUS ION CONTENT OF KIT-TYPE PREPARATIONS FOR THE PREPARATION OF Tc-99m PYROPHOSPHATE AND FOR USE IN THE LABELING OF RED BLOOD CELLS WITH Tc-99m[a]

NAME®	COMPANY	TOTAL STANNOUS ION CONTENT PER VIAL
Pyrolite	DuPont-NEN	500–950 μg
Phosphotec	Squibb Diagnostics	750 μg
TechneScan PYP	Mallinckrodt, Inc.	1680–2315 μg

[a] Suggested dosage range for RBC Labeling = 10–20 μg stannous (Sn^{+2})/kg.

the oxidized form of Tc-99m can be transported by the erythrocyte membrane (Rabito CA, et al, 1986).

In either the in vivo or the modified in vivo method, biological clearance of excess stannous pyrophosphate is the method by which extracellular stannous ions are reduced. The optimal time between the injection of stannous pyrophosphate and the administration of Tc-99m pertechnetate (in vivo method) or the incubation of the stannous ion pretreated cells (modified in vivo method) is 20–30 minutes (Callahan RJ, et al, 1982a).

With the original in vitro labeling method (Smith TD and Richards P, 1976), extracellular stannous ion could be removed by centrifugation, a step that physically separates stannous-treated cells from the noncellular stannous ions in serum.

A modification of the in vitro labeling method, known as the Brookhaven kit, uses nonpenetrating sodium hypochlorite to oxidize extracellular stannous ions, thus preventing the undesirable extracellular reduction of Tc-99m pertechnetate. With this technique, a small amount of sodium hypochlorite is added to whole blood that has been previously treated with stannous ion. Extracellular stannous ions are oxidized to the stannic form, and interference with labeling is minimized. Intracellular stannous ions are not affected by the addition of sodium hypochlorite. Unlike the centrifugation method, the chemical labeling method does not require separation of red cells and can be performed in whole blood. Avoidance of centrifugation lessens the degree of cellular damage that occurs during radiolabeling.

Addition of Tc-99m Pertechnetate to Stannous Pretreated Red Blood Cells. Actual red blood cell labeling with Tc-99m occurs whenever Tc-99m pertechnetate is brought into contact with RBCs that have been previously treated with stannous ions. This can be accomplished by either the in vivo or in vitro addition of Tc-99m pertechnetate to RBCs that have been pretreated with stannous ions.

Because the in vivo method requires only that Tc-99m pertechnetate be admin-

istered by intravenous administrations, many clinicians find this the simplest method for RBC labeling. Unfortunately, poorer quality RBC labeling is often the result (compared to the in vitro incubation of Tc-99m pertechnetate), because pertechnetate ion that is administered intravenously is subject to some degree of partitioning between the intracellular and the extracellular spaces before red blood cell labeling can be achieved. It has been shown that the rate of Tc-99m red blood cell labeling is not instantaneous (Callahan RJ, et al, 1982b); therefore, ample time exists for pertechnetate to diffuse out of the intravascular compartment.

Labeling efficiencies greater than 90% have been reported in vivo method (Pavel D, et al, 1977); however, though this figure may accurately represent the amount of radioactivity within the vascular space that is associated with red cells, it does not distinguish the amount of pertechnetate that has distributed into the extracellular space. Radioactivity within the extracellular spaces can significantly degrade image quality (Figure 13.13).

The Modified In Vivo Method. The modified in vivo method (Callahan RJ, et al, 1982a) was developed primarily as a means to avoid the poor reproducibility and inferior quality images that often resulted with the traditional in vivo method (Figure 13.14). As in the in vivo method, the modified in vivo method also requires that stannous ions (as the stannous pyrophosphate complex) be administered intravenously. However, with the modified method, the stannous ion-treated red blood cells are withdrawn directly into a syringe that contains Tc-99m pertechnetate. A dilute solution of heparin (10 units/ml) is utilized as an anticoagulant within the indwelling line. The red blood cell/Tc-99m pertechnetate mixture is allowed to incubate at room temperature for 10 minutes with gentle mixing, after which the labeled cells are reinjected. Because the entire labeling occurs within a closed system that is connected to an indwelling catheter, any likelihood of cells contamination is minimized.

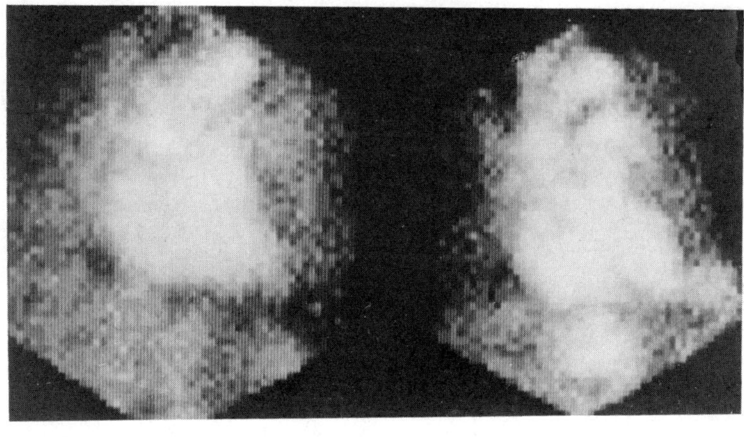

Figure 13.13   Cardiac blood pool images performed with Tc-99m labeled red blood cells showing relatively poor quality (image A) with appearance of activity in soft tissues, and typically good quality study (image B).

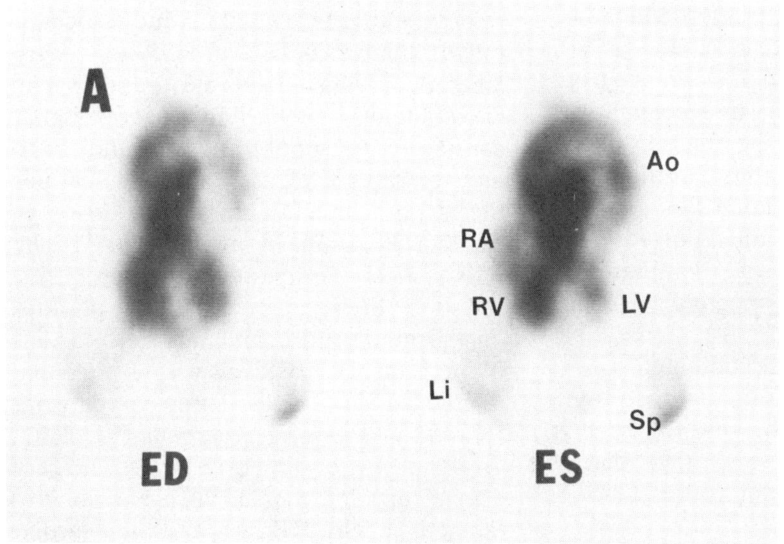

Figure 13.14   Images of cardiac blood pool obtained at end diastole (ED) and end systole (ES) with Tc-99m labeled red blood cells. Heart vessels and structures are identified, as well as liver and spleen.

With this technique, the amount of Tc-99m contained in the red cell fraction at the time of administration has been shown to be greater than 90% (Callahan RJ, et al, 1982a). Some investigators have reported slightly higher labeling efficiencies by using acid-citrate-dextrose (ACD) solution rather than heparin (Porter WC, et al, 1983). Labeling the stannous ion-treated red blood cells within a syringe prevents extravascular distribution of Tc-99m.

The labeling reaction taking place within the syringe has been well characterized. The rate of labeling is directly affected by hematocrit and temperature (Callahan RJ, 1986). In patients with low hematocrit values, for instance those with

GI bleeding, incubation time should be increased to 20 minutes. The temperature of the labeling mixture can be kept close to body temperature by using lead shields that have been stored in a warmer. The lead acts as a source of heat, lessening the rate at which blood cools after it is withdrawn from the patient.

PHARMACOKINETICS

Tc-99m Human Serum Albumin. Although the initial distribution of Tc-99m human serum albumin is intravascular, there is slow distribution to the extravascular fluid spaces (Thrall JH, et al, 1978; Yang SSL, et al, 1978; Atkins HL, et al, 1980) and some renal elimination. In dogs, the intravascular clearance half-time has been reported to be on the order of 30 minutes, compared to approximately 5 hours in humans (Atkins HL, et al, 1980).

In addition to the rate of clearance from the intravascular space, image quality is determined in part by the fraction of the administered dose remaining in the blood pool following injection. For Tc-99m HSA, this value has been reported to be 82%, 60%, and 45% at 30 minutes, 2 hours, and 4 hours, respectively (Atkins HL, et al, 1980).

Compared with radioiodinated HSA, Tc-99m HSA demonstrates a more rapid blood clearance with the rate for Tc-99m HSA, ranging from 1.5 to 2 times that of the radioiodinated product.

Tc-99m Red Blood Cells. The pharmacokinetics of Technetium-99m red blood cells has been studied in patients and normal volunteers (Hegge FN, et al, 1978; Atkins HL, et al, 1985). After intravenous injection of pertechnetate during in vivo labeling, maximum whole blood activity was not reached until at least 30 minutes after injection. This suggests that pertechnetate freely diffuses into the extracellular fluid space, then reenters the intravascular pool as blood levels of pertechnetate fall.

Up to 8 hours following injection the in vitro method resulted in higher blood levels, whereas 24-hour retention was only slightly higher for the in vivo method.

Whole-body clearance was found to be biexponential for both methods. The in vivo method of labeling resulted in a short $T_{1/2}$ component of 2.5 ± 0.7 hr (10.9 ± 6.1%) and a long $T_{1/2}$ component of 176.6 ± 163.6 hr (90.5 ± 5.0%), whereas the in vitro method resulted in whole-body retention components of 2.7 ± 1.5 hr (25.4 ± 10.4%) and 75.6 ± 25.3 hr (82.2 ± 7.7%) (Atkins HL, et al, 1985).

Comparison of Radiopharmaceuticals for Blood Pool Imaging. Several studies have compared the use of Tc-99m HSA and Tc-99m red blood cells, prepared by either the in vitro or the in vivo method of radiolabeling. H. L. Atkins and associates (1980) compared Tc-99m HSA to in vitro labeled Tc-99m RBCs and found that in vitro labeled Tc-99m RBCs have a higher cardiac blood-pool-to-background ratio and result in clearly superior cardiac blood pool imaging. In a comparison of Tc-99m HSA and in vivo labeled Tc-99m RBCs, J. H. Thrall and colleagues (1978) found a higher cardiac blood pool-to-background ratio and greater cardiac blood pool activity levels with in vitro and in vivo Tc-99m RBCs. Three comparisons (Hamilton RG and Alderson PO, 1977; Graham MM and Nelp WB, 1980; Hegge FN, et al, 1978) of in vitro and in vivo labeled Tc-99m RBCs found high cardiac bloodpool-to-background ratios and better subjective images with in vitro Tc-99m RBCs; however, the differences were not significant. The images were satisfactory with both agents and virtually identical ejection fractions were obtained.

Based upon these studies, the following conclusions can be drawn:

1. Whenever Tc-99m human serum albumin was compared to Tc-99m labeled red blood cells prepared by any method, labeled red blood cells were determined to be superior.
2. When in vivo and modified in vivo methods of labeling red blood cells were compared,

the modified in vivo method was judged to be superior.

3. When in vitro labeled red blood cells were compared to in vivo and/or modified in vivo methods and judged on labeling efficiency and image quality, in vitro labeled cells were judged superior.

4. When availability and ease of labeling were considered in comparisons among all red blood cell labeling methods, the in vitro kit was found to be inferior because of the increased manipulation required and the potential for administration of cells to the wrong patient.

5. Comparisons of all methods of red blood cell labeling showed that the modified in vivo method gave image quality approaching that of in vitro methods but is far more easily performed with readily available components.

For any given clinical situation, therefore, the selection of a blood pool agent will depend on the acceptable level of image quality, the number of studies performed daily, and the level of expertise of the technical staff.

Tc-99m Human Serum Albumin. It is not uncommon for appreciable levels of radiochemical impurities—notably, hydrolyzed, reduced (colloidal) Tc-99m, and free, unbound Tc-99m pertechnetate—to appear in this radiopharmaceutical. These impurities either remain in blood or localize in tissues that lie close to the heart (such as the liver and the stomach), creating higher than desirable levels of background activity that can seriously degrade image quality. For this reason, and because images obtained with Tc-99m RBCs are generally of higher quality and more reproducible, the use of Tc-99m HSA has given way in favor of Tc-99m labeled red blood cells.

Tc-99m Red Blood Cells. The quantity of stannous ions used for pretreatment of erythrocytes is critically important. The use of insufficient stannous ions results in very poor levels of Tc-99m radiolabeling because of the lack of adequate reducing capacity. Consequently, imaging performed with these types of poor quality cells will demonstrate high levels of blood and soft-tissue background. The use of excessively high doses of stannous ions, however, and the failure to allow for their removal from serum, may result in the reduction of Tc-99m pertechnetate in serum, which reduces the amount of radioactivity that may be transported across the red cell membrane (Rabito CA, et al, 1986). In vitro red blood cell labeling is usually accomplished with much smaller numbers of stannous ions, 1–15 micrograms. For these reasons, the number of stannous ions administered should be carefully monitored. Labeled cells were tested for adherence to intravenous lines, and no significant retention was observed (Segall GM, et al, 1986). G. H. Hinkle and coworkers (1983) have shown, however, that whenever central catheters, which are made of different materials, are used for administration, a poor-quality study often results.

Drug-Interference. Drug interference with Tc-99m red blood cells for equilibrium blood pool imaging can be classified into two general categories: (1) agents that alter, by a direct pharmacological effect, cardiac function and have the potential to interfere with the interpretation of equilibrium blood pool images, or (2) agents that inhibit or diminish the radiolabeling of red blood cells by Tc-99m.

Agents that induce an alteration in cardiac function include the beta adrenergic blockers, such as propranolol (Battler A, et al, 1979; Marshall RC, et al, 1981; Rainwater J, et al, 1982), calcium channel blockers, including verapamil (Petru MA, et al, 1983; Tan ATH, et al, 1982), and the nitrates, notably, nitroglycerin (Borer JS, et al, 1978; Pfisterer M, et al, 1983). Studies performed in patients receiving these pharmaceuticals may not detect the presence of coronary artery disease or accurately reflect its severity.

It has been proposed that these interfering drugs be withdrawn from patients prior to exercise ventriculography.

Table 13.13 PHARMACEUTICALS REPORTED TO ADVERSELY AFFECT Tc-99m RADIOLABELING OF RED BLOOD CELLS AND PROPOSED MECHANISM OF INTERFERENCE[a]

INTERFERING DRUG	ADVERSE EFFECT/PROPOSED MECHANISM OF INTERFERENCE	REFERENCE
Heparin	A Tc-99m labeled heparin complex may form when Tc-99m is injected through a heparinized catheter	Rao SA, et al, 1985 Hegge FN, et al, 1978
Methyldopa; Hydralazine	Oxidation of stannous ion, dimunition of reduction capacity	Zimmer AM, et al, 1981
Iodinated contrast media	?may involve multiple mechanisms, including lowering of Sn^{+2} reduction capacity, altered Sn^{+2} distribution, competition for RBC binding sites between Tc-99m and iodide media, or alteration in Tc-99m binding sites	Tatum JL, et al, 1983
Quinidine; Methyldopa	?may ↑ production of antibodies to red blood cells that may account for poor labeling with Tc-99m	Leitl GP, et al, 1980
Doxorubicin	Decreased labeling efficiency; mechanism unknown but effect appears related to drug concentration	Pauwels EKJ, et al, 1983 Seawright SJ, et al, 1983

[a] From Hladik WB III, et al, 1987.

J. A. Ponto suggests (1982) for beta-blocking medications a 48-hour interval between withdrawal of the drug and the nuclear medicine study. For the calcium channel blockers, the proposed interval has is 48–72 hours, whereas 12 hours has been suggested for the nitrates (Rabinovitch MA, 1985). Doxorubicin causes a dose-related cardiomyopathy that may interfere with the differential diagnosis of abnormal cardiac function. However, the radionuclide ventriculogram is often performed to monitor doxirubicin-induced cardiotoxicity (Alexander J, et al, 1979; McKillop JH, et al, 1983).

Poor radiolabeling of red blood cells with Tc-99m or early dissociation of Tc-99m from the labeled red blood cell brought about by concommitant drug therapy can adversely affect image quality (Lee HB, et al, 1983; Zanelli GD, 1982). Table 13.13 lists several of the drugs known to interfere with Tc-99m red blood cell labeling or that may be responsible for deterioration of the labeled cell.

Radiation Dosimetry. The radiation absorbed doses for these two agents are quite similar (Table 13.14).

To calculate accurate dosimetry data, detailed knowledge of the pharmacokinetics of each agent must be known and applied. For example, it is known that the initial distribution and rate of elimination of Tc-99m labeled red blood cells is a

Table 13.14 RADIATION DOSIMETRY FROM RADIOPHARMACEUTICALS EMPLOYED FOR BLOOD POOL IMAGING

ORGAN/TISSUE	RADS/MCI		
	Tc-99m RBC's[a]	Tc-99m HSA[b]	General Blood Pool Agent[c]
Total body	0.016	0.015	0.018–0.019
Spleen	0.018		0.039–0.062
Bladder wall	0.120	0.033	
Testes	0.012	0.016	
Ovaries	0.023		
Blood	0.052		
Red marrow	0.022	0.015	
Liver			0.040–0.098
Kidneys		0.013	0.043–0.066
Lungs			0.048–0.064
Heart			0.075–0.081

[a] Package inserts: TechneScan®-PYP (Mallinckrodt, Inc, St. Louis, Mo), Pyrolite® (Dupont-NEN, N. Billerica, MA).

[b] Package insert: Technetium-HSA Unit Dose (Medi-Physics, Inc, Richmond, CA)

[c] From Malamud H, 1978.

function of the method of labeling. To date, these factors have not been carefully applied to dosimetry calculations.

One factor that affects the dosimetry of blood pool imaging agents is the blood volume of the individual organs. This factor has been applied to dosimetry calculations by H. Malamud (1978). These data are shown in column 3 of Table 13.14. In these calculations, the effective half-life is assumed to be equal to the physical half-life, and the distribution to the organs is assumed to be solely a function of blood volume. The dosimetry calculated by this method results in higher values than those given from other sources.

References

Albro PC, Gould KL, Westcott RJ, et al. Noninvasive assessment of coronary stenoses by myocardial imaging during pharmacologic coronary vasodilation: III. Clinical trial. *Am J Cardiol* 1978, 42:751–760.

Alexander J, Dainiak N, Berger HJ, et al. Serial assessment of doxorubicin cardiotoxicity with quantitative radionuclide angiography. *N Engl J Med* 1979, 300:278–283.

Alfonso S. Inhibition of coronary vasodilating action of dipyridamole and adenosine by aminophyllin in the dog. *Circ Res* 1970, 26:743–747.

Aretz HT, Billingham ME, Edwards WD, et al. Myocarditis: A histopathologic definition and classification. *Am J Cardiovasc Pathol* 1986, 1:3–8.

Atkins HL, Budinger TF, Lebowitz E, et al. Thallium-201 for medical use. Part: Human distribution and physical imaging properties. *J Nucl Med* 1977, 18:133–140.

Atkins HL, Klopper JF, Ansari AN, et al. A comparison of Tc-99m-labeled human serum albumin and in vitro labeled red blood cells for blood pool studies. *Clin Nucl Med* 1980, 5:166–169.

Atkins HL, Srivastava SC, Meinken GE, Richards P. Biological behavior of erythrocytes labeled in vivo and in vitro with technetim-99m. *J Nucl Med Technol* 1985, 13:136–139.

Barreo JR, McDonald NS, Robinson GD, et al. Remote, semiautomated production of F-18 labeled 2-deoxy-2-fluoro-D-glucose. *J Nucl Med* 1981, 22:372–375.

Battler A, Ross J, Slutsky R, et al. Improvement of exercise induced left ventricular dysfunction with oral propranolol in patients with coronary heart disease. *Am J Cardiol* 1979, 44:318–324.

Becker L. Conditions for vasodilator-induced coronary steal in experimental myocardial ischemia. *Circulation* 1978, 57:1103–1110.

Berger BC, Watson DD, Burwell LR, et al. Redistribution of thallium at rest in patients with stable and unstable angina and the effects of coronary artery bypass surgery. *Circulation* 1979, 60:1114–1125.

Berger BC, Watson DD, Taylor GJ, et al. Sensitivity of quantitative thallium-201 scintigraphy following nondiagnostic exercise stress (Abst). *Circulation* 60 (Suppl): Abstracts of the 52nd Scientific Sessions. 1979, II-172.

Bergmann SR, Fox KAA, Rand AL, et al. Quantification of regional myocardial blood flow in vivo with $H_2^{15}O$. *Circulation* 1984, 70:724–733.

Bergmann SR, Fox KA, Geltman EM, et al. Positron emission tomography of the heart. *Prog Cardiovasc Dis* 1985, 28:165–194.

Bergmann SR, Hack S, Tewson T, et al. The dependence of accumulation of ^{13}N H_3 by myocardium on metabolic factors and its implication for the quantitative assessment of perfusion. *Circulation* 1980, 61:34–43.

Berman DS, Amsterdam EA, Hines HH, et al. New approach to interpretation of technetium-99m pyrophosphate scintigraphy in detection of acture myocardial infarction. *Am J Cardiol* 1977, 39:341–346.

Berman DS, Garcia, EV, Maddahi J, et al. Thallium-201 myocardial perfusion scintigraphy. In *Freeman and Johnson's Clinical Radionuclide Imaging* (3rd Ed.), Freeman LM (ed.). Orlando, FL, Grune and Stratton, 1984, pp. 479–536.

Bonte FJ, Parkey RW, Graham KD, et al. A new method for radionuclide imaging of myocardial infarcts. *Radiology* 1974, 110:473–474.

Borer JS, Bacharach SL, Gree MV, et al. Effect of nitroglycerine on exercise-induced abnormalities of left ventricular regional function and ejection fraction in coronary artery disease: Assessment by radionuclide cineangiography in symptomatic and asymptomatic patients. *Circulation* 1978, 57:314–320.

Boucher CA, Zir LM, Beller GA, et al. Increased lung uptake during exercise myocardial imaging: Clinical, hemodynamic and angiographic implications in patients with coronary artery disease. *Am J Cardiol* 1980, 46:189–196.

Bradley-Moore PR, Lebowitz E, Greene MW, et al. Thallium-201 for medical use. II. Biologic behavior. *J Nucl Med* 1975, 16:156–160.

Braunwald E. Protection of the ischemic myocardium. American Heart Association Monograph. Dallas, The American Heart Assoc., Inc., 48, 1976.

Brihaye C, Butler TA, Knapp FF, Jr, et al. A new osmium-191/iridium-191m radionuclide generator system using activated charcoal. *J Nucl Med* 1986, 27:380–387.

Britten J, Blank M. Thallium activation of Na-K-ATPase of rabbit kidney. *Biochim Biophys Acta* 1968, 159:160–166.

Brown JM, Dean RT, Kaplan P, et al. Absence of Human Antimouse (HAMA) response in patients given antimyosin Fab-DTPA monoclonal antibody (Abst) *J Nucl Med* 1988, 29:851.

Budinger TF, Derenzo SE, Gullberg GT, et al. Emission computer assisted tomography with single-photon and positron annihilation photon emitters. *J Comp Assist Tomogr.* 1977, 1:131–136.

Buja LM, Parkey RW, Dees JH, et al. Morphologic correlates of technetium-99m stannous pyrophosphate imaging of acute myocardial infarcts in dogs. *Circulation* 1975, 52:596–607.

Buja LM, Parkey RW, Stokely EM, et al. Pathophysiology of technetium-99m stannous pyrophosphate and thallium-201 scintigraphy of acute anterior myocardial infarcts in dogs. *J Clin Invest* 1976, 57:1508–1515.

Buja LM, Tofe AJ, Kulkarni PV, et al. Sites and mechanisms of localization of technetium-99m phosphorous radiopharmaceuticals in acute myocardial infarcts and other tissues. *J Clin Invest* 1977, 60:724–740.

Buja LM, Tofe AJ, Parkey RW, et al. Effect of EHDP on calcium accumulation and technetium-99m pyrophosphate uptake in experimental myocardial infarction. *Circulation* 1981, 64:1012–1017.

Burow RD, Pond M, Schafer W, et al. "Circumferential profiles," new method for computer analysis of thallium-201 myocardial perfusion images. *J Nucl Med* 1979, 20:771–777.

Callahan RJ. Radiolabeled Red Blood Cells as Diagnostic Radiopharmaceutical Vol II, p. 50. In *Radiopharmaceuticals: Progress and Clinical Prospectives*, Fritzberg AR (ed). Boca Raton, CRC Press, 1986.

Callahan RJ, Froelich JW, McKusick KA, et al. A modified method for the in vivo labeling of RBC with ^{99m}Tc. *J Nucl Med* 1982a 23:315–318.

Callahan RJ, Rabito CA. The inhibitory effect of dipyridamole on the caselins of red blood cells with technetium-99m (Abst). *Circulation* 1987, 76:(Suppl IV), 203.

Callahan RJ, Froelich JW, McKusick KA, et al. Factors affecting the rate and extent of incorporation of Tc-99m into pre-tinned red blood cells (RBC) (Abst). *J Nucl Med* 1982b, 23:109.

Carr EA, Cafruny EJ. Beierwalthes WH, et al. Evaluation of ^{203}Hg-chlormerodrin in the demonstration of human myocardial infarcts by scanning. *Univ Mich Med Cent J* 1963, 29:27.

Carr EA, Carroll M, Montes M. Effect of vitamin D_3, other drugs altering serum calcium or phosphorous concentrations, and desoxycorticosterone on the distribution of Tc-99m-pyrophosphate between target and non-target tissues. *J. Nucl. Med.* 22:526–534, 1981.

Chacko AK, Gordon DH, Bennett JM, et al. Myocardial imaging with Tc-99m pyrophosphate in patients on adriamycin treatment for neoplasia. *J Nucl Med* 1977, 18:680–683.

Chaudhuri TK. Liver uptake of ^{99m}Tc-diphosphonate. *Radiology* 119:485–486, 1976.

Cheng C, Treves S, Samuel A, et al. A new osmium-191/iridium-191m generator. *J Nucl Med* 1980, 21:1169–1176.

Coleman RE, Maturi M, Nunn AD, et al. Imaging of myocardial perfusion with

Tc-99m SQ 30217: Dog and human studies (Abst). 1986, *J Nucl Med* 27:893.

Cordova MA, Hladik WB, III, Rhodes BA. Adverse reactions associated with radiopharmaceuticals. In *Essentials of Nuclear Medicine Science*, Hladik WB, III, Saha G, Study KT (eds.). Baltimore, Williams and Wilkins, 1987, pp. 303–320.

D'Agostino AN and Chiga M. Mitochondrial mineralization in human myocardium. *Am J Clin Pathol* 1970, 53:820–824.

Delano ML, Sands H, Gallagher BM. Transport of $^{42}K^+$, $^{201}Tl^+$, and $[^{99m}Tc$-$(DMPE)_2Cl]^+$ by neonatal rat myocyte cultures. *Biochem Pharmacol* 1985, 34:3377–3380.

Deutsch E, Glavan KA, Sodd VJ, et al. Cationic Tc-99m complexes as potential myocardial imaging agents. *J Nucl Med* 1981, 22:897–907.

Dewanjee M. Binding of ^{99m}Tc ion to hemoglobulin. *J Nucl Med* 1974, 15:703–706.

Dewanjee MK, Fliegl C, Treves S, et al. ^{99m}Tc-tetracycline: A new radiopharmaceutical for renal imaging. *J Nucl Med* 1972, 13:427–428.

Dudczak R, Angelberger P, Homan R, et al. Evaluation of ^{99m}Tc-dichloro-bis(1,2-dimethylphosphino)-ethane (^{99m}Tc-DMPE) for myocardial scintigraphy in man. *Eur J Nucl Med* 1983, 8:513–515.

Dudczak R, Homan R, Zangeneh A, et al. Myocardial metabolic studies in patients with cardiomyopathy (Abst) *J Nucl Med* 1983, 24:p 20.

Dudczak R, Leitha T, Kletter K, et al. Comparison of Tc-99m-methoxypropyl-isonitrile (MPIN) and Tc-99m-methoxyisobutyl-isonitrile (MIBI) for myocardial imaging in man (Abst). *J Nucl Med* 1988, 29:794.

Dudczak R, Schmoliner R, Angelberger P, et al. Myocardial studies with I-123 p-phenylpentadecanoic acid in patients with coronary artery and idiopathic cardiomyopathy (Abst). *J Nucl Med* 1982, 23:P 35.

Dymond DS, Elliot AT, Flatman W, et al. Clinical validation of gold-195m: A new short half-life radiopharmaceutical for rapid sequential first-pass angiography in man. *J Am Coll Cardiol* 1983, 2:85–92.

Ferlin G, Borsato, N, Camerani M, et al. New prospectives in localizing enlarged parathyroids by technetium-thallium subtraction scan. *J Nucl Med* 1983, 24:438–441.

Fowler JS, MacGregor RR, Wolf AP, et al. A shielded synthesis system for production of 2-deoxy-2-[^{18}F]fluoro-D-glucose. *J Nucl Med* 1981, 22:376–380.

Francisco DA, Collins SM, Go RT, et al. Tomographic Tl-201 myocardial perfusion scintigrams after maximal coronary artery vasodilation with intravenous dipyridamole. *Circulation* 1982, 66:370–379.

Freundlieb C, Hock A, Vyska K, et al. Myocardial imaging and metabolic studies with 17-(I-123)-iodoheptadeconoic acid. *J Nucl Med* 1980, 21:1043–1050.

Garcia E, Maddahi J, Berman D, et al. Space/time quantitation of thallium-201 myocardial scintigraphy. *J Nucl Med* 1981, 22:309–317.

Gehring PJ, Hammond PB. The uptake of thallium by rabbit erythrocytes. *J Pharmacol Exp Ther* 1964, 145:215–221.

Gehring PJ, Hammond PB. The interrelationship between thallium and potassium in animals. *J Pharmacol Exp Ther* 1967, 55:187–201.

Geltman EM, Biello D, Welch MJ, et al. Characterization of non-transmural myocardial infarction by positron emission tomography. *Circulation* 1982, 65:747–755.

Gerber KH, Higgins CB: Quantitation of size of myocardial infarcts by computerized transmission tomography. Comparison with hot-spot and cold-spot radionuclide scans. *Invest Radiol* 1983, 18:238–243.

Gerundini P, Sari A, Gilardi MC, et al. Evaluation in dogs and humans of three potential technetium-99m myocardial perfusion agents. *J Nucl Med* 1986, 27:409–416.

Gorten RJ, Hardy LB, McGraw BH, et al. The selective uptake of Hg-203 chloromerodrin in experimentally produced myocardial infarcts. *Am Heart J* 1966, 72:71–78.

Gould KL. Noninvasive assessment of coronary stenoses by myocardial imaging during pharmacologic coronary vasodilation. I. Physiologic basis and experimental validation. *Am J Cardiol* 1978a, 41:267–278.

Gould KL, Schelbert HR, Phelps ME, et al. Non-invasive assessment of coronary stenoses with myocardial perfusion imaging during pharmacologic coronary vasodilation. V. Detection of 47% diameter coronary stenoses with intravenous nitrogen-13 ammonia and emission-computer transaxial tomography in intact dogs. *Am J Cardiol* 1979, 43:200–208.

Gould KL, Westcott RJ, Albro PC, et al. Noninvasive assessment of coronary stenoses by myocardial imaging during pharmacologic coronary vasodilation. II. Clinical methodology and feasibility. *Am J Cardiol* 1978b, 41:279–287.

Graham MM, Nelp WB. Cardiac blood pool activity after in vivo and in vitro red blood cell (RBC) labeling (Abst). *J Nucl Med* 1980, 21:P7.

Grover M, Schwaiger M, Hansen H, et al. Coronary artery occlusion and reperfusion alters rubidium-82 extraction fraction. *Circulation* 1984, 70:II-148 (Abst).

Hamilton GW, Narahara KA, Yee H, et al. Myocardial imaging with thallium-201: Effect of cardiac drugs on myocardial images and absolute tissue distribution. *J Nucl Med* 19:10–16, 1978.

Hamilton RG, Alderson PO. A comparative evaluation of technique for rapid and efficient in vivo labeling of red blood cells with ^{99m}Tc pertechnetate. *J Nucl Med* 1977, 18:1010–1013.

Hansen S, Stadalnik RC. Liver uptake of ^{99m}Tc-pyrophosphate. *Semin Nucl Med* 1982, 12:89–91.

Hecht HS, Chew CYC, Burnam MH, et al. Verapamil in chronic stable angina: Amelioration of pacing-induced abnormalities of left ventricular ejection fraction regional wall motion, latate metabolism and hemodynamics. *Am J Cardiol* 1981, 48:536–544.

Hegge FN, Hamilton GW, Larson SM. Cardiac chamber imaging: A comparison of red blood cells labeled with ^{99m}Tc, in vitro and in vivo. *J Nucl Med* 1978, 19:129–134.

Henkin RE, Chang W, Provus R. The effect of beta blockers on thallium scans (Abst). *J Nucl Med* 1982, 23:P63.

Hillis LD, Braunwald E. Myocardial ischemia. *N Engl J Med* 1977, 296:971–978.

Hinkle GH, Shaffer PB, Olsen JO. Radiolabeling red blood cells using a Hickman catheter. *J Nucl Med Technol* 1983, 11:69–70.

Hirth W, Jurisson S, Linder K, et al. Chloro-hydroxy substitution on technetium dioxime complexes: Chemical and biological comparison of TcCl(dioxime)$_3$Br and TcOH(dioxime)$_3$Br (Abst). *J Nucl Med* 1988, 29:800.

Hladik WB III, Ponto JA, Lentle BC, et al. Iatrogenic alterations in the biodistribution of radiotracers as a result of drug therapy: Reported instances. In *Essentials of Nuclear Medicine Science*, Hladik WB, Saha GB, Study KT. (eds.). Baltimore, Williams and Wilkins, 1987, pp. 189–219.

Hockings B, Saltissi S, Croft DN, et al. Effect of beta adrenergic blockade of thallium-201 myocardial perfusion imaging. *Br Heart J* 1983, 49:83–89.

Holman BL, Dewanjee MK, Iodine J, et al. Detection and localization of experimental myocardial infarction with ^{99m}Tc-tetracycline. *J Nucl Med*, 1973, 14:595–599.

Holman BL, Jones AG, Lister-James J, et al. A new Tc-99m-labeled-myocardial imaging agent, hexakis (t-butylisonitrile) technetium (I)[Tc-99m TBI]: Initial experience in the human. *J Nucl Med* 1984, 25:1350–1355.

Horlock P, Clark J, O'Brien HA, et al. The preparation of a rubidium-82 radionuclide generator. *J Radioanalyt Chem* 1981, 64:257–265.

Huang SC, Phelps ME, Hoffman EJ, et al. Noninvasive determination of local cerebral metabolic rate of glucose in man. *Am J Physiol* 1980, 238:E69.

ICRP Publication 52, Protection of the Nuclear Medicine Patient. Oxford, Pergamon, 1988.

Ido T, Cuan CN, Fowler JS, et al. Fluorination with F_2-A convenient synthesis of 2-deoxy-2 fluoro-D-glucose. *J Org Chem* 1977, 42:2341–2342.

Ido T, Wan CN, Casella V, et al. Labeled 2-deoxy-D-glucose analogs: ^{18}F-labeled 2-deoxy-2-fluoro-D-glucose, 2-deoxy-2-fluoro-D-mannose and ^{14}C-2-deoxy-2-fluoro-D-glucose. *J Label Compds Radiopharm* 1978, 14:175–183.

Jansen D, Gabliani G, Wolfe C, et al. Determination of viable myocardial mass with iodinated phenylpentadecanoic acid and single photon emission computed tomography (Abst). *Circulation* 1984, 70 (Suppl 11):11–449.

Jones AG, Davis MA, Uren RF, et al. In vivo red cell labeling with [99m]Tc (Abst). *J Nucl Med* 1977, 18:637.

Josephson MA, Brown BG, Hecht HS, et al. Noninvasive detection and localization of coronary artery stenoses in patients: Comparison of resting dipyridamole and exercise thallium-201 myocardial perfusion imaging. *Am Heart J*, 1982, 103:1008–1010.

Josephson MA, Hecht HS, Hopkins J, et al. Comparative effects of oral verapamil and propranolol on exercise-induced ischemia and energetics in patients with coronary artery disease–single blind–crossover evaluation using radionuclides. *Am Heart J* 1982, 103:978–985.

Kawana M, Krizek H, Porter J, et al. Use of Tl-199 as a potassium analog in scanning (Abst). *J Nucl Med* 1970, 11:333.

Kelly RJ, Chilton HM, Hackshaw BT, et al. Comparison of Tc-99m pyrophosphate and Tc-99m methylene diphosphonate in acute myocardial infarction: Concise communication. *J Nucl Med* 1979, 20:402–406.

Ketring AR, Deutsch E, Libson K, et al. The Noah's Ark experiment. A search for a suitable animal model for the evaluation of cationic Tc-99m myocardial imaging agents (Abst). *J Nucl Med* 1983, 24:P9.

Khaw BA, Beller GA, Haber E. Experimental myocardial infarct imaging following intravenous administration of iodine-131 labeled antibody (Fab)$_2$ fragments specific for cardiac myosin. 1978a, *Circulation* 57:743–750.

Khaw BA, Beller GA, Haber E, et al. Localization of cardiac myosinspecific antibody in myocardial infarction. 1976, *J Clin Invest* 58:439–446.

Khaw BA, Fallon JT, Beller GA, et al. Specificity of localization of myosin-specific antibody fragments in experimental myocardial infarction: Histologic, histochemical, autoradiographic, and scintigraphic studies. *Circulation* 1979, 60:1527–1531.

Khaw BA, Fallon JT, Strauss HW, et al. Myocardial infarct imaging with Indium-111-diethylene triamine pentaacetic acid-anticanine cardiac myosin antibodies. *Science* 1980, 209:295–297.

Khaw BA, Gold HK, Leinbach RC, et al. Early imaging of experimental myocardial infarction by intracoronary administration of ^{131}I-labeled anticardiac myosin (Fab$_2$) fragments. *Circulation* 1978b, 58:1137–1142.

Khaw BA, Gold HK, Yasuda T, et al. Scintigraphic quantification of myocardial necrosis in patients after intravenous injection of myosin specific antibody. *Circulation* 1986, 74:501–508.

Khaw BA, Mattis JA, Melincoff G, et al. Monoclonal antibody to cardiac myosin: Imaging of experimental myocardial infarction. *Hybridoma* 1984a, 3:11–15.

Khaw BA, Strauss HW, Cahill SL, et al. Sequential imaging of indium-111-labeled monoclonal antibody in human mammary tumors hosted in nude mice. *J Nucl Med* 1984b, 25:592–603.

Khaw BA, Strauss HW, Carvalho A, et al. Technetium-99m labeling of antibodies to cardiac myosin Fab and to human fibrinogen. *J Nucl Med* 1982, 23:1011–1018.

Khentigan A, Garret M, Lum D, et al.

Effects of prior administration of SN(II) complexed on in vivo distribution of ^{99m}Tc pertechnetate. *J Nucl Med* 1976, 17:380–384.

Kloner RA, Ellis SG, Lange R, et al. Studies of experimental coronary artery reperfusion. Effects on infarct size, myocardial function, biochemistry, ultrastructure and microvascular damage. (Abst). 1983, *Circulation* 68:8.

Kohler G, Milstein C. Continuous cultures of fused cells secreting antibody of predefined specificity. *Nature (Lond)* 1975, 256:495–497.

Krejcarek GE, Tucker KL. Covalent attachments of chelating groups of macromolecules. *Biochem Biophys Res Commun* 1977, 77:581–585.

Kuhl DE, Edwards RQ, Ricci AR, et al. The MARK IV system for radionuclide computed tomography of the brain. *Radiology* 1976, 121:405–413.

Kushner FG, Okada RD, Kirshenbaum HD, et al. Lung thallium-201 uptake after stress testing in patients with coronary artery disease. *Circulation* 1981, 63:341–347.

Lebowitz E, Greene MW, Fairchild R, et al. Thallium for medical use. *J Nucl Med* 1975, 16:151–155.

Lee HB, Wexler JP, Scharf SC, et al. Pharmacologic alterations in Tc-99m binding by red blood cells.: Concise communication. *J Nucl Med* 1983, 24:397–401.

Leitl GP, Drew HMN, Kelly ME, et al. Interference with Tc-99m labeling of red blood cells (RBCs) by RBC antibodies (Abst). *J Nucl Med* 1980, 21:P44.

Leppo J, Boucher CA, Okada RD, et al. Serial thallium-201 myocardial imaging after dipyridamole infusion: Diagnostic utility in detecting coronary stenoses and relationship to regional wall motion. *Circulation* 1982, 66:649–656.

Leppo JA, Moring AF. An evaluation of a technetium-labeled isonitrile analog as a myocardial imaging agent and comparison to thallium (Abst.). *Circulation* [Suppl]. 1986, 2, 74:II–297.

Liedtke JA. Alterations in carbohydrate and lipid metabolism in the acutely ischemic heart. *Prog Cardiovasc Dis* 1981, 23:321–328.

Linder KE, Treher EN, Juri PN, et al. Neutral tris oxime complexes of technetium (III): Chemistry and biodistribution of TcX(oxime)$_3$ (Abst). *J Nucl Med* 1988, 29:800.

Livini E, Elmalch DR, Barlai-Kovach M, et al. Radioiodinated beta-methyl phenyl fatty acids as potential tracers for myocardial imaging and metabolism. *Eur Heart J* 1985, 6:85–87.

Livini E, Elmalch DR, Levy S, et al. Beta-methyl (1-C-11) heptadeconoic acid: A new myocardial metabolic tracer for positron emission tomography. *J Nucl Med* 1982, 23:169–175.

Love WD, Ishihara Y, Lyon LD, et al. Differences in the relationships between coronary blood flow and myocardial clearance of isotopes of potassium, rubidium, and cesium. *Am Heart J*, 1968, 76:353–355.

Lyons KP, Olson HG, Aronow WS. Pyrophosphate myocardial imaging. *Semin Nucl Med* 1980, 10:168–177.

Makler PT, Lederman S, Charkes ND, et al. Myocardial infarct imaging with ^{99m}Tc-pyrophosphate and ^{99m}Tc diphosphonate: Lack of correlation. *Clin Nucl Med* 1979, 4:89–91.

Malamud H. Dosimetry of ^{99m}Tc labeled blood pool scanning agents. *Clin Nucl Med* 1978, 3:420–421.

Malek P, Kolc J, Zastava V, et al. Fluorescence of tetracycline analogues fixed in myocardial infarction. *Cardiologica* 1963, 42:303–318.

Malek P, Vavrejn B, Ratusky J, et al. Detection of myocardial infarction by in vivo scanning. *Cardiologica* 1967, 51:22–32.

Marshall RC, Huang SC, Nash WW, et al. Assessment of the [^{18}F] fluorodeoxyglucose kinetic model in calculations of myocardial glucose metabolism during ischemia. *J Nucl Med* 1983, 24:1060–1064.

Marshall RC, Wisenberg G, Schelbert HR, et al. Effect of oral propranolol on rest, exercise and postexercise left ventricular performance in normal subjects and patients with coronary artery disease. *Circulation* 1981, 63:572–583.

Massie B, Kramer B, Wisneski J, et al. Differences in Tl-201 washout rates with maximal and submaximal exercise: Implications for diagnosis of coronary artery disease. *Clin Res* 1982, 30:15A.

Matthews CME, Kibby PM, Gabe IT, et al. Distribution of cesium, rubidium, and potassium isotopes in the dog and measurement of coronary flow. *J Nucl Biol Med* 1969, 13:49–60.

Mazziotta JC, Phelps M. Positron emission tomography studies of the brain. In *Positron Emission Tomography and Autoradiography: Principles and Application for the Brain and Heart.* Phelps M, Mazziotta J, Schelbert H (eds). New York, Raven, 1986, pp. 493–579.

McKillop JH, Bristow MR, Goris ML, et al. Sensitivity and specificity of radionuclide ejection fractions in doxorubicin cardiotoxicity. *Am Heart J* 1983, 106:1048–1056.

McKusick KA. Comparison of 3 Tc-99m isonitriles for detection of ischemic heart disease in humans. *J Nucl Med* 1986a 27:878.

McKusick KA, Holman BL, Rigo P, et al. Human myocardial imaging with Tc-99m isonitriles. *Circulation* 1986b, 74:II–196.

McLaughlin PR, Martin RP, Doherty P, et al. Reproducibility of thallium-201 myocardial imaging. *Circulation* 1979, 55:497–503.

Meade RC, Bamrah VS, Horgan JD, et al. Quantitative methods in the evaluation of thallium-201 myocardial perfusion images. *J Nucl Med* 1978, 19:1175–1178.

Metler FA, Jr, Guiberteau MJ. Cardiovascular system. In *Essentials of Nuclear Medicine*, 2nd Ed. W.B. Saunders, Philadelphia, 1985, p. 153.

Miller DD, Gill JB, Barlai-Kovach M, et al. Identification of the ischemic border zone in reperfused canine myocardium using iodinated fatty acid analogs. *Clin Res* 1985a, 33:211A.

Miller DD, Gill JB, Barlai-Kovach M, et al. Modified fatty acid analog imaging: Correlation of SPECT and clearance kinetics in ischemic reperfused myocardium (Abst). *J Nucl Med* 1985b, 23:P84.

Miller DD, Strauss HW. Radionuclides for cardiac imaging. *Clin Cardiac Imaging*, 1988, P3.

Mueller TM, Marcus ML, Ehrhardt JC, et al. Limitations of thallium-201 myocardial perfusion scintigrams. *Circulation* 1976, 54:640–646.

Mullins LJ and Moore RD. The movement of thallium ions in muscle. *J. Gen. Physiol.* 43:759–773, 1960.

Narra RK, Kuczynski BL, Feld T, et al. A comparison of the pharmacokinetics of a new Tc-99m-labeled myocardial imaging agent, SQ 32, 014 with SQ 30, 217 (Abst.). *J Nucl Med* 1987, 28:674.

Neely JR, Morgan HE. Relationship between carbohydrate and lipid metabolism and the energy balance of heart muscle. *Ann Rev Physiol* 1974, 36:413–418.

Neirinckx RD, Kronauge JF, Gennaro GP, et al. Evaluation of inorganic absorbance for the rubidium-82 generators: I. Hydrous SnO_2. *J Nucl Med* 1982, 23:245–249.

Nelson MF, Melton RE, and Van Wazer JR. Sodium trimetaphosphate as a bone-imaging agent. I. Animal studies. *J Nucl Med* 1975, 16:1043-1048.

Nicol PD, Yasuda T, Locke E, et al. Multiple intravenous administrations of In-111 labeled antimyosin Fab: Determination of antimurine Fab response in patients with myocarditis. *Abst J Nucl Med* 1988, 29:939.

Nishiyama H, Deutsch E, Adolph RJ, et al. Basal kinetic studies of Tc-99m DMPE as a myocardial imaging agent in the dog. *J Nucl Med* 1982, 23:1093–1101.

Nunn AD, Treher EN, Feld T. Boronic acid adducts of technetium oxime complexes (BATOs): A new class of neutral complexes with myocardial imaging capabilities (Abst). *J Nucl Med* 1986, 27:893.

Nusynowitz ML, Straw JD, Benedetto AR, et al. Blood clearance rates of technetium-99m albumin preparations: Concise communication. *J Nucl Med* 1978, 19:1142–1145.

Opie L. Carbohydrates and lipids. *Heart* 1984, 10:118–123.

Opie LH, Owen P, Riemersma RA: Relative rates of oxidation of glucose and free fatty acids by ischaemic and non-ischaemic myocardium after coronary artery ligation in the dog. *Eur J Clin Invest* 1973, 3:419–422.

Osbakken MD, Okada RD, Boucher CA, et al. The effect of inderal, exercise level, and subcritical disease on the specificity of exercise thallium-201 imaging (Abst). *J Nucl Med* 1981, 22:P41.

Parkey RW, Bonte FJ, Meyer SL, et al. A new method for radionuclide imaging of acute myocardial infarctions in humans. *Circulation* 1974, 50:540–546.

Pauwels EKJ, Feitsma RIJ, Blom J. Influence of adriamycin on red blood cells labeling: A pitfall in scintigraphic blood pool imaging. *Nucl Med Commun* 1983, 4:290–293.

Pavel D, Zimmer ZM, Patterson VN. In vivo labeling of red blood cells with ^{99m}Tc: A new approach to blood pool visualization. *J Nucl Med* 1977, 18:305–308.

Petru MA, Crawford, MH, Sorenson SG, et al. Short- and long-term efficacy of high-dose oral diltiazem for angina due to coronary artery disease: A placebo-controlled, randomized, double-blind crossover study. *Circulation* 1983, 68:139–147.

Pfisterer M, Glans L, Burkart F. Comparative effect of nitroglycerin, nifedipine, and metroprolol on regional left ventricular function in patients with one-vessel coronary disease. *Circulation* 1983, 67:291–301.

Phelps ME. Emission computed tomography. *Semin Nucl Med* 1977, 7:337–315.

Phelps ME, Hoffman EJ, Huang SC, et al. ECAT: A new computerized tomographic imaging system for positron-emitting radiopharmaceuticals. *J Nucl Med* 1978, 19:635–647.

Phelps ME, Huang SC, Hoffman EJ, et al. Tomographic measurement of local cerebral glucose metabolic rate in humans with (F-18)1-fluoro-2-deoxy-D-glucose: Validation of method. *Ann, Neurol* 1979, 6:371–388.

Pohost GM, Alpert NM, Ingwall JS, et al. Thallium redistribution: Mechanisms and clinical utility. *Semin Nucl Med* 1980, 10:70–93.

Pohost GM, O'Keefe DD, Gweirtz H, et al. Thallium redistribution in the presence of severe fixed coronary stenosis (Abst). *Clin Res* 1978, 26:260A.

Pohost GM, Zir LM, Moore RH, et al. Differentiation of transiently ischemic from infarcted myocardium by serial imaging after a single dose of thallium-201. *Circulation* 1977, 55:294–302.

Ponto JA, Holmes KA. Discontinuation of beta blockers before exercise radionuclide ventriculograms. *J Nucl Med* 1982, 23:456–457.

Porter WC, Dees SM, Freitas JE, et al. Acid-Citrate-Detrose compared with heparin in the preparation of in vivo–in vitro technetium-99m RBC. *J Nucl Med* 1983, 24:383–387.

Rabinovitch MA. Pharmacologic interventions in nuclear cardiology. In *Diagnostic Interventions in Nuclear Medicine*, Thrall JH, Swanson DP (eds). Chicago, Yearbook, 1985, pp. 31–60.

Rabito CA, Callahan RJ, McKusick KA, et al. Transport of pertechnetate by human erythrocyte membrane (Abst). *J Nucl Med* 1986, 27:946.

Rainwater J, Steele P, Kirch D, et al. Effect of propranolol on myocardial perfusion images and exercise ejection fractions in men with coronary artery disease. *Circulation* 1982, 65:77–81.

Rao SA, Knobel J, Collier BD. Effect of therapeutic dose of heparin on the in vivo labeling of red blood cells with technetium-99m for blood pool imaging: Importance of stannous ion concentration (Abst). *J Nucl Med* 1985, 26:P65.

Raynaud C, Comar D, Buisson M, et al. Radioactive thallium: A new agent for scans of the renal medulla. In *Radionuclides in Nephrology*, New York,

Grune and Stratton, 1972, pp. 289–294.

Rehani MN, Sharma SK. Site of ^{99m}Tc binding to the red blood cell: Concise communication. *J Nucl Med* 1980, 21: 676–678.

Rellas JS, Corbett JR, Kulkarni P, et al. I-123 phenyl-pentadecanoic acid: Detection of acute myocardial infarction and injury in dogs using an iodinated fatty acid and SPECT. *Am J Cardiol* 1983, 52:1326–1332.

Reske SN, Knopp R, Machulla HJ, et al. Clearance patterns of 15(p-I-123-phenyl) pentadecanoic acid in patients with CAD after bicycle exercise (Abst). *J Nucl Med* 1983, 24:P13.

Reske SN, Knust EJ, Machulla HJ, et al. Comparison of cardiac C-14 palmitic acid and I-123 phenyl-pentadecanoic acid oxidation (Abst). *J Nucl Med* 1983, 24:P118.

Reske SN, Simon H, Machulla HJ, et al. Myocardial turnover of p-(I-123) phenyl-pentadecanoic acid in patients with CAD (Abst) 1982, *J Nucl Med* 23:P34.

Ritchie JL, Hamilton GW. Biologic properties of thallium. In Ritchie JL Hamilton GW, Wackers FG Th: (eds.). *Thallium-201 Myocardial Imaging*, New York, Raven Press, 1978, pp 9–28.

Rossman DJ, Rouleau J, Strauss HW, et al. Detection and size estimation of acute myocardial infarction using ^{99m}Tc-gluceptate. *J Nucl Med* 1975, 16, 980–985.

Rovetto MJ, Lamberton WF, Neely JR. Mechanisms of glycolytic inhibition of ischemic rat heart. *Circ Res* 1975, 37:742–751.

Sands H, Delano ML, Camin LL, et al. Comparison of the transport of $^{42}K^+$, $^{22}Na^+$, $^{201}Tl^+$, and $[^{99m}Tc(DMPE)_2Cl_2]^+$ using human erythrocytes. *Biochem Biophys Acta* 1985, 812:665–670.

Sands H, Delano ML, Gallagher BM. Uptake of Hexakis (t-butyl isonitrile) Technetium (I) and Hexakis-(Isopropyl Isonitrile) Technetium (I) by neonatal rat myocytes and human erythrocytes. *J Nucl Med* 1986, 27:4041–408.

Schachner ER, Oster ZH, Cicale N, et al.

The effect of diphenylhydantoin (dilantin) on thallium-201 chloride uptake (abst). *J Nucl Med* 1980, 21:P57.

Schelbert HR. Radionuclides for cardiac imaging. *Semin Nucl Med* 1987, 17: 145–181.

Schelbert HR, Phelps ME, Huang SC, et al. N-13 ammonia as an indicator of myocardial blood flow. *Circulation* 1981, 63:1259–1272.

Schelbert HR, Verba JW, Johnson AD, et al. Nontraumatic determination of left ventricular ejection fraction by radionuclide angiocardiography. *Circulation* 1975, 51:902–909.

Schelbert HR, Wisenberg G, Phelps ME, et al. Non-invasive assessment of coronary stenoses by myocardial imaging during pharmacologic coronary vasodilation. VI. Detection of coronary artery disease in many with intravenous N-13 ammonia and positron computed tomography. *Am J Cardiol* 1982, 49: 1197–1207.

Schon H, Schelbert HR, Henze E, et al. Quantification of regional C-11 palmitate kinetics by positron tomography (PET) (Abst). *Circulation* 1984, 70:11.

Seawright SJ, Maton PJ, Greenall J, et al. Factors affecting in vivo labeling of red blood cells. *J Nucl Med Technol* 1983, 11:95.

Segall GM, Gurevich N, McDougall IR. Adherence of radiopharmaceuticals and labeled cells to intravenous tubing. *Clin Nucl Med* 1986, 12:830–833.

Shah A, Schelbert HR, Schwaiger M, et al. Measurement of regional myocardial blood flow with N-13 ammonia and positron emission tomography in intact dogs. *J Am Coll Cardiol* 1985, 5:92–100.

Singh A, Usher M. Comparison of Tc-99m methylene diphosphonate with Tc-99m pyrophosphate in the detection of acute myocardial infarction: Concise communication. *J Nucl Med* 1977, 18: 790–792.

Smith TD, Richards P. A simple kit for the preparation of ^{99m}Tc labeled red blood cells. *J Nucl Med 1976*, 17:126–132.

Smith TW, Haber E, Yehtman L, et al.

Reversal of advanced digoxin intoxication with Fab fragments of digoxin-specific antibodies. *N Engl J Med* 1976, 294:797–800.

Sporn V, Perez-Balino N, Holman BL, et al. Myocardial imaging with Tc-99m CPI: Initial experience in the human (Abst). *J Nucl Med* 1986, 27:P878.

Srivastava SC, Babick JB, Richards P. A new kit method for the selective labeling of erythrocytes in whole blood with technetium-99m (Abst). *J Nucl Med* 1983, 24: P128.

Stabin M. Personal communication from the Radiopharmaceutical Internal Dose Information Center, Oak Ridge Associated Universities, Oak Ridge, TN, 1988.

Strauss HW, Harrison K, Langan JK, et al. Thallium-201 for myocardial imaging: Relation of thallium-201 to regional myocardial perfusion. *Circulation* 1975, 51:641–645.

Strauss HW, Zaret BL, Hurley PJ, et al. A scintiphotographic method for measuring left ventricular ejection fraction in man without cardiac catherization. *Am J Cardiol* 1971, 28:575–580.

Subramanian G, McAfee JG, Blair RJ, et al. Technetium-99m-methylene diphosphonate—a superior agent for skeletal imaging: Comparison with other technetium complexes. *J Nucl Med* 1975, 16:744–755.

Tamaki N, Yonekura Y, Senda M, et al. Myocardial positron computed tomography with ^{13}N-ammonia at rest and during exercise. *Eur J Nucl Med* 1985, 11:246–251.

Tan ATH, Sadic N, Kelly DT, et al. Verapamil in stable effort angina: Effects on left ventricular function evaluated with exercise radionuclide ventriculography. *Am J Cardiol* 1982, 49:425–430.

Tatum JL, Burke TS, Hirsch JI, et al. Pitfall to modified in vivo method of technetium-99m red blood cell labeling-iodinated contrast media. *Clin Nucl Med* 1983, 8:585–590.

Thrall JH, Freitas JE, Swanson D, et al. Clinical comparison of cardiac blood pool visualization with technetium-99m red blood cells labeled in vivo and with technetium-99m human serum albumin. *J Nucl Med* 1978, 19:796–803.

USP DI 1988 (8th Ed.), Drug Information for the Health Care Professional, United States Pharmacopeia, Easton, Mack Printing Company, 1988.

Wahner HK, Dewanjee MK. Drug-induced modulation of Tc-99m pyrophosphate tissue distribution: What is involved? *J Nucl Med* 1981, 22:555–559.

Wakat MA, Chilton HM, Hackshaw BT, et al. Comparison of Tc-99m pyrophosphate and Tc-99m hydroxymethylene diphosphonate in acute myocardial infarction. *J Nucl Med* 1980, 21:203–206.

Watson EE, Stabin MG, Goodman MM, et al. A comparison of radiation dosimetry for several potential myocardial imaging agents. In *Proceedings of Fourth International Radiation Dosimetry Symposium* (Conf-851113), 1985.

Wildenthal K, Morgan HR, Opie LH, et al. Regulation of cardiac metabolism. American Heart Association Monograph, Dallas, The American Heart Assn, 49, 1976.

Willerson JT, Parkey RN, Bonte FJ, et al. Pathophysiologic considerations and clinicopathological correlates of technetium-99m stannous pyrophosphate myocardial scintigraphy. *Semin Nucl Med* 1980, 10:54–69.

Wilson RA, Sullivan PJ, Okada RD, et al. The effect of eating on thallium myocardial imaging. *Chest* 1986, 89:195–198.

Wolf R, Pretschner P, Engel HJ, et al. Effect of isosorbide dinitrate on thallium-201 myocardial imaging in coronary heart disease (Abst). *Am J Cardiol* 1979, 43:432.

Yang SSL, Nickoloff EL, McIntyre PA, et al. Tc-99m human serum albumin: A suitable agent for plasma volume measurements in man. *J Nucl Med* 1978, 19:804–807.

Yasuda T, Palacios I, Dec W, et al. Indium-111 monoclonal antimyosin antibody in the diagnosis of acute myocarditis. *Circulation* 1987, 76:306–311.

Young AE, Gaunt JI, Croft DN, et al. Location of parathyroid adenomas by thallium-201 and technetium-99m subtraction scanning. *Br Med J* 1983, 286:1384–1387.

Zanelli GD. Effects of certain drugs used in the treatment of cardiovascular disease on the in vitro labeling of red blood cells with Tc-99m. *Nucl Med Commun* 1982, 3:155–161.

Zaret BL, DiCola VC, Donabedian RK, et al. Dual radionuclide study of myocardial infarction. Relationships between myocardial uptake of potassium-43, technetium-99m stannous pyrophosphate, regional myocardial blood flow and creatine phosphokinase depletion. *Circulation* 1976, 53:422–428.

Zimmer AM, Spies SM, Majewski W. Effect of drugs on in vivo labeling: A proposed mechanism of inhibition. Presented at the Second International Symposium on Radiopharmacology, Chicago, September, 1981.

Radiopharmaceuticals for Abdominal and Gastrointestinal Imaging: Reticuloendothelial, Hepatobiliary, and Intestinal

Henry M. Chilton
Manuel L. Brown

I. Radiopharmaceuticals for Liver Imaging

The two distinct cell types of the liver, the phagocytic Kupffer's cells of the reticuloendothelial (RE) system and the hepatocytes, permit the evaluation of that organ by the use of two different classes of radiopharmaceuticals. Colloidal substances, particulate matter smaller than red blood cells, pass the capillary beds of the lungs without becoming trapped, yet are rapidly removed from blood by the hepatic Kupffer's cells remaining there sufficiently long to permit the evaluation of liver morphology via scintillation imaging. Hepatocellular function, on the other hand, can be evaluated using non-particulate radiolabeled substances that are actively removed from blood by the hepatocytes (or polygonal cells) and excreted via the hepatobiliary pathway. Substances normally excreted in this manner include soluble metabolic breakdown substances and exogenous materials sufficiently lipophilic to undergo hepatocellular transport.

LIVER IMAGING: THE RETICULOENDOTHELIAL SYSTEM

The cells of the reticuloendothelial system exist principally in the liver, spleen, and bone marrow and share the common property of phagocytosis of colloidal substances in blood. In the liver, the RE cells, known as Kupffer cells, constitute approximately 85% of the RE system, while making up only 15% of the liver cell population. Approximately 5–10% are found in the spleen, with the remainder distributed in the bone marrow.

As an organ of the RE system, the liver is highly efficient for the removal of colloidal substances from blood with a single-pass extraction efficiency approaching 95% (Shaldon S, et al, 1961). Although the rate of particle clearance by the liver is affected by the number and size of the particles administered, clearance varies inversely only with the number administered within a wide range of mean particles size (Cohen Y, et al, 1968).

BACKGROUND/HISTORY

A variety of radiocolloidal preparations have been evaluated for usefulness in the study of hepatic morphology. Earliest investigations attempted to study hepatic blood flow using the Beta-emitting radionuclide P-32 as colloidal chromic phosphate (Dobson EL and Jones HB, 1952). Later, heat-denatured human serum albumin labeled with I-131 and gelatin stabilized Au-198 were investigated (Stirrett LA, et al, 1953; Vetter H, et al, 1954). For all practical purposes, the era of liver scanning began in 1954 when Stirrett and co-workers utilized Au-198 colloid and obtained the first nuclear medicine images of the liver.

Colloids are generally defined as

nonhomogeneous dispersion of particles, usually in an aqueous media, that are between 0.05–5 microns in diameter. Colloids less than 0.1 microns are taken up to a greater extent by the bone marrow whereas intermediate-sized colloids (0.3–1 microns) are predominantly removed by the liver. Relatively large colloids (greater than 1 micron) are preferentially taken up by the spleen. Colloids composed of organic substances, such as denatured proteins, are metabolized by the liver and eventually cleared. Inorganic colloids, however, do not undergo metabolism and are believed to be fixed in the RE cells indefinitely.

Au-198 colloid was for many years the agent of choice for liver imaging. Au-198 colloid could be purchased in ready-to-use form and, although its relatively high gamma photon energy (0.411 MeV) and Beta-minus decay mode were less than ideal, no other radiopharmaceuticals available at that time were suitable for liver imaging. Because of its relatively small particle size (0.02–0.04 microns), a significant proportion of this radiopharmaceutical accumulated in the bone marrow as well as the liver. The amount of Au-198 colloid that localized in the spleen (2–3%) was insufficient to permit imaging of that organ (Nelp WB, 1970).

The development of the Mo-99/Tc-99m generator during the mid-1960s made practical the use of short-lived radionuclides with highly desirable imaging properties. P. Richards (1960) noted the po-potential usefulness of Tc-99m, whereas P.V. Harper and colleagues (1964a) first employed Tc-99m sulfur colloid for liver scanning.

Initially, Tc-99m sulfur colloid was prepared by bubbling hydrogen sulfide gas through an acidified solution of Tc-99m sodium pertechnetate and gelatin. The product was sterilized by terminal membrane filtration and had an estimated particle size of 0.05–0.15 microns (Harper PV, et al, 1964b). Another method developed for preparing Tc-99m sulfur colloid utilized the acid reduction of sodium thiosulfate in the presence of Tc-99m pertechnetate (Stern HS, et al, 1966). The reaction proceeds in a boiling water bath. In both methods, thiosulfuric acid is formed that decomposes to sulfur and sulfur dioxide, with the elemental sulfur forming a colloidal coprecipitate with Tc-99m pertechnetate.

The notable difference between these two methods was the much smaller particle size of Tc-99m sulfur colloid prepared by the former method: Tc-99m sulfur colloid prepared by the hydrogen sulfide gas method is approximately 10 times smaller than that prepared by the acid reduction of thiosulfate (Atkins HL, et al, 1970). The acid reduction method, which is preferred for its relative convenience, has been the basis of the well-known kit-type formulation of this product.

Several other Tc-99m radiopharmaceuticals have attempted to replace Tc-99m sulfur colloid, including Tc-99m labeled particles of antimony sulfide, dioxide colloid (Johnson AE and Gollan F, 1970), stannous oxide colloid (Subramanian G, et al, 1970), and phytate (inositol hexaphosphate) (Subramanian G, et al, 1973). None, however, approach the reliability of Tc-99m sulfur colloid for imaging the reticuloendothelial system.

Tc-99m microaggregated albumin colloid was developed several years ago as a replacement for Tc-99m sulfur colloid (Scheffel U, et al, 1972). Its method of preparation is much like that of human albumin microspheres (HAM)—both are prepared as an albumin-oil homogenate in a hot cottonseed oil bath. Since the manufacturing steps involved the isolation of the desired particle size by mechanical sieving, it was theoretically possible to isolate a colloidal product of more uniform particle size than that produced by the existing formulations of Tc-99m sulfur colloid. Earliest formulations of Tc-99m microaggregated albumin colloid were not appealing for clinical use, however, since the labeling procedure required as much as 1 hour to perform. More recently, the Food and Drug Administration has approved a formulation of microaggregated albumin colloid that utilizes the familiar and relatively convenient stannous ion-assisted method of radiolabeling with technetium.

Compared to Tc-99m sulfur colloid, Tc-99m microaggregated albumin colloid is slightly more convenient to prepare and is handled differently by the liver following phagocytosis (see Pharmacokinetics). Tc-99m microaggregated albumin colloid, however, has not been shown to be clinically advantageous to Tc-99m sulfur colloid.

Tc-99m sulfur colloid remains the drug of choice for imaging the RE system, including the liver, spleen, and bone marrow, because of its reliability, reasonable cost, and widespread availability.

CHEMISTRY

Tc-99m Sulfur Colloid. In the preparation of Tc-99m sulfur colloid, generator-produced Tc-99m sodium pertechnetate is added to an acidic solution of sodium thiosulfate, and this mixture is heated in a boiling water bath for 5–10 minutes. Following heating, the vial is vented and a buffer is added to neutralize the acidic pH. Some formulations require at this point an additional boiling time of 2–5 minutes. Regardless, the entire preparation is usually accomplished in less than a quarter-hour.

In this reaction, elemental sulfur most likely condenses to form colloidal-sized particles that, in turn, coprecipitate Tc-99m, probably as the heptasulfide, Tc_2S_7. Acid is necessary to bring about the precipitation reaction, whereas heating (in a boiling water bath) is required to catalyze the reaction. Gelatin is utilized as a surface active agent to coat the particles as they form, thus lessening any likelihood of the particles becoming undesirably larger.

Of the several commercial formulations currently available for the preparation of Tc-99m sulfur colloid (Table 14.1), all utilize sodium thiosulfate as the source of elemental sulfur and either phosphoric acid or hydrochloric acid to generate the precipitation reaction. A buffering substance is necessarily added to the preparation in order to raise the strongly acidic pH prior to patient administration in order to prevent any likelihood of irritation during intravenous administration. Other components of commercially available formulations (and their purposes) include sodium chloride (for isotonicity) and gelatin (as a surface active protectant to prevent aggregation of colloidal particles).

Some formulations also contain disodium edetate, a chelating substance for aluminum ions that may be present in varying levels in the generator-produced eluate used to compound Tc-99m sulfur colloid. In the physical chemistry of colloidal substances, the charge that exists at the surface of colloidal substances determines their ability to either disperse (in the desirable situation) or agglomerate into much larger particles. The measure of colloidal stability to resist becoming undesirably large can be determined by measuring the in vitro migration of colloidal substances through an electric field (electrophoretic mobility). This measure, called zeta potential and expressed in millivolts, indicates greater stability with increasing negativity. When the negative charge is diminished, as occurs in the presence of highly electropositive metal ions such as aluminum (Al^{+3}), larger sized particles are likely to result that are taken up by the capillary beds of the lungs (Bell EG and McAfee JG, 1972) (see Precautions).

Whereas the vast majority of Tc-99m radiopharmaceuticals contain technetium in a reduced oxidation state, technetium in Tc-99m sulfur colloid exists in the non-reduced (+7) oxidation state. It is possible and likely, however, that some reduction of technetium does occur in the acidic environment that is required to bring about the preparation of Tc-99m sulfur colloid. Reduced technetium in the presence of disodium edetate (a component of most sulfur colloid formulations) would result in the formation of Tc-99m EDTA, a species that closely resembles Tc-99m DTPA and also undergoes renal clearance via glomerular filtration. The quantities of this impurity present in Tc-99m sulfur colloid, however, have not been shown to be clinically significant.

Tc-99m Albumin Colloid. Tc-99m albumin colloid is prepared by the stannous ion-assisted reduction of technetium with

Table 14.1 COLLOIDAL RADIOPHARMACEUTICALS FOR IMAGING RES FUNCTION AND THEIR FORMULATIONS

KITS FOR FORMULATION OF Tc-99m SULFUR COLLOID

Name®/Manufacturer	Constituent		Quantity and Compartment		
			Reaction Vial	Syringe "A"	Syringe "B"
TechneColl	Phosphoric acid		100 mg		
Mallinckrodt, Inc.	Gelatin			13.2 mg	21.6 mg
	Sodium thiosulfate			6.6 mg	
	Sodium acetate				0.544 mg
	Sodium chloride			0.99 mg	5.4 mg
	Disodium acetate				4.0 mg
		Volumes	2.0 mls	1.65 mls	1.6 mls
AN-Sulfur Colloid	Sodium thiosulfate		2.0 mg		
Syncor International	Disodium edate		2.3 mg		
	Gelatin		18.1 mg		
	HCl (0.148M)			1.5 ml	
	Sodium biphosphate				38.8 mg
	Sodium hydroxide				11.1 mg
		Volumes	(lyophilized)	1.5 mls	1.5 mls
Tesuloid	Sodium thiosulfate		12.0 mg		
Squibb Diagnostics	Gelatin		9.0 mg		
	Dibasic potassium phosphate		25.5 mg		
	Disodium edetate		2.79 mg		
	HCl (0.25M)			2.0 ml	
	Sodium biphosphate				80.0 mg
	Sodium hydroxide				20.0 mg
		Volumes	0.5 ml	1.1 mls	2.1 mls
TSC	HCl (1.0M)		0.5 ml	1.9 mg	
Medi + Physics, Inc.	Sodium thiosulfate				
	Gelatin				5.3 mg
	Sodium acetate				177.0 mg
		Volumes	0.5 ml	1.1 mls	2.1 mls

KITS FOR FORMULATION OF Tc-99m MICROAGGREGATED COLLOID

Name®/Manufacturer	Constituent	Quantity
Microlite®	Each 10 ml vial (lyophilized) contains:	
DuPont-NEN	Albumin colloid	1.0 mg
	Normal human serum albumin	10.0 mg
	Stannous chloride dihydrate	
	Min.	0.006 mg
	Max.	0.170 mg
	Polaxmer 188	1.1 mg
	Medronate sodium	0.12 mg
	Sodium phosphate anhydrous	10.0 mg

labeling occurring with the reduced (probably Tc+4) oxidation state of this transition metal.

PHARMACOKINETICS

Following intravenous administration, both Tc-99m sulfur colloid and Tc-99m albumin colloid are cleared rapidly from blood by the cells of the reticuloendothelial system with a clearance half-time of 2–3 minutes (Figure 14.1). Localization of both these radiopharmaceuticals within organs of the RE system is dependent upon blood flow rates and the functional capacity of the phagocytic cells. In normal humans, 80–90% of the administered activity localizes in the liver, 5–10% in the spleen, and the balance is taken up by the bone marrow. Saba (1970) has shown that pathophysiologic states significantly affect blood clearance and biodistribution of intravenously administered colloids. In progressively severe liver disease, for example, greater amounts of radiopharmaceutical appear in the spleen, bone marrow, and occasionally the lungs. Uptake of both these radiopharmaceuticals is essentially complete by 15 minutes following intravenous administration.

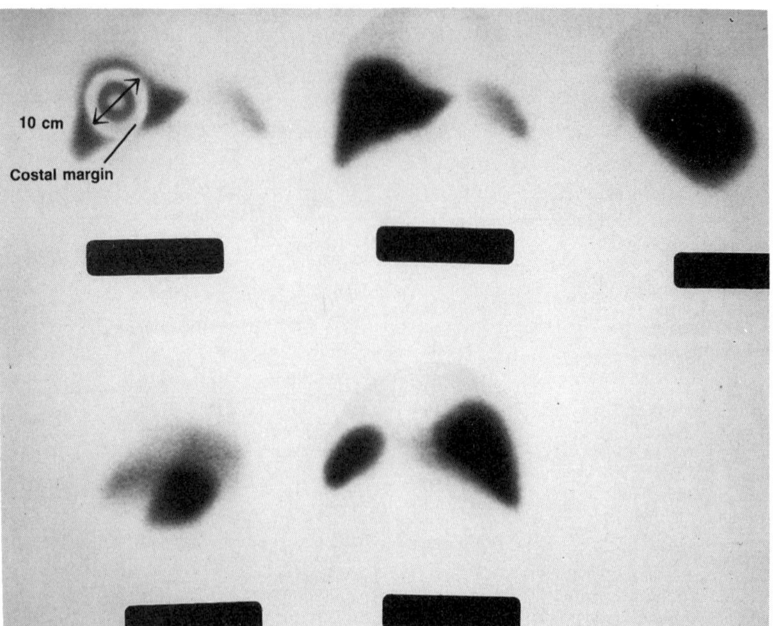

Figure 14.1   Liver-spleen scan with Tc-99m-sulfur colloid showing a normal-appearing liver and spleen.

Though lung uptake of these radiopharmaceuticals can be due to technical problems involving the presence of undesirably large particles (Saba TM, 1970), this
is not the case whenever other patients
studied with the same preparation either
before or afterwards yield satisfactory
localization of the colloid radiopharmaceutical. In these situations, a primary
mechanism appears to involve stimulation
of RES function, since studies performed
in patients that have either infection of
neoplastic diseases that are known to produce increased RE activity have correspondingly higher lung deposition of the
colloidal radiopharmaceuticals (Quinones
JD, 1973). This uptake has been attributed to phagocytosis by macrophages
in the lungs (Klingensmith WC and Ryerson TW, 1973). M.A. Mikhael and
R.G. Evens (1975) have shown in animals
that RE cells, under the influence of exogenous estrogen, endotoxin, and heparin, migrate to the lungs, are trapped in
the pulmonary capillary bed, and retain
their ability to phagocytize colloidal substances. They suggest the migration and
embolization of macrophages to the lung
as a possible mechanism to explain lung

uptake of colloidal radiopharmaceuticals
in those patients with liver disease or
other pathophysiology that stimulates the
RE system.

Following phagocytosis, Tc-99m sulfur
colloid, by virtue of its inorganic composition, is fixed in the RE cells indefinitely.
Tc-99m albumin colloid, on the other
hand, is metabolized and eventually
cleared from the RE cells. Following intravenous administration, the levels of Tc-
99m albumin colloid in the liver and
spleen remain constant for at least 4
hours. Activity is cleared from blood via
the kidneys with 4–30% of the administered dose excreted by 24 hours following
injection.

Since relatively small (e. g., trace) amounts
of either radiopharmaceutical are administered, the rate of radiopharmaceutical removal from blood is related primarily to
organ blood flow rather than the functional
capacity of the RE system. With very large
doses of colloid radiopharmaceutical, however,
progressively slower clearance of the agent
from blood occurs; that is due primarily to
the diminishing ability of the RE system to
phagocytize the larger numbers of administered particles. When extremely large amounts
of colloid particles are administered, lengthy

blood clearance often results, to the point the RE system appears to be functionally saturated with colloidal particles. It has been shown, however, that a colloid of a different substance injected under these circumstances of apparent "RES blockade" will clear immediately from blood, indicating that the cause of the blockade was the result of depletion of specific serum opsonins required only for the clearance of the initial colloidal agent (Wagner HN, Jr and Iio M, 1964). The administration of sufficiently large quantities of colloidal radiopharmaceutical to cause a "blockade" situation is rare; however, viral infections can bring about decreased RES function (Wagner HN, Jr, et al, 1963) that could be responsible for prolonged appearance of the colloidal radiopharmaceutical in blood.

PRECAUTIONS

The size and physicochemical properties of Tc-99m sulfur colloid determine biodistribution and uptake by the RE system and other tissues. As a general rule, relatively larger colloid particles clear more rapidly from blood than smaller colloids and have greater uptake in the liver and spleen. Smaller colloid particles localize to a much greater extent in bone marrow (Atkins HL, et al, 1970; Dobson EL, et al, 1949). The presence of very large particles, as can occur when excessive levels of aluminum ions are present in generator eluate used to prepare Tc-99m sulfur colloid (Haney TA, et al, 1970), can result in the lung uptake of this radiopharmaceutical. Therefore, it is recommended that Tc-99m sodium pertechnetate solutions containing more than 10 micrograms Al^{+3}/milliliter not be used in preparing Tc-99m sulfur colloid (no similar warning exists for the generator eluate used to prepare Tc-99m albumin colloid). A colorimetric test is available for the rapid determination of Al^{+3} ions above this level in generator eluate.

Another cause of excessively large particles may be heating the Tc-99m sulfur colloid in the boiling water bath for much longer than those times specified by the manufacturer. Heating times during the preparation of Tc-99m sulfur colloid should be carefully monitored. Such large particles will be taken up by the lungs before reaching the cells of the RE system. The pH value of the final product is also important, since an alkaline pH causes hydrolysis of the radiolabeled colloid with subsequent generation of free pertechnetate (U.S.P. XXI specifies a pH of 4.5–7.5).

Several techniques have been utilized for particle size determination with most involving some type of membrane filtration (Pedersen B and Kristensen K, 1981). The majority of particles in Tc-99m sulfur colloid prepared by the acid reduction of thiosulfate are 1.0 micron or less (80%). Less than 5% of particles are greater than 1.0 micron (Davis MA, et al, 1974).

Toxicity/Adverse Reactions. From 1976 through 1984, the number of adverse reactions reported in the United States that involved the use of Tc-99m sulfur colloid was 84, the largest number reported for any radiopharmaceutical during this period. The majority of adverse reactions appear to be allergic manifestations (rash, urticaria, pruritus, dyspnea) that have been attributed to the presence of potentially antigenic substances (primarily gelatin) in formulations of Tc-99m sulfur colloid (Cordova MA et al, 1987). Although the relative number of reported adverse reactions appears high, the incidence is well within the range that has been reported in the United States for radiopharmaceuticals (1–6 adverse reactions/100,000 administrations) (Cordova MA, et al, 1980; 1982).

Toxicity associated with Tc-99m sulfur colloid appears minimal since mice receiving 1000 times the usual adult dose failed to demonstrate any toxic response to the material (Haney TA, et al, 1970).

Drug–Radiopharmaceutical Interference.

Cancer Chemotherapeutic Agents. Cancer patients on short-term chemotherapy (notably the nitrosoureas) have shown transient changes in radiopharmaceutical distribution involving the inhomogencous or irregular distribution of radiocolloid in the liver and/or a shift of radiocolloid from the liver to the spleen or bone marrow (Kaplan WD, et al,

1980; Geronemus RG, et al, 1982). The mechanism is thought to involve direct chemotherapy toxicity on the liver cells. The duration of effect is not known.

Aluminum Hydroxide-Containing Antacids. Diffuse pulmonary localization of Tc-99m sulfur colloid has been noted in patients receiving aluminum hydroxide-containing antacids. It is believed that resultant hyperaluminemia secondary to very high-dose antacids therapy causes in vivo alteration of the usually negative zeta potential to cause the formation of undesirably large particles that are cleared from blood by the lungs (Staum MM, 1972; Mikhael MA and Evens RG, 1975; Bobinet DD, et al, 1974).

Androgen therapy. Androgen therapy has also been implicated as a cause of lung uptake of Tc-99m sulfur colloid. It is thought that androgen therapy (or estrogen degradation products from the androgens) may stimulate the reticuloendothelial system, resulting in the mobilization of large numbers of phagocytic cells from their storage sites with the eventual demonstration of lung activity (Sayle BA, et al, 1981).

Anesthetic Agents. General anesthetic agents, such as halothane, have been implicated as causing a shift of Tc-99m sulfur colloid activity from the liver to the spleen. It is known that anesthetic agents can cause a decrease in hepatic blood flow with a probable similar reduction in the hepatic extraction of this radiopharmaceutical (Lentle BC, et al, 1979).

Use During Pregnancy/Breastfeeding. Animal reproductive studies have not been conducted with either Tc-99m sulfur colloid or Tc-99m albumin colloid; therefore, it is not known whether these radiopharmaceuticals cause fetal harm. As a general rule, radiopharmaceuticals should not be administered during pregnancy unless clearly needed and if the benefits to be expected clearly outweigh any risks that might be reasonably anticipated to occur.

It is not known whether Tc-99m sulfur colloid or albumin colloid is secreted in human breast milk; however, Tc-99m pertechnetate that is contained in varying levels in both these radiopharmaceuticals is known to be secreted in breast milk. Therefore, it is advised that breast-feeding be withheld for 12 hours following the administration of these radiopharmaceuticals (ICRP, 1988).

Packaging/Storage Data. Manufacturers' package inserts for Tc-99m sulfur colloid specify the labeled product should be stored at room temperature and that the product should be used within 6 hours from the time of preparation. In practice, however, these products tend to be very stable and do not show the ongoing time-associated deterioration of the radiolabel, as often occurs with other Tc-99m radiopharmaceuticals. U.S.P. XXI specifies for Tc-99m sulfur colloid a radiochemical purity of 92%. For Tc-99m albumin colloid, the manufacturers' package inserts specifies storage of the radiolabeled product at 2–8 degrees centigrade and use within 6 hours of preparation.

DOSAGE/DOSIMETRY

Method. In adults, liver and spleen imaging is routinely performed with 5–8 millicuries of either Tc-99m sulfur colloid or Tc-99m albumin colloid. The radiopharmaceutical is administered intravenously, and imaging can begin 10–15 minutes later. Patients may be imaged either supine or erect; however, in the erect position the liver may appear larger, due primarily to an increase in vertical length (Jackson ML, et al, 1986). Maximal uptake of these radiopharmaceuticals in the organs of the RE system usually occurs by this time. The onset of imaging may be delayed, however, in patients with severe hepatic disease because of slower blood clearance of the colloidal radiopharmaceuticals. No patient preparation is required. Images in several projections are obtained with large field-of-view scintillation cameras in order to provide visualization of both the liver and spleen. SPECT-type imaging may be useful, particularly in the demonstration of neoplasms deep within the liver.

Pediatric patients undergoing liver and spleen imaging receive appropriately smaller doses based on proportional

Table 14.2 ABSORBED RADIATION DOSIMETRY FROM INTRAVENOUS ADMINISTRATION OF Tc-99m SULFUR COLLOID IN ADULTS WITH AND WITHOUT PARENCHYMAL LIVER DISEASE[a]

	RADS/5 MCi	
Tissue	*Normal Liver*	*Advanced Liver Disease*
Liver	1.7	0.8
Spleen	1.1	2.1
Bone marrow	0.14	0.4
Testes	0.0055	0.016
Ovaries	0.028	0.06
Whole body	0.094	0.088

[a] Modified from summary of Current Radiation Dose Estimates to Humans with Various Liver Conditions from Technetium Tc-99m Sulfur Colloid, MIRD Dose Estimate Report No. 3, *J Nucl Med*, 1975, 16, No. 1: 108 A-B.

weight tables. A suggested-dose range for liver and spleen imaging in pediatric patients is 15–75 microcuries per kilogram body weight with a usual dose of 50 microcuries/kg, except in newborns, for whom the minimum administered activity is suggested at 300–500 microcuries (Bekerman C, et al, 1979). Radiation absorbed dose estimates for Tc-99m sulfur colloid are shown in Table 14.2.

CLINICAL CONSIDERATIONS

Liver and spleen imaging is clinically beneficial in the evaluation of liver shape, size, and position and to detect the presence or extent of involvement of liver tumors. The distribution of colloidal radiopharmaceuticals, such as Tc-99m sulfur colloid or Tc-99m albumin colloid, in the liver and spleen is relatively homogeneous due to the uniform presence of RE cells in these organs. Changes in liver and spleen size, as occur in diffuse hepatic disease, such as hepatitis and cirrhosis, can be readily appreciated in liver and spleen imaging with radioactive colloids. Liver and spleen imaging is sometimes helpful in the evaluation of diffuse hepatic disease, such as hepatitis and cirrhosis. It is also useful in the evaluation of abdominal masses and to outline the organ margins in studying extrahepatic disease, such as subphrenic abscesses and retroperitoneal masses.

Whenever disease disrupts the normal architecture of the liver and spleen, however, RE function is sufficiently compromised that colloid uptake no longer occurs in that area. As a result, a "cold" spot, or hole, appears in the image of that organ (Figure 14.2). Imaging with radioactive colloids is also useful in the detection and localization of primary and metastatic lesions, abscesses, and cysts that appear as focal defects during scintillation imaging.

Space-occupying lesions of the liver must be 2–3 centimeters in size and near the liver periphery in order to be appreciated in planar images. SPECT-type images, however, often permit the visualization of smaller lesions well within the liver (Figure 14.3).

The normal liver and spleen scan shows a uniform distribution of colloid throughout the liver. The right lobe of the liver is larger than the left lobe of the liver, and

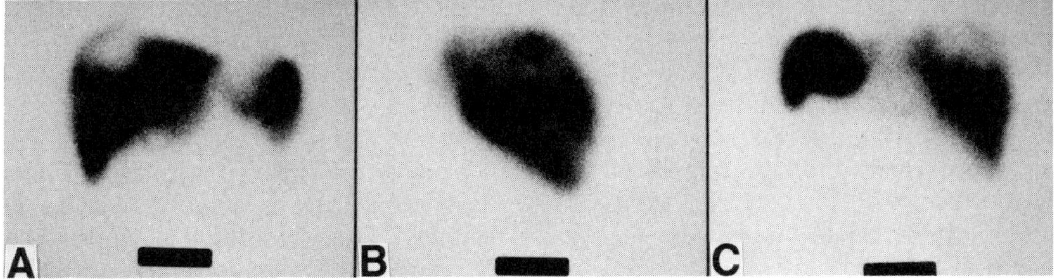

Figure 14.2 Liver-spleen scan performed with Tc-99m-sulfur colloid. Anterior (A), right lateral (B), and posterior (C) views demonstrates a large focal defect (cold area) in the dome of the right lobe of the liver and two smaller areas of decreased uptake in the lateral aspect of the right lobe of the liver and in the left lobe of the liver. These are secondary to metastatic disease.

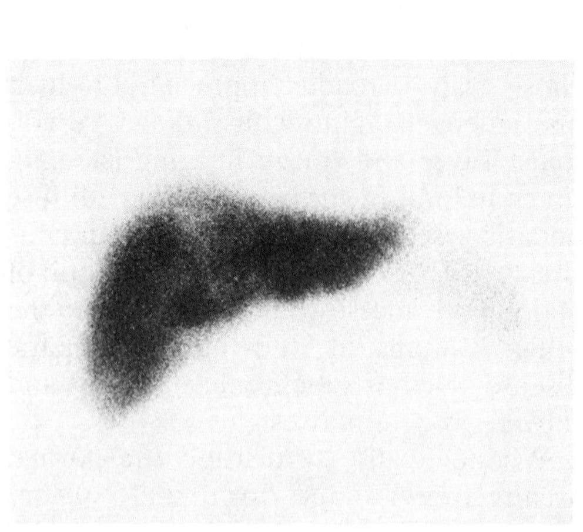

A

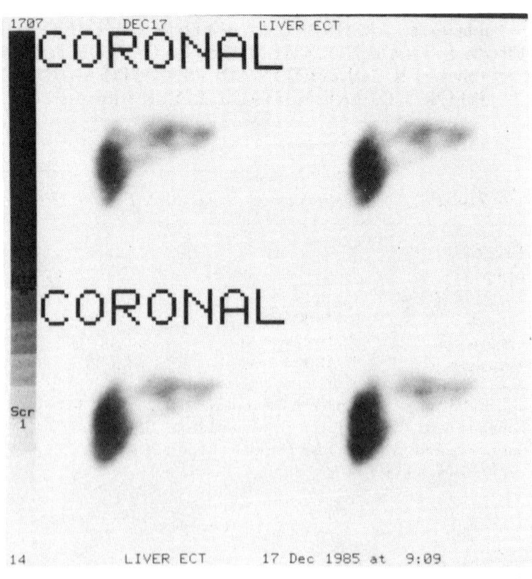

B

Figure 14.3   Liver-spleen scan with Tc-99m-sulfur colloid. The anterior planar image (Figure 14.3A) shows irregular uptake with the suggestion of a defect in the dome of the right lobe of the liver. Figure 14.3B shows four cuts of the coronal slices of a SPECT (single photon emission computed tomography) study. Note that the lesion in the dome of the right lobe of the liver is better seen and there are numerous other lesions in the left lobe of the liver not well seen on the planar images.

both lobes of the liver usually lie above the costal margin. The left lobe of the liver is a relatively thin lobe, and mild irregularities of uptake may be seen in the left lobe. The spleen is often seen on the anterior view but is better studied on the posterior view, left lateral views, and oblique projections when necessary. On the posterior view, the spleen is of equal or less intensity than the right lobe of the liver in normal cases.

Increased splenic activity compared to the right lobe of the liver is considered a colloid shift and can be secondary to a number of disease conditions (Figure 14.4). The appearance of colloid shift is more significant when bone marrow activity is seen in the spine and pelvis. Such occurence usually indicates hepatocellular dysfunction that may be secondary to either diffuse hepatic processes, such as hepatitis, cirrhosis, and chemotherapy, or may result from significant focal disease in the liver, such as occurs in diffuse metastatic disease. In cirrhosis, the right lobe of the liver will be small and the left lobe may be large or normal in size (Fig-

ure 14.4). There will be a colloid shift, and ascites may be present.

Most liver imaging is now being performed with ultrasound and x-ray computed tomography (CT). These modalities allow a survey not only of the liver but adjacent organs, and in the case of ultrasound does not involve ionizing radiation. Combined interpretation of liver spleen scans with ultrasound or CT often provides complimentary information (MacCarthy RL, et al, 1977; Sullivan DC, et al, 1978). In many institutions, liver and spleen scans are performed primarily to follow the size of metastatic lesions following various chemotherapy interventions.

An additional use of liver and spleen imaging is for the young patient with a benign-appearing mass in the liver on CT scanning. The differential diagnosis usually is between hepatic adenoma and focal nodular hyperplasia (Kerlin P, et al, 1983). Reticuloendothelial elements are usually absent in hepatic adenomas, whereas focal nodular hyperplasia may contain significant amounts of Kupffer's

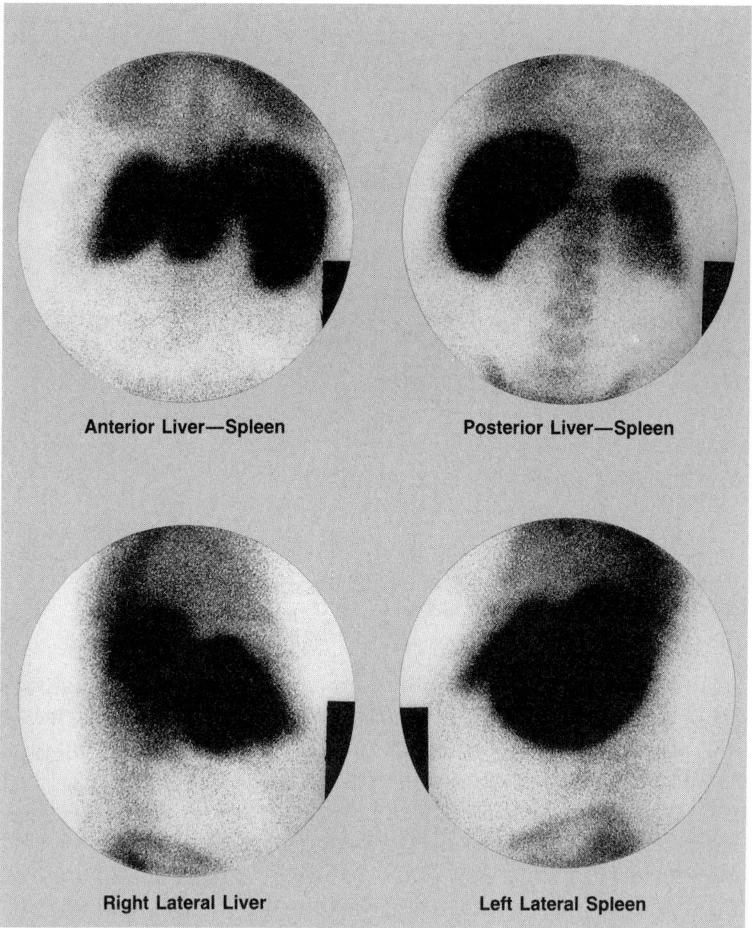

Figure 14.4 Liver-spleen scan with Tc-99m-sulfur colloid demonstrating a small right lobe of the liver with a relatively prominent left lobe of the liver. There is marked splenomegaly and a colloid shift to the spleen and marrow RES. There is also abnormal uptake in the lung fields and separation of the liver from the lateral abdominal wall and from the lung fields due to ascites. This would be a classical pattern for severe cirrhosis.

cells. When the liver and spleen scan shows normal or increased activity in the area of the CT or ultrasound lesion, the diagnosis of focal nodular hyperplasia can often be made (Rogers JV, et al, 1985; Welch TJ, et al, 1985).

RADIOPHARMACEUTICALS FOR HEPATOBILIARY IMAGING

Hepatocytes normally remove from blood a variety of soluble metabolic substances, such as red blood cell breakdown products, heme and bilirubin, that are taken up by the hepatocytes and eventually concentrated and excreted in the bile. At least four carrier-mediated transport pathways have been identified on the surface of the hepatocyte membrane that are responsible for the entry of organic anions, organic cations, neutral compounds, and conjugated bile salts. Substances transported across the membrane sites exhibit a transport maximum that can be competitively inhibited by other substances that share the transport pathway. Following hepatocellular uptake, substances may be stored within protein vesicles before being transported at the bile canaliculus into the bile. Intermediate

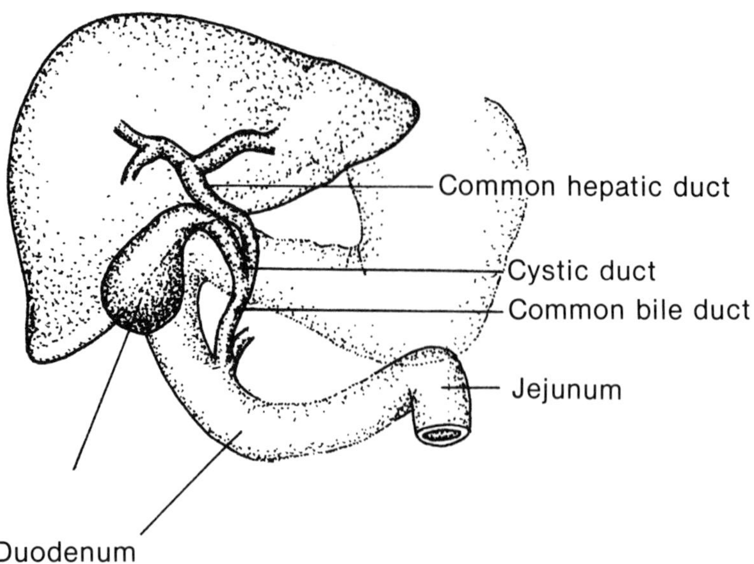

Figure 14.5 Normal liver anatomy showing liver, common hepatic duct, cystic duct, gallbladder, and common bile duct.

binding and storage sites, such as ligandin (Awasthi YC, et al, 1980), bind bilirubin and several other organic anions.

Within the gallbladder, bile is concentrated and stored for later discharge through the cystic duct into the common bile duct and into the intestines (Figure 14.5). The primary determinant of gallbladder emptying is circulating cholecystokinin (CCK) that is secreted postprandially into the blood by cells lining the upper intestinal tract. Some bile components may be resorbed from the intestines and returned to the liver via the circulation, a cyclic process known as enterophepatic circulation.

BACKGROUND/HISTORY

Radiopharmaceuticals employed to evaluate the hepatobiliary system are intended to provide information about the distribution and function of the hepatocytes, to outline the biliary tract, and to provide evidence of the pathway of bile flow or its obstruction. Radiopharmaceuticals were initially employed to study hepatobiliary function in 1955 when G.V. Taplin and colleagues demonstrated the liver appearance of I-131 rose bengal, a radiolabeled analogue of the triphenyl-

methane family of dyes that also includes bromosulphophthalein (BSP). For many years afterwards, I-131 rose bengal was the principal agent for the investigation of hepatobiliary function. The less-than-ideal Beta-minus decay mode of I-131, however, resulted in substantial patient radiation exposure and limited the amount of activity that could be safely administered to 300 microcuries or less. Also, significant amounts of I-131 rose bengal underwent renal excretion (up to 5% is normally excreted by the kidneys), while much greater amounts appeared in the urine of patients with severe liver disease or congenital biliary atresia (Ghadimi H and Sass-Kortsak A, 1961). An additional 4% of the administered activity is cleared by mechanisms that are both "extrahepatic and extrarenal" (Jones DP, et al, 1961). I-123 rose bengal was developed that had imaging properties superior to those of the I-131 product (Christy B, et al, 1974); however, clinicians still had to contend with the less-than-desirable biodistribution properties of rose bengal.

Researchers sought to improve upon the biodistribution properties of radioiodinated rose bengal and poor imaging properties of I-131 by developing a suitably labeled complex of Tc-99m that would clear predominantly by the hepatocytes. Although a variety of Tc-99m complexes were initially investigated for usefulness in hepatobiliary imaging, most had significant renal excretion (owing to the imparted hydrophilicity necessary for Tc-99m radiolabeling) and failed to demonstrate predominant hepatocellular localization.

Among the earlier radiopharmaceuticals investigated as replacements for radioiodinated rose bengal for hepatobiliary imaging were the pyridoxylindene amino acid complexes of Tc-99m. Initially, Tc-99m pyridoxylidene glutamate (PYG) was prepared by autoclaving pertechnetate, pyridoxal hydrochloride, and monosodium glutamate at 120 degrees centigrade (Baker RJ, et al, 1974). In this method, technetium is probably reduced by the pyridoxal group to the IV oxidation state and is bound by the Schiff's base ligand that is formed by the condensation of pyridoxal carbonyl group and the amino group of glutamic acid (Baker RJ, et al, 1975). The autoclave method produced several technetium labeled radiochemical impurities that degraded image quality, including hydrolyzed, reduced (colloidal) technetium and soluble species of technetium that are cleared primarily by the kidneys.

Later, M. Kato and M. Hazue (1978) developed a variation of this technique using Sn^{+2} ions as a reductant in an alkaline medium with ascorbic acid as a stabilizer. Unlike the autoclave method, the product formed in this manner demonstrated a single radiochemical component on high-performance liquid chromatography (HPLC). A predominant disadvantage remained, however, in that most of these Tc-99m labeled Schiff's base complexes underwent significant urinary excretion.

Difficulties associated with developing a compound that had sufficient hydrophilic groups for Tc-99m complexation yet possessed the necessary hepatocellular specificity were overcome with the production of the series of N-substituted iminodiacetic acid agents (Loberg MD, et al,

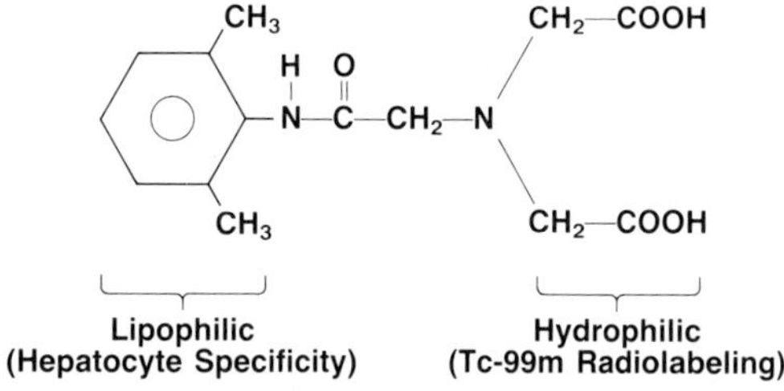

Figure 14.6 Basic chemical structure of HIDA (lidofenin) illustrating the bifunctional properties of the IDA-type hepatobiliary agents. Lipophilicity, which largely accounts for hepatocyte specificity, is influenced by the phenyl ring and substitutions that are made upon it. Tc-99m complexation occurs at the hydrophilic site.

1976). These bifunctional compounds contained both a chelating site Tc-99m (iminodiacetic acid) as well as a tissue-specific constituent that accounts for biodistribution properties. The first Tc-99m labeled N-substituted iminodiacetic acid was Tc-99m HIDA (N-2,6-dimethylacetoanilido iminodiacetic acid) (Figure 14.6). Tc-99m HIDA cleared from blood more rapidly than radioiodinated rose begal and had a nearly identical hepatobiliary clearance rate (Loberg MD, et al, 1979). A variety of Tc-99m analogues of IDA have followed that have various chemical substituents upon the aromatic ring of the basic HIDA structure (Wistow BW, et al, 1977). As a general rule, the newer analogues offer improvements in hepatocellular specificity and more rapid blood clearance.

CHEMISTRY

The mechanism for clearance of bilirubin and related compounds includes three major steps: (1) hepatocyte uptake, by an active transport system of high capacity; (2) hepatocyte binding, conjugation, and storage; and (3) excretion into the biliary canaliculus by an active membrane transport mechanism of relatively low capacity (Goresky CA, 1965). Substances cleared by the hepatocellular mechanisms probably are not dependent upon specific receptor-type interactions with these cells since so many different and diverse materials appear to share the same hepatobiliary pathways. B.W. Wistow and colleagues (1977) summarized the factors required for biliary excretion as follows: molecular size and weight, polarity (lipid solubility), molecular structure (relation of polar and nonpolar groups), and, possibly, protein binding. Substances with a molecular weight between 300 and 1000 are preferentially excreted in the bile. A strong polar group—anion, cation, or nonionized molecule with polar and lipophilic groups—is necessary for biliary excretion. Hydrophilic and lipophilic groups should not be too close together, however, since biliary excretion may be severely decreased. Protein binding may prevent the likelihood of an exogenous substance being rapidly filtered from blood by renal glomerulus (Neilsen P and Rasmussen F, 1975).

Among the radiopharmaceuticals that exhibit hepatobiliary excretion, however, reasonable structural similarities exist that can be modified to create diagnostic agents that have improved cellular specificity and rapid clearance rates, even in the face of severe hepatocellular disease. B.W. Wistow and colleagues (1977) have shown that substitutions upon the aromatic ring of the basic structure of the N-substituted IDA compounds favorably alter in vivo distribution. Increasing the molecular weight of the lipophilic moiety could be expected to increase lipophilicity as well.

As a class, the information developed on the Tc-99m IDA-type derivatives for hepatobiliary imaging has provided substantial information about mechanisms of hepatocellular clearance and function. As a result, the analogues of these compounds that were subsequently developed can be distinguished from most other radiopharmaceuticals as being derived largely from data involving structural-distribution relationships (SDR).

Structural-distribution relationships for radiopharmaceuticals employed for hepatobiliary imaging began to be apparent as early as 1976 when G. Firnau examined the Tc-99m agents employed for chole-scintigraphy and found that all had molecular weights of 300–1000, existed as organic anions, and contained at least two aromatic ring systems in the molecule. The compounds he examined also demonstrated significant binding to serum albumin. Later W.C. Eckelman and W.A. Volkert (1982) confirmed the necessary presence of at least two planar lipophilic structures plus a polar group and protein binding for hepatobiliary excretion. B.W. Wistow and co-workers (1977) had earlier observed that cyclic chemical structures arranged in different planes were preferred for biliary excretion.

Iminodiacetic acid had been known for years to be a useful chelating structure for the treatment of heavy metal poisonings and for the analytical separation of radiometals (Helffreich FP, 1961; Bjerrum J, et al, 1957). It was not until 1976, however, when Loberg et al, reported the development of Tc-99m HIDA (lidofenin) that iminodiacetic acid was employed as a chelating group for Tc-99m.

As a radiometal coordination structure, iminodiacetic acid is nearly ideal. It is relatively small and possesses sufficient nucleophilic character that permits its synthetic placement into a variety of organic compounds.

M.D. Loberg and colleagues (1976) confirmed the essential character of the aromatic ring in order for the N-substituted iminodiacetic acid complexes of Tc-99m to undergo hepatocellular uptake. When the N-substituted aromatic ring was replaced with a methyl group, for example, renal excretion predominated.

In additional to the general characteristics of polarity, structural configuration, and molecular size and weight, several specific structural characteristics have been identified for the formation of the Tc-99m IDA complexes with cholescintigraphic properties (Loberg MD, et al, 1981), including: (1) diacetate substitution on the amine nitrogen, (2) an electron withdrawing substituent beta to the amine, and (3) a lipophilic group separated by substantial distance from the hydrophilic group (Loberg MD, et al, 1981). Stable complex formation is

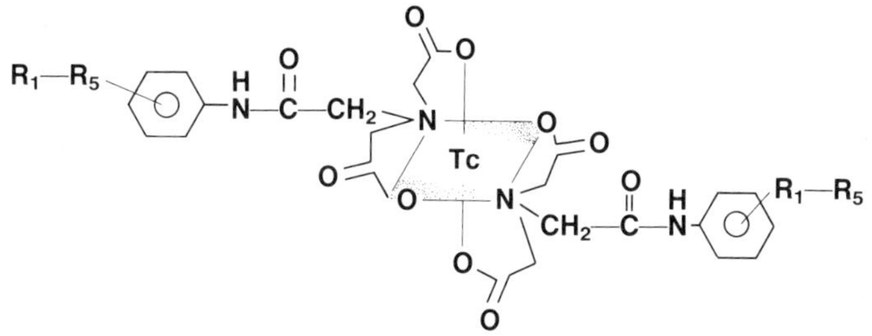

Figure 14.7 Proposed *bis*-structure of Tc-99m lidofenin-type agents, showing central configuration of Tc-99m coordinated between two molecules of the IDA-type component (from Nunn AD and Loberg MD, 1981).

achieved when the imino nitrogen is substituted with a carbamoyl group in the beta position. The carbamoyl methyl moiety appears to be crucial for the formation of stable complexes that have very high biliary clearance (Chervu LR, et al, 1982).

Long-term biodistribution studies had shown that significant differences existed in the hepatobiliary clearance of Tc-99m HIDA and C-14 labeled HIDA, suggesting the effect of the technetium metal upon the radiochemical composition of Tc-99m HIDA. Whereas greater than 75% of Tc-99m HIDA is cleared through the hepatobiliary system of animals in 4 hours, less than 1% of C-14 HIDA is found over the same time interval. In their study of the radiochemical structure of Tc-99m HIDA, M.D. Loberg and associates (1978a; 1978b) and D. Burns and co-workers (1977) showed that the molar ratio of HIDA to technetium was 2:1, suggesting that Tc-99m HIDA existed as a bis structured complex (Figure 14.7). It was also shown that tin ions are not part of the complex and that in the Tc-99m IDA complexes, technetium exists in the +3 oxidation state.

In 1983, A.D. Nunn and colleagues reported correlations between physiochemical parameters, structural effects, and in vivo distribution characteristics of Tc-99m IDA derivatives. Using reverse phase high-performance liquid chromatography (HPLC) as a measure of lipophilicity, they demonstrated that lipophilicity could be used to predict protein binding and the in vivo distribution of the Tc-99m IDA complexes. Based upon these structural-distribution relationships, they were able to develop a new radiopharmaceutical, Tc-99m mebrofenin (Nunn AD, et al, 1981) that had significantly improved hepatic specificity, hepatocellular transit time, and resistance to competitive inhibition for hepatobiliary excretion from serum bilirubin.

The literature records several different names for the many Tc-99m IDA-analogues, with the majority of the earlier researchers choosing to employ chemically derived abbreviations of the iminodiacetic complex (i. e., HIDA, DISIDA, etc.). More recently, the United States Adopted Names (USAN) Council adopted for uniformity the use of the suffix *fenin* to denote compounds of the basic IDA-type chemical structure (Table 14.3).

Presently, in the United States, three Tc-99m IDA derivatives are approved by the FDA for hepatobiliary imaging. These pharmaceuticals and information regarding their formulations are listed in Table 14.4. For these agents, the complexation of reduced Tc-99m using stannous (Sn^{+2}) as a reductant at room temperature is similar to the well-known methods involved in the preparation of various other Tc-99m radiopharmaceuticals.

PHARMACOKINETICS

Radiopharmaceuticals useful for hepatobiliary imaging are removed from blood by the hepatocytes by carrier-mediated processes that are subject to competitive inhibition by substances, such as bilirubin,

Table 14.3 OFFICIAL NAMES[a] OF SELECTED Tc-99m IDA DERIVATIVES CURRENTLY AVAILABLE IN THE UNITED STATES AND THEIR CHEMICAL NAMES AND PREVIOUSLY USED UNOFFICIAL NAMES

OFFICIAL/ UNOFFICIAL NAME	SITES OF SUBSTITUTION	CHEMCAL NAME
Lidofenin/HIDA	CH_3 / CH_3 (2,6-substituted phenyl)—N(H)—C(=O)—	[[(2,6-Xylylcarbamoyl)methyl] -imino]diacetic acid
Disofenin/DISIDA	$CH(CH_3)_2$ / $CH(CH_3)_2$ (2,6-substituted phenyl)—N(H)—C(=O)—	[[[(2,6-diisopropylphenyl)-carbamoyl]methyl]-imino]diacetic acid
Mebrofenin/BrIDA	CH_3 / CH_3 / CH_3 / Br (substituted phenyl)—N(H)—C(=O)—	[[[(3-Bromomesityl)-carbamoyl] methyl] imino] diacetic acid

[a] From USAN and the USP Dictionary of Drug Names, USP, Rockville, MD, 1989.

Table 14.4 FORMULATION OF CURRENTLY AVAILABLE Tc-99m LABELED DERIVATIVES OF IMINODIACETIC ACID (IDA)

TRADENAME® (GENERIC)	MANUFACTURER/DISTRIBUTOR	COMPOSITION/FORMULATION
TechneScan HIDA (lidofenin)	Mallinckrodt, Inc.	Lidofenin 10 mg Stannous chloride dihydrate 0.8–1.0 mg (min.–max.) pH adjusted 3.9–4.1 with HCl or NaOH (Contents are lyophilized; stored under nitrogen)
Hepatolite (disofenin)	Dupont-NEN	Disofenin 20 mg Stannous chloride dihydrate 0.24–0.6 mg (min.–max.) pH adjusted 4–5 with HCl or NaOH (Contents are lyophilized; stored under nitrogen)
Choletec (mebrofenin)	Squibb Diagnostics	Mebrofenin 45 mg Stannous fluoride dihydrate 0.54–1.03 mg (min.–max.) Methylparaben 5.2 mg Propylparaben 0.58 mg pH adjusted 4.2–5.7 with HCl or NaOH (Contents are lyophilized; stored under nitrogen)

that share the same transport and excretion pathways. As a result, the uptake and clearance of these radiopharmaceuticals, in addition to being nonlinear, are also influenced by the presence in blood of increasing levels of bilirubin (Harvey E, et al, 1979). Accordingly, enhanced renal excretion of these radiopharmaceuticals would be expected to occur in patients with incapacitated liver function.

Following intravenous administration, Tc-99m lidofenin (HIDA) shows a blood-clearance curve that is biexponential with first and second half-lives of 4.6 and 31.5 minutes, in normals, that increases to 5.3 and 118 minutes, in jaundiced patients.

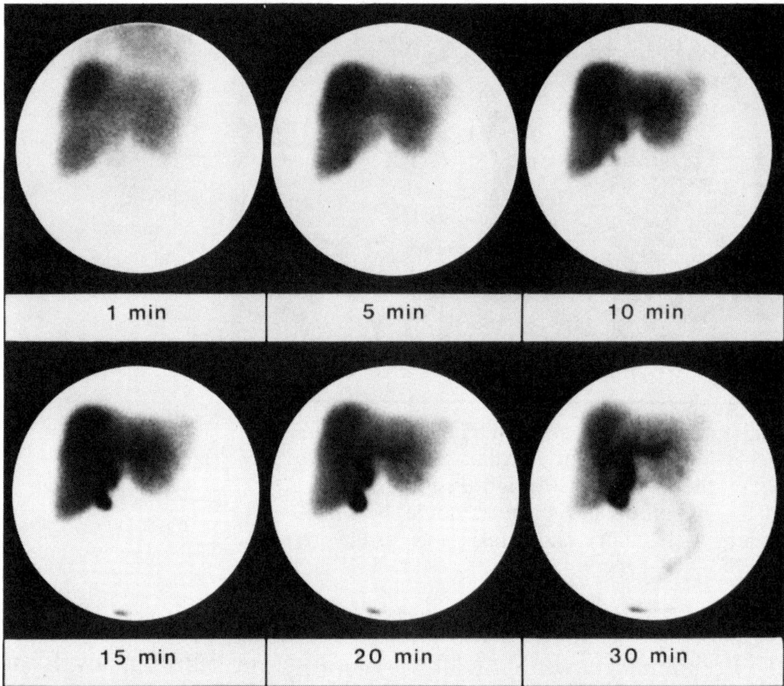

Figure 14.8 Hepatobiliary scan with Tc-99m-disofenin. This is a normal study demonstrating prompt accumulation of activity in the liver with the visualization of the intrahepatic biliary system by 10 minutes, visualization of the gallbladder (in this case by 15 minutes), and visualization of the bowel by 30 minutes.

Mean blood levels in normal subjects at 5 and 60 minutes post injection were 32% and 5% of the administered activity. In normal patients following intravenous administration, the cumulative 90-minute urinary excretion of Tc-99m lidofenin was 14.2% of the injected dose, whereas in jaundiced patients, 22% is present in the urine at 90 minutes, increasing to 53% by 18–24 hours (Ryan J, et al, 1977). In patients with serum bilirubin levels of 5–8 mg/dl, the biliary tract is usually adequately outlined in sequential imaging, however, the liver concentration and transport of this radiopharmaceutical is less rapid than in normal patients, and urinary excretion is higher.

Tc-99m disofenin clears rapidly from blood in normal patients with only 8% of the administered activity remaining in blood 30 minutes post injection. About 9% is excreted in urine over the first 2 hours post injection. Peak liver uptake occurs by 10 minutes post injection; in individuals with normal hepatobiliary function, visualization of the gallbladder and intestinal activity occurs by 60 minutes post injection (Figure 14.8). In patients with serum bilirubin levels of less than 10 mg/dL, Tc-99m disofenin provides visualization of the common duct that is at least equal to that of Tc-99m lidofenin. In comparisons with other Tc-99m IDA-type radiopharmaceuticals, Tc-99m disofenin has been shown superior for use whenever serum bilirubin is between 15–30 mg/dL (Hernandez M and Rosenthall L, 1980a; b).

Following intravenous administration in normal patients, the mean percent injected dose of Tc-99m mebrofenin remaining in blood at 10 minutes was 17%. Visualization of the liver is noted by 5 minutes with peak liver uptake occurring 5 minutes later. Hepatic duct and gallbladder visualization occurs by 10–15 minutes, and intestinal activity is visualized by 30–60 minutes in patients with normal

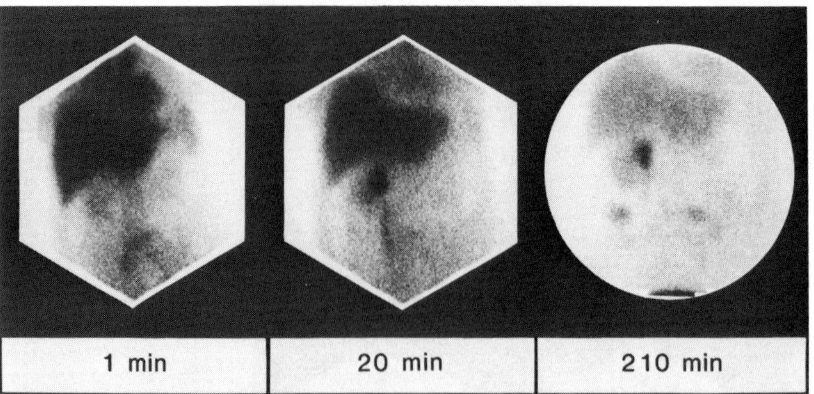

Figure 14.9 Hepatobiliary study with Tc-99m-HIDA. On the 20-minute image, there is still significant cardiac blood pool activity. The activity below the liver is in the right kidney. At 4 hours, renal activity is again noted, and there is some bowel activity. This is in a patient with biliary cholestasis and an elevated bilirubin level.

hepatobiliary function. Preliminary evidence suggests that although no significant differences exist between the hepatocyte extraction efficiency and hepatic parenchymal transit time for Tc-99m mebrofenin and Tc-99m disofenin, Tc-99m mebrofenin has lesser renal excretion in normal patients and a lower rate of increase in patients with decreasing hepatocyte function (Klingensmith WC, et al, 1982). A clinical comparison of Tc-99m mebrofenin and Tc-99m disofenin in patients with seriously elevated bilirubinemia remains to be performed.

As serum bilirubin level increases, the blood clearance of the Tc-99m IDA-analogs becomes progressively delayed, resulting in higher background-to-liver ratios and increased renal excretion. Kidney visualization becomes increasingly evident in patients with significantly compromised biliary function. Patients with complete biliary obstruction may not show any activity in the intestines, even with delayed imaging at 18–24 hours post radiopharmaceutical administration. With Tc-99m lidofenin, the biliary system is not well visualized in patients with serum bilirubin values over 7–8 mg/dL although liver and intestinal radioactivity is observed with serum bilirubin levels up to 10 mg/dL (Figure 14.9). In patients with

mean elevated serum bilirubin levels of 9.8 mg/dL, the mean percent injected dose of Tc-99m mebrofenin excreted in urine during the first 3 hours was 3.0% with 14.9% appearing in the urine by 24 hours (range 0.4–34.8%).

PRECAUTIONS

The long-term in vivo stability of Tc-99m radiopharmaceuticals intended for hepatobiliary imaging is critical since imaging with these agents may be carried out as long as 18–24 hours post injection. In vivo degradation of the radiopharmaceutical into radiochemical impurities and the subsequent distribution of these products within extrahepatic tissues would seriously degrade the scintillation image and lessen the diagnostic information that might be obtained. M.D. Loberg and colleagues (1976) have shown that Tc-99m HIDA is stable in vivo since reinjection of the contents of the urinary bladder and gallbladder in mice produced tissue distributions that were similar to Tc-99m HIDA itself. In vitro analysis of radiochemical purity using high-voltage electrophoresis and high-performance liquid chromatography (HPLC) are capable of demonstrating the presence of radiochemical impurities other than free pertechnetate and hydrolyzed, reduced (colloidal) technetium. Unfortunately, no simple and convenient paper or thin layer radiochromatography system yet exists that is capable of resolving the multiple radiochemical species that potentially exist in these preparations.

Delayed or nonvisualization of the gallbladder may occur in the immediate postprandial period or after prolonged fasting or parenteral feeding. Functional biliary obstruction may accompany chronic cholecystitis or pancreatitis. In addition, patients with hepatocellular disease may show nonvisualization or delayed visualization of the gallbladder. It has been suggested that radiopharmaceuticals that rapidly clear from the hepatobiliary tract may not permit adequate demonstration of gallbladder filling. As a result, the possibility exists that a false-positive diagnosis of acute cholecystitis may occur with the rapid clearance of an agent that fails to fill an otherwise normal gallbladder.

Drug–Radiopharmaceutical Interference

Narcotic analgesics. Opioid analgesics cause increased intrabiliary pressure and spasms of the sphincter of Oddi, preventing the movement of bile (and radiopharmaceutical) into the small intestine (Taylor A, et al, 1982; Joehl RJ, et al, 1984). Delayed biliary-to-bowel transit time results with prolonged radiopharmaceutical appearance in the gallbladder or common bile duct. No release of radiopharmaceutical into the intestine occurs, thus simulating the appearance of bile-duct obstruction. Ideally, hepatobiliary studies in patients who have received narcotic analgesics as part of their pain-management therapy should be delayed until the drug effect dissipates. (See also Interventional Techniques—Adjunctive Pharmaceuticals.)

Nicotinic Acid. In large doses, nicotinic acid has been known to cause significant hepatic dysfunction, including pruritus and jaundice with accompanying rise in blood levels of liver enzymes, including alkaline phosphatase and lactic dehydrogenase. These effects are probably due to nicotinic toxicity upon the hepatocyte (Pardue WO, 1961). P. Richards and R. Brighouse (1981) reported a case involving poor liver uptake and biliary excretion of Tc-99m lidofenin that resolved after the medication was stopped.

Total Parenteral Nutrition (TPN). Nonvisualization of the gallbladder has also been reported in patients who are receiving total parenteral nutrition (TPN) therapy (Shuman WP, et al, 1982), and also in patients undergoing hepatic artery infusion chemotherapy (Housholder DF, et al, 1985). During TPN therapy, the relative inactivity of the gallbladder results in bile stasis and the formation of a thick viscous jellylike bile that behaves as "sludge" and impedes the flow of the radiopharmaceutical into the gallbladder. In hepatic artery infusion chemotherapy, the mechanism involves a chemically induced cholecystitis that occurs from the incidental perfusion of the gallbladder with the chemotherapy agent (Carrasco CH, et al, 1983).

Use During Pregnancy/Breast Feeding. It is not known whether any of the Tc-99m IDA-type hepatobiliary agents cross the placenta or if these radiopharmaceuticals cause fetal harm. They should not be used during pregnancy, however, unless the reasonable benefits to be expected outweigh any potential risks. It is also not known whether these radiopharmaceuticals are excreted in human breast milk; however, pertechnetate, the radiochemical impurity that often occurs in variable amounts of these agents, is known to be excreted in breast milk during lactation. Therefore, it has been suggested that breastfeeding should be withheld for 12 hours following the administration of these agents (ICRP, 1988) or until levels of radioactivity in breast milk are found to be safe.

Adverse Reactions. Single cases of chills and nausea have been attributed to the use of Tc-99m lidofenin. No adverse reactions have been reported associated with the use of either Tc-99m disofenin or mebrofenin.

Dosage Dosimetry

Estimated radiation absorbed dosimetry for patients receiving either Tc-99m lidofenin, disofenin, or mebrofenin are listed in Table 14.5.

Method

Patient Preparation. Since the endogenous release of cholecystokinin secondary to a meal

Table 14.5 ESTIMATED ABSORBED RADIATION DOSE[a] IN HEALTHY, ADULT SUBJECTS FROM Tc-99m IDA-TYPE ANALOGS EMPLOYED FOR HEPATOBILIARY IMAGING

	RADS/5 MCi		
Tissue	^{99m}Tc-*lidofenin*[1]	^{99m}Tc-*disofenin*[2]	^{99m}Tc-*mebrofenin*[3]
Total body	0.05	0.08	0.09
Liver	0.15	0.2	0.9
Gallbladder wall	0.65	0.6	0.63
Small intestine	1.0	1.0	0.80
Upper large intestine wall	1.9	2.0	1.25
Lower large intestine wall	0.8	1.5	1.0
Urinary bladder wall	0.45	0.45	1.2

[a] Data from manufacturer's package inserts:

1. Mallinckrodt, Inc., November, 1986.
2. Dupont-NEN, May, 1985.
3. E.R. Squibb Diagnostics, March, 1987.

can result in failure of the gallbladder to visualize, patients should fast for 4–6 hours prior to the administration of the radiopharmaceutical. Though insufficient fasting can be a cause of false-positive studies, fasting beyond 1 day has been implicated as a cause of nonvisualization of the gallbladder despite the appearance of radioactivity in the liver, common duct, and intestine. In the case of prolonged fasting, bile is presumably concentrated to the point of a "sludgelike" consistency that prevents radiopharmaceutical entry into the gallbladder.

Imaging Technique. The usual activity administered to an adult for a routine hepatobiliary study is 3–5 millicuries of the desired Tc-99m labeled IDA derivative; patients with severely elevated bilirubin levels may require the administration of doses as large as 10 millicuries.

Patients are administered the radiopharmaceutical while in position beneath the scintillation camera. The anterior position is usually chosen, and the patient is positioned such that the liver, gallbladder, and duodenum are within the camera field of view (see Figure 14.8). Serial imaging is begun immediately following radiopharmaceutical administration at 5-minute intervals over the first 30 minutes, then at 15-minutes intervals until the gallbladder is visualized or intestinal activity is noted (Figure 14.10). Imaging in most

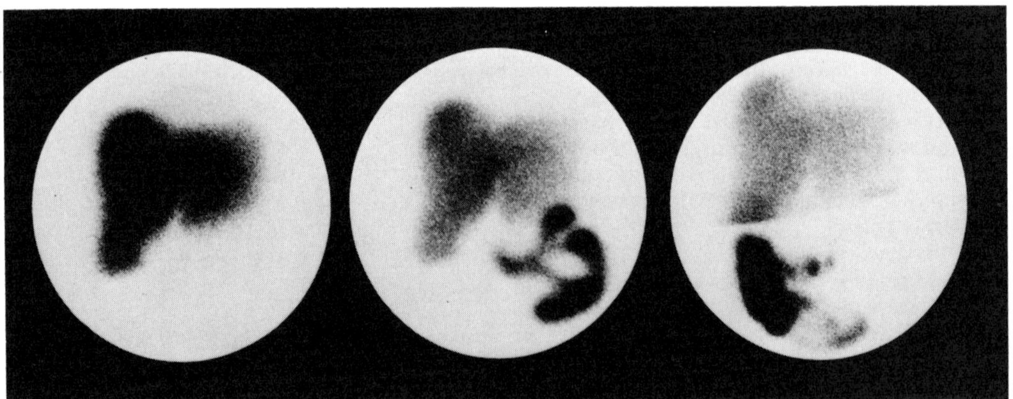

Figure 14.10 Hepatobiliary study with Tc-99m-disofenin. Five-minute image, 60-minute image, and 4-hour image demonstrates prompt visualization of the liver with normal biliary-to-bowel transit time (within 1 hour) but no visualization of the gallbladder. Four hours following the injection, gallbladder is still not visualized. The findings are consistent with cystic duct obstruction, and in this case represented acute cholecystitis.

cases is usually complete by 60–90 minutes; however, delayed imaging (up to 4 hours or longer) may be necessary if gallbladder or intestinal activity fails to appear. Imaging at 24 hours may be diagnostically significant, particularly if visualization of the biliary tract is incomplete during earlier imaging.

CLINICAL CONSIDERATIONS

Hepatobiliary imaging is of primary benefit in the differential diagnosis of the patient with right upper quadrant pain. Its utility has been well defined for the diagnosis of acute cholecystitis, and hepatobiliary imaging also plays a role in the definition of hepatobiliary leaks and in patients with post cholecystectomy pain.

The vast majority of patients with acute cholecystitis have cystic duct obstruction, most commonly due to an impacted stone as in calculus cholecystitis, although functional obstruction of the cystic duct may also occur due to edema in a calculus cholecystitis. There have been many excellent studies demonstrating the high degree of sensitivity and specificity for hepatobiliary imaging in the diagnosis of acute cholecystitis. The criteria for the diagnosis of acute cholecystitis is visualiza-

tion of the common bile duct and normal biliary-to-bowel transit time (within 1 hour) and non-visualization of the gallbladder up to 4 hours following the injection of the tracer. Patients with chronic cholecystitis, on the other hand, usually show visualization of the gallbladder by 4 hours (Figure 14.11). In one study of 296 patients, the sensitivity was 95% with a specificity of 99% and an accuracy of approximately 98% (Weissman HS, et al, 1981). Similar results were found in another study of 117 patients where the hepatobiliary test had an accuracy of 98.7% (Szlabick RE, et al, 1980). The diagnosis of acalculus cholecystitis can also be seen using the same criteria with a high degree of accuracy (Swayne LC, 1986). Patients with acute cholecystitis may show the "hyperemic rim sign" where there is increased activity on the flow study and increased activity about the gallbladder on the early images. Although this is seen frequently, it is not as definitive a sign as gallbladder nonvisualization (Colletti P, et al, 1984; Cawthon MA, et al, 1984).

In patients with abnormal liver uptake or delayed biliary to bowel transit, the ability to make the diagnosis of acute cholecystitis may be difficult. This may

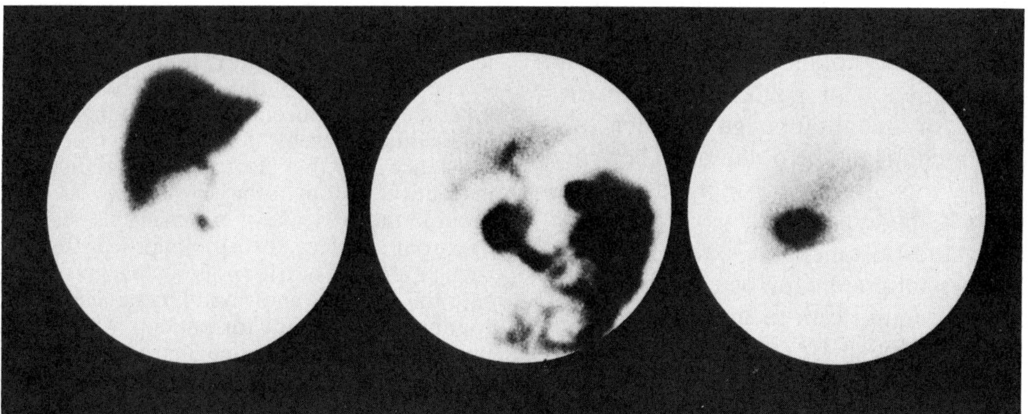

Figure 14.11 Hepatobiliary study with Tc-99m-disofenin. Images are at 10 minutes, 60 minutes, and 4 hours. There is prompt visualization of the intra- and extra-hepatic biliary ducts. There is normal bowel activity at 10 minutes and more at 60 minutes. The gallbladder is not visualized at 1 hour. The delayed images at 4 hours show visualization of the gallbladder. The findings would indicate a patent cystic duct. The findings would be most likely due to chronic cholecystitis.

occur in cases of severely compromised hepatic function or in patients with partial or complete common duct obstruction. In patients with partial common bile duct obstruction, a prominent common bile duct may be seen with activity increasing rather than decreasing in the common bile duct over time. However, the lack of this finding does not preclude the possibility of a partial common bile duct obstruction. In complete common bile duct obstruction, activity usually does not reach the bowel, although in relatively acute obstruction, activity may be seen to enter the gallbladder either within the first 4 hours or by the 24-hour image. Subacute common bile duct obstruction often shows poor radiopharmaceutical uptake by the liver and increased renal excretion.

In order to increase the sensitivity of hepatobiliary agents in the diagnosis of acute cholecystitis, cholecystokinetic agents or the narcotic analgesics may be used as described in the following subsection. Biliary leaks can be seen as areas of abnormal accumulation inferior, lateral, or superior to the liver or with free flow into the abdominal cavity. If a biliary leak is considered, then delayed images, up to 24 hours, should be obtained.

Biliary dyskinesia can be a cause for abdominal pain. Chronic acalculus cholecystitis may also be in the differential diagnosis of right upper quadrant pain. In the patient who has gallbladder filling, the use of the cholecystokinetic agents allows for the evaluation of gallbladder emptying. Visual or quantitative gallbladder ejection fractions can be obtained. There may also be impairment of gallbladder emptying in diabetic patients.

For the postoperative patient, hepatobiliary scintigraphy can be used along with other imaging tests to detect stenosis of the sphincter of Oddi. In one series, retention of activity of 2 hours in visually prominent ducts was the best predictor of abnormal biliary drainage (Zeman RK, et al, 1985). An excellent review article was written by Weissman on the evaluation of the postoperative patient with the cholescintigraphy agents (Weissman HS, et al, 1982).

Interventional Techniques—Adjunctive Pharmaceuticals

Cholecystokinetic Agents. Although the use of cholecystokinin (Topper TE, et al, 1980; Mesgarzadeh M, et al, 1983), sincalide (Freeman LM, et al, 1981; Hedner P and Lundequist A, 1972), and ceruletide (Krishnamurthy GT, et al, 1983) to induce contraction and subsequent filling of the gallbladder is well known, only sincalide is currently available in the United States. Sincalide is the synthetic C-terminal octapeptide of the hormone cholecystokinin (Sargent EN, 1976) and possesses similar pharmacologic action, causing gallbladder contraction resulting in both reduction of gallbladder size and evacuation of gallbladder contents (Rubin B, et al, 1969). To induce gallbladder emptying, an intravenous dose of 20 nanograms/kg (1.4 micrograms/70 kg adult) should be given. The duration of action of sincalide following a single IV dose is approximately 1 hour (American Society of Hospital Pharmacists, 1985). In order to prevent contraction of the neck of the gallbladder, sincalide should be injected slowly over 30–60 seconds. A wait of 15–30 minutes before administration of the radiopharmaceutical is usually sufficient if this is done to empty a full gallbladder prior to study, such as in the patient who has not eaten within 24 hours or is on TPN. Side effects appear due to the pharmacologic action of the drug and include nausea, abdominal pain or discomfort, and an urge to defecate. Dizziness and flushing have also been reported to occur. Side effects appear immediately upon administration of the drug and last only a few minutes (American Society of Hospital Pharmacists, 1985).

The rationale for the use of a cholecystokinetic agent is to empty the contents of the gallbladder, thereby lessening any functional resistance to the flow of the radiopharmaceutical through the cystic duct as may occur in the presence of extremely viscous bile in chronic cholecystitis, prolonged fasting, or total parenteral nutrition. Few clinicians advocate the use of a cholecystokinetic agent as a routine pretreatment for patients who are to undergo hepatobiliary imaging. Sincalide pretreatment causes earlier gallbladder filling during subsequent cholescintigraphy and may lessen the time required for delayed imaging. The possibility exists, however, that the routine use of these types of interventional agents would prevent the differentiation of chronic cholecystitis from normal gallbladder filling and mask the small percentage of cases in which acute cholecystitis may present as delayed gallbladder filling (Freeman LM, et al, 1981).

Another approach is the administration of sincalide only when the gallbladder does not initially fill within the first hour of imaging, followed by another injection of the radiopharmaceutical. If, after an additional hour, the gallbladder does not fill, a diagnosis of acute cholecystitis is considered; however, if the gallbladder fills, a diagnosis of chronic cholecystitis is suspected. In addition to the obvious increase in patient radiation exposure associated with the two administrations of radiopharmaceutical, this technique has not been shown superior to delayed imaging for the detection of chronic cholecystitis (Freeman LM, et al, 1981). When sincalide is used to assess gallbladder emptying or ejection fraction, images are taken after the gallbladder has filled with the radiopharmaceutical. Sincalide is given as previously noted and images are obtained up to 30 minutes. Visualization or quantitative estimation of gallbladder emptying is obtained.

Phenobarbital. Phenobarbital is used as a therapeutic aid in neonatal physiologic jaundice (Maisels, 1972) and type II chronic nonhemolytic unconjugated hyperbilirubinemia (Yaffe SJ, et al, 1966) as well as to enhance the uptake and clearance of certain substances (Sharp HL and Mirkin BL, 1972). Phenobarbital is a potent inducer of hepatic enzymes (Harvey E, 1985); however, the choleretic effect of phenobarbital is thought to be independent from enzyme induction and to be due to an effect of phenobarbital upon the whole hepatic transport system for organic anions (Majd M, et al, 1981). Phenobarbital is used in nuclear medicine in conjunction with hepatobiliary imaging primarily to distinguish neonatal jaundice occurring from hepatitis and biliary atresia (Thaler MM, 1972). Neonates are usually administered phenobarbital in doses of approximately 5 mg/kg/day (in two divided doses daily) for at least 5 days prior to the administration of the radiopharmaceutical (Majd M, et al, 1981.) Up to 1 millicurie of the radiopharmaceutical is administered, and imaging is carried out for at least 24 hours afterwards. Without the use of phenobarbital, the transport of the radiopharmaceutical through the biliary tract is very slow in neonates with hepatitis, although the biliary tract is patent.

Narcotic Analgesics. Though narcotic analgesics have been shown to result in hepatobiliary studies that simulate bile duct obstruction, their use may also serve as a beneficial pharmacologic intervention in the assessment of acute cholecystitis in the presence of chronic cholecystitis (Choy D, et al, 1984) or other conditions that usually delay or prevent gallbladder visualization (Sefczek DM, et al, 1985). The usual method involves the intravenous administration of morphine (0.04 mg/kg in 10 ml of saline given over 3 minutes) if no gallbladder filling is noted over 40–60 minutes following radiopharmaceutical administration (Choy D, et al, 1984). Morphine-stimulated contraction of the sphincter of Oddi causes a prompt elevation in biliary-tract pressure that begins within 5 minutes of administration, reaches a peak within 15 minutes, and persists for 2 hours or more (Jaffe JH and Martin WR, 1985), and that may promote gallbladder filling. The contraindications to this morphine-assisted technique are hyperamylasemia, and patients with a history of opioid addiction. Morphine intervention is probably of no benefit in patients with common bile duct obstruction and could give false-negative results in acalculous cholecystitis (Choy D, et al, 1984).

II. Spleen-Specific Radiopharmaceuticals

Although not a commonly performed procedure, spleen-specific imaging (non-colloid) may be of some usefulness in the detection of accessory splenic tissues in patients who have undergone splenectomy and still show signs of hypersplenism. It is also beneficial in the visualization of spleen only, or as an aid in the determination of a left upper quadrant mass, usually in conjuction with CT or ultrasound.

The phagocytic function of the spleen is most often utilized as the means for radiopharmaceutical uptake in order to visualize this organ. However, the reticuloendothelial cells of the liver take up the bulk of Tc-99m sulfur colloid, thus making it impossible to visualize the spleen only. This is particularly significant since accessory spleens are often located in the left upper quadrant region and may be partially obscured by the proportionally greater Tc-99m colloid activity in the liver.

Since the spleen is the principal organ for the destruction of senescent erythrocytes, spleen-specific imaging can be performed by using radiolabeled erythrocytes that have been appropriately denatured in order to undergo splenic localization (Wagner HN, Jr, et al, 1962).

A variety of techniques have been employed to modify erythrocytes' membranes for this purpose, including red cells labeled with Cr-51 and altered by immunologic sensitization (Johnson PM, et al, 1960) and chemical and heat denaturation methods that utilized red blood cells labeled with Hg-197, Hg-203, and Tc-99m (Winkelman JW, et al, 1960; Atkins HL, et al, 1972; Sodee DB, 1963; Wagner HN, Jr, et al, 1964).

RADIOPHARMACEUTICALS

Though Cr-51 was originally employed as the radionuclide of choice for erythrocyte labeling, its relatively high energy 320 keV principal photon that is formed in less than 10% abundance is less than ideal for scintillation imaging. Chromium is known to bind firmly and irreversibly to the beta polypeptide chain of globulin in the erythrocyte (Pearson H, 1963). Tc-99m, on the other hand, is well suited for imaging and a variety of methods have been developed for radiolabeling red cells with this radionuclide.

The anionic pertechnetate species (+7) of technetium that is obtained directly from the ^{99}Mo-^{99m}Tc generator will penetrate the red cell membrane; however, localization within the erythrocyte appears to require the reduction of technetium to some lower oxidation state (probably the + 4 state). Earlier investigators had shown that pertechnetate will not label erythrocytes irreversibly and in a high yield (Burdine JA and Legeay R, 1968), although some reports had shown good results (Fischer J, et al, 1967).

The majority of successful Tc-99m red cell labeling techniques have employed stannous ion-assisted reduction of technetium and have differed primarily in the manner in which red blood cells are incubated with the stannous ions and/or pertechnetate (in vivo versus in vitro). (See Chapter 13 for additional information.)

METHOD FOR HEAT DENATURATION.

Heat denaturation of erythrocytes produces spherocytes that are characterized by a loss of intracellular electrolytes and an altered cellular membrane that is more susceptible to cell lysis (Wagner HN, Jr, et al, 1963).

In order to ensure that adequate damage to the erythrocyte occurs, it is necessary to heat the Tc-99m labeled cells in a water bath at 50 degrees centigrade for 15 minutes. Alternatively, heating at 56 degrees for 10 minutes provides adequate cell damage. Insufficient heating results in incomplete denaturation with decreased sequestration by the spleen whereas excessive heating results in increased hepatic localization.

Method. One millicurie of Tc-99m-labeled autologous heat-damaged erythrocytes is administered intravenously with scintillation imaging begun at 30 minutes. Sequential imaging of the abdomen and pelvis may be necessary to monitor the clearance of the radiolabeled cells from blood pool. In the postsplenectomy patient without accessory spleen, only a faintly outlined liver should be observed. Accessory spleens may be located anywhere in the abdomen but usually are found in the left upper quadrant and are

Table 14.6 RADIATION ABSORBED DOSE ESTIMATE TO AN ADULT FOR HEAT-DAMAGED Tc-99m RED BLOOD CELLS[a]

	RADS/MCi
Total body	0.019
Spleen	2.6
Ovaries	0.0052
Testes	0.0018
Red marrow	0.016

(Assumptions: 90% of radioactivity localizes in spleen; 10% in remainder of body.)

[a] Personal communication from the Radiopharmaceutical Internal Dose Information Center, Oak Ridge Associated Universities, TN.

considerably smaller than the normal spleen. No special patient preparation is required. Drug interference with this radiopharmaceutical resulting in altered biodistribution has not been reported. Alternatively, labeled leukocytes and platelets have also been used.

RADIATION DOSIMETRY

Patient radiation absorbed dose estimates for heat-damaged Tc-99m red blood cells are listed in Table 14.6.

CLINICAL CONSIDERATIONS

Today, there is very little call clinically for spleen-specific imaging. In patients with evidence of residual splenic function, routine liver and spleen scintigraphy with Tc-99m sulfur colloid will often detect the small splenic remnant, and it is only rarely that spleen-specific imaging need be considered. Similarly, in cases of suspect polysplenia, the routine Tc-99m sulfur colloid image usually suffices and rarely would a specific label for splenic imaging be needed.

III. Other Studies of the Gastric Tract

MECKEL'S DIVERTICULUM SCINTIGRAPHY

Meckel's diverticulum is an outpouching of the distal ileum and occurs in approximately 3% of the general population. Meckel's diverticulum may contain small bowel mucosa, pancreatic mucosa, or gastric mucosa. Although most patients are not symptomatic, those patients that are symptomatic more commonly contain ectopic gastric mucosa. The cause for the symptomatology is that the gastric mucosa will produce acid and enzymes that can lead to ulceration and even perforation. Meckel's diverticulum can also cause intussusception of the small bowel.

Meckel's diverticulum scanning operates on the principle that gastric mucosa secretes Tc-99m pertechnetate (Jewett TC, et al, 1970; Berquist TH, et al, 1976).

METHOD

Meckel's diverticulum scintigraphy is performed with the patient fasting. The patient is placed supine under the scintillation camera and 5–10 mCi of Tc-99m-sodium pertechnetate is administered intravenously. Sequential images are taken at 5-minute intervals over the abdomen and pelvis. Abnormal foci of activity appear in the Meckel's diverticulum occurring at the same time that stomach activity is visualized. Meckel's diverticulum is most commonly noted in the right lower quadrant, although the right upper quadrant and midline have also been described as locations for the visualization of Meckel's diverticulum (Figure 14.12). The accuracy of scintigraphy for Meckel's diverticulum localization has been reported to be 90% for surgically proven cases and 98% when surgical or clinical criteria are used (Sfakianakis GN and Conway JJ, 1981a). Causes of a false-positive scan include peptic ulceration, intussusception, intestinal obstruction, regional enteritis, localized inflammation, arterial-venous malformations, and hemangiomata (Sfakianakis GN and Conway JJ, 1981b). Sfakianakis and Conway (1981b) also list false-negative studies, and these include insufficient ectopic gastric mucosa such as occurs after necrosis and dilution of activity by hemorrhage or hypersecretion. Other entities that contain ectopic gastric mucosa include enteric duplication, duplication cysts, and Barett's esophagus.

Interventions that have been used to

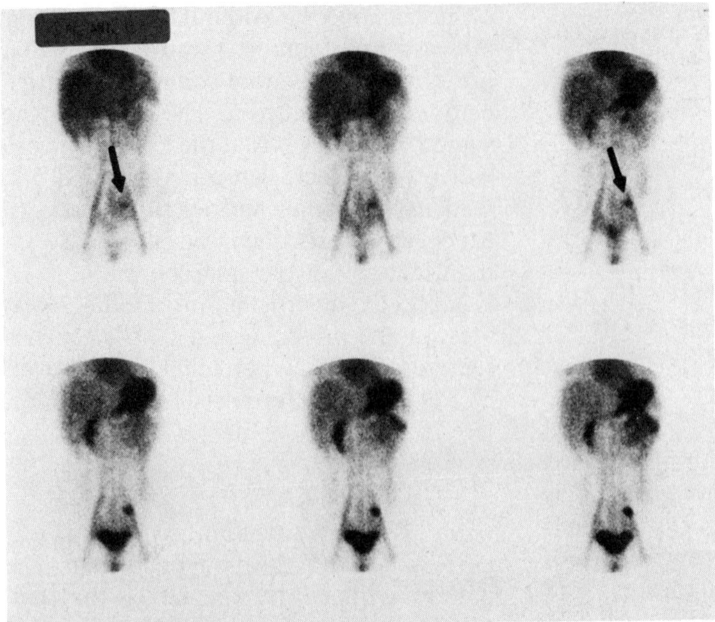

Figure 14.12   Meckel's diverticulum scan at 5-minute intervals with Tc-99m-pertechnetate. There is increasing activity to the left of midline in the pelvis (arrows). The activity begins and intensifies along with activity in the stomach. This is a Meckel's diverticulum. The location is somewhat atypical as Meckel's diverticulum usually occurs in the right lower quadrant.

increase the sensitivity of Meckel's diverticulum scintigraphy include the administration of pentagastrin (Treves S, et al, 1978) and cimetidine (Petrokubi RJ, et al, 1978). Cimetidine is a histamine H2-receptor antagonist that inhibits gastric acid secretion. Since pertechnetate is normally secreted by gastric mucosa, however, the intraluminal release of pertechnetate is inhibited in the presence of cimetidine (Sagar VV and Piccone JM, 1980) with an accumulation of pertechnetate by these cells. Pentagastrin enhances pertechnetate localization in the gastric mucosa (Treves S, et al, 1978). On the other hand, perchlorate has been shown to suppress pertechnetate localization (Oldendorf WH, et al, 1970), and atropine has been shown to block pertechnetate uptake by the gastric mucosa (Hofmeyr NG, 1967).

STUDIES OF ESOPHAGEAL REFLUX

Esophageal reflux studies are useful to detect and quantitate gastroesophageal reflux in patients who present with heartburn and regurgitation and are suspected of having pulmonary aspiration secondary to reflux. Other methods of evaluating patients with these symptomatologies include the barium upper GI series, endoscopy, lower esophageal sphincter pressure measurements, and the acid reflux test (which requires intubation).

METHOD

L.S. Malmud and R.S. Fisher (1988) perform esophageal reflux studies in the morning following an overnight fast by giving the patient, in an upright position, 150 ml of orange juice, 150 ml of 0.1 N HCl, and 300 uCi of Tc-99m-sulfur colloid. The patient is instructed to drink an additional 30 ml of water to clear any residual activity from the esophagus. They use an abdominal binder with the ability to increase pressure in 20 mm of Hg increments from 0 to 100 mm of Hg. The patient is placed supine under a large-field-of-view scintillation camera, and 30-second images are obtained at each pressure gradient from 0 to 100 mm Hg. All data is stored on a small on-line computer, and esophageal reflux is calculated using the following formula:

$$R = E_t - E_b \times \frac{100}{G_o}$$

where R equals the percentage gastroesophageal reflux index, E_t equals the esophageal counts at time t, E_b is esophageal background counts (although in their studies, background was negligible in all cases), and G_o is gastric counts at the beginning of the study.

In the study by R.S. Fisher and associates (1976), 2 out of 20 normal controls had abnormal studies using a G-E reflux index of 4% or more as abnormal, and 27 out of 30 patients with confirmed gastrointestinal reflux had abnormal results. In this group, the G-E reflux index was significantly greater in reflux patients averaging approximately 12% for patients compared with approximately 3% for controls. In that study, the sensitivity for varying tests were as follows: radiographic definition of a hiatal hernia, 60%; fluoroscopic reflux, 50%; lower esophageal sphincter pressure of less than 10 ml of Hg, 57%; lower esophageal sphincter pressures of less than 15 ml of Hg, 77%; phenol red reflux test, 47%; acid perfusion test, 63%; endoscopic esophagitis, 40%; histologic evidence of esophagitis, 47%; whereas the gastroesophageal scintigraphic study had a sensitivity of 90%. L.S. Malmud and colleagues (1988) also reported on the use of the gastroesophageal reflux study to evaluate the effects of various treatments for heartburn (Table 14.7).

In infants, esophageal reflux studies and evaluation of pulmonary aspiration are performed somewhat differently than in adults. Children should not eat for approximately 4 hours prior to the study. Approximately 200 uCi of Tc-99m-sulfur colloid is mixed with formula (or milk or orange juice) followed by approximately 15 cc of water to assure that all of the activity has left the mouth and esophageal areas. An abdominal binder is not used with children but, if necessary, intra

Table 14.7 EFFECTS OF THERAPIES FOR REFLUX[a]

	GE REFLUX INDEX (%)	
	Before	*After*
Bethanechol	12	6–8
Atrophine	8	10–13
Antacid	11	8
Gaviscon	10	7
Position change to erect	15	8
Nissen fundoplication	17	3

[a] Modified from LS Malmud and RS Fisher, 1988.

abdominal pressure can be increased by leg raising. The patient is studied under the gamma camera for approximately 30 minutes with the data acquired with a small on-line computer. Quantitation is performed as previously described. When pulmonary aspiration is suspected, the patient is brought back the next morning and images of the chest are obtained in order to detect the presence of lung activity that would indicate pulmonary aspiration.

ESOPHAGEAL TRANSIT STUDIES

Patients presenting with dysphagia or difficulty swallowing may require assessment of esophageal motor function. The studies that can be performed include barium swallows, esophageal manometry, and the acid clearance test. While each test provides different information, each also has significant limitations including the need for intubation (the acid clearance test and esophageal manometry) and a relatively high radiation burden and a lack of quantitative information (barium swallows). Radionuclide esophageal transit studies, on the other hand, provide minimal radiation exposure, are noninvasive, and yield quantitative information in patients with dysphagia and other esophageal motor disorders.

METHOD

A variety of methods have been described for esophageal transit studies. Each institution should standardize the methodology used for this procedure since considerable variation may exist. For example, some techniques require the patient to be fasting overnight while others will perform esophageal imaging any time so long as the patient is not immediately postprandial. Patients can be studied supine or upright. Several radiopharmaceuticals have been used including Tc-99m-sulfur colloid in water (Klein KA and Wald A, 1987) and Tc-99m-sulfur colloid in varying consistencies in jello or pudding (O'Connor MK, et al, 1988a).

The most commonly employed technique includes studying the patient in the morning following an overnight fast. The patient is placed supine over a large or jumbo field-of-view scintillation camera with a parallel hole low-energy collimator. Imaging is begun immediately as the patient swallows 15 ml of water containing 300 uCi of Tc-99m-sulfur colloid in a single swallow who is then instructed to swallow dry at 15-second intervals for 10 minutes. The data is recorded on a computer where regions of interest are drawn over the esophagus and stomach area. Esophageal transit rates are calculated using the formula below:

$$C_t = \frac{(E_{max} - E_t)}{E_{max}} \times 100$$

where C_t is the percent esophageal transit at time t, E_{max} is the maximal count rate in the esophagus immediately after the swallow, and E_t is the esophageal count rate at time t (Tolin RD, et al, 1979; Malmud LS and Fisher RS, 1988).

Esophageal activity is determined at each second for the first 15 seconds of the study and then at each succeeding 15-second interval for the 10 minutes of the examination.

In normal subjects, esophageal activity decreases rapidly with less than 10% of activity remaining after the first 15-second interval. After eight swallows, esophageal transit in patients with achalasia was 27 ± 11%; for patients with scleroderma, 24 ± 15%, compared to 93 ± 1% in normals. Patients with diffuse spasm had esophageal transit of 76 ± 11% after eight swallows (Tolin RD, et al, 1979).

M.K. O'Connor and colleagues (1988b) studied normal subjects with Tc-99m-sulfur colloid in water in the supine position and with varying consistencies of jello or pudding labeled with Tc-99m-sulfur colloid, which ranged from watery to solid. Measured mean transit times (MTT) were calculated. Mean transit time for water was 6.6 ± 1.8 seconds, whereas for the semisolid boluses the MTT increase from 5.2 ± 0.9 seconds to 6.1 ± 1.2 seconds as the semisolid bolus viscosity increased. These investigators also noted an increase in MTT for the water bolus, but not for the semisolid boluses, with increasing age. They noted no effects of sex on MTT. It should be noted that in the study, the patients swallowed the bolus of water in the supine position, but the five semisolid boluses were swallowed in the erect-position.

Esophageal transit studies have also demonstrated abnormalities in patients with symptomatic gastroesophageal reflux both with and without motor disorders as demonstrated by manometry (Malmud LS and Fisher RS, 1988). Both manometry and acid clearance tests require intubation, which in some individuals may adversely affect esophageal function.

Esophageal transit studies provide an excellent means of evaluating esophageal transit of a physiologic marker. Although the most common methodology involves the swallowing of a liquid marker and the observation of its transit, any liquid or solid marker that can be labeled with a radionuclide can be used to study esophageal function.

GASTRIC EMPTYING, SMALL BOWEL AND COLONIC TRANSIT, AND RECTAL-EMPTYING STUDIES

Radionuclide techniques for the evaluation of gastric emptying have been used since the early 1970s. Measurement of small bowel and colonic transit began in the 1980s, and the use of radiotracers for the evaluation of rectal emptying began in the mid 1980s. A central requirement for all these studies is the use of a suitably labeled physiologic marker that stays in the appropriate compartment sufficiently long for the measurement or transit period. Examples would include tracers

Table 14.8 CAUSES OF DELAYED GASTRIC EMPTYING

Diabetes mellitus
Nausea of any cause
Atrophic gastritis
Gastric ulcers
Amyloidosis
Myotonic dystrophy
Postsurgical
Functional or idiopathic
Medications:
  Beta adrenergic agonists (e.g., isoproterenol)
  Cholinergic antagonists (e.g., tricyclic antidepressants)
  Dopamine and dopaminergic D_2 agonists (e.g., apomorphine, Levo-dopa, opioid agents)

Table 14.9 CAUSES OF RAPID GASTRIC EMPTYING

Postsurgical
Duodenal ulcers
Hyperthyroidism
Celiac sprue
Medications:
  Cholinergic agonists (e.g., bethanechol)
  Dopaminergic antagonists (e.g., metoclopramide, domperidine)

that remain in either the liquid or solid phase during gastric-emptying studies or a tracer that would maintain the consistency of stool for rectal-emptying studies. Additionally, tracers must maintain their integrity throughout the study and be immune to the effects of the various chemical and enzymatic environments to which they will be subjected. As an example, gastric-emptying agents must maintain their integrity in the acid and pepsin environment of the stomach, agents used for small bowel transit must remain stable at a neutral-to-alkaline pH, and agents that are used for colonic transit must not be digestible by the bacterial environment of the colon. The agents must not be absorbed to any degree in the gastrointestinal tract, nor should they be excreted through the GI mucosa.

Gastric-emptying studies complement other tests for the evaluation of patients with various signs and symptoms of gastric dysfunction including delayed gastric emptying or gastroparesis (Table 14.8) or increased gastric emptying (Table 14.9). The most common presentation for patients with disturbances of gastric emptying include nausea and vomitting, abdominal pain, post-prandial bloating, malnutrition or anorexia.

Method

Gastric emptying is a complex mechanism that involves mixing, grinding, and emptying of the components of an ingested meal. The components of a mixed meal include the solid phase, which usu-

ally refers to particles in the millimeter-or-larger range, and the liquid phase. Pressure from the fundus of the stomach forces the liquid portion of the meal and gastric juices into the antrum and through the pylorus. The liquid phase of a mixed meal empties in an exponential fashion (Figure 14.13). The solid phase of a mixed meal needs to be reduced to approximately 2 millimeters in size to be emptied through the pylorus (Meyer JH, et al, 1982; Mayer EA, 1985). There is often a "lag

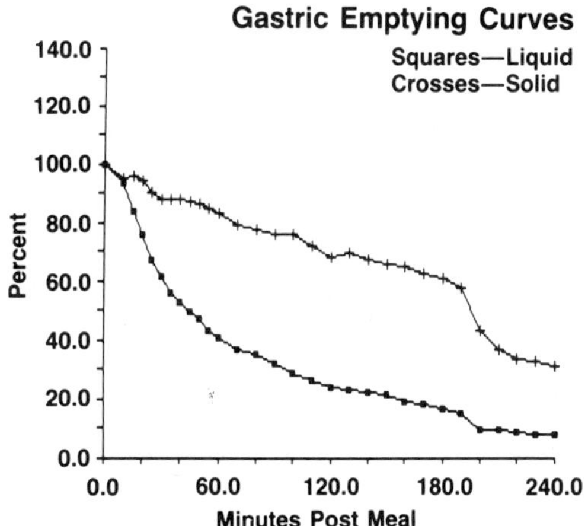

Figure 14.13 Gastric emptying curve with the percent remaining in the stomach plotted on the *y*-axis and the minutes following the meal on the *x*-axis. Squares represent the liquid component of the mixed meal, and crosses represent the solid component of the mixed meal. Note that the liquid component empties in an exponential fashion whereas the solid component empties in a linear fashion. The $T_{1/2}$ for liquid emptying of 40 minutes and the $T_{1/2}$ for solid emptying of 190 minutes in this case is within normal limits for this mixed meal.

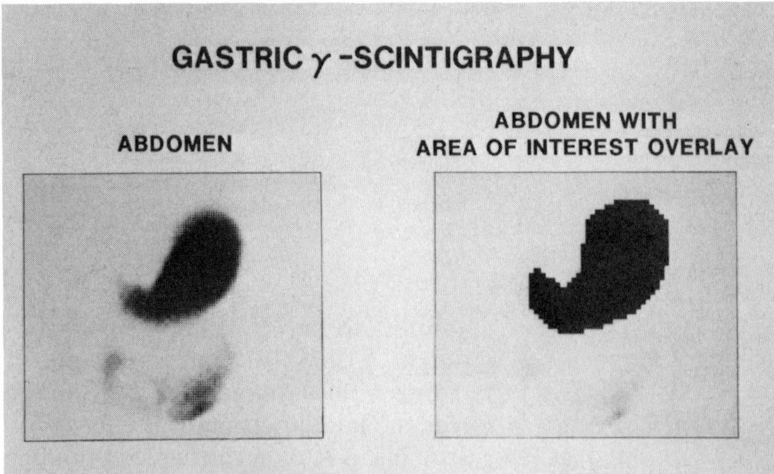

Figure 14.14   Activity in the stomach and small bowel with the gastric region of interest (right panel) used for generating time activity curves in gastric-emptying studies.

phase" while the solids are being broken down, and this lasts approximately 20–30 minutes. The solid phase of the mixed meal then empties in a linear fashion (Figure 14.14).

There have been many agents used for gastric emptying. The most elegant is the use of Tc-99m-sulfur colloid chicken liver. The method was described by J.H. Meyer and colleges (1976) and involves the injection of Tc-99m-sulfur colloid into a live chicken, sacrificing the chicken after approximately 20 minutes, removing the liver, and cooking it to a firm consistency. This is truly an intracellular label of a physiologic solid marker. More commonly, the solid marker used for gastric emptying studies is Tc-99m-sulfur colloid in eggs which are then scrambled and cooked to a firm consistency and eaten with other components of a mixed meal such as bread and meat. The liquid component of the mixed meal is usually In-111 DTPA in water or milk (Chaudhari TK, 1974; Heading RC, et al, 1971). The choice of these markers is that they are easy to prepare, they do not break down in the stomach, and they maintain their relationship to their appropriate phase (Knight LC, et al, 1982; Thomforde GM, et al, 1985).

In the setting up of gastric-emptying tests, it is important to carefully standardize the meal used for gastric emptying. One of the important determinants of the rate of gastric emptying is the meal composition (Table 14.10). One standardized meal includes 1 mCi of Tc-99m-sulfur colloid in two eggs scrambled and cooked to a firm consistency and placed between two slices of white bread and 250 uCi In-111 DTPA in 200 ml of water. An alternative marker of liquid and solid emptying would be 500 uCi Tc-99m-sulfur colloid in 60 gm of Egg Beaters® cooked to a firm consistency, 30 gm of Canadian bacon, a slice of white bread with 5 gm of margarine and 20 gm of grape jelly; and the liquid component of the mixed meal containing 250 uCi In-111 DTPA in 60 gm of Ensure and 60 gm of skim milk. This meal yields a composition of 57% carbohydrates, 25% protein, and 18% fat with 293 calories.

Before a new marker is used for gastric emptying, it should be tested in an in vitro system. One such system (Thomforde GM, et al, 1985) uses an in vitro model consisting of a 1-liter beaker with 500 ml of isotonic saline kept at 37° C. Large fragments of the solid marker being tested are added to the beaker. A solution of 0.2 N HCl and pepsin at a concentration of 1200 ug/ml is infused at a rate of

Table 14.10 FACTORS AFFECTING THE RATE OF GASTRIC EMPTYING[a]

A. Accelerate Emptying
  Smaller particles of a solid marker
  Liquid markers
  Increased gastric pressure
B. Delayed Emptying
  Larger particles of a solid meal
  Larger meal volume (size)
  Meal composition:
    Increased caloric content (energy density)
    Increased osmolality
    Increased fatty acid chain length
    Increased acidity
  Supine versus upright position

[a] Modified from LS Malmud and RS Fisher. 1988.

0.7 mls/min into the beaker. During the process, an overhead motor agitates the mixture at approximately 120 rpm. Aliquots are removed at 30-minute intervals for 4 hours, centrifuged at 640 g for 10 minutes, and samples of the supernatant are counted to determine how much tracer dissociates from the solid marker. In order to test the liquid component, the above method is used except that no label is used on the solid component and the liquid marker is added to the beaker. Other models include incubating the marker with gastric juices that have been aspirated during endoscopy.

The patient is asked to eat the meal in approximately 10 minutes and imaging is begun immediately afterwards. Studies can be performed with the patient either supine, reclining, or upright, and this should also be standardized, as it will influence gastric emptying (Table 14.10). One standard approach is to have the patient eat the meal in a sitting position and then stand in front of a gamma camera where images are obtained at 10-minute intervals. If a mixed meal with labels of both the solid and liquid components is used, then a medium energy collimator is needed with imaging using the Tc-99m window (140 keV ± 10%) and the upper peak of In-111 (247 keV ± 10%). Some laboratories take both anterior and posterior images to correct for the attenuation. Other corrections that are required include the scatter from Indium into the Tc-99m window (based on phantom studies) and correction for decay. Activity

within the stomach and small bowel is defined on the first image as 100%. Regions of interest are then generated for the area of the stomach (see Figure 14.14) on all subsequent times. Gastric-emptying studies are usually carried out for 3–4 hours. The data is plotted as the percent activity remaining in the stomach over time (see Figure 14.13). For the second meal noted above, the normal values for the liquid half-time are 43 minutes (33–75 minutes, tenth and ninetieth percentile) and for the solid half-time 129 minutes (71–190 minutes, tenth and ninetieth percentile). It is important to remember that these half-times apply only to an exact duplication of the gastric-emptying methodology noted above and that each laboratory should set up its own standard for meal composition, position, imaging times, and corrections, and have a subset of normal volunteers to define normal values.

Various disease states will give different patterns of gastric emptying. As noted above, the normal patients will have an exponential emptying of the liquid phase and a more linear emptying of the solid phase. Patients with gastroparesis may show normal emptying of the liquid phase with significantly delayed emptying of the solid phase or may show significant abnormalities in emptying of both the liquid and solid components of the mixed meal (Figure 14.15). Patients with a dumping-type syndrome may show very rapid emptying of the liquid phase with up to 50% of the material emptying in the first 10 minutes followed by little, if any, emptying of either the liquid or solid phases following this initial period (Figure 14.16). Small bowel transit studies have been performed with several radiolabeled markers including I-131-labeled fiber (Malagelada JR, et al, 1980). This technique yields results that are similar to the hydrogen breath technique (Caride VJ, et al, 1984). Studies show that changes in small bowel transit can occur independent of changes in gastric emptying (Read NW, et al, 1982). Ileal cecal transit times have been measured using Tc-99m-labeled bran (Trotman IF and Price CC, 1986). Whole-bowel transit studies have been performed using Tc-99m- and In-111-labeled resin beads (Hardy JG, et al, 1986) and with Cr-51 and Tc-99m sulfur colloid (Jain R, et al, 1984). These techniques are primarily research studies but may yield important information on the physiology of small bowel and colonic transit and the pathophysiology of irritable

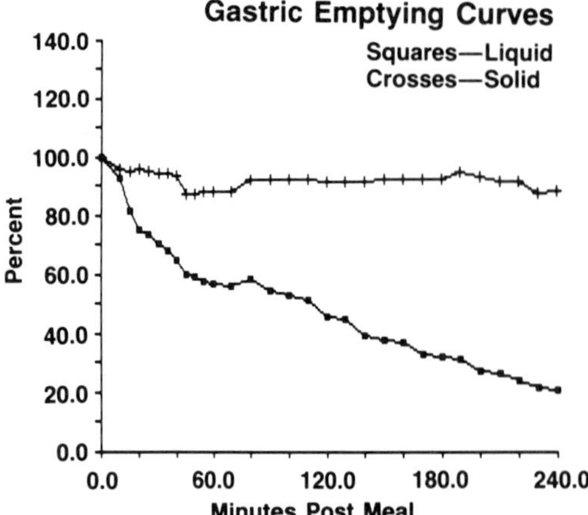

Figure 14.15 Gastric emptying shows delayed emptying of the liquid component with almost no emptying of the solid component of the mixed meal during the 4 hours of the study. The patient had diabetic gastroparesis.

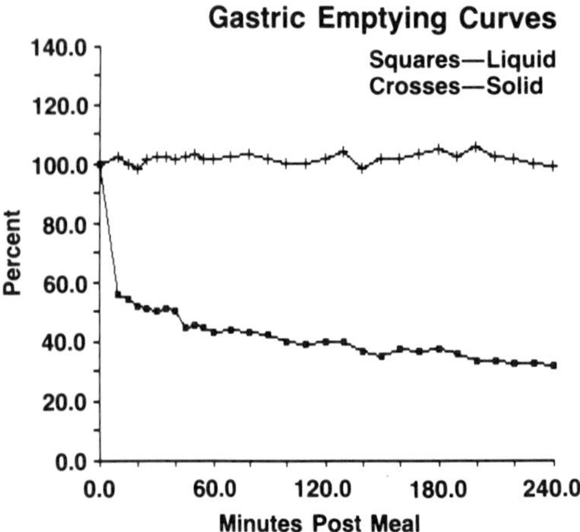

Figure 14.16 Gastric emptying of a mixed meal demonstrates very rapid emptying of the liquid component in the first 10 minutes with delayed emptying of the remainder of the liquid component of the mixed meal. There is essentially no emptying of the solid component of the mixed meal during the 4 hours of the study. This patient was status post Billroth II anastomosis and had impaired gastric emptying following the vagotomy and pyloroplasty. This can be considered an initial "dumping syndrome" followed by delayed emptying of the remainder of the meal.

bowel syndrome and various causes of diarrhea and constipation (Figure 14.17).

RADIATION DOSIMETRY

Radiation dosimetry values for the radiopharmaceuticals commonly employed for gastric emptying and GI transit studies are shown in Table 14.11.

Rectal emptying studies are also primarily a research tool. Other studies used for the evaluation of problems in defecation in patients with constipation or with severe diarrhea include anorectal manometry, recto-anal inhibitory reflex measurements, distention of a rectal balloon with air, defecating protocogram using barium, and a new test using a radiolabeled stool analogue. The advantage of the nuclear medicine technique (O'Connell PR, et al, 1986) is the ability to quantitate the rate of emptying and the percentage emptying of the radiolabeled stool analogue.

References

American Society of Hospital Pharmacists, Monograph on Sincalide, 1987.

Atkins HL, Eckelman WC, Hauser W, et al. Splenic sequestration of Tc-99m labeled red blood cells. *J Nucl Med* 1972, 13:811–814.

Atkins HL, Hauser W, Richards P. Factors affecting the distribution of technetium-sulfur colloid. *J Reticuloendothel Soc* 1970, 8:176–184.

Awasthi YC, Dao DD, Saneto RP. Interrelationships between anionic and cationic forms of glutathionine S-transferases of human liver. *Biochem J* 1980, 191:1–10.

Baker RJ, Bellen JD, Ronai PM. Tc-99m-pyridoxylidene glutamate: A new rapid cholescintigraphic agent. *J Nucl Med* 1974, 15:476.

Baker RJ, Bellen JC, and Ronai PM. Technetium-99m pyridoxylidene glutamate: A new hepatobiliary radiopharmaceutical. I. Experimental aspects. *J Nucl Med* 1975, 16:720–727.

Bekerman C, Conway J, Pinsky S, et al.

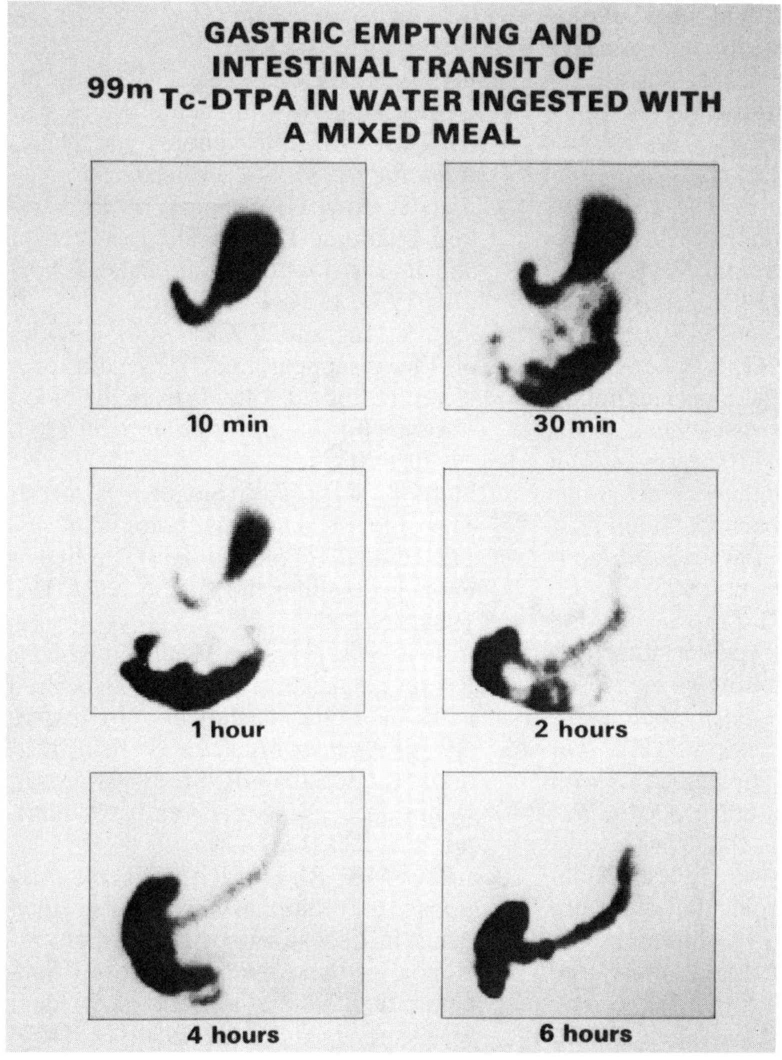

Figure 14.17   Gastric emptying of Tc-99m-DTPA in water in a mixed meal. The scans demonstrate the ability to do gastric emptying and small-bowel transit of a meal.

Table 14.11   RADIATION ABSORBED DOSE ESTIMATES FOR GASTRIC EMPTYING AND GI TRANSIT STUDIES[a]

	ORGAN ABSORBED DOSE (RADS)						
AGENT	*Stomach*	*SI*[b]	*ULI*[c]	*LLI*[d]	*Ovary*	*Testis*	*TB*[e]
Tc-99m sulfur colloid (300 μ Ci) in liquid	0.028	0.083	0.160	0.097	0.029	0.002	0.005
In-111 DTPA (250 μCi) in liquid	0.110	0.490	1.100	2.000	0.420	0.027	0.060
Tc-99m sulfur colloid (500 μCi) in solid	0.120	0.120	0.230	0.140	0.042	0.002	0.009

[a] Modified from Siegel JA, et al, 1983.
[b] SI =   Small intestine.
[c] ULI = Upper large intestine.
[d] LLI = Lower large intestine.
[e] TB = Total body.

Manual of pediatric and unusual nuclear medicine procedures, February 1979, "Liver/spleen and/or pertechnetate." Chicago, Central Chapter, Society of Nuclear Medicine, 1979.

Bell EG, McAfee JG. Concepts of colloid chemistry. In *Hematopoietic and Gastrointestinal Investigations with Radionuclides*, Gilson AJ, Smoak WM, Weinstein MB (eds.). Springfield, IL, Charles C Thomas, 1972, pp. 66–84.

Berquist TH, Nolan NG, Stephens DH, et al. Specificity of ^{99m}Tc-pertechnetate in scintigraphy diagnosis of Meckel's diverticulum: Review of 100 cases. *J Nucl Med* 1976, 17:465–469.

Bjerrum J, Schwarzenbach G, Sillen LG. Stability constants. Part I. London, London Chemical Society, 1957.

Bobinet DD, Sevrin R, Zurbriggen MT, et al. Lung uptake of Tc-99m sulfur colloid in patient exhibiting presence of Al^{+3} in plasma. *J Nucl Med* 1974, 15:1220–1222.

Burdine JA, Legeay R. Spleen scans with ^{99m}Tc-labeled heated erythrocytes. *Radiology* 1968, 91:162–164.

Burns D, Marzilli L, Sowa D, et al. Relationship between molecular structure and biliary excretion of technetium-99m HIDA and HIDA analogs. *J Nucl Med* 1977 (Abst), 18:624.

Carrasco CH, Freny PC, Chuang VP, et al. Chemical cholecystitis associated with hepatic artery infusion chemotherapy. *Am J Roentgenol* 1983, 141:703–706.

Caride VJ, Prokop EK, Troncale FJ, et al. Scintigraphic determination of small intestinal transit time: Comparison with the hydrogen breath technique. *Gastroenterology* 1984, 86:714–720.

Cawthon MA, Brown DM, Hartshorne MF, et al. Biliary scintigraphy, the "hot rim" sign. *Clin Nucl Med* 1984, 9:619–621.

Chaudhari TK. Use of ^{99m}Tc-DTPA for measuring gastric emptying time. *J Nucl Med* 1974, 15:391–395.

Chervu LR, Nunn AD, Loberg MD. Radiopharmaceuticals for hepatobiliary imaging. *Semin Nucl Med* 1982, 12:5–17.

Choy D, Shi EC, McLean RG, et al. Cholescintigraphy in acute cholecystitis: Use of intravenous morphine. *Radiology* 1984, 151:203–207.

Christy B, King G, Smoak WM. Preparation of iodine-123 labeled rose bengal and its distribution in animals. *J Nucl Med* 1974, 15:484.

Cohen Y, Ingrand J, Caro RA. Kinetics of the disappearance of gelatin protected radiogold colloids from the blood stream. *Int J Appl Radiat Isot* 1968, 19:703–705.

Colletti P, Ralls PW, Siegel ME, et al. The role of scintiangiography in suspected acute cholecystitis: "The hyperemic gallbladder fossa." *J Nucl Med* 1984, 15:P95.

Cordova MA, Hladik WB III, Rhodes BA, et al. Adverse reactions associated with radiopharmaceuticals. In *Essentials of Nuclear Medicine Science*, Hladik WB III, Saha GB, Study KT (eds.), Baltimore, Williams and Wilkins, pp. 303–320, 1987.

Cordova MA, Rhodes BA. Adverse reactions to radiopharmaceuticals: Incidence in 1978 and associated symptoms. Report of the Adverse Reactions Subcommittee of the Society of Nuclear Medicine. *J Nucl Med* 1980, 21:1107–1110.

Cordova MA, Rhodes BA, Atkins HL, et al. Adverse reactions to radiopharmaceuticals. *J Nucl Med* 1982, 23:550–551.

Davis MA, Jones AG, Trinade H. A rapid and accurate method for sizing radiocolloid. *J Nucl Med* 1974, 15:923–928.

Dobson EL, Gofman JW, Jones HB, et al. Studies with colloids containing radioisotopes of yttrium, zirconium, columbium, and lanthanum. II. The controlled selective localization of radioisotopes of yttrium, zirconium, and columbium in the bone marrow, liver, and spleen. *J Lab Clin Med* 1949, 34:305–309.

Dobson EL, Jones HB. The behavior of

intravenously injected particulate material: Its rate of disappearance from the blood stream as a measure of liver blood flow. *Acta Med Scand* 1952, 144 (Suppl 273):1–71.

Eckelman WC, Volkert WA. In vivo chemistry of Tc-99m chelates. *Int J Appl Radiat Isot* 1982, 33:945–952.

Firnau G. Why do ^{99m}Tc-chelates work for cholescintigraphy? *Eur J Nucl Med* 1976, 1:137–139.

Fischer J, Wolf R, Leon A. Technetium-99m as a label for erythrocytes. *J Nucl Med* 1967, 8:229–232.

Fisher RS, Malmud LS, Roberts GS, et al. Gastroesophageal (GE) scintiscanning to detect and quantitate GE reflux. *Gastroenterology* 1976, 70:301–308.

Freeman LM, Sugarman LA, Weissman HS. Role of cholecystokinetic agents in ^{99m}Tc-IDA cholescintigraphy. *Semin Nucl Med* 1981, 11:186–193.

Geronemus RG, Auerbach R, Tobias H. Liver biopsies vs. liver scans in methotrexate-treated patients with psoriasis. *Arch Dermatol* 1982, 118:649–651.

Ghadimi H, Sass-Kortsak A. Evaluation of the radioactive rose bengal test for the differential diagnosis of obstructive jaundice in infants. *N Engl J Med* 1961, 265:351–358.

Goresky CA. The hepatic uptake and excretion of sulfobromophthalein and bilirubin. *Can Med Assoc J* 1965, 92:851–857.

Haney TA, Ascanio I, Gigliotti JA, et al. Physical and biological properties of a Tc-99m sulfur colloid preparation containing disodium edetate. *J Nucl Med* 1970, 12:64–68.

Hardy JG, Wood E, Clark AG, et al. Whole-bowel transit in patients with irritable bowel syndrome. *Eur J Nucl Med* 1986, 11:393–396.

Harper PV, Beck R, Charleston D, et al. Optimization of a scanning method using Tc-99m. *Nucleonics* 1964a, 22:50–54.

Harper PV, Lathrop KA, Richards P. Tc-99m as a radiocolloid. *J Nucl Med* 1964b, 5:382.

Harvey SC. Hypnotics and sedatives. Barbiturates. In *Goodman and Gilman's The Pharmacological Basis of Therapy*, Seventh Edition, New York, Macmillan, 1985, pp. 356–360.

Harvey E, Loberg M, Ryan J, et al. Hepatic clearance mechanism of Tc-99m-HIDA and its effect on quantitation of hepatobiliary function: Concise communication. *J Nucl Med* 1979, 20:310–313.

Heading RC, Tothill P, Laidlaw AJ, et al. An evaluation of [113m]Indium DPTA chelate in the measurement of gastric emptying by scintiscanning. *Gut* 1971, 12:611–615.

Hedner P, Lundequist A. Use of the C-terminal octapeptide of cholecystokinin for gallbladder evacuation in cholecystokinin. *Am J Roentgenol* 1972, 116:320–326.

Helffreich F. Ligand exchange: A novel separation technique. *Nature* 1961, 189:1001–1002.

Hernandez M, Rosenthall L. A crossover study comparing the kinetics of Tc-99m-labeled diisopropyl and P-butyl IDA analogs in patients. *Clin Nucl Med* 1980a, 8:159–165.

Hernandez M, Rosenthall L. A crossover study comparing the kinetics of Tc-99m-labeled diethyl- and diisopropyl-IDA. *Clin Nucl Med* 1980b, 8:352–358.

Hofmeyr NG. Stomach scanning after intravenous ^{99m}Tc administration. A preliminary report. *S Afr Med J* 1967, 41:572–575.

Housholder DF, Hynes HE, Dakhil SR, et al. Hepatobiliary scintigraphy in patients receiving hepatic artery infusion chemotherapy. *J Nucl Med* 1985, 26:474–477.

ICRP Publication 52, Protection of the patient in nuclear medicine, Oxford, Pergamon, 1988.

Jackson ML, Zuckier L, Goldfarb CR, et al. Effect of patient positioning on liver size. *J Nucl Med* 1986, 27:1632–1634.

Jaffe JH, Martin WR. Opioid analgesics and antagonists. In *Goodman and Gilman's The Pharmacological Basis of*

Therapeutics, Seventh Edition, New York, Macmillan, 1985, pp. 491–531.

Jain R, Najean Y, Bernier JJ. Measurement of intestinal progression of a meal and its residues in normal subjects and patients with functional diarrhea by a dual isotope technique. *Gut* 1984, 25:728–731.

Jewett TC, Duszynski DO, Allen JE. The visualization of Meckel's diverticulum with ^{99m}Tc-pertechnetate. *Surgery* 1970, 68:567–570.

Joehl RJ, Koch KL, Nahrwold DL. Opioid drugs cause bile duct obstruction during hepatobiliary scans. *Am J Surg* 1984, 147:134–138.

Johnson AE, Gollan F. ^{99m}Tc-technetium dioxide for liver scanning. *J Nucl Med* 1970, 11:564–565.

Johnson PM, Herion JC, Mooring SL. Scintillation scanning of the normal human spleen utilizing sensitized radioactive erythrocytes. *Radiology* 1960, 74:99–101.

Jones DP, Terz J, Lawrence W, et al. Extrahepatic clearance of I-131 rose bengal. *Am J Physiol* 1961, 201:1025–1029.

Kaplan WD, Drum DE, Lokich JJ. The effect of cancer chemotherapy agents on the liver–spleen scan. *J Nucl Med* 1980, 21:84–87.

Kato M, Hazue M. Tc-99m (Sn) pyridoxylideneaminates: Preparation and biologic evaluation. *J Nucl Med* 1978, 19:397–406.

Kerlin P, Davis GL, McGill DB, et al. Hepatic adenoma and focal nodular hyperplasia: Clinical, pathologic, and radiologic features. *Gastroenterology* 1983, 84:994–1002.

Klein HA, Wald A. Normal variation in radionuclide esophageal transit studies. *Eur J Nucl Med* 1987, 13:115–120.

Klingensmith WC, Ryerson TW: Lung uptake of ^{99m}Tc-sulfur colloid. *J Nucl Med* 1973, 14:201–204.

Klingensmith WC, Fritzberg AR, Spitzer VM, et al. Clinical evaluation of Tc-99m-trimethylbromo-IDA and comparison with Tc-99m-diisopropyl-IDA

for hepatobiliary imaging. *J Nucl Med* 1982 (Abst), 23:P73.

Knight LC, Fisher RS, Malmud LS. Comparison of solid food markers in gastric emptying studies. In *Nuclear Medicine and Biology: Proceedings of the Third World Congress of Nuclear Medicine and Biology*. Paris, New York, Pergamon Press, 1982, Vol. III, pp. 2407–2410.

Krishnamurthy GT, Turner FE, Mangham D, et al. Optimization of ceruletide intravenous dose for gallbladder (GB) emptying. *J Nucl Med* 1983 (Abst) 24:P38–39.

Lentle BC, Scott JR, Noujaim AA, et al. Iatrogenic alterations in radionuclide biodistributions. *Semin Nucl Med* 1979, 9:131–143.

Loberg MD. Radiolabeled drug analogs based upon N-substituted imino diacetic acid. In *The Chemistry of Radiopharmaceuticals*, Heindel ND, Burns HD, Honda T, Brady LW (eds.). New York, Masson, 1978b, pp. 191–204.

Loberg MD, Cooper MD, Harvey EB, et al. Development of a new radiopharmaceutical based on N-substituted iminodiacetic acid. *J Nucl Med* 1976, 17:633–638.

Loberg MD, Fields AT. Chemical structure of Tc-99m-labeled N-(2,6-dimethyl carbamoylmethyl) iminodiacetic acid (Tc-HIDA). *Int J Appl Radiat Isot* 1978a, 29:167–173.

Loberg MD, Nunn AD, Porter DS. Development of hepatobiliary imaging agents. In *Nuclear Medicine Annual 1981*, Freeman LM, Weissman HS (eds.). New York, Raven, 1981, pp. 1–33.

Loberg MD, Porter DW, Ryan JW. Review and current status of hepatobiliary imaging agents. In Sorenson JA (ed.), Radiopharmaceuticals II: Proceedings of the Second International Symposium on Radiopharmaceuticals, New York, Society of Nuclear Medicine, 1979, 519–543.

MacCarthy RL, Wahner HW, Stephens DH, et al. Retrospective comparison of radionuclide scans and computed tomography of the liver and pancreas. *AJR* 1977, 129:23–28.

Maisels MJ. Bilirubin. On understanding and influencing its metabolism in the newborn infant. *Pediatr Clin North Am* 1972, 19:447–501.

Majd M, Reba RC, Altman RP. Effect of phenobarbital on ^{99m}Tc-IDA scintigraphy in the evaluation of neonatal jaundice. *Semin Nucl Med* 1981, 11:194–204.

Malagelada JR, Carter SE, Brown ML, et al. Radiolabeled fiber: A physiologic marker for gastric emptying and intestinal transit of solids. *Dig Dis Sci* 1980, 25:81–87.

Malmud LS, Fisher RS. Scintigraphic evaluation of esophageal transit, gastroesophageal reflux, and gastric emptying. In *Diagnostic Nuclear Medicine*, Gottschalk A, Hoffer PH, Potchen EJ (eds.), Volume 2, Chapter 40, Baltimore, Williams and Wilkins, 1988, pp. 663–686.

Mayer EA, Thomson JB, Jen D, et al. Gastric emptying in sieving of solid food and pancreatic and biliary secretion after solid meals in patients with truncal vagotomy and antrectomy. *Gastroenterology* 1982, 83:184–192.

Meyer JH, Dressman J, Fink A, et al. Effect of size and density on canine gastric emptying of nondigestible solids. *Gastroenterology* 1985, 89:805–813.

Meyer JH, McGregor IL, Gueller R, et al. ^{99m}Tc-tagged chicken liver as a marker of solid food in the human stomach. *Dig Dis* 1976, 21:296–304.

Mezgarzadeh M, Krishnamurthy GT, Bobba VR, et al. Filling, postcholecystokinin emptying, and refilling of normal gallbladder: Effects of two different doses of CCK on refilling: Concise communication. *J Nucl Med* 1983, 24:666–671.

Mikhael MA, Evens RG. Migration and embolization of macrophages to the lung—A possible mechanism for colloid uptake in the lung during liver scanning. *J Nucl Med* 1975, 16:22–27.

Neilsen P, Rasmussen F. Relationships between molecular structure and excretion of drugs. *Life Sci* 1975, 17:1495–1512.

Nelp WB. Distribution and radiobiological behavior of colloids and macroaggregates. In *Medical Radionuclides: Radiation Dose and Effects*, Cloutier RJ, Edwards CL, Snyder WS (eds.). Springfield, VA, USAEC Symposium Series 20, 1970, pp. 239–245.

Nunn AD, Loberg MD, Conley RA. The development of a new cholescintigraphic agent, Tc-SQ 26,962, using a structure-distribution relationship approach. *J Nucl Med* 1981 (Abst), 22:P51.

Nunn AD, Loberg MD, Conley RA. A structure-distribution-relationship approach leading to the development of Tc-99m mebrofenin: An improved cholescintigraphic agent. *J Nucl Med* 1983, 24:423–430.

O'Connell PR, Kelly KA, Brown ML. Scintigraphic assessment of neorectal motor function. *J Nucl Med* 1986, 27:460–464.

O'Connor MK, Kim CH, Hung JCY, et al. Personal communication, 1988a.

O'Connor MK, Kim CH, Hung JCY, et al. The effects of age, sex, and bolus composition on esophageal transit. Personal communication, 1988b.

Oldendorf WH, Sisson WB, Iisaka Y. Compartmental redistribution of ^{99m}Tc-pertechnetate in the presence of perchlorate ion and its relation to plasma protein binding. *J Nucl Med* 1970, 11:85–88.

Pardue WO. Severe liver dysfunction during nicotinic acid therapy. *JAMA* 1961, 175:137–138.

Pearson H. The binding of Cr^{51} to hemoglobin. I. In vitro studies. *Blood* 1963, 22:218–230.

Pedersen B, Kristensen K. Evaluation of methods for sizing of colloidal radiopharmaceuticals. *Eur J Nucl Med* 1981, 6:521–526.

Petrokubi RJ, Baum S, Rohrer GV. Cimetidine administration resulting in improved pertechnetate imaging of Meckel's diverticulum. *Clin Nucl Med* 1978, 3:385–388.

Quinones JD. Localization of technetium sulfur colloid after RES stimulation. *J Nucl Med* 1973, 14:443–446.

Read NW, Cammack J, Edwards C, et al. Is the transit time of a meal through the small intestine related to the rate at which it leaves the stomach? *Gut* 1982, 23:824–828.

Richards AG, Brighouse R. Nicotinic acid—a cause of failed HIDA scanning. *J Nucl Med* 1981, 22:746–747.

Richards P. A survey of the production at Brookhaven National Laboratory of radioisotopes for medical research. In *V. Congresso Nucleare, Rome, 1960.* Rome Comitato Nazional Ricerche Nuclari, 1960, Vol. 2, pp. 223–244.

Rogers JV, Mack LA, Freeny PC, et al. Hepatic focal nodular hyperplasia: Angiography, CT, sonography, and scintigraphy. *AJR* 1981, 137:983–990.

Rubin B, Engel SL, Drungis AM, et al. Cholecystokinin-like activities of C-terminal octapeptide of cholecystokinin in guinea pigs and dogs. *J Pharm Sci* 1969, 58:955–959.

Ryan J, Cooper M, Loberg M, et al. Technetium-99m labeled N-(2,3-dimethylphenyl carbamoylmethyl) iminodiacetic acid (Tc-99m HIDA): A new radiopharmaceutical for hepatobiliary imaging studies. *J Nucl Med* 1977, 18:997–1002.

Saba TM. Physiology and physiopathology of the reticuloendothelial system. *Arch Intern Med* 1970, 126:1031–1050.

Sagar VV, Piccone JM. The gastric uptake and secretion of Tc-99m pertechnetate after H_2 receptor blockage in dogs. *J Nucl Med* 1980, 21:P67.

Sargent EN. Cholecystokinetic cholecystography: Efficacy and tolerance of sincalide. *Am J Roentgenol* 1976, 127:267–271.

Sayle BA, Helmer RE III, Balachandran S, et al. Lung uptake of Tc-99m sulfur colloid secondary to androgen therapy in patients with anemia. *Nucl Med Commun* 1981, 2:1289–1293.

Scheffel U, Rhodes BA, Natarajan TK, et al. Albumin microspheres for study of the reticuloendothelial system. *J Nucl Med* 1972, 13:498–503.

Sefczek DM, Sharma P, Isaacs GH, et al. Effect of narcotic premedication on scintigraphic valuation of gallbladder perforation. *J Nucl Med* 1985, 26:51–53.

Sfakianakis GN, Conway JJ. Detection of ectopic gastric mucosa in Meckel's diverticulum and in other aberrations by scintigraphy: I. Pathophysiology and 10-year clinical experience. *J Nucl Med* 1981a, 22:647–654.

Sfakianakis GN, Conway JJ. Detection of ectopic gastric mucosa in Meckel's diverticulum and in other aberrations by scintigraphy: II. Indications and methods—a 10-year experience. *J Nucl Med* 1981b, 22:732–738.

Shaldon S, Chiandussi L, Guevara L, et al. The measurement of hepatic blood flow and intrahepatic shunted blood flow by colloidal heat denatured serum albumin labeled with I-131. *J Clin Invest* 1961, 40:1346–1354.

Sharp HL, Mirkin BL. Effect of phenobarbital on hyperbilirubinemia, bile acid metabolism, and microsomal enzyme activity in chronic intrahepatic cholestasis of childhood. *J Pediatr* 1972, 81:116–126.

Shuman WP, Gibbs P, Rudd TG, et al. PIPIDA scintigraphy for cholecystitis: False positives in alcoholism and total parenteral nutrition. *Am J Roentgenol* 1982, 138:1–5.

Siegel JA, Wu RK, Knight LC, et al. Radiation dose estimates for oral agents used in upper gastrointestinal disease. *J Nucl Med*, 1983, 24:835–837.

Sodee DB. A new scanning isotope, mercury-197. A preliminary report. *J Nucl Med* 1963, 4:335–344.

Staum MM. Incompatibility of phosphate buffer in ^{99m}Tc-sulfur colloid containing aluminum ion. *J Nucl Med* 1972, 13:386–387.

Stern HS, McAfee JG, Subramanian G. Preparation, distribution, and utilization of technetium-99m sulfur colloid. *J Nucl Med* 1966, 7:655–675.

Stirrett LA, Yuhl ET, Libby RL. The hepatic radioactivity survey. *Radiology* 1953, 61:930–932.

Stirrett LA, Yuhl ET, Cassen B. Clinical applications of hepatic radioactivity surveys. *Am J Gastroenterol* 1954, 21:310–315.

Subramanian G, McAfee JG. Stannous oxide colloid labeled with ^{99m}Tc or ^{113m}In for bone marrow imaging. *J Nucl Med* 1970, 11:365.

Subramanian G, McAfee JG, Mehter A, et al. A new in vivo colloid for imaging the reticuloendothelial system. *J Nucl Med* 1973, 14:459.

Sullivan DC, Taylor KJW, Gottschalk A. The use of ultrasound to enhance the diagnostic utility of the equivocal liver scintigraph. *Radiology* 1978, 128:727–733.

Swayne LC. Acute acalculus cholecystitis. Sensitivity in detection using technetium-99m iminodiacetic acid cholescintigraphy. *Radiology* 1986, 160:33–38.

Szlabick RE, Catto JA, Fink-Bennett D, et al. Hepatobiliary scanning in the diagnosis of acute cholecystitis. *Arch Surg* 1980, 115:540–544.

Taplin GV, Meredith OM, Kade H. The radioactive (^{131}I-tagged) rose bengal uptake: Excretion test for liver function using external gamma-ray scintillation counting techniques. USAEC Report UCLA-319, University of California, Los Angeles, 1954.

Taylor A, Kipper MS, Witztum K, et al. Abnormal Tc-99m-PIPIDA scans mistaken for common bile duct obstruction. *Radiology* 1982, 144:373–375.

Thaler MM. Effect of phenobarbital on hepatic transport and excretion of ^{131}I-rose bengal in children with cholestasis. *Pediatr Res* 1972, 6:100–110.

Thomforde GM, Brown ML, Malagelada JR. Practical solid and liquid phase markers for studying gastric emptying in man. *J Nucl Med Tech* 1985, 13:11–14.

Tolin RD, Malmud LS, Reilley J, et al. Esophageal scintigraphy to quantitate esophageal transit (quantitation of esophageal transit). *Gastroenterology* 1979, 76:1402–1408.

Topper TE, Ryerson TW, Nora PF. Quantitative gallbladder imaging following cholecystokinin. *J Nucl Med* 1980, 21:694–696.

Treves S, Grand RJ, Eraklis AJ. Pentagastrin stimulation of technetium-99m uptake by ectopic gastric mucosa in a Meckel's diverticulum. *Radiology* 1978, 128:711–712.

Trotman IF, Price CC. Bloated irritable bowel syndrome defined by dynamic ^{99m}Tc bran scan. *Lancet* 1986, 2:364–366.

Vetter H, Falkner R, Neumayr A. The disappearance rate of colloidal gold from the circulation and its application to the estimation of liver blood flow in normal and cirrhotic subjects. *J Clin Invest* 1954, 33:1594–1602.

Wagner HN, Jr. Radioisotope scanning of the spleen. In *Progress in Medical Radioisotope Scanning*, Kniseley RM, Wagner HN, Jr, Andrews GA, Harris CC (eds). Proceedings of a Symposium, Oak Ridge, TN, 1962, USAEC Report TID-7673:1963, p. 468.

Wagner HN, Jr, Iio M. Studies on the reticuloendothelial system (RES). III. Blockade of the RES in man. *J Clin Invest* 1964, 43:1525–1530.

Wagner HN, Jr, Iio M, Hornick RB. Studies of the reticuloendothelial system (RES) II. Changes in the phagocytic capacity of the RES in patients with certain infections. *J Clin Invest* 1963, 42:427–430.

Wagner HN, Jr, Razzak MA, Gaertner RA, et al. Removal of erythrocytes from the circulation. *Arch Intern Med* 1962, 110:90–97.

Wagner HN, Jr, Weiner IM, McAfee JG, et al. 1-mercuri-2-hydroxypropane (MHP). A new pharmaceutical for visualization of the spleen by radioisotope scanning. *Arch Intern Med* 1964, 113:696–701.

Weissman HS, Badia J, Sugarman LA, et al. Spectrum of 99m-Tc-IDA cholescintigraphic patterns in acute cholecystitis. *Radiology* 1981, 138:167–175.

Weissman HS, Gliedman ML, Wilk PJ, et al. Evaluation of the postoperative patient with [99mTc]-IDA cholescintigraphy. *Semin Nucl Med* 1982, 12:27–52.

Welch TJ, Sheedy PF, Johnson CM, et al. Focal nodular hyperplasia and hepatic adenoma: Comparison of angiography, CT, US, and scintigraphy. *Radiology* 1985, 156:593–595.

Winkelman JW, Wagner HN, Jr, McAfee JG, et al. Visualization of the spleen in man by radioisotope scanning. *Radiology* 1960, 75:465–466.

Wistow BW, Subramanian G, Van Heertum RL, et al. An evaluation of [99mTc]-labeled hepatobiliary agents. *J Nucl Med* 1977, 18:455–461.

Yaffe SJ, Levy G, Matsuzawa T, et al. Enhancement of glucoronide conjugating capacity in a hyperbilirubinemic infant due to apparent enzyme induction by phenobarbital. *N Engl J Med* 1966, 275:1461–1466.

Zeman RK, Burrell MI, Dobbins J, et al. Post cholecystectomy syndrome: Evaluation using biliary scintigraphy and endoscopic retrograde cholangiopancreatography. *Radiology* 1985, 156:787–792.

Radiopharmaceuticals for Genitourinary Imaging: Glomerular and Tubular Function, Anatomy, Urodynamics, and Testicular Imaging

James A. Ponto
Henry M. Chilton
Nat E. Watson, Jr.

Earliest radiopharmaceuticals for assessment of renal function (Oeser H and Billion H, 1952) were radioiodinated (I-131) preparations of selected radiographic contrast agents that underwent renal excretion, including acetotrizoate (Urokon), iodopyracet (Diodrast®), diatrizoate (Hypaque®), and iothalamate (Conray®). The first clinical use of radioactive tracers to measure quantitative differences in renal function occurred in 1956 when G.V. Taplin and co-workers used I-131 labeled Diodrast and collimated external scintillation detectors to evaluate the time-related clearance functions of the kidney. I-131 Diodrast, like most of the other radioiodinated contrast media-type renal agents, was unsatisfactory because a significant fraction of the injected dose also underwent nonrenal excretion.

In 1960, M. Tubis and colleagues substituted I-131 for stable iodine in ortho-iodohippurate (I-131 OIHA), an agent previously used in nonradioactive form to measure renal plasma flow, and developed the first radiopharmaceutical for functional studies of the kidney. Although the renal clearance of this radiopharmaceutical was too rapid for adequate imaging with the rectilinear scanner, time-activity curves of radiopharmaceutical appearance and excretion could be generated with the assistance of a strip-chart recorder and probe-type detectors that were placed over the kidneys. Although of limited value initially, this time-activity curve (called a "renogram") later proved useful in the detection of asymmetrical renal disease and in the diagnosis of some forms of obstructive disease.

Also in 1960, J.G. McAfee and H.N. Wagner, Jr, were first to perform renal imaging with Hg-203 labeled chlormerodrin, a previously employed brain imaging radiopharmaceutical. Hg-203 chlormerodrin bound within the tubular cells of the renal cortex and, because of its long-term renal disposition, could be used with the rectilinear scanning device to obtain static images of the kidney.

In 1967, a method for labeling diethylenetriaminepentaacetic acid (DTPA) with Tc-99m was developed (Richards P and Atkins HL, 1967). Soon afterward, a variety of Tc-99m radiolabeled chelates followed with varying degrees of usefulness in the evaluation of renal morphology and/or function. In direct contrast to the earlier radiodiagnostic renal agents that were radiolabeled substitution products of compounds known to be excreted by the kidneys (such as radiolabeled contrast media and the diuretic chlormerodrin), most of the Tc-99m agents were developed by trial and error.

Localization of radiopharmaceuticals in the kidneys is based on the normal renal function, primarily the removal from blood and excretion of substances that are bodily waste products or foreign materials. Thus, several substances have been

Table 15.1 RADIOPHARMACEUTICALS UTILIZED FOR RENAL IMAGING CLASSIFIED ACCORDING TO RENAL HANDLING MECHANISMS

RENAL MECHANISM	COMMENTS
I. Radiopharmaceuticals cleared predominantly by glomerular filtration:	
Cr-51 EDTA	Not available in the United States. Poor nuclear imaging properties
Tc-99m DTPA (pentetate)	Nearly 100% filtered in glomerulus
Tc-99m sodium pertechnetate	Significant serum protein binding and tubular reabsorption. Limited to imaging renal blood flow only
I-125 iothalamate	Useful in the determination of GFR; not useful for imaging (poor imaging properties of I-125)
II. Radiopharmaceuticals that are predominanlty tubular secreted:	
Radioiodinated (I-123 or I-131) ortho-iodohippuric acid (OIHA)	Approximately 80% secreted, 20% filtered in glomerulus
Tc-99m Mercaptoacetyltriglycine (MAG$_3$)	Kit-type Tc-99m agent, closely resembles biodistribution of radioiodinated OIHA. Currently limited to investigational use only (USA)
III. Radiopharmaceuticals that localize in renal cortex:	
Tc-99m gluceptate	Significant retention in renal cortex. Primary usefulness as renal cortical imaging agent
Tc-99m succimer (dimercaptosuccinic acid, or DMSA)	Very slowly cleared by the kidneys; about 25% of dose localizes in cortex at 1 hour and 40% at 6 hours

identified, radiolabeled, and found to localize, at least transiently, in the kidneys. Depending upon the renal mechanism, various parameters of renal function can be evaluated by the time-related appearance and/or distribution of these radiolabeled substances in the kidney or urine.

The two mechanisms of renal excretion are glomerular filtration and tubular secretion. The amount of substance excreted by glomerular filtration is limited to the non–protein-bound portion in the plasma. The fraction of renal plasma flow normally passing through the glomerular membrane is about 20%. On the other hand, the amount of substance excreted by tubular secretion may in some cases approach the total renal plasma flow. Some substances that enter the tubular transport system, however, bind in the tubular renal cells and are secreted only very slowly into the urine, if at all.

Renal handling mechanisms largely determine the suitability of radiopharmaceuticals for clinical indications and can be generally described as (1) agents excreted by glomerular filtration (2) agents excreted by tubular secretion, and (3) agents that are either slowly excreted or bound within the renal cortex and are useful for imaging renal anatomy (Table 15.1).

I. Radiopharmaceuticals Excreted by Glomerular Filtration

RADIOLABELED COMPLEXES OF SOLUBLE CHELATES

BACKGROUND/HISTORY

Radiopharmaceuticals excreted by glomerular filtration are useful in (1) the measurement of glomerular filtration rate (GFR), (2) the evaluation of renal artery perfusion, and (3) the visualization of the collecting system. Ideally, substances utilized to measure GFR must (1) be completely filtered by the glomerulus; (2) not be metabolized, destroyed, reabsorbed, or secreted by renal tubular cells; (3) be physiologically and pharmacologically inert; and (4) not be protein bound. Additionally, they should possess desirable physical decay characteristics, including gamma rays suitable for detection and/or imaging and low patient radiation exposure.

Determination of GFR. The classic method for determining GFR involves measuring the clearance of inulin, a fructose polysaccharide (Shannon JA and Smith HW, 1935). However, because techniques for determining inulin concentrations are too laborious to be practical, this method is rarely offered as a routine diagnostic aid. (Attempts at developing a suitable radiolabeled form of inulin have been largely unsuccessful, although several radiolabeled substances have been evaluated as potential replacements for radiolabeled inulin [Bianchi C, 1972].) Measurement of creatinine clearance to estimate GFR is the most common means of assessing renal function clinically. Creatinine clearance is dependent upon accurate urine collection. Also, the relatively long time required to complete the study and the inability to determine relative GFR for each kidney without an invasive technique involving selective ureteral catheterization contribute to its less-than-ideal nature.

Advantages of radiometric methods for determination of GFR include the relative ease of measuring radioactivity and the ability to calculate GFR from plasma disappearance following a single intravenous injection (Cohen ML, et al, 1969).

In 1964, W.B. Nelp and associates showed that the renal excretion of non–protein-bound Co-57 cyanocobalamin (vitamin B_{12}) correlated with that of inulin. However, substantial variability in plasma protein binding was noted, in spite of pretreatment with nonradioactive cyanocobalamin.

Radioiodinated iothalamate was first used to measure GFR by E.M. Sigman and colleagues (1965a; b). Numerous investigators found its clearance to agree with that of inulin over a wide range of GFR values. More recently, however, B. Odlind and co-workers (1985) have reported that the clearance of nonradiolabeled iothalamate substantially exceeds that of simultaneous inulin clearance (Maher FT, et al, 1971), indicating the probability of tubular secretion. Thus, it is possible that the observed agreement between inulin and I-125 iothalamate clearances may result from a balancing overestimation based on tubular secretion and underestimation based on the small degree of protein binding. Although not widely used, I-125 iothalamate is commercially available in the United States.

In addition to I-125 iothalamate, other radiotracers that have been employed for GFR measurement include Cr-51 EDTA (ethylenediamine tetraacetic acid) and DTPA (diethylenetriamine pentaacetic acid, also known as *pentetate*) labeled with Yb-169, In-113m, In-111, and Tc-99m (Bianchi C, 1972; McAfee JG, et al, 1979; Stacy BD and Thorburn GD, 1966; Hosain F, et al, 1969). Of these, the pharmacokinetic properties of Cr-51 EDTA have been studied in most detail. Cr-51 EDTA underestimates GFR, as determined by inulin clearance, by as much as 5–15% (Stacy BD and Thorburn GD 1966). Why this occurs is not clear; no significant protein binding or complexation with blood components or any secretion or absorption by renal tubules has been detected. All these radiopharmaceuticals, however, and in particular the previously mentioned chelates of the transition metals, can be used for glomerular filtration measurement as well as for the imaging of renal blood flow and visualization of the urinary collecting system.

The first complex of Tc-99m DTPA was prepared using ferrous ion to reduce pertechnetate in the presence of DTPA. Attempts to accelerate the ferrous reduction by adding ascorbic acid resulted in the formation of an altogether different product that belongs to the class of renal radiopharmaceuticals that bind in the renal cortex (Hauser W, et al, 1970, 1971) rather than those that undergo glomerular filtration (Atkins HL, et al, 1971). Today, Tc-99m DTPA prepared by the ascorbic acid–ferrous ion reduction method is known as Tc-99m *ferpentetate*. Tc-99m DTPA prepared by the stannous ion reduction method (Eckelman WC and Richards P, 1970) is known as Tc-99m *pentetate* and is cleared almost entirely by glomerular filtration (Eckelman WC, et al, 1971).

Method of Determining GFR. The traditional plasma clearance method for calculating GFR required multiple blood samples obtained over a period of several hours following intravenous injection of the radiopharmaceutical. C. Russell and associates (1985b) have shown, however, that simple one-sample or two-sample methods give results that closely approximate those derived from multisampling techniques. It is also possible to use direct scintigraphic estimation of GFR using a computer-linked gamma camera (Russell C, et al, 1985a). Several methods have been proposed, including those of A. Piepsz and colleagues (1978), J. Assailly and colleagues (1977), S.P. Nielsen and colleagues (1977), and G.F. Gates (1982; 1983). In general, these methods appear to be less accurate than plasma clearance methods. However, they may have a place in situations that do not require great accuracy. Their primary advantage is their ability to determine relative (differential) kidney function noninvasively. Adequate hydration is necessary for accurate determination of GFR.

Imaging Renal Filtration. Renal imaging with radiopharmaceuticals excreted by glomerular filtration typically consists of first-transit images (1–3-second frames over 30–60 seconds) following bolus injection (Figure 15.1A) and then sequential 1–3-minute frames over 20–30 minutes (Figure 15.1B). Simultaneous computer acquisition allows for generation of "renogram" curves and quantitation of parameters such as kidney/aorta blood flow ratios and relative (differential) kidney function (Figure 15.1C). These quantitative data are of special value for comparisons between initial and subsequent studies on the same patient.

The approximately 10–15% of Tc-99m pertechnetate ions that exist freely in plasma are filtered by the glomerulus; approximately 87% of these filtered ions are reabsorbed in the proximal tubule. Consequently, only about

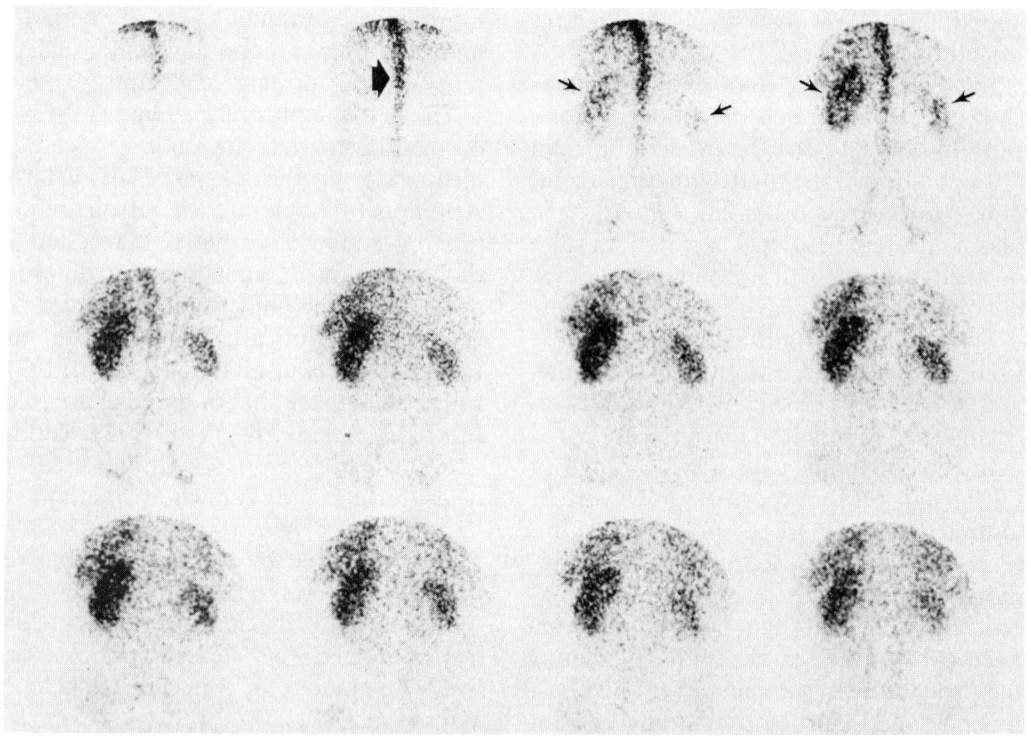

Figure 15.1A Images obtained every 2 seconds during the first transit of Tc-99m DTPA following bolus injection shows early visualization of the aorta (larger arrow) and kidneys (small arrows). The decreased perfusion to the right kidney in this patient is due to renovascular disease. Right kidney to aorta and left kidney to aorta ratios are 0.57 and 0.77, respectively. Integration of 1–3-minute data shows relative (differential) kidney function of 23% and 77% for the right kidney and left kidney, respectively.

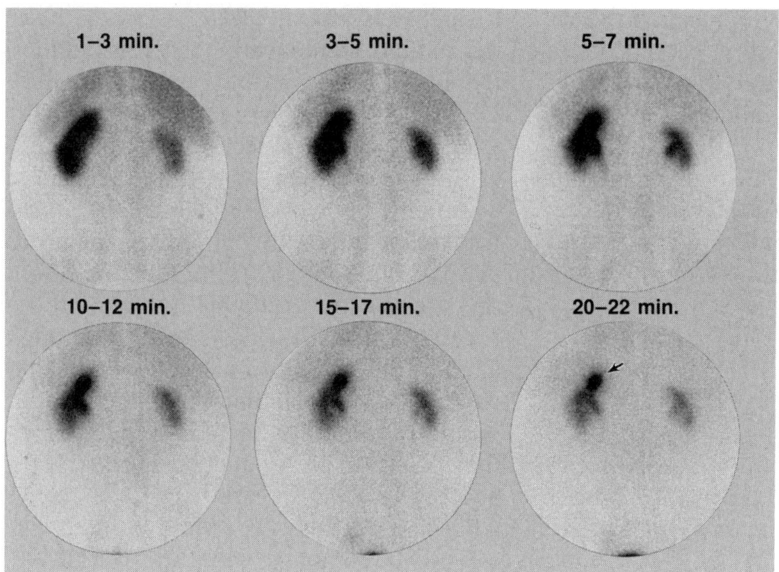

Figure 15.1B Images obtained sequentially following Tc-99m DTPA injection show transit of the radiopharmeceutical from the renal parenchyma (1–3-min. image) into the collecting system. Renal pelvis activity is first seen on the 3–5-minute and 5–7-minute images, and bladder activity is partially seen at the extreme bottom of images obtained after 10 minutes. Although the right kidney is affected by renovascular disease, radiopharmaceutical excretion is noted in its collecting system. Moderate retention of calyceal activity in the left kidney (arrow) probably represents urine stasis, confirmation of which can be achieved with furosemide diuresis.

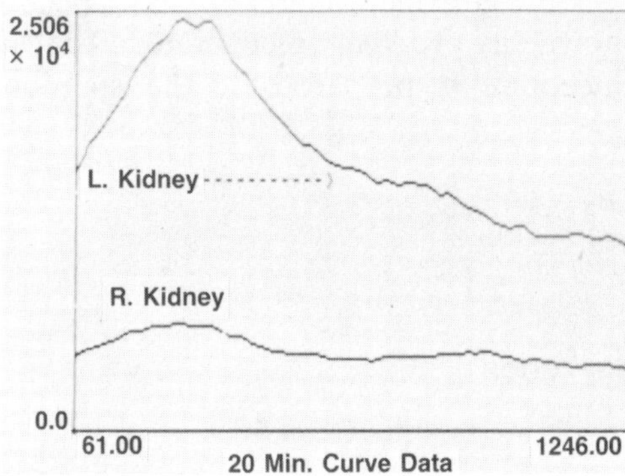

Figure 15.1C "Time-activity" curves (i.e., renogram) for both kidneys obtained following injection of Tc-99m pentetate. Note decreased function of right kidney.

3% of the activity in plasma appears in the urine (Lathrop KA and Harper PV, 1972). Thus, although Tc-99m pertechnetate has been used to assess arterial perfusion to the kidneys, its low urinary concentration as a result of both serum protein binding and tubular reabsorption precludes any usefulness in the evaluation of the collecting system.

Tc-99m DTPA is the "glomerular agent" of choice and should be used whenever quantitation of GFR or visualization of renal filtration function is desired (Klopper JF, et al, 1972). Its rapid renal clearance permits visualization of the pelvocalyceal collecting system and ureters and simulates the morphological information obtained by intravenous urography. Because of its low retention by the renal cortex, it may fail to delineate small cortical lesions and may not reveal abnormalities involving only tubular function without changes in GFR.

Another Tc-99m radiopharmaceutical, Tc-99m gluceptate, is often considered a general-purpose renal imaging agent because its use permits visualization of renal blood flow and imaging of renal cortical anatomy. This is possible because a fraction of the injected dose is promptly excreted in the urine that enables visualization of renal blood flow and the pelvocalyceal collecting system (Lee HB and Blaufox MD, 1985). A smaller amount localizes in the renal tubular cells and is retained there sufficiently long to permit cortical visualization after the activity in the collecting system has cleared.

CHEMISTRY

Iodine-125 iothalamate is monosodium 5-acetamido-2,4,6-triiodo-N-methylisophzoic acid, 3-(acetylamino)-2,4,6-triiodo-5[(methylamino)-carbonyl)]-, monosodium salt (Figure 15.2). In the United States, I-125 iothalamate is commercially available under the trade name Glofil®-125 (Iso-Tex Diagnostics, Inc., Friendswood, TX). Each vial contains sodium iothalamate I-125 in a concentration of approximately 1 mg/ml sodium iothalamate, with an activity concentration of 250–300 microcuries/ml at the time of calibration. Benzyl alcohol, 0.9% concentration, is added as a preservative, and sodium bicarbonate or hydrochloric acid may be added for pH adjustment. The product should contain only minimal (i.e., less than 2%) free I-125. I-125 iothalamate should be stored at 2–8 °C.

Tc-99m pentetate (DTPA or diethylenetriamine pentaacetic acid) is sodium [N,N-bis [2-bis (carbamoxymethyl)amino]-ethyl]-glycinato (5-)-technetate (1-)-Tc-99m. The chemical structure of pentetate is shown in Figure 15.2. Although most commonly known as Tc-99m DTPA, its official name is Tc-99m pentetate. The product obtained by Tc-99m labeling using the stannous ion reduction appears to be a radiochemically pure species although among different commercially available formulations, variability has been noted in their suitability for GFR determinations (Carlsen JE, et al, 1980; Russell CD, et al, 1983; 1986). Although it was originally believed that Tc-99m pentetate was a Tc(IV) complex with an overall −1 charge, it has recently been suggested (Russell CD, et al, 1980) that a Tc(III) complex predominates, and the product has an overall −2 charge. As with most other Tc-99m radiopharmaceuticals, oxidation of reduced technetium can occur under certain conditions (Sampson CB, 1984)

Tc-99m gluceptate (glucoheptonate) is the technetium-99m complex of D-glycero-D-gulo-heptonic acid (Figure 15.2). Although commonly referred to as Tc-99m glucoheptonate, it is officially known as Tc-99m gluceptate. Tc-99m gluceptate is prepared by the stannous

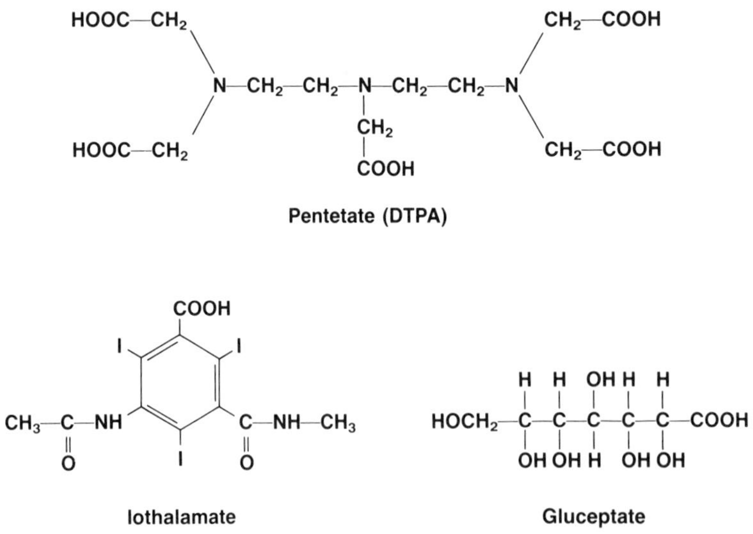

Figure 15.2 Chemical structures of iothalamate, pentetate (DTPA), and gluceptate.

ion reduction of Tc-99m in the presence of gluceptate. The structure of Tc-99m has been established by W. de Kieviet (1981) as a 1:2 Tc(V) complex, with two gluceptate molecules coordinated to the metal atom by the oxygens of the end carboxyl group and the adjacent hydroxyl group. Tc-99m gluceptate is susceptible to oxidative degradation with resultant formation of radiochemical impurities (Zbrzeznj D and Khan RAA, 1981). Both Tc-99m pentetate and Tc-99m gluceptate are prepared by the onsite addition of Tc-99m sodium pertechnetate to vials containing the lyophilized reagents. Commercially available pentetate and gluceptate kits and their formulations are listed in Table 15.2.

PHARMACOKINETICS

I-125 Iothalamate. Following intravenous injection, the peak plasma concentration of I-125 iothalamate is achieved almost immediately and then rapidly declines with at least a biexponential clearance. The extremely fast component represents initial mixing in the vascular compartment, whereas the somewhat slower component is dependent on equilibrium with the extravascular, extracellular fluid space (ECF) and concomitant excretion by the kidney. Complete equilibrium with the ECF is normally achieved after 80–120 minutes. In humans, binding to plasma proteins is usually no more than 2–3% of the injected dose (Sigman EM, et al, 1965; Cattell WR, 1970).

I-125 iothalamate is rapidly cleared from blood by glomerular filtration, which was originally thought to be the sole means of excretion. Recent reports, however, indicate that a small fraction of I-125 iothalamate may undergo tubular secretion (Odlind B, et al, 1985). Cumulative urine elimination is approximately 38% at 1 hour and 94–100% at 24 hours.

Tc-99m Pentetate. Following intravenous injection, Tc-99m pentetate is rapidly distributed throughout the ECF space. About 2 hours are required, however, to penetrate all parts of the ECF and, in the presence of edema, even more time is necessary. Tc-99m pentetate does not enter cells, being excluded both by its lipid insolubility and by its net negative charge. Plasma clearance is multiexponential with biological half-lives of 3.8 minutes (58%), 16 minutes (24%), 2 hours (16%), and 14 hours (2%). The extremely fast component represents diffusion into the extravascular ECF space, whereas the slowest component probably represents plasma protein binding. Tc-99m pentetate is rapidly and nearly completely eliminated from the body by glomerular filtration, with only traces found in the bile (concentration of Tc-99m pentetate in bile is lower than in plasma).

Table 15.2 FORMULATION DATA FOR CURRENTLY AVAILABLE Tc-99m PENTETATE (DTPA) AND GLUCEPTATE KITS

TRADENAME/MFG		FORMULATION
Pentetate (DTPA)		
AN-DTPA®	CIS-US, Inc.	Calcium trisodium DTPA 20.6 mg $SnCl_2 \cdot 2\ H_2O$ 0.15 mg (min)–0.3 mg (max) pH adjusted 3.9–4.1 prior to lyophilization with HCl/NaOH
MPI DTPA	Medi-Physics, Inc.	Sodium DTPA 5.0 mg $SnCl_2$ 0.25 mg pH adjusted 4.0–7.5 prior to lyophilization with HCl/NaOH
TechnePlex®	Squibb Diagnostics	Calcium trisodium DTPA 10 mg $SnCl2 \cdot 2\ H_2O$ 0.5 mg pH adjusted prior to lyophilization with HCl
Gluceptate		
Glucoscan®	Dupont	Gluceptate sodium 200 mg $SnCl_2 \cdot 2\ H_2O$ 0.5 mg pH adjusted 8.5–9.1 prior to lyophilization with HCl/NaOH
TechneScan® Gluceptate	Mallinckrodt, Inc.	Gluceptate calcium 50 mg $SnCl_2 \cdot H_2O$ 0.7 mg (min)–1.1 mg (max) pH adjusted prior to lyophilization with HCl/NaOH

Tc-99m pentetate reaches a peak concentration in the kidneys normally 3–4 minutes after injection. About 5% of the administered dose remains in the two kidneys at 15 minutes, about 3–4% at 1 hour, and less than 1% at 24 hours (Klopper JF, et al, 1972; McAfee JG, et al, 1979).

The fraction of the administered dose remaining in the plasma is approximately 15–20% after 1 hour, 10–12% after 2 hours, and 4% after 6 hours. Plasma clearance may be delayed in patients with renal disease. Approximately 2–6% of the injected dose is bound to plasma proteins. There is negligible binding to red blood cells (Arnold RW, et al, 1975; McAfee JG, et al, 1979).

The rate of renal clearance is unaffected by either urine flow rate (a test for resorption) or the administration of probenecid (a test for weak-acid tubular secretion). Whole-body clearance is biexponential with biological half-lives of 1.0 hour (58%) and 9.2 hours (42%), resulting in an overall effective half-life of about 2.2 hours. Approximately 50% of the injected dose is eliminated in the urine in the first 2 hours and about 95% at 24 hours (McAfee JG, et al, 1979; Thomas SR, et al, 1984).

Tc-99m Gluceptate. Following intravenous injection, Tc-99m gluceptate is rapidly cleared from blood with triexponential biological half-lives of 5 minutes (84%), 1 hour (10%), and 24 hours (6%). The fraction of the administered dose remaining in the blood pool is approximately 10–15% after 1 hour, 6–10% after 2 hours, and 5% after 6 hours. Blood-pool clearance may be delayed in patients with renal disease. Approximately 98% of the blood-pool activity occurs in the plasma; only 2% is associated with red blood cells. From an initial value of about 50%, plasma protein binding increases to 75% at 6 hours and 87% at 24 hours (Arnold RW, et al, 1975).

In view of its high degree of serum protein binding, glomerular filtration alone cannot be responsible for the rapid clearance of Tc-99m gluceptate from blood; some degree of tubular secretion must occur in order to account for the observed rate of excretion. Whole body clearance is triexponential, with biological half-lives of 20 minutes (35%), 2.4 hours (30%), and 8.9 hours (35%), resulting in an overall effective half-life of about 2.6 hours. An estimated 27–29% of Tc-99m gluceptate in blood is extracted on each passage through healthy kidneys. Activity in the renal collecting system is usually first visualized about 5–15 minutes after injection. Approximately 50% of the injected dose is eliminated in the urine in the first 2 hours and about 70% at 24 hours (Arnold RW, et al, 1975).

Much of the portion of Tc-99m gluceptate that undergoes tubular secretion is retained in the renal cortex. By 3 hours, approximately 15% of the injected dose localizes in the kidneys, probably bound to the proximal convoluted tubules. The biological half-life of this cortical localization is about 45 minutes. Kidney uptake has been significantly reduced by probenecid blockade and paraminohippuric acid (PAH) competition, indicating that it is actively concentrated by the tubular weak acid transport system (Vanlic-Razumenic N, et al, 1979).

The hepatobiliary system represents a normal alternate route of excretion for Tc-99m gluceptate (Tyler JL and Powers TA, 1982; Wilson MA and Pastakia B, 1980). Imaging studies occasionally demonstrate hepatic uptake, gallbladder visualization or intestinal activity (Figure 15.3). Gallbladder visualization has been reported to occur more frequently in healthy patients who are fasting. With renal insufficiency, relatively more Tc-99m gluceptate is expected to be excreted via the biliary system.

PRECAUTIONS

I-125 Iothalamate. Patients receiving I-125 iothalamate should be pretreated with a suitable agent (Appendix B) to block thyroid uptake of any free radioiodine present in the preparation and, accordingly, to reduce exposure to that organ.

Since decreased urine production in states of dehydration may result in decreased GFR, adequate hydration of the patient is recommended.

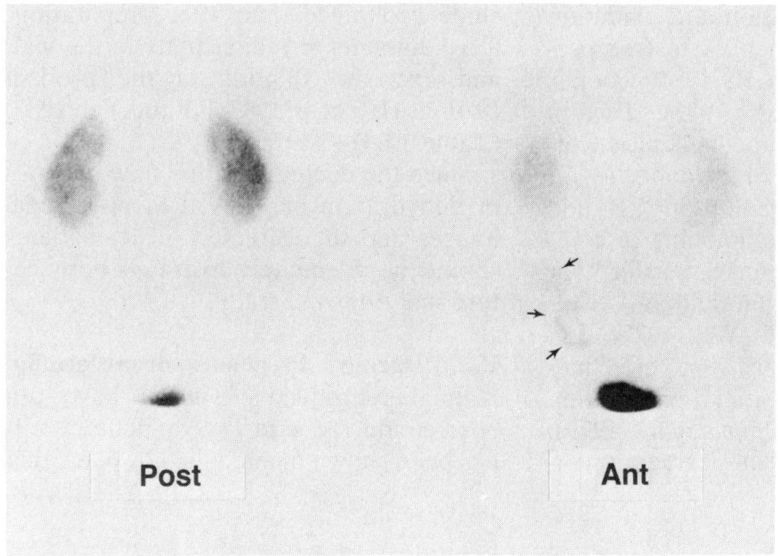

Figure 15.3 Tc-99m gluceptate renal study performed 2 hours following intravenous administration of 15 mCi. Intestinal activity is seen in anterior views (arrows) due to biliary excretion of radiopharmaceutical.

Use During Pregnancy/Breastfeeding. Animal reproductive studies have not been conducted with I-125 iothalamate. It is not known whether I-125 iothalamate crosses the placenta. Unbound radioiodine, however, crosses the placenta and is taken up by the fetal thyroid (Hibbard B and Herbert R, 1960). Since varying amounts of this radiochemical impurity exist in this radiopharmaceutical, it is advisable that this radiopharmaceutical not be given during pregnancy. No adverse reactions specifically attributable to the use of I-125 iothalamate have been reported.

It is not known whether I-125 iothalamate is excreted in breast milk. However, iodide is excreted in breast milk and, since varying levels of free iodide are known to occur in this radiopharmaceutical, it has been recommended that nursing be discontinued whenever this radiopharmaceutical is administered to patients who are breastfeeding (ICRP, 1988).

Tc-99m Pentetate. When Tc-99m pentetate is employed for measuring GFR, quality control analyses may be advisable to ensure that levels of radiochemical impurities or radiolabeled by-products are minimal. It has been shown that small yet statistically significant differences in the rates of renal clearance occur with Tc-99m pentetate products from different manufacturers (Carlsen JE, et al, 1980). These differences are thought to be related to the presence of unidentified impurities that bind to plasma proteins, thus reducing the clearance rate of radioactivity from blood. C. D. Russell and colleagues (1986) noted similar variations in protein binding among products from the same manufacturer. Unfortunately, no simple quality assurance technique is available for the routine determination of anticipated protein binding in vivo. In vivo protein binding can be predicted using anion-exchange paper chromatography and gel filtration; however, the techniques are relatively complex and are not always practical in the routine clinical setting.

Another quality control consideration is that levels of free, unbound Tc-99m pertechnetate be kept as low as possible. (Cooper PA and Zimmer AM, 1975). Significant levels of free pertechnetate may arise from either incomplete reduction and complexation of technetium to pentetate during the labeling process or from subsequent decomposition and oxidation of reduced technetium back to free pertechnetate (Sampson CB, 1984; Cooper PA and Zimmer AM, 1975). Factors associated with low labeling efficiencies include the presence of oxidants (e. g., hydrogen peroxide) (Sampson CB and Keegan J, 1985), large amounts of competing radiometals such as "carrier" (or "pseudo-stable") technetium-99 (Colombetti LG and Barnes WE, 1977), and very large increases in Tc-99m pertechnetate activity during on-site kit preparation (Robbins PJ and Williams CC, 1979). Other causes of significant degradation include prolonged time after preparation, large amounts of radioactivity in the vial, and excessive dilution of the product (Collins HR, et al, 1983; Ponto, et al, 1987) (Table 15.3).

Since the decreased urine flow in states of dehydration may result in poor renal images and/or decreased GFR, patients should be adequately hydrated both before and after the study.

Use During Pregnancy/Breastfeeding. Animal reproductive studies have not been conducted with Tc-99m pentetate. It has been shown in animals, however, that

Table 15.3 CAUSES OF POOR QUALITY IMAGES AND/OR ALTERED BIODISTRIBUTION OF RADIOPHARMACEUTICALS USED FOR RENAL IMAGING

CLINICAL APPEARANCE	CAUSE	REFERENCE
GLUCEPTATE		
↑ Free pertechnetate	Improper pH during preparation	Chi SL, et al, 1978
	Radiolytic decomposition	Zbrzeznj D and Khan RAA, 1981
	Oxidative degradation	Collins HR, et al, 1983
Enhanced biliary excretion	Penicillin, acetaminophen	Hinkle GH, et al, 1982
	Trimethoprim-sulfamethoxazole (involves transchelation of Tc-99m with formed species eliminated by hepatobiliary mode)	
	Fasting	Tyler JL and Powers TA, 1982
↓ Renal accumulation and excretion	Probenecid (inhibits tubular transport of organic acids)	Lee HB and Blaufox MD, 1984
PENTETATE (DTPA)		
↑ Free pertechnetate	Improper formulation	Colombetti LG and Barnes WE, 1977
	-Excessive carrier Tc-99	
	-Inadequate Sn^{+2} levels	Robbins PJ and Williams CC, 1979
		McKusick KA, et al, 1973
	-Radiolytic decomposition and/or oxidative degradation	Sampson CB and Keegan J, 1985
		Sampson CB, 1984
	-Hyperaluminemia	Specht HD, et al, 1987
SUCCIMER (DMSA)		
↑ Renal clearance rate	Preparation at alkaline pH	Krejcarek GE, et al, 1976
		Ikeda I, et al, 1977
↓ Renal, ↑ liver uptake	Radiolytic decomposition and/or oxidative degradation	Taylor A, et al, 1980
	Ammonium chloride (acidosis of urine)	Yee CA, et al, 1981
↓ Renal, ↑ bone uptake	Inadequate incubation time	Ikeda I, et al, 1977
↓ Distribution to kidney	Sodium bicarbonate (alkalination of urine), mannitol (? cause dehydration)	Yee CA, et al, 1981
I-123/I-131 OIHA		
↑ Thyroid uptake, ↓ urinary excretion	Radiolytic decomposition and/or oxidative degradation	Hatte CE and Ice RD, 1979
		Hammermaier A, et al, 1986
↓ ERPF	Iodinated contrast media (directly affects renal function)	Gates GF, et al, 1981
	Gentamicin, tobramycin (nephrotoxicity)	Keyes TF, et al, 1981
↓ Renal uptake, ↓ excretion	Probenecid (inhibits renal tubular function)	Antar MA and Jones AN, 1985
↓ Tubular function	Cyclosporine (nephrotoxicity)	Kim EE, et al, 1983
		Klintmalm GBG, et al, 1981

Tc-99m pentetate can cross the placenta (Wegst A, 1988). Therefore, Tc-99m pentetate should be given during pregnancy only if clearly needed and if benefits outweigh any potential risks.

A small fraction of the administered activity is excreted in breast milk following injection of Tc-99m pentetate. The concentration of radioactivity present in breast milk has been observed to decrease exponentially, with an effective half-life of about 4 hours (Ahlgren L, et al, 1985). L. Ahlgren and co-workers (1985) and P. J. Mountford and co-workers (1985) recommend that breast feeding be interrupted for 4 hours following injection of 2.4 mCi Tc-99m pentetate and that milk produced during this time be collected and discarded. Based upon these findings, ICRP (1988) recommends that breast-feeding be withheld for 4 hours following administration of Tc-99m pentetate.

Adverse Reactions. A total of fourteen adverse reactions were reported from 1976–1984 that were indicated to have occurred in association with the use of Tc-99m pentetate (Cordova MA, et al, 1987). These reports have usually involved apparent allergic and/or pyrogenic reactions.

Storage/Preparation. Tc-99m pentetate is a sterile solution of pentetic acid that is complexed with Tc-99m in sodium chloride injection. It is intended for intravenous injection and may contain buffers for pH adjustment. It contains not less than 90% and not more than 110.0% of the labeled amount of Tc-99m as the pentetic acid complex expressed in microcuries or millicuries per ml at the time indicated in the labeling. Other chemical forms of radioactivity should not exceed 10% of the total radioactivity. Tc-99m pentetate should be preserved in single-dose or multiple-dose containers. Although the United States Pharmacopeia (U.S.P.) XXI specifies storage at 2–8 degrees centigrade, at least one manufacturer's package insert specifies storage of Tc-99m pentetate at room temperature.

Tc-99m Gluceptate. The primary quality control consideration with Tc-99m gluceptate is that levels of radiochemical impurities be kept as low as possible. Signi-

ficant levels of free pertechnetate may arise either from incomplete reduction and complexation of technetium to gluceptate during the radiolabeling process or from subsequent decomposition and oxidation of reduced technetium back to free pertechnetate. Factors associated with low radiolabeling efficiencies include the presence of excessive oxidants in Mo-99/Tc-99m generator eluate and the addition, during radiolabeling, of excessive amounts of Tc-99m sodium pertechnetate. Significant decomposition of Tc-99m gluceptate to form radiochemical impurities increases with time and may be hastened by placing large amounts of radioactivity in the vial during on-site kit preparation (Zbrzeznj D and Kahn RAA, 1981). Compendial requirements and techniques for the determination of radiochemical purity of Tc-99m pentetate and Tc-99m gluceptate are listed in Table 15.4.

Since the decreased urine flow in states of dehydration may result in poor renal images and/or decreased GFR, adequate hydration of the patient before and after the study is recommended.

Use During Pregnancy/Breastfeeding. Animal reproductive studies have not been conducted with Tc-99m gluceptate. It has not been established whether Tc-99m gluceptate crosses the placenta; however, Tc-99m pertechnetate, a radiochemical impurity that is often present in varying amounts in all Tc-99m radiopharmaceuticals, is known to undergo placental transfer (Wegst A, et al, 1983). Therefore, Tc-99m gluceptate should be given during pregnancy only if the benefits to be expected clearly outweigh potential risks.

It is not known if Tc-99m gluceptate is excreted in breast milk. However, the radiochemical impurity Tc-99m sodium pertechnetate that is often found in varying levels in Tc-99m gluceptate is known to be excreted in breast milk. It has been advised (ICRP, 1988), therefore, that formula feedings be discontinued for 12 hours following administration of the radiopharmaceutical.

Table 15.4   COMPENDIAL REQUIREMENTS (U.S.P. XXI) FOR Tc-99m PENTETATE (DTPA) AND GLUCEPTATE, AND TECHNIQUES FOR DETERMINATION OF RADIOCHEMICAL PURITY

A. Compendial Requirements (U.S.P. XXI)

	Tc-99m pentetate (DTPA)	Tc-99m gluceptate
pH	3.8–7.5	4.0–8.0
Radiochemical purity	≥90%	≥90%

B. Radiochemical Analysis Technique

	System #1	System #2
Radiochemical component:	Free unbound pertechnetate	Hydrolyzed, reduced technetium
Mobile phase:	Methyl ethyl ketone (MEK) or acetone	Normal saline
Stationary phase:	Whatman 31 ET (or ITLC-SG)	Whatman 31 ET (or ITLC-SG)

R_f VALUES OF PRINCIPLE RADIOCHEMICAL COMPONENTS

	System #1	System #2
Bound chelate	0.0	1.0
Free pertechnetate	1.0	1.0
Hydrolyzed, reduced Tc-99m	0.0	0.0

Adverse Reactions. Allergic dermatologic manifestations (erythema) have been reported in association with the use of Tc-99m gluceptate. The incidence of reported reactions, however, is low. Sixteen adverse reactions were reported from 1976–1984 that involved Tc-99m gluceptate (Cordova MA, et al, 1987). In 1979, the incidence of adverse reactions reported for Tc-99m gluceptate was 0.25/100,000 administrations (Cordova MA and Rhodes BA, 1980).

Storage/preparation. Tc-99m gluceptate is a clear and colorless sterile, apyrogenic solution that is prepared of sodium (or calcium) gluceptate and stannous chloride. It contains not less than 90% and not more than 110% of the labeled amount of Tc-99mm as stannous gluceptate complex expressed as microcuries or millicuries per milliliter at the time of calibration. It may contain antimicrobial agents and buffers. Other chemical forms of radioactivity should not exceed 10% of the total radioactivity. Tc-99m gluceptate should be preserved in single-dose or in multiple-dose containers. Although U.S.P. XXI specifies storage at 2–8 degrees centigrade, at least one manufacturer's package insert specifies storage of the reconstituted (radiolabeled) gluceptate at room temperature (15–30 degrees centigrade).

DOSAGE/DOSIMETRY

I-125 Iothalamate. I-125 iothalamate may be administered as a single intravenous injection of 10–30 microcuries (using the method of Cohen ML, et al, 1969) or as a continuous infusion of 20–100 microcuries (using the method of Sigman EM, et al, 1965a; b). A. H. Israelit and associates (1973) suggested that, as an alternative to a continous infusion, a single subcutaneous injection of I-125 iothalamate with epinephrine can be used to obtain a relatively constant plasma level (currently in the United States, subcutaneous injection is not an approved route of administration). The radiation absorbed dose from I-125 iothalamate is summarized in Table 15.5.

Tc-99m Pentetate. The suggested dose range for renal imaging studies with intravenously administered Tc-99m pentetate in the average adult patient (70 kg) is 10–15 mCi. Administered doses for pediatric patients are individualized as a proportion of the adult dose based either on body weight or body surface area (see Chapter 9). Optimum perfusion or first-transit images are obtained when the radiopharmaceutical is injected as a bolus (<1.5 ml).

Images of native kidneys are usually obtained posteriorly with the patient supine over the face of a large-field-of-view scintillation camera with a low-energy, all-purpose (LEAP) parallel hole collimator. Imaging of transplanted kidneys is usually performed as an anterior

Table 15.5 RADIATION DOSE ESTIMATES IN ADULTS FOR I-125 IOTHALAMATE, Tc-99m PENTETATE, AND Tc-99m GLUCEPTATE[a]

| | ESTIMATED RADIATION DOSE (RAD/mCi) | | |
Organ	*I-125 Iothalamate*	*Tc-99m Pentetate*	*Tc-99m Gluceptate*
Bladder wall	0.59[b]	0.28[a]	0.28
Kidneys	0.02	0.022	0.16
Liver	0.015	—	0.012
Ovaries	0.01	0.019	0.021
Red marrow	0.067	0.012	0.015
Testes	0.022	0.013	0.013
Total body	0.0078	0.0091	0.011

[a] Personal communication from the Radiopharmaceutical Internal Dose Information Center, Oak Ridge Associated Universities, Oak Ridge, TN.
[b] Assumes voiding interval of 4.8 hours.

view with the patient positioned so that the distal aorta, renal transplant, and urinary bladder are in the same field of view. Typically, 3–6-second images are obtained over the first 1–2 minutes after bolus injection. Sequential 1–3-minute images are then obtained for 20–30 minutes. Prevoid and postvoid bladder images are also frequently obtained. Simultaneous computer acquisition allows subsequent quantitative evaluation of flow and function.

Tc-99m Gluceptate. The suggested adult dose of Tc-99m gluceptate is 15–20 millicuries, with dynamic perfusion imaging obtained as 3–6 second images taken over the first 1–2 minutes. Subsequent static images of renal anatomy are optimally taken up to 1–3 hours later, when most of the filtered activity has cleared, permitting visualization of the fraction of the administered dose that has localized within the renal cortex.

Radiation absorbed doses from both Tc-99m pentetate and Tc-99m gluceptate are summarized in Table 15.5. With both radiopharmaceuticals, the radiation dose to the bladder may be reduced by voiding at the completion of the study and frequently thereafter for the next 4–6 hours.

CLINICAL CONSIDERATIONS

In the functional evaluation of organ status, radiopharmaceutical quality is of paramount importance in that the presence of radiochemical impurities in all but the smallest amounts can lead to erroneous assumptions regarding organ function. When Tc-99m pentetate is employed for the determination of GFR, manufacturers' package inserts caution that Tc-99m pentetate should be formulated within 1 hour prior to its clinical use, presumably to avoid the use of a product that might otherwise contain significant levels of free, unbound pertechnetate and/or other types of radiochemical impurities that result from the time-associated radiochemical degradation of Tc-99m pentetate. In the past, such assumptions have been based primarily upon empirical observations, largely without scientific evaluations. In this regard, it is interesting to note that C. D. Russell and associates (1983) measured radiochemical impurities in Tc-99m pentetate over time and observed a significant decrease in the amounts of impurities in Tc-99m pentetate during the first hour after its preparation. Their findings suggest that optimal radiochemical purity for Tc-99m pentetate does not occur for at least 30–60 minutes after its reconstitution with Tc-99m pertechnetate. P. J. Robbins and C. C. Williams (1979) investigated low efficiency yields for Tc-99m pertechnetate kits and found that low yields (high levels of pertechnetate) were caused by (1) high levels of oxidant in the generator eluate used to prepare the kit, (2) time-associated deterioration of the radiolabel, and (3) "kit-to-kit" (lot) variability. In this regard, it may be prudent to perform radiochromatographic analysis of radiochemical purity prior to patient use.

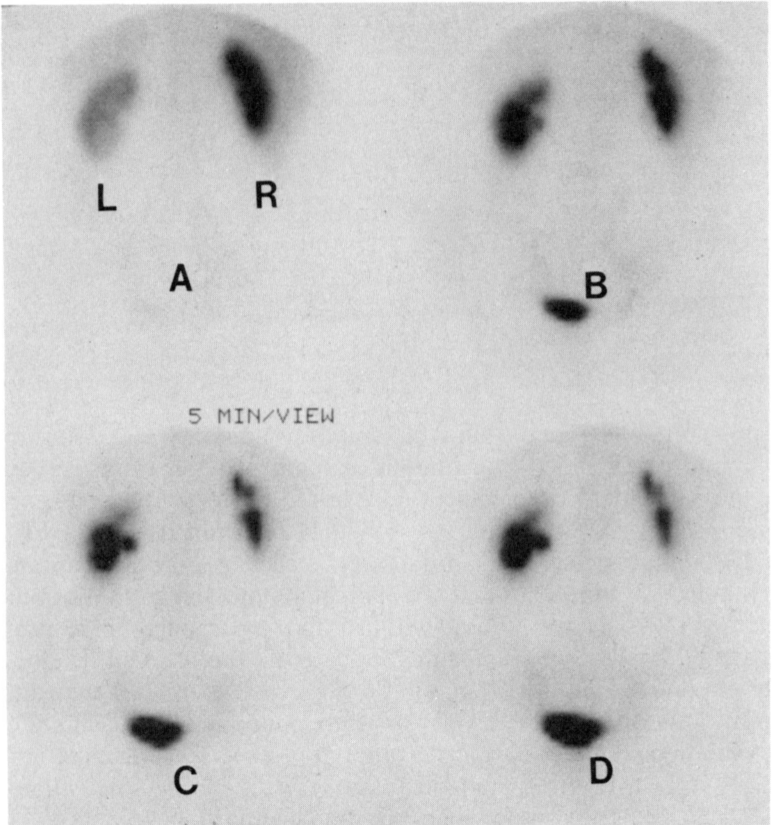

Figure 15.4 Sequential 5-minute images from a Tc-99m pentetate (DTPA) renal study in a patient with left ureteropelvic junction obstruction. There is delayed function in the left kidney (A) followed by visualization of dilated collecting structures (B) and a failure of washout following administration of Lasix (furosemide) (C and D).

Pharmacologic Intervention

Lasix® (Furosemide). In the evaluation of a dilated collecting system, the distinction between mechanical obstruction and dilation without obstruction is a critical diagnostic concern that can often be facilitated by diuresis renography (O'Reilly PH, et al, 1978; Koff SA, et al, 1979).

The fundamental hypothesis underlying the diuretic renogram is that prolonged retention of radioactivity seen in nonobstructed dilation is due to a pooling effect that should promptly clear with increased urine flow following diuretic administration (Figure 15.4). In cases of mechanical obstruction, however, the narrowed and fixed luminal cross-sectional area at the ureteropelvic or ureterovesical junction prevents any greater washout, resulting in continued, prolonged retention of the radiopharmaceutical proximal to the obstruction. Central to this hypothesis is the ability of the kidneys to promote a significant diuresis in the face of a diuretic and the patient's state of hydration (Thrall JH, et al, 1981).

The diuretic of choice for diuresis renography is the anthranilic acid derivative, furosemide. This "high-ceiling" diuretic has a peak effect far greater than that observed with other diuretics. Its mechanism of action is inhibition of sodium and chloride reabsorption from the proximal and distal tubules and from the ascending loop of Henle. Following intravenous administration, the onset of action is prompt, often occurring in as little as 30–60 seconds (U.S.P. DI, 1989).

Typically, furosemide is administered 15–30 minutes after radiopharmaceutical administration, and data collection is continued for an additional 15–30 minutes thereafter. The usual adult dose of furosemide is 0.3–0.5 mg/kg (20–40 mg); infants and children should receive 1.0 mg/kg up to 20 mg in a single dose (Koff SA, et al, 1979; MacGregor RJ, et al, 1983). Furosemide should be administered by slow intravenous injection over a period of 1–2 minutes. More rapid administration appears to cause some degree of nausea.

Captopril. Interventional renography with angiotensin converting enzyme inhibitors, such as captopril, has shown considerable promise in the diagnosis of renal artery stenosis (including potentially curable renovascular hypertension) (Wenting GJ, et al, 1984). Given prior to radionuclide renography, angiotensin converting enzyme inhibitors induce a striking depression of radiopharmaceutical transit in ipsilateral kidneys affected by renal artery stenosis (Majd M, et al, 1986). Although a single 50 mg dose of captopril may be given 1 hour before the renal scintigraphy, some clinicians choose to have patients stabilized on a therapeutic captopril regimen.

II. Radiopharmaceuticals that Undergo Tubular Secretion

While Tc-99m pentetate is highly useful in the evaluation of conditions that affect renal arterial blood flow or glomerular function, its lack of tubular secretion prevents usefulness in the diagnostic evaluation of conditions that affect renal tubular function. Reasonably, other radiopharmaceuticals, such as the radioiodinated derivatives of ortho-iodohippurate, are necessary.

Clinically, the clearance of a tubular-secreted compound could provide a measure of renal plasma flow if tubular secretion were complete. Such a physiologic measurement is based on the application of the Fick principle, which states that the rate of blood flow to the kidney is directly proportional to the rate of excretion and inversely proportional to the arteriovenous difference of the concentration of the agent in question. If the radiopharmaceutical is completely extracted in a single pass through the kidneys, the calculated clearance would give the total renal plasma flow. Since no radiopharmaceutical currently available is excreted entirely via tubular secretion, calculated clearances using radiopharmaceuticals such as radioiodinated ortho-iodohippurate (OIHA) provide a measure of the effective renal plasma flow (ERPF) rather than total renal plasma flow (Blaufox MD, et al, 1967).

RADIOIODINATED ORTHO-IODOHIPPURATE

BACKGROUND/HISTORY

The use of radioiodinated OIHA in the late 1950's and early 1960's by G. V. Taplin and colleagues (1956, 1963) and others (Haynie TP, et al, 1960; Nordyke RA, et al, 1960; Rosenthall L, 1966) lead to the first practical application of radionuclides for studies of renal function. Since the renal clearance of radioiodinated OIHA was too rapid to permit imaging by the rectilinear scanner, probe-type scintillation detectors were necessarily employed to determine renal clearance. (Taplin GV, et al, 1956). These detectors were placed over each kidney while a third detector was usually placed over the bladder in order to record the appearance of the radiopharmaceutical in the urine (Blaufox MD, et al, 1966). This study was called radionuclide renography (Taplin GV, et al, 1956; Blaufox MD, et al, 1963). The clinical value of OIHA radionuclide renography (or the "renogram") was not fully appreciated initially; however, it eventually proved useful in the evaluation of several types of obstructive disease and in the detection of asymmetrical renal disease (Figure 15.5). With the development of the scintillation camera and computer-assisted image analysis techniques, modern-day renography is useful in the determination of renal function, effective renal plasma flow, and imaging of urinary tract obstruction.

CHEMISTRY

The chemical names of ortho-iodohippurate are glycine, N-(2-iodo-benzoyl)-, monosodium salt or monosodium ortho-iodo-hippurate ($C_9H_7{}^{123/131}I\text{-}NaO_3$). Radiolabeling of ortho-iodohippurate is accomplished by simple exchange reactions first described by M. Tubis and associates (1960) and later modified by K. E. Scheer and W. Meier-Borst (1962) and

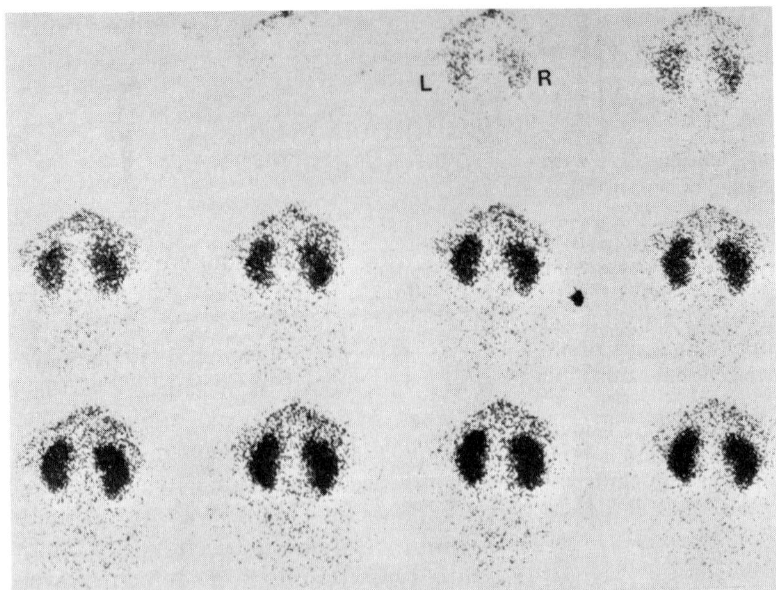

A

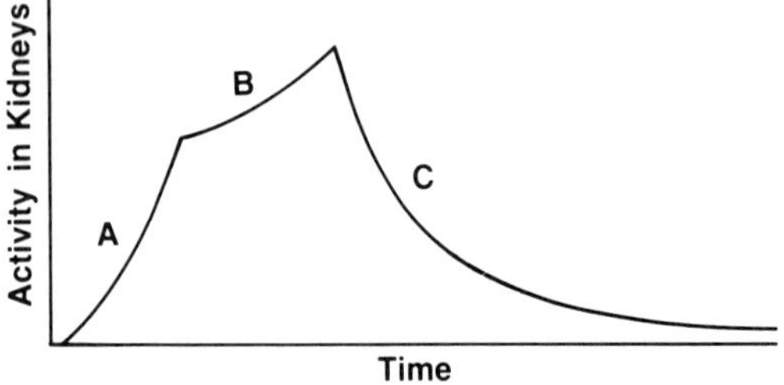

A Radiopharmaceutical appearance phase
B The vascular phase
C The excretory (or drainage) phase

B

Figure 15.5 Renogram obtained with I-123 OIHA showing dynamic renal appearance of the radiopharmaceutical over 2-second intervals (image A). Image B is a "tracing" renogram showing normal radiopharmaceutical localization and clearance from the kidneys. The time-activity curve (e. g., renogram) for appearance and excretion of radiopharmaceutical by the kidneys provides qualitative information about renal function. Depending upon the radiopharmaceutical employed (Tc-99m pentetate or radioiodinated OIHA), the data derived will provided diagnostic information involving either glomerular filtration (Tc-99m pentetate) or tubular function (radioiodinated OIHA).

The first phase of the renogram reflects appearance of the radiopharmaceutical in both renal and extrarenal blood flow. It occurs within the first 30 seconds following radiopharmaceutical administration. The second phase demonstrates relative renal blood flow. The latter phase, known as the excretory phase, reflects the degree of radioactivity that remains in the kidney as activity is being excreted.

Renal clearance of substances is almost exclusively influenced by factors that govern the excretory competence of the kidney, including dehydration, ureteral spasms, ureteral obstruction due to stone, and strictures. Patient positioning during imaging is also an important consideration in the renogram since drainage can be affected by position. Upright or sitting positions are avoided since partial ureteral obstruction can occur.

A. E. A. Mitta and colleagues (1961). Generally, the radioiodination process occurs by heating radioiodine and orthoiodohippuric acid at pH 6.0 at 100 °C for 2 hours. Reduction in overall reaction time has been made possible by the use of iodination catalysts. However, such preparations are likely to contain radiochemical impurities, such as radioiodinated ortho-benzoic acid and radioiodinated sodium 2,4,6-triiodohippurate.

Initially, only orthoiodohippurate radiolabeled with I-131 was available in the United States; however, methods for preparation of I-123 radiolabeled orthoiodohippurate have been developed (Wellman HN, et al, 1972). This agent was recently approved for routine use (Nephroflow®, Medi-Physics, Inc.). I-131 OIHA provides relatively poor spatial resolution since only low amounts of the β^- emitting radionuclide can be safely administered ($\approx$300 microcuries), and relatively poor resolution medium energy collimators are required to image the 364 keV emissions of I-131. As a general rule, the preferential imaging properties of I-123 account for its radiopharmaceutical superiority (Stadalnik RC, et al, 1980). Disadvantageous properties of I-123 OIHA include its relatively short physical half-life (13 hrs) that requires daily air-freight shipments. Additionally, depending upon the I-123 production method, some I-123 OIHA preparations may contain significant amounts of radioisotopic impurities of iodine (Bijl JA, et al, 1977). One previously available commercial preparation utilized I-123 produced by the (p,2n) reaction on Te-124 that contained up to 13% I-124 at the time of calibration. This radionuclide impurity has relatively high-energy photons (0.511, 0.605, and 1.7 MeV) that contribute substantially to patient radiation exposure and may necessitate the use of a medium energy collimator for adequate imaging.

Formulations of radioiodinated OIHA (Table 15.6) may contain preservatives (propylene glycol, methyl parabens, and/or benzyl alcohol), stabilizers (sodium citrate, edetate disodium, sodium phosphate, or potassium phosphate), and sodium hydroxide and/or hydrochloric acid for pH adjustment. Both I-131 and I-123 iodohippurate sodium injections are clear, colorless, sterile, nonpyrogenic solutions intended for intravenous administration. Commercially available I-131 orthoiodohippurate sodium injection is available in the United States from several companies and in strengths of 200–250 microcuries per milliliter and a specific activity of 300 microcuries per milligram at the time of calibration. I-123 orthoiodohippurate is available in a strength of 1.0 millicurie per milliliter at the time of calibration.

Table 15.6   PRODUCT FORMULATION OF COMMERCIALLY AVAILABLE RADIOIODINATED OIHA PRODUCTS

	MANUFACTURER	FORMULATION
I-131 OIHA		
Hippuran®	Mallinckrodt, Inc.	Contains propylene glycol 37.5%, methylparaben 0.1%, and propylparaben 0.03% as preservatives, and sodium citrate 0.015% and edetate disodium 0.005% as stabilizers. pH adjusted with HCl/NaOH (7.0–8.5). Specific activity 0.3 mCi/mg OIHA at time of calibration
Hipputope®	Squibb Diagnostics	Contains methylparaben 0.18% and propylparaben 0.02% as preservatives, and sodium citrate 0.015% and edetate disodium 0.005%. pH adjusted with HCl, NaOH, and citric acid (7.0–8.5)
Iodohippurate Sodium I-131	CIS-US, Inc.	Contains benzyl alcohol 0.9% as a preservative, sodium phosphate 1.6 mg/ml, and potassium phosphate 0.76 mg/ml. pH adjusted with NaOH and/or HCl.
I-123 OIHA		
Nephroflow®	Medi-Physics, Inc.	Contains benzyl alcohol 1%, alcohol 0.1%, sodium phosphate monobasic and dibasic 0.12 and 0.005%, respectively. pH adjusted with HCl and NaOH (7.0–8.5). Specific activity 0.5 mCi/mg OIHA at time of calibration

Stability. Radioiodinated OIHA is generally stored at temperatures less than 4 degrees centigrade, unless otherwise specified by the manufacturer. Upon standing, both the solution and the glass vial container may darken as a result of the effects of radiolysis. Change in color, however, does not indicate that product integrity has been adversely affected. Radiochemical purity has been shown to depend upon the stability of the radioiodinated OIHA as a function of time, temperature, pH, and internal irradiation (Hotte CE and Ice RD, 1979; Hammermaier A, et al, 1986). The radiopharmaceutical preparation should be protected from light since exposure to light has been shown to hasten decomposition (Magnusson G, 1962). Compendial requirements (U.S.P. XXI) and methods to check the amount of radiochemical impurities in radioiodinated OIHA are shown in Table 15.7.

I-123 OIHA products specify an expiration time of 24 hours after the time of calibration. However, I-123 OIHA should be administered as soon as possible after receipt (i.e., as close to the calibration time as possible) in order to minimize radiation exposure that would occur from the administration of increasingly larger amounts of the longer-lived radionuclidic contaminants (e.g., I-124: $T_{1/2phy}$ 4.2 days).

Table 15.7 COMPENDIAL REQUIREMENTS FOR RADIOIODINATED (I-131) OIHA (U.S.P. XXI) AND TECHNIQUES FOR THE ASSESSMENT OF RADIOCHEMICAL PURITY

A. Compendial Requirements (U.S.P. XXI)
Packaging/Storage —single or multi-dose vials, refrigeration not specified
pH —7.0–8.5
Radiochemical purity—≥97%

B. Radiochemical Analysis Techniques
Mobile phase —Chloroform/glacial acetic acid (90:10)
Stationary phase —ITLC-SG (Gelman)

Radiochemical Components	R_f Value
1. Free iodide	0.0
2. Radioiodinated OIHA	0.4
3. Ortho-iodobenzoic acid	0.8–0.9

PHARMACOKINETICS

Radioiodinated OIHA exists both freely and protein-bound in plasma, red blood cells, and extracellular fluid (Maher FT and Tauxe WN, 1969). Following intravenous administration, radioiodinated OIHA is excreted predominantly via the kidneys with approximately 80% cleared by tubular secretion and 20% by glomerular filtration. The biologic half-life in the body (excluding the bladder) is approximately 1 hour or less. In normal patients, 50–75% of the administered dose is excreted within 25 minutes, with upwards of 90–95% excreted within 8 hours of administration. More than 98% and less than 0.2% of the administered dose is excreted in the urine and bile, respectively, within 24 hours.

Within 15–30 seconds after intravenous administration, approximately 10% of the injected dose arrives at each kidney as a bolus. The mean renal artery to vein transit time is about 6 seconds, and since 83% of the radioiodinated OIHA is taken up with each passage of blood, the quantity in the kidney rises rapidly and then more slowly as recirculated radioiodinated OIHA in lower concentrations enters the kidney. Peak concentration of radioiodinated OIHA occurs in the kidneys approximately 3–6 minutes post injection (Tauxe WN, et al, 1962; 1964; 1971).

Enterohepatic excretion normally accounts for less than 1% of the administered activity, and distribution in red blood cells is also less than 1%.

PRECAUTIONS

Patients administered radioiodinated pharmaceuticals should be given Lugol's solution or saturated solution of potassium iodide (SSKI) prior to the administration of this radiodiagnostic agent and for several days afterwards in order to prevent thyroidal uptake of any free iodide contained in the product (see Appendix B for specific dosages of these thyroid blocking agents). The presence of significant amounts of free iodine may account for slower-than-usual blood clearance rates for radioiodinated OIHA.

Use in Children. The use of radioiodinated OIHA has been reported in pediatric patients; however, potential risk-to-benefit must be addressed in view of the fact that overall determinations of safety and effectiveness of these radiopharmaceuticals in pediatric patients has not been clearly established.

Use During Pregnancy/Breastfeeding. Since radioiodinated radiopharmaceuticals contain varying amounts of unbound radioiodine that can cross the placenta (Hibbard B and Herbert R, 1960), the use of these radiopharmaceuticals during pregnancy should be carefully evaluated (Hodges R, et al, 1955). It is advised that I-131-containing radiopharmaceuticals not be used during pregnancy since severe and irreversible hypothyroidism may result in the developing fetus. The use of I-123 OIHA in pregnancy should be carefully weighed against possible risks.

Radioactive iodine is excreted into breast milk; therefore, women who are administered radioiodinated OIHA during lactation should substitute formula feedings for breast milk for approximately 3 days or 5 days for I-123 OIHA and I-131 OIHA, respectively (Mountford PJ and Coakley AJ, 1986; Romney BM, et al, 1986).

Storage/Preparation. The common radiochemical impurity is inorganic iodide, the content of which increases during storage, being adversely influenced by various factors such as light, temperature, specific activity, and pH (Hammermaier A, et al, 1986). Proper storage conditions are critical, and materials should be used prior to expiration dates to ensure that levels of free iodide are less than 2% (Chervu LR and Blaufox MD, 1982). Radiochromatographic techniques are available for ascertaining the levels of free iodide in radioiodinated OIHA prior to

patient administration (Hammermaier A, et al, 1986). Additionally, commercial radioiodinated OIHA products that contain up to 37.5% propylene glycol should be carefully monitored to ensure that no patient administration (Hammermaier A, propylene glycol per kilogram of body weight.

Adverse Reactions. Relatively few adverse reactions have been reported with the use of radioiodinated OIHA (Cordova MA and Rhodes BA, 1980; Cordova MA, et al, 1987). These include nausea, vomiting, and dizziness. As with the use of all organic iodine-containing compounds, the possibility of hypersensitivity should be kept in mind and appropriate supportive treatment should be nearby.

DOSAGE/DOSIMETRY

The average amount of radioactivity of I-131 and I-123 OIHA administered to adults and the radiation dosimetry estimates are shown in Table 15.8.

CLINICAL CONSIDERATIONS

Substances that undergo tubular secretion and that are of clinical significance are primarily organic acids and certain aromatic compounds that are neither normal body constituents nor metabolic by-products. The clinical gold standard for

Table 15.8 ESTIMATED RADIATION DOSE IN ADULTS WITH NORMAL RENAL FUNCTION FOR I-123/I-131 ORTHOIODOHIPPURIC ACID (OIHA).

| | ESTIMATED RADIATION DOSE[a] | |
Organ	I-123 OIHA[b] (Rads/1.0 mCi)	I-131 OIHA (Rads/300 uCi)
Bladder	1.46	1.63
Kidneys	0.046	0.05
Ovaries	0.050	0.027
Testes	0.031	0.017
Total body	0.023	0.01
Thyroid	3.0	11.7

[a] Calculations from data provided as personal communication from Radiopharmaceutical Internal Dose Information Center, Oak Ridge Associated Universities, Oak Ridge, TN.
[b] Radiation dose estimates are for I-123 OIHA that contains up to 4.8% I-124 at time of calibration.

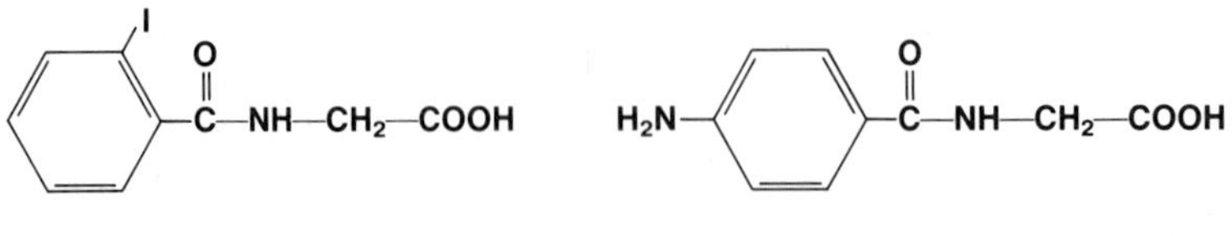

Ortho-iodohippuric acid (OIHA)   **Para-aminohippuric acid (PAH)**

Figure 15.6 Chemical structures of para-aminohippuric acid (PAH) and ortho-iodohippuric acid (OIHA).

measuring effective renal plasma flow is paraaminohippuric acid (PAH) that has a renal extraction rate from arterial plasma of approximately 90%. Unfortunately, no technique has been developed to radiolabel PAH with a suitable gamma-emitting radionuclide. As a result, the greatest advantage of radioiodinated OIHA over PAH for determining ERPF is its ability to be detected externally by the use of scintillation detectors. Although the structures of PAH and OIHA are similar (Figure 15.6), the substitution of an iodide ion atom in the ortho position for the para amino group affects renal tubular transport. For example, the extraction efficiency for OIHA is only about 0.7, whereas that of PAH is about 0.85 (McAfee JG, et al, 1981).

NEW TC-99M RADIOPHARMACEUTICALS

Tc-99m MAG3. Tc-99m mercaptoacetyltriglycine (MAG3) (also known as Tc-99m mertiatide, or TechneScan MAG3®, Mallinckrodt, Inc, St. Louis, MO) (Figure 15.7) is a relatively new radiopharmaceutical for renal imaging developed largely as a result of the earlier work of

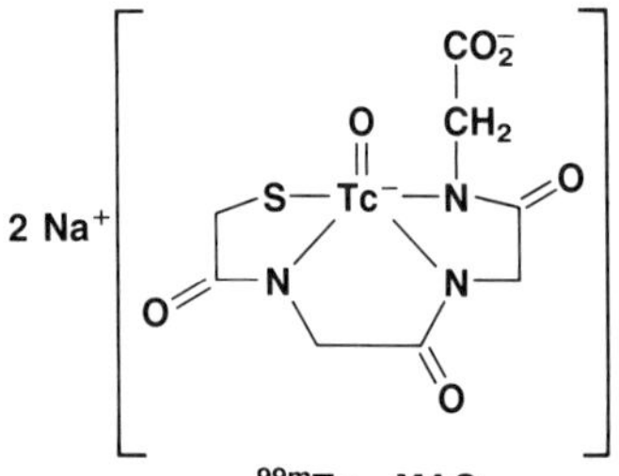

Figure 15.7 Proposed chemical structure of Tc-99m MAG3 (mercaptoacetyltriglycine, also known as mertiatide) (from Taylor, et al, 1982).

A. Davison and colleagues (1981) and their efforts to develop chelating agents for technetium based upon amide nitrogen and thiolate sulfur donor groups. In the initial report, one member of that series, Tc-99m N,N'-bis(mercaptoacetyl)-ethylenediamine (Tc-99m DADS), demonstrated rapid renal excretion in animals. Studies comparing Tc-99m DADS and radioiodinated OIHA in animals (Fritzberg AR, et al, 1981) and humans (Klingensmith WC III, et al, 1982) confirmed that Tc-99m DADS was excreted and cleared by the kidneys, but that the rate of renal excretion was not as rapid as OIHA and biliary excretion was significant. The carboxyl derivative of Tc-99m DADS was subsequently synthesized by A. R. Fritzberg and colleagues (1982). However, this agent has two isomers, only one of which is potentially useful as an OIHA replacement, and high-pressure liquid chromatography is required for their separation. Continuing efforts by the Fritzberg group (Eshima D, et al, 1985) led to the synthesis of the non-isomeric triamide mercaptide (N_3S) ligand, Tc-99m mercaptoacetyltriglycine (MAG3, or mertiatide) that has shown considerable promise in animal models and recent clinical trials as a replacement for radioiodinated OIHA. A. T. Taylor and associates (1986) have shown in normal volunteers that urinary excretion of Tc-99m mertiatide is more rapid than radioiodinated OIHA, and times to peak concentration values for Tc-99m mertiatide and radioiodinated OIHA are approximately the same. The superior quality with Tc-99m mertiatide is due to the preferential nuclear properties of Tc-99m. At this time, Tc-99m mertiatide is classified as an investigational agent.

III. Radiopharmaceuticals Employed in the Evaluation of Space-Occupying Diseases

Scintigraphic evaluation of renal anatomy is useful for localizing space-occupying lesions (e. g., cysts, abscesses, tumors), often in conjunction with other diagnostic modalities, and for the determination of renal cortical abnormalities such as pyelonephrotic scars, infarcts, and congenital abnormalities.

Static renal imaging has also been reported useful in the assessment of kidney size and position prior to biopsy. It has also been used in the planning of radiotherapy to confirm the position of the kidneys in order to shield them to reduce the incidence of radiation nephritis.

RENAL CORTICAL AGENTS

BACKGROUND/HISTORY

For all practical purposes, the first radiopharmaceutical with demonstrated usefulness for renal cortical imaging was Hg-203 chlormerodrin, which was originally employed for brain imaging by Blau and Bender in 1959. Hg-203 chlormerodrin (or Neohydrin®) was developed by R.R.M. Borghgraef and associates (1956) when they labeled chlormerodrin with Hg-203 in order to study the pharmacologic activity of the mercurial diuretics. Renal scanning with Hg-203 chlormerodrin was performed by McAfee and Wagner in 1960. Later, Hg-197 chlormerodrin was introduced. It was preferable to the Hg-203 labeled product because of its physical half-life of 2.7 days with no beta emissions, compared to a 46.6-day half-life and significant beta emissions with Hg-203. Both radiomercurial labeled chlormerodrin compounds have identical pharmacologic behavior, binding to the cytoplasm of the proximal tubular cells with eventual excretion into the tubular lumen (Cafruny EJ and Gussin RG, 1963). Since radiochlormerodrin is almost totally bound to plasma proteins after intravenous injection, essentially no activity appears in the glomerular filtrate.

Static renal imaging was also attempted using the rectilinear scanner and radioiodinated OIHA, an agent that undergoes both tubular secretion and glomerular filtration. In general, radioiodinated OIHA was unsuccessful for use with the rectilinear scanner because of its rapid renal transit.

Recent developments in radiochemistry and the availability of short-lived radionuclides, notably technetium-99m with its superior imaging and dosimetric properties, make it difficult to justify use of the radiomercurial compounds today. Among the renal-specific Tc-99m radiopharmaceuticals that exhibit significant retention in the renal cortex to permit static imaging are Tc-99m gluceptate and Tc-99m succimer (DMSA) (Lin TH, et al, 1974) Figure 15.8).

CHEMISTRY

Tc-99m Gluceptate. Gluceptate, previously best known by its unofficial name glucoheptonate, is a simple carbohydrate that forms a clear, colorless soluble complex with reduced technetium. Commercially available reagent kits for the preparation of Tc-99m gluceptate contain either sodium or calcium gluceptate and stannous ions as a lyophilized powder. Prior to lyophilization, the pH is adjusted using hydrochloric acid and/or sodium hydroxide to 8.5–9.1 (sodium gluceptate) or 6.9–7.1 (calcium gluceptate). Lowering of the

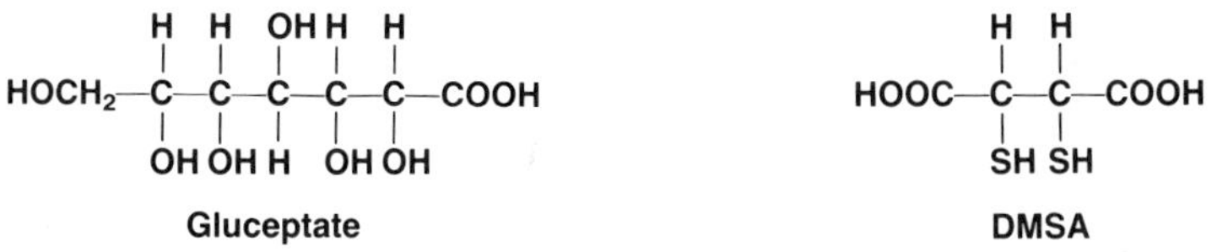

Figure 15.8 Chemical structures of gluceptate and succimer (DMSA).

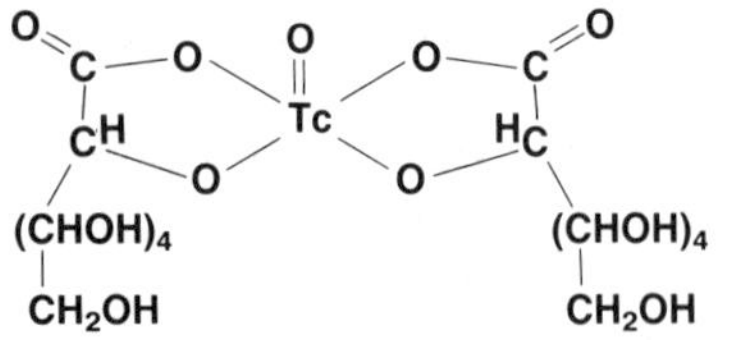

Figure 15.9 Proposed chemical structure of Tc-99m gluceptate showing coordination of technetium and the formation of two five-membered ring systems (from de Kieviet W, 1981).

Table 15.9   FORMULATION INFORMATION ON CURRENTLY AVAILABLE SUCCIMER (DMSA) PRODUCT

Reagent kit name—MPI DMSA Kidney Reagent
Manufacturer   —Medi-Physics, Inc.
Kit formulation: Reagent kit consists of: sterile, apyrogenic heat-sealed ampoules containing 2.2 mls. reagent solution [succimer (1.2 mg) and anhydrous stannous chloride (0.42 mg)], and sterile, apyrogenic mixing vials. The on-site preparation of Tc-99m succimer is by mixing one part of reagent solution with one to two parts of Tc-99m sodium pertechnetate. No more than 2.0 mls of the reagent solution should be used for each administered dose.

pertechnetate oxidation state is brought about by stannous-ion reduction to form the Tc-99m gluceptate complex. Tc-99m gluceptate is thought to contain technetium in the +5 oxidation state with a Tc=O oxytechnetium core and two five-membered gluceptate rings (Figure 15.9). Specific information on the formulation of commercially available gluceptate kits is listed in Table 15.2.

Tc-99m Succimer. Tc-99m succimer, also known as DMSA (2,6-dimercaptosuccinic acid), is a clear colorless, aqueous solution of succimer and Tc-99m. The commercially available reagent for the on-site preparation of Tc-99m succimer contains more than 90% of the *meso* isomer of succimer and less than 10% *d,l* isomer. Following addition of Tc-99m pertechnetate, technetium is reduced to a lower oxidation state, and the Tc-99m succimer complex is formed. At least four Tc-99m succimer complexes have been identified (Ikeda I, et al, 1977). Although differing biodistribution properties have been observed among these complexes, their exact structures have not been determined. It has been shown that pH, stannous ion concentration, and the concentration and volume of sodium pertechnetate added during on-site preparation affect the production of the different complexes (Ikeda I, et al; 1976, Ohta H, et al, 1984; Ramamoorthy N, et al, 1987). The optimal Tc-99m succimer complex for cortical renal imaging is formed at an acid pH and in the presence of a stannous ion : succimer molar ratio of 1 : 3 (this product is not the Tc-99m complex of DMSA that has been employed for imaging medullary carcinoma of the thyroid). In the on-site preparation of Tc-99m succimer by the addition to a reagent kit (Table 15.9) of generator-produced Tc-99m sodium pertechnetate, it appears that the formation of the desirable renal imaging complex occurs by a two-step process (Ikeda I, et al, 1977). The initial complex that is rapidly formed exhibits decreased renal localization and increased liver uptake; however, this complex is slowly transformed to the more desirable complex for renal imaging. The manufacturer's package insert cautions that Tc-99m succimer should be allowed to "incubate" for 10 minutes after reconstitution with Tc-99m sodium pertechnetate prior to its use. Additionally, Tc-99m succimer must be used within 30 minutes after the incubation period because the desirable renal imaging complex is stable only for short periods of time. Exposure to oxygen either during radiolabeling or immediately afterwards will cause significant quantities of the Tc-99m succimer complex that localizes in the liver to form (Taylor A Jr, et al, 1980).

PHARMACOKINETICS

Tc-99m Gluceptate. Following intravenous administration, Tc-99m gluceptate is rapidly distributed throughout the body and into the renal cortex where it is actively concentrated in the proximal renal tubular cells. Maximal distribution into the renal cortex occurs 3–6 hours after intravenous administration, with about 5–15% of the administered dose being retained in the kidneys.

Blood clearance is rapid and appears to occur by both tubular secretion (involving the protein-bound fraction) and glomerular filtration. Following IV administration in patients with normal renal function, about 25–40% of the dose is excreted in urine within 1 hour, 65% within 6 hours, and 70% within 24 hours. About 15% of the dose remains in the blood at 1 hour post injection, 5% after 6 hours, and 3% after 24 hours (Arnold RW, et al, 1975).

The hepatobiliary tract normally accounts for only a small percent of the excretion of Tc-99m gluceptate; however, in patients with severe renal disease, relatively greater amounts of Tc-99m gluceptate may be excreted via the biliary system.

Tc-99m Succimer. Biologically, Tc-99m succimer behaves similarly to chlormerodrin, showing high cortical and low medullary concentration, and low urinary excretion (Enlander D, et al, 1974). Following intravenous administration, Tc-99m succimer is eliminated from blood with a triphasic pattern in patients with normal renal function, with biologic half-lives of 20 minutes (44%), 50 minutes (44%), and 18 hours (12%). The effective half-life of Tc-99m succimer in blood is around 1 hour or less. About 30% of the administered activity remains in circulation after 1 hour, about 10% after 6 hours, and less than 5% after 24 hours. Serum protein binding accounts for about 75% of the activity in blood during the first 6 hours, with about 90% bound after 24 hours. In some patients, up to 10% of activity in blood is bound to erythrocytes during the first 1–2 hours after administration (Enlander D, et al, 1974).

Tc-99m succimer localizes in high concentrations in the renal cortex, where it is taken up almost exclusively by the cortical tubular cells (Moretti JL, et al, 1982). Maximal localization of Tc-99m succimer into the renal cortex occurs within 3–6 hours after intravenous administration, with about 40–50% of the dose retained in the kidneys. Tc-99m succimer is slowly excreted into the urine, with 5–20% of the activity appearing in the urine within 2 hours, 10–30% by 6 hours, and usually no more than 40% in the urine by 24 hours after radiopharmaceutical administration (Arnold RW, et al, 1975; Enlander D, et al, 1974). As a result of the slow urinary excretion, dynamic imaging of the renal collecting system is usually not possible with Tc-99m succimer. Imaging of renal blood flow is usually not possible either, since patients typically receive 5.0 mCi or less because of the relatively high radiation absorbed dose to the kidneys associated with the use of this radiopharmaceutical (see Dosage/Dosimetry).

Tc-99m succimer may also be filtered since it has been shown that renal artery stenosis treated with captopril has decreased Tc-99m succimer localization in the affected kidney probably due to the diminished GFR (Kremer Hovinga TK, et al, 1984). Similarly, patients receiving captopril have been noted to have decreased appearance of Tc-99m pentetate and radioiodinated OIHA in the kidney with the stenotic artery (Sfakianakis GN, et al, 1987). Radiopharmaceutical accumulation and excretion appear unaffected by captopril therapy in patients with essential hypertension (Wenting GJ, et al, 1984). It has been shown that tubular secretion is not a significant route for the excretion of Tc-99m succimer since probenecid has no effect on the renal handling of this radiopharmaceutical (Yee CA, et al, 1980).

A.P. Provoost and M. Van Aken (1985) studied the renal handling of Tc-99m succimer in rats before and after treatment with sodium maleate, a substance known to decrease both GFR and effective renal plasma flow and to cause a generalized proximal tubular dysfunction. They found that sodium maleate treatment resulted in significantly less renal uptake of Tc-99m succimer and increased urine activity; however, it is not clear whether this observed effect is due to inhibition of tubular reabsorption or diminished filtration of Tc-99m succimer associated with the lowered GFR.

Typically, less than 3% of an administered dose of Tc-99m succimer localizes in the liver; however, this amount can be increased significantly, and renal distribution decreased, in patients with impaired renal function (Handmaker H, et al, 1975; Taylor A, et al, 1980).

PRECAUTIONS

Patients receiving either Tc-99m gluceptate or succimer should be adequately hydrated prior to radiopharmaceutical administration because adequate hydration may enhance radiopharmaceutical excretion, thus lowering background ratios and reducing patient radiation absorbed dose (Taylor A, 1982).

As with all technetium radiopharmaceuticals that contain Tc-99m in a reduced-oxidation state (other than the +7 state of pertechnetate), care should be taken to avoid the introduction of room air into the reagent vial or to use bacteriostatic-containing diluent during radiopharmaceutical preparation. Either action adversely affects radiochemical purity and radiopharmaceutical stability. Tc-99m succimer tends to deteriorate rapidly and must be used within 30 minutes following a 10-minute incubation period from the time of Tc-99m radiolabeling. Compared to Tc-99m succimer, the in vitro stability of Tc-99m gluceptate appears greater with relatively higher radiochemical purities over longer periods of time.

Techniques for the determination of radiochemical purity of Tc-99m succimer are listed in Table 15.10, along with compendial requirements (U.S.P. XXI) for this radiopharmaceutical. Methods for radiochemical analysis of Tc-99m gluceptate may be found in Table 15.4.

Use in Pediatrics. Manufacturers' package inserts state that the safety and efficacy of either Tc-99m gluceptate or succimer in children have not been established. In clinical practice, however, the use of both of these radiopharmaceuticals has not been associated with any unusual adverse reactions or side effects. Because of the lower radiation absorbed dose to the kidneys from Tc-99m gluceptate, this radiopharmaceutical is usually preferred for cortical renal imaging in pediatric patients (Ash JM, et al, 1982).

Use During Pregnancy/Breast-feeding. Animal reproductive studies have not been performed with either Tc-99m gluceptate or succimer. It is not known whether these radiopharmaceuticals can cause fetal harm when administered during pregnancy. Neither is it known whether Tc-99m gluceptate or succimer cross the placenta; however, both these radiopharmaceuticals typically contain varying amounts of Tc-99m pertechnetate, a radiochemical impurity that is known to cross the placenta (Wegst A, et al, 1983). As a general rule, radiopharmaceuticals should be used during pregnancy only when potential benefits outweigh expected risks.

Adverse Reactions. Allergic dermatologic manifestations have been reported

---

Table 15.10   COMPENDIAL REQUIREMENTS (U.S.P. XXI) for Tc-99m SUCCIMER ACID (DMSA) AND TECHNIQUES TO DETERMINE RADIOCHEMICAL PURITY

A. Compendial Requirements (U.S.P. XXI)—Tc-99m succimer

Packaging/storage	—Preserve in single-dose containers, between 15–30°C. Do not freeze or store above 30°. Protect from light
pH	—2.0–3.0
Radiochemical purity	—≥85%

B. Radiochemical Analysis Technique

Mobile phase	—n-butanol saturated with 0.3 N HCl
Stationary phase	—ITLC-SA (silicic acid) (Gelman Co.)

Radiochemical Components	R_f Value
1. Hydrolyzed, reduced ^{99m}Tc	0.0–0.15
2. Tc-99m succimer	0.45–0.7
3. Free Tc-99m pertechnetate	1.0

infrequently in patients who have received gluceptate. Rare instances of syncope, fever, nausea, and maculopapular skin rash have been associated with the use of Tc-99m succimer (Cordova MA, et al, 1980; 1984; 1987).

DOSAGE/DOSIMETRY

Tc-99m Gluceptate. Adult patients undergoing renal imaging with Tc-99m gluceptate are administered intravenously 10–15 millicuries with dynamic imaging of renal perfusion performed immediately afterwards. Static images of renal anatomy are obtained approximately 1–3 hours later, when optimal kidney-to-background ratios occur.

Tc-99m Succimer. Tc-99m succimer is administered slowly by the intravenous route, with adult patients receiving 5 millicuries. Static imaging of renal anatomy is usually begun 1–3 hours later (Figure 15.10). Dynamic images of renal perfusion cannot be obtained with Tc-99m succimer, since the relatively larger activities required to perform dynamic imaging would provide an unacceptable level of radiation exposure to the patient. Table 15.11 lists radiation absorbed doses for both Tc-99m gluceptate and succimer.

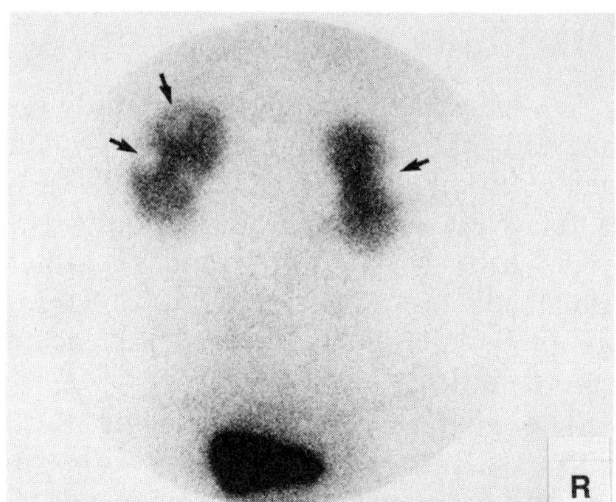

Figure 15.10 Static view (posterior projection) obtained 2 hours post administration of Tc-99m succimer (DMSA) reveals multiple cortical photon deficient areas due to renal cysts.

Table 15.11 ESTIMATED RADIATION DOSE IN ADULTS FOR Tc-99m GLUCEPTATE AND Tc-99m SUCCIMER (DMSA)[a]

| | ESTIMATED RADIATION DOSE (RADS/ADULT DOSE)[b] | |
Organ	Tc-99m Gluceptate[b] (Rads/15 mCi)	Tc-99m Succimer (Rads/5 mCi)
Bladder	4.2	0.35
Kidney	2.4	3.2
Renal cortex	3.6	4.3
Liver	0.18	0.16
Ovaries	0.32	0.07
Red marrow	0.23	0.11
Testes	0.20	0.034
Total body	0.17	0.075

[a] Personal communication from Radiopharmaceutical Internal Dose Information Center, Oak Ridge Associated Universities, Oak Ridge, TN.

[b] Estimated radiation dose assumes 4.8 hours bladder voiding interval.

CLINICAL CONSIDERATIONS

Clinical indications for the use of cortical imaging radiopharmaceuticals are (1) determination of parenchymal scarring in patients with vesico-ureteral reflux, and (2) evaluation of previously discovered mass lesions. In the evaluation of scarring in patients with vesico-ureteral reflux, surgery is generally felt to be advisable only if renal damage can be demonstrated. When mass lesions have been demonstrated by other diagnostic modalities (IVP, ultrasound, or computed tomography), imaging with cortical agents may allow one to distinguish between pseudo-tumors due to compensatory hypertrophy or fusion abnormalities, which normally demonstrate radiopharmaceutical uptake, and true tumors of the kidney (space-occupying pathological lesions), which fail to localize the radiopharmaceutical. Renal parenchymal imaging has achieved a "back-up" status as a primary diagnostic modality in patients who are allergic to contrast media (Daly MJ, et al, 1978).

Radionuclide studies of renal anatomy have shown that Tc-99m gluceptate is at least as useful as Tc-99m succimer for the scintigraphic evaluation of renal parenchymal disorders and may be preferred, especially whenever evaluation of renal perfusion is also desired or whenever visualization of the renal-collecting

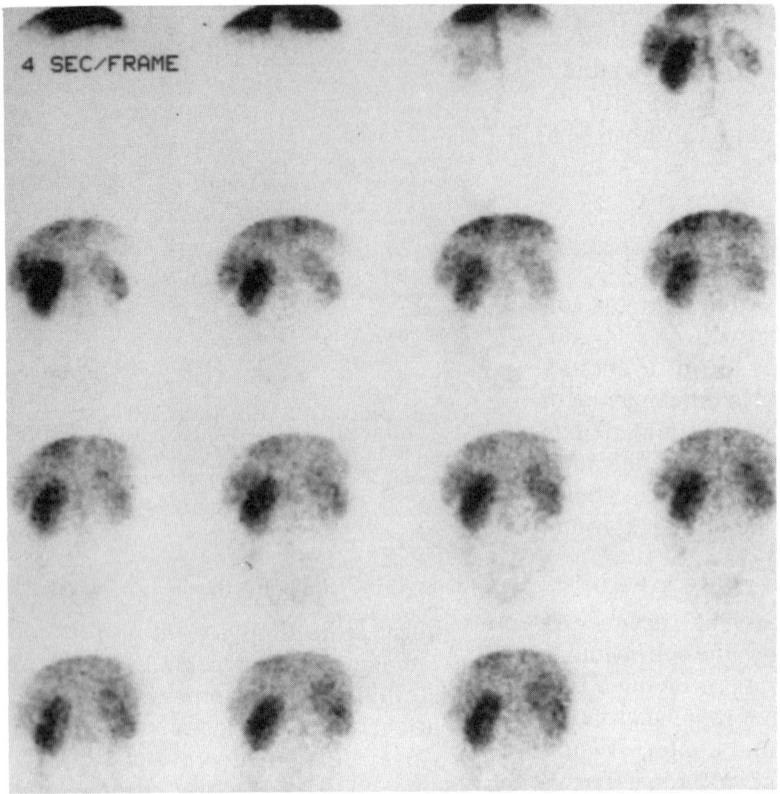

Figure 15.11 Dynamic flow study with Tc-99m gluceptate reveals marked renal asymmetry in a patient with hypertension due to chronic pyelonephritis.

system may complement the diagnosis. In the evaluation of renal trauma, Tc-99m gluceptate is the radiopharmaceutical of choice because it provides information on renal perfusion, function, and morphology in a single study (Figure 15.11).

OTHER (NON-APPROVED)
CLINICAL USES

Tc-99m Gluceptate. In addition to its approved use as a brain-imaging radiopharmaceutical, Tc-99m gluceptate has also been employed in animals to image acute myocardial infarction. However, comparative clinical evaluations performed with Tc-99m pyrophosphate have shown Tc-99m gluceptate to be inferior (Holman BL, et al, 1976). The use of Tc-99m gluceptate to detect lung tumors has also been reported (Vorne M, et al, 1982).

Tc-99m Succimer. A complex of Tc-99m succimer formed at alkaline pH has been investigated for use in the scintigraphic evaluation of medullary thyroid carcinoma and in the detection and evaluation of malignant soft-tissue tumors and lung metastases of osteosarcoma

(Ohta H, et al, 1984, 1985). Cortical renal imaging, however, is optimally performed with Tc-99m succimer that has been prepared at an acid pH.

IV. Testicular Imaging

Testicular scintigraphy is frequently requested when young men present with acute scrotal pain (Nadel N, et al 1973). It is relatively easy to perform (Datta NS and Mishkin FS, 1975), and no other diagnostic test is better in the differentiation of testicular torsion and acute epididymitis.

The goal of testicular imaging is to allow early surgery in patients with epididymitis. In one study that involved the procedure in a total of 410 patients with acute scrotal pain, the technique was found to yield a 96% sensitivity rate for torsion and a specificity for exclusion of 98% (Tanka T, et al, 1981). Scrotal imaging has little application in diagnosing non-acute processes. Testicular imaging usu-

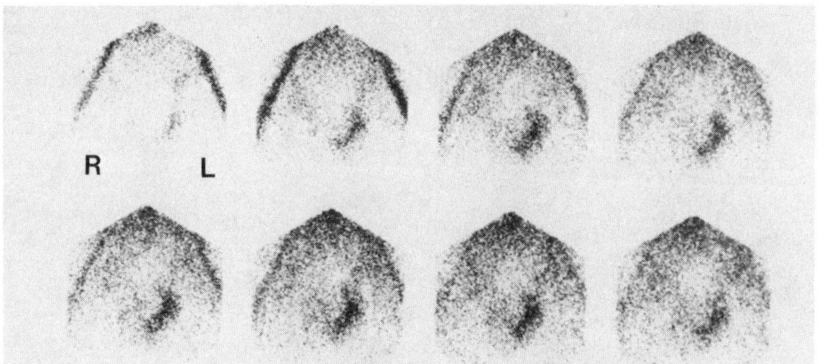

Figure 15.12   Dynamic radionuclide angiogram of the scrotum obtained with 20 millicuries Tc-99m pertechnetate in a patient complaining of pain on the left. The study illustrates intense hyperemia of the left epididymus.

ally offers no significant advantage over other modalities, notably sonography.

In neonates, the testicular study is of only low efficacy since: (1) the defect sought is near the lower limit of resolution for most imaging devices, and (2) the statistical likelihood is that torsion accounts for swelling in the neonate (provided that hydrocele has already been ruled out clinically) (Lutzker LG, 1982).

METHOD

The procedure is relatively easy to perform and should be performed as soon after the patient presents himself to the medical care facility as is possible. Failure to perform the procedure in a timely fashion may place the patient with torsion at risk for developing a testicular infarct should some degree of perfusion exist that could be salvaged via surgery.

The patient is positioned supine with the scrotum placed parallel to the face of the collimator by using a "tape sling." This serves to elevate the scrotal junction at the center of the collimator in order to faithfully reproduce a symmetrical image with the scrotum in the center and with visualization of both iliac arteries laterally (Holder LE, et al, 1981). The penis is taped back of the pubis in order to avoid extraneous source of activity. The patient's thighs may be abducted slightly in order to remove soft tissue background (Freund J, et al, 1980).

The adult patient is injected via bolus in-

travenous administration with 15–20 millicuries of Tc-99m sodium pertechnetate and ten serial images of 2–5 seconds duration are obtained immediately as the radiopharmaceutical transits the scrotal area (Figure 15.12). For children, L.E. Holder and associates (1981) utilize a minimum dose of 5 millicuries.

Static imaging is begun immediately afterwards in order that scintigraphic appearance of bladder accumulation of the radiopharmaceutical might be avoided (Figures 15.13 and 15.14A, B).

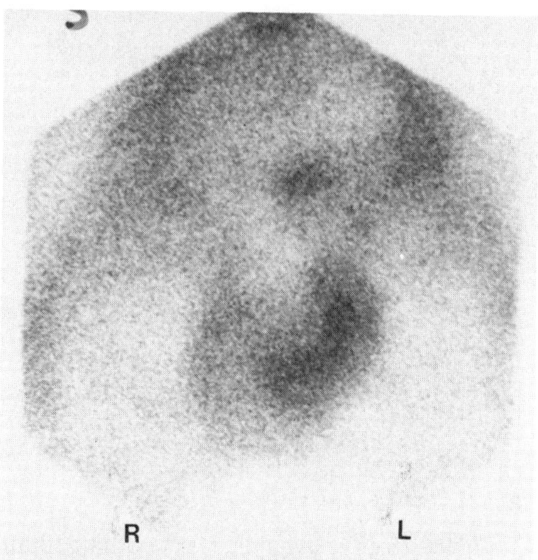

Figure 15.13   Immediate static image in the same patient (Figure 15.12) that confirms finding of left scrotal hyperemia and reveals no area of decreased uptake. Dynamic and static image findings are classic for epididymitis.

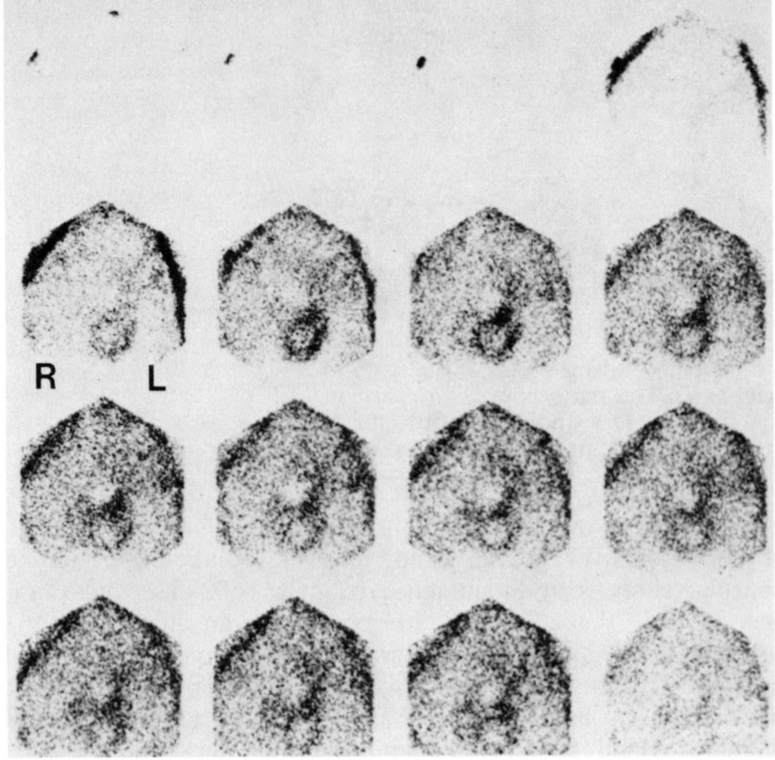

A

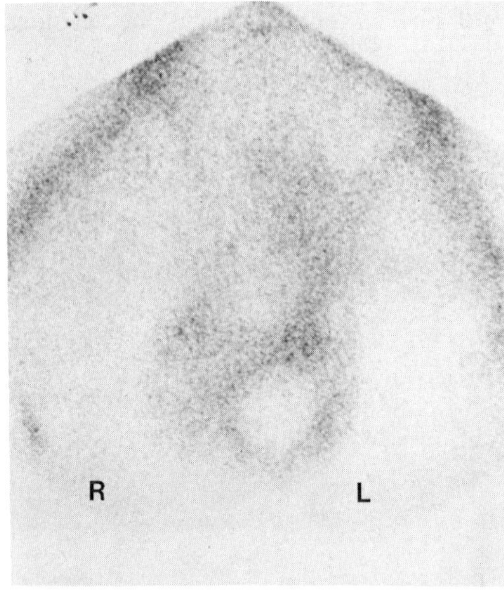

B

Figure 15.14 Dynamic (A) and immediate static (B) images of the scrotum reveal focally decreased perfusion of the left testicle with a hyperemia "halo" around it. This pattern is most commonly seen in subacute torsion and may also be seen with testicular abscesses and hematoma.

PHARMACOKINETICS

Following intravenous administration, Tc-99m pertechnetate distributes rapidly into the vascular space where it is reversibly bound to serum proteins, notably albumin (Hayes MT and Green FA, 1973). Pertechnetate demonstrates a rapid plasma clearance with equilibrium levels achieved between the vascular compartment and interstitial fluid in less than 3 minutes. While tissue distribution and blood clearance of Tc-99m pertechnetate are, for the most part, similar to iodide, the excretion of this radiopharmaceutical is different. Overall renal clearance of Tc-99m pertechnetate appears to be about one-half that of iodide, with urinary excretion accounting for approximately 30% of the administered dose within the first 24 hours (Dayton DA, et al, 1969; Lathrop KA and Harper PV, 1972).

V. Radionuclide Cystography

Unremitting reflux from the bladder into the ureters and intrarenal-collecting structures leads to renal damage. When the changes are severe enough they can lead to hypertension and even chronic renal failure. Urinary tract infection is an important cause of reflux in children. With adequate antibiotic therapy vesico-ureteral reflux usually resolves and does not require surgery. The detection and grading of reflux are important in patient management. Radionuclide methods have become increasingly accepted in the evaluation of vesico-ureteral reflux especially in children where there is a significant advantage with respect to radiation dose. The radionuclide technique is also more sensitive than the radiographic technique in detecting small amounts of reflux due to the high contrast resolution in the scintigraphic image.

RADIOPHARMACEUTICAL

METHOD

Radionuclide cystography may be performed as either an antegrade (indirect) or retrograde (direct) study. However, antegrade studies share some of the same limitations as antegrade contrast pyelography due to incremental filling from above. The potential confusion has made the retrograde approach the procedure of choice. The study is typically performed in three phases to study bladder filling, emptying, and postvoiding residual.

The patient is positioned so that the field of view of a gamma camera includes

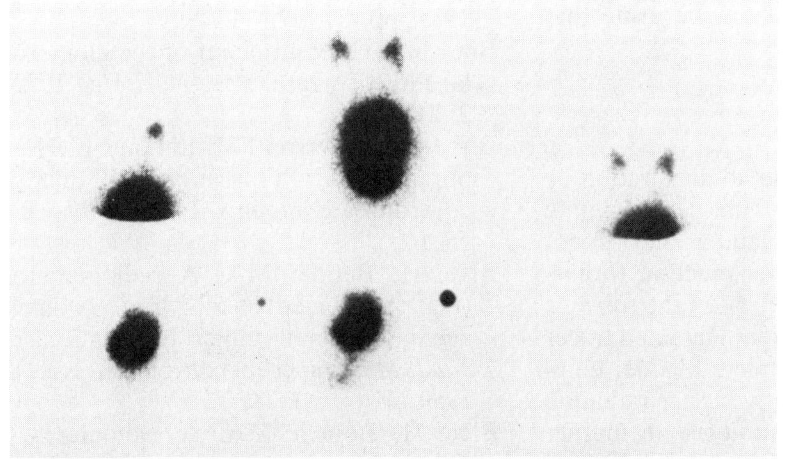

Figure 15.15 Multiple images from a retrograde (direct) cystogram demonstrating reflux during all three phases: filling, full, and voiding. Note also significant post voiding residual activity in the bladder.

the bladder, ureters, and kidneys. Technetium-99m as sodium pertechnetate, sulfur colloid or other nonabsorbable preparation is used as the radiotracer. A formulation of one millicurie technetium-99m per 500 ml normal saline provides a reasonable concentration.

After catheterization, the radioactive solution is slowly instilled in the bladder. Continuous monitoring is accomplished using a nuclear medicine computer system with a frame rate of 1 frame every 5 or 10 seconds. This permits a complete evaluation of the filling, voiding, and postvoiding phases.

In normal subjects, no radiotracer is seen outside of the bladder. In younger children voiding may be spontaneous as bladder capacity is reached, and again no tracer should be demonstrated in the region of the ureters or kidneys. In patients with vesico-ureteral reflux the tracer may be seen in the ureter at any time from early filling to late in the imaging sequence. The ability to continuously monitor the area of the ureters without additional radiation dose to the patient is a singular advantage of the radionuclide technique.

By measuring the count rate in the bladder before voiding occurs and again at the end of voiding, it is possible to calculate the postvoiding residual volume in the bladder. The count rate is simply normalized for the volume of urine that the patient has voided.

PHARMACOKINETICS

Following retrograde administration by catheter, technetium 99m pertechnetate remains within the bladder and is not absorbed by the bladder mucosa. In normal subjects, essentially all of the tracer is excreted with micturition. Retained tracer in patients with incomplete bladder emptying results in a slightly higher radiation dose than in normal subjects. In the absence of other contraindications this can be minimized by increased fluid intake with dilution and excretion of retained tracer.

References

Ahlgren L, Ivarsson S, Johansson L, et al. Excretion of radionuclides in human breast milk after the administration of radiopharmaceuticals. *J Nucl Med* 1985, 16:1085–1090.

Antar MA, Jones AN. Effect of probenecid on renal extraction of three renal radiopharmaceuticals at 15 and 30 minutes. *J Nucl Med* 1985, 26:P131.

Arnold RW, Subramanian G, McAfee JG, et al. Comparison of ^{99m}Tc complexes for renal imaging. *J Nucl Med* 1975, 16:357–367.

Ash JM, Antico VF, Gilday DL, et al. Special considerations in the pediatric use of radionuclides for kidney studies. *Semin Nucl Med* 1982, 12:345–369.

Assailly J, Pavel GP, Bader C, et al. Noninvasive experimental determination of the individual kidney filtration fraction by means of a dual-tracer technique, *J Nucl Med* 1977, 18:684–691.

Atkins HL, Cardinale KG, Eckelman WC, et al. Evaluation of ^{99m}Tc-DTPA prepared by three different methods. *Radiology* 1971, 98:674–677.

Atkins HL, Thomas SR. Dosimetry of radiopharmaceuticals used in nephrologic investigation. In *Nuclear Medicine in Clinical Urology and Nephrology*. (Tauxe WN, Dubovsky EV, eds.) Appleton-Century-Crofts, Norwalk, CT, 1985, pp. 31–37.

Bianchi C. Measurement of the glomerular filtration rate. *Prog Nucl Med* 1972, 2:21–53.

Bijl JA, Kasperson FM, Lindner L. Hippuran I-123: Preparation and quality control. *J Radioanal Chem* 1977, 35:55–62.

Blau M, Bender MA. A radiomercury (Hg^{203}) labeled Neohydrin: A new agent for brain tumor localization. *J Nucl Med* (special convention issue), 1959, 35 (abst).

Blau M, Bender MA. A radiomercury (Hg^{203}) labeled Neohydrin: A new agent for brain tumor localization. *J Nucl Med* 1962, 3:83–93.

Blaufox MD, Merril JP. Simplified hippuran clearance measurement of renal function in man with simplified hippuran clearance. *Nephron* 1966, 3:274–282.

Blaufox MD, Orvis A, Owen CA Jr. Compartmental analysis of the radiorenogram and distribution of ^{131}I-hippuran in dogs. *Am J Physiol* 1963, 204:1059–1064.

Blaufox MD, Potchen E, Merrill JP. Measurement of effective renal plasma flow in man by external counting methods. *J Nucl Med* 1967, 8:77–85.

Borghgraef RRM, Kessler RH, Pitts RF. Plasma regression, distribution and secretion of radiomercury in relation to diuresis following the intravenous administration of Hg-203 labeled chlormerodrin to the dog. *J Clin Invest* 1956, 35:1055–1066.

Cafruny EJ, Gussin RG: Renal mechanisms for excretion of mercury in the dog. *Pharmacologist* 1963, 5:266 (abst).

Carlsen JE, Moller ML, Lund JO, et al. Comparison of four commercial Tc-99m(Sn) DTPA preparations used for the measurement of glomerular filtration rate. Concise communication. *J Nucl Med* 1980, 21:126–129.

Cattell WR. Excretory pathways for contrast media. *Invest Radiol* 1970, 5:473–486.

Chervu LR, Blaufox MD. Renal radiopharmaceuticals—update. *Semin Nucl Med* 1982, 12:224–245.

Chi SL, Hoag SG, Yanchick VA. Electrolytic complexing of glucoheptonate and technetium-99m. *J Nucl Med* 1978, 19:520–524.

Cohen ML, Smith FG, Mindell RS, et al. A simple, reliable method of measuring glomerular filtration rate using single, low-dose sodium iothalamate I[131]. *Pediatrics* 1969, 43:407–415.

Collins, HR, Kavula M, Solomon AC. Stability of unit-dose technetium-99m radiopharmaceuticals: Radiochemical purity of multidose syringe. *Pharm Pract* 1983, 18:A-12 (abst).

Colombetti LG, Barnes WE. Effect of chemical and radiochemical impurities from eluants on Tc-99m-labeling efficiency. *Nuklearmedizin* 1977, 16:271–274.

Cooper PA, Zimmer AM. Radiochemical purity and stability of commercial ^{99m}Tc-stannous DTPA kits using a new chromatography technique. *J Nucl Med Tech* 1975, 3:208–209.

Cordova MA, Hladik WB, Rhodes BA. Validation and characterization of adverse reactions to radiopharmaceuticals. *Noninvasive Med Imag* 1984, 1:17–24.

Cordova MA, Rhodes BA. Adverse reactions to radiopharmaceuticals: Incidence in 1978 and associated symptoms. Report of the Adverse Reactions Subcommittee of the Society of Nuclear Medicine. *J Nucl Med* 1980, 21:1107–1110.

Daly MJ, Milutinovic J, Rudd TG, et al. Normal Tc-99m DMSA image. *Radiology* 1978, 128:701–704.

Datta NS, Mishkin FS. Radionuclide imaging in intrascrotal lesions. *JAMA* 1975, 231:1060–1062.

Davison A, Jones AG, Orvig C, et al. A new class of oxotechnetium (5+) chelate complexes containing a $TcON_2S_2$ core. *Inorg Chem* 1981, 20:1629–1632.

Dayton DA, Maher FT, Elveback LR. Renal clearance of technetium (Tc-99m) as pertechnetate. *Mayo Clin Proc* 1969, 44:549–553.

de Kieviet W. Technetium radiopharmaceuticals: Chemical characterization and tissue distribution of Tc-glucoheptonate using Tc-99m and carrier Tc-99. *J Nucl Med* 1981, 22:703–709.

Eckelman WC, Richards P. Instant ^{99m}Tc-DTPA. *J Nucl Med* 1970, 11:761.

Eckelman WC, Richards P, Hauser W, et al. ^{99m}Tc-DTPA preparations. *J Nucl Med* 1971, 12:699.

Enlander D, Weber PM, dos Remedios LV. Renal cortical imaging in 35 patients: Superior quality of ^{99m}Tc-DMSA. *J Nucl Med* 1974, 15:743–749.

Eshima D, Fritzberg AR, Kasina S, et al. Comparison of a new Tc-99m renal function agent, Tc-99m mercaptoacetyltriglycine with I-131 OIH. *J Nucl Med* 1985, 26:P56–57 (abst).

Freund J, Handelsman DJ, Bautovich GJ, et al. Detection of varicocele by radionuclide blood-pool imaging. *Radiology* 1980, 137:227–230.

Fritzberg AR, Kuni CC, Klingensmith WC III, et al. Synthesis and biological evaluation of Tc-99m N,N'-Bis(mercaptoacetyl)-2,3-diaminopropanoate: A potential replacement for [^{131}I] O-iodohippurate. *J Nucl Med* 1982, 23:592–598.

Fritzberg AR, Klingensmith WC III, Whitney WP, et al: Chemical and biological studies of Tc-99m N,N'-Bis-(mercaptoacetamido)-ethylenediamine: A potential replacement for I-131 iodohippurate. *J Nucl Med* 1981, 22:-258-263.

Gates GF. Glomerular filtration rate: Estimation from fractional renal accumulation of ^{99m}Tc-DTPA (stannous). *Am J Roentgenol* 1982, 138:565–570.

Gates GF. Split renal function testing using Tc-99m DTPA: A rapid technique for determining differential glomerular filtration. *Clin Nucl Med* 1983, 8:400–407.

Gates GF, Green GS. Transient reduction in renal function following arteriography and contrast enhanced CT scanning. Scientific exhibit presented at 28th Annual Meeting of the Society of Nuclear Medicine, Las Vegas, June, 1981.

Gillet R, Cogneau M, Mathy G. The preparation of I-123 labeled sodium-ortho-iodo-hippurate for medical research. *Int J Appl Radiat Isot* 1976, 27:61–62.

Hammermaier A, Reich E, Bogl W. Radiochemical purity and in vitro stability of commercial hippurans. *J Nucl Med* 1986, 27:850–854.

Handmaker H, Young BW, Lowenstein JM. Clinical experience with ^{99m}Tc-DMSA (dimercaptosuccinic acid), a new renal-imaging agent. *J Nucl Med* 1975, 16:28–32.

Hauser W, Atkins HL, Nelson KG, et al. Technetium-99m DTPA: A new radiopharmaceutical for brain and kidney scanning. *Radiology* 1970, 94:679–684.

Hauser W, Atkins HL, Richards P. Renal uptake of ^{99m}Tc iron ascorbic acid complex in man. *Radiology* 1971, 101:637–641.

Hayes MT, Green FA. In vitro studies of pertechnetate-99m binding by human serum and tissues. *J Nucl Med* 1973, 14:149–158.

Haynie TP, Nofal M, Carr EA Jr, et al. Scintillation scanning of the kidney and radioiodinated contrast media. *Clin Res* 1960, 8:288–295.

Hibbard B, Herbert R. Foetal radiation dose following administration of radioiodinated albumin. *Clin Sci* 1960, 19:337–344.

Hinkle GH, Basmadjian GP, Peek C, et al. Effects of concurrent drug therapy on technetium Tc-99m gluceptate biodistribution. *Am J Hosp Pharm* 1982, 39:1930–1933.

Hodges R, Evans T, Bradbury J, et al. Accumulation of radioactive iodine by human fetal thyroids. *J Clin Endocrinol* 1955, 15:661–667.

Holman BL, Tanaka TT, Lesch M. Evaluation of radiopharmaceuticals for the detection of acute myocardial infarction in man. *Radiology* 1976, 121:427–430.

Holder LE, Melloul M, Chen D. Current status of radionuclide scrotal imaging. *Semin Nucl Med* 1981, 11:232–249.

Hosain F, Reba RC, Wagner HN. Measurement of glomerular filtration rate using chelated ytterbium-169. *Int J Appl Radiat Isot* 1969, 20:517–521.

Hotte CE, Ice RD. The in vitro stability of [I-131]O-iodohippurate. *J Nucl Med* 1979, 20:441–447.

Ikeda I, Inoue O, Kurata K. Chemical and biological studies on ^{99m}Tc-DMS. II. Effect of Sn(II) on the formation of various Tc-DMS complexes. *Int J Appl Radiat Isot* 1976, 27:681–688.

ICRP Publication 52, Protection of the Nuclear Medicine Patient, Oxford, Pergamon, 1988.

Israelit AH, Long DL, White MG, et al. Measurement of glomerular filtration rate utilizing a single subcutaneous injection of ^{125}I-iothalamate. *Kidney Int* 1973, 4:346–349.

Keyes TF, Kurtz SB, Jones JD, et al. Renal toxicity during therapy with gentamicin or tobramycin. *Mayo Clin Proc* 1981, 56:556–559.

Kim EE, Gutierrez C, Sandler CM, et al. Radionuclide detection of cyclosporin: A nephrotoxicity in renal transplant patients. *J Nucl Med* 1983, 24:P129 (abst).

Klingensmith WC, Gerhold JP, Fritzberg AR, et al. Clinical comparison of Tc-99m N,N[1]-bis-(mercaptoacetamido)-ethylenediamine and [I-131] orthoiodohippurate for evaluation of renal tubular function: Concise communication. *J Nucl Med* 1982, 23:377–380.

Klintmalm GBG, Klingensmith WC III, Iwatsuki S, et al. Tc-99m DTPA and I-131 hippuran findings in cyclosporin: A nephrotoxicity in liver transplant recipients. *J Nucl Med* 1981, 22:P37–38 (abst).

Klopper JF, Hauser W, Atkins HL, et al. Evaluation of ^{99m}Tc-DTPA for the measurement of glomerular filtrate rate. *J Nucl Med* 1972, 13:107–110.

Koff SA, Thrall JH, Keyes JW Jr. Diuretic radionuclide urography: A noninvasive method for evaluating nephroureteral dilation. *J Urol* 1979, 122:451–454.

Kremer Hovinga TK, Beukhof JR, Van Luyk WHJ, et al. Reversible diminished renal ^{99m}Tc-DMSA uptake during converting-enzyme inhibition in a patient with renal artery stenosis. *Eur J Nucl Med* 1984, 9:144–146.

Lathrop KA, Harper PV. Biologic behavior of ^{99m}Tc from ^{99m}Tc-pertechnetate ion. *Prog Nucl Med* 1972, 1:145–162.

Lee HB, Blaufox MD. Tc-99m glucoheptonate (GHA) renal uptake: Influence of biochemical and physiologic factors. *J Nucl Med* 1984, 25:P75–P76 (abst).

Lee HB, Blaufox MD. Mechanism of renal concentration of technetium-99m glucoheptonate. *J Nucl Med* 1985, 26:1308–1313.

Lin TH, Khentigan A, Winchell HS. A ^{99m}Tc-chelate substitute for organomercurial renal agents. *J Nucl Med* 1974, 15:34–35.

Lutzker LG. The fine points of scrotal scintigraphy. *Semin Nucl Med* 1982, 12:387–393.

MacGregor RJ, Konnoak JW, Thrall JH, et al. Diuretic radionuclide urography in the diagnosis of suspected ureteral obstruction following renal transplantation. *J Urol (Paris)* 1983, 125:710–718.

Magnusson G. Purity and stability of commercial sodium iodohippurate labeled with I-131. *Nature (London)* 1962, 195:591–592.

Maher FT, Nolan NG, Elveback LR. Comparison of simultaneous clearances of ^{125}I-labeled sodium iothalamate (Glofil) and inulin. *Mayo Clin Proc* 1971, 46:690–691.

Maher FT, Tauxe WN. Renal clearance in man of pharmaceuticals containing radioactive iodine: Influence of plasma binding. *JAMA* 1969, 207:97–102.

Majd M, Potter BM, Guzzetta PC, et al. Captopril enhanced renal scintigraphy for detection of renal artery stenosis—an uptake. *J Nucl Med* 1986, 27:962 (abst).

McAfee JG, Gagne G, Atkins HL, et al. Biological distribution and excretion of DTPA labeled with Tc-99m and In-111. *J Nucl Med* 1979, 20:1273–1278.

McAfee JG, Grossman ZD, Gagne GR, et al. Comparison of renal extraction efficiencies for radioactive agents in the normal dog. *J Nucl Med* 1981, 22:333–338.

McAfee JG, Wagner HN. Visualization of renal parenchyma by scintiscanning with Hg^{203} Neohydrin. *Radiology* 1960, 75:820–821.

McKusick KA, Malmud LS, Kirchner PT, et al. An interesting artifact in radionuclide imaging of the kidneys. *J Nucl Med* 1973, 14:113–114.

Mitta AEA, Fraga A, Veall N. A simplified method for preparing I-131 labeled hippuran. *Int J Appl Radiat Isot* 1961, 12:146–147.

Moretti JL, Rapin JR, Saccaarini JC. 2,3 Dimercaptosuccinic acid chelates: Their structure and biological behaviour. In

Nuclear Medicine and Biology II. Raynound C (ed.). Paris, Pergamon Press, 1982, pp. 1651–1654.

Mountford PJ, Coakley AJ. Radiopharmaceuticals in breast milk. In *Proceedings of the fourth International Radiopharmaceutical Dosimetry Symposium*, Schlafke-Stelson AT, Watson EE (eds.), Oak Ridge, TN, pp. 167–180, CONF-85111, April 1986.

Mountford PJ, Coakley AJ, Hall FM. Excretion of radioactivity in breast milk following injection of ^{99m}Tc-DTPA. *Nucl Med Commun* 1985, 6:341–345.

Nadal NS, Gitter MH, Hahn LC, et al. Preoperative diagnosis of testicular torsion. *Urology* 1973, 1:478–479.

Nelp WB, Wagner HN, Reba RC. Renal excretion of vitamin B_{12} and its use in measurement of glomerular filtration rate in man. *J Lab Clin Med* 1964, 63:480–491.

Nielsen SP, Moller ML, Trap-Jensen J. ^{99m}Tc-DTPA scintillation camera renography: A new method for estimation of single-kidney function. *J Nucl Med* 1977, 18:112–117.

Nordyke RA, Tubis M, Blahd WH. Use of radioactive hippuran for individual kidney function tests. *J Lab Clin Med* 1960, 55:438–445.

Odlind B, Hallgren R, Sohtell M, et al. Is ^{125}I iothalamate an ideal marker for glomerular filtration? *Kidney Int* 1985, 27:9–16.

Oeser H, Billion H. Funktionelle strahlenediagnostik durch etikettierte rontgenkontrastmittel. *Fortschr Geb Rontgenstr Nuklearmed Erganzungsband*, 1952, 76, 431–442.

Ohta H, Ishii M, Hoshizumi M, et al. A comparison of the tumor-seeking agent Tc-99m(V) dimercaptosuccinic acid and the renal imaging agent Tc-99m imercaptosuccinic acid in humans. *Clin Nucl Med* 1985, 10:167–170.

Ohta H, Yamamoto K, Endo K, et al. A new imaging agent for medullary carcinoma of the thyroid. *J Nucl Med* 1984, 25:323–325.

O'Reilley PH, Testa HJ, Lawson RS, et al. Diuresis renography in equivocal urinary tract obstruction. *Br J Urol* 1978, 50:76–80.

Piepsz A, Denis R, Ham HR, et al. A simple method for measuring separate glomerular filtration rate using a single injection of ^{99m}Tc-DTPA and the scintillation camera. *J Pediatr* 1978, 93:769–774.

Ponto JA, Swanson DP, Freitas JE. Clinical manifestations of radiopharmaceutical formulation problems. In *Essentials of Nuclear Medicine Science*, Hladik WB III, Saha G, Study KT (eds.). Baltimore, Williams and Wilkins, 1987, pp. 268–289.

Provoost AP, Van Aken M. Renal handling of technetium-99m DMSA in rats with proximal tubular dysfunction. *J Nucl Med* 1985, 26:1063–1067.

Ramamoorthy N, Shetye SV, Pandey PM, et al. Preparation and evaluation of ^{99m}Tc(V)-DMSA complex: Studies in medullary carcinoma of thyroid. *Eur J Nucl Med* 1987, 12:623–628.

Robbins PJ, Williams CC. An investigation of low tagging yields of Tc-99m DTPA kits. *J Nucl Med* 1979, 10:653 (abst).

Romney BM, Nickoloff EL, Esser PD, et al. Radionuclide administration to nursing mothers. *Radiology* 1986, 160:549–554.

Rosenthall L: Ortho-iodohippurate-I^{131} kidney scanning in renal failure. *Radiology* 1966, 87:298–304.

Russell CD, Bischoff PG, Kontzen FN, et al. Measurement of glomerular filtration rate: Single-injection plasma clearance method without urine collection. *J Nucl Med* 1985a, 26:1243–1247.

Russell CD, Bischoff PG, Kontzen FN, et al. Measurement of glomerular filtration rate using ^{99m}Tc-DTPA and the gamma camera: A comparison of the methods. *Eur J Nucl Med* 1985b, 10:519–521.

Russell CD, Bischoff PG, Rowell KL, et al. Quality control of Tc-99m DTPA for measurement of glomerular filtration: Concise communication. *J Nucl Med* 1983, 24:722–727.

Russell CD, Crittenden RC, Cash AG. Determination of net ionic charge on Tc-99m DTPA and Tc-99m EDTA by a column ion-exchange method. *J Nucl Med* 1980, 21:354–360.

Russell CD, Rowell K, Scott JW. Quality control of technetium-99m DTPA: Correlation of analytic tests with in vivo protein binding in man. *J Nucl Med* 1986, 27:560–562.

Sampson CB. Instability of commercial ^{99m}Tc-DTPA kits—effect of dilution and delay before injection. *Nucl Med Commun* 1984, 5:239.

Sampson CB, Keegan J. Stability of Tc-99m-DTPA injection: Effect of delay after preparation, dilution, generator oxidant, and oxygen. *Nucl Med Commun* 1985, 6:313–318.

Scheer KE, Meier-Borst W. Die Darstellung Von I-131 orthoiodohippursaure durch Austauch-markierung. *Nucl Med (Stuttg)* 1962, 2:193–197.

Shannon JA, Smith HW. The excretion of inulin and urea by normal and phlorizinies man. *J Clin Invest* 1935, 14:393–401.

Sigman EM, Elwood CM, Knox F. The measurement of glomerular filtration rate in man with sodium iothalamate ^{131}I (Conray). *J Nucl Med* 1965a, 7:60–68.

Sigman EM, Elwood CM, Reagan ME, et al. The renal clearance of I^{131} labeled sodium iothalamate in man. *Invest Urol* 1965b, 2:432–438.

Specht HD, Belsey R, Hanada J. Aluminemic disturbance of technetium-99m DTPA renal function measurement. *J Nucl Med* 1987, 28:383–386.

Stacy BD, Thorburn GD. Chromium-51 ethylenediaminetetraacetate for estimation of glomerular filtrate rate. *Science* 1966, 152:1076–1077.

Stadalnik RC, Vogel JM, Jansholt AL, et al. Renal clearance and extraction parameters of ortho-iodo hippurate (I-123) compared with OIH (I-131) and PAH. *J Nucl Med* 1980, 21:168–170.

Tanaka T, Mishkin FS, Datta NS: Radionuclide imaging of the scrotal contents. In: Freeman LM, Weissman HS (eds): *Nuclear Medicine Annual 1981*. New York, Raven Press, 1981, pp. 195–221.

Taplin GV, Meredith OM, Kade H, et al. The radioisotope renogram: An external test for individual kidney function and upper urinary tract patency. *J Lab Clin Med* 1956, 48:886–901.

Taplin GV, Dore EK Johnson DE: The quantitative radiorenogram for total and differential renal blood flow measurement. *J Nucl Med* 1963, 4:404–407.

Tauxe WN, Burbank MK, Maher FT, et al. Renal clearances of radioactive orthoiodohippurate and diatrizoate. *Mayo Clin Proc* 1964, 39:761–766.

Tauxe WN, Hunt JC, Burbank MK. The radioisotope renogram (ortho-iodohippurate-I-131): Standardization and techniques of expression of data. *Am J Clin Pathol* 1962, 37:567–583.

Tauxe WN, Maher FT, Taylor WF. Effective renal plasma flow estimation from theoretical volumes of distribution of intravenously injected ^{131}I-orthoidohippurate. *Mayo Clin Proc* 1971, 46:524–551.

Taylor A, Lallone RL, Hagan PL. Optimal handling of dimercaptosuccinic acid for quantitative renal scanning. *J Nucl Med* 1980, 21:1190–193.

Taylor AT, Eshima D, Fritzberg AR, et al. Comparison of iodine-131 OIH and technetium-99m MAG$_3$ renal imaging in volunteers. *J Nucl Med* 1986, 27:795–803.

Thomas SR, Atkins HL, McAfee JG, et al. Radiation absorbed dose from Tc-99m diethylenetriamepentaacetic acid (DTPA). *J Nucl Med* 1984, 25:503–505.

Thrall JH, Koff SA, Keyes JW. Diuretic radionuclide renography and scintigraphy in the differential diagnosis of hydroureteronephrosis. *Semin Nucl Med* 1981, 11:89–104.

Tubis M, Posnick E, Nordyke RA. Preparation and use of I^{131} labeled sodium iodohippurate in kidney function tests. *Proc Soc Exp Biol Med* 1960, 103:497–498.

Tyler JL, Powers TA. Gallbladder visualization with technetium-99m glucoheptonate: Concise communicaton. *J Nucl Med* 1982, 23:870–871.

The United States Pharmacopeia, Twenty-First Revision, and the National Formulary, Sixteenth Edition. United States Pharmacopeial Convention, Inc., Rockville, 1984.

USP DI, Volume I, Drug Information for the Health Care Provider, Ninth Edition. United States Pharmacopeial Convention, Inc., 1989.

Vanlic-Razumenic N, Malesevic M, Stefanovic VJ. Comparative chemical, biological, and clinical studies of ^{99m}Tc-glucoheptonate and ^{99m}Tc-dimercaptosuccinate as used in renal scintigraphy. *Nuklearmedizin* 1979, 18:40–45.

Vorne M, Sakki S, Jarvi K, et al. Tc-99m glucoheptonate in detection of lung tumors. *J Nucl Med* 1982, 23:250–254.

Wegst, A. Personal communication, 1988.

Wegst A, Goin J, Robinson R. Cumulated activities determined from biodistribution data in pregnant rats ranging from 13–21 days gestation. I. Tc-99m pertechnetate. *Med Phys* 1983, 10(6): 841–845.

Wellman HN, Berke RA, Robbins PJ, Anger RT Jr: Dynamic quantitative renal imaging with ^{123}I-Hippuran–A possible salvation of the renogram *J Nucl Med* 1972, 12:405 (abst).

Wenting GJ, Tan-Tjiong HL, Derkx FMH. Split renal function after captopril in unilateral renal artery stenosis. *Br Med J* 1984, 288:886–890.

Wilson MA, Pastakia B. Biliary excretion of Tc-99m-glucoheptonate in poor renal function. *Clin Nucl Med* 1980, 5:448–449.

Yee CA, Lee HB, Blaufox MD. Tc-99m DMSA renal uptake: Influence of biochemical and physiologic factors. *J Nucl Med* 1981, 22:1054–1058.

Yee CA, Lee HB, Blaufox MD. The effect of various pathophysiologic conditions on the excretion and renal localization of Tc-99m DMSA. *J Nucl Med* 1980, 21:P40 (abst).

Zbrzeznj D, Khan RAA. Factors affecting the labeling efficiency and stability of technetium-99m labeled glucoheptonate. *Am J Hosp Pharm* 1981, 38: 1499–1502.

Radiopharmaceuticals for Bone and Bone Marrow Imaging

Henry M. Chilton
Marion D. Francis
James H. Thrall

I. Skeletal Imaging

In addition to primary neoplasms of bone, destructive bone lesions also occur in a variety of pathologic conditions including metastatic disease, metabolic disorders, and infections that invade bone tissues and alter normal skeletal activity. In diseases that metastasize to bone (lung, prostate, kidney, and thyroid cancers), the frequency of skeletal involvement is quite high. Although the detection of skeletal lesions may be accomplished in a large percentage of patients by roentgenograms, the early detection of most skeletal lesions by routine x-rays is difficult because bone demineralization changes of 30–50% must occur before density changes can be distinguished on x-ray film with high statistical significance (Borak J, 1942; Ardran GM, 1951). Skeletal lesions less than 1–2 cm are particularly difficult to detect by standard x-ray techniques.

Nuclear medicine skeletal imaging is considerably more sensitive than conventional x-rays for identifying the presence and extent of skeletal lesions because bone-seeking radiopharmaceuticals usually localize in skeletal lesions very early in the pathological process. In fact, a primary advantage of skeletal imaging is that it often shows abnormalities in bone at an early stage and more definitively than is possible using routine x-ray films. This highly sensitive diagnostic nature of skeletal imaging, coupled with its relative convenience to perform, makes the technique useful in a variety of clinical situations (Table 16.1).

Table 16.1 INDICATIONS FOR SKELETAL IMAGING

1. Screen preoperative patients with malignancies known to metastasize early to bone (e. g., breast, lung, prostate)
2. Detect metastatic bone lesions prior to x-ray changes
3. Determine the extent of known primary and metastatic lesions
4. Localize lesions prior to bone biopsies
5. Assist in the planning of radiotherapy portals
6. Assess benefit of therapy upon bone cancer
7. Detect infective bone lesions
8. Diagnose stress fractures, assessment of trauma
9. Detection of Paget's disease
10. Detect loosening of hip/knee prostheses

RADIOPHARMACEUTICALS FOR SKELETAL IMAGING

BACKGROUND/HISTORY

Knowledge that radionuclides localize in bone came at the turn of this century from observations on the pathologic effects of ingested radium salts in workers who painted luminous watch dials. In these workers, the effect of radium deposited in the osseous system was bone necrosis and neoplasia that occurred as a result of the localized deposition of the highly ionizing alpha radiation.

The first physiologic evaluation of radionuclides in bone occurred in 1935 when Chiewitz and Hevesy used sodium phosphate P-32 to study bone metabolism in animals. In the 1940s and 1950s, other bone-seeking radionuclides were examined for this same purpose. These included radioisotopes of strontium (Treadwell AdeG, et al, 1942; Percher C, 1942; Bauer GCH, 1958), gallium (Dudley HC, et al, 1956; Desgrez MH, et al, 1954), and calcium (Bauer GCH, 1958).

Table 16.2 NUCLEAR AND PHYSICAL PROPERTIES OF NON-Tc-99m BONE-SEEKING RADIOPHARMACEUTICALS

AGENT	$T_{1/2}$ PHY	DECAY MODE	PRIMARY PHOTON	γ EMISSION ABUNDANCE
Sr-85 chloride	64 days	E.C.	513 keV	100%
Sr-87m citrate or bicarbonate	2.8 days	I.T.	388 keV	99%
F-18 sodium fluoride	111 minutes	β^+	511 keV	97%

E.C. = Electron capture
I.T. = Isomeric transition
β^+ = Beta-plus

Of these, the radioisotopes of strontium (Sr-85 and Sr-87m) attained the most notriety for skeletal imaging in patients using rectilinear scanners (Bauer GCH and Wendebert B, 1959; Charkes ND, et al, 1964) (Table 16.2). These radioisotopes localize in bone by exchanging surface calcium ions in both amorphous calcium phosphate and crystalline hydroxyapatite in newly forming bone (Neuman WF and Neuman MW, 1958). However, because of either relatively high radiation dosimetry (Sr-85) or undesirably short physical half-life (Sr-87m) that required imaging when blood background levels were still high, neither of these two radioisotopes of strontium proved ideal for skeletal imaging.

In 1961, W.H. Fleming and associates found that Fluorine-18, as sodium fluoride, was taken up by the skeleton in proportion to bone metabolic activity. F-18 has approximately the same uptake in bone as radiostrontium (near 50% of the dose localizes in bone within 2 hours post administration) (Weber WG, et al, 1969); however, unlike radiostrontium, the rapid renal excretion of F-18 enables skeletal imaging to be performed within a few hours of administration of this radionuclide (Blau M, et al, 1962). Fluoride ions localize in bone by exchanging for the hydroxyl group in hydroxyapatite on the surface of the bone crystal, then pass into the interior of the crystal by heterionic exchange (Costeas A, et al, 1970). A primary drawback, however, is the short physical half-life of Fluorine-18 (111 minutes) that limited its use to hospitals within a few hours travel time of radionuclide production facilities.

Other radionuclides have been shown to localize in bone to a variable degree, including radioisotopes of the lanthanide series and rare earth elements (Table 16.3) that also exchange for calcium to form the insoluble phosphate on bone surface. A few of these have been used clinically for bone imaging; however, most have been limited to experimental use at a few medical centers (O'Mara RE and Subramanian G, 1972; O'Mara RE, et al, 1969; Jowsey J, et al, 1958).

Chemistry

The radionuclide Tc-99m has near-ideal imaging properties; however, little, if any, bone uptake occurs when the simple anionic species of this radionuclide, Tc-99m sodium pertechnetate, is administered intravenously (Francis MD, et al, 1976). Consequently, for Tc-99m to be useful for bone imaging, the generator-produced species of Tc-99m must be reduced to a lower oxidation state and bound to some bone-specific ligand.

During the early 1970s, G. Subramanian and J.G. McAfee (1971a) reported the preparation and evaluation of the first bone-seeking complex of Tc-99m that was formed between reduced Tc-99m and sodium tripolyphosphate. Soon afterwards, they radiolabeled a synthetic long-chain polyphosphate with Tc-99m and found it a superior skeletal imaging agent having

Table 16.3 OTHER RADIONUCLIDES AND COMPOUNDS KNOWN TO LOCALIZE IN BONE

Ca-45, Ca-47
Ga-72 citrate, Ga-68 citrate
Er-171 HEDTA, Cy-157 HEDTA
Ba-131, Ba-133m, Ba-135m
In-113m chloride

greater bone uptake, more rapid blood clearance than Tc-99m tripolyphosphate, and faster urinary excretion of the fraction of the dose not taken up by bone (Subramanian G, et al, 1972). Stannous ions were employed in both reports to reduce the usually nonreactive pertechnetate ion (Tc VII) to a lower oxidation species that radiolabels the bone. Stannous ions are generally preferred over all other methods for reduction of Tc-99m pertechnetate due to the relative convenience and reliability of this technique. Today, the stannous ion-assisted method is employed universally for the reduction of Tc-99m. While stannous ions are required for radiolabeling, they play no other role in the bone-seeking properties of these agents (Deutsch E, et al, 1980). However, stannous ions have been shown to deposit on bone (Tofe AJ and Francis MD, 1974).

It appears by most analytical methods (e. g., end point potentiometry, polarography) that the majority of technetium in the Tc-99m bone-seeking radiopharmaceuticals exists as the Tc(IV) state, with lesser amounts in the III and V oxidation states (Russell CD and Cash AG, 1979).

Although the imaging properties of Tc-99m polyphosphate were clearly superior to those of all other bone seekers used until that time (Dewanjee MK, et al, 1972), the slower blood clearance than F-18 and slight hepatic uptake of Tc-99m polyphosphate compromised the advantageous imaging properties. Unfortunately, polyphosphates tend to be broken down in vivo by phosphatase hydrolysis (Van Wazer JR, 1958) resulting in the release of the Tc(IV) from the complex and subsequent oxidation to a higher state. This results in significant levels of free, unbound technetate (VI) and/or pertechnetate that seriously lessened image quality (Figure 16.1).

Pyrophosphate (PPi), a normally occurring metabolic product found in a variety of tissues, is composed of only two phosphate moieties and is the simplest polyphosphate constituent (MW200). PPi can also be labeled with Tc-99m, using the

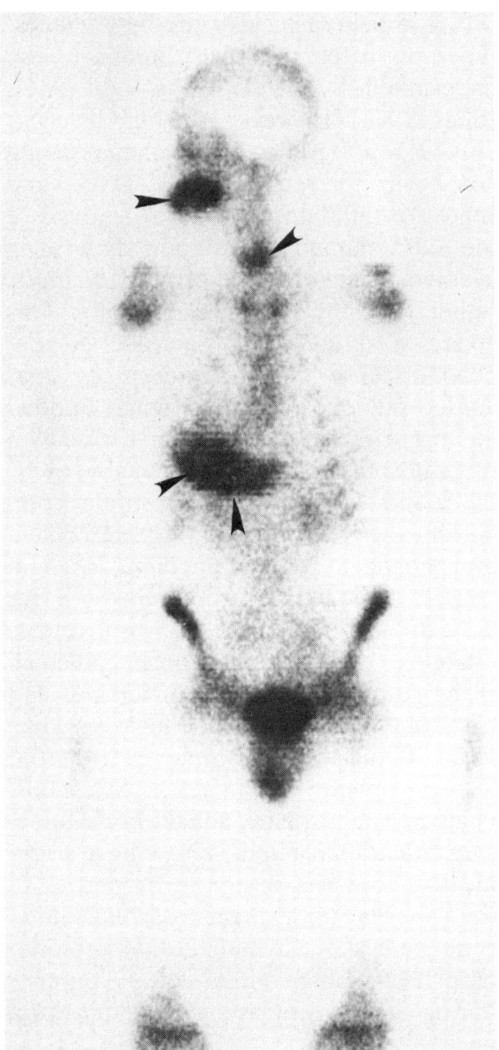

Figure 16.1 Tc-99m polyphosphate (PYP) bone scintigram demonstrating presence of free pertechnetate (arrows) in oropharynx, thyroid gland, and stomach.

stannous ion reduction technique, to form a technetium phosphate complex that is bone-avid. The development of Tc-99m pyrophosphate as a diagnostic radiopharmaceutical for skeletal imaging can be attributed to observations and investigations made involving the use of Tc-99m polyphosphate. Investigations into the optimum polyphosphate chain length to achieve highest bone-to-background ratios indicated (Subramanian G, et al, 1971b) that a linear configuration (rather than side branching) with a chain length of 46-repeating phosphate units

(PP₄₆) appeared to give the best images. Attempts to confirm these findings were undertaken by M.A. Davis and A.G. Jones (1976). However, the high levels of uptake reported by Subramanian could not be confirmed with the Davis and Jones formulation. End point analysis of the Subramanian formulation showed an average chain length of 18–20 units, rather than the 46 repeating units. This apparent discrepancy was due to depolymerization of long-chained condensed polyphosphates on aging. Following the clinical introduction of Tc-99m pyrophosphates for skeletal imaging by R. Perez and co-workers (1972), studies comparing the skeletal uptake of Tc-99m polyphosphate as a function of chain length demonstrated that the relative bone uptake of these agents was inversely related to the length of the linear chain (King AG, et al, 1973; Schumichen C and Nakken KF, 1974). Subsequently, when the original PP₄₆ sample was tested for phosphate impurities, orthophosphate, pyrophosphate, and the cyclic molecule trimetaphosphate were detected, indicating that the desirable properties of the original long-chain polyphosphates could be largely attributed to the presence of pyrophosphate either as an impurity during synthesis or as a degradation product.

Whereas the fraction of Tc-99m pyrophosphate that localizes in bone is only slightly greater than that of Tc-99m polyphosphate (approximately 10% more of the injected dose), the smaller Tc-99m complex has more rapid blood clearance and urinary excretion that results in generally superior target-to-nontarget ratios than the Tc-99m polyphosphate images (Fletcher JW, et al, 1973; Hosain P, 1973). Tc-99m pyrophosphate is also utilized for myocardial infarct imaging—see Chapter 13—and the nonradioactive form of pyrophosphate is utilized for labeling red blood cells with Tc-99m for quantification of left ventricular function and the evaluation of GI bleeding (Chapter 14). Unfortunately, Tc-99m pyrophosphate, like Tc-99m polyphosphate, is subject to in vivo enzymatic destruction. Subsequently diphosphonate analogues were synthesized that had a P-C-P central structure rather than the P-O-P configuration of pyrophosphate. These analogues could also be labeled with Tc-99m and proved to be stable chemically and resistant to the effect of in vivo phosphatases.

The Diphosphonates. Organic analogues of the phosphate complexes labeled with Tc-99m also exhibit bone uptake. These complexes, known as *diphosphonates* (or bis-phosphonates), contain a central P-C-P structure (rather than the phosphate P-O-P spine) that affords greater resistance to in vivo phosphatase hydrolysis. As a result, Tc-99m diphosphonate bone seekers generally exhibit more rapid blood clearance and somewhat higher skeletal uptake than Tc-99m pyrophosphate (approximately 50–55% for the Tc-99m diphosphonates versus 45–50% for Tc-99m pyrophosphate). Additionally, the central carbon configuration of the diphosphonates permits development of a variety of diphosphonate derivatives, several of which have been shown useful for skeletal imaging (Figure 16.2).

Disodium 1-hydroxyethylidene-1,1-diphosphonate (etidronate or HEDP) was the first Tc-99m diphosphonate to be employed clinically for bone imaging (Castronovo FP Jr and Callahan RJ, 1972; Tofe AJ and Francis MD, 1972). In comparison with Tc-99m polyphosphate and pyrophosphate, Tc-99m HEDP demonstrated more rapid blood clearance and superior bone visualization.

In 1975, G. Subramanian and colleagues introduced Tc-99m methylene diphosphonate (MDP, or *medronate*) for skeletal imaging. Approximately 50–60% of the administered dose of Tc-99m MDP localizes in bone. The blood clearance of Tc-99m MDP approximates that of F-18 (Figure 16.3). Tc-99m diphosphonate analogues soon followed as it became apparent that different substituents onto the central carbon structure might lead to radiopharmaceuticals with improved blood clearance rates and bone uptake. The presence of a hydroxyl group at this site, for example, increases bone uptake probably by altering favorably the manner of radiopharmaceuti-

Pyrophosphoric Acid

$$HO-\underset{\underset{OH}{|}}{\overset{\overset{O}{\|}}{P}}-O-\underset{\underset{OH}{|}}{\overset{\overset{O}{\|}}{P}}-OH$$

Diphosphonic Acid

$$HO-\underset{\underset{OH}{|}}{\overset{\overset{O}{\|}}{P}}-\underset{\underset{R_2}{|}}{\overset{\overset{R_1}{|}}{C}}-\underset{\underset{OH}{|}}{\overset{\overset{O}{\|}}{P}}-OH$$

R1	R2	
—OH	—CH₃	. . . etidronic acid (EHDP or 1-hydroxy ethylidene diphosphonic acid)
—H	—H	. . . medronic acid (MDP or methylene diphosphonic acid)
—H	—OH	. . . oxidronic acid (HMDP or hydroxy methylene diphosphonic acid)

Figure 16.2 Chemical structures of pyrophosphate and diphosphonate ligands used in the preparation of Tc-99m bone-seeking radiopharmaceuticals.

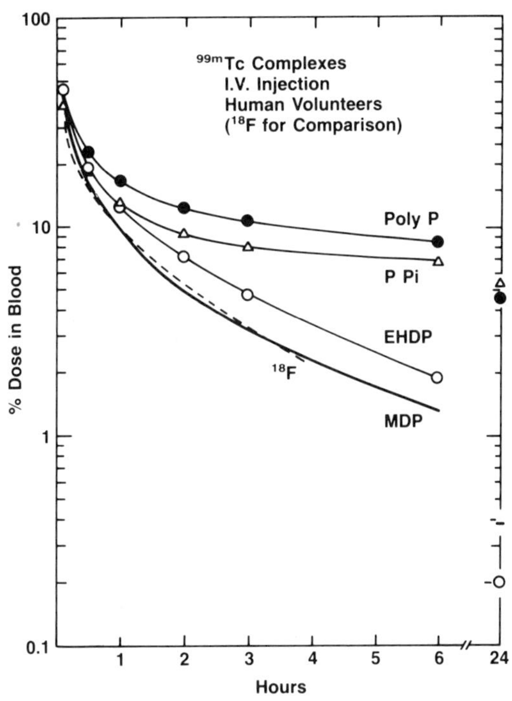

Figure 16.3 Blood clearance of MDP in humans compared with three other Tc-99m complexes and F-18 (all values corrected for physical decay), assuming blood volume was 7% of body weight. *PPi* indicates pyrophosphate and *Poly P* denotes polyphosphate. From Subramanian G, et al, 1975.

cal attachment to bone (Deutsch E and Barnett BL, 1980) (see Pharmacokinetics). The hydroxyl substituted diphosphonate, Tc-99m HMDP (hydroxymethane diphosphonate or *oxidronate*), has shown faster blood clearance and higher skeletal uptake than MDP.

The precise structures of the stannous reduced Tc-99m diphosphonate complexes are not known. Because the reduction of technetium and radiolabeling is accompanied by hydrolysis, complexation, and oxidation, it is likely that a complex mixture of oligomeric and polymeric species may form. In any given reaction, such as occurs with the stannous ion-assisted radiolabeling of Tc-99m diphosphonates, complexes formed are governed by competing reactions that are dependent upon the technetium concentration, chelate-to-metal ratio, reductant to metal ratio, oxidizing conditions, pH, temperature, and reaction time. The formation of these species is favored by the tendency of the diphosphonate ligand to promote polymer formation by bridging metal centers, as well as by the presence of excess stannous ions that may also participate in bridging reactions.

Stability/Storage. Presently, commercial formulations of MDP and HDP that are currently available in the United States are lyophilized and contain adequate amounts of ligand and reducing agent to prepare multiple doses of the radiolabeled product. The amount of Sn^{+2} ions in these "kits" is critical—sufficient tin must be present to ensure reduction of Tc-99m atoms and counteract the effects of oxygen and oxidants upon the stability of the formed radiopharmaceutical. A large excess of tin can be detrimental, however, because stannous hydrolysis products may form that compete with the phosphorous ligand for the reduced Tc-99m species (Tofe AJ and Francis MD, 1974). Excessive tin, although an inhibitor of oxidation of reduced technetium, would be expected with progressive oxidation and/or hydrolysis to form insoluble hydrated SnO or SnO_2 that would bind rather than coordinate reduced Tc-99m and form colloidal species of technetium that localize within the reticuloendothelial system (Francis MD, et al, 1981). Generally, most formulations contain no less than 20:1 ratios of ligand to stannous ions. Additionally, since stannous ions are inherently unstable and readily convert (via oxidation) to the undesirable stannic (Sn^{+4}) form, most manufacturers routinely flush and package each vial "head" space with inert nitrogen, rather than air.

One method for the protection of reduced Tc-99m diphosphonates from the effects of oxidation (from oxygen) involves the use of antioxidant stabilizers, such as ascorbic acid or gentisic acid (2,5-dihydroxybenzoic acid). Both ascorbic acid (Tofe AJ and Francis MD, 1976) and gentisic acid (Tofe AJ, et al, 1980) are effective inhibitors of in vitro oxidation that adversely affect radiopharmaceutical stability. When employed in relatively low amounts (usually less than 0.6 mg), these stabilizers are safe and without toxicity (Abt AF and Farmer CJ, 1938; Demole V, 1934; Bradley DW, et al, 1972; Nash JF, et al, 1953). Radiochemical purity analysis of low-tin Tc-99m diphosphonates formulated with gentisic acid have shown free, unbound Tc-99m levels consistently lower than 2% when tested as long as 6 hours from the time of preparation (Tofe AJ, et al, 1980). Because the complexation of reduced Tc(IV) by gentisate or ascorbate is minimal, neither antioxidant alters osseous specificity or causes the formation of secondary radiolabeled species taken up by soft tissues or organs other than bone (Tofe AJ and Francis MD, 1976; Tofe AJ, et al, 1980). D.E. Heggli and associates (1988) evaluated the biodistribution of four formulations of Tc-99m medronate containing either gentisic acid, paraminobenzoic acid, or ascorbic acid (two formulations) and found higher bone/muscle ratios with even higher gentisic acid formulations, again confirming the advantageous use of an antioxidant and indicating no adverse complexation of gentisic acid with reduced Tc-99m.

Tc-99m medronate and Tc-99m oxidronate can be refrigerated or stored at room temperature when not in use but should be discarded within 6–10 hours following reconstitution. The stability of these Tc-99m bone-seeking radiopharmaceuticals (Table 16.4) is improved by maintaining, as nearly as possible, the nitrogen atmosphere in the reaction vial. Introduction of room air into the reaction vial during kit preparation should be avoided, but during withdrawal of a patient dose, it is difficult to prevent entry of room air and oxygen, which contributes to the short shelf-life of these preparations after making them up for use. In vitro stability has also been improved by use of the antioxidants ascorbic acid or gentisic acid.

Mechanism of Localization. The mechanism by which Tc-99m diphosphonate complexes localize within bone is not fully known (Jones AG, et al, 1976). Evidence has been developed over the past several years, however, that explains some of the factors involved in their biodistribution. Central to the bone localization of these radiopharmaceuticals is their delivery to bone, and it has been shown that increased radiopharmaceutical uptake does occur in association with increased vascularity that results from either trauma or disease (Figure 16.4). However, it has been shown that hypervascularity alone does not account for the increased uptake of these radiopharmaceuticals (Francis MD and Fogelman I, 1987). Other factors are involved in their binding and interaction with bone (Lavender JP, et al, 1979).

One explanation for bone uptake is that the Tc-99m phosphorous complex reaches the bone surface intact, then dissociates because of the higher affinity of the phosphorous-containing compound for calcium phosphate. In this hypothesis, the dissociation would then allow reduced Tc-99m to deposit as the hydrolyzed oxide

Table 16.4   CURRENTLY AVAILABLE Tc-99m DIPHOSPHONATE BONE-SEEKING RADIOPHARMACEUTICALS

	TRADEMARK	MANUFACTURER	FORMULATION		
			Ligand	*Reductant*	*Other*
Medronate (MDP)	AN-MDP®	Syncor International	medronic acid 10 mg	stannous chloride 0.6–1.1 mg	—
	MDI MDP kit	Medi-Physics, Inc	medronic acid 10 mg	stannous chloride 0.17 mg	ascorbic acid 2.0 mg
	Osteolite®	Dupont-NEN	medronate disodium 10 mg	stannous and stannic chloride 1.0 mg (0.5 mg minimum stannous chloride)	—
	MDP-Squibb®	Squibb Diagnostics	medronic acid 20 mg	stannous fluoride 0.33 mg	sodium hydroxide 11.0 mg ascorbic acid 1.0 mg
	TechneScan MDP	Mallinckrodt, Inc	medronate 10 mg	stannous chloride 0.8 mg (min.)-1.15 (max.)	—
	Amerscan-MDP®	Amersham	methylene diphosphonate 15.6 mg	stannous fluoride 0.85 mg	—
Oxidronate (HDP)	Osteoscan-HDP®	Mallinckrodt, Inc	oxidronate disodium 2.0 mg	stannous chloride 0.16 mg	gentisic acid 0.56 mg

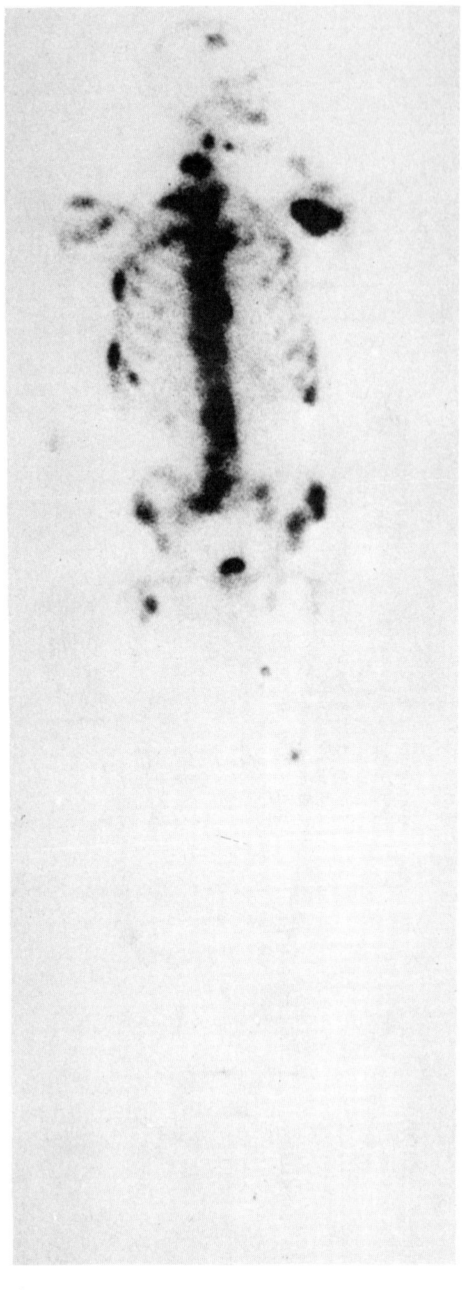

A

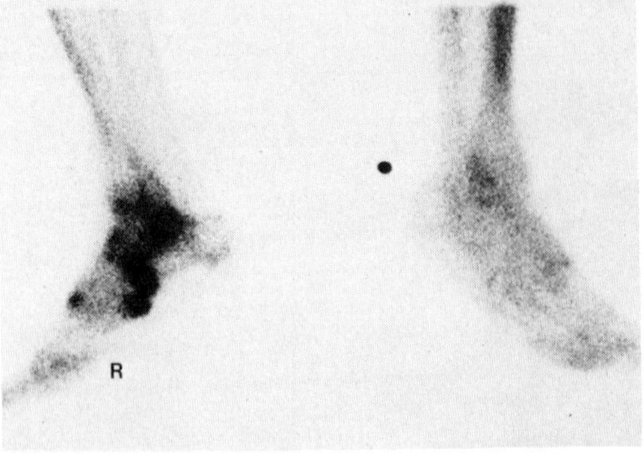

B

Figure 16.4 *Two cases illustrating the utility of bone scanning.*
A. Tc-99m medronate bone scintigram in a patient with prostatic carcinoma illustrating widespread skeletal metastases in classic random distribution throughout the axial skeleton with relative sparing of the appendages.
B. Selected "spot" image illustrating intense tracer localization in torsal fracture.

(Francis MD and Fogelman I, 1987) or as a slightly soluble phosphate. To date, efforts to detect by physical techniques Tc-99m dioxide or Tc-99m phosphates in apatite or amorphous calcium phosphate have failed. Alternatively, the likelihood that the soluble Tc-99m phosphorous complex adsorbs bone as an entity has not yet been determined.

Another theory (Zimmer AM, et al, 1975) suggests that phosphatase enzymes (particularly alkaline phosphatase) may be the localizing factor for bone uptake of these radiopharmaceuticals. Most researchers have concluded, however, that evidence to support this mechanism is lacking because the original report measured enzyme inhibition with levels of diphosphonates several orders of magnitude above those that occur clinically (Francis MD, et al, 1979).

The prevalent explanation for skeletal localization of the Tc-99m diphosphonates is that adsorption occurs onto the mineral phase (hydroxyapatite) of bone with insignificant binding to the organic phase (Francis MD, et al, 1979). Within the mineral phase, it has been shown that Tc-99m diphosphonate bone seekers localize to a much higher degree in amorphous calcium phosphate than crystalline hydroxyapatite. Clinically, areas of increased osteogenic activity secondary to disease or trauma contain higher concentrations of amorphous calcium phosphate than otherwise normal bone. Higher uptake of the Tc-99m bone seekers in amorphous calcium phosphate has been postulated to be due to the presence of a crystal-growing face that provides in its immature phase optimal chemical configuration properties for radiopharmaceutical attachment (Francis MD, et al, 1979; 1980).

The effect of slight alterations in the basic diphosphonate chemical structure have been shown to affect the specificity of these agents for osseous tissues. I. Fogelman and co-workers (1981) found in their comparison of skeletal uptakes of Tc-99m HEDP, MDP, and HDP in normal volunteers that average whole-body retention at 24 hours (reflecting skeletal uptake) was 18.4%, 30.3%, and 36.6%, respectively, for these radiopharmaceuticals. Kinetic studies by J. S. Arnold and associates (1979) suggests that variations in molecular structure may account for the higher uptake of Tc-99m HDP onto bone by leading to tighter binding of this radiopharmaceutical at the osseous binding site. B. L. Barnett and L. C. Strickland (1976) and V. A. Uchtman (1972) have shown by x-ray diffraction studies that with the hydroxyl group on the central carbon of HDP, tridentate chelation is possible because the unshared electrons of the oxygen of the hydroxyl group and an oxygen atom of each phosphonate group exist in the same planar configuration (Figure 16.5). This tridentate alignment is closely similar to that of the three oxygens that coordinate with calcium in the 001-crystal interface. X-ray diffraction and atomic configuration studies have shown that Tc-99m MDP must exist only in a bidentate configuration and, thus, bidentate–bidentate configuration pertains for Tc-99m MDP compared to the higher bidentate–tridentate binding possible with Tc-99m HDP. The dramatic difference in bone uptake and retention between HEDP and HDP is less understood because both radiopharmaceuticals bear a hydroxyl group on the central carbon and are apparently capable of bidentate–tridentate binding. It has been suggested that steric hindrance associated with the methyl group on the central carbon of HEDP prevents

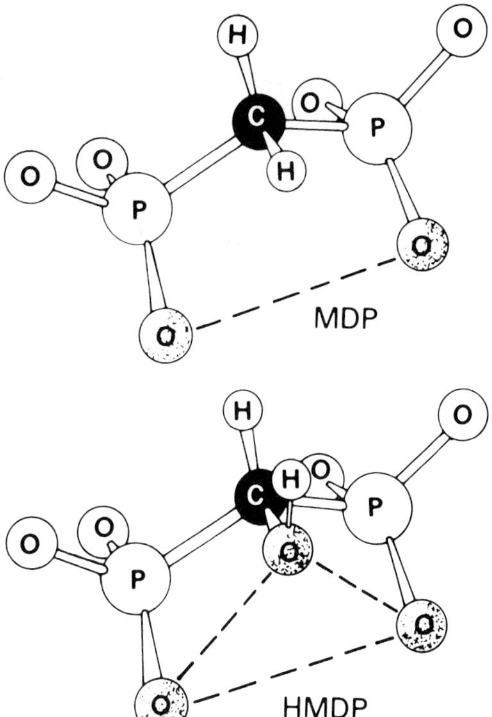

Figure 16.5 Structures of HMDP and MDP compared. Phosphate oxygen atoms are shown unprotonated. Tridentate binding potential of hydroxylated molecules is emphasized in heavy print. From Bevan JA, et al, 1980.

electronic configuration of all three oxygens in the planar geometric alignment or that obscured differences may be a function of altered hydrophilicity/lipophilicity (Francis MD and Fogelman I, 1987).

Among the Tc-99m disphosphonates observed, dissimilarities in bone uptake rates may be due to differences in molecular sizes as well as the occasional formation of diphosphonate polymeric complexes with varying bone specificity and renal execretory rates (Francis MD and Fogelman I, 1987). In an attempt to resolve the mechanism for these observations, the Tc-99m diphosphonate bone-seeking radiopharmaceuticals have recently been the subject of a number of chemical investigations using a variety of techniques. Using high-performance liquid chromatography, a number of different radiolabeled complexes have been isolated from Tc-99m diphosphonates (Pinkerton TC, et al, 1980; 1982). These radiolabeled species have markedly different biodistribution properties that may be manifested as differences in bone uptake and renal clearance, which may explain observed variations in skeletal imaging quality. It is likely that complex coordination of diphosphonate and metal ions (Tc and Sn) results in a complex mixture of oligomeric and polymeric components rather than a single radiolabeled entity. The number and relative concentrations of these components are determined as a function of time, technetium concentration, temperature, and the presence of oxygen.

R.E. Henkin and co-workers (1980) have reported that contrasts in femur to soft-tissue ratios of Tc-99m MDP could be increased by about 20% by increasing the incubation time (from kit reconstitution with Tc-99m sodium pertechnetate until injection) to more than 30 minutes. U. Buell and colleagues (1982) report similar findings with Tc-99m MDP and Tc-99m DPD (dicarboxypropane diphosphonate), another bone-seeking diphosphonate. The precise mechanism which explains their observations has not been determined. R.E. Henkin and associates (1980) raise the possibility that more than one labeling reaction occurs during incubation with compounds formed that have different rates of renal clearance. The kinetics of these reactions may not be as great as the principal reaction, requiring several minutes before equilibrium is attained and the formation of the desired complex, in higher amounts, is favored.

The potential effect of technetium concentration on the radiochemical purity of the diphosphonates was shown by T.C. Pinkerton and associates (1982) and Deutsch and colleagues (1982) when they prepared and tested technetium $(NaBH_4) \cdot HEDP$ prepared from "no-carrier-added" Tc-99m pertechnetate and pertechnetate containing millimolar amounts of Tc-99. HPLC analysis of these reaction mixtures from the "no-carrier-added" pertechnetate exhibited primarily one peak containing over 95% of the radioactivity; however, $Tc(NaBH_4) \cdot HEDP$

prepared from millimolar amounts of Tc-99 yields HPLC chromatograms exhibiting at least seven peaks (Pinkerton TC, et al, 1980). These results indicate that at low metal concentrations (i.e., borohydride reduction of "no-carrier-added" Tc-99m pertechnetate), the formation of polymeric species is disfavored. However, at higher metal concentrations (i.e., ether borohydride reduction of millimolar concentrations of a pseudo-stable Tc-99m or stannous ion reduction of "no-carrier-added" Tc-99m), polymer formation is favored and a range of radiolabeled components occurs that is likely to have varying biodistribution properties and differing elimination characteristics.

PHARMACOKINETICS

During the initial 4–6 hours following intravenous administration, about 50% of both Tc-99m oxidronate and medronate is retained in the skeleton, and about 50% is excreted by the kidneys, primarily by glomerular filtration. Maximal uptake by the skeleton usually occurs within the first hour following injection. Both oxidronate and medronate have similar urinary excretion values showing cumulative urinary excretion of approximately 20%, 40%, and 60% of the injected dose by 2, 4, and 24 hours, respectively (Figure 16.6).

The Tc-99m diphosphonate complexes are cleared from blood in a triphasic manner (Subramanian G, et al, 1975; Mele M, et al, 1983). For Tc-99m medronate the initial rapid tissue distribution phase represents approximately 78% of the injected dose with a biological half-life of 2.4 minutes, the second component represents 20% and a half-life of 51 minutes, and the third represents 1.5% of the dose with a half-life of 14.5 hours. At 1, 4, and 24 hours post injection, the blood levels of Tc-99m medronate are 9.21%, 4.0%, and 0.4% of the administered dose, respectively (Subramanian G, et al, 1975; Littlefield JL and Rudd TG, 1983; Silberstein EB, 1980). At 1 and 4 hours post injection, the blood levels of Tc-99m oxidronate are 8.3% and 3% of the administered dose.

The slightly faster blood clearance of Tc-99m oxidronate may be due to altera-

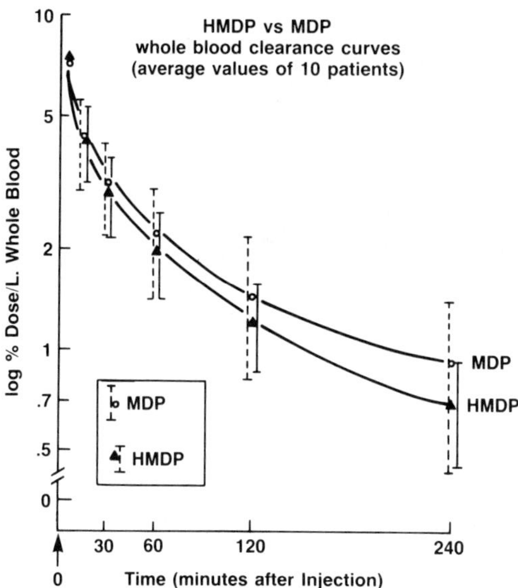

Figure 16.6 Comparative wholebody blood clearance of Tc-99m HMDP (oxidronate) and MDP (medronate). From Littlefield JL and Rudd TG, 1983.

tions in lipophilicity. It has been shown that the presence of the hydroxyl group on the central carbon of HMDP reduces lipophilicity and increases hydrophilicity (compared to MDP), causing, at least in part, the more rapid blood clearance of HMDP (Francis MD and Fogelman I, 1987).

Because significant amounts of these two radiopharmaceuticals are normally excreted by the kidneys, any compromise in renal function and/or the state of hydration of the patient can result in slower-than-normal blood clearance of these agents and, likewise, images that reflect lower bone-to-background ratios.

PRECAUTIONS

Diphosphonates are known to complex cations, such as calcium ions at basic pH, and inhibit both the formation and dissolution of this mineral in vitro at physiological pH. Nonradioactive forms of the diphosphonates are employed therapeutically in patients undergoing total joint replacement to prevent ectopic ossification and to reduce bone turnover in Paget's disease and resorption in bone tumor diseases. Caution would seem appro-

priate and in order whenever radiolabeled forms of these agents are used in patients who have or may be disposed to hypocalcemia; however, in practice, no untoward effects have been reported associated with their use. Calculation of the potential lowering of ionized calcium by chelation with diphosphonate in commercially available products indicates a drop of less than 0.02 mg Ca^{++}/dL is possible.

Rarely, instances of allergic reactions have been reported following the administration of Tc-99m diphosphonate bone seekers (incidence less than 1–6 cases per 100,000 administrations) (Cordova MA, et al, 1987). Similar incidences of a delayed onset rash localized at the site of administration have been reported to appear at 2–24 hours post injection and attributed to the administration of these radiopharmaceuticals (Cordova MA, et al, 1987; Spicer JA, et al, 1985). Other reported adverse reactions include flushing, headache, swelling of the extremities, and nausea and vomiting (Cordova MA, et al, 1984). Reactions involving localized tissue irritation (erythema and pain at the injection site) have been observed with Tc-99m oxidronate that may be allergic in nature or center upon infiltration of the administered dose with a secondary irritation response.

Since bacteriostatic agents have oxidant properties, only preservative-free saline should be used if dilution is necessary during the preparation of these agents (Study KT, et al, 1981). Air should not be injected into the vial during dose preparation (Coupal JJ, et al, 1981). The rubber septum should not be cleaned with an iodinated antiseptic because iodinated antiseptic remaining on the septum may enter the vial by needle puncture and act to oxidize reduced Tc-99m radiopharmaceuticals (Fisher SM, et al, 1977). Radiochemical contaminants (generally free pertechnetate and colloidal Tc-99m species) formed in this manner localize in nonosseous tissues resulting in serious degradation of the skeletal image (Billinghurst MW, et al, 1979; Der M, et al, 1981; Dhawan V and Yeh DJ, 1979). Radiolytic

Table 16.5   SELECTED DRUG-INDUCED AND PATHOLOGY-ASSOCIATED CHANGES IN BIODISTRIBUTION FOR Tc-99m DIPHOSPHONATE RADIOPHARMACEUTICALS EMPLOYED FOR SKELETAL IMAGING

RADIOPHARMACEUTICAL OBSERVED ALTERATION	RESPONSIBLE DRUG OR CONDITION	PROBABLE MECHANISM	REFERENCES
Renal uptake	Vincristine, cyclophosphamide, and doxorubicin, either alone or in combination. Also, amphotericin-B, gentamycin, iron therapy	Direct effect upon renal tubule due to nephostoxic or vascular damage	Lutrin CL, et al, 1978 Trackler RT and Chinn RYW, 1982
Generalized decrease in skeletal uptake of radiopharmaceutical	Long-term steroid therapy in post-menopausal, elderly and debilitated patients	Bone mineral depletion	Powell ML, 1977
Accumulation in breast	Diethylstilbestrol (DES)	Unknown	RamSingh PS, et al, 1977 McRae J, et al, 1976 Choy D, et al, 1981 Parker, et al, 1976
Decrease skeletal uptake, increased renal activity	Supplemental iron therapy	Iron facilitates dissociation of Tc-99m from phosphonate to form a renal specific ligand	
Decreased skeletal uptake	Phospho-Soda	Saturation of bone-binding sites by endogenous phosphorous ions	Saha GB, et al, 1977
Visualization of liver	Aluminum containing antacids (particularly in patients with GI obstructions or impaired renal functions)	Formation of insoluble Tc-99m complex	Chaudhuri TK, 1976a Chaudhuri TK, 1976b Jaresko GS, et al, 1980
Marked renal and hepatic uptake	Sodium diatrizoate	Renal activity due to osmotic effect; ? pH change stimulated hepatic uptake?	Crawford JA, and Gumerman LW, 1978
Extraosseous accumulation	Various-regional chemoperfusion agents heparin, meperidine, iron dextran	Resutant hyperemia with possible complexation to substance administered or deterioration of radiolabled species	Planchon CA, et al, 1983 Sorkin SJ, et al, 1977 VanAntwerp JD, et al, 1975 Balsam D, et al, 1980
Accumulation at injection site (intramuscular iron therapy)	Iron therapy	Formation of insoluble iron complex with Tc-99m diphosphonate	Duong RB, et al, 1984 Mazzola AL, et al, 1976

decomposition (Billinghurst MW, et al, 1979), the presence of oxidizing substances (Tofe AJ, et al, 1980), the presence of Al^{+3} ions (Chaudhuri TK, 1976a), improper pH (Chaudhuri TK, 1976b), time-associated degradation (Tofe AJ et al, 1980) and inadequate incubation of the formed radiopharmaceutical prior to use (Henkin RE, et al, 1980; Buell U, et al, 1982) have all been mentioned as causes of poor-quality images involving these bone-seeking radiopharmaceuticals.

Drug-Related Alterations in Biodistribution. W. B. Hladik III and colleagues (1982; 1987), in their comprehensive review of alterations in radiopharmaceutical biodistribution, have detailed a variety of pharmacological causes of biodistribution changes for the Tc-99m diphosphonate agents (Table 16.5).

Use During Pregnancy/Breastfeeding. The use of these radiopharmaceuticals during pregnancy is contraindicated. It is not known whether Tc-99m medronate or oxidronate are distributed in breast milk; however, Tc-99m pertechnetate, a radiochemical impurity often found in varying quantities in most Tc-99m radiopharmaceuticals, is secreted in breast milk. Therefore, it is generally advisable that following the administration of these radiopharmaceuticals, breastfeeding should be discontinued for at least 4 hours (ICRP, 1988), or until levels of radioactivity in breast milk are considered safe.

DOSAGE/DOSIMETRY

In adults, bone imaging is accomplished by the intravenous administration of 15–20 mCi of either Tc-99m MDP or HMDP (Figure 16.7). Images are obtained 2–3 hours later. Because a significant fraction of either radiopharmaceutical that is not taken up by bone is rapidly cleared from blood by renal filtration, patients should be adequately hydrated and instructed to void frequently before imaging. Activity

in the bladder may interfere with visualization of pelvic lesions.

Use in Children. The safety and efficacy of either Tc-99m medronate or oxidronate in children have not been established. However, in practice, these radiopharmaceuticals are often routinely employed in pediatrics with appropriate adjustment of the administered activity based on weight and/or body surface area (see Chapter 9).

Radiation dosimetry for both Tc-99m MDP and HMDP is shown in Table 16.6.

CLINICAL CONSIDERATIONS

Uptake of the bone-seeking radiopharmaceuticals occurs due to localized increases in both skeletal blood supply and bone metabolic activity. Blood flow has the greatest effect upon bone uptake of the Tc-99m diphosphonates, both when circulation is restricted or slightly increased. Large increases in localized blood flow does not in itself cause a proportional increase in bone uptake of these radiopharmaceuticals. As a general rule, localized increased radiopharmaceutical accumulation almost always indicates pathology or trauma by identifying sites of bone repair. Less frequently, however, areas of skeletal destruction appear as photon-deficient (i. e., photopenic) lesions wherein radiopharmaceutical uptake fails to occur (Figure 16.8). In bone imaging, photopenic regions usually are the manifestations of large lytic lesions with locally diminished blood supply, which prevents subsequent delivery of the bone-seeking radiopharmaceutical.

The Tc-99m bone-seeking radiopharmaceuticals may, under certain conditions, localize in extraosseous lesions such as dystrophic calcification (as in hyperparathyroidism, heterotopic bone formation), calcifying lesions such as neuroblastoma, metastatic soft-tissue calcification, skeletal muscle necrosis, and myocardial infarction (Figure 16.9). Although the Tc-99m diphosphonate complexes are clearly superior to Tc-99m pyrophosphate for

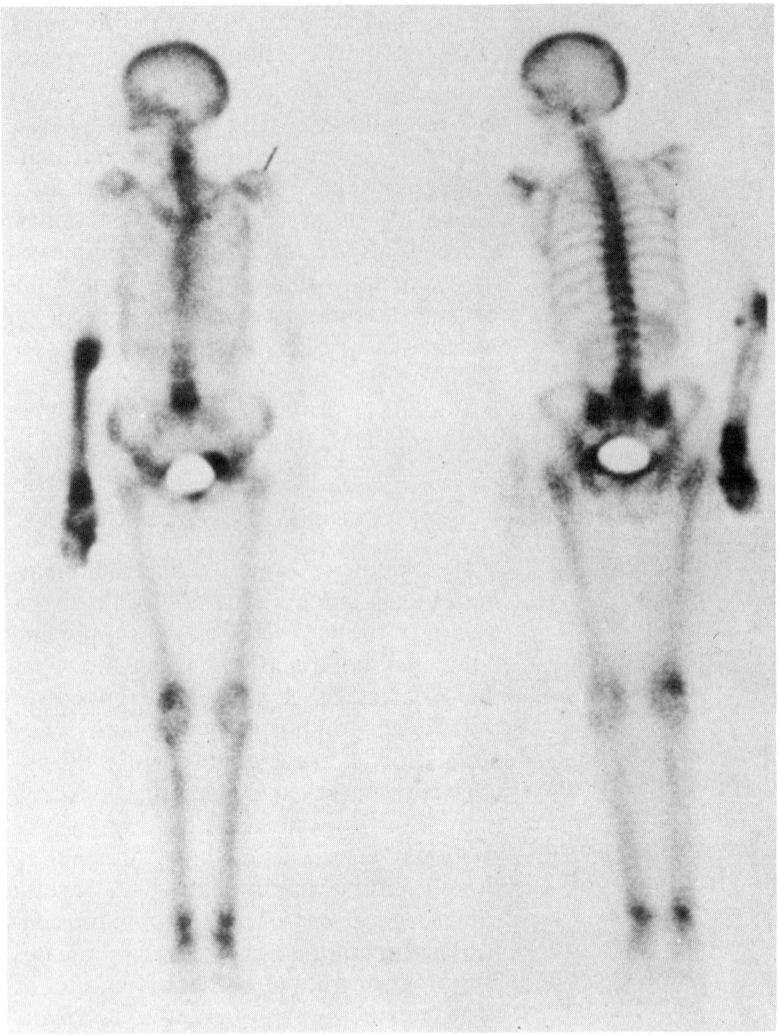

Figure 16.7 Inadvertent arterial injection of Tc-99m MDP that results in the "gauntlet" appearance on subsequent imaging. The pattern of distribution illustrates a high first-transit extraction of the radiopharmaceutical.

Table 16.6 ESTIMATED RADIATION ABSORBED DOSE IN AN ADULT FOR Tc-99m MEDRONATE (MDP) AND Tc-99m OXIDRONATE (HMDP)[a]

	RADS/MCI	
ORGAN	*Tc-99m MDP*	*Tc-99m HMDP*
Bone surface	0.2	0.29
Red marrow	0.029	0.040
Bladder wall	0.18	0.12
Kidneys	0.013	0.012
Ovaries	0.012	0.010
Testes	0.0079	0.0075
Total body	0.0085	0.011

[a] Personal communication from Radiopharmaceutical Internal Dose Information Center, Oak Ridge Associated Universities, Oak Ridge, TN.

skeletal imaging, direct comparative studies have shown that Tc-99m pyrophosphate is superior to all other Tc-99m diphosphonate complexes for the detection of myocardial infarction (see Chapter 13).

Whether Tc-99m oxidronate or Tc-99m medronate is the superior Tc-99m diphosphonate for skeletal imaging has not been clearly resolved, although a number of clinical studies have addressed this issue. The majority of studies found no difference in image quality between these two

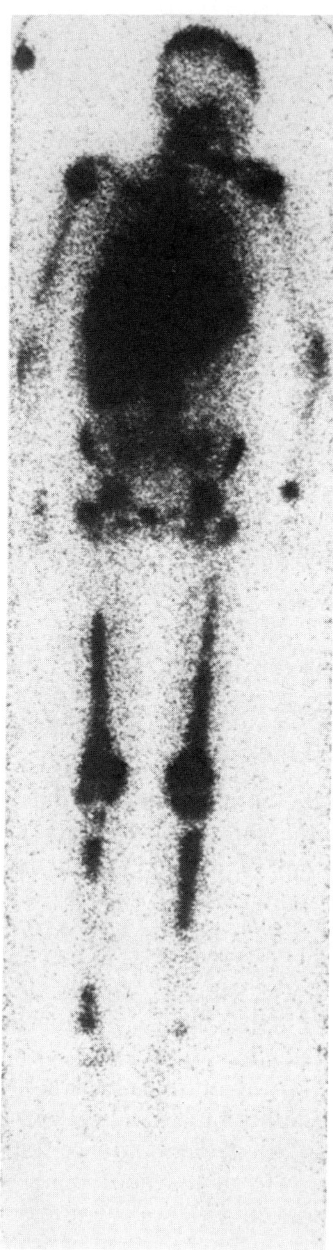

Figure 16.8 Anterior whole-body view from a Tc-99m sulfur colloid bone marrow scan in a patient with sickle cell anemia. There is abnormal expansion of marrow activity into the extremities and intense skull activity characteristic of this disease. Note the multiple "cold" areas in the long bones resulting from prior bone marrow infarctions. The intense abdominal activity is due to Tc-99m sulfur colloid uptake in the liver.

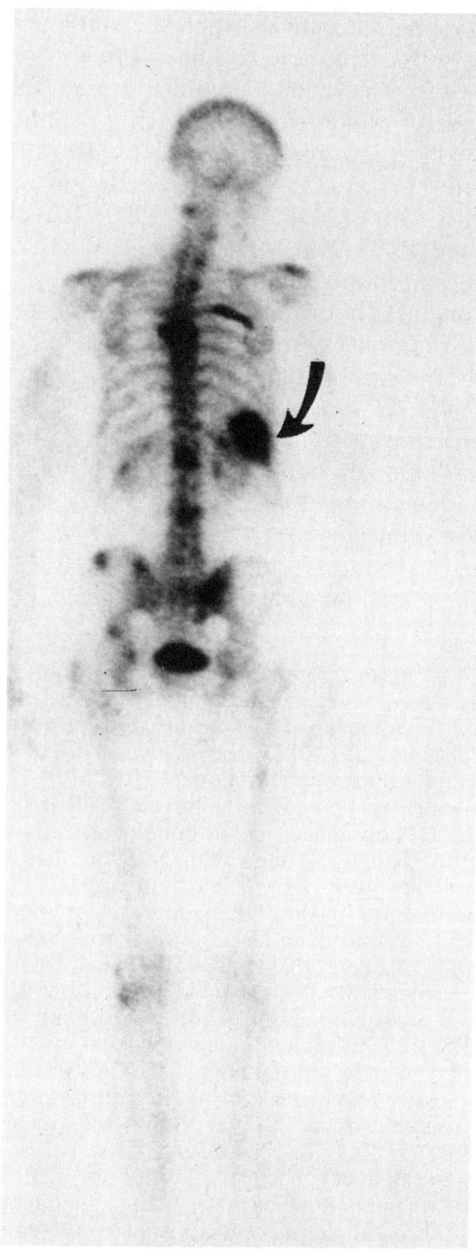

Figure 16.9 Tc-99m MDP bone scintigram in a patient with breast cancer metastatic to bone and liver. There is intense localization of the radiopharmaceutical in the liver metastasis (liver) in addition to skeletal lesions.

radiopharmaceuticals when skeletal imaging was performed at 2 and 4 hours following intravenous administration (the times at which skeletal imaging is most usually performed) (Littlefield JL and Rudd TG, 1983; Van Duzee BF, et al, 1984; Domstad PA et al, 1980). Compared to Tc-99m MDP, bone-to-soft tissue ratios are higher with Tc-99m oxidronate at both of these times, however, the differences were not statistically significant. Most studies found the quality of the Tc-99m oxidronate image superior; however, no study has found that Tc-99m oxidronate has any greater ability to detect skeletal lesions. As a result, most clinicians feel that these two radiopharmaceuticals offer comparable utility for skeletal imaging.

The newest research involving radiopharmaceuticals for skeletal imaging includes the diphosphonates, Tc-99m dicarboxypropane diphosphonate (DPD) and Tc-99m di-methyl-amino-methane diphosphonate (DMAD). Limited clinical investigation has shown that Tc-99m DPD produces higher bone-to-soft tissue ratios than those seen with Tc-99m medronate; however, lesion detection appears no greater with Tc-99m DPD since Tc-99m medronate shows higher lesion-normal bone ratios (Mele M, et al, 1983; Pauwel EKJ, et al, 1983).

Tc-99m DMAD also provides significant uptake in *osseous* lesions; however, unlike all other Tc-99m skeletal imaging agents investigated to date, only minimal amounts of this radiopharmaceutical localize in normal bone (Rosenthall L, et al, 1982; Smith ML, et al, 1984). Though Tc-99m DMAD may be capable of delineating skeletal lesions not seen in Tc-99m medronate scans (since the low uptake of this radiopharmaceutical in normal bone results in very high lesion-to-bone ratios), it remains to be seen how sensitive DMAD is for skeletal lesions and whether the slightly higher muscle uptake mentioned by G. Subramanian and associates (1983) may be disadvantageous. Also, many clinicians may find the failure to visualize the skeleton during Tc-99m DMAD imaging highly undesirable because normal anatomic markers would no longer be visible. Likewise, photon-deficient lesions may not be readily appreciated with Tc-99m DMAD imaging in the absence of normal bone visualization. Still unexplored, however, is whether the formulation of two or more scanning agents in some yet-to-be-determined ratio of a lesion-only bone seeker with an existing bone-seeking radiopharmaceutical would result in superior lesion definition while permitting visualization of normal bone for anatomic reference.

II. Bone Marrow Imaging

Bone marrow imaging has been shown potentially useful in a variety of clinical disorders that affect marrow and hematological function, including tumor invasion, leukemia, and lymphomas. Today, bone marrow imaging is primarily of benefit in the diagnosis of bone infarction, especially in patients with sickle cell anemia when bone pain may due to either infarction or infection (DeNardo SJ, et al, 1975). It also has usefulness in the localization of sites for bone marrow biopsy.

RADIOPHARMACEUTICALS FOR BONE MARROW IMAGING

BACKGROUND/HISTORY

During the 1950s, fundamental clinical and experimental work involving the biodistribution of Au-198 colloid (Zilversmit DB, et al, 1952; Dobson EL and Jones HB, 1952; Root SW, et al, 1954; Krook HG, 1956) showed that intravenously injected Au-198 was cleared rapidly and efficiently from blood by the phagocytic cells of the reticuloendothelial system. Although most of the administered activity localized within the liver and spleen, a small amount of Au-198 colloid was trapped by the RE cells of the bone marrow that could be imaged with scintillation devices. The relatively long physical half-life (2.7 days) and Beta-minus decay mode of Au-198 limited the amount of activity that could be safely administered to less than 0.5–1.0 mCi. These activities still provided a radiation-absorbed dose to the liver (the critical organ) of around 50 rads.

Because in normal subjects marrow erythropoiesis accounts for 80–90% of plasma iron turnover, radioisotopes of iron can also be employed for bone marrow imaging utilizing this localization pathway. Radioisotopes of iron that have

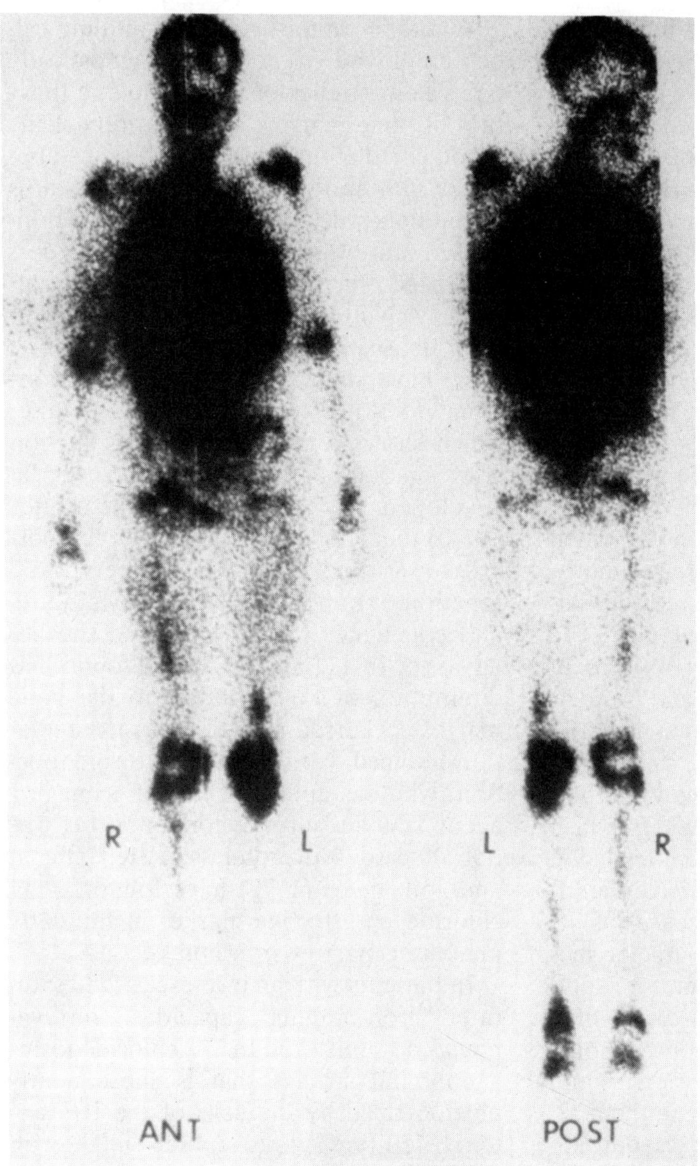

Figure 16.10   Anterior and posterior whole-body bone marrow scans performed with 10 millicuries Tc-99m sulfur colloid in patient with sickle cell anemia. Images show marrow expansion into extremities with photon deficient foci due to previous infarcts. Note increased marrow uptake in skull. Intense activity in liver is normally expected due to prominent distribution within RE system.

been utilized for this purpose include Fe-59 and the accelerator product Fe-52. A primary advantage of radioiron imaging over reticuloendothelial imaging of the bone marrow is that erythropoietically active marrow can be identified in contrast to the active RE portions. The clinical significance lies in the fact that expansion and contraction of the erythropoietic system is not always accompanied by a corresponding change in the reticuloendothelial cell activity (Van Dyke D, et al, 1967). From a physiologic standpoint, therefore, radioiron is ideal since the capacity to evaluate the functional marrow is realized. Of the radioisotopes of iron available, however, none have satisfactory imaging properties. Fe-59 is unsatisfactory due to its relatively high principal gamma energies of 1.1 and 1.3 MeV and its decay by Beta-minus emission. Fe-52, on the other hand, is limited in availability since its 8-hour physical half-life requires nearby cyclotron production facilities. As a result of the limited availability of Fe-52, this agent is rarely employed for marrow imaging. Fe-59, as ferrous citrate, is occasionally employed for marrow imaging, however, instrumentation necessary to adequately image the high energy emissions of Fe-59 is not commonly available.

Marrow localization is also noted when radioisotopes of indium are administered intravenously as the chloride salt (Mishkin F and Reese IC, 1968). The sites of localization appear to closely mimic that of iron (Lilien DL and Bennett L, 1973). Indium injected at a low pH binds transferrin in exactly the same manner as iron with a competitive inhibition demonstrated between the two (Beamish MR and Brown EB, 1974a). Biologically, however, indium does not behave identically to iron, probably because of its markedly different redox characteristics compared to iron. Ionic indium, for example, clears more slowly from blood than does iron (physical half-life of 6–10 hours versus 1–2 hours for iron transferrin) and accumulates to a lesser degree in the marrow (McIntyre PA, et al, 1973; Rayudu VS, et al, 1973; Staub RF and Gaston E, 1973). Erythrocyte localization is also markedly different with up to 80% of the injected dose of iron appearing in the circulating erythrocytes by 12–24 days (Harris JW and Kellermeyer RW, 1970) compared to only 4% for indium (Farrer PA, et al, 1973). Indium does show, however, greater liver uptake. M.R. Beamish and E.B. Brown (1974a;b) found that indium binding to red blood cells is reversible and that indium does not bind to hemoglobin, binding instead to the cell membrane. Of the radioisotopes of indium available, In-111 offers imaging properties that are most desirable.

Whether radioisotopes of indium can be employed to obtain diagnostically equivalent studies of hematopoietic function of bone marrow is not entirely clear. Good correlations have been reported between indium scans and the clinical status of patients with aplastic anemia, myelofibrosis, and other hematological disorders (Horn NL, et al, 1980; Sayle BA, et al, 1982; McNeil BJ, et al, 1974). Indium-111 chloride scans of irradiated bone, however, have shown that localization of indium does not follow radioiron uptake, which shows a marked uptake reduction after irradiation. Using an animal model developed by W.B. Nelp and associates (1970) that showed that radiation temporarily disassociates the RES and erythroid function of bone marrow, P.A. McIntyre and colleagues (1974) compared the behavior of In-111 and Fe-59 and found that diminution of Fe-59 uptake in the bone marrow occurred secondary to the radiation-induced depression of erythroid function, whereas uptake of the RES imaging agent Tc-99m sulfur colloid or In-111 was not affected. Nevertheless, M.K. Jeffcoat and colleagues (1978) have found In-111 chloride an effective marker in the early phases of marrow iron uptake.

In patients with an iron excess and saturated iron-binding capacities, intravenously administered In-111 chloride forms a colloidal species that is subsequently phagocytized by the cells of the RE system (McIntyre PA, 1977; McNeil BJ, et al, 1974). Transferrin saturation can be a contributing factor, therefore, to explain the RES behavior of In-111 chloride in these patients.

The development of Tc-99m sulfur colloid provided a nearly ideal radiopharmaceutical for imaging the RE system (Richards P, 1960; Harper PV, et al, 1964). Tc-99m sulfur colloid is relatively convenient to prepare and offers ready availability. The principal gamma emission of Tc-99m at 140 keV is well suited for imaging with conventional scintillation instrumentation and its highly desirable decay by isomeric transition results in relatively low radiation dosimetry. Like Au-198 colloid, the small fraction of the administered activity that localizes in the RE cells of the bone marrow enables scintillation detection of reticuloendothelial activity.

Due to its relative convenience and highly desirable nuclear properties, Tc-99m sulfur colloid has for many years been the most widely employed radiopharmaceutical for bone marrow imaging. Investigators have tried to improved upon this agent for bone marrow imaging by developing other Tc-99m labeled agents that are intended to have specificity for bone marrow localization. Tc-99m stannous phytate (inisitol hexaphosphate) (Subramanian G, et al, 1973) showed biodistribution values in the marrow of rats as high as 30% of the injected dose but did not give the same results in humans. More recently, Tc-99m microaggregated albumin, another colloid of Tc-99m, has been employed for imaging the RE system. The particle size of this radiopharmaceutical is well within the colloid size range, although it has been reported that Tc-99m microaggregated albumin colloid shows bone marrow-to-liver ratios that are approximately 60% higher than those seen with Tc-99m sulfur colloid (Klingensmith WC, et al, 1982). It is known that the RE cells of the bone marrow preferentially phagocytize smaller sized colloids than the cells of liver and spleen, indicating that the Tc-99m microaggregated albumin colloid possesses greater numbers of such particles. Attempts have been made to develop a formulation of Tc-99m sulfur colloid that contains a larger proportion of smaller sized colloid particles than other preparations. H.L. Atkins, et al (1969) reported the use of the hydrogen sulfide method for preparing Tc-99m sulfur colloid for bone marrow imaging. This method, which involves the bubbling of H_2S gas in an acidified solution of Tc-99m pertechnetate and gelatin, yields particles approximately one-tenth the size of the commercially available sulfur colloid formulations that utilize sodium thiosulfate and acid to generate sulfur colloid.

Millipore filtration (0.22 micron pore diameter) of Tc-99m sulfur colloid prior to injection is useful to remove the undesirably larger colloid particles that would localize to a greater extent in the liver and spleen.

CHEMISTRY

Tc-99m Sulfur Colloid (SC). Tc-99m sulfur colloid, the most commonly used radiopharmaceutical for bone marrow imaging, exists as an insoluble heptasulfide (Tc_2S_7), which is co-precipitated with colloidal sulfur and technetium with gelatin (see Chapter 14 for a greater detailed explanation of the production of Tc-99m sulfur colloid). Kit-type formulations used to prepare Tc-99m sulfur colloid contain an acid (either phosphorous or hydrochloric), sodium thiosulfate, a buffer, and gelatin. In the preparation of Tc-99m sulfur colloid, generator-produced Tc-99m sodium pertechnetate is added to an acidic solution of sodium thiosulfate, and this mixture is heated in a boiling water bath for approximately 5–12 minutes. Following heating, the vial is briefly vented and a buffer is added to the mixture to neutralize pH. Certain commercial formulations require at this point an additional boiling for 5–8 minutes. Gelatin is used in many formulations as a surface-active stabilizer to prevent colloid particles from becoming undesirably large. The range of particle sizes of Tc-99m sulfur colloid prepared by this technique is 0.1–2 microns (Kniseley RM, 1972).

Tc-99m Albumin Colloid (AC). This radiopharmaceutical is prepared from human serum albumin that has been heat denatured in an acidified media. Particle size range is 0.1–3 microns. Technetium-99m radiolabeling of albumin colloid occurs via the stannous ion-mediated reduction of generator-produced pertechnetate to a lower oxidation state (probably IV). Heating is not a requirement for the preparation of Tc-99m AC. In the United States, the only commercially available formulation of Tc-99m AC is Microlite™ (Dupont-NEN, North Billerica, MA). A description of the components of this formulation can be found in Chapter 14.

PHARMACOKINETICS

Following intravenous administration, both Tc-99m SC and Tc-99m AC are rapidly cleared from blood by the RE system with a clearance rate of 2–3 minutes. In normal patients, both radiopharmaceuticals demonstrate 80–85% of the administered activity localizing in the liver,

5–10% in the spleen, and the remainder of the dose localizing primarily in the bone marrow. Slightly greater bone marrow uptake has been reported with Tc-99m AC (Klingensmith WC, et al, 1982). Lung uptake of Tc-99m colloidal radiopharmaceuticals has been reported and often involves the activation of pulmonary reticuloendothelial cells in severe disease. A primary distinction between these two radiopharmaceuticals is that Tc-99m AC is catabolized following RE cell localization due to its protein nature. Tc-99m SC is believed to remain fixed within the RE cells and does not undergo any form of metabolic degradation. Tc-99m AC is not metabolized so rapidly, however, to cause any defect in image quality during RE imaging. Localization of both radiopharmaceuticals in the principal organs of the RE system is essentially complete by 15 minutes after injection, and Tc-99m AC levels in the organs of the RE system remain constant for at least 4 hours afterwards.

PRECAUTIONS

Because Tc-99m AC contains human serum albumin and many Tc-99m SC formulations include gelatin, it is possible that hypersensitivity reactions may occur whenever these foreign proteins are administered in humans. Cardiopulmonary arrest, bronchospasm, anaphylactic shock, seizures, flushing, nausea, vomiting, dizziness, weakness, hypertension, and hypotension have all been reported with the use of Tc-99m SC. Although rare, deaths have occurred following intravenous administration of Tc-99m SC containing gelatin. Severe adverse reactions have also been reported following the use of Tc-99m AC. Over a 5 year period from 1976–1981, the incidence of adverse reactions associated with the use of Tc-99m sulfur colloid has been reported to be less than 19 per 100,000 administrations. The frequency of adverse reactions for Tc-99m microaggregated albumin colloid has not been established because the product has only been available for a short period of time. Anaphylactoid reactions, however, have been associated with the use of this product (Cordova MA, et al, 1987).

Because severe hypersensitivity reactions have been associated with the use of these products, prompt medical treatment, including corticosteroids, pressor agents, and a means for providing cardiopulmonary support should be readily available.

Use During Pregnancy and Breastfeeding. Tc-99m (as the radiochemical impurity-free, unbound pertechnetate) is excreted into human breast milk during lactation. Because varying amounts of Tc-99m pertechnetate can be expected to occur in both Tc-99m sulfur colloid and Tc-99m microaggregated albumin, it is suggested that formula feedings should be substituted for breast feedings for 12 hours following the intravenous administration of both these radiopharmaceuticals (ICRP, 1988).

Animal reproductive studies have not been conducted with either Tc-99m sulfur colloid or microaggregated albumin. It is not known whether either of these radiopharmaceuticals can cause fetal harm when administered during pregnancy. V. Hahn and associates (1980) has estimated that less than 0.05% of activity from Tc-99m sulfur colloid crosses the placenta. Whether this represents Tc-99m sulfur colloid or a freely diffusible Tc-99m radiochemical impurity (i. e., pertechnetate) is not clear. These radiopharmaceuticals should be given during pregnancy only if the benefits to be expected clearly outweigh any risks that might reasonably be anticipated to occur.

Storage Data. Prior to use, the kits of these products may be stored at room temperature. Following radiolabeling with generator-produced Tc-99m sodium pertechnetate, Tc-99m sulfur colloid may be stored at room temperature. Tc-99m microaggregated albumin colloid should be stored at 2–8 degrees centigrade following radiolabeling. Both radiopharmaceuticals should be protected from excessive exposure to light.

Dosage/Dosimetry

For bone marrow imaging, it is necessary to administer doses of Tc-99m sulfur colloid and Tc-99m microaggregated albumin colloid that are considerably larger than those employed for routine liver and spleen imaging. Doses of 10–12 mCi are required for bone marrow imaging (versus 3–5 mCi for liver and spleen imaging) in order to visualize the marrow. The procedure calls for the radiopharmaceutical to be administered intravenously, with imaging to begin 15 minutes later. No special patient preparation is required.

Radiation dosimetry figures for both these radiopharmaceuticals are listed in Chapter 14.

Clinical Considerations

Bone marrow imaging is a useful procedure for defining the location and extent of functioning marrow in a variety of hematoalogic disorders including lymphoma, leukemias, anemias, and myelofibrosis. It can also be helpful in localizing sites for bone marrow biopsy and will demonstrate (as cold regions) areas of marrow invasion by metastatic disease. Bone marrow imaging with Tc-99m sulfur colloid or microaggregated albumin colloid can be used to define areas of decreased marrow function secondary to radiation therapy and as a crude measure of functional marrow reserve in patients on chemotherapy. The presence and extent of bone marrow infarctions in patients with sickle cell anemia may be depicted by bone marrow imaging.

Bone marrow imaging with RES-type agents, such as Tc-99m sulfur colloid, is limited, however, in that the marrow distribution of functional hematopoietic cells is not always uniform, particularly in disease. The considerable variations that exist in marrow distribution patterns of many hematologic disorders require that bone marrow studies performed with Tc-99m sulfur colloid or microaggregated albumin colloid be interpreted in light of the existing clinical situation.

At this time, In-111 chloride has not received approval by the Food and Drug Administration for routine use in bone marrow imaging.

References

Abt AF, Farmer CJ. Vitamin C: Pharmacology and therapeutics. *JAMA* 1938, 111:1555–1565.

Ardran GM. Bone destruction not demonstrable by radiography. *Br J Radiol* 1951, 24:107–109.

Arnold JS, Barnes WF, Khedkar N, et al. Kinetic studies of a new and superior Tc-99m diphosphonate bone imaging agent. *J Nucl Med* 1979, 20:653–654.

Atkins HL, Hauser W, Richards P. Factors affecting distribution of Tc-99m sulfur colloid. *J Nucl Med* 1969, 10:319–322.

Balsam D, Goldfarb CR, Stringer B, et al. Bone scintrigraphy for neonatal osteomyelitis: Simulation by extravasation of intravenous calcium. *Radiology* 1980, 135:185–186.

Barnett BL, Strickland LC. Structure of disodium dihydrogen-1-hydroxyethylidene diphosphonate tetrahydrate: A bone growth regulator. *Acta Cryst* 1976, B35:1212–1214.

Bauer GCH. Skeletal metabolism in humans studied with body surface coating of Sr-85 and Ca-47. In Extermann RC (ed.), U.N.E.S.C.O. International Conference on Radioisotopes, Paris, 1957, Vol. 4, New York, Pergamon Press, p. 232, 1958.

Bauer GCH, Wendeberg B. External counting of Ca-47 and Sr-85 in studies of localized skeletal lesions in man. *J Bone Joint Surg (Br)* 1959, 41B:558.

Beamish MR, Brown EB. A comparison of the behavior of In-111 and Fe-59 labeled transferrin on incubation with human and rat reticulocytes. *Blood* 1974a, 43:703–711.

Beamish MR, Brown EB. The metabolism of transferrin bound ^{111}In and ^{59}Fe in the rat. *Blood* 1974b, 43, 693–701.

Bevan JA, Tofe AJ, Benedict JJ, et al. Tc-99m HMDP (Hydroxymethylene Diphosphonate): A radiopharmaceutical for skeletal and acute myocardial infarction imaging. I. Synthesis and distribution in animals. *J Nucl Med* 1980, 21:961–966.

Billinghurst MW, Rempel S, Westendorf BA. Radiation decomposition of ^{99m}Tc radiopharmaceuticals. *J Nucl Med* 1979, 20:138–143.

Blau M, Nagler W, Bender MA. Fluorine-18. A new isotope for bone scanning. *J Nucl Med* 1962, 3:332.

Borak J. Relationships between the clinical and roentgenological findings in bone metastases. *Surg Gynecol Obstet*, 1942, 75:599–612.

Bradley DW, Maynard JE, Emery G. Comparison of ascorbic acid concentrations in whole blood obtained by venipuncture and by finger prick. *Clin Chem* 1972, 18:968–970.

Buell U, Kleinhans E, Zorn-Bopp E, et al. A comparison of bone imaging with Tc-99m DPD and Tc-99m MDP: Concise communication. *J Nucl Med* 1982, 23:214–217.

Castronovo FP, Jr, Callahan RJ. New bone scanning agent: ^{99m}Tc-labeled 1-hydroxy-ethylidene-1, 1-disodium phosphonate. *J Nucl Med* 1972, 13:823–827.

Charkes ND, Sklaroff DM, Bierly J. Detection of metastatic cancer to bone by scintiscanning with strontium-87m. *Am J Roentgenol* 1964, 91:1121.

Chaudhuri TK. The effect of aluminum and pH on altered body distribution of Tc-99m EHDP. *Int J Nucl Med Biol* 1976a 3:37.

Chaudhuri TK. Liver uptake of Tc-99m-diphosphonate. *Radiology* 1976b, 119:485–486.

Chiewitz O, Hevesy G. Radioactive indicators in the study of phosphorous metabolism in rats. *Nature* 1935, 13:754.

Choy D, Murray IPC, Hoschl R. The effect of iron on the biodistribution of bone scanning agents in humans. *Radiology* 1981, 140:197–202.

Cordova MA, Hladik WB III, Rhodes BA. Validation and characterization of adverse reactions to radiopharmaceuticals. *Noninvasive Med Imag* 1984, 1:17–24.

Cordova MA, Hladik WB III, Rhodes BA. Adverse reactions associated with radiopharmaceuticals. In *Essentials of Nuclear Medicine Science*, Hladik WB, III, Saha GB, Study KT (eds). Baltimore, Williams and Wilkins, 1987, 303–320.

Cordova MA, Rhodes BA, Atkins HL, et al. Adverse reactions to radiopharmaceuticals. (Letter) *J Nucl Med* 1982, 23:550–551.

Costeas A, Woodward HQ, Laughlin J. Depletion of 18-F from blood flowing through bone. *J Nucl Med* 1970, 11:43–48.

Coupal JJ, Kim EE, Deland FH. Effects of dissolved oxygen on ^{99m}Tc methylene diphosphonate: Concise communication. *J Nucl Med* 1981, 22:153–156.

Crawford JA, Gumerman LW. Alteration of body distribution of ^{99m}Tc-pyrophosphate by radiographic contrast material. *Clin Nucl Med* 1978, 3:305–307.

Davis MA, Jones AG. Comparison of ^{99m}Tc-labeled phosphate and phosphonate agents for skeletal imaging. *Semin Nucl Med* 1976, 6:19–31.

Demole V. On the physiological action of ascorbic acid and some related compounds. *Biochem J* 1934, 28:770–773.

DeNardo SJ, Hamel CF, Lewis AP, et al. Assessment of the bone and marrow in sickle cell disease. *J Nucl Med* 1975, 13:425–426.

Der M, Ballinger JR, Bowen BM. Decomposition of ^{99m}Tc pyrophosphate by peroxides in pertechnetate used in preparation. *J Nucl Med* 1981, 22:645–646.

Desgrez MH, Guerin RA, Guerin MT. Le test au 72-gallium dans les tumeurs malignes des os. *Presse Med* 1954, 62;997-1006.

Deutsch E, Barnett BL. Inorganic chemistry in biology and medicine. ACS Symposium Series 140, Martell AE (ed.), Washington, American Chemical Society, 1980, pp. 103–120.

Deutsch E, Heineman WR, Zodda JP, et al. Preparation of "no-carrier added" Technetium-99m complexes: Determination of the total technetium content of generator elutions. *Int J Appl Radiat Isot* 1982, 33:843–848.

Deutsch E, Libson K, Becker CB, et al. Preparation and biological distribution of technetium diphosphonate radiotracers synthesized without stannous ion. *J Nucl Med* 1980, 21:859–866.

Dewanjee MK, Fletcher JW, Davis MA. Chemical properties and biologic distribution of technetium-tin-polyphosphates (abst). *J Nucl Med* 1972, 13:427.

Dhawan V, Yeh DJ. Labeling efficiency and stomach concentration in methylene diphosphonate bone imaging. *J Nucl Med* 1979, 20:791–793.

Dobson EL, Jones HB. The behavior of intravenously injected particulate material: Its rate of disappearance from the bloodstream as a measure of liver blood flow. *Acta Med Scand* 1952 (Suppl), 273:8–12.

Domstad PA, Coupal JJ, Kim EE, et al. ^{99m}Tc-hydroxymethane diphosphonate: A new bone imaging agent with a low tin content. *Radiology* 1980, 136:209–211.

Dudley HC, Markowitz HA, Mitchell TG. Studies on the localization of radioactive gallium (Ga-72) in bone lesions. *J Bone Joint Surg* 1956, 38A:627.

Duong RB, Volarich DT, Fernandez-Ulloa M, et al. Tc-99m MDP bone scan artifact-Abdominal soft-tissue uptake secondary to subcutaneous heparin injection. *Clin Nucl Med* 1984, 9:47.

Farrer PA, Saha GB, Katz M. Further observations of the use of In-111-transferrin for the visualization of bone marrow in man. (Abst) *J Nucl Med* 1973, 394–495.

Fisher SM, Brown RG, Greyson ND. Unbinding of Tc-99m by iodinated antiseptics. *J Nucl Med* 1977, 18:1139–1140.

Fleming WH, McIlraith JD, King ER. Photoscanning of bone lesions utilizing strontium-85. *Radiology* 1961, 77:635.

Fletcher JW, Solaric-George E, Henry RE, et al. Evaluation of ^{99m}Tc-pyrophosphate as a bone imaging agent. *Radiology* 1973, 109:467–469.

Fogelman I, Pearson DW, Bessent RG, et al. A comparison of skeletal uptakes of three diphosphonates by whole body retention: Concise communication. *J Nucl Med* 1981, 22:880–883.

Francis MD, Ferguson DL, Tofe AJ, et al. Comparative evaluation of three diphosphonates: In vivo adsorption (C^{14}-labeled) and in vivo osteogenic uptake (Tc-99m complexed). *J Nucl Med* 1980, 21:1185–1189.

Francis MD, Fogelman I. ^{99m}Tc Diphosphonate uptake mechanism on bone. In *Bone Scanning in Clinical Practice.* London, Springer-Verlag, 7–18, 1987.

Francis MD, Slough CL, Tofe AJ. Factors affecting uptake and retention of Tc-99m-diphosphonate and 99m-technetate in osseous connective and soft tissue. *Calcif Tissue Res*, 1976, 20:303–311.

Francis MD, Tofe AJ, Benedict JJ, et al. Imaging the skeletal system. In Radiopharmaceuticals II. Proceedings of the Second International Symposium on Radiopharmaceuticals, Sodd VJ, Allen DR, Hoogland DR, Ice RD (eds), New York, Society of Nuclear Medicine, pp 603–614, 1979.

Francis MD, Tofe AJ, Hiles RA, et al. Inorganic tin: Chemistry, disposition, and role in nuclear medicine diagnostic skeletal imaging agents. *Int J Nucl Med* 1981, 8:145–152.

Hahn V, Brod K, Wolf R. The radiation dose to the fetus during isotope investigations of the mother. *Fortschr Roentgentsr* 1980, 132(3):326–330.

Harper PV, Lathrop KA, Richards P. Tc-99m as a radiocolloid. *J Nucl Med* 1964, 5:382–385.

Harris JW, Kellermeyer RW. The red cell. Cambridge, MA, Harvard University, 1970, p. 309.

Heggli DE, Franco P, Nobygaard E. Differences in biodistribution in rats injected with ^{99m}Tc-MDP preparations with different stabilizing agents. *Eur J Nucl Med* 1988, 14:105–107.

Henkin RE, Woodruff A, Chang W, et al. The effect of radiopharmaceutical incubation time on bone scan quality. *Radiology* 1980, 135:463–466.

Hladik WB III, Nigg KK, Rhodes BA. Drug induced changes in the biologic distribution of radiopharmaceuticals. *Semin Nucl Med* 1982, 12:184–218.

Hladik WB III, Ponto JA, Lentle BC, et al. Inatrogenic alterations in the biodistribution of radiotracers as a result of drug therapy: Reported instances. In *Essentials of Nuclear Medicine Science*, Hladik WB III, Saha G, Study KT, (eds). Baltimore, Williams and Wilkins, 189–219, 1987.

Horn NL, Bennett LR, Marciano D. Evaluation of aplastic anemia with indium chloride In-111 scanning. *Arch Intern Med* 1980, 140:1299–1303.

Hosain P. Technetium-99m labeled pyrophosphate: A simple and reproducible bone scanning agent. *Br J Radiol* 1973, 46:724–728.

ICRP Publications 52, Protection of the Nuclear Medicine Patient, Oxford, 1988.

Jaresko GS, Zimmer AM, Pavel DG, et al. Effect of circulating aluminum on the biodistribution of Tc-99m-Sn-diphosphonate in rats. *J Nucl Med Technol* 1980, 8:160–161.

Jeffcoat MK, McNeil BJ, Davis MA. Indium and iron as tracers for erythroid precursors. *J Nucl Med* 1978, 19:496–500.

Jones, AG, Francis, MD, Davis, MA: Bone scanning: radionuclide reaction mechanisms. *Semin Nucl Med* 1976, 6:3–18.

Jowsey J, Rowland RE, Marshall JH. The deposition of the rare earths in bone, *Radiat Res*, 1958, 8:490.

King AG, Christy B, Hupf HB, et al. Polyphosphates: A chemical analysis of average chain length and the relationship to bone deposition in rats. *J Nucl Med* 1973, 14:695–698.

Klingensmith WC, Spitzer VM, Fritzberg AR, et al. Normal reproducibility of Tc-99m-sulfur colloid (Tc-SC) and Tc-99m-microalbumin colloid (Tc-MAC) liver–spleen studies. (Abst) *J Nucl Med* 1982, 23:90.

Kniseley RM: Marrow studies with radiocolloids. *Semin Nucl Med* 1972, 2:71–85.

Krook HG. Measurement of liver circulation by means of the disappearance of colloidal radiogold from the blood. *Acta Med Scand* 1956 (Suppl), 318:38–44.

Lavender JP, Khan RAA, Hughes SPF. Blood flow and tracer uptake in normal and abnormal canine bone: Comparisons with Sr-85 microspheres, Kr-81m and Tc-99m MDP. *J Nucl Med* 1979, 20:413–418.

Lilien DL, Bennett L. A comparison of the uptake and disposition of radioiron and ^{111}In-chloride in human erythrocytes. *J Nucl Med* 1973, 14:184–186.

Littlefield JL, Rudd TG. Tc-99m hydroxymethylene diphosphonate and Tc-99m methylene diphosphonate: Biological and clinical comparison: Concise communication. *J Nucl Med* 1983, 24:463–466.

Lutrin CL, McDougall IR, Goris ML. Intense concentration of technetium-99m pyrophosphate in the kidneys of children treated with chemotherapeutic drugs for malignant disease. *Radiology* 1978, 128:165–167.

Mazzola AL, Barker MH, Belliveau RE. Accumulation of Tc-99m diphosphonate at sites of intramuscular iron therapy: Case report. *J Nucl Med Technol* 1976, 4:133–135.

McIntyre PA. Newer developments in nuclear medicine applicable to hematology. In *Progress in Hematology*, Brown EB (ed). Vol. 10, Orlando, Grune & Stratton, 1977, pp. 361–409.

McIntyre PA, Larson SM, Eikman EA, et al. Comparison of the metabolism of iron labeled transferrin (Fe-TF) and indium labeled transferrin (In-TF) by the erythropoietic marrow. *J Nucl Med* 1974, 15:856–862.

McIntyre PA, Larson SM, Scheffel U, et al. Comparison of metabolism of iron-transferrin and indium-transferrin by erythropoietic marrow. *J Nucl Med* 1973, 14:425–426.

McNeil BJ, Holman BL, Button LN, et al. Use of indium chloride scintigraphy in patients with myelofibrosis. *J Nucl Med* 1974, 15:647–651.

McRae J, Hambright P, Valk, P, et al. Chemistry of Tc-99m tracers. II. In vitro conversion of tagged HEDP and pyrophosphate (bone-seekers) into gluconate (renal agent). Effects of CA and Fe(II) on in vivo distribution. *J Nucl Med* 1976, 17:208–211.

Mele M, Conte E, Fratello A, et al. Computer analysis for Tc-99m DPD and Tc-99m MDP kinetics in humans: Concise communication. *J Nucl Med* 1983, 24:334–338.

Mishkin F, Reese IC. ^{113m}In for scanning bone and kidney. *J Nucl Med* 1968, 9:462–463.

Nash JF, Bope FW, Christensen BV. Esters of gentisic acid and their toxicities. III. Toxicities of new gentisic acid esters. *J Am Pharmacol Assoc* 1953, 42:254–257.

Nelp WB, Gohil MN, Larson SM, et al. Long-term effects of local irradiation of the marrow on erythron and red cell function. *Blood* 1970, 36:617–622.

Neuman, WF, Newman MW. The chemical dynamics of bone mineral. University of Chicago Press, Chicago, 1958.

O'Mara RE, McAfee JG, Subramanian G. Rare earth nuclides as potential agents for skeletal imaging. *J Nucl Med* 1969, 10:49.

O'Mara RE, Subramanian G. Experimental agents for skeletal imaging. *Semin Nucl Med* 1972, 2:38.

Parker JA, Jones AG, Davis MA, et al. Reduced uptake of bone-seeking radiopharmaceuticals related to iron excess. *Clin Nucl Med* 1976, 1:267–268.

Pauwels EKJ, Blom J, Camps JAJ, et al. A comparison between the diagnostic efficacy of Tc-99m MDP, Tc-99m DPD, and Tc-99m HDP for the detection of bone metastases. *Eur J Nucl Med* 1983, 25:266–269.

Percher C. Biological investigation with radioactive calcium and strontium: Preliminary report on the use of radioactive strontium in the treatment of metastatic bone cancer. *Univ Calif Publ Pharmacol* 1942, 2:117.

Perez R, Cohen Y, Henry R, et al. A new radiopharmaceutical for ^{99m}Tc-bone scanning (Abst). *J Nucl Med* 1972, 13:788.

Pinkerton TC, Ferguson DL, Deutsch E, et al. In vivo distributions of some component fractions of Tc(NaBH$_4$)-HEDP mixtures separated by anion-exchange high-performance liquid chromatography. *Int J Appl Radiat Isot* 1982, 33:907–915.

Pinkerton TC, Heineman WR, Deutsch E. Separation of technetium hydroxyethylidene diphosphonate complexes by anion-exchange high-performance liquid chromatography. *Anal Chem* 1980, 52:1106–1110.

Planchon CA, Donadieu A, Perez R, et al. Calcium heparinate induced extraosseous uptake in bone scanning. *Eur J Nucl Med* 1983, 8:113–117.

Powell ML. Bone imaging. In *Handbook of Clinical Nuclear Medicine*, Matin P (ed), Flushing NY, Medical Examination Publishing, pp 238–262, 1977.

RamSingh PS, Pujara S, Logic JR. Tc-99m pyrophosphate uptake in drug-induced gynecomastia. *Clin Nucl Med* 1977, 2:206.

Rayudu VS, Shirazi PH, Friedman A, et al. An evaluation of ^{52}Fe II-citrate and ^{111}In-chloride for hematopoietic marrow scanning. (Abst) *J Nucl Med* 1973, 14:397.

Richards P. A survey of the production at Brookhaven National Laboratory of radioisotopes for medical research. In: V. Congresso Nucleare, Rome, 1960. Rome Comitato Nazionale Ricerche Nucleari, 1960, Vol. 2, pp. 223–224.

Root SW, Andrews GA, Kniseley RM, et al. The distribution and radiation effects of intravenously administered colloidal Au-198 in man. *Cancer* 1954, 7:856–866.

Rosenthall L, Stern J, Arzoumanian A. A clinical comparison of MDP and DMAD. *Clin Nucl Med* 1982, 7:403–406.

Russell CD, Cash AG. Oxidation state of technetium in bone scanning agents. In Radiopharmaceuticals II. Proceedings, Second International Symposium on Radiopharmaceuticals, Sodd VJ, Allen DR, Hoogland DR, Ice RD (eds). New York, Society of Nuclear Medicine, pp. 627–636, 1979.

Saha GB, Herzberg DL, Boyd CM. Unusual in vivo distribution of Tc-99m diphosphonate. *Clin Nucl Med,* 1977, 2:303–305.

Sayle BA, Helmer E III, Birdsong BA, et al. Bone marrow imaging with indium-III chloride in aplastic anemia and myelofibrosis: Concise communication. *J Nucl Med* 1982, 23:121–125.

Schumichen C, Nakken KF. A comparison of the bone seeking properties of short-chained ^{99m}Tc-Sn-polyphosphates. *Nucl Med (Stuttg)* 1974, 139–143.

Silberstein EB. A radiopharmaceutical and clinical comparison of Tc-99m-Sn-hydroxymethylene diphosphonate with Tc-99m-Sn-hydroxyethylidene diphosphonate. *Radiology* 1980, 136:747–751.

Smith ML, Martin W, McKillop JH, Fogelman I. Improved lesion detection with dimethyl-amino-diphosphonate: A report of two cases. *Eur J Nucl Med* 1984, 9:519–520.

Sorkin SJ, Horii SC, Passalaqua A, et al. Augmented activity on bone scan following local chemoperfusion. *Clin Nucl Med* 1977, 2:451.

Spicer, JA, Preston DF, Stephens RL. Adverse allergic reaction to technetium-99m methylene diphosphonate. *J Nucl Med* 1985, 26:373–374.

Staub RF, Gaston E. ^{111}In-chloride distribution and kinetics in hematologic disease. (Abst) *J Nucl Med* 1973, 14:456–457.

Study KT, Schultz HW, Laven DL. The effect of bacteriostatic saline on ^{99m}Tc-radiopharmaceuticals. *J Nucl Med Technol* 1981, 9:115–116.

Subramanian G, McAfee JG. A new complex of ^{99m}Tc for skeletal imaging. *Radiology* 1971a, 99:192–196.

Subramanian G, McAfee JG, Bell EG, et al. ^{99m}Tc-labeled polyphosphate as a skeletal imaging agent. *Radiology* 1972, 102:701–704.

Subramanian G, McAfee JG, Blair RJ, et al. Technetium-99m-methylene diphosphonate—A superior agent for skeletal imaging: Comparison with other technetium complexes. *J Nucl Med* 1975, 16:744–755.

Subramanian G, McAfee JG, Mehta A, et al. Tc-99m stannors phytate: A new in-vivo colloid for imaging the reticuloendothelial system. *J Nucl Med* 1973, 14:459–463.

Subramanian G, McAfee JG, O'Mara RE, et al. ^{99m}Tc-polyphosphate, PP$_{46}$: A new radiopharmaceutical for skeletal imaging. *J Nucl Med* 1971b, 12:399–404.

Subramanian G, McAfee JG, Thomas FD, et al. New diphosphonate compounds for skeletal imaging: Comparison with methylene diphosphonate. *Radiology* 1983, 149:823–828.

Tofe AJ, Bevan JA, Fawzi MB. et al. Gentisic acid: A new stabilizer for low tin skeletal imaging agents: Concise communication. *J Nucl Med* 1980, 21:366–370.

Tofe AJ, Francis MD. In vitro optimization and organ distribution studies in animals with the bone scanning agent ^{99m}Tc-Sn-EHDP. *J Nucl Med* 1972, 13:472.

Tofe AJ, Francis MD. Optimization of the ratio of stannous tin, ethane-1-hydroxy-1, 1-diphosphonate for bone scanning with Tc-99m pertechnetate. *J Nucl Med* 1974, 15:69–74.

Tofe AJ, Francis MD. In vitro stabilization of a low tin bone imaging agent (Tc-99m Sn-HEDP) by ascorbic acid. *J Nucl Med* 1976, 17:820–825.

Trackler RT, Chinn RYW. Amphotericin B therapy—A cause of increased renal uptake of Tc-99m MDP. *Clin Nucl Med* 1982, 7:293.

Treadwell AdeG, Low-Beer VL, Friedell

HL, et al. Metabolic studies on the neoplasm of bone with the aid of radioactive strontium. *Am J Med Sci* 1942, 204:521.

Uchtman VA. Structural investigations of calcium binding molecules. II. The crystal and molecular structures of calcium dihydrogen ethane-1-hydroxy-1, 1-diphosphonate dihydrate: CaC(CH$_3$)-(OH)(PO$_3$H)$_2$2H$_2$O); Implications for polynuclear complex formation. *J Phy Chem* 1972, 76:1304–1310.

VanAntwerp JD, Hall JN, O'Mara RE, et al. Bone scan abnormality produced by interaction of Tc-99m diphosphonate with iron dextran (Imferon). (Abst) *J Nucl Med* 1975, 16:577.

Van Duzee BF, Schaeffer JA, Ball JD, et al. Relative lesion detection ability of Tc-99m HMDP and Tc-99m MDP: Concise communication. *J Nucl Med* 1984, 25:166–169.

Van Dyke D, Shkurkin C, Price D, et al. Differences in the distribution of erythropoietic and reticuloendothelial marrow in hematologic disease. *Blood* 1967, 30:364–369.

Van Wazer JR. *Phosphorous and Its Compounds.* New York, Interscience, 1958.

Weber WG, Greenberg EJ, Dimich A, et al. Kinetics of radionuclides uses for bone studies. *J Nucl Med* 1969, 10:8.

Zilversmit DB, Boyd GA, Brucer M. The effect of particle size on blood clearance and tissue distribution of radioactive gold colloids. *J Lab Clin Med* 1952, 40:255–260.

Zimmer AM, Isitman AT, Holmes RA. Enzymatic inhibition of diphosphonate: A proposed mechanism of tissue uptake. *J Nucl Med* 1975, 16:352–356.

Radiopharmaceuticals for Imaging Tumors and Inflammatory Processes: Gallium, Antibodies, and Leukocytes

Henry M. Chilton
Scott W. Burchiel
Nat E. Watson, Jr.

Tumor Imaging

The early detection of neoplastic disease has been one of nuclear medicine's major goals, and a variety of agents have been investigated for this purpose. Two different radiopharmaceutical localization approaches for tumor detection have been explored. In the first, radiopharmaceutical localization in normal tissues occurs by some specific function not shared by malignant tissues. In this manner, tumorous tissues appear as areas of relatively low radioactivity (i.e., "cold" spots) within the organ to be imaged (e.g., Tc-99m sulfur colloid localization occurs only within normal cells of the reticuloendothelial system). This approach for tumor detection is discussed within the various chapters addressing organ-specific radiopharmaceutical localization.

The other tumor-imaging approach involves the direct visualization of tumor itself, using unique tumor characteristics as localization mechanisms. With this approach, only tumor concentrates the radiopharmaceutical and, therefore, appears as an area of relatively intense activity (i.e., a "hot" spot) against normal tissues that fail to concentrate the radiopharmaceutical. Several different radiopharmaceuticals have been developed that use this latter approach to detect tumor, including gallium Ga-67 citrate, radiolabeled bleomycin and, more recently, radiolabeled monoclonal antibodies reactive against tumor-associated antigens.

To date, an ideal radiopharmaceutical with appropriate tumor specificity and sensitivity and suitable nuclear properties has not been found. Though it is the subject of debate whether, in the future, the role of Ga-67 tumor imaging (Silberstein EB, 1976) may be sharply reduced if the promise of radiolabeled antitumor antibodies is realized, Ga-67 citrate remains today the most useful tumor-avid radiopharmaceutical. (Radiolabeled antibodies for tumor imaging are discussed later in this chapter.)

I. GALLIUM-67 CITRATE

BACKGROUND/HISTORY

The use of gallium in medicine can be traced to early studies by H.C. Dudley and co-workers (1949a;b; 1950; 1952) in their investigation of gallium toxicity and biodistribution. Initially, they studied the tissue distribution of stable gallium and later evaluated the biodistribution of Ga-72, a carrier-containing reactor product. In their studies, they noted gallium deposition in high concentrations in bone and sites of osteogenic activity and suggested that Ga-72 might be useful in the detection of osteogenic sarcoma and other metastatic skeletal lesions. Because Ga-72 had poor nuclear properties (β-decay mode, principal photon emission at 835 keV) other radioisotopes of gallium were investigated, including Ga-67.

Compared to Ga-72, Ga-67 uptake and deposition in bone was decreased, and Ga-67 localization in the liver and other soft tissues was much higher. Gallium-67 demonstrated slower blood clearance than Ga-72 and reversed urinary and fecal excretion patterns (urinary excretion of Ga-67 is prominent in the first 24 hours only; subsequent excretion occurs by the fecal route only) (Bruner HD, 1953a). Further studies revealed that this difference in biodistribution was attributable to the carrier state of these radioisotopes of gallium. The addition of stable gallium to Ga-67 (accelerator-produced Ga-67 is essentially "carrier-free") produced Ga-67 tissue distribution and excretion patterns that matched those of carrier-containing Ga-72 (Bruner HD, 1953b).

Clinical investigations were performed using carrier-free Ga-67 as a potential bone-scanning agent. While performing a Ga-67 bone scan on a patient with Hodgkin's disease, C.L. Edwards and R.L. Hayes (1969) noted the localization of radioactivity in afflicted lymph nodes. Subsequent clinical studies confirmed the tumor-localizing properties of Ga-67 and investigations in tumor-bearing animals

bore out the relationship of carrier levels of gallium to bone uptake. Gallium-67 citrate localization in sites of inflammation was also demonstrated.

Gallium-67 citrate is useful in the localization of both inflammatory and malignant foci in many clinical situations (Table 17.1) and may be advantageous when the primary lesion or the extent of pathology are unknown (Teates CD and Bray ST, 1978; Levitt RG, et al, 1979). Gallium imaging is of particular value in the diagnosis and staging of lymphomas and Hodgkin's disease. Gallium-67 localization in lymphomas is influenced by several factors including the size and location of the neoplasm. Tumor visualization is also influenced by imaging technique, including the type of instrumentation and collimation employed and the amount of radioactivity administered (see Dosage).

CHEMISTRY

Gallium-67 is produced in a cyclotron by the (p,2n) reaction on Zinc-68. It decays by electron capture with a physical half-life of 78 hours, and has four principal photopeaks (93, 185, 300, and 394 keV) that are present in sufficient abundance for imaging (Table 17.2). The several commercial formulations of Ga-67 citrate available in the United States are shown in Table 17.3.

Gallium is a member of Group III of the periodic chart, which includes the elements aluminum and indium. Although gallium possesses the toxicity common to other members of this periodic group, accelerator-produced Ga-67 contains minimal amounts of elemental gallium (e.g., a patient dose contains less than 10^{-7} mg/kg).

Table 17.1 TYPES OF NEOPLASTIC AND NON-NEOPLASTIC PATHOLOGIES THAT RESULT IN Ga-67 LOCALIZATION

Neoplasms

Hodgkin's disease
Non-Hodgkin's lymphoma
Carcinoma of the lung
Malignant melanoma
Hepatoma
Bone sarcoma
Malignant fibrous histiocytoma
Leukemia (AML, CML)
Testicular tumors

Non-neoplastic conditions

Pyogenic abscess
Subacute thyroiditis
Acute inflammation
Radiation pneumonitis
Acute tuberculosis
Rheumatoid arthritis
Recent surgical trauma
Sarcoid
Renal amyloidosis
Osteomyelitis
Pyelonephritis
Bacterial pneumonia

Table 17.2 NUCLEAR PROPERTIES OF Ga-67

Physical half-life: 78 Hours
Decay mode: Electron capture (to Zn-67, stable)

PHOTON ENERGY (KEV)	(ABUNDANCE %/DISINTEGRATION)
93	38.0
185	23.9
300	16.1
394	4.3

Table 17.3 CURRENTLY AVAILABLE FORMULATIONS OF Ga-67 CITRATE[a]

MANUFACTURER	CITRATE CONC. (SOD. CITRATE/ML)	pH	RADIONUCLIDIC IMPURITIES (AT CALIBRATION)	PRESERVATIVES
Mallinckrodt, Inc	1.9 ngm	5–8	<0.02% Ga-66, <0.2% Zn-65	0.9% Benzyl alcohol
Medi-Physics	25 mg	4.5–7.5	<0.9% Ga-66, <0.1% Zn-65	1.0% Benzyl alcohol
Dupont-NEN	2.0 ngm	5–8	"Negligible"	—

[a] U.S. only.

Gallium mimics the ferric ion in that it distributes in tissues much like iron, forms many analogues of iron-containing compounds, and complexes several iron-binding molecules in serum, including transferrin, lactoferrin, ferritin, and siderophores. Gallium is dissimilar to iron, however, in that it is not reduced in vivo and therefore not incorporated into hemoglobin.

PHARMACOKENETICS

Following intravenous administration of Ga-67 citrate, radioactivity clearance from blood occurs at an exponential rate with three components. The rapid clearance phase, which accounts for elimination of approximately 48% of the administered activity, has a half-life of about 30 minutes; the intermediate component (12% of administered activity) has a half-life of 4 hours; and the prolonged phase (40% of administered activity) has a half-life of nearly 40 hours (Larson SM, et al, 1978). At 48 and 72 hours post injection, about 10% and 5% of administered dose, respectively, remains within the body bound to plasma proteins, primarily transferrin and possibly haptoglobulins (Gunasekera SW, et al, 1972). As high as 90% of the injected dose may be bound to serum transferrin immediately after administration. The non–protein-bound fraction diffuses throughout the extravascular, extracellular space and is excreted by the kidney. However, less than 25% of an injected dose of Ga-67 citrate is normally excreted by the kidneys during the first 24 hours after injection. Another 10% of the dose is excreted in the stool over the next 7-days, and the remaining 65% is distributed within the body (Nelson B, et al, 1972). Studies have shown that total

body elimination of Ga-67 involves two components, the first component of excretion (comprising 17% of administered activity) having a half-life of 30 hours and the long component (83%) having a half-life of 25 days (Watson EE, et al, 1973).

At 2–3 days after injection, the highest concentrations of Ga-67 are seen in the liver (5% of administered dose), spleen (1%), kidney, (2%), and skeleton (including marrow, 24%). In the spleen, Ga-67 is accumulated in the phagocytic cells, while in the liver both Kupffer's cells and hepatocytes show gallium uptake (Larson SM, et al, 1975). Normal images show the greatest accumulation of Ga-67 in the liver and throughout the skeleton and bone marrow (Figure 17.1). The spleen, which shows minimal uptake of Ga-67, is frequently not visualized. Other sites of normal activity include Ga-67 uptake in the nasopharynx, lacrimal glands, salivary

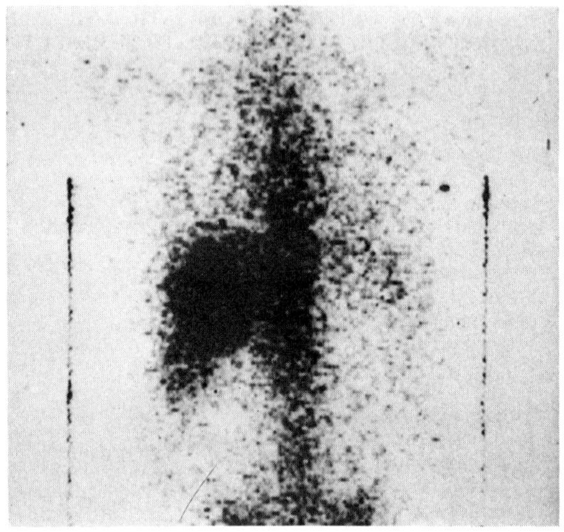

Figure 17.1 Normal biodistribution of Ga-67 at 48 hours following the injection of Ga-67 citrate. Note intense activity in the liver, skeleton, and bone marrow.

glands, and external genitalia. Gallium-67 uptake has been noted in human breast and it is secreted in breast milk during pregnancy, lactation, and estrogen therapy (see Clinical Considerations). The high concentration of lactoferrin in these latter tissues is believed to be responsible for the respective localization of Ga-67. Lactoferrin, a protein that closely resembles transferrin, is capable of binding gallium.

The mechanisms of Ga-67 localization in tumors and sites of inflammation are not completely understood but appear to involve the transfer of gallium to intracellular components, possibly by one or more mechanisms. Whether or not the actual uptake mechanism involves a carrier-mediated transport system whereby gallium binds to serum protein complexes (mainly transferrin) in order to cross cell membranes is not clearly resolved. There is some agreement, however, that specific transport mechanisms may play a role in the tumor uptake of Ga-67 because many hypervascular tumorous lesions fail to concentrate gallium at all. One theory is that tumor uptake of Ga-67 requires the initial formation in serum of a gallium-transferrin complex. The importance of transferrin to the uptake of Ga-67 in tumors was first described by R.G. Sephton and A.W. Harris (1975) in their experiments involving tumor tissue cultures. Later, S.M. Larson and associates (1978) confirmed that transferrin enhanced Ga-67 uptake into in vitro tumor slices and suggested the role of a tumor associated transferrin receptor in the tumor uptake of both Ga-67 and Fe-59. The "transferrin receptor hypothesis" has not identified an active cellular component with specific binding properties and physical characteristics but is an operational concept that refers to a high affinity, saturable component of the intracellular transferrin transport system. Following cellular entry, gallium appears to bind to other iron-binding macromolecules such as lactoferrin, ferritin, or a siderophorelike growth factor (Fernandez-Pol JA, 1978).

Variations in Ga-67 uptake may relate not only to the concentration of iron-binding molecules in tumor but also to the presence of compounds that enhance the transfer of gallium from transferrin to the other iron-binding compounds (Weiner RE, et al, 1985) or that affect the availability of unoccupied serum transferrin binding sites. For example, methotrexate therapy in animal studies has been shown to reduce the number of occupied serum transferrin binding sites (and alter normal Ga-67 biodistribution) by temporarily inhibiting the erythrocyte incorporation of iron and thereby increasing serum iron levels (Chilton HM, et al, 1981a). In animals, whole-body irradiation produced a similar alteration of Ga-67 biodistribution (increased Ga-67 uptake in bone and renal excretion) that was secondary to increasing serum iron levels and decreasing available serum transferrin binding sites (Bradley WP, et al, 1978).

In opposition to the "transferrin receptor hypothesis," R.L. Hayes and D.H. Brown (1974) suggest that tumor uptake of Ga-67 requires the free, ionic state of gallium and that any complexation of this radionuclide with serum proteins (such as transferrin) lowers its tumor uptake.

PRECAUTIONS

Relatively few precautions are associated with the use of Ga-67 citrate. Attention should be given, however, to situations that may result in an altered biodistribution of Ga-67.

Causes of Altered Biodistribution. Surgical wound sites result in increased Ga-67 localization for several weeks, whereas previous radiation may cause decreased Ga-67 tumor uptake. As outlined in Table 17.4 and below, several drugs administered concurrently with Ga-67 citrate may also influence the biodistribution of Ga-67 (Hladik WB III, et al, 1987).

An alteration in the ability of serum transferrin to bind iron can profoundly affect gallium biodistribution, blood clearance, and whole-body retention. Both disease states and drugs can affect iron levels

Table 17.4 CONCOMITANT DRUG THERAPY AND OTHER CAUSES OF ALTERED Ga-67 BIODISTRIBUTION[a]

CAUSATIVE DRUG(S)/CONDITION(S)	ALTERED BIODISTRIBUTION/MECHANISM	REFERENCE(S)
Phenytoin	Lymphoma-like pattern (25% patients)	Lentle BC, et al, 1983
Cyclophosphamide-vincristine chemotherapy	Abnormal lung uptake	MacMahon H and Beckerman C, 1978
Bisulfan; Bleomycin	Diffuse lune uptake/Drug-induced interstitial inflammation	Manning DM, et al, 1980; Richman SD, et al, 1975
Radiopaque contrast media (water insoluble)	Abnormal lung uptake	Lentle BC, et al, 1975
Antibiotics (ampicillin, clindamycin, cephalosporins)	Colonic uptake/Drug-induced pseudomembraneous colitis	Tedesco RS, et al, 1976
Ampicillin, sulfonamides, ibuprofen, hydrochlorothiazide, cephlexin, sulfin-pyrazone	Avid renal uptake/Drug-induced interstitial nephritis	Linton AL, et al, 1980
Post-partum, pregnancy	Breast uptake/Normal variant	—
Reserpine, phenothiazines, metoclopromide, oral contraceptives, DES	Breast uptake/Drug-induced gynecomastia and hyperprolactinemia	Beckerman C, et al, 1980, Stephanas AV and Maisey YC, 1976; Kim MN et al, 1977
Steroids	Decreased localization in CNS tumors /Drug-induced stabilization of blood-brain barrier alterations.	Waxman AD, et al, 1978

[a] See Hladik WB, III, et al, 1987.

and hence gallium binding capacity by serum proteins. For example, in patients receiving parenteral iron therapy the binding capacity of serum transferrin may become saturated, resulting in an alteration in the distribution (i. e., increased bone uptake and renal excretion) of concomitantly administered Ga-67. As a rule, oral iron therapy does not totally saturate transferrin because of a negative feedback system at the respective intestinal absorption site (Fletcher JW, et al, 1975). Similar effects on Ga-67 biodistribution have been observed following irradiation or chemotherapy with methotrexate, vincristine, nitrogen mustard, and possibly cisplatinum, although in the latter case the interference may be due to effects on protein synthesis rather than an effect on the ability of transferrin to bind gallium (Noujaim AA, 1981). B. Englestad and colleagues (1982) report similar alterations in Ga-67 biodistribution (increased kidney and bone uptake with decreased liver and colon localization) in four patients who received multiple red blood cell transfusions. Their findings are suggestive of competition with iron for receptor binding.

Altered biodistribution of Ga-67 can be caused by pathological conditions distinct from the pathological processes (e. g., tumor, abscess) that lead to its focal localization. In severe hepatocellular disease, for example, increased renal excretion of Ga-67 occurs presumably due to a decreased synthesis of gallium binding serum proteins.

Adverse Reactions. To date, both the number and types of adverse reactions associated with the use of Ga-67 citrate have been minor with most involving mild skin rashes and nausea.

Use during Pregnancy/breastfeeding. Ga-67 has been shown in animals to cross the placenta (Hayes RL and Byrd B, 1981). Its use during pregnancy, therefore, is not advised. Because gallium is secreted in breast milk (Tobin RE and Schneider PB, 1976), patients who are breastfeeding should be told to discontinue feeding until levels in breast milk are considered safe. It has been suggested that following intravenous administration of a 3 millicurie dose, a wait of at least 2 weeks is advisable before Ga-67 levels in breast milk fall to levels that are considered safe for a resumption of breast feeding (Tobin RE and Schneider PB, 1976). Others have suggested a delay of 3–4 weeks before resuming breastfeeding (Romney BM, et al, 1986; Coakley JL and Mountford PJ, 1985).

CLINICAL CONSIDERATIONS.

In the early period of its clinical use, Ga-67 citrate was investigated in virtually all human tumors as clinicians sought to evaluate its potential as a universal tumor-localizing radiopharmaceutical.

Gallium-67 has been found to be of primary benefit for the detection of lymphoma. Nearly 90% of untreated patients with Hodgkin's disease have positive Ga-67 uptake in one or more lesions (Figure 17.2). Lymphomas other than Hodgkin's disease show variability in their affinity for Ga-67. For example, patients with histiocytic lymphoma have positive Ga-67 studies in approximately 80% of cases, while patients with mixed cell types approach a 90% detection rate. The accuracy of Ga-67 imaging is also dependent upon several additional factors, such as lesion size and location, amount of radiopharmaceutical administered, as well as the imaging equipment and technique employed (See Dosage/Dosimetry). Lesions most reliably detected are around 4 cm or larger in diameter; lesions less than 1 cm are not routinely visualized. Abdominal lesions may be difficult to localize because of their proximity to the

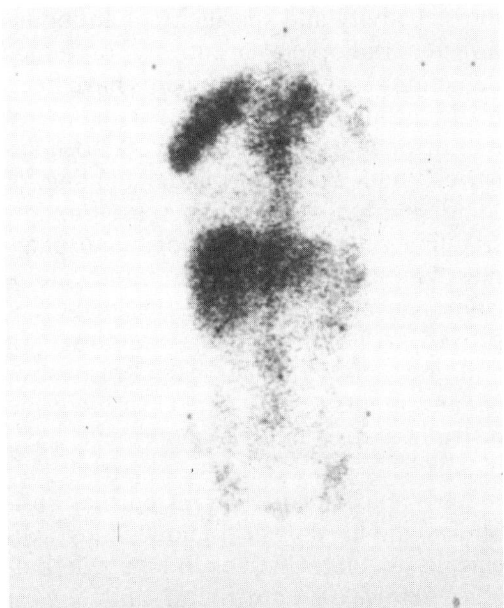

Figure 17.2 Abnormal Ga-67 localization in the involved lymph nodes of a patient with Hodgkin's disease.

liver and bowel and the normal Ga-67 distribution in these tissues. It has also been shown that Ga-67 detection rates are lower in lymphoma patients who have already had radiotherapy and/or chemotherapy (Johnston GS, et al, 1977). The efficacy of Ga-67 imaging as an aid in the clinical management of these patients and their follow-up is, however, without question.

For other tumors, the use of Ga-67 imaging becomes somewhat controversial since not all tumors concentrate Ga-67, and among those that do, tumor location and differences in tumor histology can be significant factors that affect Ga-67 uptake.

A large number of clinical studies have been directed at defining the optimal use of Ga-67, particularly in comparing the diagnostic benefits of this procedure to other imaging techniques. Despite the numerous original reports and the more recent reviews, considerable debate exists as to the most efficacious use of Ga-67 vis-a-vis other imaging techniques. Central to this controversy is the fact that many of the original reports utilized imaging techniques presently deemed suboptimal. The majority of these studies have not been repeated with the currently available imaging instrumentation and higher dosages (Anderson KC, et al, 1983). Presently, it is generally accepted that greater diagnostic sensitivity for tumor results whenever higher millicurie amounts of Ga-67 are administered (e.g., 7–10 millicuries versus 3 millicuries).

DOSAGE/DOSIMETRY

Because it is generally felt that greater diagnostic sensitivity results with larger administered activities of Ga-67 citrate, most clinicians now inject "standard" adult doses of 3–8 mCi for inflammatory lesions and as much as 10 millicuries for tumor imaging in patients with known malignancies. Pediatric dosages are calculated by body weight and range from 30–50 uCi per kg, when there is no known

Table 17.5 RADIATION-ABSORBED DOSE ESTIMATES FOR ^{67}Ga-CITRATE[a]

ORGAN	RADS/MCI
Lower large intestine	4.5
Upper large intestine	2.8
Spleen	2.7
Liver	2.3
Kidneys	2.1
Small intestine	1.8
Ovaries	1.4
Testes	1.2
Whole body	1.3

[a] From MIRD Dose Estimate Report No 2, *J Nucl Med* 1973, 14:755–756.

malignancy, to 50–100 uCi per kg in patients with known tumor. Radiation dosimetry estimates for Ga-67 citrate are summarized in Table 17.5.

Tumor imaging is usually initiated 48 hours after Ga-67 citrate injection in order to allow for adequate clearance of the radiopharmaceutical from blood and soft tissues. Imaging may be carried out to 4–5 days, if necessary, to permit adequate tumor visualization. When imaging either tumor or inflammatory processes, it is advisable to utilize a bowel-cleansing preparation prior to imaging because normal colonic activity can mask areas of abnormal Ga-67 uptake in the pelvis. In some cases, repeat studies at a later time may be advisable in order to differentiate normal gallium activity in the bowel from pathological uptake.

Although imaging may be performed with either a rectilinear scanner or scintillation camera, the latter instrumentation is usually preferred. Newer systems that permit multiple photopeak acquisition of the relatively abundant 93, 185, and 300 keV photopeaks are most desirable. Recently, tomographic scintillation imaging, using the SPECT-type devices or linear tomography (Kirkwood JA, et al, 1982), have been reported to yield clinically superior images compared to the standard scintillation camera. In either case, collimators should be of the medium- to high-energy type in order to prevent undesirable septal penetration by the 394 keV photons of Ga-67. Spot views of 500,000 counts each are recommended for increased sensitivity in the detection of tumors.

II. RADIOLABELED ANTIBODIES

Scott W. Burchiel

Radiolabeled antibodies have undergone evaluation over the past several years for the detection of a variety of tumors and occult masses (Goldenberg DM, 1980; Sfakianakis GN and DeLand FH, 1982; Burchiel SW and Rhodes BA, 1983; Larson SM, 1985). Although numerous radiolabeled antibody products are under development and being investigated clinically, no approved agents of this type currently exist in the United States. Therefore, the properties of these agents relating to their use as radiopharmaceuticals will be discussed as a group rather than focusing on individual products. This section will primarily discuss the use of radiolabeled antibodies for tumor detection (i. e., radioimmunoimaging or radioimmunodetection) and therapy (i. e., radioimmunotherapy), since the greatest amount of experience has been obtained in these areas.

BACKGROUND/HISTORY

Over the past decade, extensive efforts have been directed at methods to improve the sensitivity and specificity of antibody-directed radiopharmaceuticals for tumor detection. Many improvements have been made through the development and use of monoclonal antibodies, new radiochemistries, and a greater understanding of tumor immunology. An increased understanding of the pharmacologic and pharmacokinetic properties of antibody molecules has also led to the design of improved radioimmunopharmaceuticals. In addition, there have been respective advancements related to nuclear medicine instrumentation and enhancement techniques.

Early experiments suggested that antibodies might deliver radionuclides specifically to target tissues like "magic bullets." However, preclinical and clinical experience with radiolabeled antibodies have not realized the expectations regarding specificity and sensitivity of tumor localization with these agents. In fact, quantitative experiments have demonstrated that only a small proportion of the total administered activity associated with radiolabeled antibodies localizes at tumor sites (Mach JP, et al, 1980; Colcher D, et al, 1987a). It now appears that several factors may limit the current usefulness of radiolabeled antibodies for tumor detection. Factors such as tumor biology and immunology, antibody pharmacology and pharmacokinetics, and the radioimmunochemical properties of anti-tumor antibodies appear to be important in the radioimmunodetection of tumors. The overall significance of these factors with regard to tumor imaging via antibody-targeted radiopharmaceuticals is discussed in the following sections.

CHEMISTRY

Immunochemistry. Perhaps the greatest advancements that have been made in the development of antibody-targeted radiopharmaceuticals have come in the areas of tumor biology and immunochemistry.

In recent years, a number of tumor-associated molecules that can be recognized by antibodies have been described, and the characterization of these relatively specific tumor-associated antigens has been a major area of advancement. In addition, the discovery of monoclonal antibody technology (Kohler G and Milstein C, 1975) has led to a wide array of immunoglobulin reagents that have shown specificity for various tumor types (Table 17.6).

Based upon animal and human data, tumor-associated antigens (TAA) can be generally categorized into three groups based on their origin. In this regard, TAA may occur as a result of: (1) inappropriate cellular expression during cancer (i. e., differentiation antigens); (2) transformation with oncogenic viruses; and (3) random mutations spontaneously induced or under the influence of radiation or chemical carcinogens. Most of the TAA that have proven useful for tumor detection with radiolabeled antibodies belong to the first class of differentiation TAA. Since no single TAA has been shown to be expressed by all human tumors, no individual radiolabeled antibody has proven to be sufficient for general tumor imaging. Rather, certain types of tumors known to express specific TAA can be reasonably effectively matched with specific antibody reagents (Table 17.6). Despite such matching of specific tumors with select antibody reagents, investigators have found that most tumors are quite heterogeneous in their expression of TAA; leading to a concern about whether tumor cells expressing low levels of TAA may escape detection (Burchiel SW, et al, 1982a).

Table 17.6   REPRESENTATIVE HUMAN TUMOR ASSOCIATED ANTIGENS IDENTIFIED USING MONOCLONAL ANTIBODIES

ANTIGEN	MOLECULE	ANTIBODY[a]	REPRESENTATIVE TUMOR TYPE
CEA	200K glycoprotein	Several	Lung, colon, and breast carcinoma
hCG	38K glycoprotein	Several	Choriocarcinoma
AFP	68K glycoprotein	Several	Hepatoma
Ferritin	600K glycoprotein	Several	Hepatoma
T65	65K glycoprotein	T101	T-cell leukemias and CTCL
P97	97K glycoprotein	8.2 & 96.5	Melanoma
HMW MAA	280K glycoprotein/ 400K proteoglycan	9.2.27 and 225.28	Melanoma
Mucin	310K glycoprotein	B72.3	Lung, colon, breast, and ovarian carcinoma
Milk fat globule	400K glycoprotein (68K glycoprotein)	HMFG1/HMFG2	Breast cancer
?	?	791T/36	Osteogenic sarcoma
?	?	1D6 & UJ13A	Glioma/Neuroblastoma

[a] All monoclonal antibodies are derived from murine hybridomas with the exception of the 1D6, which is a human monoclonal antibody.

Other issues relating to TAA expression and detection have also surfaced during the past few years. For example, TAA secreted from tumor cells and circulating in blood may compete with cell-associated TAA for binding of the radiolabeled antibody. In the case of carcinoembryonic antigen (CEA), however, free circulating antigen has not appeared to inhibit tumor localization of radiolabeled anti-CEA antibodies (Goldenberg, DM, et al, 1978). The problem of antigenic modulation has also been observed in the detection of certain leukemias and lymphomas (Miller RA, et al, 1981). Antigenic modulation refers to activation of a cellular membrane following antibody binding to cell surface antigens. This results in either a shedding or an internalization of the antigen-antibody complex. In this fashion, the radiolabeled antibody actually clears from tumor following complexation with TAA, causing potential problems in tumor detection.

Finally, the problem of cross reactivity of certain antibody reagents with normal antigens on normal cells has also become apparent. Such binding of antibodies to normal cells can lead not only to false positives for tumor detection but may also be injurious to the normal cells or tissues. For example, it has been shown that NCA and other CEA-like molecules are expressed on normal human granulocytes (Kuroki M, et al, 1981). Radioimmunodetection studies have shown that monoclonal antibodies that cross-react with NCA do not localize tumors in patients, but they do produce systemic toxicity (Dillman RD, et al, 1984). These findings demonstrate the need for extensive in vitro screening of antibody reagents for cross reactivity with normal human cells and tissues before the introduction of radiolabeled antibodies into clinical trials.

Radiochemistry—General. Three important criteria are necessary for the development of antibody radiolabeling methodologies. First, labeling must be achieved under nondenaturing conditions that preserve the immunoreactivity of the antibody. Second, the radiolabeled antibody or conjugate must be stable, and not susceptible to rapid breakdown or cleavage. Third, significant amounts of impurities that may affect the activity of the radiolabeled antibody should not be generated during the radiolabeling process. These considerations will be briefly discussed with regard to the specific radioisotopes and radiolabeling procedures listed in the following subsection.

Radionuclides for the radiolabeling of antibodies can be conveniently grouped according to nuclear properties and their associated utility for either diagnosis or therapeutic applications (Table 17.7). The use of short-lived radioisotopes for labeling antibodies for diagnostic applications has been made possible by the commercial availability of new radionuclides with highly desirable imaging properties. The use of these radionuclides has been facilitated by the development of simplified radiolabeling procedures and the preparation

Table 17.7 RADIONUCLIDES EMPLOYED FOR ANTIBODY RADIOIMMUNOIMAGING (RII) OR RADIOIMMUNOTHERAPY (RIT)[a]

RADIONUCLIDE	PHYSICAL HALF-LIFE	DECAY MODE	PRINCIPAL EMISSION TYPE/ENERGY (YIELD)	TYPE OF ANTIBODY BINDING	USE
Iodine-123	13 h	E.C.	γ 159 keV, (83%)	Covalent	RII
Iodine-131	8.1 d	β^-	γ 364 keV, (82%) β^- 606 keV	Covalent	RII, RIT
Technetium-99m	6.0 h	I.T.	γ 140 keV, (90%)	Chelation	RII
Indium-111	67 h	E.C.	γ 173 keV, (89%) γ 247 keV, (94%)	Chelation	RII
Yttrium-90	64 h	β^-	β^- 2.3 MeV	Chelation	RIT
Rhenium-186	90 h	β^-	β^- 1.1 MeV Multiple γ 137–768 keV	Chelation	RIT

[a] Source of information: *Radiological Health Handbook*, 1970 Edition; U.S. Dept of Health, Education, & Welfare, Food and Drug Administration, Rockville, MD.

Table 17.8 QUALITY ASSURANCE PARAMETERS FOR RADIOLABELED ANTIBODIES[a]

1. Radiolabeling efficiency
2. Percent immunoreactive radioactivity
3. Percent aggregated antibody activity
4. Stability of radiolabeled antibody
5. Sterility and pyrogenicity of radiolabeled antibody product

[a] Note: A more complete description of quality assurance tests for radiolabeled antibodies can be obtained from the U.S. Food and Drug Administration under the title of "Points to Consider in the Manufacture and Testing of Monoclonal Antibody Products for Human Use (1987)."

of antibody labeling kits. Antibody labeling with short-lived radioisotopes requires completion within a relatively short time period in order to minimize any significant loss of radioactivity due to physical decay. Ideally, methods should be developed that permit labeling to be accomplished within a clinical setting a few hours before the intended use. It is equally important that appropriate quality assurance control measures be developed that are capable of being performed quickly and efficiently. A list of commonly used quality assurance tests for radiolabeled antibodies is shown in Table 17.8.

Radiochemistry—radioiodines (I-131, I-125, I-123). Early studies by S.A. Berson and associates (1953) demonstrated that tracer levels of covalently bound I-131 can be used to monitor the in vivo behavior of proteins. Several methods have been developed for radioiodinating proteins including procedures that utilize chloramine T (Hunter WM and Greenwood FC, 1962), lactoperoxidase (Marchalonis JJ, 1969; Thorell JI and Johansson BG, 1971), iodogen (Fraker PJ and Speck JC, 1978), or iodobeads (Markwell MAK, 1982). In each of these methods, radioiodine is covalently bound to tyrosine residues that occur naturally in most proteins. In an iodinated method developed by A.E. Bolton and W.M. Hunter (1973), radioiodine is covalently bound to lysine residues of proteins.

An important question related to the therapeutic and/or diagnostic use of radioiodinated antibodies pertains to the stability of the radiolabel. Previously, it has been suggested that radioiodine may be removed from antibody molecules by tissue dehalogenase enzymes (Stern P, et al, 1982). In these experimental studies, the rapid appearance of radioiodine in the urine combined with the observed increase in tumor uptake of the In-111 versus I-131 labeled antibody provided evidence that a radioiodine label was unstable. However, substantial clinical data comparing behavior of radioiodinated antibodies with antibodies labeled by various other techniques is lacking. It has been demonstrated that the rapid excretion of radioiodine in the urine may not be due to nonspecific antibody deiodination, but may rather reflect the true catabolism of antibody molecules (DeNardo GL, et al, 1986). Recent studies by M. Hylarides and colleagues (1987) have demonstrated that antibodies may be radiolabeled with iodophenyl conjugates to achieve greater stability of the radioiodine on the protein. Although it is clear that the overall stability of radioiodinated antibodies will depend upon the method of iodination used and the particular antibody that is radiolabeled, further studies are necessary to determine whether radioiodinated antibodies will be appropriate for tumor imaging and/or tumor therapy.

Iodine-131 labeled antibodies have been employed for many years for the detection of tumors; however, the poor imaging properties of its 364 keV gamma radiation and the associated high radiation exposure from its β^- decay make I-131 less than ideal for radioimmunodetection. In addition, studies have determined that I-131 may damage antibody immunoreactivity when too many atoms of this radionuclide are covalently bound to the protein (Larson SM, 1985). Clinical studies with I-131 labeled antibodies have shown that tumor imaging can be achieved but image quality is usually not sufficient to permit detection of lesions less than 1 cm in diameter. Some groups have experimented with image enhancement and background-subtraction techniques in order to increase the sensitivity of tumor detection (Goldenberg DM, et al, 1978); however, any use of background-subtraction techniques for image enhancement has the potential for artifact generation.

The beta decay mode of I-131 is well suited for therapy; therefore antibodies labeled with this radionuclide have been investigated for the radioimmunotherapy of hepatomas (Order SE, et al, 1980; 1981), and melanomas (Larson SM, et al, 1983). In Larson's studies, patients successfully imaged with I-131 antitumor antibodies received as much as 340 mCi in a single injection and as much as 830 mCi total activity over several injections. These investigators calculated that in patients with good antibody uptake in tumor, a dose of 100 mCi delivered 1040 rads to the tumor, 325 rads to the liver, and 30 rads to the bone marrow. While some studies have reported partial remissions using I-131 radioimmunotherapy, the overall therapeutic benefit of these procedures is yet to be established.

Other isotopes of radioiodine, such as I-125 and I-123 (Tabe 17.7), have received only limited use for tumor imaging with antibodies. The 25-35 keV photon emissions of I-125 are inadequate for scintillation imaging, and its 60-day half-life limits the amount of activity that can be safely administered. Iodine-123, with its monoenergetic 159 keV gamma emission and 13-hour physical half-life, is well suited for scintillation imaging. Iodine-123 radiolabeled antibodies have been used successfully for the clinical detection of tumors by some investigators (Epenetos AA, et al, 1982). The varying radionuclidic purity of I-123 produced by different methods, its relatively low specific activity, and the uncertain availability of this radionuclide have, however, been major limitations to the development of I-123 radiolabeled antibodies. A suitable commercial source of I-123 with high purity and high specific activity has recently become available, which may permit more widespread use and development of this radionuclide for diagnostic imaging.

Radiochemistry—Radiometals (Tc-99m, In-111, Y-90). During recent years, numerous attempts have been directed at radiolabeling proteins for diagnostic use with short-lived isotopes of various radio-metals, most importantly Technetium-99m (Tc-99m) and Indium-111 (In-111). For radioimmunotherapy applications, Yttrium-90 (Y-90), Copper-67 (Cu-67), and Rhenium-186 (Re-186) have also been explored. Diagnostic and therapeutic experiences with a select number of these radiometals are discussed briefly here.

Technetium-99m is nearly ideal for the radiolabeling of antibodies for diagnostic imaging purposes because of its optimal imaging properties, widespread availability, and relatively low cost. Unlike radioiodine, however, Tc-99m does not covalently bind to proteins and, hence, different approaches such as direct chelation (Pettit WA, 1980; Rhodes BA, et al, 1986) and chelation through covalently bound conjugates are needed for radiolabling antibodies. Technetium-99m binds with relatively high affinity to chelating agents, such as diethylenetriamine pentaacetic acid (or DTPA) (Khaw BA, et al, 1982), ethylenediamine tetraacetic actic (or EDTA) (Scheinberg DA, et al, 1982), metallothionein (Brown BA, et al, 1988), or N_2S_2 ligands (Fritzberg AR, et al, 1986). Each of these conjugates must be convalently linked to protein or carbohydrate moieties on the antibody to permit radiolabeling. Because new and improved radiometal binding conjugates are being continually described in the literature, it would be premature at this time to speculate as to which chelating technique may be optimal for the radiometal labeling of antibodies.

It is not entirely clear that Tc-99m will prove to have the same degree of utility for radioimmunodetection that it currently enjoys for other diagnostic nuclear medicine studies. Two historic limitations exist with regard to the use of Tc-99m. First, most of the methods developed for coupling Tc-99m to antibodies suffer from a lack of in vivo stability resulting in rapid loss of the radiolabel from the protein and its rapid urinary excretion (Burchiel SW, et al, 1985). Second, because optimal tumor-to-blood radioactivity ratios may not occur for up to 2–3 days after injection of the radiolabeled antibody, the 6-hour half-life of Tc-99m may be too short. Therefore, further studies are needed with Tc-99m labeled antibodies to determine their usefulness for tumor imaging.

Several of the conjugates and bifunctional chelating agents developed for Tc-99m antibody labeling have also proven useful for radiolabeling antibodies wth In-111. Of these, DTPA conjugates (Halpern SE, et al, 1983; Paxton RJ, et al, 1985; Carasquillo JA, et al, 1986; Keenan AM, et al, 1987; Murray JL, et al, 1987), bifunctional EDTA conjugates (Yeh SM, et al, 1979), and cyclic anhydrides of DTPA (Hnatowich DJ, et al, 1983; 1985) have proven most useful. Experience with In-111 DTPA conjugated antibodies has shown that liver uptake is a primary limitation to their use. However, in one study, In-111 DTPA conjugated antibodies were found to be advantageous to the respective I-131 labeled antibody in the detection of cancer (Stern P, et al, 1982). Again, further studies with In-111 conjugates are needed to determine whether suitable radiochemistries can be developed to permit routine labeling of antibodies for accurate tumor detection.

An antibody labeled with Y-90 has recently been evaluated as a therapeutic agent for cancer (Order SE, et al, 1986). Like the In-111 conjugates, Y-90 is coupled to antibodies via bifunctional chelation with DTPA. Yttrium-90 does, however, present special problems to investigators with regard to its radiochemical purity, because the principal trace contaminant, Strontium-90 (beta emission = 546 keV; $t_{1/2}$ = 28.6 yrs), localizes in bone and produces significant radiation exposure to the bone marrow. The high energy beta emission of Y-90 also presents concerns to personnel who handle the radionuclide or conduct the studies. Finally, Y-90 decays purely by beta emission; therefore, external imaging can be achieved only by using its Bremsstrahlung radiations. As a result, the difficulties associated with accurately imaging Y-90 rendering inaccurate any dosimetry calculations based upon imaging distri-

bution data. Clinical experience thus far is inadequate to judge the success of radioimmunotherapy with Y-90 labeled antibodies. The use of radionuclides that decay by alpa emissions (such as Astatine-211; see Zalutsky MR, et al, 1988) represents another potentially significant area of research for radioimmunotherapy.

Pharmacokinetics

The basic two-heavy-chain and two-light-chain structure of antibody molecules has been known since the mid-1960s. (Figure 17.3) The Fab portion of the antibody is important for the binding of antigen, whereas the Fc portion is associated with binding of complement proteins and interactions with specific cell surface Fc receptors. There is a relative paucity of information regarding antibody structure-activity relationships and how such factors influence in vivo biodistribution and metabolism. Various domains on the antibody molecule (such as the CH_2 and CH_3 domains) may be important in antibody biodistribution and catabolism and could be, in part, responsible for the pharmacokinetic differences seen between antibodies derived from different animal species (Burchiel SW, et al, 1987). The

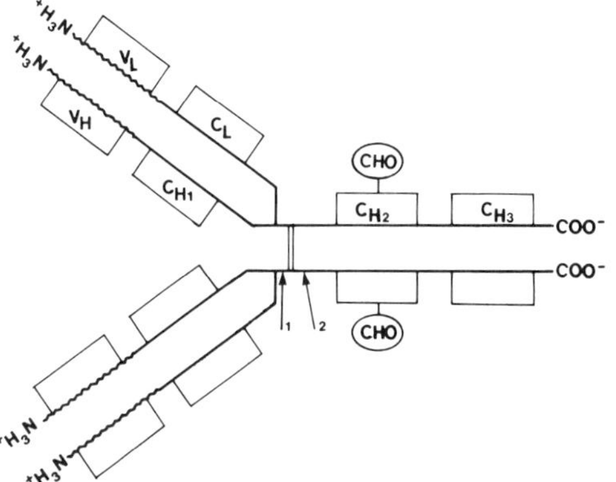

Figure 17.3 Diagram of an IgG antibody demonstrating sites of papain (site 1) and pepsin (site 2) cleavage to produce Fab and F(ab')$_2$ fragments, respectively. CHO = carbohydrate, V = variable region, C = constant region, H = heavy chain, L = light chain.

carbohydrate moieties associated with immunoglobulins may also play a role in antibody biodistribution and metabolism, but there has been little work to define how carbohydrate influences the in vivo behavior of immunoglobulins.

Of the several classes of antibodies synthesized by plasma cells (i. e., IgM, IgG, IgA, and IgD), the IgG class has received the most attention in the development of antibody-targeted radiopharmaceuticals. IgG antibodies are readily obtained following host immunization with tumor cells or antigens, can be produced using monoclonal antibody technology, and have reasonably high affinity for antigens. Additionally, the immunochemistry of IgG has been relatively well studied. Several animal species synthesize two or more subclasses of IgG, which may have slightly different immunologic and pharmacokinetic properties. In humans, four subclasses of IgG (designated IgG_1, IgG_2, IgG_3, and IgG_4) have been demonstrated, and they are known to have slightly different rates of metabolism following intravenous injection (Morrell A, et al, 1970).

Studies of endogenous immunoglobulins directed at understanding the normal biodistribution and metabolism of antibody molecules have found that IgG is distributed in highest concentrations in the blood, with slightly lower concentrations in the extracellular fluid. IgG is present in reduced concentrations in ultrafiltrates (such as in the cerebrospinal fluid), and IgG does not efficiently penetrate the blood-brain barrier. Specific Fc receptors are associated with the transplacental transfer of IgG into fetal blood to form a passive immunity against infections. Intravenous injection of IgG usually results in a biphasic or triphasic pattern of blood elimination, representing the distribution of the antibody from the intravascular to the extravascular compartments, followed by protein metabolism and clearance (Waldmann TA and Strober W, 1968). Some antibodies demonstrate a dose-dependent clearance from blood (Larson SM, et al, 1983; Caras-

quillo JA, et al, 1988), whereas other antibodies do not show this effect (Rosenblum MG, et al, 1987).

Early studies have shown that different families of immunoglobulin molecules have significantly different blood elimination kinetics when administered intravenously (Waldmann TA and Strober W, 1968). Antibodies of the IgG class were found in most species to clear slowly from blood following intravenous injection. As previously mentioned, due to the macromolecular size of antibodies, there is little penetration into the central nervous system (Goldman A, et al, 1984). However, antibody localization (in particular, uptake of antibody fragments) in brain tumors can occur when there has been significant disruption of the blood-brain barrier (Day ED, et al, 1965).

In animals, optimal imaging with radiolabeled IgG antibodies is achieved several days after injection, when the circulating antibody declines to sufficiently low levels to permit reasonable tumor-to-blood ratios. This observation promoted several investigations to evaluate techniques that accelerate the blood elimination of antibodies; techniques that may permit the use of short-lived isotopes for imaging studies. These experiments have led to the widespread use of antibody fragments for in vivo imaging.

Antibody fragments, such as the bivalent $F(ab')_2$ or the univalent Fab molecules, clear more rapidly from blood than whole antibody molecules (Burchiel SW, et al, 1982b). $F(ab')_2$ molecules are prepared using a pepsin digest that cleaves the Fc portion of the antibody molecule at Site 2 (see Figure 17.3). Fab fragments are made using the enzyme papain that clips IgG at Site 1 on both heavy chains. A procedure to make Fab' antibody fragments involves the production of $F(ab')_2$ fragments with pepsin, followed by a mild reduction step to separate the intra-heavy chain disulfide bonds.

The choice of a whole IgG antibody versus an $F(ab')_2$ or Fab fragment depends upon the intended use of the radiolabeled antibody. Since vascular permeability influences the uptake of antibodies by tumors (Sands H, et al, 1988), antibody fragments may penetrate tumors more efficiently than whole IgG molecules. However, though antibody fragments may penetrate tumors better, some studies have shown that they may also have a reduced residence time in tumors (Wahl RL, et al, 1983). For imaging studies with short-lived radioisotopes, antibody fragments may be preferred because of their rapid blood clearance. However, for radioimmunotherapy studies, the whole IgG antibody with its longer blood half-time and potentially longer tumor residence time may be advantageous.

It has only recently been realized that heterologous antibodies (antibodies of one species studied in another species) have quite variable blood half-lives. For example, it has been found that mouse monoclonal antibodies have much shorter half-lives in the blood of humans and primates than they do in mice (Burchiel SW, et al, 1987). Therefore, in some studies the localization of tumors with IgG has been sufficiently rapid that the use of antibody fragments has not been necessary.

Another issue relating to antibody pharmacokinetics and clearance involves potential changes in in vivo antibody behavior in immune individuals. Since most of the antitumor antibodies that have been used in humans in recent years were derived from animal sources, antibody immunogenicity has proven to be an important consideration in imaging and therapy studies. Patients developing antibodies to the foreign antitumor antibody exhibit marked differences in the patterns of foreign antibody distribution and clearance. In most of these cases, intravenously administered antibodies are cleared rapidly from the blood stream in the form of immune complexes that deposit in the organs of the reticuloendothelial system (i.e., liver, spleen, or bone marrow). Since immune complexes are removed quickly from blood, the anti-tumor antibody bound in this manner is no longer effective in reaching the tumor target. In most cases the presence of even a weak immune response against a heterologous antibody will effectively neutralize the activity of the antitumor antibody. These findings have prompted investigators to develop other sources of antibodies, such as human monoclonal antibodies and chimeric antibodies. The latter are usually a combination of mouse variable regions and human constant regions. An alternative approach has been to chemically modify antibodies to reduce their immunogenicity in patients (Tomasi TB, et al, 1983).

PRECAUTIONS

Specific limitations and precautions to be observed for the use of antibody-targeted radiopharmaceuticals are yet to be defined and will undoubtedly vary somewhat for the various agents developed. In general, there has been a relatively low incidence of side effects associated with the parenteral administration of most antibody reagents. The development of an immune response against foreign antibody molecules has been a common observation that limits the number of times that an individual can receive a given species or class of an antibody molecule. Although the incidence of acute allergic reactions to antibody molecules is relatively low, many investigators skin test patients with a small intradermal injection of antibody or antibody conjugate before proceeding with a radiolabeled antibody study. The skin test, however, does not usually detect the presence of circulating antibodies reactive with the antibody-directed radiopharmaceutical. Such reactivity must usually be identified using an in vitro immunoassay.

Another general precaution that must be observed pertains to the prevention of protein aggregation that can occur with antibody labeling procedures. Protein aggregates can produce rapid and profound hypotension if injected intravenously. Quality assurance techniques must be developed to ensure that protein aggregates are not formed, or that they are appropriately removed. Ultracentrifugation (approximately 100,000 × g for 30 min) of antibody solutions is effective for the removal of most protein aggregates. In addition, the administration of antibodies by slow intravenous infusion can minimize the related side effects seen with a bolus injection.

CLINICAL CONSIDERATIONS

Because no radiolabeled antibodies are currently approved for routine use in the United States, only general comments can be made regarding the clinical use and particular contraindications for radioimmunodetection and/or therapy. Little is known about the in vivo behavior of antibodies (particularly mouse monoclonal antibodies) in normal versus cancer patients. Several investigators have reported a relatively high incidence of false positives and false negatives in antibody imaging studies (Sullivan DC, et al, 1982), and the general sensitivity and specificity of tumor detection with antibodies has thus been questioned. As greater experience is gained in the use of particular radiolabeled antibodies, normal patterns of biodistribution and metabolism will become better understood and anomalous patterns of uptake are likely to be better recognized. Further improvements in the radiolabeled antibody products themselves are also likely to help improve the sensitivity and specificity of tumor localization.

With regard to the use of radiolabeled antibodies, several general contraindications exist. Patients should not be entered into any diagnostic or therapeutic study involving antibody-targeted radiopharmaceuticals if they have either known or suspected allergies or sensitivities to the type of antibody to be used. Second, patients with circulating antibodies to the antibody-targeted radiopharmaceutical are likely to receive little clinical benefit and should be excluded from the study. Because most patients given antibodies develop an immune response against the foreign protein within 2–4 weeks, repeat studies in patients must be cautiously conducted. Third, because the effects of radiolabeled antibodies on germ cells or developing tissues are not known, pregnant women should not be studied until further data is obtained.

Additional clinical considerations and contraindications for the use of radiolabeled antibodies for imaging and therapy will become available as more experience is gained with specific agents. Clearly, great potential exists for the development of new and improved antibody-targeted radiopharmaceuticals for diagnostic and therapeutic applications; however, only further studies will determine whether the potential for using radiolabeled antibodies will be realized.

DOSAGE/DOSIMETRY

Route of Administration. Though most clinical studies with radiolabeled antibodies have utilized the intravenous route of injection, several recent studies have demonstrated the feasibility of administering antibodies subcutaneosuly, via the intraperitoneal cavity, or into an afferent vessel to enhance a more regional distribution. The technique of lymphoscintigraphy has been used to identify tumor cells in lymph nodes of patients following subcutaneous administration of a radiolabeled antibody (DeLand FH, et al, 1979; 1980; Weinstein JN, et al, 1986; Keenan AM, et al, 1987). However, the specificity of antibody uptake in involved lymph nodes has been questioned (Nelp WB, et al, 1987). Colorectal tumors have been successfully identified with anti-tumor antibodies given by the intraperitoneal route (Colcher D, et al, 1987a;b; Ward BG, et al, 1987) and intercarotid administration has been used to localize neuroblastomas and gliomas in the brain (Day ED, et al, 1965; Moseley R, et al, 1987).

Dosage. When determining the dose of a radiolabeled antibody that should be used in a clinical study, several different factors require consideration. First, the total amount of protein to be administered is dependent on the particular antibody to be used as well as the tumor type to be imaged or treated. In contrast to most nuclear medicine studies that involve the administration of radiolabeled substances in tracer amounts, antibody studies may require the use of pharmacologic concentrations of protein (.01 to 1 mg/kg body weight) to permit successsful imaging. One explanation for these findings is that circulating antigen that is either shed or excreted by tumor cells complexes the antibody in serum before it has an opportunity to reach tumor. The administration of large amounts of antibody saturates the circulating antigen and allows free antibody to reach tumor sites. Alternatively, the presence of a dose response for antibody clearance may relate to saturation of an uptake or elimination process associated with antibody metabolism. Further studies are necessary to resolve which of these explanations is responsible for the observed dose-related changes in antibody biodistribuution and metabolism.

Second, the radionuclide and the radioactivity to be administered for imaging/therapy will depend upon the particular radiolabeled antibody studied and its kinetics for localization. An advantage to the use of radiolabeled antibody chelates is that a diagnostic radionuclide (such as Tc-99m or In-111) can be used to determine the percnt uptake of the radiolabeled antibody in the tumor versus other tissues. If sufficient uptake in the tumor is detected, then a therapeutic radionuclide (such as Y-90 and Re-186) may be substitued for tumor therapy with minimal concern in regard to an associated alteration in antibody biodistribution. Based upon the imaging study, calculations can be made of the dose of radiation that will be delivered to the tumor with the therapeutic radionuclide. The amount of activity targeted to the tumor will likely be limited by the amount of absorbed dose that normal tissues and organs will receive. Because antibodies normally distribute to the liver, bone marrow, and kidneys, these organs or tissues are likely to receive significant radiation exposure during an antibody study.

III. Imaging Inflammatory Processes Abscesses

GA-67 CITRATE

Background/History

Until recently, the tumor-seeking radiopharmaceutical, Ga-67 citrate, was also the agent of choice for the detection of inflammatory processes and pelvic and abdominal abscesses; demonstrating, in the latter conditions, a sensitivity and specificity approaching 90% (Staab EV and McCartney WH, 1978).

Chemistry

See previous section on Ga-67 citrate for tumor imaging.

Pharmacokinetics

(See previous section on Ga-67 citrate for tumor imaging.)

The mechanism of Ga-67 localization in abscesses and other inflammatory processes is not fully understood. Lactoferrin, a protein for which Ga-67 has greater avidity than transferrin, is found intracellularly in leukocytes. It has been postulated that transferrin-bound Ga-67 can pass into the leukocyte, whereupon the gallium becomes bound to intracellular lactoferrin (Hoffer PB, 1978). Hence, gallium localization in inflammatory lesions may be related to its internal labeling of leukocytes that are already present at, or will subsequently migrate to, the respective site. Gallium-67 uptake in inflammatory processes does not appear to be totally dependent on leukocyte activity, however, because gallium localization will also occur in the presence of leukopenia.

Because a variety of microorganisms will take up gallium, it is possible that a high local concentration of bacteria in the abscess or at the site of inflammation may be partly responsible for the respective localization of Ga-67 (Tsan M, et al, 1978; Menon S, et al, 1978; Camargo EE, et al,

1979). Intracellular iron-binding substances other than lactoferrin have also been suggested as being responsible for Ga-67 uptake in bacteria. Ferritin, the intracellular iron-storage protein, and siderophores, iron-binding molecules synthesized by bacteria, have been shown to have a great affinity for Ga-67. Because these intracellular iron-binding substances have higher affinity for Ga-67 than transferrin, it is possible that Ga-67 is transported to an abscess bound to transferrin with subsequent translocation to these intracellular proteins (Weiner RE, et al, 1985).

Reasonably, the localization of Ga-67 in abscesses and other inflammatory processes may also involve other or multiple pathways. The localization mechanism may be as simplistic as abnormal passive diffusion of the bulky transferrin-Ga-67 complex through the altered vascular endothelium of inflamed tissue.

Clinical Considerations. Although in clinical practice Ga-67 citrate is often preferred over other radiopharmaceuticals or imaging modalities for the localization of sites of inflammation, particularly when whole-body scanning is indicated, a primary disadvantage to its use is the normal localization of Ga-67 in the liver and its excretion in the bowel. This normal distribution of Ga-67 activity can complicate the diagnosis of abdominal abscess and often requires that bowel cleansing be performed. More recently the use of Ga-67 citrate for the evaluation of abdominal inflammation has diminished in favor of the alternate imaging modalities of computed body tomography and ultrasound, or the nuclear medicine application of radiolabeled leukocytes (In-111 leukocytes), the latter having a reported higher sensitivity for the detection of acute processes. Ga-67 citrate imaging remains preferable to In-111 leukocytes for the detection and evaluation of chronic inflammatory processes (Figure 17.4).

DOSAGE/DOSIMETRY

The amount of Ga-67 citrate administered for abscess imaging is typically lower (i. e., 3–5 mCi) than the dosage used for tumor imaging (i. e., 8–10 mCi). Because Ga-67 localization in abscesses or other inflammatory processes is relatively rapid, imaging may commence at 24 hours following administration rather than at the 48–96-hour interval suggested for tumor imaging. Imaging at earlier than 24 hours post Ga-67 citrate injection is undesirable because it has been associated with diminished sensitivity and specificity. The dosimetry of Ga-67 citrate associated with imaging sites of abscess/inflammation is the same as for tumor imaging (Table 17.5).

IN-111 LABELED LEUKOCYTES

BACKGROUND/HISTORY

Body defense mechanisms, which are activated during infection to immobilize, phagocytize, and kill the causative bacterial agent, utilize white cells, or leukocytes, to play the major role in this defense process. White cells are made up of three classes: granulocytes, mononuclear phagocytes, and lymphocytes. The granulocytic functions, which include chemotaxis, ingestion, and/or inhibition of bacterial replication are performed by three distinct cell types: neutrophils, eosinophils, and basophils, whose names are derived from their staining characteristics. Neutrophils are the principal cells in the localization and removal of microorganisms, immune complexes, and damaged cells. Mononuclear phagocytes (monocytes and tissue macrophages) serve a secondary defense mechanism in more severe infections by ingesting causative organisms to control their proliferation and spread. In severe infections of a chronic nature, the lymphoid system may also be activated.

Because leukocytes comprise the primary defense mechanism against infection, researchers have attempted to image

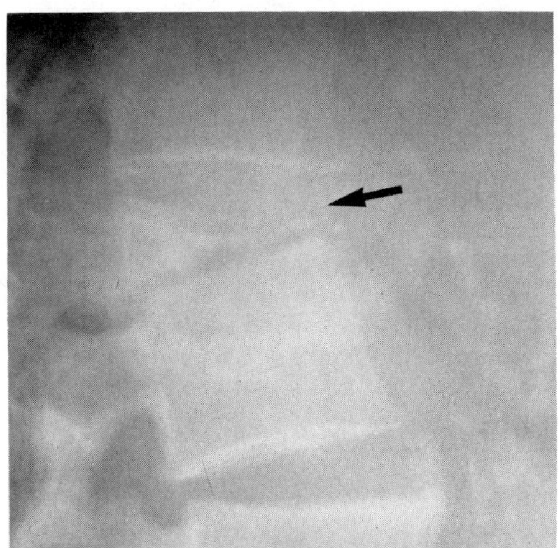

Figure 17.4A Lateral radiograph of the spine reveals collapse of the third lumbar vertebral body (arrow) resulting from chronic arthritis.

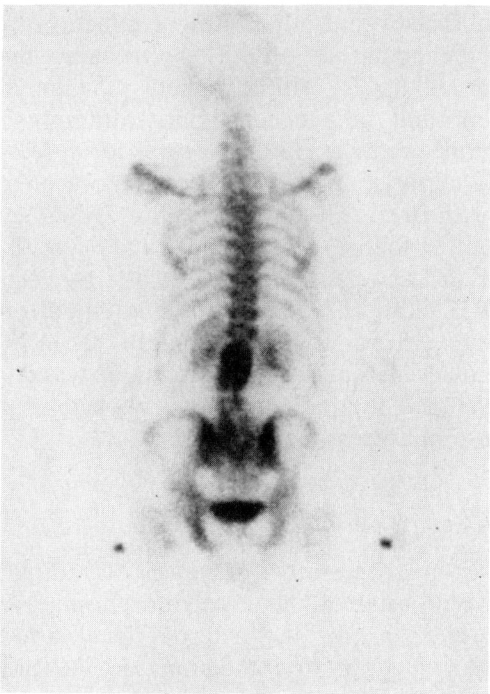

Figure 17.4B Tc-99m medronate skeletal scintigram in the same patient demonstrates markedly increased tracer uptake in the mid-lumbar spine. The skeletal tracer localizes in reactive bone but does not reveal the soft tissue extent of inflammation.

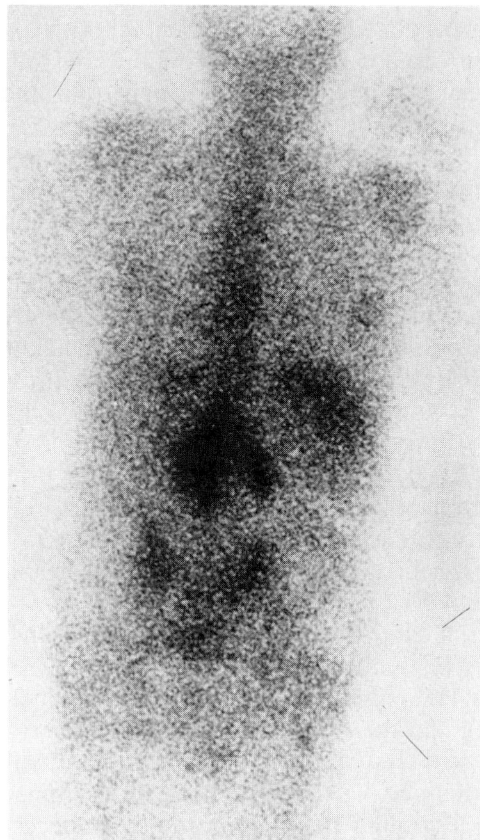

Figure 17.4C Ga-67 citrate study (posterior view) in same patient demonstrates intense uptake in skeletal and paravertebral tissues involved in the inflammatory process.

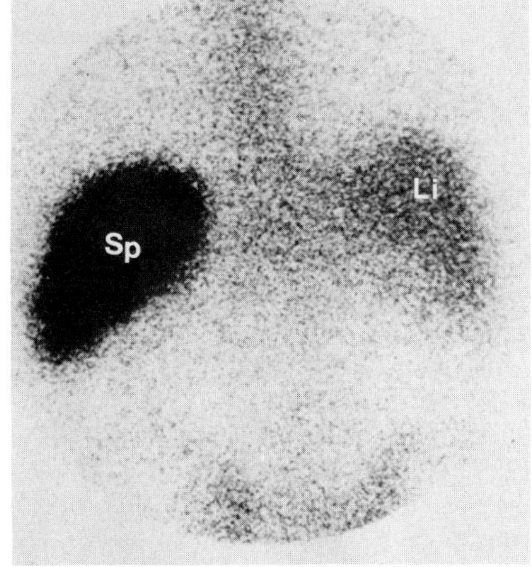

Figure 17.4D In-111 leukocyte study (posterior view) in same patient demonstrates negative localization in the involved region apparently due to the chronic nature of this inflammatory process. Li = liver, Sp = spleen.

abscesses and other sites of infection by labeling these cells (in particular the granulocytes) with a variety of gamma-emitting radionuclides. Early attempts to utilize radiolabeled leukocytes for abscess localization involved their radiolabeling with Cr-51, Ga-67, or Tc-99m (as Tc-99m sulfur colloid) (McMillan R and Scott JL, 1968; Deysine M, et al, 1970; Burleson RL, et al, 1975; English D and Andersen BR, 1975). It was not until recently, however, that a reliable technique was developed for radiolabeling leukocytes for use in abscess localization.

CHEMISTRY

The successful application of radiolabeled autologous polymorphonuclear leukocytes for the external localization of infections and inflammatory lesions centered upon work performed by J.G. McAfee and M.L. Thakur (1976c) when they examined a large variety of soluble and particulate substances for cellular radiolabeling suitability. Among substances they examined, nonpolar, lipid-soluble reagents were found preferable, and of these, In-111 oxine (or 8-hydroxy-quinoline) provided excellent properties for cellular labeling. Technetium-99m oxine was also investigated and found useful; however, Indium-111 was preferred to Tc-99m because its longer half-life (2.8 days) permitted imaging at 24 hours following administration of the labeled leukocytes when blood and background levels are low.

The cyclotron-produced radionuclide, In-111, decays by electron capture with a physical half-life of 2.8 days. Its decay is accompanied by the emission of a 172 keV (90% abundance) and a 247 keV (94% abundance) gamma photons. Hence, each disintegration of In-111 results in the release of 1.8 photons with energies suitable for nuclear medicine imaging. C.S. Marcus and colleagues (1985) caution that because the radionuclide contaminants In-114 and In-114m contribute substantially to radiation dose, In-111 radiopharmaceuticals in general (includ-

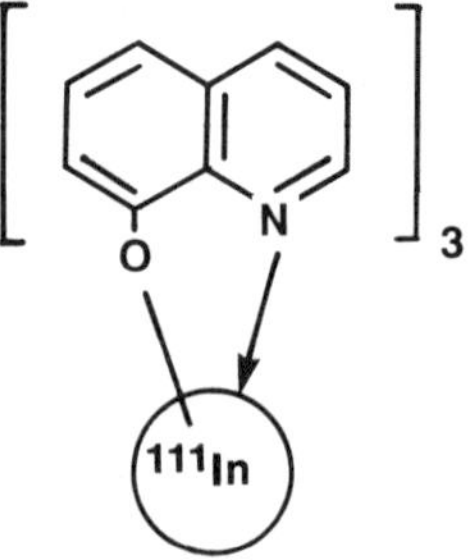

Figure 17.5 Neutral lipophilic 1:3 complex of In-111 with oxine (8-hydroxyquinoline).

ing In-111 oxine) should not be used much later than about 3 days after the time of calibration.

Oxine (molecular weight 145) is a lipophilic chelating agent that has been used for many years as a topical fungicide, antiperspirant, and spermicide. Indium forms a saturated (1:3) complex with oxine (Figure 17.5) that is neutral and sufficiently lipid soluble to penetrate the leukocyte membrane. Once within the cell, the complex dissociates and the indium binds firmly to nuclear and cytoplasmic proteins. Such intracellular binding occurs because the stability constant of the In-111 oxine complex is relatively low compared to the higher affinity of the cytoplasmic proteins for In-111 (Thakur ML, et al, 1977b). Oxine remains diffusible and is removed in subsequent cell washings (Mathias CJ and Welch MJ, 1979). During the leukocyte labeling procedure (Table 17.9) it is important to remove plasma because In-111 also possesses higher affinity for serum transferrin than for oxine. The dissociation of In-111 from oxine and its binding to serum transferrin significantly lowers the amount of In-111 oxine available for leukocyte labeling and the resultant labeling efficiency.

In-111 oxine is nonspecific for leukocytes and will label almost all cell types indiscriminately. Therefore, it is necessary during cell labeling (Table 17.9) to separate from whole blood the desired cellular fraction (in this case, the leukocytes) in order to assure optimum In-111 labeling of this specific cellular component (Thakur ML et al, 1977c). Even with

Table 17.9   STEPS IN THE PREPARATION OF [111]IN-OXINE LABELED LEUKOCYTES (MIXED)

A. Leukocyte Collection/Isolation
  1. Collect approximately 40 ml whole blood into a syringe containing 1000–2000 U heparin (or 7 ml ACD solution).
  2. Add 3 ml of 6% Hetastarch (optional), to blood and incubate with needle up at 30°–45° angle for 30–60 minutes at room temperature.
  3. Express equal volumes of leukocyte-rich plasma (LRP) into 2 disposable, sterile centrifuge tubes.
    a. Centrifuge LRP at 150–300 G for 5 minutes.
    b. Remove leukocyte-poor plasma (LPP) and *save*.
  4. Resuspend leukocyte pellets in 5 ml of 0.9% Sodium Chloride Injection, U.S.P. and combine.
    a. Centrifuge combined leukocyte suspension at 150–300 G for 5 minutes.
    b. Remove saline wash and resuspend leukocytes in 5 ml 0.9% Sodium Chloride Injection, U.S.P.
    c. Repeat steps 4a and 4b.
B. Leukocyte Labeling
  1. Add ^{111}In-oxine dropwise to the leukocyte suspension.
  2. Incubate for 15 minutes at room temperature with frequent mild agitation.
  3. Add 5 ml of LPP (step 3b.) to ^{111}In-leukocyte suspension.
    a. Centrifuge at 150–300 G for 5 minutes.
    b. Remove supernatant (i. e., non-^{111}In-leukocyte activity).
  4. Resuspend ^{111}In-leukocyte pellet in 5 ml of LPP (step 3b.)
  5. Perform assay and quality assurance procedures.

---

extreme care in separation, contamination by other cell types does occur. Studies of the relative labeling of granulocytes and red blood cells by In-111 oxine indicates that red blood cells take up only a small fraction of In-111. In practice, whenever red blood cells constitute less than 10% of the total cell population, the red-blood-cell-associated radioactivity is negligible (Weiblen BJ, et al, 1979). However, studies performed in the presence of an unusually large number of radiolabeled red blood cells demonstrate persistent blood pool activity and poor abscess to background ratios.

Leukocyte Separation and Collection. Erthyrocyte separation by gravity sedimentation of anticoagulated whole blood is the often-employed method of obtaining mixed leukocyte suspensions for In-111 labeling (Table 17.9). Although heparin is the most commonly employed anticoagulant, J.G. McAfee and associates (1984) suggest the use of ACD solution because ACD anticoagulated leukocytes show less tendency to adhere to disposable plastic centrifuge tubes and syringes used in the radiolabeling procedure. After gravity sedimentation for about 1 hour, most platelets and about 70% of the leukocytes remain suspended in the supernatant plasma. Adjunctive erythrocyte-aggregating agents, including 2% methylcellulose in saline, 6% dextran, or 6% hydroxyethyl starch (HES), are fre-

quently employed in the sedimentation process (Table 17.9). Of these, HES is preferred because it induces more rapid red cell sedimentation and greater leukocyte recovery. HES is cleared from the body after administration, and its use has not been associated with allergic reactions (Roy AJ, et al, 1971). HES is commercially available as a 6% sterile, apyrogenic solution.

A variety of cell-separation techniques, including density gradient centrifugation with Ficoll-Hypaque and Percoll, centrifugal elutriation, and flow cytometry have been employed in leukocyte labeling, each requiring varying degrees of sophisticated equipment and expertise. Although Ficoll-Hypaque gradients are popular for separation of neutrophils, studies have shown that Ficoll-Hypaque may have an adverse metabolic effect upon leukocytes (Dooley DC, et al, 1982). Separation by the use of Percoll gradients has shown no detrimental effects on human cells. Pure neutrophils, obtained by a gradient-separation technique followed by hypotonic lysis of erythrocytes, have been shown to accumulate in liver in higher quantities than those obtained similarly but without hypotonic lysis (Thakur ML, et al, 1977b).

In-111 Oxine Formulations. Originally, the preparation of In-111 oxine involved solvent extraction of the radiolabeled complex using chloroform or methylene chloride, followed by solvent evaporation and by dissolution in ethanol. The product prepared in this manner was subsequently added to mixed leukocytes suspended in approximately 5 ml of plasma-free medium (Thakur ML, 1981). Ethanol is undesirable, however, because even in dilute concentrations it demonstrates cytotoxicity. Concentrations of ethanol as low as 0.125% have been shown to induce structural changes in neutrophils (Lichtman M, et al, 1976).

Ethanol is avoided entirely by formulating In-111 oxine in an aqueous surfactant solution (Goedemens WTH, 1981) or by using the soluble salt, oxine sulfate, in TRIS or HEPES buffer (Ducassou D, et al, 1978). Presently, the only In-111 oxine preparation commercially available in the United States is an ethanol-free formulation that contains 50 μg/ml oxine dissolved in HEPES-saline buffer with Polysorbate 80 (Table 17.10).

Comparisons of leukocyte labeling efficiencies using either In-111 oxine in ethanol or the aqueous surfactant formulation have shown that In-111 oxine in aqueous solution yields significantly higher labeling efficiencies (Marcus CS, 1984b). Chemotaxis of labeled cells has also been shown to be reduced in those preparations that contain greater than 1% ethanol (Weiblen BJ, et al, 1979).

Trace-element contamination of the In-111 chloride used to form the oxine complex can significantly lower leukocyte-labeling efficiencies or cause harmful effects on neutrophils. Trace amounts of the metals, Zn, Cd, Cu, or Fe, which may be present in concentrations as high as 3 μg/ml, compete with In-111 by forming 2:1 or 3:1 complexes with the relatively small amount of oxine utilized. Cadmium ions are derived from the cadmium target used in In-111 production. The manufacturer of the currently available commercial preparation of In-111 oxine specifies that not more than 0.5 μg/ml cadmium or other metal ion impurities are present. Whether cadmium in this relatively small amount is harmful to leukocytes is not known. However, concentrations of zinc as low as 0.3 μg/ml have been reported to be harmful to neutrophils (Chvapil M, et al, 1977).

PHARMACOKINETICS

B. J. Weiblen and colleagues (1979) found the mean intravascular survival time of an essentially pure In-111 granulocyte preparation to be approximately 5 hours. In this study the level of radioactivity in the circulation did not reach its maximum until 1/2–2 hours after injection. M. L. Thakur and colleagues (1977a; b) studied granulocyte kinetics using a mixed leukocyte suspension contaminated with red blood cells and noted recovery results of 50–75%. Unfortunately, whole-blood radioactivity did not accurately represent granulocyte survival time.

In-111 activity from labeled leukocytes normally localizes only in the spleen, liver, marrow, and transiently in the lungs (Figure 17.6). Immediately after injection of the labeled leukocytes, radioactivity distributes throughout the lungs, with approximately one-half of this activity cleared by 15 minutes (Thakur ML, et al, 1977b). Lung uptake is often evident in images taken 1–2 hours post injection but usually clears entirely by 4 hours. Accumulation of radioactivity in the liver and spleen reaches a plateau within the first 75 minutes, then decreases gradually during the following 24 hours (Figure 17.6). At 4 hours, approximately 12% and 19% of the administered activity is in the liver and spleen, respectively. The liver and spleen activity appears to represent margination

Table 17.10   CURRENTLY AVAILABLE[a] FORMULATION OF ^{111}IN-OXINE FOR LEUKOCYTE LABELING

CONSTITUENTS	CONCENTRATION
Oxine (8-hydroxyquinoline)	50 μg/ml
Polysorbate 80	100 ppm
HEPES buffer	25 mM
Sodium chloride	0.75% w/v
Indium-111	1 mCi/ml[b]

[a] U.S. market, Amersham, Inc.
[b] At calibration.

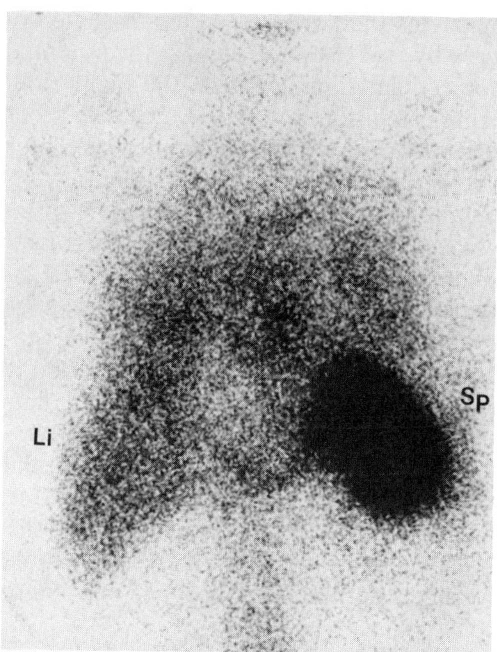

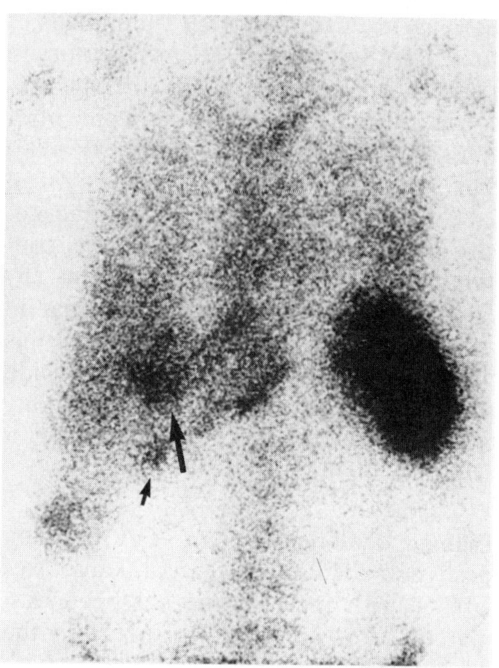

Figure 17.6A Anterior chest and abdominal image obtained with In-111 leukocytes at 4 hours post injection. The image reveals a normal degree of lung activity for this time period and residual tracer in the cardiac blood pool. The relative activities of the liver (Li) and spleen (Sp) are also normal. No focal abnormalities are apparent.

Figure 17.6B Corresponding view in the same patient obtained at 24 hours post tracer administration reveals normal clearing of lung and blood pool activity. Note (arrows) that at least two focal areas of In-111 leukocyte uptake can now be discerned in the liver associated with hepatic abscesses.

of the viable labeled cells as well as removal of damaged cells or cell fragments. The distribution of radioactivity between the liver and spleen seems influenced by parameters involved in the preparation of the radiolabeled leukocytes. Cells with lowered viability give high levels of activity in the liver, whereas preparations with higher viability but contaminated with red cells and lymphocytes result in high levels of splenic radioactivity (Thakur ML, et al, 1977b).

PRECAUTIONS

It is possible that the viability of the radiolabeled leukocytes can be adversely affected by an excess concentration of oxine or by cellular radiation effects. Other factors that can affect the accuracy of the respective imaging study include leukocyte count and radiolabeling efficiency.

Oxine Concentration. The LD_{50} of oxine in mice by subcutaneous and intraperitoneal administration is 30 mg/kg and 88.8 mg/kg, respectively (Albert A, et al, 1954). This toxicity is no apparent concern, however, because oxine released from the cell following radiolabeling is probably removed from the preparation by subsequent cell washings. Whether oxine is directly cytotoxic is not entirely clear. A. W. Segal and associates (1978) found that concentrations of oxine as low as 7.5 $\mu g/10^7$ cells reduced the random migration and chemotaxis of polymorphonuclear leukocyte by almost 50%. In another report no loss of leukocyte function was observed with oxine concentrations up to 10 $\mu g/10^7$ cells (Zakhireh B, et al, 1979), whereas J. E. T. Burke and coworkers (1982) found that oxine markedly depressed leukocyte chemotaxis and phagocytosis in concentrations as low as 3 μg/ml. (The reported differences of toxic thresholds for oxine may be due, in part, to differences in cell labeling protocols.) Reduction of oxine concentrations to nontoxic levels (0.5 μg/10^7 cells), was reported to reduce the In-111 cell labeling efficiency by 80%. In practice, commercially available preparations containing 0.5–1.0 mCi of In-111 in 25–50 μg oxine generally exhibit no apparent adverse effects, thus suggesting that this preparation still permits a relatively wide safety margin (i. e., maintenance of functionally normal leukocyte function) with relatively high labeling efficiency.

Cellular Radiation Effects. The radiation dose delivered to individual leukocytes labeled with In-111 oxine has been estimated. In a typical study involving the labeling of 100 million leukocytes with 0.5 mCi In-111 oxine, the integrated dose/cell has been calculated to be approximately 8500 rads. Although this radiation dose seems high, polymorphonuclear leukocytes are very resistant to any damaging effects by ionizing radiation (Selvaraj RJ, et al, 1967; Holley RH, et al, 1974). In in vitro studies involving external irradiation with 50,000 rads, little or no effect on polymorphonuclear phagocytic or metabolic functions was observed (Selvaraj RJ and Sbarra AJ, 1966), and doses of less than 75,000 rads did not cause any ultrastructural damage (Holley RH, et al, 1974). B. Zakhireh and associates (1979) showed no detectable effects on the random migration or chemotaxis of leukocytes labeled with doses of In-111 up to six times the upper limit per million leukocytes and tested at 4 hours after radiolabeling.

Of potentially greater concern is the radiation dose to lymphocytes. Controversy exists as to whether lymphocytes labeled with In-111 may result in transformed cells that, after proliferation, may trigger a malignant process (ten Berge RJM, et al, 1983). Central to this concern is (1) the observation that mixed leukocyte suspensions contain up to 20% lymphocytes that will be labeled to some degree by In-111 oxine, and (2) the potential for cellular damage from the highly ionizing radiation of the Auger electrons emitted by In-111. Whether complex cytogenetic abnormalities in mature, circulating lymphocytes are indicators of increased risk of leukemogenesis and lymphomagenesis is not entirely clear. Evidence of increased risk certainly can be found in atomic bomb survivors who received a significant amount of whole-body irradiation. C. S. Marcus (1984a) points out, however, that mature lymphocytes are not subject to division and that the increased incidence of leukemia noted in the population that received this whole-body irradiation is most likely attributable to radiation-induced oncogenesis of stem cells.

Leukocyte Count. The number of leukocytes to be administered is a significant parameter that affects image quality. M. K. Loken and colleagues (1985) suggested that when autologous leukocytes are used for abscess localization studies, approximately 1×10^8 leukocytes are adequate for imaging, with corresponding fewer leukocytes required in pediatric patients. When nonautologous cells must be used, it is suggested that no fewer than 2–4×10^8 cells be given because histocompatibility factors in some patients can reduce the intravascular survival of the nonautologous cells such that less than 5% of the administered cells remain in the vascular compartment at 1 hour following injection (McCullough J, et al, 1981).

Quality Control of In-111 Leukocytes. Because to achieve an adequate labeling efficiency the leukocytes must be removed from plasma during the In-111 oxine radiolabeling procedure, a loss of cellular viability may result (Thakur ML, et al, 1984). The early, transient lung uptake of In-111 leukocytes has been suggested to be due to cell damage sustained in the labeling process (Saverymuttu MU, et al, 1983). F.L. Datz and coworkers (1984) did not, however, find any statistically significant correlation between early diffuse lung uptake (a possible sign of decreased cell viability) and decrease in sensitivity of leukocytes for diagnosing infection at early imaging times (<4 hrs), thus indicating that sufficient numbers of cells apparently survive the labeling process. It has been suggested that lung uptake may represent the natural physiology of polymorphonuclear leukocytes in the lungs (Weisberger AS, et al, 1950).

In consideration of the rigors of the In-111 oxine labeling procedure and the detrimental effects of free In-111 (i. e., distributes in blood as In-111 transferrin) on subsequent images, quality-assurance procedures should be developed that are relatively convenient to perform and that permit a rapid evaluation of leukocyte viability and the quantification of cell-associated radioactivity. Prior to reinjection of the labeled leukocytes, their viability can be evaluated by a number of procedures including the Ficoll-Hypaque distribution analysis (Clay ME and McCullough J, 1978), trypan blue exclusion test (Table 17.11), dual-filter radiochemotaxis assay (English D and Clanton JA, 1984) and others. The Ficoll-Hypaque distribution analysis and other similar cell viability tests are time extensive and have not been good predictors of clinical utility. Therefore, it has been suggested that routinely performed white cell counts, microscopic examinations, and determinations of labeling efficiency are adequate for quality control of In-111 labeled leukocytes (Baker WJ and Datz FL, 1984).

Indium-111 leukocyte labeling procedures (see Table 17.9) typically employ a final centrifugation and washing step to remove any In-111 (oxine or transferrin) not incorporated within the cells. If this step is not included, a quantification of cell-associated radioactivity should be performed to ensure that an adequate labeling efficiency has been achieved. Using a hematocrit tube, a small aliquot of the labeled cell suspension is sampled. Following centrifugation at 300 G or greater, the hematocrit tube is broken at the cell-supernatant interface and the radioactivity of each portion quantified by assay in a scintillation well counter. The fraction of cell-associated activity is determined by dividing the activity asociated with the cellular portion by the total activity (i. e., supernatant plus cellular activity) in the tube.

CLINICAL CONSIDERATIONS

Utrasound, computed tomography, and In-111 leukocytes have all been shown to be excellent methods for localizing abscesses with reported accuracies ranging from 80–95%. Ultrasound has some advantages over CT and leukocyte imaging in that it is the fastest and least expensive mode of abscess imaging. It can distinguish fluid from solid masses, and sagittal and transverse scans can be obtained for accurate lesion localization. Ultrasound does, however, require considerable expertise and may be compromised when open wounds, drain lines, or tubes exist. Unfortunately, it is also of low specificity since a variety of conditions (seromas, hematomas, lymphoceles, urinomas, and cysts) mimic the sonographic appearance of abscess.

Computed tomography also permits the precise localization of abscesses and is not hindered by tubes, drains, or the presence

---

Table 17.11   EVALUATION OF GRANULOCYTE VIABILITY BY TRYPAN BLUE EXCLUSION

Materials and Reagents
Cell suspension (2–5 × 10^8 cells ml)
Trypan Blue solution (0.2% w/v)
Sodium chloride solution (4.25% w/v)

Procedure
1. On day of test, mix 4 parts Trypan Blue solution with 1 part Sodium chloride solution.
2. Add 1 part of Cell suspension (1:2 dilution)[a] to 12 parts of Trypan Blue-Sodium chloride solution (step 1).
3. Place sample of Cell suspension (step 2) onto hemocytometer. Count the number of unstained (viable) and stained (nonviable) leukocytes separately[b,c].

[a] Since Trypan Blue has a great affinity for proteins, removal of serum from cell dilution permits more accurate determination.

[b] Cells must be counted within 3 minutes after staining with Trypan Blue. After this time, viable cells will begin to accumulate dye.

[c] A combined total of at least 200 cells should be counted for greater accuracy.

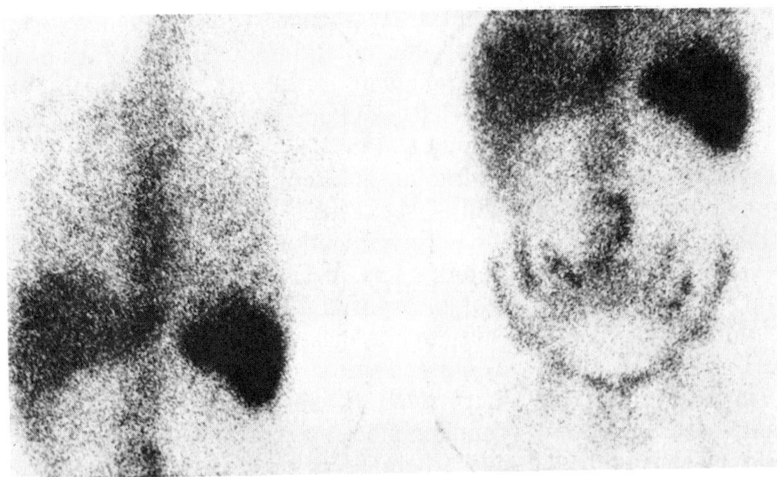

Figure 17.7 Anterior chest (left panel) and abdomen (right panel) views from an In-111 leukocyte study in a patient with regional enteritis. There are multiple crescentric areas of abnormal uptake in the abdomen corresponding to active inflammatory disease of the gastrointestinal tract.

of open wounds. Computed tomography is a relatively fast procedure that can be performed with a minimum of patient discomfort. Whole-body screening with CT is, however, time extensive and results in a high radiation dose to the patient. Indium-111 leukocyte scanning of the whole body, on the other hand, is very sensitive for the detection of abscess and may be relatively easily performed. However, some degree of expertise is necessary for the cell labeling procedure.

The imaging procedure to be utilized for the diagnosis of abscess is dependent upon an analysis of the underlying clinical features. Most clinicians suggest that patients who are not critically ill and/or who have no localizing signs should be studied first with In-111 leukocytes. Patients requiring prompt intervention or who have localizing signs should be initially evaluated with either CT or ultrasound. In-111 leukocyte imaging appears to be of particular value in the evaluation of inflammatory bowel disease (Figure 17.7 and 17.8). Its noninvasive nature and ability to discern active from remissive disease make In-111 leukocyte imaging advantageous over colonoscopy and barium enema studies, respectively.

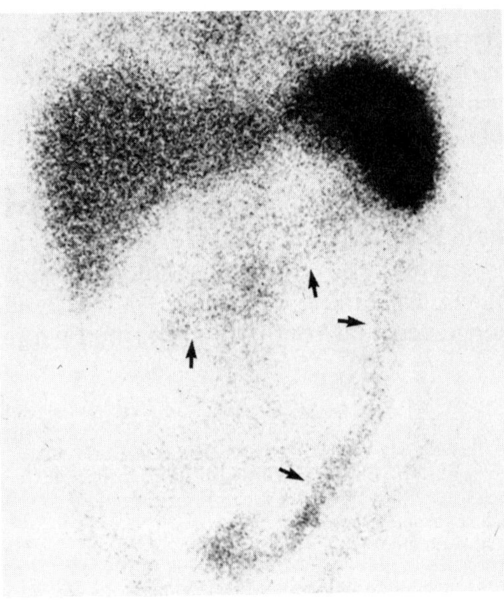

Figure 17.8 Anterior view of the abdomen obtained in a patient with active ulcerative colitis following the administration of In-111 leukocytes. Abnormal tracer localization is seen (arrows) from the mid-transverse colon to the rectum.

Though the value of In-111 leukocyte scanning is well known, it appears that the sensitivity of labeled leukocytes for chronic or low-level infective or inflammatory processes is often lower than for acute lesions. This is probably due to the fact that chronic infections often have well-defined marginal walls without a significant inflammatory response, thus resulting in a lesser attraction and accumulation of leukocytes than occurs in acute lesions. Ga-67 citrate imaging, therefore, appears to be preferable to In-111 leukocytes for the detection and evaluation of chronic inflammatory processes (see Figure 17.4). Although it has been reported that antibiotic therapy may adversely affect the accumulation of In-111 leukocytes and that discontinuance of antibiotic therapy may be necessary to adequately image the site of inflammation (Knochel JQ, et al, 1980), such a strategy is not a practical clinical consideration.

Reports of false-positive diagnoses with In-111 leukocytes involve the swallowing of labeled cells that have accumulated in infective processes in the mouth, throat, or lungs (Marcus CS, 1984b). Other pitfalls (Coleman RE and Welch D, 1980) include the reinjection of cellular clumps that subsequently localize as "hot spots" in the lungs (Figure 17.9). The latter problem can be minimized by mildly agitating the syringe containing the labeled cells just prior to their reinjection and by incorporating an infusion set containing an in-line filter.

Imaging Technique. The In-111 labeled leukocytes are administered via slow intravenous injection using a 18–19 gauge needle. Small needles may lead to cellular damage. If venous access is limited, the labeled cells can be injected through an existing intravenous line. Hyperalimentation lines should be avoided because these solutions have been reported to impair neutrophil function (Ascher NJ, et al, 1979). Whenever IV lines are used to administer leukocytes, the lines should be flushed immediately prior to and following injection using 10–20 milliliters of

A

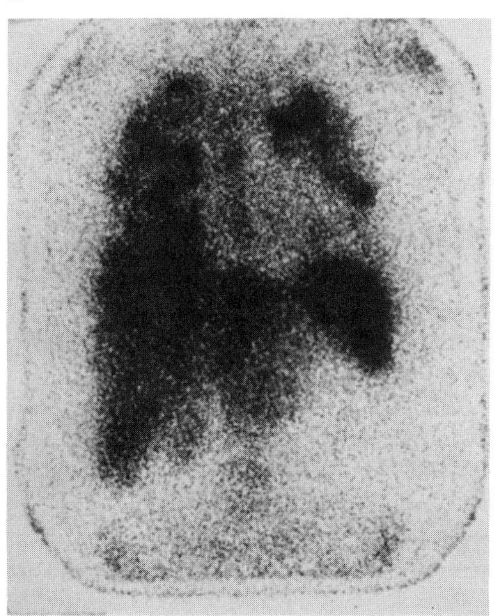

B

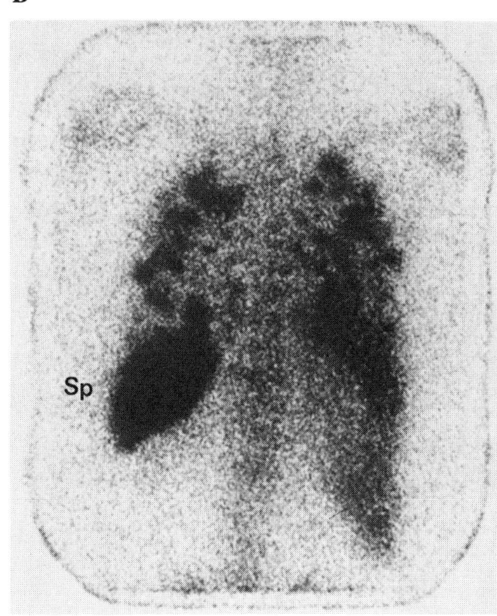

Figure 17.9 Anterior (A) and posterior (B) chest and abdomen images obtained with In-111 leukocytes at 4 hours post injection. The images reveal multiple foci of intense activity in lungs due to the injection of cellular clumps. The intense uptake in the spleen (Sp) is normal.

normal saline. In all cases, labeled cells should be injected as soon after preparation as possible, certainly within 60 minutes, since cellular viability outside the body diminishes with time (Loken MK, et al, 1985), especially if the labeled cells are resuspended in a plasma-poor environment.

Imaging for abscesses or inflammatory processes is optimally performed 24 hours after the administration of labeled leukocytes (see Figure 17.6). Preliminary images may be obtained at 4–6 hours; however, diagnostic specificity in almost all cases is greater at 24 hours (Datz FL, et al, 1984). Images obtained at 48 hours may be beneficial if intestinal activity visualized at 24 hours is suspected to originate from the swallowing of leukocytes rather than an inflammatory lesion.

Imaging should preferably be performed with a large-field-of-view scintillation camera with multiple photopeak capabilities. A parallel hole, medium-energy collimator, preferably designed for Ga-67 (rather than I-131), is optimally employed to image the 172 and 247 keV emissions of In-111.

DOSAGE/DOSIMETRY

Most clinical studies with In-111 labeled leukocytes employ a maximum adult dose of 500 microcuries. Radiation dosimetry from this activity is shown in Table 17.12.

Table 17.12 RADIATION-ABSORBED DOSE ESTIMATES[a] **FOR In-111 LEUKOCYTES (MIXED)**

ORGAN	RADS/$500\,\mu$Ci
Spleen	20
Liver	2.7
Red marrow	2.0
Skeleton	0.45
Testes	0.014
Ovaries	0.20
Total body	0.37

[a] Assumes radionuclidic purity of 99.75% (0.25% In-114/114m) and an in vivo distribution to the liver (30% injected dose), spleen (30%), red marrow (34%), and remainder of body (6%) with no excretion.

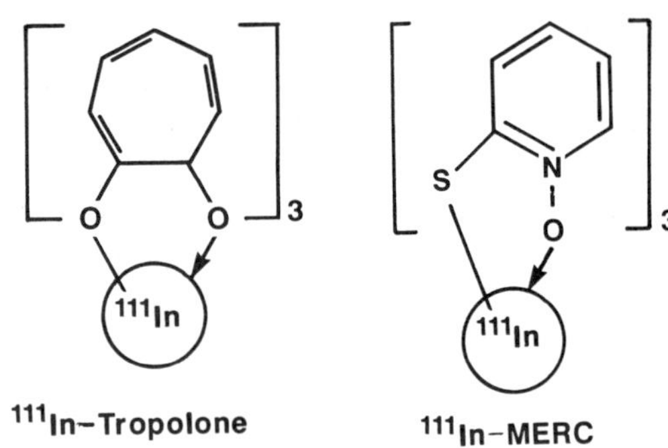

Figure 17.10 Neutral, lipophilic 1:3 complexes of In-111 with tropolone and with MERC (2-mercapto-pyridine-1-oxide).

INDIUM-111 TROPOLONE AND MERC

Other chelating agents of indium have been investigated for labeling blood cellular components. These include tropolone (Dewanjee MK, et al, 1981, 1982) and mercaptopyridine-n-oxide (MERC).

Tropolone, (2-hydroxy-2, 4, 6-cyclohepta-trien-1-one), 122), and MERC (2-mercapto-pyridine-1-oxide) (Figure 17.10) are lipophilic chelating agents that label leukocytes by the same basic mechanism as In-111 oxine: passive cellular entry with subsequent labeling of intracellular ligands (Danpure HJ, et al, 1982; Thakur ML, et al, 1985). Compared to oxine, the primary difference is that both tropolone and MERC bind In-111 strongly enough to prevent the plasma transchelation of In-111 to transferrin. Thus, leukocyte labeling with either tropolone or MERC does not require total separation of leukocyte from plasma (Burke JET, et al, 1982; Thakur ML, et al, 1985). Whether this results in In-111 leukocytes that are less damaged during labeling and more suitable for abscess localization is not clear, although the likelihood for such a case certainly exists. Leukocytes labeled in plasma with tropolone were shown by in vitro chemotaxis assays and electron microscopy to be morphologically and functionally intact and superior to most other In-111 leukocyte preparations (Mortelemans L, et al, 1986). Although In-111 tropolone labeled leukocytes proved slightly more sensitive than those labeled with oxine for the detection of abscesses in early images (obtained 1–4 hours post administration), superior lesion detectability was noted with both agents at 24 hours and little difference appeared to exist in the ability of either chelating agent to permit the detection of abscesses at this time (Datz FL, et al, 1985). Currently (i.e., at the time of this writing)

In-111 oxine is the only radiopharmaceutical approveed in the United States for the purpose of leukocyte labeling.

References

Albert A, Hampton A, Selbie FR, et al. The influence of chemical constitution on antibacterial activity. Part VII. The site of action of 8-hydroxy-quinoline (oxine). *Br J Exp Path* 1954, 35:75–84.

Anderson KC, Leonard RCG, Canellos GP, et al. High-dose gallium imaging in lymphoma. *Am J Med* 1983, 75:327–331.

Ascher NJ, Ahrenholz DH, Simmons RL, et al. Indium-111 autologous tagged leukocytes in the diagnosis of intraperitoneal sepsis. *Arch Surg* 1979, 114:386–392.

Baker WJ, Datz FL. Preparation and clinical utility of In-111 labeled leukocytes. *J Nucl Med Technol* 1984, 12:131–136.

Beckerman C, Hoffer PB, Bitran JD, et al. Gallium-67 citrate imaging studies of the lung. *Semin Nucl Med.* 1980, 10:286–301.

Berson SA, Yalow RS, Schreiber SS, et al. Tracer experiments with ^{131}I-labeled human serum albumin: Distribution and degradation studies. *Clin Invest* 1953, 32:746–768.

Bolton AE, Hunter WM. The labeling of proteins to high specific radioactivities by conjugation to a ^{125}I-containing acylating agent. *Biochem J* 1973, 133:529–539.

Bradley WP, Alderson PO, Eckelman WC, et al. Decreased tumor uptake of gallium-67 in animals after whole-body irradiation. *J Nucl Med* 1978, 19:204–209.

Bradley WP, Alderson PO, Weiss JF. Effect of iron deficiency on the biodistribution and tumor uptake of Ga-67 citrate in animals. Concise communication. *J Nucl Med* 1979, 20:243–247.

Brown BA, Drozynski CA, Dearborne CD, et al. Conjugation of metallothionein to a murine monoclonal antibody. *Anal Biochem* 1988, in press.

Bruner HD, Perkinson JD, Jr, King ER, et al. Distribution studies on gallium in rats. *Radiology* 1953a, 61:555–570.

Bruner HD, Hayes RL, Perkinson JD, Jr. Preliminary data on gallium[67]. *Radiology* 1953b, 61:602–613.

Burchiel SW, Martin JC, Imai K, et al. Heterogeneity of HLA-A,B,Ia-like and melanoma-associated antigen expression by human melanoma cell lines analized with monoclonal antibodies and flow cytometry. *Cancer Res* 1982a, 42:4110–4115.

Burchiel SW, Khaw BA, Rhodes BA, et al. Immunopharmacokinetics of radiolabeled antibodies and their fragments. In *Tumor Imaging: The Radioimmunochemical Detection of Cancer*, Burchiel SW, Rhodes BA (eds), New York, Masson Publishers, 1982b, pp. 125–139.

Burchiel SW, Rhodes BA. *Radioimmunoimaging and Radioimmunotherapy*, New York, Elsevier Science Publishers, 1983.

Burchiel SW, Knight R, Christie JH, et al. Biodistribution and kinetic modeling of labeled murine monoclonal antibodies in normal Rhesus monkeys. *J Nucl Med* 1985, 26(abst):p. 112.

Burchiel SW, Pollock R, Covell D, et al. Pharmacokinetic analysis of biosynthetically labeled murine monoclonal antibodies in normal Rhesus monkeys. *Int J Immunopharmacol* 1987, 9:913–918.

Burke JET, Roath S, Ackery D, et al. A comparison of 8-hydroxyquinoline, tropolone, and acetylacetone as mediators in the labeling of polymorphonuclear leukocytes with indium-111. A functional study. *Eur J Nucl Med* 1982, 7:73–76.

Burleson RL, Holman BL, Tow DE. Scintigraphic demonstration of absceses with radioactive gallium labeled leukocytes. *Surg Gynecol Obstet*, 1975, 142:379–382.

Camargo EE, Wagner HN, Tsan M, Jr. Gallium accumulation in inflammatory lesions: Role of polymorphonuclear leukocytes in the distribution of gallium in experimental inflammatory exudates. *Nuklearmedizin* 1979, 18:147–150.

Carasquillo JA, Abrams PG, Schroff RW, et al. Effect of antibody dose on the imaging and biodistribution of indium-111 9.2.27 anti-melanoma monoclonal antibody. *J Nucl Med* 1988, 29:39–47.

Carasquillo JA, Bunn PA, Keenan AM, et al. Radioimmunodetection of cutaneous T-cell lymphoma with ^{111}In-labeled T101 monoclonal antibody. *N Engl J Med* 1986, 315:673–680.

Chilton HM, Witcofski RL, Watson NE, Jr, et al. Alteration of gallium-67 distribution in tumor-bearing mice following treatment with methotrexate: Concise communication. *J Nucl Med* 1981, 22:1064–1068.

Chvapil M, Stankova L, Zukoski E, et al. Inhibition of some functions of polymorphonuclear leukocytes by in vitro zinc. *J Lab Clin Med* 1977, 89:135–146.

Clay ME, McCullough J. Studies of the granulocyte cytotoxicity assay. *Transfusion* 1978, 18:395.

Coakley JL, Mountford PJ. Nuclear medicine and the nursing mother. *Br Med J* 1985, 291:159–160.

Colcher D, Esteban JM, Carasquillo JA, et al. Quantitative analyses of selective radiolabeled monoclonal antibody localization in metastatic lesions of colorectal cancer patients. *Cancer Res* 1987a, 47:1185–1189.

Colcher D, Esteban J, Carasquillo JA, et al. Complementation of intracavitary and intravenous administration of a monoclonal antibody (B.2.3) in patients with carcinoma. *Cancer Res* 1987b, 47:4218–4224.

Coleman RE, Welch D. Possible pitfalls with clinical imaging of indium-111 leukocytes: Concise communication. *J Nucl Med* 1980, 21:122–125.

Danpure HJ, Osman S, Brady F. The labeling of blood cells in plasma with In-111 tropolonate. *Br J Surg* 1982, 55:247–249.

Datz FL, Bedont RA, Baker WJ, et al. No difference in sensitivity for occult infection between tropolone and oxine-labeled Indium-111 leukocytes. *J Nucl Med* 1985, 26:469–473.

Datz FL, Jacobs J, Baker W, et al. Decreased sensitivity of early imaging with In-111 oxine-labeled leukocytes in detection of occult infection: Concise communication. *J Nucl Med* 1984, 25:303–306.

Day ED, Lassiter S, Woodhall B, et al. The localization of radioantibodies in human brain tumors. I. Preliminary exploration. *Cancer Res* 1965, 25:773–778.

DeLand FH, Kim EE, Corgan RL, et al. Axillary lymphoscintigraphy by radioimmunodetection of carcinoembryonic antigen in breast cancer. *J Nucl Med* 1979, 20:1243–1250.

DeLand FH, Kim EE, Goldenberg DM. Lymphoscintigraphy with radionuclide-labeled antibodies to carcinoembryonic antigen. *Cancer Res* 1980, 40:2997–3000.

DeNardo GL, Young WC, DeNardo SJ, et al. Urinary metabolites after injection of monoclonal antibodies (MAb) or fibrinogen (F) radioiodinated with a small and large number of iodine atoms. *J Nucl Med* 1986, 27 (abst):958.

Dewanjee MK, Rao SA, Didisheim P. Indium-111 tropolone, a new high-affinity platelet label: Preparation and evaluation of labeling parameters. *J Nucl Med* 1981, 22:981–987.

Dewanjee MK, Rao SA, Rosemark JA, et al. Indium-111 tropolone, a new tracer for platelet labeling. *Radiology* 1982, 145:149–153.

Deysine M, Robinson RG, Winder JR. Abscess detection by radioactive chromium labeled autologous white blood cells. *Surg Gynecol Obstet* 1970, 131:216–220.

Dillman RO, Beauregard JC, Sobol RE, et al. Lack of radioimmunodetection and complications associated with monoclonal anticarcinoembryonic antigen antibody: Cross reactivity with an antigen on circulating cells. *Cancer Res* 1984, 44:2213–2218.

Dooley DC, Simpson JF, Meryman HT.

Isolation of large numbers of fully viable human neutrophils: A preparative technique using Percoll density gradient centrifugation. *Exp Hematol* 1982, 10: 591–599.

Ducassou D, Nouel JP, Brendel A. Le marquages des elements figures du sang par l'indium radioactif-methodology-resultants-indications. *Radiol Isot in Klinik und Forschung* 1978, 13:91–96.

Dudley HC, Levin MD. Mechanisms of localization of Gallium-67 in tumor. *J Pharmacol Exp Ther*, 1949a, 95:487–493.

Dudley HC, Maddox GE, La Rue HC. Studies of the metabolism of gallium. *J Pharmacol Exp Ther*. 1949b, 96:135–144.

Dudley HC, Munn JI, Henry KE. Studies of the metabolism of gallium. II. *J Pharmacol Exp Ther* 1950, 98:105–110.

Dudley HC, Marrer HH. Studies of the metabolism of gallium III. Deposition in and clearance from bone. *J Pharmacol Exp Ther* 1952, 106:129–134.

Edwards CL, Hayes RL. Tumor scanning with Ga-67 citrate. *J Nucl Med* 1969, 10:103–105.

Engelstad B, Luk SS, Haltner RS. Altered Ga-67 citrate distribution in patients with multiple red cell transfusions. *AJR* 1982, 139:755–759.

English D, Andersen BR. Labeling of phagocytes from human blood with Tc-99m sulfur colloid. *J Nucl Med* 1975, 16:5–10.

English D, Clanton JA. Evaluation of neutrophil labeling techniques using the chemotaxis radioassay. *J Nucl Med* 1984, 25:913–916.

Epenetos AA, Mather S, Granowska M, et al. Targeting of iodine-123-labeled tumor-associated monoclonal antibodies to ovarian, breast, and gastrointestinal tumors. *Lancet* 1982, 6 Nov.: 999–1006.

Fernandez-Pol JA. Isolation and characterization of a siderophore-like growth factor from mutants of SV40-transformed cells adapted to picolinic acid. *Cell* 1978, 14:489–499.

Fletcher JW, Herbig FK, Donati RM.

Ga-67 citrate distribution following whole-body irradiation or chemotherapy. *Radiology* 1975, 117:709–712.

Fraker PJ, Speck JC. Protein and cell membrane iodinations with a sparingly soluble chloroamide, 1,3,4,6-tetrachloro-3a,6a-diphenylglycoluril. *Biochem Biophys Res Commun* 1978, 80: 849–857.

Fritzberg AR, Kasina S, Reno JM, et al. Radiolabeling of antibodies with Tc-99m using N_2S_2 ligands. *J Nucl Med* 1986, 27(abst):957.

Goedemens WTH. Simplified cell labeling with Indium-111 acetylacetonate and Indium-111 oxinate. *Br J Radiol* 1981, 54:636–637.

Goldenberg DM, Deland FH, Kim EE, et al. Use of radiolabeled antibodies to carcinoembryonic antigen for the detection and localization of diverse cancers by external photoscanning. *N Engl J Med* 1978, 298:1384–1388.

Goldenberg DM. An introduction to the radioimmunodetection of cancer. *Cancer Res* 1980, 40:2957–2959.

Goldman A, Vivan G, Gordon I, et al. Immunolocalization of neuroblastoma using radiolabeled monoclonal antibody UJ13A. *J Ped* 1984, 105:252–256.

Gunasekera SW, King LJ, Lavender PJ. The behavior of tracer gallium-67 towards serum protein. *Clin Chim Acta* 1972, 39:401–406.

Halpern SE, Hagan PL, Garver PR, et al. Stability, characterization, and kinetics of ^{111}In-labeled monoclonal antitumor antibodies in normal animals and nude mouse–human tumor models. *Cancer Res* 1983, 43:5347–5355.

Hayes R, Byrd B. Transfer of Ga-67 from hamster dam to fetus and offspring. In Watson EE, Schlakfe-Stelson A, Coffey J, Cloutier R (eds). Third International Radiopharmaceutical Dosimetry Symposium, *HHS Publication FDA-81-8166.* Rockville, MD, BRH, June 1981, pp. 447–453.

Hayes RL, Brown DH, Carlton JE. Comparison of the subcellular distribution of the tumor-localizing agents,

^{67}Ga, ^{111}In, ^{206}Bi, and ^{167}Tm. *J Nucl Med* 1974, 15:501.

Hladik WB III, Ponto JA, Lentle BC. Iatrogenic alterations in the biodistribution of radiotracers as a result of drug therapy: Reported instances. In: *Essentials of Nuclear Medicine*, Hladik WB III, Saha GB, Study KT (eds), Williams and Wilkins, Baltimore, 1987, pp. 189–219.

Hnatowich DJ, Childs RL, Lanteigne D, et al. The preparation of DTPA-coupled antibodies radiolabeled with metallic radionuclides: An improved method. *J Immunol Methods* 1983, 65:147–157.

Hnatowich DJ, Griffin TW, Kosciuczk C, el al. Pharmacokinetics of an indium-111-labeled monoclonal antibody in cancer patients. *J Nucl Med* 1985, 26:849–858.

Hoffer PB. Mechanisms of localization. In, Hoffer PB, Beckerman C, Henkin RE (eds). *Gallium-67 Imaging* New York, Wiley, 1978, p. 3.

Holley RH, Van Epps DE, Harvey RL, et al. Effect of high doses of radiation on human neutrophil chemotaxis, phagocytosis, and morphology. *Am J Pathol* 1974, 75:61–72.

Hunter WM, Greenwood FC. Preparation of iodine-131 labeled growth hormone of high specific activity. *Nature* 1962, 194:495–596.

Hylarides M, Jones D, Seubert J, et al. Synthesis and radioiodination of iodophenyl conjugates for protein labeling. *J Nucl Med* 1987, 28(abst):560.

Johnston GS, Go MF, Benua RS, et al. Gallium-67 citrate imaging in Hodgkin's disease: Final report of cooperative group. *J Nucl Med* 1977, 18:692–698.

Keenan AM, Weinstein JN, Mulshine JL, et al. Immunolymphoscintigraphy in patients with lymphoma after subcutaneous injection of Indium-111-labeled T101 monoclonal antibody. *J Nucl Med* 1987, 28:42–46.

Khaw BA, Strauss HW, Carvalho A, et al. Technetium-99m labeling of antibodies to cardiac myosin Fab and

to human fibrinogen. *J Nucl Med* 1982, 23:1011–1019.

Kim YC, Brown ML, Thrall JH. Scintigraphic patterns of Gallium-67 uptake in the breast. *Radiology* 1977, 124:169–175.

Kirkwood JM, Myers JE, Vlock DR, et al. Tomographic gallium-67 citrate scanning: Useful new surveillance for metastatic melanoma. *Ann Intern Med* 1982, 97:694–699.

Knochel JQ, Koehler PF, Lee TG, et al. Diagnosis of abdominal abscesses versus computed tomography, ultrasound, and In-111 labeled leukocyte scans. *Radiology* 1980, 137:425–432.

Kohler G, Milstein C. Continuous cultures of fused cells secreting antibody of predefined specificity. *Nature* 1975, 256:494–497.

Kuroki M, Koga Y, Matsuoka Y. Purification and characterization of carcinoembryonic antigen-related antigens in normal adult feces. *Cancer Res* 1981, 41:713–720.

Larson SM. Mechanisms of localization of Gallium-67 in tumor. *Semin Nucl Med* 1978, 8:193–204.

Larson SM. Radiolabeled monclonal antitumor antibodies in diagnosis and therapy. *J Nucl Med* 1985, 26:538–545.

Larson SM, Carasquillo JA, Krohn KA, et al. Localization of ^{131}I-labeled p97-specific Fab fragments in human melanoma as a basis for radiotherapy. *J Clin Invest* 1983, 72:2101–2114.

Lentle BC, Castor WR, Khaliq A, et al. The effect of contrast lymphangiography on localization of 67 Ga-citrate. *J Nucl Med* 1975, 16:374–376.

Lentle BC, Starreveld E, Catz Z, et al. Abnormal biodistribution of radiogallium in persons treated with phenytoin. *J Can Assoc Radiol* 1983, 34:114–115.

Levitt RG, Biella DR, Sagel SS, et al. Computed tomography and Ga-67 citrate radionuclide imaging for evaluating suspected abdominal abscess. *AJR* 1979, 132:529–534.

Lichtman M, Santillo PA, Kearney EA, et al. The shape and surface morphology of human leukocytes. The in vitro effect of temperature, metabolic inhibitions, and agents that influence membrane structure. *Nouv Rev Fr Hematol; Blood Cells* 1976, 17:507–532.

Linton AL, Clark WF, Driedger AA, et al. Acute interstitial nephritis due to drugs. *Ann Intern Med* 1980, 93:735–741.

Loken MK, Clay ME, Carpenter RT, et al. Clinical use of indium-111 labeled blood products. *Clin Nucl Med* 1985, 10:902–911.

Mach JP, Carrel S, Forni M, et al. Tumor localization of radiolabeled antibodies against carcinoembryonic antigen in patients with carcinoma: A critical evaluation. *N Engl J Med* 1980, 303:5–10.

MacMahon H, Beckerman C. The diagnostic significance of gallium lung uptake in patients with normal chest radiographs. *Radiology* 1978, 127:189–193.

Manning DM, Strimlan CV, Turbiner EH. Early detection of busulfan lung: Report of a case. *Clin Nucl Med* 1980, 5:412–414.

Marchalonis JJ. An enzymatic method for the trace iodination of immunoglobulin and other proteins. *Biochem J* 1969, 113:299–305.

Marcus CS. Re: Labeling with indium-111 has detrimental effects on human lymphocytes (Letter). *J Nucl Med* 1984a, 25:406.

Marcus CS. The status of indium-111 oxine leukocyte imaging studies. *Noninvasive Med Imag* 1984b, 3:213–226.

Marcus CS, Stabin MG, Watson EE, et al. Contribution of contaminant Indium-114m/Indium-114 to Indium-111 oxine blood dosimetry. *J Nucl Med* 26:1091–1093, 1985.

Markwell MAK. A new solid-state reagent to iodinate proteins. *Anal Biochem* 1982, 125:427–432.

Marrack D, Kubala M, Corry P, et al. Localization of intracranial tumors. Comparative study with ^{131}I-labeled antibody to human fibrinogen and neohydrin-[203]Hg. *Cancer* 1967, 20:751–755.

Mathias CJ, Welch MJ. Labeling mechanism and localization of indium-111 in human platelets. *J Nucl Med* 1979, 20:659 (Abst).

McAfee JG, Thakur ML. Survey of radioactive agents for in vitro labeling of phagocytic leukocytes. I. Soluble agents. *J Nucl Med* 1976, 17:480–487.

McAfee JG, Subramanian G, Gagne G. Technique of leukocyte harvesting and labeling: Problems and perspectives. *Semin Nucl Med* 1984, 14:38–106.

McCullough J, Weiblen BJ, Clay ME, et al. Effect of leukocyte antibodies on the fate in vivo of indium-111 labeled granulocytes. *Blood* 1981, 58:164–170.

McMillan R, Scott JL. Leukocyte labeling with chromium-51. I. Technique and results in normal subjects. *Blood* 1968, 32:738–754.

Menon S, Wagner HN, Tsan M. Studies on gallium accumulation in inflammatory lesions. II. Uptake by staphylococcus aureus: Concise communication. *J Nucl Med* 1978, 19:44–47.

Miller RA, Maloney DG, McKillop J, et al. In vivo effects of murine hybridoma monoclonal antibody in a patient with T-cell leukemia. *Blood* 1981, 58:78–86.

MIRD Dose Estimate Report No. 2, *J Nucl Med* 1973, 14:755–756.

Morrell A, Terry WD, Waldmann RA. Metabolic properties of IgG subclasses in man. *J Clin Invest* 1970, 49:673–680.

Mortelemans L, Verbruggen A, Bogaerts M, et al. In vitro evaluation of granulocyte labeling with In-111 chelated to three different agents. *J Nucl Med* 1986, 27:1014 (Abst).

Moseley R, Zalutsky MR, Cockham RE, et al. Distribution of I-131 81C6 monoclonal antibody (Mab) administered via carotid artery in patients with glioma. *J Nucl Med* 1987, 28(abst):603.

Murray JL, Rosenblum MG, Lamki L, et al. Clinical parameters related to optimal tumor localization on In-111-labeled mouse antimelanoma antibody ZME-018. *J Nucl Med* 1987, 28:25–33.

Nelp WB, Eary JF, Jones RK, et al. Preliminary studies of monoclonal antibody lymphoscintigraphy in malignant melanoma. *J Nucl Med* 1987, 28:34–41.

Nelson B, Hayes RL, Edwards CL, et al. Distribution of gallium in human tissues after intravenous administration. *J Nucl Med* 1972, 13:92–100.

Noujaim AA, Ferner UK, Turner CJ, et al. Alterations of gallium-67 uptake in tumors by cis-platinum. *Int J Nucl Med Biol* 1981, 8:289–293.

Order SE, Klein JL, Alderson P, et al. Use of isotopic immunoglobulin in therapy. *Cancer Res* 1980, 40:3001–3007.

Order SE, Klein JL, Leichner, PK. Antiferritin IgG antibody for isotopic cancer therapy. *Oncology* 1981, 38:154–160.

Order SE, Klein JL, Leichner, PK, et al. [90]Yttrium antiferritin—a new therapeutic radiolabeled antibody. *Int J Radiat Oncol Biol Phys* 1986, 12:277–281.

Paxton RJ, Jakowatz JG, Beatty JD, et al. High-specific-activity ^{111}In-labeled anticarcinoembryonic antigen monoclonal antibody: Improved method for the synthesis of diethylenetriaminepentaacetic acid conjugates. *Cancer Res* 1985, 45:5694–5699.

Pettit WA, DeLand FH, Bennett SJ, et al. Improved protein labeling by stannous tartrate reduction of pertechnetate. *J Nucl Med* 1980, 21:59–62.

Rhodes BA, Zamora PO, Newell KD, et al. Technetium-99m labeling of murine monoclonal antibody fragments. *J Nucl Med* 1986, 27:685–693.

Richardson RB, Davies AG, Bourne SP, et al. Radioimmunolocalization of human brain tumors: Biodistribution or radiolabeled antibody UJ13A. *Eur J Nucl Med* 1986, 12:313–320.

Richman SD, Levenson SM, Bunn PA, et al. 67 Ga accumulation in pulmonary lesions associated with bleomycin toxicity. *Cancer* 1975, 36:1966–1972.

Romney BM, Nickoloff EL, Esser PD, et al. Radionuclide administration to nursing mothers: Mathematically derived guidelines. *Radiology* 1986, 160:549–554.

Rosenblum MG, Murray JL, Lamki L, et al. Comparative clinical pharmacology of ^{111}In-labeled murine monoclonal antibodies. *Cancer Chemother Pharmacol* 1987, 20:41–47.

Roy AJ, Franklin A, Simmons WB, et al. A method of separation of granulocytes from normal human blood using hydroxyethyl starch. *Pre Biochem* 1971, 1:197–203.

Sands H, Jones PL, Shah SA, et al. Correlation of vascular permeability and blood flow with monoclonal antibody uptake by human Clouser and renal cell xenografts. *Cancer Res* 1988, 48:188–193.

Saverymuttu MU, Peters AM, Danpure HJ, et al. Lung transit of In-111 labeled granulocytes: Relationship to labeling techniques. *Scand J Haematol*, 1983, 30:151–160.

Scheinberg DA, Strand M, Gansow OA. Tumor imaging with radioactive metal chelates conjugated to monoclonal antibodies. *Science* 1982, 215:1511–1513.

Segal AW, Detrix P, Garcia R, et al. Indium-111 labeling for leukocytes: A detrimental effect on neutrophil and lymphocyte function and an improved method of cell labeling. *J Nucl Med* 1978, 19:1238–1244.

Selvaraj RJ, Sbarra AJ. Effects on X-irradiation on the metabolic changes accompanying phagocytosis. *Nature* 1966, 210:158–161.

Selvaraj RJ, McRipley RJ, Sbarra AJ. The effect of phagocytosis and X-irradiation on human leukocyte metabolism. *Cancer Res* 1967, 27:2280-2286.

Sephton RG, Harris AW. Brief communication: Gallium-67 citrate uptake by cultured tumor cells, stimulated by serum transferrin. *J Natl Cancer Inst* 1975, 54:1263–1266.

Sfakianakis GN, DeLand FH. Radioimmunodiagnosis and radioimmunotherapy, 1982. *J Nucl Med* 1982, 23:840-850.

Silberstein EB. Cancer diagnosis. The role of tumor imaging radiopharmaceuticals. *Am J Med* 1976, 60:226–237

Silvester DJ. Consequences of indium-111 decay in vivo: Calculated absorbed radiation dose to cells labeled by indium-111 oxine. *J Labeled Comp Radiopharmaceuticals*, 1979, 1:16 (Abst).

Staab EV, McCartney WH. Role of gallium-67 in inflammatory disease. *Semin Nucl Med* 1978, 8:219–234.

Stephanas AV, Maisey MN. Hyperprolactinaemia as a cause of gallium-67 uptake in the breast. *Br J Radiol* 1976, 49:379–380.

Stern P, Hagan P, Halpern S, et al. The effect of radiolabel on the kinetics of monoclonal anti-CEA in a nude mouse–human colon tumor model. In *Hybridomas in Cancer Diagnosis and Treatment*, Mitchell MS, Oettgen HF (eds). *Prog Cancer Res Ther*, Vol 21, New York, Raven Press, 1982, pp 245–253.

Sullivan DC, Silva JS, Cox CE, et al. Localization of I-131-labeled goat and primate anti-carcinoembryonic antigen (CEA) antibodies in patients with cancer. *Invest Radiol* 1982, 17:350–355.

Teates CD, Bray ST. Tumor detection with ^{67}Ga-citrate: A literature survey (1970–1978). *Clin Nucl Med* 1978 3:456–460.

Tedesco FJ, Coleman RE, Siegel BA. Gallium citrate GA-67 accumulation in pseudomembranous colitis. *JAMA* 1976, 235:59–60.

Ten Berge RJM, Natarajan AT, Hardeman MR, et al. Labeling with indium-111 has detrimental effects on human lymphocytes. Concise communication. *J Nucl Med* 1983, 24:615–620.

Thakur ML. Cell Labeling: Achievements, challenges and prospects. *J Nucl Med* 1981, 22:1011–1014.

Thakur ML, Coleman RE, Welch MJ, et al. Indium In-111 labeled leukocytes for the localization of abscesses: Preparation, analysis, tissue distribution, and comparison with gallium-67 citrate in dogs. *J Lab Clin Med* 1977a, 89:217–228.

Thakur ML, Lavender JP, Arnot RN, et al. Indium-111 labeled autologous leukocytes in man. *J Nucl Med* 1977b, 18:1014–1021.

Thakur ML, McKenney SL, Park CH. Evaluation of indium-111-1-mercaptao-pyridine-N-oxide for labeling leukocytes in plasma: A kit preparation. *J Nucl Med* 1985, 26:518–523.

Thakur ML, Segal AW, Louis L, et al. Indium-111-labeled cellular blood compounds. Mechanisms of labeling and intracellular location in human neutrophils. *J Nucl Med* 1977c, 18:1022–1024.

Thakur ML, Siefert CL, Madsen MT, et al. Neutrophil labeling: Problems and pitfalls. *Semin Nucl Med* 1984, 14:107–117.

Thorell JI, Johansson BG. Enzymatic iodination of polypeptides with ^{125}I to high specific activity. *Biochem Biosphys Acta* 1971, 251:363–369.

Tobin RE, Schneider PB. Uptake of Ga-67 in the lactating breast and its persistence in milk. Case report. *J Nucl Med* 1976, 17:1055–1056.

Tomasi TB, Spellman C, Anderson WD. Clinically applicable procedures for producing tolerance to foreign proteins. In *Radioimmunoimaging and Radioimmunotherapy*, Burchiel SW, Rhodes BA (eds). New York, Elsevier, 1983, pp. 63–69.

Tsan M, Chen W, Scheffel U, et al. Studies on gallium accumulation in inflammatory lesions. I. Gallium uptake by human polymorphonuclear leukocytes. *J Nucl Med* 1978, 19:36–43.

Tzen KY, Oster ZH, Wagner HN, Jr, et al. Role of iron-binding proteins and enhanced capillary permeability on the accumulation of gallium-67. *J Nucl Med* 1980, 21:31–35.

Wahl RL, Parker CW, Philpott GW. Improved radioimaging and tumor localization with monoclonal F(ab')2. *J Nucl Med* 1983, 24:316–325.

Waldmann TA, Strober W. Metabolism of immunoglobulins. *Prog Allergy* 1968, 13:1–110.

Ward BG, Mather SJ, Hawkins LR, et al. Localization of radioiodine conjugated to the monoclonal antibody HMFG2 in human ovarian carcinoma: Assessment of intravenous and intraperitoneal routes of administration. *Cancer Res* 1987, 47:4719–4723.

Watson EE, Cloutier RJ, Gibbs WD. Whole-body retention of Ga-67 citrate. *J Nucl Med* 1973, 14:840–842.

Waxman AD, Beldon JR, Richli W, et al. Steroid-induced suppression of gallium uptake in tumors of the central nervous system: Concise communication. *J Nucl Med* 1978, 19:480–482.

Weiblen BJ, Forstrom L, McCullough J. Studies of the kinetics of Indium-111 labeled granulocytes. *J Lab Clin Med* 1979, 94:246–255.

Weiner RE, Schreiber GJ, Hoffer PB, et al. Compounds which mediate gallium-67 transfer from lactoferrin to ferritin. *J Nucl Med* 1985, 26:908–916.

Weinstein JN, Steller MA, Keenan AM, et al. Monoclonal antibodies in the lymphatics: Selective delivery to lymph node metastases of a solid tumor. *Science* 1986, 222:423–426.

Weisberger AS, Heinle RW, Storaasli JP, et al. Transfusion of leukocytes labeled with radioactive phosphorus. *J Clin Invest* 1950, 29:336–341.

Yeh SM, Sherman DG, Meares CF. A new route to "bifunctional chelating agents." *Anal Biochem* 1979, 100:152–159.

Zakhireh B, Thakur ML, Malech HL, et al. Indium-111-labeled human polymorphonuclear leukocytes: Viability, random migration, chemotaxis, bactericidal capacity, and ultrastructure. *J Nucl Med* 1979, 20:741–747.

Zalutsky MR, Narula AS. Astatination of proteins using an N-succimidyl-N-butyl-stanyl-benzoate intermediate. *J Appl Rad Isotopes* 1988, 39:227–232.

Therapeutic Applications of Radiopharmaceuticals: Thyroid Disease, Polycythemia Vera, and Malignant Effusion

James A. Ponto
Henry M. Chilton

In the therapeutic management of certain diseases, radionuclides may be a desirable alternative or adjunctive to either chemotherapy or surgery. A principal requirement for radiopharmaceutical therapy is not unlike that with diagnostic applications of radiopharmaceuticals; both require selective uptake of radioactivity in organs or tissues soon after radiopharmaceutical administration. With therapeutic applications, however, radionuclides that emit highly ionizing radiation are used to deliver therapeutic amounts of radiation to the target tissues.

Therapeutic radiopharmaceuticals (Table 18.1) are intended to provide lethal doses of radiation to the selected tissues, while producing only minimal levels of damage to nearby organs or tissues. The radiobiologic effects of highly ionizing radiations at the cellular and subcellular levels are due to disruptions of intracellular bonds. Resultant chromosomal damage in the nucleus prevents cellular replication. More rapidly dividing cells, such as those that are malignant, are more susceptible to radiation damage than are otherwise healthy cells.

Generally, radiopharmaceuticals composed of beta-emitting radionuclides are preferred for therapeutic applications because beta particles emitted during decay are confined largely to the target tissues and do not pose any significant external radiation hazard to nursing staff, other patients, and family members. In some cases, however, therapeutic radiopharmaceuticals that produce both beta and gamma emissions may be desirable because the gamma emissions may be used for imaging in order to determine whether desired localization of the therapeutic agent has been achieved.

In all cases involving therapeutic ra-

Table 18.1 SELECTED THERAPEUTIC RADIOPHARMACEUTICALS, CLINICAL INDICATIONS, DECAY MODES, AND ROUTES OF ADMINISTRATION

THERAPEUTIC RADIOPHARMACEUTICAL AND SELECTED CLINICAL INDICATIONS	DECAY MODE	ROUTE OF ADMINISTRATION
I-131 Sodium Iodide · Hyperthyroidism · Thyroid carcinoma (including metastases)	Beta$^{(-)}$, gamma	Oral
P-32 Sodium Phosphate · Polycythemia vera · Relief of pain from skeletal metastases	Beta$^{(-)}$	Intravenous
P-32 Chromic Phosphate · Malignant effusions · Cystic brian tumors	Beta$^{(-)}$	Intracavitary

diopharmaceuticals, it is a requirement that radiopharmaceutical uptake occurs in the target tissue soon after administration in order to reduce radiation doses to non-target tissues. Occasionally, where target uptake may be slowed or prohibited by standard administration techniques (i. e., IV, PO), it may be desirable to place the radiopharmaceutical directly into target tissue (e. g., via intracavitary instillation).

I. Treatment of Thyroid Disease with I-131 Sodium Iodide

Treatment of hyperthyroidism and some forms of thyroid carcinoma with radioiodine is a convenient and highly effective complement to surgery. The rationale underlying the use of radio-iodine for therapy is directly from the role of iodine in thyroid metabolism. Following oral administration, radioiodine is rapidly absorbed from the gastrointestinal tract, removed from blood, and concentrated in the thyroid follicle. Selective irradiation of thyroid cells by radioiodine causes cessation of cell division and eventual cell death with loss of thyroid hormone production. Depending upon the type and amount of radiation employed, the extent of loss of thyroid function can be controlled and a measured therapeutic response obtained.

For example, in the treatment of hyperthyroidism, the therapeutic goal is to render the patient euthyroid in a reasonable length of time from a single dose of radioiodine. With thyroid carcinoma, the objective is to ablate neoplastic tissues by giving relatively large amounts of radioiodine, occasionally in multiple doses. In the treatment of thyroid carcinoma, radioiodine treatment is usually employed as an adjunct following surgical thyroidectomy.

Of the four types of thyroid cancer (papillary, follicular, medullary, and anaplastic), only papillary and follicular cancers arise from thyroid follicular cells and retain their ability to concentrate radioio-

dine. However, because these two types of cancers represent the majority of thyroid neoplasms (estimated at 50–80% and 10–20% of thyroid cancers, respectively), radioiodine is a highly useful treatment modality.

RADIOPHARMACEUTICALS FOR TREATMENT OF THYROID DISEASE

BACKGROUND/HISTORY

The original application of radioiodine for the treatment of thyroid disease was reported in 1942 when S. Hertz and A. Roberts treated hyperthyroid patients with the beta-emitting radionuclide I-131. Presently, there is universal agreement on the effectiveness and overall safety of I-131 sodium iodide for treating hyperthyroidism and thyroid carcinoma. Another radioisotope of iodine, I-125, has also been utilized for treating thyroid disease. With I-125, the therapy dose is delivered by a combination of the relatively long physical half-life of I-125 (60 days) and its low-energy characteristic x-rays and gamma photons. Unlike I-131, I-125 has no primary particulate emissions. Researchers once hoped that the low-energy nature of the electromagnetic emissions of I-125 might permit selective irradiation of the apical portion of follicular cells of the thyroid, thus effecting a cure for hyperthyroidism without inducing hypothyroidism. No substantive clinical evidence for this likelihood has developed, however, and I-125 sodium iodide is not commonly used at this time for treating thyroid disease. Today, I-131 sodium iodide is the radiopharmaceutical of choice for the treatment of thyroid disease, including hyperthyroidism and iodine-concentrating carcinoma.

CHEMISTRY

The original I-131 radionuclide employed for studies of iodine metabolism was produced by bombarding stable tellurium with deuterons. Today, I-131 is obtained primarily as a reactor by-product from fissioning Uranium-235. The nuclear

Table 18.2 NUCLEAR PROPERTIES OF IODINE-131

Physical half-life:	8.05 days
Decay mode:	Beta$^{(-)}$ with gamma emissions
Mean Beta$^{(-)}$ energy (abundance):	192 keV (89.8%)
Gamma energy (abundance):	364 keV (82%)

and physical properties of I-131 are listed in Table 18.2.

Sodium iodide I-131 is available in either capsular or liquid form. Sodium iodide I-131 therapeutic capsules are prepared by absorbing a solution of carrier-free sodium iodide I-131 onto an inert filler that is contained within a gelatin capsule (Table 18.3). Capsules are available from several manufacturers and are calibrated in various activities.

Sodium iodide I-131 therapeutic solution is an aqueous solution with some formulations containing stabilizers and buffering agents (Table 18.3).

PHARMACOKINETICS

Following oral administration, sodium iodide I-131 is rapidly absorbed from the gastrointestinal tract and is distributed primarily within the body's extracellular fluid. It is actively trapped by the thyroid gland, where it is rapidly converted to protein-bound iodine. It is also distributed to the stomach and salivary glands. Excretion is primarily by the kidneys. Following oral administration, about 40% of the activity has an effective half-life of 0.3 days and 60% has an effective half-life of 7.61 days (Childs DS, et al, 1950).

PRECAUTIONS

Uptake of sodium iodide I-131 by the thyroid gland will be adversely affected by recent intake of stable iodide in any form, or by the use of thyroid, antithyroid, or certain other drugs (see Table 11.3, Chapter 11). Patient histories should include a review of concurrent medications and previous procedures involving iodinated radiologic contrast media.

Whenever therapeutic oral solutions of sodium iodide I-131 are diluted before use, the recommended diluent is purified water buffered to pH 7.5–9.0 that contains 0.2% sodium thiosulfate, an antioxidant. Tap water should be avoided as a diluent because its generally acidic nature may cause the pH to drop below 7.5, thus stimulating the volatilization of Iodine-131 hydriodic acid. Open vials of sodium iodide I-131 therapeutic solution should be handled in an atmospheric exhaust hood in order to lessen the likelihood of airborne radiocontamination in the immediate environment. Depending upon the types and the amounts of I-131 and the manner in which it is handled, bioassay of personnel may be required (Table 18.4).

Adverse Reactions. Adverse reactions and reported complications of radioiodine therapy are listed in Table 18.5. While symptoms of radiation sickness, includ-

Table 18.3 COMMERCIALLY AVAILABLE FORMULATIONS OF THERAPEUTIC I-131 SODIUM IODIDE

MANUFACTURER	FORMULATION INFORMATION
Mallinckrodt, Inc.	Capsule (gelatin-white): Sodium iodide I-131 absorbed onto sodium phosphate dibasic (approx. 500 mg/capsule)
Squibb Diagnostics	Capsule (gelatin-blue/buff): Sodium iodide I-131 bound to Carbowax-4000 (approx. 240 mg/capsule)
CIS-US, Inc.	Capsule (gelatin-white opaque): Sodium iodide I-131 absorbed onto an inert filler
Mallinckrodt, Inc.	Sodium Iodide I-131 Oral Solution: 0.1% sodium bisulfite and 0.2% edetate disodium (stabilizers), 0.5% sodium phosphate (buffer), sodium hydroxide or hydrochloric acid (pH adjustment: 7.5–9.0)
Squibb Diagnostics	Sodium Iodide I-131 Oral Solution: 0.01% sodium thiosulfate (antioxidant), 0.85% potassium phosphate dibasic (buffer), 0.01% edetate disodium (stabilizer), sodium hydroxide or hydrochloric acid (pH adjustment: 7.5–9.0)
CIS-US, Inc.	Sodium Iodide I-131 Oral Solution: 2.48 mg/ml sodium thiosulfate (antioxidant), 4.2 mg/ml phosphate buffer, sodium hydroxide (pH adjustment: 7.5–9.0)

Table 18.4 BIOASSAY REQUIREMENTS FOR PERSONS HANDLING RADIOIODINE (I-125 AND I-131)

Due to the inherent volatility of radioiodine and the concern that airborne radioactivity potentially constitutes a hazard to personnel who handle these materials, the Nuclear Regulatory Commission has adopted guidelines requiring the routine bioassay of individuals who handle specific amounts of unsealed quantities of volatile I-125 and I-131. The levels of radioactivity above which bioassay is necessary and the conditions under which handling occurs are shown below.

MODE OF HANDLING	ACTIVITY IN VOLATILE/DISPERSIBLE FORM[a]
1. Open room or bench	1 millicurie
2. Fume hood	10 millicuries
3. Glove box	100 millicuries

The activities shown apply to single events involving the specific amounts of activities, or to the total amounts of radioactivity handled by an individual in a 3 month period. (From: 10 CFR Part 20, Section 20.108, Applications for Bioassay For I-125 and I-131.)

[a] When using I-125 or I-131 in a nonvolatile form, the activities are higher by a factor of 10.

Table 18.5 REPORTED ADVERSE REACTIONS AND COMPLICATIONS OF I-131 SODIUM IODIDE THERAPY

Acute radiation sickness
Radiation thyroiditis
Sialoadenitis
Thyroid storm
Swelling and hemorrhage of metastases
Bone marrow suppression
Radiation pneumonitis and fibrosis

ing fatigue, headache, nausea, and vomiting, have been reported, the occurrence of radiation sickness attributable to radioiodine therapy is infrequent at doses of 200 millicuries and less. Generally, nausea and vomiting are intratherapeutic in origin, occur soon after the oral administration of radioiodine, and can be managed effectively by the employment of suitable antinausea medications.

Radiation thyroiditis, sialoadenitis, exacerbation of hyperthyroidism (thyroid crisis or storm), bone marrow depression, and swelling and hemorrhage of metastases have also been reported. Symptoms of radiation thyroiditis include swelling, tenderness, and increased firmness of the gland with erythemia of the skin over the thyroid. This condition is relatively low in incidence and usually subsides spontaneously in a few days after therapy has been given. Sialoadenitis is frequently noted following radioiodine therapy and can be averted by increasing salivary flow using hard candies or lozenges. Thyroid storm occurs relatively infrequently although it is a potential complication in patients who are hyperthyroid from functioning metastatic disease. Bone marrow suppression to some degree can be observed in practically all patients receiving radioiodine therapy; however, serious and permanent depression of bone marrow function has not been observed in patients receiving less than 200 rads exposure to hematopoietic tissues (Edmonds CJ, 1979; Benua RS, et al, 1962). Although a low incidence of swelling in metastatic deposits has been reported (Benua RS, et al, 1962), it is occasionally desirable in patients with significant tumor load to employ corticosteroid pretreatment in order to avoid potential complications of therapy, particularly in patients with brain metastases. In patients with large goiters, thyroid swelling can lead to symptomatic tracheal compression that requires administration of corticosteroids for relief.

Pneumonitis and pulmonary radiation fibrosis are other complications that have been rarely observed to be associated with radioiodine therapy.

Pediatric Considerations. Whether or not sodium iodide I-131 therapy should be employed for the treatment of hyperthyroidism in patients who are either children or young adults in the childbearing years is a matter of debate. The principal concern is the potential for oncogenesis in the treated subjects and birth defects in their offspring. The occurrence of neither, however, has been borne out in recent studies as associated with I-131 therapy. In fact, patients with hyperthyroidism have a 50% higher than expected incidence of leukemia compared to the general population, an occurrence that is most likely related to the disease itself and not the mode of treatment (Saenger EL, et al, 1968). The National Center for Radiological Health found the incidence of leukemia to be the same in 22,000 patients treated with I-131 and 14,000 patients treated surgically or with antithyroid drugs. In that study, the incidence of thyroid cancer actually was lower in the radioiodine treated group (0.1%) than in the surgical (0.5%) or medical (0.3%) groups (Saenger EL, et al,

1968). This finding was probably due to the radiation-induced damage to the thyroid cells that inhibited replication (Dobyns BM, et al, 1974).

Considerations of long-term infertility in patients who have undergone radioiodine therapy have been raised since it has been reported that ovarian failure and azospermia have been observed in patients after treatment for thyroid cancer. S.D. Sarker and co-workers (1976) found no significant decrease in fertility in patients treated with radioiodine.

CLINICAL CONSIDERATIONS/ CONTRAINDICATIONS

In patients being treated for hyperthyroidism, the most common consequence of radioiodine therapy involves the development of hypothyroidism. Although several treatment protocols have attempted to define I-131 dosage regimens that avoid this complication, all to date have been unsuccessful, and subsequent hypothyroidism is now considered an essentially unavoidable consequence of I-131 therapy. In most studies of I-131 treatment for hyperthyroidism, the greatest incidence of hypothyroidism occurs within 6 months of treatment. From 5–70% of patients will be hypothyroid by 1 year, and the cumulative incidence varies from 2–6% per year thereafter (Beierwaltes WH, 1978).

Contraindications. The major contraindication to I-131 therapy is pregnancy. Radioiodine crosses the placenta and the fetal thyroid attains an iodine-concentrating ability after approximately the twelveth week of gestation. As a result, treatment of a female in the second trimester of pregnancy or later may result in her infant developing cretinism or congenital hypothyroidism. Prior to the twelveth week of gestation, the lack of concentrating ability protects the fetal thyroid; however, I-131 is still contraindicated.

As an additional consideration, radioiodine and radiolabeled thyroid hormones are concentrated and excreted in breast milk, requiring that nursing be discontinued following I-131 administration.

DOSAGE/DOSIMETRY

Hyperthyroidism. In the treatment of hyperthyroidism, it is clearly established that between 5,000–10,000 rads to the thyroid gland are required. This amount of radiation is delivered to the thyroid when 80–100 microcuries of I-131 are retained by the gland per gram of tissue. Table 18.6 illustrates a typical calculation of an individualized treatment dose based upon estimated thyroid gland weight and measurement of the 24-hour radioiodine uptake.

The use of such individualized treatment doses may not always correlate with response due to (1) difficulties in accurately determining the size of the gland; (2) differences in the biological half-life of the therapeutic dose of I-131 versus the diagnostic dose (Miller ER and Sheline GE, 1957); (3) inhomogenous distribution of the radionuclide in the gland; and (4) differences in the radiosensitivity of diseased thyroid tissue from one patient to another. As a result of these difficulties, some treatment centers have abandoned the approach of individualized therapy in favor of a standard dose of 5–10 millicuries of I-131 to all patients with diffuse toxic goiter. Patients with one or more toxic nodules (Plummer's disease) are generally administered twice the amount of I-131 that is given patients with diffuse goiters because nodular disease is regarded as being more difficult to treat. The relative radio-resistance of toxic

Table 18.6   SAMPLE CALCULATION OF INDIVIDUALIZED I-131 SODIUM IODIDE DOSAGE FOR THE TREATMENT OF HYPERTHYROIDISM

Clinical Data
- Estimated weight of the patient's thyroid gland: 60 gm
- ^{131}I-sodium iodide uptake value (at 24 hours): 80% of the admin. dose
- Required I-131 concentration to deliver 8,000–10,000 rads: 100 μCi/Gm

Dosage Calculation

$$\text{Required dose (microcuries)} = \frac{60 \text{ gm} \times 10\mu\text{Ci/gm}}{0.80}$$

$$= 7,500\mu\text{Ci}$$

nodules may be due to faster turnover of radioiodine (as a result of its short biologic half-life in nodular tissues) or to inhomogenous distribution of radioiodine in the nodules due to existing necrosis and ischemia.

Thyroid carcinoma. Following surgical removal of all identifiable normal and neoplastic tissues, radioiodine therapy is employed for the ablation of thyroid remnants and/or treatment of metastatic disease. In order to detect the presence of thyroid remnants, a dose of 0.5–10 millicuries of I-131 sodium iodide is employed as a scanning dose with images of the neck and chest obtained 24–72 hours later If radioiodine uptake is noted in the thyroid bed only, between 75–100 millicuries

of sodium iodide I-131 is given orally. The US Nuclear Regulatory Commission (NRC) requires that the patient be hospitalized until the activity in the body is less than 30 millicuries or until the measured dose rate from the patient is less than 5 millirems per hour at a distance of one meter. (I-131 body activity is generally halved every 12–24 hours.) A whole-body scan of I-131 activity may be desirable 3–7 days after therapeutic dosing in order to search for regional or distant metastases not seen in the original whole-body I-131 scan (Figure 18.1).

The amount of I-131 sodium iodide to be given for treatment of thyroid carcinoma is determined based upon empirical decisions involving the extent of disease and the site(s) of involvement. Usually, a

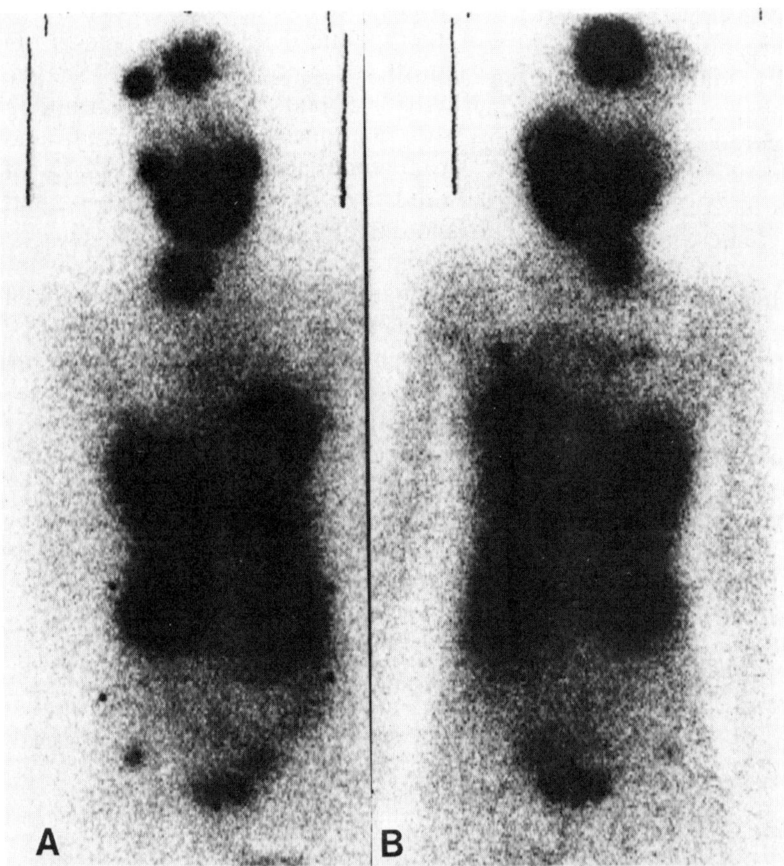

Figure 18.1 Anterior (A) and posterior (B) upper body images obtained 48 hours following administration of 150 mCi sodium iodide I-131 for treatment of metastatic thyroid carcinoma. Note normal uptake in salivary glands, kidneys, liver, colon, and bladder. Foci of metastatic disease appear in skull, neck, chest, and abdomen.

single dose of 100–200 millicuries of sodium iodide I-131 is employed. Approximately 50–80% of patients with distant metastases will develop sufficient uptake to allow treatment. Several studies (Freitas JE, et al, 1985), have shown that doses in the range of 200 millicuries of sodium iodide I-131 are efficacious in the treatment of patients with lung metastases (lung metastases are eradicated more easily than are bone metastases). Occassionally, however, it is necessary that patients must be given cumulative doses of I-131 sodium iodide as large as 1 curie in order to obtain adequate therapeutic results. The administered dose at each therapeutic intervention should be individualized so that the radiation dose to the blood (and bone marrow) does not exceed 200 rads. According to one report (Leeper RD, 1983), 200 rads are delivered to blood by doses of 70–650 mCi, with the average activity being 300 mCi. The radiation dose to blood is typically estimated using the Marinelli formulae (Marinelli LD, et al, 1948), which assumes that all of the energy from the beta-emissions is absorbed in whole blood and that both I-131 and the critical organ (bone marrow) are uniformly distributed in the body.

Since increasing thyroid-stimulating hormone (TSH) levels have been shown to augment I-131 uptake by well-differentiated thyroid carcinoma, it is desirable to maximize radioiodine uptake by a 4–6 week abstinence from thyroid hormone (i. e., thyroxine) in order to expose thyroid tissues and metastases to elevated TSH levels. Verification of elevated TSH blood levels can be readily obtained from a routine lab test.

II. Treatment of Polycythemia Vera with P-32 Sodium Phosphate

RADIOPHARMACEUTICALS

BACKGROUND/HISTORY

For nearly 50 years, P-32 sodium phosphate has been employed as a therapeutic aid in the management of a variety of

Table 18.7   REPORTED THERAPEUTIC APPLICATIONS OF P-32 SODIUM PHOSPHATE

Polycythemia vera[a]
Essential thrombocythemia
Chronic myelogenous leukemia[a]
Chronic lymphocytic leukemia[a]
Hodgkin's disease
Non-Hodgkin's lymphoma
Multiple myeloma
Intractable bone pain secondary to skeletal metastases[a]

[a] Indications are listed in respective product insert information.

pathologies (Table 18.7). Its first use for the treatment of polycythemia vera and leukemia occurred soon after it was noted to localize in bone, bone marrow, and leukemic tissue (Lawrence JH, et al, 1939; 1940). Concentration of P-32 sodium phosphate in cells occurs in relation to cell growth rates; hence, the bone marrow exhibits a higher concentration of P-32 than does muscle or other slower growing tissues.

Although it is still debatable whether radiation and/or chemical-induced myelosuppression is superior for the treatment of polycythemia vera, a number of uncontrolled studies have shown P-32 sodium phosphate to be an efficacious treatment modality. Excellent therapeutic responses have been achieved with P-32 sodium phosphate with some reports of median survival as long as 13–16 years following treatment. (Van Nostrand D and Silberstein E, 1985). Currently, a multifaceted study is underway by the Polycythemia Vera Study Group to evaluate and define the relationship between P-32 sodium phosphate and alternate therapies. Because no other therapeutic radiopharmaceutical has been developed that is superior to this agent, P-32 sodium phosphate remains the agent of choice for radiation-induced myelosuppression.

Because P-32 sodium phosphate is incorporated into sites of new bone formation, this radiopharmaceutical has also found therapeutic usefulness in the palliation of bone pain in patients with extensive skeletal metastases (Friedell HL and Storaasli JP, 1950). In the treatment of pain from skeletal metastases, P-32 destroys metastatic cells by three potential mechanisms. First, rapidly growing tumors concentrate P-32 sodium phosphate to a greater degree and hence receive greater irradiation than normal tissues. Second, tumor cells in the skeleton are irradiated from P-32 localization in neighboring sites of new bone formation. Third, tumor cells may be destroyed from the disruption of chemical bonds when P-32 atoms, which have been previously incorporated into DNA and RNA, decay to Sulfur-32. The actual mechanism for the relief of pain from skeletal metastases, is, however, less clear. Because relief of pain may occur as early as 3–5 days following treatment with P-32 sodium phosphate, intraosseous tumor destruction in an incomplete explanation. Perhaps decreased pressure in perineural lymphatics contributes to amelioration of pain. Also, it cannot be ruled out that a placebo effect or response to concurrent drugs (e. g, testosterone) may be responsible for some degree of analgesia experienced by some patients.

Given in small doses, P-32 sodium phosphate can also be used safely as a diagnostic aid for the detection of ocular malignant melanoma. The procedure involves the intravenous administration of P-32 sodium phosphate and the detection several days later of its uptake in the choroidal lesion. Since no gamma emissions are produced by the beta decay of P-32, the presence of radioactivity is necessarily determined using a hand-held probe detector rather than a standard scintillation camera.

CHEMISTRY

The nuclear and physical properties of Phosphorous-32 are shown in Table 18.8.

P-32 sodium phosphate is the sodium salt of dihydrogen P-32 phosphate and forms a clear, colorless solution. In the United States, P-32 sodium phosphate is available in 10 milliliter single-dose glass vials (containing no bacteriostatic agents or preservatives) that contain 5 millicuries of P-32 on the day of calibration. The intravenous solution contains approximately 1.6 mg/ml of sodium acetate as a buffer, sodium chloride for isotonicity, and hydrochloric acid or sodium hydroxide for pH adjustment. Total phosphorous content is less than 0.5 mg/ml.

PHARMACOKINETICS

Following oral administration in fasting patients, P-32 sodium phosphate is readily and completely absorbed from the gastrointestinal tract. However, since food can cause variability in the gastrointestinal absorption of P-32 sodium phosphate, the intravenous route of administration is preferred. Within 6–24 hours after parenteral administration, the bone activity is 4–6 times greater than muscle, fat, or skin, with this ratio increasing to 6–10 at 3 days (Silberstein EB, 1979). The liver and spleen exhibit P-32 uptake that is similar to muscle, fat, and skin.

Studies in patients with polycythemia suggest biexponential blood pool clearances with mean half-lives of 1.7 and 22.5 days for whole blood and 0.8 and 20.0 days for plasma. Whole-body retention appears to be monoexponential with a mean biological half-life of 39 days. Biological half-lives in other organs include iliac marrow—9 days; sternal marrow—7 days; and trabecular bone—27 days (Spiers FW, et al, 1976).

Body clearance is primarily by renal excretion, with normal patients excreting 5–10% of the administered dose in urine within 24 hours and about 20% being excreted by the end of the first week (U.S.P.-DI, 1989). A very small percentage of P-32 sodium phosphate is excreted in the feces.

PRECAUTIONS

Handling. Since P-32 decays exclusively by beta emission, the plastic syringe or

Table 18.8 NUCLEAR PROPERTIES OF PHOSPHORUS-32

Physical half-life:	14.3 days
Decay mode:	Beta[-]
Mean Beta [-] energy (abundance):	695 keV (100%)

glass vial in which P-32 is contained is usually sufficient shielding. When handling beta-emitting radionuclides, the greatest source of radiation exposure to occupational workers is from the production of Bremsstrahlung radiation. Because the amount of Bremsstrahlung radiation produced is proportional to the increasing density of shielding materials, low-density materials, such as Lucite or other plastics, are recommended instead of lead for shielding of beta-emitting radionuclides.

Adverse Reactions in the Treatment of Polycythemia Vera. The leukemogenic effects of P-32 sodium phosphate therapy have not been clearly defined. Although the risk of neoplasia in polycythemia vera patients treated with myelosuppression has been reported to be as high as 20–40 times that of controls, polycythemia vera patients treated only with drugs or phlebotomy also develop acute leukemia. One study found that the risk of acute leukemia in patients treated with chlorambucil was 2.3 times that in patients given P-32 sodium phosphate, and 13 times that in patients treated with phlebotomy alone (Berk PD, et al, 1981). It has been suggested (Lawrence JH, et al, 1969) that the incidence of leukemia observed in patients treated with P-32 sodium phosphate could be primarily the result of prolonged survival, permitting the natural evolution of polycythemia vera into acute leukemia. The possible carcinogenic action of P-32 may also be associated with irradiation of a susceptible population. The incidence of acute leukemia reported in polycythemia vera patients treated with P-32 sodium phosphate ranges from 2–9.6%, increasing to approximately 15% in patients surviving more than 10 years of therapy (Van Nostrand D and Silberstein E, 1985; Najean Y, et al, 1980).

Singular cases of angioimmunoblastic lymphadenopathy and Hodgkin's disease have also been reported in polycythemia vera patients treated only with P-32 sodium phosphate. In addition, there appears to be a slight increase in the number of skin and intestinal malignancies reported in this patient treatment group.

Another problem encountered in P-32 sodium phosphate treatment of polycythemia vera is the secondary appearance of resistance to subsequent treatments. It has been shown that with treatment, the mean duration of successive remissions progressively decreases. Complete resistance has seldom been observed, however, since other complications or death ensue earlier.

Adverse Reactions in the Treatment of Bone Pain. A number of frequent and significant complications have been reported with the use of P-32 sodium phosphate for metastatic bone pain. The majority of treated patients exhibits myelosuppression, typically occurring 4–8 weeks after initiation of therapy, with many patients (as high as 40–60% in some studies) requiring blood transfusions. Symptoms associated with pancytopenia include low-grade fever, nausea, vomiting, and gastroenteritis. Only one death has been reported that was attributable to aplastic anemia induced by P-32 treatment. Complications more commonly reported include transient elevations in blood urea nitrogen (BUN) and mild increases in serum calcium levels.

Occasionally, patient pretreatment with pharmacological adjuncts is performed in an attempt to stimulate bone uptake of P-32 sodium phosphate (Table 18.9). In patients given P-32 sodium phosphate treatment and who received testosterone either alone or in combination with parathyroid hormone (PTH), it was noted that exacerbation of bone pain occurred in nearly two-thirds of patients with the pain typically improved or resolved on the completion of the P-32 treatment (Van Nostrand D and Silberstein E, 1985). However, when testosterone was not used, no exacerbation of bone pain was reported. Patients receiving certain pharmaceutical adjuncts have also been reported to have additional complications. For example, patients receiving testosterone showed a six-fold increase in the incidence of spinal cord compression (2.5%) as compared to those patients who did not receive testosterone (0.4%). No cases of spinal cord compression have been reported in patients pre-treated with PTH.

Regardless of the treatment indication, care must be exercised during intravenous administration of P-32 sodium phosphate because infiltration of the radiopharmaceutical may cause local tissue necrosis. Overdosage of P-32 may produce serious depressive effects on the hematopoietic system.

**Table 18.9 SUGGESTED P-32 SODIUM PHOSPHATE TREATMENT
PROTOCOLS FOR THE RELIEF OF BONE PAIN DUE TO
METASTATIC INVOLVEMENT**

Protocol 1 (Maxfield JR, et al, 1958)		
Androgens[a]		Days 1–15
P-32 Sodium phosphate	1.5–3 mCi	Days 5–10
Protocol 2 (Tong ECK, et al, 1973)		
Parathyroid hormone	300 I.U./day IM	Days 1–7
	(3 divided doses)	
P-32 Sodium phosphate	3 mCi	Day 9
	2 mCi	Days 10, 11, 14, 17, 21, 24
	1 mCi	Days 28, 31, 35, 38, 42
Protocol 3 (Rodriguez-Atunez A, et al, 1973)		
Parathyroid hormone	300 I.U./day IM	Days 1–7
	(3 divided doses)	
Androgens[a]		Days 4–13
P-32 Sodium phosphate	3 mCi	Day 9
	2 mCi	Days 10, 11, 14, 17, 21, 24
	1 mCi	Days 28, 31, 35, 38, 42

[a] Aqueous testosterone (testosterone proprionate, cypionate), 100 mg/day IM; Fluoxymester-one, 40–60 mg/day oral (4 divided doses).

Use During Pregnancy/Breastfeeding.
The use of this radiopharmaceutical is contraindicated in patients who are either pregnant or breastfeeding.

CLINICAL CONSIDERATIONS/
CONTRAINDICATIONS

In the Treatment of Polycythemia Vera.
A number of uncontrolled studies have shown P-32 sodium phosphate therapy to be highly efficacious in the treatment of polycythemia vera; excellent therapeutic responses and prolonged median survival of 13–16 years have been reported. However, the relationship between P-32 and alternate therapies is not yet fully defined. Therapeutic trials comparing the efficiency and complications of P-32, alkylating agents, and phlebotomy are yet to be completed.

In the Treatment of Bone Pain. A large number of studies have been published reporting the use of P-32 sodium phosphate in the treatment of bone pain associated with skeletal metastases. A collective therapeutic response was observed in 78% of treated patients. The therapeutic response in patients with metastases from prostate cancer was somewhat lower than in patients with metastases from breast and other cancers (73% versus 86%). The collective mean duration of response was 1.5–11.3 months, with the longest duration of response being 36 months. Therapeutic response was achieved for 37–68% of follow-up months, with many patients dying without pain (Van Nostrand D and Silberstein E, 1985).

The role of pharmacological adjuncts in P-32 therapy for metastatic bone pain is unclear. Data regarding the benefit of pretreatment with testosterone and/or PTH in terms of therapeutic response are inconclusive. If pharmacological adjuncts are to be employed, special caution should be exercised in those patients who have advanced renal failure or who have had extensive prior external-beam therapy. Testosterone should be used with care in patients with severe and/or diffuse vertebral involvement. If PTH is to be used, skin testing should be considered to determine patients' hypersensitivity, and special care should be taken in patients having abnormal calcium levels or myocardial dysrhythmias.

Contraindications. P-32 sodium phosphate treatment is contraindicated if the platelet count is less than 100,000 per microliter or the leukocyte count is less than 3,000 per microliter. All patients treated with P-32 sodium phosphate should be followed with complete blood counts, serum calcium levels, and renal function tests. P-32 sodium phosphate is contraindicated during pregnancy and breastfeeding.

DOSAGE/DOSIMETRY

Treatment of Polycythemia Vera. An initial dose of P-32 sodium phosphate (3.5–5.0 mCi) is given intravenously with subsequent doses given every 12–24 weeks as needed to control the elevated hematocrit. The dosage regimen recommended by the Polycythemia Vera Study Group is as follows:

1. Induction is performed with intravenous P-32 sodium phosphate; 2.3 mCi/m^2 not to exceed 5 millicuries.
2. If, at twelve weeks following the induction dose, the hematocrit is still greater than 45% and the platelet or leukocyte count has decreased less than 25%, or if the platelet count still exceeds 600,000 per microliter, a second P-32 dose is given. This dose may be increased at 12-week intervals by 25% of the initial dose, to a limit of 7 millicuries/dose. P-32 is no longer given when the hematocrit has stabilized without phlebotomy.
3. For relapses (i. e., hematocrit greater than 45%), phlebotomy is employed, and P-32 is given at the previous effective dose.

Treatment of Metastatic Bone Pain. For the treatment of bone pain, P-32 sodium phosphate has been given in various schedules of single doses, multiple continuous doses, or multiple intermittent doses with or without pharmacological adjuncts. The single doses range from 3–10 millicuries and the total doses for multiple treatments range from 5–20 millicuries depending on schedule and patient response. Pretreatment with pharmacological adjuncts may also be employed in an attempt to enhance bone localization of P-32 (Table 18.9).

As a Diagnostic Aid in the Localization of Ocular Melanoma. For the diagnosis of choroidal melanoma, the usual dose of P-32 sodium phosphate is 10 μCi/kg (up to 700 microcuries) given intravenously. Forty-eight hours later, probe counting

Table 18.10 RADIATION DOSIMETRY FOR INTRAVENOUS P-32 SODIUM PHOSPHATE[a]

ORGAN	RADS/MCI
Skeleton	63
Marrow	24
Liver	6.2
Spleen	7.3
Brain	3.0
Testes	1.0
Ovaries	0.8
Whole body	10.0

[a]From Spiers FW and colleagues, 1976 and respective product insert information, Mallinckrodt, Inc.

over the tumor and over a normal (control) area of the eye is performed. Typically, triplicate counts over 1–2 minutes are obtained. Results are expressed as % uptake where:

$$\% \text{ uptake} = \frac{(\text{average tumor counts}) - (\text{average control counts})}{(\text{average control counts})} \times 100\%$$

Uptakes of greater than 50–60% are considered positive.

Radiation Dosimetry. The estimated radiation dosimetry for P-32 sodium phosphate is summarized in Table 18.10. Typically, marrow doses between 80–200 rads have been employed for myelosuppression in patients with polycythemia vera, whereas doses used for the treatment of skeletal metastases have resulted in even greater marrow irradiation.

III. Treatment of Malignant Effusion with P-32 Chromic Phosphate

Malignant effusions frequently occur in the natural history of many cancers, especially breast cancer (pleural effusion) and ovarian cancer (peritoneal effusion). Treatment is often warranted to improve either the quality of life (by reducing discomfort, frequency of fluid drainage, and frequency of hospitalization) or the rate of survival (by reducing respiratory compromise and recurrent infections). Since thoracentesis and paracentesis often do not prevent the reaccumulation of fluid, alternative treatments, including radiation, must be considered.

Direct radiation treatment of effusions can be accomplished by the intracavitary instillation of beta-emitting radiopharmaceuticals. The therapeutic radiopharmaceuticals used for this purpose are colloidal in nature; therefore, they remain confined sufficiently long in the pleural or peritoneal cavity into which they are directly instilled to permit the delivery of therapeutic doses of radiation.

RADIOPHARMACEUTICALS

BACKGROUND/HISTORY

The treatment of malignant effusion with radiation from radionuclides instilled into the pathogenic body cavity was first described by J.H. Müller in Zurich in 1945 using colloidal preparations of Zn-63 and later Au-198. In 1958, M.L. Jacobs reported the efficacious use of intracavitary P-32 chromic phosphate.

P-32 chromic phosphate possesses several advantageous properties related to its use in the treatment of malignant effusions. First, because P-32 decays purely by beta-emission it is relatively easy to shield and provides minimal occupational radiation exposure. Also, significant radiation doses to adjacent normal organs such as the bowel mucosa do not occur because no gamma emissions are produced. Second, the physical half-life for P-32 of 14.3 days facilitates radiopharmaceutical shipping and storage. Third, the relatively high-energy beta emission of P-32 allows treatment of cells that are underlying the cavity surface. Finally, the particle size of P-32 chromic phosphate is sufficiently large to prevent leakage of the radiopharmaceutical from the treatment cavity. As a result of these advantageous properties, P-32 chromic phosphate is the preferred radiopharmaceutical for the treatment of malignant effusions.

Though the primary application of P-

Table 18.11 REPORTED THERAPEUTIC APPLICATIONS OF P-32 CHROMIC PHOSPHATE

THERAPEUTIC APPLICATION	ROUTE OF ADMINISTRATION
Malignant pericardial effusion	Intraperitoneal
Malignant pleural effusion[a]	Intrapleural
Malignant pericardial effusion	Intrapericardial
Synovial effusion	Intraarticular
Prevention of hepatic metastases from colorectal carcinoma	Intraarterial
Ovarian carcinoma	Intraperitoneal
Endometrial adenocarcinoma	Intraperitoneal
Cystic astrocytoma, craniopharyngioma	Intracystic
Cystic astrocytoma	Intracystic
Prostate carcinoma[a]	Intrastitial
Bladder carcinoma[a]	Intrastitial

[a] Indications listed in respective product insert information.

32 chromic phosphate has been in the treatment of cancers of the chest and abdomen, instillations have also been made in other closed cavities and the interstitium of some tumors. Reported clinical indications for P-32 chromic phosphate are listed in Table 18.11.

CHEMISTRY

P-32 chromic phosphate is a greenish-blue suspension that is prepared by the chemical precipitation method. The colloid particles are clumps or aggregates of hundreds or thousands of chromic phosphate molecules. The size of the majority of the particles (greater than 90%) is between 0.6–2.0 microns.

The nuclear properties of P-32 are listed in Table 18.8.

Chromic phosphate P-32 is commercially available (Phosphocol®, Mallinckrodt, Inc.) as a sterile aqueous suspension in a 30% dextrose solution with 2% benzyl alcohol as a preservative. The product also contains 1 mg/ml sodium acetate and sodium hydroxide or hydrochloric acid for pH adjustment. It is available in 10 ml vials containing 10 or 15 mCi with a concentration of 5 mCi/ml and a specific activity of up to 5 mCi/mg at the time of calibration.

PHARMACOKINETICS

Immediately after peritoneal instillation, P-32 chromic phosphate rapidly disperses in the abdomen; however, within only a few minutes, the distribution becomes nonuniform, frequently localizing in the abdomen to the side of the catheter. After 6 hours, the localization becomes even more inhomogeneous, often with regional and/or serpiginous distribution. Focal areas of aggregated activity and particulate settling with gravity may also occur. Despite changing the patient positioning frequently during the initial few hours after radiopharmaceutical instillation, activity often localizes around the bladder and cul-de-sac. By 24 hours, less than 10% of the P-32 chromic phosphate remains in the intracavitary fluid with most of the radioactivity fixed (by phagocytosis or adsorption) onto the mesothelial membranes where it remains unchanged for weeks. Minor alterations in radioactivity localization observed after 24 hours may be secondary to the movement of abdominal organs (Kaplan WD, et al, 1981).

Although poorly characterized in humans, P-32 chromic phosphate appears to be slowly removed from the peritoneal cavity and distributed systemically. The amount of radioactivity in blood shows a biphasic increase for about 7 days and thereafter shows a slow gradual decline. Once in the vascular system, colloid particles are rapidly removed by organs of the reticuloendothelial system. Localization in various organs reported at autopsy include the liver (0.9–13%), spleen (0.02–0.14%), and bone marrow (0.23–4.09%) (Root SW, et al, 1954). Because a small fraction of the administered dose has been recoved in the urine (approximately 5% at 11 days), it has been suggested that P-32 may also be distributed systemically as the phosphate ion (Root SW, et al, 1954). Gel chromatography of blood samples has shown that about one-third of the activity is high molecular weight (colloid) and the remaining two-thirds of the activity is low molecular weight materials that are probably physiologic degradation products (Boye E, et al, 1984). P-32 chromic phosphate is also removed, in part, from the peritoneal cavity by the lymphatics. Localization in intrathoracic nodes, which has been observed as early as the first day

post treatment, commonly occurs (Kaplan WD, et al, 1981).

The biodistribution of P-32 chromic phosphate administered intrapleurally has not been well characterized.

Following intraarticular administration, most of P-32 chromic phosphate remains in the joint cavity for at least 14 days with only minute amounts of radioactivity being detected in blood and urine (Van Nostrand D and Silberstein E, 1985). Rarely does the radiopharmaceutical migrate to the inguinal nodes.

No significant blood, urine, or liver and spleen activity has been observed following intracystic administration of P-32 chromic phosphate (Taasan V, et al, 1985).

PRECAUTIONS

Adverse reactions reported with the use of P-32 chromic phosphate are summarized in Table 18.12. Although some minor absorption and systemic distribution have been observed, no hematological complications have been reported following therapy with P-32 chromic phosphate.

Low-density shielding materials such as glass or Lucite are recommended to shield beta-emitting radionuclides such as P-32.

CLINICAL CONSIDERATIONS/ CONTRAINDICATIONS

The efficacy of P-32 chromic phosphate in the treatment of malignant ascites and

Table 18.12 REPORTED ADVERSE REACTIONS FOR P-32 CHROMIC PHOSPHATE

ROUTE OF ADMINISTRATION	ADVERSE REACTIONS
Intraperitoneal[a]	Small bowel obstruction
	Fever (transient, low-grade)
	Nausea, vomiting
	Abdominal cramping, diarrhea
	Delayed wound healing
Intrapleural[a]	Fever
	Radiation sickness (minor)
	Pleuritis
	Shortness of breath, cyanosis
Intrapericardial[b]	Constrictive pericarditis
Intraarticular[a]	Synovitis (acute)
	Fever (transient)
	Radiation dermatitis
	Flexion deformity
	Cartilage necrosis

[a] Van Nostrand D and Silberstein E, 1985..
[b] Martini N and associates, 1977.

pleural effusion is somewhat variable with reported response rates averaging 46% (Van Nostrand D and Silberstein E, 1985). The duration of response is not well described but was reported in one study as 15.6 ± 2.9 weeks (O'Bryan RM, et al, 1968).

The limited data available describing P-32 chromic phosphate therapy for pericardial effusion indicate a response rate of 71% with a mean remission of 6 months (Martini N, et al, 1977).

Most studies of radiocolloid therapy for chronic synovitis report an improvement rate of 50–60% with a duration of months to years (Winston MA, 1979).

Insufficient data exist to describe the efficacy of P-32 chromic phosphate for cystic brain tumors. Preliminary reports, however, indicate that therapy is beneficial in terms of prolonging the interval between cyst decompressions and, in some patients, reducing cyst size (Taasan V, et al, 1985).

Contraindications.   Contraindications for P-32 chromic phosphate therapy are few. In the postoperative patient, the surgical wound should be adequately healed to prevent mechanical leakage of the radiopharmaceutical from the administration site. With intracavitary therapy, it should be determined that loculation is not present that would prevent desirable dispersion of the therapeutic radiopharmaceutical in the treatment cavity. P-32 chromic phosphate should not be administered to either pregnant women or children unless the expected benefits of therapy far outweigh the risk of irradiation. Finally, because maximum effects of P-32 chromic phosphate therapy may not be achieved for several months post radiopharmaceutical administration, it is desirable that candidates for treatment have a life expectancy of at least 3 months.

DOSAGE/DOSIMETRY

Doses of P-32 chromic phosphate required to deliver the desired radiation for treatment of most clinical indications are shown in Table 18.13. These doses have generally been determined empirically in conjunction with intended radiation dosimetry estimates.

Following catheter placement, it may be desirable to perform peritoneal scintigraphy in order to verify catheter patency and position and to determine that no loculation exists. Peritoneal scintigraphy is performed by the intraperitoneal administration of Tc-99m sulfur colloid with scintiphotos of radiopharmaceutical distribution in the peritoneal spaces obtained soon afterwards. Because Tc-99m sulfur colloid administered intraperitoneally exhibits distribution similar to P-32 chromic phosphate, Tc-99m peritoneal scintigraphy can be employed to predict whether adequate distribution of the subsequently administered P-32 chromic phosphate can be expected. Additionally, direct imaging of the P-32 Bremsstrahlung may be performed after administration of P-32 chromic phosphate to verify distribution. The energy spectrum of Bremsstrahlung from P-32 in simulated tissue medium has been reported to be from 40 keV to 1.5 MeV with a peak at 40–81 keV (Kaplan WD, et al, 1981). Recomendations for imaging include the use of a high-energy collimator (in order to prevent septal penetration of

Table 18.13   TYPICAL DOSAGES OF P-32 CHROMIC PHOSPHATE FOR VARIOUS THERAPEUTIC APPLICATIONS

THERAPEUTIC APPLICATION	ROUTE OF ADMINISTRATION	DOSAGE RANGE
Malignant peritoneal effusion	Intraperitoneal	10–20 mCi
Malignant pleural effusion	Intrapleural	5–15 mCi
Maligant pericardial effusion	Intrapericardial	5–10 mCi
Synovial effusion	Intraarticular	1–2 mCi
Cystic astrocytoma, craniopharyn-gioma	Intracystic	0.06 mCi/ml cyst volume
Prostate, bladder carcinoma	Intrastitial	0.1–0.5 mCi/gram

the very high energy Bremsstrahlung) and an imaging window centered at approximately 80 keV.

Treatment of Intraperitoneal Effusions. P-32 chromic phosphate is instilled by direct bolus or is combined with additional fluids for volume. A preinfusion of 500 ml of normal saline is occasionally employed to improve the dispersion of the P-32 suspension. Other methods involve mixing the P-32 chromic phosphate in 250–500 ml of normal saline prior to infusion. Because the particles may settle with time, it is important to resuspend the radiopharmaceutical immediately prior to administration. P-32 chromic phosphate particles in normal saline do not significantly stick to glass or plastic, so premixing is acceptable.

Treatment of Intrapleural Effusions. The technique for intrapleural administration of P-32 chromic phosphate is similar to that for intraperitoneal administration. Intrapleural therapies should be preceded by pleuroscintigraphy to aid in identifying loculations, potential pulmonary misadministrations or other complications such as bronchopleural communications.

Intraarticular Therapy. Recommendations for intraarticular administration of P-32 chromic phosphate include (1) pretherapy articuloscintigraphy (to demonstrate that adequate distribution can be obtained), and (2) pretreatment with intraarticular steroids.

Treatment of Cystic Brain Tumor. Prior to performing P-32 chromic phosphate therapy of cystic brain tumor, the volume of the cyst should be determined by standard radioisotope dilution techniques (e.g., using Tc-99m sulfur colloid). The required dose of P-32 chromic phosphate, based upon cyst volume, is then injected with barbotage, using aspirations to ensure homogenous mixing.

Radiation Dosimetry. Radiation dosimetry for P-32 chromic phosphate admin-

Table 18.14 RADIATION DOSIMETRY ASSOCIATED WITH THE INTRAPERITONEAL AND INTRAPLEURAL ADMINISTRATION OF P-32 CHROMIC PHOSPHATE[a]

	RADS/10 MCI	
TISSUE DEPTH (MM)	Peritoneal membrane[b]	Pleural membrane[b]
0.04	9,000	11,500
0.08	7,500	9,500
0.12	7,000	8,500
0.16	6,000	7,500
0.20	5,500	7,000
1.0	2,150	2,700
2.0	850	1,050

[a] From respective product insert information, Mallinckrodt, Inc.
[b] Assumes surface area of 5,000 cm^2.
[c] Assumes surface area of 4,000 cm^2.

istered intraperitoneally and intrapleurally is summarized in Table 18.14. The maximum doses received by the blood and bone marrow from intraperitoneal administration have been estimated to be 0.12 and 0.6 rad/mCi, respectively (Boye E, et al, 1984). Administered intraarticularly, P-32 chromic phosphate delivers approximately 10,000 rads/mCi to the synovial surface (Winston MA, 1979). A target dose of 20,000 rads is typically the goal with P-32 chromic phosphate administration into cystic brain tumors (Taason V, et al, 1985). Administered intrastitially, P-32 chromic phosphate delivers approximately 730,000 rads/mCi/gram of tissue (Blahd WH, 1971).

References

Beierwaltes WH. The treatment of hyperthyroidism with I-131. *Semin Nucl Med* 1978, 8:95–103.

Benua RS. Consultant's Corner. *J Nucl Med* 1985, 26:8.

Benua RS, Cicale NR, Sonenberg M, et al. The relation of radioiodine dosimetry to results and complications in the treatment of metastatic thyroid cancer. *AJR* 1962, 87:171–182.

Berk PD, Goldberg JD, Silverstein MN, et al. Increased incidence of acute leukemia in polycythemia vera associated with chlorambucil therapy. *N Engl J Med* 1981, 304:441–447.

Blahd WH. *Nuclear Medicine*, Second

Edition. New York, McGraw-Hill, 1971, p. 118.

Boye E, Lindegaard MW, Paus E, et al. Whole body distribution of radioactivity after intraperitoneal administration of ^{32}P colloids. *Br J Radiol* 1984, 57:395–402.

Card RY, Cole DR, Henschke UK. Summary of ten years of the use of radioactive colloids in intracavitary therapy. *J Nucl Med* 1960, 1:195–198.

Cheung A, Driedger AA. Evaluation of radiophosphorous in the palliation of metastatic bone lesions from carcinoma of the breast and prostate. *Radiology* 1980, 134:209–212.

Childs DS, Keating FR, Rall JE, et al. The effect of varying quantities of inorganic iodide (carrier) on the urinary excretion and thyroidal accumulation of radioiodine in exophthalmic goiter, *J Clin Invest* 1950, 29:726–738.

Croll MN, Brady LW. Intracavitary uses of colloids. *Semin Nucl Med* 1979, 9:108–113.

Dobyns BM, Sheline GE, Workman JB, et al. Malignant and benign neoplasms of the thyroid in patients treated for hypertension: A report of the cooperative thyrotoxicosis follow-up study. *J Clin Endocrinol Metab* 1974, 38:976–998.

Edmonds CJ. Treatment of thyroid cancer. *Clin Endocrinol Metab* 1979; 8:223–243.

Friedell HL, Storaasli JP. The use of radioactive phosphorous in the treatment of carcinoma of the breast with widespread metastases to bone. *Am J Roentgenol Rad Ther Nucl Med* 1950, 64:559–575.

Frietas JE, Gross MD, Ripley S, et al. Radionuclide diagnosis and therapy of thyroid cancer: Current status report. *Semin Nucl Med* 1985, 15:106–131.

Hertz S, Roberts A. Application of radioactive iodine in therapy of Graves' disease. *J Clin Invest* 1942, 21:624.

Hertz S, Roberts A, Evens RD. Radioactive iodine as an indicator in the study of thyroid physiology. *Proc Soc Exp Biol Med* 1938, 38:510.

Hurley RD, Becker DV. The use of radioiodine in the management of thyroid cancer. In *Nuclear Medicine Annual 1983* Freeman LM, Weissman HS (eds), New York, Raven Press, 1983.

Jacobs ML. Radioactive colloidal chromic phosphate to control pleural effusion of ascites. *JAMA* 1958, 166:597–599.

Kaplan WD, Zimmerman RE, Bloomer WD, et al. Therapeutic intraperitoneal ^{32}P: A clinical assessment of the dynamics of distribution. *Radiology* 1981, 138:683–688.

Lawrence JH. Nuclear physics and therapy: Preliminary report on a new method for the treatment of leukemia and polycythemia. *Radiology* 1940, 35:51–60.

Lawrence JH, Scott KG, Tuttle LW. Studies on leukemia with the aid of radioactive phosphorous. *Int Clin* 1939, 3:33–58.

Lawrence JH, Winchell HS, Donald WB. Leukemia in polycythemia vera—relationship to splenic myeloid metaplasia and therapeutic radiation dose. *Ann Intern Med* 1969, 70:763–771.

Leeper RD. Treatment of thyroid cancer. In *New Concepts in Thyroid Disease*, New York, Liss, 1983, p. 139.

Leff A, Hopewell PC, Costello J. Pleural effusion from malignancy. *Ann Intern Med* 1978, 88:532–537.

Marinelli LD, Quimby EH, Hine GH. Dosage determination with radioactive isotopes. II. Practical considerations in therapy and protection. *AJR* 1948, 59:260–280.

Martini N, Freiman AH, Watson RC, et al. Intrapericardial instillation of radioactive chromic phosphate in malignant pericardial effusion. *AJR* 1977, 128:639–641.

Maxfield JR, Maxfield JGS, Maxfield WS. The use of radioactive phosphorous and testosterone in metastatic bone lesions from breast and prostate. *South Med J* 1958, 51:320–328.

Miller ER, Sheline GE. Studies with radioiodine. III. Problem of dosage in the treatment of hyperthyroidism. *Radiology* 1957, 69:527–545.

Müller JH. Uber die verwendung von kunstilichen radioaktiven isotopen zur erzielung von lokalisierten biologishen strahlenwirkungen. *Experientia* 1945, 1:199–200.

Najean Y, Triebel F, Dresch C. P-32 therapy of polycythemia: A review and reappraisal. *Clin Nucl Med* 1980, 5:275–280.

National Council on Radiation Protection and Measurements. Precautions in the Management of Patients Who Have Received Therapeutic Amounts of Radionuclides. NCRP Number 37, 1970.

O'Bryan RM, Talley RW, Brennan MJ, et al. Critical analysis of the control of malignant effusions with radioisotopes. *Henry Ford Hosp Med J* 1962, 16:1–14.

Rodriguez-Antunez A, Cook SA, Jelden GL, et al. Management of primary and metastatic carcinoma of the prostate by the radiotherapist. *Am J Roentgenol Rad Ther Nucl Med* 1973, 118:876–880.

Root SW, Tyor MP, Andrews Ga, et al. Distribution of colloidal radioactive chromic phosphate after intracavitary administration *Radiology* 1954, 63:251–257.

Rosenshein NB, Leichner PK, Vogelsang G. Radiocolloids in the treatment of ovarian cancer. *Obstet Gynecol Surv* 1979, 34:708–720.

Saenger EL, Thoma GE, Tompkins EA. Incidence of leukemia following treatment of hyperthyroidism: Preliminary report of the cooperative thyrotoxicosis therapy follow-up study. *JAMA* 1968; 205:855–862.

Sarker SD, Beierwaltes SH, Gill SP, et al. Subsequent fertility and birth histories of children and adolescents treated with I-131 for thyroid cancer. *J Nucl Med* 1976, 17:460–464.

Sheline GE, Miller ER. Studies with radioiodine. IV. Evaluation of radioiodine treatment of carcinoma of the thyroid based on the experience at the University of California from 1938 to 1954. *Radiology* 1957, 69:527–545.

Shields JA, Packer S. Radioactive phosphorous uptake test for the diagnosis of malignant melanoma of the choroid. *Semin Nucl Med* 1984, 14:31–34.

Silberstein EB. Radionuclide therapy of hematologic disorders. *Semin Nucl Med* 1979, 9:100–107.

Sullivan DC, Harris CC, Currie JL, et al. Observations on the intraperitoneal distribution of chromic phosphate (^{32}P) suspension for intraperitoneal therapy. *Radiology* 1983, 146:539–541.

Silver S. Radioactive nuclides in medicine and biology. In *Medicine* Third Edition, Philadelphia, Lea & Febiger, 1968.

Spiers FW, Beddoe AH, King SD, et al. The absorbed dose to bone marrow in the treatment of polycythemia by ^{32}P. *Br J Radiol* 1976, 49:133–140.

Taasan V, Shapiro B, Taren JA, et al. Phosphorous-32 therapy of cystic grade IV astrocytomas: Technique and preliminary application. *J Nucl Med* 1985, 26:1335–1338.

Tong ECK, Finkelstein P. The treatment of prostatic bone metastases with parathormone and radioactive phosphorous. *J Urol* 1973, 109:71–75.

U.S.P.-DI, Volume I, *Drug Information for the Health Care Provider*, Ninth Edition. Rockville, MD, United States Pharmacopeial Convention, Inc., 1989; pp. 808–809, 2181–2184, 2190–2191.

Van Nostrand D, Silberstein E. Therapeutic uses of ^{32}P. In *Nuclear Medicine Annual 1985* Freeman LM, Weissman HS (eds), New York, Raven Press, 1985, pp. 285–344.

Walton RJ, Sinclair WK. Intracavitary irradiation with radioactive colloidal gold in the palliative treatment of malignant pleural and peritoneal effusions. *Br Med Bull* 1952, 8:165–172.

Winston MA. Radioisotope therapy in bone and joint disease. *Semin Nucl Med* 1979, 9:114–120.

Radiopharmaceuticals for Hematological Applications

I. Blood Volume Measurements

Dennis P. Swanson

Radionuclide dilution techniques can be used to accurately quantitate the volume of blood or blood components within the vascular compartment. These techniques are based on the equation, $Vc = ViCi/Cd$, where Vi and Ci represent the initial volume (e. g., mL) and specific concentration (e. g., $\mu Ci/mL$) of a radiotracer introduced into a given body compartment, Cd is the specific concentration of the radiotracer following its dilution within the compartment, and Vc is the volume of the compartment.

Such measurements of body compartment volumes require that the radiotracer mix with the substance(s) within the compartment and that it distribute uniformly throughout the compartment. During the duration of the measurement, the radiotracer should be confined solely to the compartment being analyzed. Of course, the radiotracer should exert no effect on the volume of the compartment and should be nontoxic. The radionuclidic properties of radiotracers utilized for dilution studies must permit convenient and accurate detection and quantification at very low concentrations.

Blood within the vascular compartment is a heterogenous substance consisting of plasma and cellular elements, predominantly red blood cells. Hence, a determination of total blood volume using radionuclide dilution techniques should employ the combined use of a radiotracer that mixes with and distributes uniformly in the plasma volume and a radiotracer that mixes with and distributes uniformly in the red cell volume. Although they do not optimally fulfill the aforestated criteria, radioiodinated (i. e., I-131 or I-125 labeled) human serum albumin and Cr-51 labeled red blood cells can provide accurate quantifications of the plasma volume and the red cell volume, respectively, and a determination of total blood volume.

Because a relationship between plasma volume and red cell volume can be derived from a knowledge of the patient's hematocrit, it is possible to extrapolate a total blood volume measurement from a single determination of the plasma volume or the red cell volume. However this method for quantitating total blood volume is potentially erroneous due to variations between central and peripheral hematocrit values and inaccuracies in the hematocrit measurement. Accurate quantifications of total blood volume therefore require a determination of both the plasma volume and the red cell volume (Price DC and McIntyre PA, 1984; Alazraki NP and Mishkin FS, 1984).

CHEMISTRY

Radioiodinated Human Serum Albumin (RISA). I-125 and I-131 human serum albumin (HSA) are commercially available as sterile, pyrogenic-free solutions containing, in addition to the RISA, benzyl alcohol as a preservative and stabilizing quantities (i. e., > 10 mg/mL) of normal HSA. Various buffering agents (e. g., phosphates, guanidine HCl) may also be present to maintain a pH of 7.0–8.5. The I-125 HSA is currently available in unit-dosage syringes (Isojex®, Mallinckrodt, Inc.) containing, at calibration, 10 μCi in a volume of 1.5 mL. The I-131 HSA is distributed in a multiple-dose vial (Albumotope®, Squibb Diagnostics) containing, at calibration, 1 mCi in a volume of 5 mL.

RISA is prepared using mild radioiodination techniques so as to introduce less than 1 gram-atom of iodine per gram-molecule of HSA (U.S.P. XXI, 1984). Excessive iodination (or a nonphysiological pH) risks denaturation of the RISA, which can result in an accelerated rate of plasma clearance. Pharmacopeial specifications require a radiochemical purity in excess of 97% at calibration. The preparations should be stored at 2–8° C to minimize the potential for radiolytic decomposition and bacterial growth (especially with use of the multiple-dose vial).

Iodine-125 decays by electron capture with a half-life of 60 days. This decay is accompanied by the emission of a 35 keV gamma radiation (6.7% abundance) and 27–32 keV characteristic x-rays (140% abundance). Although not suitable for external imaging, these I-125 emissions can be conveniently and accurately quantitated in in vitro samples. Iodine-131 decays by beta-particle (i. e., negatron) emission with a half-life of approximately 8.1 days. The 364 keV gamma radiation (82% abundance) that accompanies this decay can also be accurately quantitated in in vitro samples, and it can be imaged externally. However, the in vivo biodistribution of I-131 HSA is seldom evaluated by imaging.

Cr-51 Red Blood Cells (RBCs). Cr-51 labeled RBCs are prepared using the radiopharmaceutical Sodium Chromate (Cr-51) Injection, U.S.P. This radiolabeling reagent is commercially available (Mallinckrodt, Inc., Chromitope Sodium®, Squibb Diagnostics) as a sterile, pyrogen-free solution containing 0.9% benzyl-alcohol as a preservative and sodium bicarbonate as a buffering agent (pH 7.5-8.5). Both manufacturers supply a 0.5 mCi multiple-dose vial that at calibration has a specific concentration of 100 μCi/mL (Mallinckrodt, Inc.) or 200 μCi/mL (Squibb Diagnostics). To avoid toxic effects on the RBCs (Weinstein IM, et al, 1971), the initial specific activity and expiration dating of these preparations must be such to guarantee a pharmacopeial

(U.S.P. XXI, 1984) requirement of greater than 10 mCi/mg sodium chromate at the end of the expiry period. Greater than 90% of the Cr-51 activity must be in the chromate chemical form.

In the chemical form of sodium chromate (Na_2CrO_4), the chromium atom exists in a +6 valence state. When added to a mixture of RBCs and acid-citrate-dextrose (ACD) solution, these hexavalent chromium atoms are capable of readily penetrating the erythrocyte membrane. Within the red cell, the chromium atoms are enzymatically reduced to a +3 valence state and rapidly bind to hemoglobin. It has been shown that at a pH of 6.7–6.9, 90% of the added Cr-51 chromate activity becomes bound to intracellular hemoglobin within 10 minutes (Phan T and Wasnich R, 1981). The Cr-51 is minimally eluted from the tagged RBCs at a rate of approximately 1% per day (Weinstein IM, et al, 1971). The eluted chromium atoms remain in the trivalent state and as such are incapable of repenetrating the erythrocyte membrane.

Table 19.1 outlines the basic steps involved in the labeling of RBCs using sodium chromate (Cr-51) injection. The addition of ascorbic acid (step 3) to reduce the hexavalent chromium atoms to the trivalent state and thus terminate the labeling process is optional because washing of the tagged cells (steps 4 and 5) will also serve to remove any unbound Cr-51 chromate activity. As previously discussed, Cr-51 in the trivalent state is not incorporated into RBCs and if injected into the patient would be expected

Table 19.1 BASIC STEPS INVOLVED IN THE Cr-51 LABELING OF RED BLOOD CELLS

Using aseptic techniques:
1. Inject (18G needle) whole blood (e. g., 30–50 mL) into a sterile vial containing ACD solution (e. g., 5–10 mL).
2. Add Cr-51 chromate (e. g., 50–200 μCi) and incubate for 30–60 minutes with frequent swirling.
3. Terminate labeling by adding ascorbic acid (e. g., 50–100 mg).
4. Centrifuge Cr-51 RBCs and remove supernatant activity.
5. Resuspend Cr-51 RBCs in normal saline solution. Repeat step 4.
6. Resuspend Cr-51 RBCs in normal saline solution to known volume. Assay and reinject.

to undergo fairly rapid renal excretion. It is advised, however, that the washing steps be included even if the ascorbic acid is added. If not washed, the activity associated with the trivalent Cr-51 in the plasma must be determined prior to reinjection in order to accurately quantitate the activity associated with the tagged RBCs. Moreover, if the washing step is not performed, the collected blood samples should be evaluated for plasma Cr-51 activity to ensure that adequate excretion of the trivalent Cr-51 has indeed occurred so as to not interfere with the measurement of red cell volume.

The Cr-51 radionuclide decays by electron capture with a half-life of 27.7 days. Although the 320 keV gamma radiation that accompanies this decay is appropriate for external imaging, it only occurs with a 10.2% abundance. Hence, the administered activity required for adequate imaging count densities imposes substantial dosimetry concerns. However, the Cr-51 radionuclide is useful for in vitro counting procedures, which are not limited by a time constraint for data collection.

PHARMACOKINETICS

RISA. A problem associated with the use of RISA for the determination of plasma volume is related to the fact that the radiotracer is not confined solely to the vascular compartment following intravenous injection. RISA normally diffuses into the extravascular, extracellular (i.e., interstitial) space at a fractional rate of 6–10% per hour (Albert SN, 1971; Phan T and Wasnich R, 1981). The rate of albumin loss from the vascular compartment may be even greater in the presence of diseases that alter vascular permeability or involve protein loss. Hence, determination of total plasma volume requires the collection and quantification of a minimum of two timed blood samples post RISA injection. A semi-log plot of this data with extrapolation to time zero will provide a relatively accurate estimate of the total plasma volume.

Uniform distribution of RISA in the vascular compartment normally occurs within 10–20 minutes following intravenous injection. However, a longer period for uniform vascular distribution may be required in patients with volume-modification or circulation disorders (e. g., congestive heart failure, severe dehydration, shock) (Phan T and Wasnich R, 1981). Clearance of RISA from the plasma is multiexponential. An initial rapid clearance component that occurs as a result of its distribution to the interstitial space is followed by a slow component that demonstrates a half-life of approximately 20 days (Bell EG, et al, 1975). Virtually all of the administered activity is eventually excreted via the kidneys, with less than 2% of the dose appearing in the feces (Phan T and Wasnich R, 1981).

Cr-51 Red Blood Cells (RBCs). Uniform mixing of the Cr-51 RBCs in the vascular compartment is normally complete within 10–20 minutes post injection. Prolonged mixing times again may be expected in patients with blood volume disorders, circulatory problems, or splenomegaly. Although the true life-span of erythrocytes is approximately 120 days, the normal half-life of Cr-51 RBCs is only 25–30 days (Sisson JC, 1983). This discrepancy occurs because Cr-51 chromate nonspecifically labels both newly released and mature erythrocytes. Whole-body counting studies have shown that the retention of Cr-51 in the body is substantially longer than that suggested by the quantification of blood samples, thus indicating that dead (or damaged) Cr-51 RBCs are sequestered in the reticuloendothelial cells of the spleen and liver for a period of time prior to their release of the trivalent Cr-51 (Baker WJ and Datz FL, 1987).

As previously discussed (see Chemistry), Cr-51 is normally eluted from the tagged red cells at a rate of approximately 1% per day. The trivalent Cr-51 that is eluted from the radiolabeled cells or recovered following their death undergoes rapid renal excretion.

PRECAUTIONS

RISA

Patient Preparation. Thyroid blockage is usually recommended for patients undergoing RISA plasma volume studies. An oral dosage of Lugol's solution (i. e., contains 100 mg potassium iodide/mL) or Saturated Solution of Potassium Iodide (SSKI, contains 1 gm potassium iodide/mL) corresponding to 30–130 mg of potassium iodide per day should be initiated prior to the study and continued for several days (Stathis VJ, et al, 1987). In the presence of an iodine allergy, potassium perchlorate may be substituted at an oral dosage of 200 mg per day. (See also Appendix B.)

Physical Incompabilities. RISA can readily adhere to glassware. Therefore, in the preparation of standard solutions for the plasma volume study, dilute HSA or detergent solution should be utilized for the dilution procedures or siliconized glassware should be employed. For the same reason, RISA should not be injected through polyethylene tubing or catheters.

Pregnancy/Breastfeeding. Following the administration of RISA, radioactivity can cross the placenta to expose the fetus and will appear in the breast milk of lactating patients. Hence caution should be observed in ensuring that the patient is not pregnant prior to injection. Consideration should also be given to a discontinuance of breastfeeding.

CR-51 RED BLOOD CELLS (RBCs)

Preparation/Handling. Extreme care should be taken in the blood withdrawal and labeling procedure to ensure that the RBCs are not damaged. Damaged Cr-51 RBCs will be rapidly sequestered by the reticuloendothelial cells of the spleen and liver resulting in erroneous red cell volume and survival determinations. Care should also be taken to avoid blood clot formation. The reinjection of blood clots is not only hazardous to the patient but will interfere with uniform mixing of the Cr-51 RBCs in the vascular compartment.

Drug–Radiopharmaceutical Interactions. It is possible that the patient's blood may contain certain drugs (e. g., polyvitamins, antibiotics) that can reduce the hexavalent Cr-51 chromate to a trivalent state and thereby decrease the RBC labeling efficiency (Albert SN, 1971). Circulating stannous ions associated with the prior administration of Tc-99m radiopharmaceuticals can produce a similar effect, as can excess calcium ions or prolonged incubation of the Cr-51 chromate with ACD (Price DC and McIntyre PA, 1984). If labeling difficulties are encountered, prewashing of the RBCs to remove any such reducing agents may overcome the problem.

Pregnancy/Breastfeeding. Sodium chromate will appear in the breast milk of lactating patients. Therefore consideration should be given to a discontinuance of breastfeeding if the red cell volume study is warranted. Because the reinjection of Cr-51 RBCs will result in fetal radiation exposure, care should be taken to ensure that the patient is not pregnant prior to initiating the study.

CLINICAL CONSIDERATIONS

CLINICAL INDICATIONS

Total Blood Volume. The combined determinations of plasma volume and red cell volume for the quantification of total blood volume are frequently performed on patients with an elevated hematocrit in order to determine the relative contribution of erythrocytosis to this observation. In patients with polycythemia rubra vera there is an absolute increase in red cell volume with a normal or slightly elevated plasma volume. In contradistinction, the findings of a normal red cell volume and decreased plasma volume constitute relative polycythemia.

Plasma Volume. In addition to its contribution to the quantitation of total blood volume, RISA plasma volume studies may be singularly performed to evaluate plasma losses in patients with severe burns and fluid losses in postsurgical patients or patients with severe diarrhea or other dehydrating diseases. The results of these studies often form the basis for subsequent volume replacement therapy.

Red Cell Survival/Sequestration. In patients with anemia of unknown origin, a Cr-51 RBC survival study may be singularly performed to provide a direct measurement of extramedullary hemolysis. This half-life determination is typically combined with external counting (i.e., using a scintillation probe) over the spleen and liver to evaluate the relative contribution of these organs to the hemolytic process.

Red cell survival studies may also provide evidence of nonapparent bleeding sites post trauma or surgery. When combined with the collection and counting of fecal samples, a Cr-51 RBC study can detect chronic intestinal blood loss at rates as low as 3 ml/day, a value that minimally exceeds the normal rate of intestinal blood loss (McIntyre P, 1975).

RADIOPHARMACEUTICAL
CONSIDERATIONS

I-125 versus I-131 RISA. For plasma volume determinations, the commercially available I-125 RISA provides several advantages compared to the I-131 RISA. In addition to the convenience of its unit-dosage packaging, the considerably longer physical half-life of the I-125 radionuclide permits longer on-site storage and increased efficiency of utilization. I-125 RISA preparations typically have an expiration dating of 4 months post calibration, whereas I-131 RISA has only a 1-month dating. Finally, the low-energy photon emissions of I-125 are substantially different from the 320 keV emission of Cr-51, thus permitting (with correction for scatter into the I-125 energy window)

the simultaneous quantification of plasma and red cell volumes.

DOSAGE/DOSIMETRY

STUDY PROCEDURES—DOSAGE

The accurate performance of plasma volume and red cell volume and survival studies requires careful attention to technique. The measurement of volumes and the preparation of counting standards must be exact. Care must be taken to avoid extravasation of the radiopharmaceuticals upon their injection into the vascular compartment, and the respective syringes must be thoroughly flushed with blood to ensure complete delivery of the activity. Withdrawal of blood samples should be performed from the extremity opposite to the site of injection.

Plasma Volume. Plasma volume studies are performed following the intravenous injection of 10 μCi of I-125 or I-131 RISA. Blood samples are typically collected at 10 and 20 minutes post injection. If there is no significant difference in activity between these samples, an average of their values may be used for the quantification of plasma volume. However, if a difference does exist, the activity values should be plotted as a function of their time of collection post injection on semi-log paper. Extrapolation of this data to time zero will provide an activity value to be used for the quantification of total plasma volume.

Red Cell Volume. The determination of red cell volume typically involves the rejection of approximately 50 μCi of Cr-51 labeled autologous RBCs. When performed stimultaneous to the plasma volume study, blood samples for red cell volume quantification are collected at the same time intervals post injection (i.e., 10min., 20 min.). If performed as a single study, a blood sample is collected at 20 minutes post injection of the Cr-51 RBCs.

Red Cell Survival/Sequestration. Approximately 200 μCi of Cr-51 RBCs are reinjected for red cell survival and sequestration studies. To evaluate survival, blood samples are collected and counted at 24 hours and then at alternate-day intervals until the count rate falls to 50% that of the initial (i. e., 24-hour) value. A semi-log plot of this data will provide an estimate of the vascular half-life of the Cr-51 RBCs.

To evaluate splenic and hepatic sequestration of the Cr-51 RBCs, external counting is performed over the approximate midpoint of these organs and over the precordium using a collimated scintillation probe. The exact sites of external counting should be marked (e. g., indelible ink) to ensure counting reproducibility on subsequent measurements. Multiple determinations are made at time intervals corresponding to the sampling for survival analysis.

STUDY INTERPRETATION

Total Blood Volume. Normal blood volume is dependent on the height, weight, and sex of the patient and can be obtained from published nomograms. It must be noted, however, that these published values are approximate average volumes; the normal blood volume for any given patient may vary by up to 20% from these expected values (Sisson JC, 1983). Normal plasma or red cell volumes can be readily determined from these published total blood volumes and their hematocrit relationship.

Red Cell Survival. The normal half-life of Cr-51 RBCs in the vascular compartment is 25–30 days. A demonstrated half-life of less than 20 days provides a clinically significant indication of accelerated red cell destruction or blood loss (Sisson JC, 1983).

Red Cell Sequestration. A comparison of count rates over the spleen and precordium and over the spleen and liver should normally reveal ratios of approximately 1:1 (Sisson JC, 1983). Abnormal splenic sequestration of red cells is indicated by a spleen-to-precordium count rate ratio in excess of 2:1 or spleen-to-liver ratio of greater than 2.5:1 with progressive and gradual increases over time. Because the liver may also be involved in red cell sequestration, the spleen-to-precordium ratio tends to more accurately reflect splenic involvement (McIntyre P, 1975). Note that in the presence of splenomegaly, the spleen-to-liver count rate ratio may approach 2:1 without a corresponding abnormal degree of sequestration. Spleen-to-liver ratios of substantially less than 1:1 may be indicative of hemolytic anemia.

DOSIMETRY

Radiation dosimetry estimates for various organs following the intravenous administration of RISA and Cr-51 RBCs are listed in Table 19.2 and Table 19.3, respectively.

II. Schilling Test
James A. Ponto

The test of a patient's ability to absorb orally administered Vitamin B_{12} has important implications for the diagnosis and treatment-planning in patients exhibiting

Table 19.2 RADIATION ABSORBED DOSE ESTIMATES FOR I-125 and I-131 HUMAN SERUM ALBUMIN[a]

ORGAN	mRADS/10 μCi	
	I-125 HSA	*I-131 HSA*
Blood	18	50–200
Liver	—	12
Spleen	59	—
Gonads	2.8–3.4	20–90
Thyroid (blocked)	3.8	250–500
Whole body	3.8	10

[a] From respective product information.

Table 19.3 RADIATION ABSORBED DOSE ESTIMATES FOR Cr-51 LABELED RED BLOOD CELLS[a]

ORGAN	mRADS/50 μCi	mRADS/200 μCi
Blood	50	200
Spleen	660	2,640
Ovaries	16	66
Testes	16	66
Whole Body	14	55

[a] From respective product information.

Table 19.4   ADVANTAGES AND DISADVANTAGES OF VITAMIN B$_{12}$ ABSORPTION TESTS[a]

	URINARY EXCRETION	FECAL EXCRETION	PLASMA CONCENTRATION	LIVER UPTAKE	WHOLE-BODY RETENTION
Counting technique	in vitro	in vitro	in vitro	in vivo	in vivo
Counting sample	urine	feces	blood	liver	whole body
Required time (days)	2	7–10	0.5	5–7	7–10
Quantitation	indirect	direct	indirect	indirect	direct
Common errors	lost urine	lost feces	—	lack of geometry reproducibility	—
Interfering diseases	renal disease	—	—	liver disease	—

[a] Adapted from International Committee for Standardization in Hematology, 1981.

Vitamin B$_{12}$ deficiency. The five methods used involve radioactivity measurements of urine, feces, plasma, liver, or whole body following oral administration of radiolabeled Vitamin B$_{12}$ (cyanocobalamin). Advantages and disadvantages of these methods are summarized in Table 19.4. The most popular method is the urinary excretion test originally described by Schilling, hence called the "Schilling Test." All modifications of this test are also loosely called Schilling Tests. Because of its reliability and convenience, the Schilling Test has become the selected method for the measurement of Vitamin B$_{12}$ absorption.

HISTORY

In 1953 Schilling demonstrated the utility of the urinary excretion test in patients with pernicious anemia following the oral administration of Co-60 Vitamin B$_{12}$ and human gastric juice (intrinsic factor). L. Ellenbogen and colleagues (1955) later modified this test to use Co-57 instead of Co-58 for the radiolabel. In 1963, J.H. Katz and associates introduced a dual isotope Schilling Test (DIST) for simultaneous measurement of the absorption of free Co-60 Vitamin B$_{12}$ and Co-57 Vitamin B$_{12}$ bound to intrinsic factor. To reduce the radiation dose, T.K. Bell (1965) modified the DIST by substituting Co-58 for Co-60.

Currently, the agents of choice are Co-57 Vitamin B$_{12}$ for the single tracer Shilling Test and Co-58 Vitamin B$_{12}$/Co-57 Vitamin B$_{12}$ bound to intrinsic factor for DIST.

CHEMISTRY

Radiolabeled Vitamin B$_{12}$ products consist of cyanocobalamin molecules wherein radioisotopes of cobalt are substituted for the stable cobalt atoms. The principal emission characteristics of the three radioisotopes of cobalt used are summarized in Table 19.5. Radiolabeled Vitamin B$_{12}$ is commercially obtained from fermentation of *Streptomyces griseus* (Rosenblum C, 1966).

Vitamin B$_{12}$ is water soluble. It crytallizes as small red needles or prisms. At pH 4–7, it is stable at room temperature but decomposes when autoclaved at 115°C for 30 minutes (Silber R and Moldow CF, 1970). Exposure to sunlight results in photolysis and loss of vitamin activity

Table 19.5   PRINCIPAL EMISSION DATA FOR Co-57, Co-58, AND Co-60

ISOTOPE	HALF-LIFE	DECAY	EMISSION	ENERGY	ABUNDANCE (%)
Co-57	270 days	Electron capture	gamma-2	122 keV	85.9
Co-58	71 days	Electron capture; positron	gamma-1	810 keV	99.4
			beta-plus-1	204 keV	15.0
			annihilation	511 keV	30.0
Co-60	5.26 years	Beta-minus	beta-1	94 keV	99.8
			gamma-1	1.17 MeV	99.8
			gamma-2	1.33 MeV	100.0

Table 19.6 COMMERCIALLY AVAILABLE RADIOLABELED VITAMIN B_{12} PRODUCTS

RADIOPHARMACEUTICAL	NAME®	MANUFACTURER	RADIOACTIVITY	AMOUNT OF VITAMIN B_{12}
Co-57 cyanocobalamin	Rubratope-57	Squibb Diagnostics, Inc.	0.5–1.0 μCi	0.5–1.0 μg
Co-57 cyanocobalamin	—	Mallinckrodt, Inc.	~ 0.5 μCi	0.5–1.0 μg
Co-58 cyanocobalamin and	Dicopac[a]	Amersham	~ 0.8 μCi	0.25 μg
Co-57 cyanocobalamin bound			~ 0.5 μCi	0.25 μg
to human gastric juice				

[a] Not currently available. Re-release date uncertain.

(Rosenblum C, 1966). Radiolytic decomposition, a problem with high specific cencentrations of radiolabeled Vitamin B_{12} solutions, is minimized by dry capsule formulation (Rosenblum C, 1966).

Since the intrinsic factor-mediated absorption process becomes saturated above 2 μg of Vitamin B_{12}, radiolabeled Vitamin B_{12} products should contain only physiologic (2 μg or less) amounts (Corcino JJ, et al, 1970; Herbert V, 1972; McIntyre PA, 1975). Commercially available products are described in Table 19.6.

PHARMACOKINETICS

Gastrointestinal Absorption. The absorption of orally administered radiolabeled Vitamin B_{12} ($^*B_{12}$) occurs through a complex series of steps. In the presence of stomach acid, $^*B_{12}$ is initially bound to R-proteins present in saliva and gastric juice. Once in the small intestine, pancreatic proteolytic enzymes (primarily trypsin and chymotrypsin) partially degrade the R-proteins and free the $^*B_{12}$ (Allen RH, et al, 1978; Parmentier Y, et al, 1979). Free $^*B_{12}$ then binds to the intrinsic factor (IF) of Castle, a glycoprotein with a molecular weight of 50,000–60,000 that is secreted by the parietal cells in the fundal region of the stomach (Corcino JJ, et al, 1970; Herbert V, 1972; Allen RH, et al, 1978; Hilman RS, 1980). The $^*B_{12}$-IF complex, in the form of a dimer, is carried to specific receptors in the distal ileum (Corcino JJ, et al, 1970; Herbert V, 1972; Hilman RS, 1980). On the surface of these ileal mucosal cells, the $^*B_{12}$-IF complex undergoes dissociation, a process enhanced by the presence of bile (Teo NH, et al, 1980). The IF remains on the epithelial cell surface whereas the $^*B_{12}$, after a delay of several hours, is absorbed into the blood stream (Herbert V, 1972, Hilman RS, 1980). Peak absorption occurs at about 12 hours (Herbert V, 1972). In addition to IF, the absorption of $^*B_{12}$ also requires ionic calcium (or magnesium) and a pH in excess of 6 (Carmel R, et al, 1969; Corcino JJ, et al, 1970; Herbert V, 1972).

The amount of $^*B_{12}$ absorbed is inversely related to the amount ingested. For example, the absorption from 0.25 μg and 1.0 μg doses averages about 75% and 50%, respectively (Herbert V, 1972). The absorption from routine dosages of $^*B_{12}$ containing 1.0 μg or less ranges from 20–97% (Herbert V, 1972). At masses greater than 2 μg, the physiologic IF-dependent absorption system becomes saturated, and the percentage absorbed decreases markedly (Corcino JJ, et al, 1970; Herbert V, 1972; McIntyre PA, 1975). Only approximately 1% of orally administered $^*B_{12}$ is absorbed by a passive diffusion process (Corcino JJ, et al, 1970; Herbert V, 1972).

The absorption of $^*B_{12}$ has been observed to follow a circadian rhythmicity. Significantly better absorption occurs at 1300 (early afternoon) whereas the poorest absorption is in the nocturnal early morning (Markiewicz A, et al, 1981).

Distribution. In the plasma, $^*B_{12}$ is highly (90–99%) protein bound with the remaining fraction free or loosely bound. It is transported throughout the body mainly bound (90%) to a specific B_{12}-binding β-globulin (transcobalamin II) and to a lesser extent (10%) to a specific B_{12}-binding α_1-glycoprotein (transcobalamin I) and to an inter-α-glycoprotein (transcobalamin III) (Hilman RS, 1980). Liver uptake peaks at 5–7 days past oral administration (Herbert V, 1972).

Radiolabeled Vitamin B_{12} rapidly accumulates in the placenta and is slowly transported to the fetus. Placental and fetal uptake is related to gestational age with the greatest uptake late in pregnancy (Luhby AL, et al, 1961; Graber SE, et al, 1971; Nishimura Y, et al, 1978). Placental uptake peaks at 8–10% of the administered dose within 24–48 hours and then slowly decreases to 1–2% over the next 2–3 weeks (Luhby AL, et al, 1961, Ullberg S, et al, 1967). The $*B_{12}$ slowly accumulates in the fetus over 14–20 days, peaking at a maximum of 35–45% of the administered dose (Luhby AL, et al, 1961). Fetal distribution is nonspecific to all fetal tissues but with highest concentrations in the endocrine organs, renal cortex, and gastric mucosa (Ullberg S, et al, 1967).

Elimination. Protein-bound $*B_{12}$ is primarily excreted in the bile and undergoes enterohepatic recirculation (Corcino JJ, et al, 1970; Hilman RS, 1980). Free $*B_{12}$ is excreted in the urine by glomerular filtration with a clearance approximately that of inulin (Nelp WB, et al, 1964: Hilman RS, 1980). However, because $*B_{12}$ is highly protein bound, urinary excretion is negligible in the absence of a "flushing dose" of cyanocobalamin (Schilling RF, 1953). Whole-body clearance is monoexponential with a half-life of 76 weeks in normal subjects (Amin S, et al, 1980). Patients with pernicious anemia show a faster whole-body clearance (half-life = 61 weeks) because of their failure to reabsorb biliary $*B_{12}$ (Amin S, et al, 1980).

The urinary elimination of $*B_{12}$ can be markedly affected by saturation of plasma protein binding sites with a "flushing dose" of cyanocobalamin. A 1.0 mg flushing dose of cyanocobalamin administered a few hours after $*B_{12}$ results in urinary excretion of 6–48% of administered $*B_{12}$ (or about one-third of absorbed $*B_{12}$) in the first 24 hours (Herbert V, 1972). A second flushing dose of cyanocobalamin given 24 hours after the first results in a cumulative excretion of about 50% of the absorbed $*B_{12}$ (Herbert V, 1972).

PRECAUTIONS

Bioavailability. The bioavailability of encapsulated $*B_{12}$ may be less than an oral solution. In one report (Baun DC, et al, 1975), the average absorption from a liquid dosage form was 23% greater than from a capsule. The capsule tended to collapse into a stringy mass and dissolve slowly, thus retarding the dissolution of $*B_{12}$ and inhibiting or delaying binding with IF. Similarly, spuriously low absorption has been reported using encapsulated $*B_{12}$ and IF as compared with premixed solution of $*B_{12}$ and IF (McDonald JWD, et al, 1975).

The use of the dual-isotope method (i. e., simultaneous administration of $*B_{12}$ and $*B_{12}$ bound to IF prepared with different isotopes of cobalt) for assessing $*B_{12}$ absorption has been associated with a high frequency of spurious results (Briedis D, et al, 1973; Fairbanks VF, et al, 1983; Zuckier LS and Chervu LR, 1984). Exchange of $*B_{12}$ isotopes bound to IF has been demonstrated in vitro, with equimolar concentrations achieved within 10 minutes in simulated gastric juice (Fairbanks VF, et al, 1983). Exchange occurs more slowly and less completely at near-neutral pH values (Donaldson RM and Katz JH, 1963; Fairbanks VF, et al, 1983). Administration of the two components 2 hours apart has been suggested as a method to avoid this problem of isotope exchange (Briedis D, et al, 1973; Zuckier LS and Chervu LR, 1984).

Drug Interactions. A number of drugs have been reported to interfere with the oral absorption of $*B_{12}$ (Table 19.7). In most cases, the malabsorption is associated with chronic drug therapy and is reversible upon discontinuation of the drug. Reversal of the malabsorption caused by

Table 19.7   DRUGS THAT INTERFERE WITH THE ABSORPTION OF RADIOLABELED VITAMIN B$_{12}$

DRUG	PROPOSED MECHANISM	REFERENCE
Vitamin B$_{12}$—large parenteral doses	Dilution of *B$_{12}$ and saturation of ileal binding sites by high concentrations of B$_{12}$ in the bile	Chow and Okuda, 1955 Ellenbogen, et al, 1955 Mailloux and Streeto, 1965 Breuel and Fischer, 1979
Aminosalicylic acid (PAS)—chronic, high-dose therapy Anticonvulsants (phenobarbital with or without phenytoin and primidone)	Direct effect on ileal transport of B$_{12}$, probably by disturbing a folate-dependent enzyme system	Heinivaara and Palva, 1964 Heinivaara and Palva, 1965 Paaby and Norvin, 1966 Halsted and McIntyre, 1972 Palva, et al, 1972a Toskes and Deren, 1972 Lees, 1961 Reynolds, et al, 1965
Biguanides (phenformin, metformin)—chronic therapy Colchicine Cyclohexamide Ethanol—chronic intake for greater than 2 weeks	Direct effect on ileal transport of B$_{12}$	Willms and Creutzfeldt, 1970 Berchtold, et al, 1971 Tomkin, et al, 1971 Tomkin, 1973 Jounela, et al, 1974 Yeh and Shils, 1966 Webb, et al, 1968 Faloon and Chodos, 1969 Race, et al, 1970 Yeh and Shils, 1969 Lindenbaum and Lieber, 1969 Findlay, et al, 1976
Calcium-chelating agents (e.g., EDTA)	Sequestration of ionic calcium	Gräsbeck and Nyberg, 1958 Okuda and Sasayama, 1965
Antibiotics (neomycin, others)	Probably causes decreased ileal mucosal binding of B$_{12}$ secondary to inflammatory reactions (i. e., enteritis). Other possible mechanisms include gastritis (decreased IF production and release), increased intestinal motility, chelation of calcium ions, and bacterial superinfection	Faloon and Chodos, 1969 Jacobsen, et al, 1960 Herbert, 1972
Slow-release potassium tablets	Acidification of intestinal pH	Salokannel, et al, 1970 Palva, et al, 1972b Palva, et al, 1974
Cholesytramine	Binds to IF and prevents formation of B$_{12}$-IF complex	Coronato and Glass, 1973
Dactinomycin Methotrexate Oral contraceptives Pyrimethamine		Yeh and Shils, 1966 Squibb, 1978 Herbert, 1972 Squibb, 1978

aminosalicylic acid and anticonvulsants can be achieved by the coadministration of folic acid (Palva IP, et al, 1972; Lee F, 1961). Although cimetidine reduces secretion of IF, *B$_{12}$ absorption is rarely affected by cimetidine (Fielding LP, et al, 1978; Steinberg WM, et al, 1980).

Laboratory Test Interferences. If examinations of bone marrow morphology are to be performed, they should precede a Schilling Test because the parenteral "flushing dose" of cyanocobalamin may alter the bone marrow picture (Herbert V, 1982; McIntyre PA, 1975). Similarly, the "flushing dose" of cyanocobalamin will make a subnormal serum B$_{12}$ level normal for a period up to 6 months (Herbert V, 1972; McIntyre PA, 1975).

Breastfeeding. Radiolabeled Vitamin B$_{12}$ is excreted in breast milk. A study in rats showed that 1–2% of the maternal dose was transferred to the suckling via milk (Nishimura Y, et al, 1978). Although the radiation dose to a breastfeeding infant would be exceedingly small, it is generally recommended that formula feedings be considered as a substitute for breastfeedings.

Adverse Reactions. At present, no adverse reactions have been reported following the administration of *B$_{12}$, with or without intrinsic factor. Adverse reactions reported with nonradioactive cyanocobalamin include mild transient diarrhea, polycythemia vera, peripheral vascular thrombosis, itching, transitory exanthema, feeling of swelling of the entire body, pulmonary edema, congestive heart failure, anaphylactic shock, and death (Squibb, 1978).

CLINICAL CONSIDERATIONS

Clinical Indications. The Schilling test is indicated for the diagnosis of Vitamin B$_{12}$ malabsorption due to lack of intrinsic factor (i. e., pernicious anemia), and as a diagnostic adjunct in other defects of intestinal Vitamin B$_{12}$ absorption. Causes of Vitamin B$_{12}$ malabsorption are outlined in Table 19.8. Intrinsic factor may be co-administered with radiolabeled Vitamin B$_{12}$ to aid in differentiating the cause of malabsorption (Schilling RF, 1953; Schilling RF, 1955; Herbert V, 1972; McIntyre PA, 1975).

The Stage I Schilling Test consists of urinary excretion measurements following the oral administration of *B$_{12}$. Normal 24-hour urinary excretion is 7–10% or greater of the administered dose (U.S.P.-DI, 1988). Less than this indicates some type of malabsorption. The Stage II Schilling Test consists of urinary excretion measurements following the oral administration of *B$_{12}$ and IF. A normal result indicates that the malabsorption demonstrated in the Stage I test is due to lack of IF secretion. An abnormal result indicates a problem with intestinal absorption. Repeat of a Stage I test following a course of antibiotic therapy is sometimes referred to as a Stage III Schilling Test. A normal result indicates that the malabsorption demonstrated in the initial Stage I test was due to bacterial competition (Herbert V, 1972; McIntyre PA, 1975).

Patient Preparation. The patient should be fasting for at least 2 hours and preferably overnight. For patients who have been receiving Vitamin B$_{12}$ supplements, it is advisable to wait at least 24 hours before beginning the test. It is essential to obtain radioactivity measurements of a pretest urine sample prior to starting the test (Herbert V, 1972; International Committee for Standardization in Hematology, 1981).

Table 19.8   CAUSES OF MALABSORPTION OF VITAMIN B$_{12}$[a]

A. *Inadequate secretion of gastric intrinsic factor*
1. Failure of stomach to adequately secrete intrinsic factor
   - Addisonian pernicious anemia
     —hereditary failure of intrinsic factor secretion
     —hereditary degenerative gastric atrophy
     —gastric atrophy following superficial inflammatory gastritis
     —autoimmune gastric atrophy (?)
   - Lesions that destroy the gastric mucosa
   - Endocrine disorders (hypothyroidism, polyendocrinopathy, etc.)
2. Intrinsic factor inhibitor in upper GI secretions
   - Blocking and/or binding antibodies

B. *Small intestinal disorders (especially of ileum)*
1. Gluten-induced enteropathy (celiac disease, nontropical sprue, etc.)
2. Tropical sprue
3. Regional ileitis
4. Strictures or anastomoses
5. Intestinal resection
6. Therapeutic abdominal irradiation
7. Malignancies and granulomatous lesions
8. Pregnancy
9. Severe nutritional deficiencies
   - Vitamin B$_{12}$ deficiency
   - Folic acid deficiency
   - Pyridoxine deficiency
   - Iron deficiency
   - Protein or protein-calorie malnutrition (kwashiorkor, marasmus)
10. Drugs (PAS, colchicine, neomycin, etc.)
11. Radiation
12. Specific malabsorption for Vitamin B$_{12}$
   - Long-term ingestion of calcium-chelating agents
   - Inadequate alkaline pH in ileum (Menetrier's syndrome, Zollinger-Ellison syndrome)
   - Inadequate pancreatic exocrine secretion
   - Unknown causes
     —congenital (Imerslund-Gräsbeck syndrome)
     —acquired (from fruste of sprue)

C. *Competition for Vitamin B$_{12}$*
1. Fish tapeworm
2. Bacteria (blind loop syndrome)

---

[a] Adapted from Corcino JJ, et al, 1980, Herbert V, 1972.

Table 19.9 ADVANTAGES AND DISADVANTAGES OF DUAL-ISOTOPE SCHILLING TESTS[a]

ADVANTAGES	DISADVANTAGES
Shortened study time	Possibility of isotope exchange in vivo
Equivalent test conditions for both stages	Unnecessary cost/radiation exposure in patients with normal absorption of $*B_{12}$
Salvable results if incomplete urine collection	Increased technical difficulty/calculations for dual-isotope counting

[a] Adapted from Zuckier LS and Chervu LR, 1984.

Radiopharmaceutical Considerations. The dual-isotope Schilling Test (DIST) allows simultaneous performance of Stage I and Stage II tests. Advantages and disadvantages of the DIST over the single isotope test are indicated in Table 19.9. In addition to percent urinary excretion results for free $*B_{12}$ and IF-bound $*B_{12}$, the DIST also generates a bound-to-free (B/F) ratio (Katz JH, et al, 1963). Theoretically, the B/F ratio should be independent of renal excretion and completeness of urine collection. Using the manufacturer's recommendations for interpretation of B/F ratios, however, several clinical studies have reported a relatively high incidence of false-negative results because of overlap between controls and patients with pernicious anemia (Zuckier LS and Chervu LR, 1984). These results may reflect minor degrees of malabsorption, a physiologic "gray area" of graduation from normal to clearly deficient IF secretion, or spurious results owing to experimental difficulties (e. g., isotope exchange between IF-$*B_{12}$ and free $*B_{12}$).

Note that the commercial DIST product, Dicopac® (Amersham) has not been available for at least two years prior to this writing. Whether this agent will be re-released is uncertain.

Fundamental to the performance of the Schilling Test is the intramuscular administration of a 1000 μg "flushing dose" of nonradioactive Vitamin B_{12} (Schilling RF, 1953). This "flushing dose" saturates plasma protein and tissue binding sites so that the $*B_{12}$ is filtered out in the urine. Although the "flushing dose" may be administered simultaneously with or as late as 12 hours after $*B_{12}$ administration, a delay of 2 hours post $*B_{12}$ administra-tion is recommended (Herbert V, 1972; McIntyre PA, 1975; International Committee on Standardization in Hematology, 1981). This ensures that receptor sites are saturated just prior to the absorption of the $*B_{12}$ and that none of the nonradioactive Vitamin B_{12} gets into the bile until the $*B_{12}$ has already reached the ileum. It should be emphasized that the "flushing dose" may influence or interfere with subsequent diagnostic studies (Herbert V, 1972; McIntyre PA, 1975). For example, it will normalize a subnormal serum B_{12} level for a period of up to 6 months. Also, it will produce a hematologic response even if the patient is deficient in folic acid, rather than B_{12}.

Limitations. The accuracy of the Schilling Test depends a great deal upon the proper performance of the test (Streeter AM, et al, 1981). This includes avoiding common pitfalls such as incomplete urine collection, omission of the nonradioactive Vitamin B_{12} "flushing dose", and isotope exchange. The test also depends on the patient's physiologic function. For example, in a smooth, dry, achlorhydric stomach, dissolution of the capsule may be delayed and the $*B_{12}$ then exposed to a suboptimal concentration of IF (Baun DC et al, 1975). Also, impaired renal function will decrease the rate of $*B_{12}$ excretion (Rath CE, et al, 1957; International Committee for Standardization in Hematology 1981; Streeter AM, et al, 1981).

Another limitation involves the radiopharmaceutical itself. The normal ileum is capable of handling a maximum of approximately 1.5 μg of Vitamin B_{12} in a single bolus. If the radiopharmaceutical contains less than this quantity, the maximal capacity of the ileum will not be tested. For example, when only 0.5 μg *B_{12} (the usual quantity) is administered, it is theoretically possible that two-thirds of the ileum could be missing, and yet absorption of the *B_{12} will be normal (Herbert V, 1972). A further limitation of the radiopharmaceutical is related to the fact that, unlike dietary B_{12}, which is complexed via peptide bonds to proteins, *B_{12} is administered in the free, crystalline form. Hence, a normal Schilling Test may occur in some patients who cannot absorb dietary B_{12} because of failure to cleave B_{12} from food proteins (Herbert V, 1972; Streeter AM, et al, 1981). This may be seen in conditions such as partial gastrectomy, pancreatic insufficiency, long-term cimetidine therapy, and other disorders involving decreased secretion of acid, pepsin, and/or other enzymes.

Contraindications. Although there are no absolute contraindications for the Schilling Test, the test may be invalid in the presence of renal dysfunction (i. e., GFR of less than 20 ml/min.) (Rath CE et al, 1957; International Committee for Standardization in Hematology, 1981; Streeter AM, et al, 1981).

DOSAGE/DOSIMETRY

Dosage. Following appropriate patient preparation (described previously), 0.5– 1.0 μCi in 0.5–1.0 μg Vitamin B_{12} is administered orally. If the co-administration of IF is desired, the usual dose of IF is one capsule containing the equivalent of 1 NF XI unit or 60 mg. To avoid problems with capsule dissolution, the contents of the capsule(s) may be mixed in water prior to oral administration (McDonald JWD, et al, 1975). The problem of isotope exchange with use of the dual-isotope method may be avoided by administering the components 2 hours apart (Briedis D, et al, 1973). The usual "flushing dose" of nonradioactive cyanocobalamin is 1000 μg injected intramuscularly 2 hours after the oral dose of *B_{12}. Resumption of eating may also begin at this time. All urine voided in the subsequent 24 hours should be collected and saved. If renal function is impaired, urine collection for 48 hours is recommended (Corcino JJ, et al, 1970; Herbert V, 1972). Urine samples and a radioactive standard (i. e., to accurately quantitate % administered dose excreted) should be counted with identical geometry in an appropriate counting device (e. g., scintillation well counter). When the dual-isotope method is used, the contribution of counts at the Co-57 setting from Co-58 radioactivity must be determined and taken into account.

Dosimetry. Radiation dosimetry estimates are summarized in Table 19.10.

Table 19.10   ESTIMATED RADIATION DOSES TO AN AVERAGE PATIENT FOLLOWING ORAL ADMINISTRATION OF RADIOACTIVE VITAMIN B_{12}[a]

Organ	RADS/1.0 μCi CO-57		RADS/1.0 μCi CO-58		RADS/1.0 μCi CO-60	
	Normal	Pernicious Anemia	Normal	Pernicious Anemia	Normal	Pernicious Anemia
Liver[b]	0.13	0.026	0.175	0.0375	3.4	0.65
Stomach	0.00008	0.00011	0.00034	0.00053	0.00085	0.0013
Small intestine	0.00013	0.00040	0.00054	0.0016	0.0013	0.0039
Upper Large intestine	0.00025	0.00076	0.00088	0.0026	0.0022	0.0066
Lower large intestine	0.00060	0.0018	0.0023	0.0067	0.0055	0.167
Testes[b]	0.0052	0.00012	0.0093	0.00046	0.18	0.0052
Ovaries[b]	0.0065	0.00057	0.0125	0.0026	0.24	0.020
Whole body[b]	0.0099	0.0013	0.015	0.0028	0.32	0.040

[a] From respective product information.
[b] The administration of a "flushing dose" of cyanocobalamin will decrease the dose to the liver, gonads, and whole body by about 30%.

III. Radioferrokinetic Studies

Dennis P. Swanson

Radioactive iron, in the chemical form of Fe-59 ferrous citrate, can be administered orally or intravenously to evaluate several aspects of iron kinetics and metabolism including gastrointestinal absorption, plasma clearance and turnover rates, extent of erythrocyte incorporation and turnover, and patterns of tissue storage and release. In addition to providing an understanding of the mechanism for anemia in several disease states, radioferrokinetic studies have proven clinically useful in the evaluation of bone marrow failure and hematological problems associated with extramedullary sites of erythropoiesis.

CHEMISTRY

Ferrous (Fe-59) citrate is commercially available (Mallinckrodt, Inc., St. Louis, MO) as a sterile, pyrogen-free solution suitable for intravenous administration. The commercial formulation contains the preservative, benzyl-alcohol (0.9% v/v), and trace amounts of a reducing agent, ascorbic acid. The pH of the preparation is adjusted to a final range of 5–7.

The manufacturer's specifications for Fe-59 ferrous citrate include a specific activity in excess of 5 mCi/mg iron and a specific concentration of 25 μCi/mL at calibration. Expiration dating is typically 2 months post calibration. The Fe-59 decays by beta-minus emission (average energy = 0.081 MeV (45.2%), 0.149 MeV (53.1%)) to stable Co-59 with a half-life of approximately 46 days. This decay is accompanied by high-energy gamma emissions at 1.1 MeV (56%) and 1.3 MeV (43.2%).

PHARMACOKINETICS

The kinetics and distribution of Fe-59 ferrous citrate in the body following its oral or intravenous administration reflect the metabolic pathways for iron following its dietary intake and systemic absorption, respectively.

Gastrointestinal Absorption. The average daily diet contains 10–20 mg of iron; however, only approximately 1–1.5 mg is normally absorbed systemically per day. In order to undergo systemic absorption, the dietary iron must be in or converted to the ferrous state. Excess dietary iron, rather than undergoing direct fecal excretion, is stored within intestinal epithelial cells. In the event of increased body demands for iron (e. g., accelerated erythropoiesis, depleted systemic iron stores), the rate of iron absorption from these epithelial storage sites is accelerated via an undefined feedback mechanism. With a normal rate of erythropoiesis and adequate systemic iron stores, the iron stored within the intestinal epithelial cells is excreted in the feces as a function of cellular lifespan and sloughing. Via this latter process, the average loss of dietary iron (i. e., 1–1.5 mg/day) approaches its rate of systemic absorption (Weinstein IM, 1971).

Systemic Kinetics/Biodistribution. Following its systemic absorption (or intravenous administration), iron binds to the beta-1 globulin, transferrin. Plasma transferrin, which has two specific iron-binding sites per molecule, is normally only one-third saturated with iron (i. e., at 100 μgm%). Hence, the iron-binding capacity of plasma transferrin typically approaches 200 μgm% (Weinstein IM, 1971).

Under normal conditions, 80–90% of the plasma iron is transported by transferrin to a labile pool within the bone marrow for use primarily in hemogloblin synthesis and erythropoiesis. The remaining 10–20% of the transferrin-bound iron is transported to labile pools in the liver and spleen for eventual incorporation into ferritin and subsequently into hemosiderin for long-term storage. Plasma iron is in constant equilibrium with these labile iron pools; as a result, 25–40% of iron enters and leaves the plasma per day (Price DC and McIntyre PA, 1984).

Mature erythrocytes within the circulation retain their full complement of hemoglobin-iron throughout their lifespan of approximately 120 days. Upon their death, erythrocytes are sequestered by reticuloendothelial cells of the liver, spleen, and bone marrow. Iron associated with the hemoglobin of these sequestered erythrocytes eventually becomes available for plasma transferrin binding and reutilization (Price DC and McIntyre PA, 1984).

Of the total body iron content of 5 grams (males), approximately 1.5 grams are found within liver, spleen, and marrow storage sites and 3 Gm are associated with circulating and noncirculating erythrocyte hemoglobin. The remaining body iron is incorporated into various protein (e. g., transferrin, myoglobin) or enzyme (e. g., cytochromes, catalase, peroxidase) systems (Weinstein IM, 1971; Price DC and McIntyre PA, 1984).

PRECAUTIONS

Plasma Iron-Binding Capacity. In order to accurately perform radioferrokinetic studies, the intravenously administered Fe-59 must be completely bound to plasma transferrin. This is normally accomplished by incubating the Fe-59 ferrous citrate with autologous plasma prior to injection. If, however, the specific activity of the Fe-59 or the iron-binding capacity of the patient's plasma is low, the radioiron may not totally bind to transferrin. Non–transferrin-bound iron is rapidly eliminated from the circulation and does not reflect the various metabolic pathways involved in erythropoiesis (Price DC and McIntyre PA, 1984).

Based on this discussion, it becomes apparent that the unsaturated iron-binding capacity (UIBC) of the patient's plasma should be evaluated prior to the ferrokinetic study. If the UIBC is less than 75 μgm%, heterologous, ABO-matched plasma of suitable UBIC should be utilized for incubation with the Fe-59 ferrous citrate prior to patient injection (Weinstein IM, 1971). A significantly reduced UIBC is frequently encountered in patients with hemochromatosis, hemosiderosis, hemolytic anemia, or aplastic anemia, and in patients receiving iron therapy or blood transfusions. Furthermore, to ensure an adequate specific activity for complete transferrin binding, the Fe-59 ferrous citrate should not be used beyond its indicated expiration dating.

Gastrointestinal Absorption. The gastrointestinal storage and absorption of iron may be inhibited by the presence of food in the stomach. Therefore, patients should be advised to fast for a period of 6–8 hours prior to the oral administration of Fe-59 ferrous citrate for gastrointestinal absorption studies.

Drug–Radiopharmaceutical Interactions. Cytotoxic drugs (e. g., cytarabine, methotrexate, vinblastine, bisulfan, cyclophosphamide) can alter hematopoiesis and the normal biodistribution of iron (Lee F, 1978). Hence, abnormal radioferrokinetic studies may be observed or be expected (i. e., to evaluate hematopoietic effects) in patients undergoing such therapy. Iron chelating agents, such as desferroxamine and pyrophosphate, would also be expected to alter the normal kinetics and metabolism of iron and the results of radioferrokinetic studies (Dimopoulou CS and Soulpi C, 1983).

Increased amounts of iron are frequently found in the livers of alcoholics independent of the severity of any hepatic dysfunction. The mechanism for increased hepatic deposition of iron in alcoholics is unclear; however, it may be related to a direct or indirect effect of alcohol on the rate of gastrointestinal iron absorption (Chapman RW, et al, 1982; 1983; Friedman BI, et al, 1966).

Pregnancy/Breastfeeding. It has been shown that Fe-59 will cross the placenta to expose the fetus and does appear in breast milk following maternal administration. Therefore, radioferrokinetic studies should be limited to nonpregnant women, as best determined by a pregnancy test. If a radioferrokinetic study is required, a discontinuation of breastfeeding should be considered.

CLINICAL CONSIDERATIONS

Systemic Kinetics/Biodistribution. A ferrokinetic study performed following the intravenous administration of Fe-59 ferrous citrate typically involves three components: (1) the rate of Fe-59 clearance from the plasma, (2) the extent of Fe-59 incorporation into circulating erythrocytes, and (3) the kinetics of Fe-59 distribution to organs involved in erythropoiesis and iron storage. Although no single component of this ferrokinetic study is of significant clinical value by itself, the study as a whole can provide important information on effective erythropoiesis, including the relative contribution of bone marrow versus extramedullary sites, in various hematological disorders.

Plasma Iron Clearance. A determination of plasma iron clearance involves sampling of the plasma for radioactivity content at multiple time intervals (e. g., 10 minutes—4 hours) following the intravenous injection of Fe-59 ferrous citrate (see Dosage/Dosimetry). A semilog plot of this data should yield a multicomponent disappearance curve with an initial clearance half-life (normal) of 1.5 ± 0.5 hours (Weinstein IM, 1971). Assuming that the injected Fe-59 was totally bound to transferrin, extrapolation of the initial component of this plasma disappearance curve to time zero will also provide an estimate of total plasma volume (Price DC and McIntyre PA, 1984). Disease entities involving a reduced rate of erythropoiesis (e. g., aplastic anemia, myelofibrosis, myeloid metaplasia) or iron overload conditions (e. g., hemachromatosis, iron therapy) will demonstrate a prolonged clearance half-life. Conversely, disorders characterized by an increased rate of erythropoiesis (e. g., hemolytic anemia, pernicious anemia, polycythemia vera, chronic blood loss) or iron deficiency will demonstrate an accelerated clearance half-life.

A problem associated with the determination of plasma iron clearance is that this information by itself does not provide a measure of effective erythropoiesis. As previously discussed (see Pharmacokinetics), not all of the iron leaving the plasma is used for erythrocyte production. Moreover, although the iron may be incorporated into developing red blood cells, they may be destroyed before entering the circulation (i. e., intramedullary hemolysis). Plasma iron clearance data may also be misleading in cases of myelofibrosis with extramedullary sites of erythropoiesis. Although plasma iron clearance data can be combined with a knowledge of the plasma volume and serum iron level to yield metabolic information on plasma and erythrocyte iron turnover rates (Weinstein IM, 1971), these latter indices are also of limited clinical value.

Erythrocyte Iron Incorporation. Perhaps the best method to evaluate effective erythropoiesis is to determine the extent of incorporation of Fe-59 into newly formed erythrocytes released into the circulation. Normally, approximately 80–90% of the administered Fe-59 will appear in circulating erythrocytes within 7–10 days post injection (Weinstein IM, 1971; Price DC and McIntyre PA, 1984). Although this measurement is clinically useful in detecting decreased erythrocyte production and release, especially in the face of equivocal bone marrow findings, it is less beneficial in determining accelerated erythropoiesis. This measurement of effective erythropoiesis also fails to provide information on the site of erythrocyte production; therefore, it is best used when combined with external organ counting over potential sites of erythropoiesis and iron storage.

The determination of erythrocyte iron incorporation has a high potential for errors due to the very low concentrations of Fe-59 radioactivity in the respective blood cell samples. Even minor amounts of hemolysis in the collection procedure can lead to a large variation in results.

Organ Kinetics. The use of a well-collimated, external probe to quantitate the kinetics of intravenously administered

Fe-59 in the blood (i. e., with placement over the precordium), bone marrow, liver, and spleen can provide useful adjunct information on the site(s) of erythropoiesis and iron storage. Organs actively involved in erythrocyte production (e. g., bone marrow) demonstrate a rapid, substantial uptake of radioiron, which continues for 1–2 days, followed by a gradual clearance. In comparison, iron storage sites demonstrate a slow, progressive accumulation of the Fe-59 with negligible release (Weinstein IM, 1971; Price DC and McIntyre PA, 1984).

Summary. Because most disorders of iron metabolism and erythrocyte kinetics can be diagnosed by alternate methods, the technically demanding radioferrokinetic studies have, in general, found only limited clinical use. These studies have been recognized as an important tool in the evaluation of ineffective erythropoiesis disorders such as thallasemia, pernicious anemia, and glucose-6-phosphate deficiency. In such conditions, there is typically an increased delivery and retention of iron in the bone marrow with an accompanying decrease in erythrocyte release to the circulation due to intramedullary hemolysis (Price DC and McIntyre PA, 1984).

A radioferrokinetic study combined with an analysis of splenic sequestration (see I. Blood Volume Studies, Cr-51 Sodium Chromate) can also provide clinically unique information in patients with myelofibrotic disorders. In such patients, the site of effective erythropoiesis gradually shifts from the bone marrow to the spleen and liver. Coincidently, as the disease progresses, the development of splenomegaly leads to an increased rate of erythrocyte sequestration and destruction. The use of the radioferrokinetic study to evaluate the relative contribution of the spleen to erythrocyte production and the Cr-51 sequestration study to evaluate splenic erythrocyte destruction can contribute information upon which to base a decision regarding splenectomy (Price DC and McIntyre PA, 1984).

Gastrointestinal Absorption. Absorption of iron from the gastrointestinal tract can be quantitated following the oral administration of Fe-59 ferrous citrate. Although the original method of measuring the amount of radioiron appearing in the blood and the amount excreted in the feces appears simplistic, it suffers from several problems. Not all of the absorbed iron is incorporated into circulating erythrocytes; some is deposited in long-term storage sites. Moreover, the amount of iron in the patient's diet and the accuracy of stool collections can substantially affect the results of the study. More recently, whole-body counting and dual isotope (e. g., intravenous Fe-59, oral Fe-55) techniques have been employed to facilitate the evaluation of iron absorption. However, the study remains tedious and has, in general, provided less clinical information than the intravenous studies (Weinstein IM, 1971).

DOSAGE/DOSIMETRY

Systemic Kinetics/Biodistribution. Ferrokinetic studies to evaluate plasma iron clearance, erythrocyte iron incorporation, and organ kinetics are performed following the intravenous injection of 10–20 μCi of Fe-59 ferrous citrate. As previously discussed (see Precautions), for accurate ferrokinetic evaluations it is important that the Fe-59 be completely bound to transferrin. Hence, the dosage of Fe-59 ferrous citrate is incubated with citrated (ACD) autologous plasma for 15–30 minutes prior to injection. If the patient's plasma has an unsaturated iron-binding capacity (UIBC) of less than 75 μgm %, heterologous plasma of suitable UBIC should be used for this incubation procedure (Weinstein IM, 1971). Upon reinjection of the Fe-59 transferrin/ACD plasma mixture, it is important to save a calibrated sample for use as standard for plasma volume and erythrocyte iron incorporated measurements.

For plasma iron clearance studies, blood samples are typically obtained at 10, 30, and 60 minutes and then at hourly intervals until 4 hours post injection. Radioactive counting is performed on calibrated plasma samples. For an analysis of erythrocyte iron incorporation, additional blood samples are typically obtained at 1, 3, 5, 7, 10, and 14 days post injection. For this portion of the study, radioactive counting can be performed on whole blood. External probe counting of organ kinetics involves the use of a well-collimated scintillation detector positioned over the precordium, sacrum (i. e., for bone marrow evaluation), spleen, and liver. Measurements are typically obtained at hourly intervals for the first 6 hours post Fe-59 administration, and then at intervals corresponding to the erythrocyte iron incorporation studies. Care must be taken in placement of the probe to ensure reproducibility and accuracy of the results.

Gastrointestinal Absorption. Studies to specifically evaluate iron absorption incorporate an oral dosage of 5–10 μCi of Fe-59 ferrous citrate. Fasting prior to radioiron administration will avoid potential problems associated with the inference of food on the absorption process and/or the influence of dietary iron variations on study results.

Dosimetry. Dosimetry estimates for Fe-59 ferrous citrate, administered intravenously, are presented in Table 19.11. For oral administration, the estimated radiation doses are 10–25% of the intravenous estimate.

Table 19.11 RADIATION DOSIMETRY ESTIMATES (ADULT) FOR Fe-59 FERROUS CITRATE[a,b]

ORGAN	RADS/10 μCi
Liver	0.29
Kidney	0.45
Spleen	0.58
Bone marrow	0.65
Testes	0.34
Ovaries	0.33
Total body	0.27

[a] Intravenous administration.
[b] From respective product insert information, Mallinckrodt, Inc.

IV. Venous Thrombosis Detection

Dennis P. Swanson

The formation of an intravascular thrombus involves initially the adhesion of circulating platelets at a site of blood flow stasis and/or injury to a vessel wall. This platelet adhesion is accompanied by the respective release of adenosine diphosphate (ADP) and an associated stimulation of platelet–platelet interactions and aggregation. However, the viscous mass formed as a result of ADP-stimulated platelet aggregation is unstable. Venous thrombus production requires, in addition, the formation of an insoluble fibrin network (O'Reilly RA, 1985).

The precursor of fibrin, fibrinogen, circulates in blood as a soluble protein. The conversion of fibrinogen to fibrin is mediated by the protease enzyme, thrombin. Thrombin is formed at the site of the platelet mass via the activation and interaction of multiple proteolytic enzymes and cofactors that constitute the intrinsic and extrinsic systems of the coagulation process. In addition to promoting the formation of a fibrin network, thrombin stimulates further platelet aggregation by inducing platelet synthesis and release of additional ADP and tromboxane A2, a prostaglandin with potent aggregating properties.

The ability to radiolabel substrates (e. g., fibrinogen, platelets) for this thrombogenic process has led to methods for the scintigraphic detection of intravascular thrombi. As might be expected, however, these radionuclide techniques have been limited by relatively low thrombus-to-blood radioactivity ratios resulting from the normal circulatory properties of these substrates. Moreover, the utility of these radiolabeled substrates is restricted to actively forming thrombi; they demonstrate negligible incorporation into already formed or aged thrombi. Although various thrombolytic substrates and inducers (e. g., plasminogen, streptokinase, urokinase) have been radiolabeled in an attempt to image established thrombi, these agents have, to date, not recognized substantial clinical use or utility (Charkes ND, et al, 1975).

I-125 FIBRINOGEN

Chemistry. I-125 fibrinogen is commercially available (IBRIN®, Amersham, Inc.) in sterile, pyrogen-free unit-dosage vials containing, in addition to the radiolabeled protein (1 mg), various buffering agents (i. e., sodium citrate, glycine; pH 6.5–8.5) and human serum albumin (22 mg) in a lyophilized state. The human-derived proteins are obtained from plasmapheresis of selected donors who have undergone extensive and repeated screening for potential viral and bacterial contaminants. The lyophilized formulation is reconstituted with 1 ml of Sterile Water for Injection, U.S.P., immediately prior to patient administration.

The commercial unit dosage vials of I-125 fibrinogen contain approximately 150 μCi at calibration. The fibrinogen is radiolabeled with I-125 so as to result in less than 0.38 micrograms of iodine per milligram of protein. Such limitation of the number of iodine atoms (i. e., 0.5–1) per molecule of protein helps to ensure that the behavior of I-125 fibrinogen is similar to the native substance in regard to its rate of catabolism and blood clearance (Welch MJ and Krohn KA, 1975). Although clottability alone is not a good indicator of biological effectiveness, the radioiodination procedures currently utilized for the production of I-125 fibrinogen typically result in greater than 90% of the labeled fibrinogen being clottable. At calibration, the radiochemical purity of I-125 fibrinogen exceeds 95% (i. e., less than 5% non-protein-bound radio-iodine).

The I-125 fibrinogen has an expiratory dating of approximately 4 weeks post calibration when stored at the recommended temperature of 4° C. Storage at elevated temperatures results in an accelerated rate of deiodination. For example, the rate of deiodination of I-125 fibrinogen at 37° C is 2% per day (Phan T

and Wasnich R, 1981). Therefore, if the I-125 fibrinogen has encountered prolonged delays in its shipment or if it appears discolored upon receipt, it should not be administered to patients unless its radiochemical purity has been reexamined.

The I-125 radiolabel decays by electron capture with a physical half-life of 60 days. This decay is accompanied by the emission of a 35 keV gamma (6.7% abundance) and 27–32 keV characteristic x-rays (140% abundance). Although these photons are acceptable for external counting procedures, they have a suboptimal energy for external imaging. Thrombus imaging studies with I-131 and I-123 fibrinogen have been reported; however, these radiolabeled derivatives are not commercially available.

PHARMACOKINETICS

Intravenously administered I-125 fibrinogen demonstrates biodistribution and physiological properties similar to endogenous fibrinogen. In this regard, over 80% of the body's fibrinogen pool is associated with the circulating plasma. The normal plasma half-life of I-125 fibrinogen is in the range of 4 days, although an initial rapid ($T_{1/2}$ = 12 hours) component of plasma disappearance accounting for up to 30% of the administered activity may be observed (Saha GB, 1987). In addition to blood, major organs of radioactivity localization include the liver and stomach (Loberg M, et al, 1975).

Under the influence of thrombin, I-125 fibrinogen is converted to fibrin and incorporated into actively forming venous thrombi. Thrombus-to-serum radioactivity ratios in the range of 10:1 have been reported following the injection of radioiodinated fibrinogen (Coleman RE, et al, 1974; Loberg M, et al, 1975).

PRECAUTIONS

DRUG-PROCEDURE INTERACTIONS

Due to their hyperosmolarity and direct chemical toxicity, intravascular radiopaque contrast media can produce alterations in vascular permeability and irritation of the intima of blood vessels, particularly in areas of blood flow stasis. As a result, abnormal I-125 fibrinogen studies have been observed in the absence of a venous thrombus in patients who have undergone a prior venography (i. e., phlebography) procedure (Gjolberg T, et al, 1983). False positive I-125 fibrinogen results may also occur at the sites of injection of iron-dextran (Shaw SM and Faint J, 1981) or other irritative drugs.

Pregnancy/Lactation. In vivo degradation of I-125 fibrinogen results in the release of "free" I-125 iodide, which is capable of placental transmission and secretion into breast milk. Hence, I-125 fibrinogen should ideally not be administered to pregnant or possibly pregnant women, as best determined by appropriate testing. It must be noted, however, that pregnant women occasionally develop thrombophlebitis during their pregnancy or within the immediate postpartum period. In the event of respective signs and symptoms, the potential benefit to be gained from I-125 fibrinogen detection of a developing thrombus must be weighed against the potential risk.

Peak I-125 activity in the breast milk occurs at 1–3 days following the administration of I-125 fibrinogen (Mattsson S, et al, 1981). Hence, consideration should be given to discontinuing breastfeeding until radioactivity in the breast milk is at a negligible level. In this regard, it has been determined that discontinuing breastfeeding for a period of 3 weeks post I-125 fibrinogen injection will reduce the child's thyroid exposure to about 7 rads (Mattsson S, et al, 1981).

CLINICAL CONSIDERATIONS

Clinical Indications. The injection of I-125 fibrinogen is indicated for the detection of actively forming thrombi within the veins of the lower extremities, particularly in the calf region. The study is typically performed to rule out acute venous

Table 19.12 PATIENT CONDITIONS THAT REPRESENT A HIGH RISK FOR THE DEVELOPMENT OF LOWER EXTREMITY VENOUS THROMBOSIS

Acute myocardial infarction
Cancer (certain)
Congestive heart failure
Immobility
Major surgical procedure
Stroke

thrombi in the presence of equivocal signs and symptoms of thrombophlebitis and/or with known pulmonary embolism. It may also be used prospectively for the detection of developing lower extremity thrombi in high-risk patients (Table 19.12).

Because the I-125 fibrinogen demonstrates negligible uptake in established thrombi, false-negative results may be encountered if the test is initiated at some length (i. e., greater than 7 days) post the onset of symptoms (Kline RC, 1983). The usefulness of the I-125 fibrinogen test decreases greatly with venous thrombi in the regions of the upper thigh or pelvis due to tissue attenuation of the low-energy I-125 photons and bladder activity.

Patient Preparation. Patients undergoing an I-125 fibrinogen test should be administered a stable iodide preparation (e. g., Lugol's Solution, Saturated Solution of Potassium Iodide) to block thyroidal uptake of free radioiodide occurring as a radiochemical impurity or a byproduct of in vivo degradation. An effective thyroid-blocking dosage should provide 30–130 mg of potassium iodide per day commencing prior to I-125 fibrinogen injection and continued for 10 days (Stathis VJ, et al, 1987). In patients who cannot tolerate iodide preparations, potassium perchlorate may be substituted at an oral dosage of 200 mg daily. (See also Appendix B.)

DOSAGE/DOSIMETRY

Study Procedure. The recommended dosage of I-125 fibrinogen for a 70 kg adult is 100 μCi administered intravenously. External counting using a collimated, thin-window scintillation probe may commence as early as 1 hour post injection; however, an interval of 4 hours is typically employed to ensure systemic equilibration of the radiotracer.

Counting is performed with the patient supine and legs raised above the heart to minimize extremity blood pooling. Because reproducibility of measurements is critical to study interpretation and accuracy, counting points should be designated (e. g., using an indelible marker) at 5 cm intervals over the deep veins of the medial thighs, popliteal fossae, and calves. Count rates are measured over each point on both legs and over the precordium. Extremity readings are expressed as a percentage of the precordium activity.

Study Interpretation. In a normal study (i. e., no venous thrombi), there should be a gradual, symmetrical decrease in count rate with time over each of the extremity counting points. Slightly greater count rates may be observed in the region of the knee compared to the other counting sites. Venous thrombosis is indicated if the radioactivity measurement at any extremity counting point exceeds by 20% the measurement over an adjacent point on the same extremity or the corresponding point on the opposite extremity. Note that false-positive studies commonly occur with conditions (Table 19.13) that lead to localized blood pooling or hyperemia in the extremity counting region. Positive studies should be repeated at 24 hours for confirmation (Kline RC, 1983; Carretta RF and Matin P, 1981).

Table 19.13 CONDITIONS THAT MAY LEAD TO A FALSE-POSITIVE I-125 FIBRINOGEN DIAGNOSIS OF VENOUS THROMBUS

Arthritis
Cellulitis
Fracture
Gross edema
Hematoma
Surgical incision
Trauma
Ulcer
Varicose veins
Venous stasis

Table 19.14 ESTIMATED RADIATION ABSORBED DOSIMETRY FOR INTRAVENOUS I-125 FIBRINOGEN[a]

ORGAN	RADS/100 μCi
Thyroid (unblocked)	1.3
Thyroid (blocked)	0.02
Kidneys	0.06
Liver	0.08
Lungs	0.04
Testes	0.03
Ovaries	0.03
Whole body	0.02

[a] From respective package insert information.

If the initial counting study is negative, it may be repeated at daily (or every other day) intervals for up to 10–14 days. A positive study for a developing thrombi may demonstrate, in addition to the previously described criteria, a 20% increase in the radioactivity measurement over a given counting point when compared to the previously performed measurement. If the patient remains at risk, a second injection of I-125 fibrinogen should be administered at the end of the initial 10-day interval or when the precordium count rate falls below 100 counts/second.

Dosimetry. Table 19.14 lists estimated radiation absorbed doses to various organs following the intravenous administration of I-125 fibrinogen.

IN-111 PLATELETS

Autologous platelets can be radiolabeled with Indium-111 to permit the external imaging of acute thrombi. The commercially available radiopharmaceutical used for this procedure, In-111 oxine, is currently indicated for the preparation of In-111 leukocytes (see Chapter 17: Radiopharmaceuticals for Imaging Tumors and Inflammatory Processes.) However, In-111 oxine will label blood cells in a nonspecific manner based on its high degree of lipid solubility and related ability to passively diffuse through the cell wall. Once within the blood cell, the Indium-111 is displaced from the oxine as a result of its greater affinity for cytoplasmic proteins. The noncomplexed oxine (8-hydroxyquinoline) remains lipid soluble and subsequently diffuses from the cell. Hence, by isolating platelets from the other blood cells, it is possible to specifically label them with In-111.

The In-111 radiolabel has ideal nuclidic properties for the external imaging of platelet kinetics, biodistribution, and pathophysiology. Its decay, which occurs by electron capture with a physical half-life of 2.8 days, is accompanied by the emission of two gamma radiations (172 keV, 89.6% abundance; 247 keV, 93.9% abundance) with energies suitable for currently available imaging instrumentation. Because platelets are the initiating substrate for thrombogenesis and are incorporated into actively forming thrombi, the administration of In-111 platelets should permit the external detection of acute thrombi provided they retain their normal physiological functions.

In-111 platelets have not been utilized extensively in the clinical setting for the diagnosis of venous or arterial thrombi. This may be related to the previously described limitations of a low thrombus-to-blood radioactivity ratio and the minimal incorporation of platelets into established or aged thrombi. Or, it may be due to the fact that the In-111 oxine is not currently indicated for this purpose, or that the labeling procedure is fairly tedious. Another problem is related to the extreme fragility of platelets and the inherent rigors of the In-111 oxine labeling technique. In order to obtain an adequate radiolabeling efficiency, the platelets must be separated from serum. This requirement stems from the fact that the Indium-111 has a greater affinity for serum transferrin than it does for oxine. Failure to remove the serum transferrin results in less In-111 oxine available to penetrate the cell wall. Separation of the platelets from their normal source of nutrients, the serum, results in a rapid loss of their viability. Whether new labeling reagents (i.e., In-111 tropolone, In-111 MERC; see Chapter 17) that permit platelet labeling in the presence of a small amount of

plasma will result in an increased clinical utility of In-111 platelets awaits further investigation.

RADIONUCLIDE VENOGRAPHY

An alternate method to the use of radiolabeled thrombogenic substrates for the detection of venous thrombi involves an evaluation of lower extremity venous blood flow following the injection of a radiotracer into a superficial vein of the foot. Any high photon yield (e. g., Technetium-99m) radiopharmaceutical may be utilized for this study; however, Tc-99m macroaggregated albumin (Tc-99m MAA) is commonly employed because it can provide additional information on lung perfusion in these patients at high risk for pulmonary embolism (See Chapter 12: Radiopharmaceuticals for Lung Imaging).

Typically, 1–2 mCi of Tc-99m MAA is injected simultaneously into a dorsal vein of each foot. During injection and imaging, tourniquets are placed on each leg at the calf level to force radiotracer distribution to the deep veins. Using a large field-of-view gamma camera, multiple overlapping images are obtained to visualize the flow of the Tc-99m MAA through the deep veins of both legs, particularly in the region from the knee to the pelvis. Alternately, a scanning camera may be utilized with scanning speed adjusted to correspond with the rate of venous flow of the Tc-99m MAA bolus. Subsequent imaging of the lungs and reimaging of the legs may be performed to respectively evaluate pulmonary perfusion and retention of the radiotracer in areas of venous stasis. The absorbed radiation doses associated with this study are essentially the same as those which occur with a Tc-99m MAA pulmonary perfusion study (see Chapter 12).

A normal radionuclide venogram should demonstrate uniform, symmetrical filling of the deep veins of both legs from the level of the knees to above the bifurcation of the inferior vena cava (Figure 19.1). No evidence of obstruction or

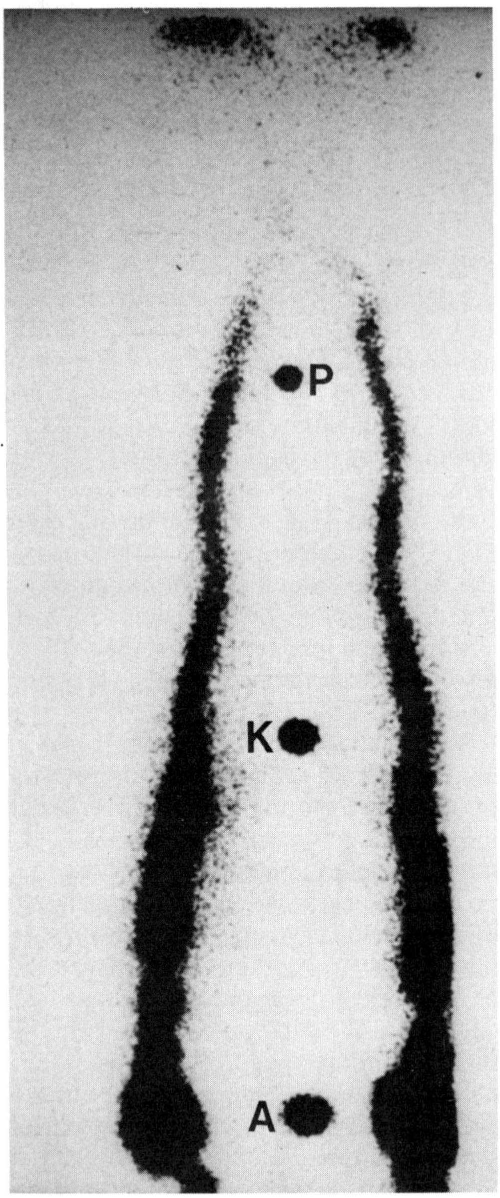

Figure 19.1 Normal, bilateral radionuclide venography study demonstrating uniform filling and flow in the deep veins of the leg. Radioactive markers are positioned at the ankle (A), knee (K), and pubis (P).

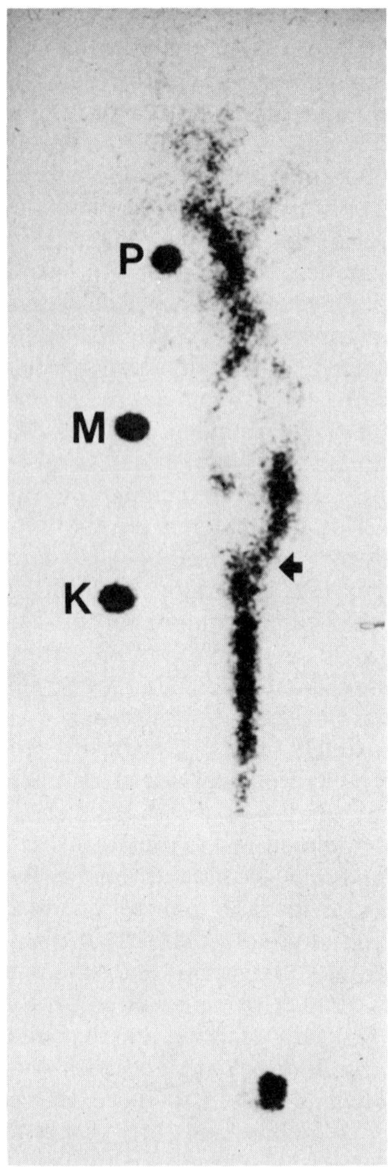

Figure 19.2 Unilateral radionuclide venography study demonstrating (arrow) an abrupt termination of deep venous flow with abnormal filling of collateral veins. Radioactive markers are positioned at the knee (K), mid-thigh (M), and pubis (P).

tortuosity of flow should be observed. Delayed imaging should reveal rapid clearance of the Tc-99m MAA from the extremity veins with no areas of substantial radiotracer retention. An abrupt termination of the venous flow is indicative of a venous thrombus (Figure 19.2). This ob-

structive pattern may be accompanied by the appearance of collateral blood vessels and vessel tortuosity.

Compared to the use of I-125 fibrinogen or In-111 platelets for the detection of venous thrombosis, the radionuclide venography study has the advantage of being able to demonstrate established thrombi. Unlike I-125 fibrinogen, the relatively high energy gamma emissions of Tc-99m will permit accurate evaluations of venous flow in the inguinal and pelvic regions. However, due to the multiplicity and variability of veins below the knee, the radionuclide venography study is of very limited value for evaluation of the calf region where many thrombi develop. Based on this discussion, it becomes apparent that radionuclide venography is frequently performed as a complementary study to the I-125 fibrinogen procedure.

References

Alazraki NP, Mishkin FS, eds. Non-imaging procedures. In *Fundamentals of Nuclear Medicine*. Society of Nuclear Medicine, Inc., New York, 1984, pp 140–142.

Albert SN. Blood volume. In *Nuclear Medicine, Second Edition*, Blahd WH (ed). New York, McGraw-Hill Book Co., 1971, pp 593–619.

Allen RH, Seetharam B, Podell E. Effect of proteolytic enzymes on the binding of cobalamin to R protein and intrinsic factor. *J Clin Invest* 1978, 61:47–54.

Amersham. Dicopac® package insert. Arlington Heights, IL: September, 1979.

Amin S, Spinks T, Ranicar A, et al. Long-term clearance of [^{57}Co] cyanocobalamin in vegans and pernicious anemia. *Clin Sci* 1980, 58:101–103.

Baker WJ, Datz FL. Preparation and clinical utility of labeled blood products. In *Essentials of Nuclear Medicine Science*, Hladik WB, Saha GB, Study KT, (eds). Baltimore, Williams and Wilkins, 1987, pp 90–98.

Baun DC, Bowen BM, Wood DE. Comparison of the bioavailability of cyanocobalamin from capsule and liquid dosage forms. *Am J Hosp Pharm* 1975, 32:1047–1049.

Bell EG, Maher B, McAfee JG, et al. Radiopharmaceuticals for gamma cisternography. In *Radiopharmaceuticals*, Subramanian G, Rhodes BA, Cooper JF, Sodd VJ (eds). New York, Society of Nuclear Medicine, Inc., 1975, p 405.

Bell TK, Bridges JM, Nelson MG. Simultaneous free and bound radioactive vitamin B$_{12}$ urinary excretion test. *J Clin Pathol* 1965, 18:611–613.

Berchtold P, Dahlqvist A, Gustafson A, et al. Effects of a biguanide (metformin) on vitamin B$_{12}$ and folic acid absorption and intestinal enzyme activities. *Scand J Gastroenterol* 1971, 6:751–754.

Breuel HP, Fischer P. [The influence of vitamin B$_{12}$ premedication on the results of the Schilling test (author's transl)]. *Nuklearmedizin* 1979, 18:186–188.

Briedis D, McIntyre PA, Judisch J, et al. An evaluation of a dual-isotope method for the measurement of vitamin B$_{12}$ absorption. *J Nucl Med* 1973, 14:135–141.

Carmel R, Rosenberg AH, Lau KS, et al. Vitamin B$_{12}$ uptake by human small bowel homogenate and its enhancement by intrinsic factor. *Gastroenterology* 1969, 56:548–555.

Carretta RF, Matin P. Thrombus detection with radionuclides. In *Clinical Nuclear Medicine*, Matin P (ed). Garden City, NY, Medical Examination Publ. Co., Inc., 1981, pp 293–306.

Chapman RW, Morgan MY, Boss AM, et al. Acute and chronic effects of alcohol on iron absorption. *Dig Dis Sci* 1983, 28:321–327.

Chapman RW, Morgan MY, Laulicht M, et al. Hepatic iron stores and markers of iron overload in alcoholics and patients with hemochromatosis. *Dig Dis Sci* 1982, 27:909–916.

Charkes ND, Malmud LS, Stern H. Comparative evaluation of current scanning agents for thrombus detection. In *Radiopharmaceuticals*, Subramanian G, Rhodes BA, Cooper JF, Sodd VJ (eds). New York, Society of Nuclear Medicine, Inc., 1975; pp 525–534.

Chow BF, Okuda K. Urinary excretion test for vitamin B$_{12}$. *Fed Proc* 1955, 14:430.

Coleman RE, Krohn KA, Metzger JM et al. An in-vivo evaluation of

*I-fibrinogen labeled by four different methods. *J Lab Clin Med* 1974, 83: 977–982.

Corcino JJ, Waxman S, Herbert V. Absorption and malabsorption of vitamin B$_{12}$. *Am J Med* 1970, 48:562–569.

Coronato A, Glass GBJ. Depression of the intestinal uptake of radio-vitamin B$_{12}$ by cholestyramine. *Proc Soc Exp Biol Med* 1973, 142:1341–1344.

Dimopoulou CS, Soulpi C. Alterations of Fe-59 ferric citrate biodistribution in hyperferremic mice after the administration of pyrophosphate and desferroxamine. *J Pharmacol Exp Ther* 1983, 224:415–418.

Donaldson RM, Katz JH. Exchange between free and gastric juice-bound cyanocobalamin. *J Clin Invest* 1963, 42:534–545.

Ellenbogen L, Williams WL, Rabiner SF, et al. An improved urinary excretion test as an assay for intrinsic factor. *Proc Soc Exp Biol Med* 1955, 89:357–362.

Faloon WW, Chodos RB. Vitamin B$_{12}$ absorption studies using colchicine, neomycin and continuous ^{57}Co B$_{12}$ administration. *Gastroenterology* 1969, 56:1251.

Fairbanks VF, Wahner HW, Valley TB, et al. Spurious results from dual-isotope (Dicopac®) vitamin B$_{12}$ absorption test are due to rapid or variable rates of exchange of ^{58}Co-B$_{12}$ for ^{57}Co-B$_{12}$ bound to intrinsic factor. *Nucl Med Commun* 1983, 4:17–23.

Fielding LP, Chalmers DM, Chanarin I, et al. Inhibition of intrinsic factor secretion by cimetidine. *Br Med J* 1978, 1:818–819.

Findlay J, Sellers E, Forstner G. Lack of effect of alcohol on small intestinal binding of the vitamin B-12 intrinsic factor complex. *Can J Physiol Pharmacol* 1976, 54:469–476.

Friedman BI, Schaefer JW, Schiff L. Increased iron-59 absorption in patients with hepatic cirrhosis. *J Nucl Med* 1966, 7:594–602.

Gjolberg T, Andrew E, Enge I. Iohexol in phlebography of the leg. *Acta Radiol* 1983, 366(Suppl):65–69.

Graber SE, Scheffel U, Hodkinson B, et al. Placental transport of vitamin B$_{12}$ in the pregnant rat. *J Clin Invest* 1971, 50:1000–1004.

Grasbeck R, Nyberg W. Inhibition of radiovitamin B$_{12}$ absorption by ethylenediaminetetraacetate (EDTA) and its reversal by calcium ions. *Scand J Clin Lab Invest* 1958, 10:448.

Halsted CH, McIntyre PA. Intestinal malabsorption caused by aminosalicylic acid therapy. *Arch Intern Med* 1972, 130:935–939.

Heinivaara O, Palva IP. Malabsorption of vitamin B$_{12}$ during treatment with para-aminosalicylic acid. *Acta Med Scand* 1964, 175:469–471.

Heinivaara O, Palva IP. Malabsorption and deficiency of vitamin B$_{12}$ caused by treatment with para-aminosalicylic acid. *Acta Med Scand* 1965, 177:337–341.

Herbert V. Detection of malabsorption of vitamin B$_{12}$ due to gastric or intestinal dysfunction. *Semin Nucl Med* 1972, 2:220–234.

Hilman RS. Vitamin B$_{12}$, folic acid, and the treatment of megaloblastic anemias. In *Goodman and Gilman's The Pharmacological Basis of Therapeutics*, sixth Edition, AG Gilman, L Goodman, A Gilman (eds). New York, Macmillan Publishing Company, 1980, 1331–1346.

International Committee for Standardization in Hematology. Recommended methods for the measurement of vitamin B$_{12}$ absorption. *J Nucl Med* 1981, 22:1091–1093.

Jacobsen ED, Chodos RB, Faloon WW. An experimental malabsorption syndrome induced by neomycin. *Am J Med* 1960, 28:524–533.

Jounela AJ, Pirttiaho H, Palva IP. Drug-induced malabsorption of vitamin B$_{12}$. VI. Malabsorption of vitamin B$_{12}$ during treatment with phenformin. *Acta Med Scand* 1974, 196:267–269.

Katz JH, DiMase J, Donaldson RM. Simultaneous administration of gastric juice-bound and free radioactive cyanocobalamin: Rapid procedure for differentiating between intrinsic factor deficiency and other causes of vitamin B_{12} malabsorption. *J Lab Clin Med* 1963, 61:266–271.

Kline RC. Venous thrombosis (Iodine-125 fibrinogen) scanning. In *Manual of Nuclear Medicine Procedures, Fourth Edition*, Carey JE, Kline RC, Keyes JW, Jr (eds). Boca Raton, FL, CRC Press, 1983, pp. 121–122.

Lee EW. Fe-59 uptake method to differentiate between proliferation-dependent and non-dependent cytotoxic agents. *Toxicol Appl Pharmacol* 1978, 43:485–491.

Lees F: Radioactive vitamin B_{12} absorption in the megaloblastic anaemia caused by anticonvulsant drugs. *QJ Med* 1961, 30:231–248.

Lindenbaum J, Lieber CS. Alcohol-induced malabsorption of vitamin B_{12} in man. *Nature* 1969, 224:806.

Loberg M, Miller I, Cooper M. Radioiodinated autologous fibrinogen: A rapid method of preparation for clinical use. In *Radiopharmaceuticals*, Subramanian G, Rhodes BA, Cooper JF, Sodd VJ (eds), New York, Society of Nuclear Medicine, Inc., 1975, pp. 503–513.

Luhby AL, Cooperman JM, Stone ML, et al. Physiology of vitamin B_{12} in pregnancy, the placenta, and the newborn. *Am J Dis Child* 1961, 102:753–754.

Mailloux LU, Streeto JM. The effect of prior vitamin B-12 administration on the Schilling test. *Am J Med Sci* 1965, 250:697–699.

Markiewicz A, Gomoluch T, Marek E, et al. Circadian absorption of vitamin B_{12}. *Scand J Gastroenterol* 1981, 16:541–544.

Mattsson S, Johansson L, Nosslin B, et al. Excretion of radionuclides in human breast milk following administration of ^{125}I-fibrinogen, ^{99m}Tc-MAA, and ^{51}Cr-EDTA. In *Third International Radiopharmaceutical Dosimetry Symposium*. Watson EE, Schlafke-Stetson AT, Coffey JL, Cloutier RJ (eds), Rockville, MD, H.H.S. Publication FDA 81–8166, Bureau of Radiological Health, 1981, pp. 102–110.

McDonald JWD, Barr RM, Barton WB. Spurious Schilling test results obtained with intrinsic factor enclosed in capsules. *Ann Intern Med* 1975, 83:827–829.

McIntyre P. The blood and blood-forming organs. In *Nuclear Medicine*, Wagner HN (ed). New York, HP Publishing Co., 1975, pp. 191–199.

McIntyre PA. Use of radioisotope techniques in the clinical evaluation of patients with megaloblastic anemia. *Semin Nucl Med* 1975, 5:79–94.

Nelp WB, Wagner HN, Reba RC. Renal excretion of vitamin B_{12} and its use in measurement of glomerular filtration rate in man. *J Lab Clin Med* 1964, 63:480–491.

Nishimura Y, Inaba J, Ichikawa R. Fetal uptake of ^{60}CoCl$_2$ and ^{57}Co-cyanocobalamin in different gestation stages of rats. *J Radiat Res* 1978, 19:236–245.

Okuda K, Sasayama K. Effects of ethylenediaminetetraacetate and metal ions in intestinal absorption of vitamin B_{12} in man and rats. *Proc Soc Exp Biol Med* 1965, 120:17–20.

O'Reilly RA. Anticoagulant, anti-thrombotic, and thrombolytic drugs. In *The Pharmacological Basis of Therapeutics*. Gilman AG, Goodman LS, Rall TW, Murad F (eds), New York, Macmillan Publishing Co., 1985, pp. 1338–1339.

Paaby P, Norvin E. The absorption of vitamin B_{12} during treatment with para-aminosalicylic acid. *Acta Med Scand* 1966, 180:561–564.

Palva IP, Rytkonen V, Alatulkkila M, et al. Drug-induced malabsorption of vitamin B_{12}. V. Intestinal pH and absorption of vitamin B_{12} during treatment with para-aminosalicylic acid. *Scand J Haematol* 1972a, 9:5–7.

Palva IP, Salokannel SJ, Timonen T, et al. Drug-induced malabsorption of vitamin B_{12}. IV. Malabsorption and deficiency of B_{12} during treatment with slow-release potassium chloride. *Acta Med Scand* 1972b, 191:355–357.

Palva IP, Salokannel SJ, Palva HLA, et al. Drug-induced malabsorption of vitamin B_{12}. VII. Malabsorption of B_{12}

during treatment with potassium citrate. *Acta Med Scand* 1974, 196:525–526.

Parmentier Y, Marcoullis G, Nicolas JP. The intraluminal transport of vitamin B_{12} and the exocrine pancreatic insufficiency. *Proc Soc Exp Biol Med* 1979, 160:396–400.

Phan T, Wasnich R, eds. *Practical Nuclear Pharmacy*, second edition, Honolulu, Banyan Enterprises, Ltd., 1981, pp. 62–63, 75–78.

Price DC, McIntyre PA. The hematopoietic system. In *Textbook of Nuclear Medicine. Volume II. Clinical Applications, Second Edition*, Harbert J, DaRocha AFG (eds). Philadelphia, Lea and Febiger, 1984, pp. 535–605.

Race TF, Paes IC, Faloon WW. Intestinal malabsorption induced by oral colchicine. Comparison with neomycin and cathartic agents. *Am J Med Sci* 1970, 259:32–41.

Rath CE, McCurdy PR, Duffy BJ. Effect of renal disease on the Schilling test. *N Engl J Med* 1957, 256:111-114.

Reynolds EH, Hallpike JF, Phillips BM, et al. Reversible absorptive defects in anticonvulsant megaloblastic anaemia. *J Clin Pathol* 1965, 18:593–598.

Rosenblum C. Production and metabolism of cobalt-labeled cyanocobalamin. In *Radioactive Pharmaceuticals,* Andrews GA, Kniseley R, et al (eds). US Atomic Energy Commission, Oak Ridge, TN, 1966:455–476 (AEC symposium series, #6 USAEC publications # CONF-651111).

Saha GB. Normal biodistribution of diagnostic radiopharmaceuticals. In *Essentials of Nuclear Medicine Science*, Hladik WB, Saha GB, Study KT (eds), Baltimore, Williams and Wilkins, 1987, p. 13.

Salokannel SJ, Palva IP, Takkunen JT. Malabsorption of vitamin B_{12} during treatment with slow-release potassium chloride. *Acta Med Scand* 1970, 187:431–432.

Schilling RF. Intrinsic factor studies. II. The effect of gastric juice on the urinary excretion of radioactivity after the oral administration of radioactive vitamin B_{12}. *J Lab Clin Med* 1953, 42:860–866.

Schilling RF. Intrinsic factor studies. III. Further observations utilizing the urinary radioactivity test in subjects with achlorhydria, pernicious anemia, or a total gastrectomy. *J Lab Clin Med* 1955, 45:926–934.

Shaw SM, Faint J, eds. *Factors and Medications Affecting the Distribution of Radiopharmaceuticals in Nuclear Medicine Procedures*, St. Louis, Mallinckrodt, Inc., 1981, pp. 15–29.

Silber R, Moldow CF. The biochemistry of B_{12}-mediated reactions in man. *Am J Med* 1970, 48:549–554.

Sisson JC. Red blood cell survival including red blood cell sequestration. In *Manual of Nuclear Medicine Procedures, Fourth Edition*, Carey JE, Kline RC, Keyes JW, Jr (eds). Boca Raton, FL, CRC Press, Inc., 1983, pp. 134–136.

Squibb ER & Sons, Inc. Rubratope®-57, Rubratope®-60 package insert. Princeton, NJ, August, 1978.

Stathis VJ, Cantrell DW, Cantrell TJ. Patient preparation for nuclear medicine studies. In *Essentials of Nuclear Medicine Science*, Hladik WB, Saha GB, Study KT (eds). Baltimore, Williams and Wilkins, 1987, p. 413.

Steinberg WM, King CE, Toskes PP. Malabsorption of protein-bound cobalamin but not unbound cobalamin during cimetidine administration. *Dig Dis Sci* 1980, 25:188–192.

Streeter AM, Bathur FA, Arnold BJ, et al. Limitations of the Schilling test. *Lancet* 1981, 1:39–40.

Teo NH, Scott JM, Neale G, et al. Effect of bile on vitamin B_{12} absorption. *Br Med J* 1980, 281:831.

Tomkin GH, Hadden DR, Weaver JA, et al. Vitamin-B_{12} status of patients on long-term metformin therapy. *Br Med J* 1971, 2(5763):685–687.

Tomkin GH. Malabsorption of vitamin B_{12} in diabetic patients treated with phenformin: A comparison with metformin. *Br Med J* 1973, 3:673–675.

Toskes PP, Deren JJ. Selective inhibition of vitamin B_{12} malabsorption by para-aminosalicylic acid. *Gastroenterology* 1972, 672:1232–1237.

Ullberg S, Kristoffersson H, Flodh H, et al. Placental passage and fetal accumulation of labeled vitamin B_{12} in the mouse. *Arch Int Pharmacodyn Ther* 1967, 67:431–449.

USP DI, Volume I, Drug Information for the Health Care Provider, eighth edition, The United States Pharmacopeial Convention, Inc., Rockville, MD, 1988:827–828.

U.S.P. XXI, United States Pharmacopeia Convention, Inc., Rockville, MD, 1984, pp 545–547.

Webb DI, Chodos RB, Mahar CQ, et al. Mechanisms of vitamin B_{12} malabsorption in patients receiving colchicine. *N Engl J Med* 1968, 279:845–850.

Weinstein IM. Measurement of iron metabolism and erythropoiesis. In Chapter 15, Disorders of hepatopoiesis, the reticuloendothelial system, and the spleen. *Nuclear Medicine, Second Edition*, Blahd WH, (ed), New York, McGraw-Hill, 1971, pp. 416–424.

Weinstein IM, Blahd WH, Schilling RF. Disorders of hematopoiesis, the reticuloendothelial system, and the spleen. In *Nuclear Medicine, Second Edition*, Blahd WH (ed), New York, McGraw-Hill Book Co., 1971, pp. 430–435.

Welch MJ, Krohn KA. Critical review of radiolabeled fibrinogen: Its preparation and use. In *Radiopharmaceuticals*, Subramanian G, Rhodes BA, Cooper JF, Sodd VJ (eds), New York, Society of Nuclear Medicine, Inc., 1975, pp. 493–502.

Willms B, Creutzfeldt W. Contribution to the intestinal resorption of vitamin B-12 (Schilling test) and of d-xylose in biguanide treatment. *Diabetologia* 1970, 6:652.

Yeh SDJ, Shils ME. Cycloheximide effect on vitamin B_{12} absorption and intrinsic factor production in the rat. *Proc Soc Exp Biol Med* 1969, 130:1260–1264.

Yeh SDJ, Shils ME. Effect of actinomycin D and cholchicine on intestinal absorption in rats. *Fed Proc* 1966, 25(2):322.

Zuckier LS, Chervu LR. Schilling evaluation of pernicious anemia: Current status. *J Nucl Med* 1984, 25:1032–1039.

ENHANCEMENT AGENTS FOR MAGNETIC RESONANCE AND ULTRASOUND IMAGING

▼▼▼

Enhancement Agents for Magnetic Resonance Imaging: Fundamentals

Susan C. Jackels

Proton nuclei, and other nuclei with nonzero nuclear spin and odd mass number, possess a nuclear magnetic moment and therefore interact with an external field to produce several nulcear spin energy states. For protons two states exist—one corresponding to the proton nuclear moment aligned with the field, and the other antiparallel to it. With magnetic fields on the order of 0.002 to 2 Tesla, the energy required to produce transitions between the two states is in the radio frequency region, 0.1 to 80 MHz. It is important to realize that in order for absorption of energy to occur, the magnetic field must produce an energy separation between nuclear spin levels that exactly matches the energy of the applied radio frequency radiation. This condition is called resonance.

The proton nuclei of tissue water molecules are responsible for the signal imaged by MRI. To produce an image based on the magnetic resonance signal, a linearly increasing magnetic field gradient is applied, in addition to a static magnetic field, to "spatially encode" the nuclei with different resonant frequencies. This causes the selection of a resonant slice approximately 1 centimeter thick in the subject (Figure 20.1). Within the slice, applied pulses of radiation separated by time intervals produce a signal that may be either an "echo" or a "free induction decay" depending upon the details of the pulse sequence. This signal, which is monitored by a receiver coil, is fourier transformed by a computer to produce a one-dimensional projection of signal amplitude along a line across the slice of subject. When this process is repeated several times along different lines and with the aid of computer algorithms (similar to those used in x-ray CT), a number of projections may be reconstructed to provide a two-dimensional image of the signal arising from the tissue water protons in the

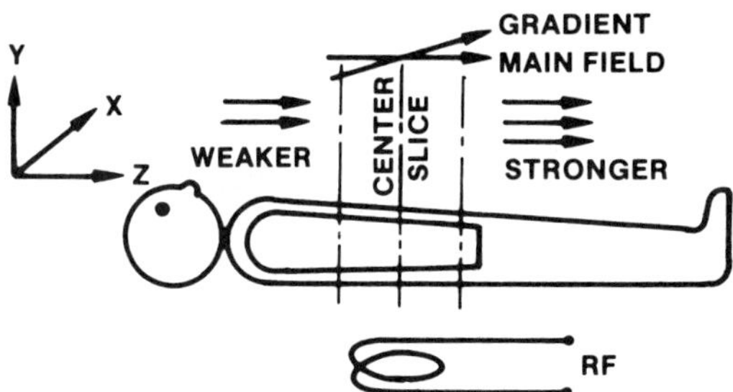

Figure 20.1   MR images of slices are obtained by imposing a magnetic field gradient in addition to the main field. Only one section approximately 1 cm thick satisfies the field condition for proton resonance.

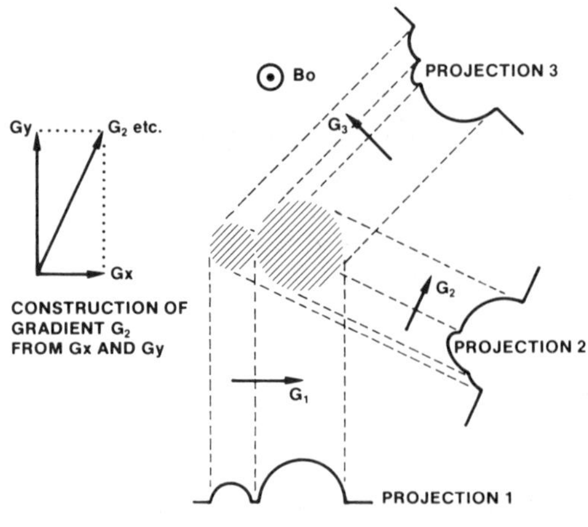

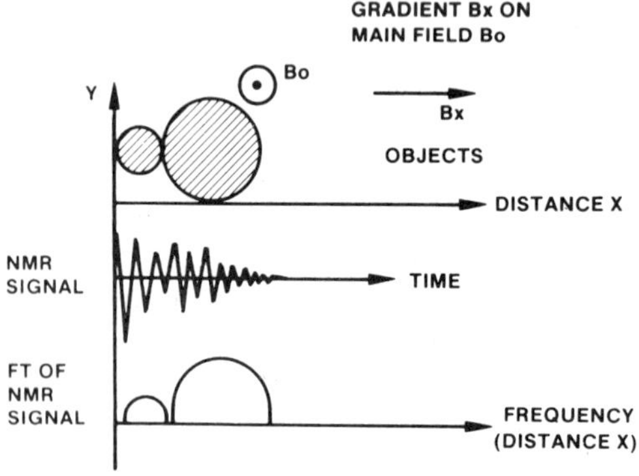

Figure 20.2 A. Within the selected slice, a series of gradients are applied in separate pulse data-collection sequences followed by fourier transformation to obtain a projection of the signal intensity through the slice along the line of the gradient.
B. A series of projection images is used to reconstruct the image via computer. Typically 180 projections are used.

slice (Figure 20.2). A more detailed description of MRI techniques is available in a number of excellent monographs and review articles (Mansfield P and Morris PG, 1982; Partain GL, et al, 1988; Wolf GL and Popp C, 1984; Beall PT, et al, 1984; Bottomley PA, 1984).

In order to understand the dependence of the MRI signal intensity upon the properties of tissue proton nuclei, one must visualize the effects of radio frequency pulses upon the slight magnetization pro-

duced in the subject by the static magnetic field.

Magnetization in the static field can be represented by a vector that points in the direction of the applied magnetic field (defined as the z axis, see Figure 20.3). Whenever this magnetization vector is pertubed by radio frequency (Rf) radiation directed at the subject along the x axis, for example, the direction of magnetization is "tipped," after some time, into the xy plane along the y axis (90° pulse) or, after a longer pulse, to the $-z$ direction (180° pulse). After the Rf radiation is turned off, the magnetization soon returns to its equilibrium orientation along the z axis. This regrowth of the z component of the magnetization vector is approximately exponential and is characterized by the time constant T_1 (the time at which it has returned to $1/e$ of its equilibrium value). Similarly, the decay of the component along the x or y axis follows a slightly different exponential behavior given by time constant T_2. T_1 and T_2 are called the longitudinal and transverse relaxation times. T_2 can be equal in length to T_1, but never longer. Sometimes the relaxation behavior is represented as the longitudinal relaxation rate, $1/T_1$, or the transverse relaxation rate, $1/T_2$.

The signal intensity in an MR image depends upon the details of the pulse sequence used to generate the image. Pulse sequences can be selected that yield images with signal intensity weighted by either T_1, T_2, or proton concentration in tissue. Protons in nonstationary tissue such as blood or CSF also influence signal intensity. Proton concentration is always a multiplicative factor in the signal intensity of MR images. Bone, because it contains no protons, is invisible in MR images. Fat tissue, though containing less water than other tissues, has a high concentration of methylenic hydrogens that contribute to signal intensity because of their proximity in resonant frequency to water hydrogen and their very short T_1 and T_2. A peculiar result in higher field MR imagers is that fat tissue appears bright and slightly spatially displaced due to this "chemical

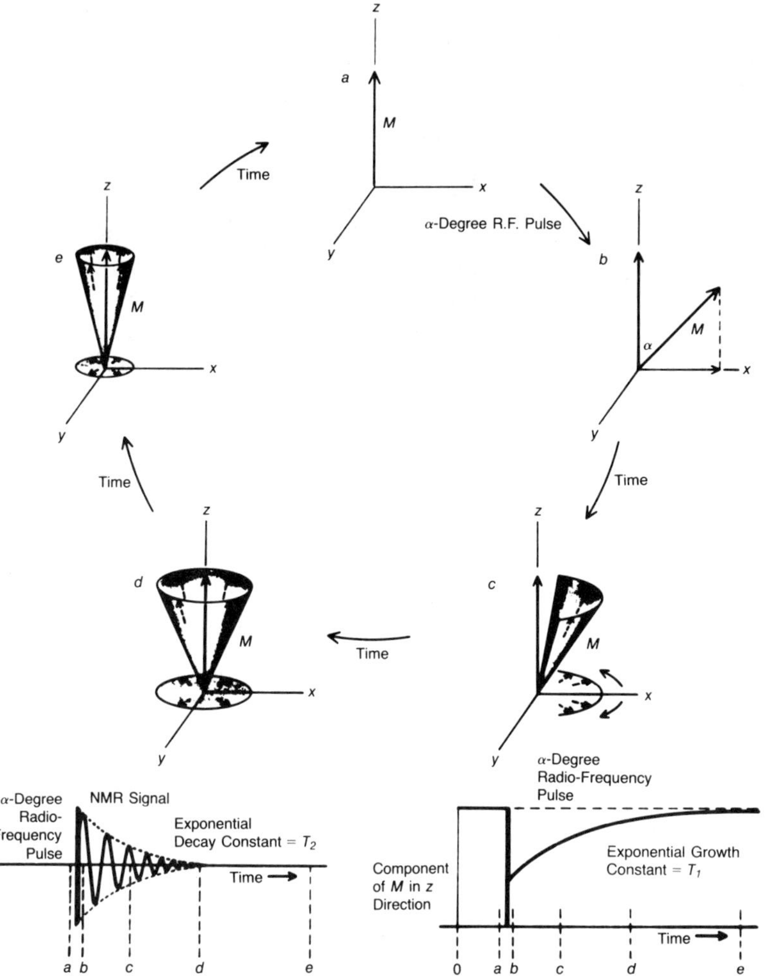

Figure 20.3 In a pulsed NMR experiment the emitted signal is observed after the radio-frequency energy that induces precession is turned off. In these diagrams the frame of reference is assumed to be rotating at the average Larmor frequency. After a radio-frequency pulse tips the vector of net magnetic moment M through some angle, a, there will be a component of M in the x-y plane (b). For a brief instant the NMR signal is at a maximum (*curve at bottom left*). Nuclei immediately begin to precess, however, at slightly different rates because of magnetic interaction between nuclei and slight nonuniformities in the magnetic field. The net component of M in the x-y plane therefore diminishes, and the signal amplitude decays exponentially with a time constant T_2 (c, d). If the magnetic field B_0 is perfectly uniform, the signal decay time is longer, and the time constant is T_2, called the spin-spin relaxation time. Simultaneously the longitudinal component of magnetization increases as M returns to its equilibrium position, aligned with the z axis (e). This relaxation, designated T_1 (spin-lattice relaxation time), measures the time needed for the spin system to return to thermal equilibrium (*curve at bottom right*).

Table 20.1   RELAXATION TIMES OF NORMAL HUMAN TISSUES AT 20 MHz (0.5 T) AND 40° C[a]

TISSUE	T_2 (ms)	T_1 (ms)
Liver	397	96
Muscle (skeletal)	629	45
Muscle (heart)	644	75
Kidney	765	124
Spleen	760	140
Brain (white matter)	687	107
Brain (grey matter)	825	110
Adipose	192	108
Lung	756	139
Blood	893	362
Pancreas	572	189
Prostate	808	98
Testis	974	153

[a] From Bottomley PA et al, 1984.

shift" effect. Blood and CSF often appear dark in MR images because of their long T_1 and T_2. Among other tissues such as brain, liver, and muscle there is a range of T_1 and T_2 values (see Table 20.1). MR images can be generated which give exquisite anatomical detail as seen in Figure 20.4.

The major advantages of MRI as a diagnostic imaging modality include the use of nonionizing radiation, modest magnetic fields, and its noninvasive nature. Primary disadvantages include the expensive instrumentation, relatively lengthy data col-

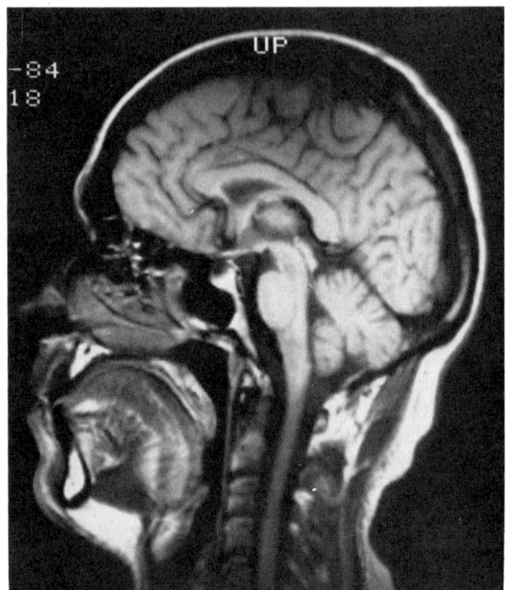

Figure 20.4   A transverse cranial MR image.

lection, and the occasional lack of diagnostic specificity, in spite of excellent anatomical detail. An illustration of the latter disadvantage is that most pathologic lesions produce regions of lengthened T_1 regardless of their nature. Thus, a region visualized on MRI with long T_1 may represent either tumor, edema, hemorrhage, inflammation, or necrosis. It is hoped that MR contrast agents which selectively alter T_1 values between tissues will provide a means of obtaining images of greater diagnostic specificity and enhanced anatomical detail. Also, MRI contrast agents have the potential to lower T_1 values of tissues, enabling image acquisition over shorter periods of time, with an additional potential improvement in cost effectiveness. More important for the future, MR contrast agents permit extensions of imaging conditions into regions that currently have poor tissue contrast. For example, in tissues that have low magnetization, rapid pulsing sequences and/or small tip angles may not produce adequate discrimination. These agents permit image acquisition. The ability to perform dynamic imaging with contrast agents will also enable potential assessment of organ function parameters including perfusion. These potential advantages cannot be realized without some risk to the patient or loss of invasiveness. Thus, MR contrast agents must possess low toxicity and a high margin of safety. Several excellent reviews of MRI contrast agents are available elsewhere. (Lauffer RB, 1987; Tweedle MF, et al, 1988; Runge VM, et al, 1986; Wolf GL, et al, 1985; Ogan MK and Brasch RC, 1985).

History of Contrast Agents in MRI

The use of paramagnetic metal ions as relaxation rate enhancers to facilitate acquisition of MR data dates back to the discovery of the NMR phenomenon. In 1946 F Bloch and colleagues reported the use of ferric nitrate to enhance the relaxation rate of water protons. The rate enhancement was found to depend linearly upon the concentration of the paramagnetic ion. Over the following decade extensive studies of rate enhancements by each of the paramagnetic first-row transition metal ions led to the formulation of the Solomon–Bloembergen–Morgan (SBM) theory (Solomon I, 1955; Bloembergen N, 1957; Bloembergen N and Morgan LO, 1961) that predicts the relaxation rates of solutions of the aquoions of the first-row transition metal and their frequency dependence. An introduction to this theory will be presented in the following section because of its established value for contrast agents both in vivo and in aqueous solution.

The first MR images (of test tubes filled with water) were made by Lauterbur in 1973. Human images were produced in 1977 (Hinshaw WS, et al, 1977; Andrew, et al, 1977; Damadian R, et al, 1977). Lauterbur, Mendonca-Dias, and Rudin first demonstrated the use of paramagnetic ions in tissue (1978) when they injected Mn(II) salts into dogs with myocardial infarcts produced by coronary artery occlusion and found differential uptake of Mn(II) by normal and infarcted tissue and observable differences in tissue relaxation rates. Thirty minutes after injection of 0.1 mmol/kg of Mn(II), the relaxation rate of normal myocardium had increased from 3.2 to 16.3 s^{-1} whereas infarcted myocardium increased from 2.9 to 6.0 s^{-1} (in vitro measurement). They also injected various amounts of Mn(II) into rats and analyzed for Mn content in liver and T_1 relaxation rate. The results indicated a linear relationship between the T_1 relaxation rate and Mn concentration in liver tissue over the range of 0–2 mmols/kg. Thus, the same general relationship between paramagnetic ion concentration and relaxation rate enhancement exists for tissue as for aqueous solution.

Although the aquoions of Mn(II) and Gd(III) were found to be extremely effective for enhancing proton relaxation rates, their relative toxicities were too great for routine human use. More recently, the search for contrast agents has centered upon chelated forms of paramagnetic ions

that clear more rapidly from the body and possess lesser toxicities than the unchelated metal ions. In addition to paramagnetic chelates, organic paramagnetic nitroxides and preparations of insoluble paramagnetic substances such as magnetite (Fe_3O_4) and magnetite-albumin microspheres are under investigation as potential contrast agents (Brasch RC, et al, 1983; Mendonca-Dias MH and Lauterbur PC, 1986; Widder DJ, et al, 1987). Also being investigated is the use of paramagnetic chelates that are covalently bound to serum proteins or monoclonal antibodies against tumor associated antigens (Lauffer RB, and Brady JJ, 1985; Shreve P and Aisen AM, 1986). Specialized delivery systems and paramagnetic species within liposomes are also under investigation (Navon G, et al, 1986).

The first paramagnetic chelate to be approved for clinical use is the Gd(III) complex of diethylenetriaminepentaacetate, Gd-DTPA (H-J Weinmann, et al, 1984). The clinical utility of Gd-DTPA was demonstrated (Carr DH, et al, 1984) who administered the agent intravenously to patients with intracranial tumors and

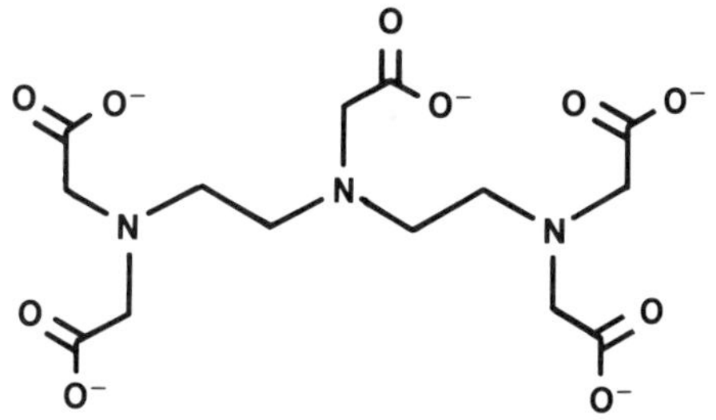

DTPA⁵⁻

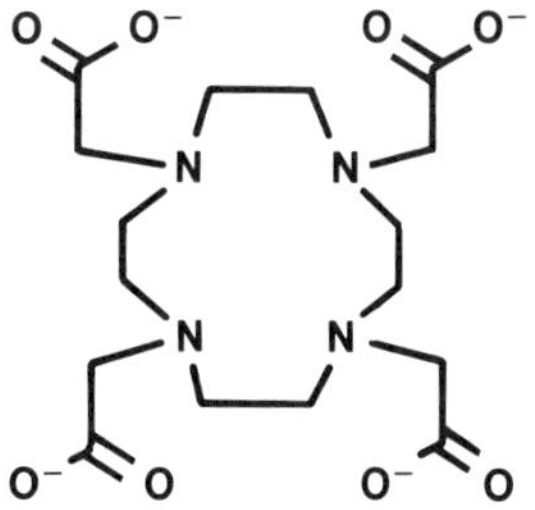

DOTA⁴⁻

obtained contrast-enhanced MR images showing bright rings around the tumors where the blood-brain barrier was disrupted. Another chelate of Gd(III), Gd-DOTA (1,4,7,10-tetraazacyclododecane-1,4,7,10-tetraacetate), has a macrocyclic tetraamine ligand substituted by carboxymethyl groups, has recently been developed as a MRI contrast agent (Geraldes CFGC, et al, 1986; Magerstadt, et al, 1986; Meyer D, et al, 1987), and is currently in clinical trials in Europe. Other promising chelates of Mn(II) and Fe(III) are under investigation (see Lauffer RB, 1987). The following section on the chemistry of contrast agents emphasizes the requirements to be met in the design of MRI contrast agents.

CHEMISTRY

OVERVIEW OF REQUIREMENTS FOR MRI CONTRAST AGENTS

The two basic requirements for a MRI contrast agent are (1) that it is biocompatible and (2) that it sufficiently enhances the proton relaxation rate of tissue-water protons. Biocompatibility is governed by several interrelated properties of the paramagnetic compound: stability, toxicity, biodistribution, and pharmacokinetics. For the chelated species of any paramagnetic element, stability with respect to release of the metal ion (both thermodynamic and kinetic) is an important consideration. The efficacy of the compound to affect proton relaxation rate enhancement is related to the magnetic moment and electron spin relaxation rate of the metal ion, and the complex of the ion with its ligand molecule, through the number of exchanging coordinated water molecules in the complex. Also important are the effect of the ligand on the metal–water interaction and the microenvironment of the complex in vivo. Specifically, the rotational motion of the complex and whether this motion is influenced by binding of the complex to macromolecular components of the biomatrix can have an important effect on relaxation enhance-

ment. In the following sub-sections, each aspect of the chemistry related to biocompatibility and efficacy of the contrast agent is discussed.

SOLUTION EQUILIBRIA AND THERMODYNAMIC STABILITY OF METAL CHELATES

The formation of a complex between a metal ion and a chelating ligand can be represented by the equation:

$$M^{N+}(aq) + L^{n-}(aq) = (ML)^{N-n}(aq) \quad (1)$$

The equilibrium constant expression for the reaction, written in simplified form omitting charges, is

$$K^{ML} = \frac{[ML]}{[M][L]} \quad (2)$$

where the brackets denote concentrations in moles/liter. K^{ML} is called the stability constant or formation constant of the complex. It is important to remember that L is the ligand in its fully deprotonated form and the stability constant is applicable, therefore, to conditions most favorable for chelate formation: optimum pH (often very basic) and the absence of competing ions or ligands. Comparisons of stability constants to give a measure of the relative tendencies for complex formation under physiological conditions is not rigorously correct and can be very misleading because apparent binding often has a very strong pH dependence (see following).

The chelating efficacy of a ligand can be reduced considerably by competing ions. In human blood plasma, for example calcium ion $(10^{-3}\ M)$, hydrogen ion $(10^{-7}\ M)$ and a host of other metal cations Cu^{2+}, Mn^{2+}, Zn^{2+} and Fe^{3+} (total concentration range from 10^{-7} to $5 \times 10^{-5}\ M$ and ligand-free metal concentration 10^{-9} to $10^{-3}\ M$) compete with the paramagnetic metal ion for binding to the ligand sites. Anions such as carbonate $(0.02\ M)$, phosphate $(4 \times 10^{-4}\ M)$, hydroxide $(10^{-7}\ M)$ and a host of small molecule species such as amino acids, organic oxyacids, and ascorbate all compete with the chelating ligand for binding sites on the metal ion. Proteins such as albumin have a significant tendency to bind metal ions. Thus, a means is necessary for evaluating equilibrium constants under near physiological conditions and for further evaluating the effect of many competing ions on the chelation equilibrium. In fact, two approaches greatly simplify this seemingly impossible task. First, equilibrium constants are measured under conditions of constant ionic strength, with 0.1 molar or greater concentrations of an inert salt present. The reason for this is that equilibrium constants are true constants only when the concentrations of the species are expressed in terms of their activities. The activity of a species is proportional to the concentration, and the proportionality factor is called the activity coefficient. At ionic strengths of $0.1\,M$ or above, activity coefficients are independent of ionic strength. Thus, the activity coefficients can be incorporated into the equilibrium constant so that the constant can be expressed in terms of the concentrations of the species rather than their activities. The second approach simplifies the problem of quantifying the effect of interfering species on equilibria by the definition of the conditional stability constant. This approach is illustrated below using hydrogen ion as an interferrent due to its effect on the concentration of deprotonated ligand, which through protonation reduces the apparent coordinating ability.

Chelating ligands that have n potentially coordinating groups have a degree of affinity for protons as well as for metal cations. Stepwise protonation constants can be defined for the ligand as follows:

$$H^+ + L^{n-} = HL^{(n-1)-} \qquad K_1$$
$$\vdots$$
$$H^+ + H_{n-2}L^{2-} = H_{n-1}L^- \qquad K_{n-1}$$
$$H^+ + H_{n-1}L^- = H_nL \qquad K_n$$

$$\text{(3)}$$

where the K's are the equilibrium constants for each step expressed in terms of concentrations. It is also useful to define the protonation stability products:

Table 20.2   PROTONATION EQUILIBRIUM CONSTANTS FOR EDTA, DTPA AND DOTA

LOG K_n	EDTA[a]	DTPA[a]	DOTA[b]
$n = 1$	10.21	10.59	11.08
2	6.11	8.65	9.23
3	2.60	4.28	4.24
4	2.00	2.73	4.18
5		2.06	

[a] $0.1\,M$ KNO$_3$, from Letkeman and Martell, 1979.
[b] $1.0\,m$ NaCl, from Desreux, et al, 1981.

$$\beta_1 = K_1,\ \beta_2 = K_1 K_2,\ \ldots\ \beta_n = K_1 K_2 \ldots K_n$$

where $\beta_n = [H_n L]/[L^{n-}][H^+]^n$. The K's and β's are usually expressed as their log values. Alternately, the reversed reactions of those shown in Equation 3, called the acid dissociation constants, are listed in the opposite order and as negative log values with pK_1 referring to the dissociation of the first proton from the fully protonated acid. Experimentally, these constants are determined by potentiometric titration of the acid form of the ligand with hydroxide. The K_n's are adjusted to give a good fit to the titration data such that the difference between the calculated and observed pH is minimized. The resulting pK_a's for DTPA, DOTA and EDTA are listed in Table 20.2. These can be used to compute the distribution of various protonated species of the ligand at any pH. Diagrams showing the distribution of species for DTPA and DOTA are given in Figures 20.5 and 20.6.

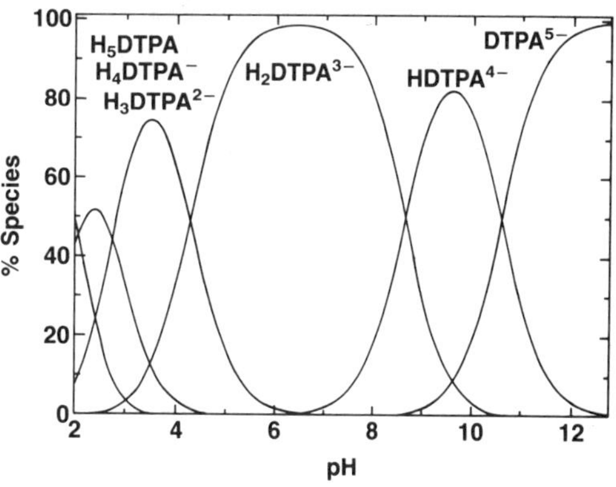

Figure 20.5 Distribution of various protonated forms of the DTPA ligand in aqueous solution as a function of pH.

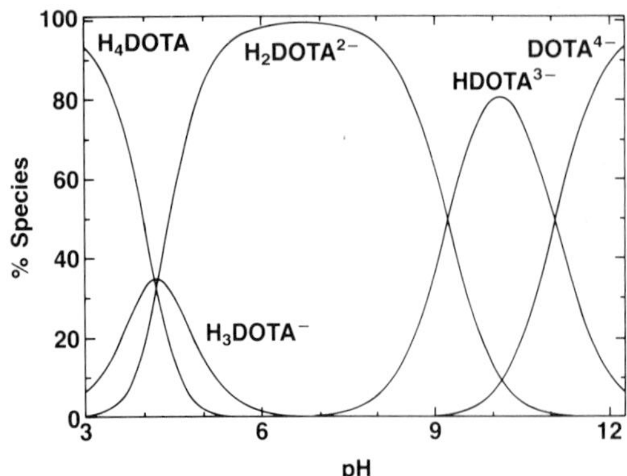

Figure 20.6 Distribution of various protonated forms of the DOTA ligand in aqueous solution as a function of pH.

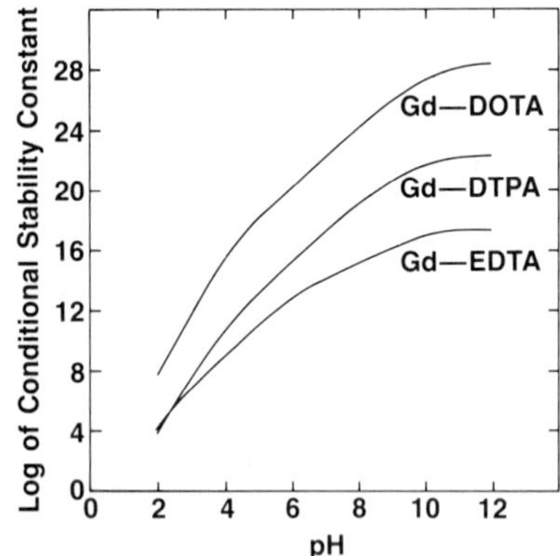

Figure 20.7 Plot of the conditional stability constant for the formation of gadolinium complexes of EDTA, DTPA, and DOTA as a function of pH.

Although it would appear a very complicated matter to express the effect of n protonation equilibria upon the stability of a metal complex involving the same ligand, in fact a very simple approach has been developed. It involves the definition of a conditional or effective stability constant (Ringbom A, 1958). Using proton interferrence as an example, α_L represents the fraction of free ligand L in its completely deprotonated form, L^{n-}, under the specified conditions. If T_L is the total concentration of uncomplexed ligand, then the actual concentration of L^{n-} is

$$[L^{n-}] = T_L \alpha_L \qquad (4)$$

α_L can be computed from the protonation stability products of the ligand and the hydrogen ion concentration as follows:

$$\alpha_L = (1 + [H^+]\beta_1 \\ + [H^+]^2\beta_2 + \ldots [H^+]^n\beta_n)^{-1} \qquad (5)$$

Since T_L is a known quantity, the conditional stability constant is defined as

$$K_{cond}^{ML} = \frac{[ML]}{[M]T_L} = \frac{[ML]}{[M][L^{n-}]} \cdot \alpha_L \qquad (6)$$

$$\log K_{cond}^{ML} = \log K^{ML} + \log(\alpha_L) \qquad (7)$$

Since α_L is always less than one, $\log(\alpha_L)$ is negative and the conditional stability constant is less than K^{ML}. This conditional stability constant is an approximation be-

cause complexation of any protonated forms of the ligand are neglected. Plots of pK_{cond}^{ML} versus pH for the Gd^{3+} complexes of DOTA, DTPA, AND EDTA are shown in Figure 20.7.

Similar expressions can be derived for metal ion interference (Pitt and Martell, 1980); for example, for Ca^{2+}:

$$K^{CaL} = [CaL]/[Ca^{2+}][L] \qquad (8)$$

and from the above equation

$$\alpha_M = [M]/T_M = (1 + [Ca^{2+}]K_{CaL})^{-1} \qquad (9)$$

Similarly, a K_{cond} can be written as:

$$\log K_{cond}^{ML} = \log K^{ML} + \log(\alpha_M) \qquad (10)$$

Finally, considering both the effects of hydrogen ion and calcium interference,

$$\log K_{cond}^{ML} = \log K^{ML} + \log(\alpha_L) + \log(\alpha_M) \qquad (11)$$

In order to avoid exchange of the metal ion between the ligand and the binding sites in the biological milieu, the stability constant of the contrast agent complex must be very high, greater than 10^{15}. Thus, the formulation of principles for the design of ligands having high stability constants with Gd^{3+} is very important. Because Gd^{3+} is a lanthanide ion with a $4f^7$ electron configuration having a half-filled

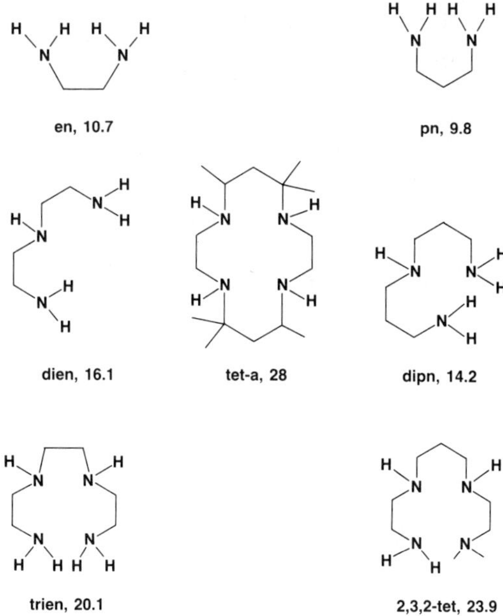

Figure 20.8 Log K^{CuL} for Cu^{2+} complexes of some multidentate ligands at 25° C.

shell, there are no ligand field stabilization effects that predispose Gd^{3+} toward certain coordination numbers or geometries. Gd^{3+} behaves most like an alkaline earth ion with ionic radius comparable to Ca^{2+} but with +3 charge. Thus, ligands interact with Gd^{3+} by coulombic attraction. Mn^{2+} and Fe^{3+} are similar in their ligand preferences. High stability is achieved by maximizing the enthalpy (ΔH) of attraction by using charged donor groups such as carboxylate and by incorporating these into a ligand that is a single molecule and wraps around the metal ion coordinating to it without undue steric strain and interligand charge repul-

sions. A further advantage of a chelating ligand is found in the entropy term of the free energy, which is more favorable for a chelate complex compared to a complex with similar monodentate ligands. This is the "chelate effect" and is illustrated in Figure 20.8 for some copper complexes (Hanzlik, 1976). The chelate effect can be extended to cyclic ligands (macrocycles). An additional stabilization is seen when the ends of a linear ligand are connected, hence the term "macrocyclic effect" (see Figure 20.8). In addition there are myriad more subtle factors that contribute to high stability. Some are summarized in Table 20.3. Among these factors, the size of the chelate ring seems to be quite important in maximizing the enthalpy of binding. The five-membered chelate ring shows enhanced stability over both smaller and larger ring sizes. This effect is illustrated in Table 20.4, which gives the stabilities and thermodynamic changes for Ca^{2+} complexes of EDTA-like ligands that vary the ring size in the alkylenediamine unit.

All of the effects described in Table 20.4 contribute to the relative stabilities of Gd(DOTA), Gd(DTPA), and Gd-(EDTA). A comparison of the characteristics of these ligands related to thermodynamic stability of the complexes is given in Table 20.5.

It is notable that DOTA and DTPA have the same number of coordinating groups all connected by five-membered rings. The ligands differ by one charge unit and one chelate ring because DOTA replaces one carboxylate with an amine donor atom that is part of the macrocyclic structure. The higher stability of the

Table 20.3 FACTORS INFLUENCING SOLUTION STABILITIES OF COMPLEXES[a]

ENTHALPY EFFECTS	ENTROPY EFFECTS
Number, charge, and basicity of coordinating groups	Number of chelate rings
Variation of bond strength with electronegativities of metal ions and ligand donor atoms	Size of the chelate rings
Ligand field effects	Arrangement of the chelate rings
Effects related to the conformation of the uncoordinated ligand	Changes in solvation upon complex formation
Steric and electrostatic repulsions between ligand donor groups in the complex	Entropy effects in the uncoordinated ligand
Size and arrangement of the chelate rings	Effects resulting from differences in configurational entropies of the free ligand and the complexed ligand (rigidity of the ligand)

[a] From Pitt CG and Martell AE, 1980.

Table 20.4   VARIATION OF THERMODYNAMIC CONSTANTS AS A FUNCTION OF CHELATE RING SIZE[a]

$$CA^{2+}(AQ) + (^-OOCCH_2)_2N—(CH_2)_n—N(CH_2COO^-)_2 = [CA\ CHELATE]^{2-}$$

n	Ring Size	log K^{ML}	$-\Delta H°$ (kcal/mol)	$\Delta S°$ (cal/deg mol)
2	5	10.7	6.55	26.6
3	6	7.28	1.74	27.4
4	7	5.66	0.9	29.7

[a] From Andregg G, 1964.

Table 20.5   THERMODYNAMIC CHARACTERISTICS OF GADOLINIUM CHELATES

GADOLINIUM CHELATE	LIGAND CHARGE	LOG K^{ML}	COORDINATION NUMBER	NUMBER OF FIVE-MEMBERED RINGS	SUM OF LIGAND pK_a's
$[Gd(DOTA)]^-$	4–	28.5	8	8	30.6
$[Gd(DTPA)]^{2-}$	5–	22.4	7 or 8	6 or 7	27.7
$[Gd(EDTA)]^-$	4–	17.4	6	5	20.8

DOTA complex is related to the added chelate ring and the structure of the macrocyclic ligand (macrocyclic effect). In addition, the sum of the pK_a's for DOTA is higher than for the other two ligands. A correlation has been made between log K^{ML} for aminocarboxylate ligands and the sum of the pK_a's (Figure 20.9). Rigidity also is important in enhancing the binding to metals such as Gd^{3+} and in determining the specificity of binding of various metals. The DOTA ligand is remarkably rigid in comparison with DTOA and EDTA. Thus, DOTA is also more specific in its

Table 20.6   SPECIFIC AFFINITY OF LIGANDS FOR GADOLINIUM

METAL	LOG $K^{Gd\text{-}DOTA}$ – LOG $K^{M\text{-}DOTA}$	LOG $K^{Gd\text{-}DTPA}$ – LOG $K^{M\text{-}DTPA}$
Ca^{2+}	11.3	11.6
Zn^{2+}	7.4	3.9
Cu^{2+}	6.3	0.9
Fe^{3+}	—	–5.0

binding than is DTPA, as can be seen from the data in Table 20.6.

KINETIC STABILITY OF METAL COMPLEXES

To minimize toxicities and to achieve optimal tissue localization capabilities, metal ions should remain firmly bound to the ligand and not dissociate. High thermodynamic stability ensures that the fraction of time a paramagnetic ion spends in the unbound state will be small but places no restriction on the rate of exchange between the two environments. The rates of formation (k_f) and dissociation (k_d) are related to the stability constant by the following equation:

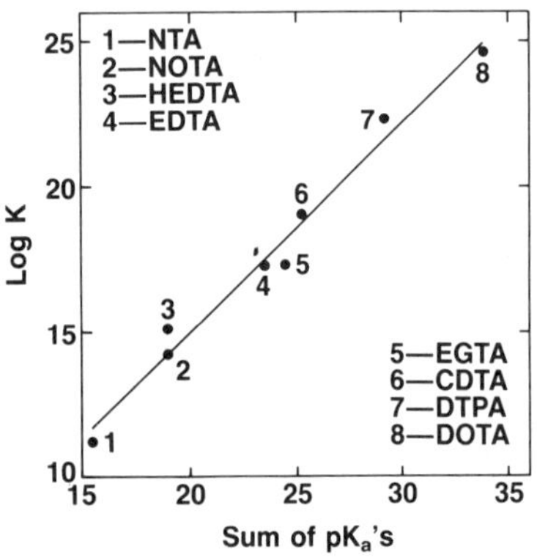

Figure 20.9 Plot of Gd^{3+} stability constants versus the sum of the pK_a's for a variety of polyamino polycarboxylate ligands.

$$K^{ML} = \frac{k_f}{k_d} \qquad (12)$$

Table 20.7   FORMATION AND DISSOCIATION RATES FOR CU^{2+} COMPLEXES[a]

LIGAND	k_f (M sec)$^{-1}$ (0.5 M OH^-)	k_d (sec^{-1}) (ACID)
en	3.8×10^9	[b]
trien	1.0×10^7	4.1
tet-a	1.6×10^3	3.6×10^{-7}
porphyrin	2.0×10^{-2}	[c]

[a] From Hanzlik RP, 1976.
[b] Not measured under these conditions.
[c] Too slow to be measured.

Table 20.8   MAGNETIC MOMENTS AND ESTIMATED ELECTRON SPIN RELAXATION TIMES FOR SOME PARAMAGNETIC METAL IONS COMMONLY USED IN NMR

METAL ION	MAGNETIC MOMENT (BM)	τ_s (sec)[a]
Ti^{3+}	1.7–1.8	10^{-9}–10^{-10}
V^{2+}	3.8	5×10^{-10}
V^{3+}	2.6–2.8	5×10^{-12}
VO^{2+}	1.7	10^{-8}–10^{-9}
Cr^{3+}	3.8	10^{-11}
Cr^{2+}	4.9	10^{-11}
Mn^{3+}	4.9	10^{-10}–10^{-11}
Mn^{2+}	5.9	10^{-8}–10^{-9}
Fe^{3+} (H.S.)	5.9	10^{-10}–10^{-11}
Fe^{3+} (L.S.)	2.0	10^{-11}–10^{-12}
Co^{2+} (H.S.)	4.1–5.2	10^{-11}–10^{-12}
Co^{2+} (L.S.)	3.8	10^{-9}–10^{-10}
Ni^{2+}	2.8–4.0	10^{-9}–10^{-12}
Cu^{2+}	1.7–2.2	1–3×10^{-9}
Ru^{3+}	0–3	10^{-11}–10^{-12}
Re^{3+}	0–2	10^{-11}
Gd^{3+}	7.94	10^{-8}–10^{-9}
Dy^{3+}	10.63	8×10^{-13}
Ho^{3+}	10.60	7.5×10^{-13}
Tb^{3+}	9.72	8×10^{-13}
Tm^{3+}	7.3	8×10^{-13}
Yb^{3+}	4.5	1×10^{-12}

[a] Electron spin relaxation time (from Bertini and Luchinat, 1986).

Thus, for a stable complex, the ratio of the rates of formation and dissociation is large, but the rates themselves may be large as well, depending on the nature of the ligand. The data in Table 20.7 show that the chelate and macrocyclic effects for complexes of Cu^{+2} are important with respect to the rates as well as the stability.

The tet-a macrocyclic complex (see Figure 20.8 for structure of tet-a) forms orders of magnitude more slowly than the open chain ligands, but the effect is even more pronounced on the dissociation kinetics, due to the fact that dissociation of a macrocyclic ligand may involve simultaneous breaking of more than one bond. The rigidity of the macrocyclic or chelating ligand is important in slowing down the exchange kinetics.

Nuclear Relaxation Enhancement by Paramagnetic Complexes

Paramagnetic metal complexes can be placed in two categories—shift reagents or relaxation agents—based upon their effect on the NMR behavior of nearby nuclei. "Shift reagents" cause large changes in the resonant frequency, by up to hundreds of ppm, but small changes in the relaxation rate. Prime examples are the lanthanide shift reagents and Ni^{2+} ion and other ions with short electron spin relaxation time (see Table 20.8). "Relaxation agents," on the other hand, cause little shift in resonant frequency but large enhancement in the nuclear relaxation rate. Exemplary complexes are those of Gd(III), Mn(II) and Fe(III), all ions having half-filled f or d electronic shells and long electron spin relaxation time. NMR contrast agents, because they function by relaxation rate enhancement, are among the second class of complexes. This subsection discusses the means by which relaxation enhancement occurs and the relationship between the magnitude of the enhancement and the physicochemical properties of the complex.

The longitudinal relaxation time of water proton nuclei T_1 is shortened by dissolving a relaxation-enhancing paramagnetic complex in the water. A plot of T_1 versus concentration of the metal complex typically has the form shown in Figure 20.10. If the relaxation *rate*, $1/T_1$, is plotted versus the concentration, a linear relationship is revealed as shown in Figure 20.11. The slope of the straight line is the relaxation rate enhancement per unit concentration of complex and is called the relaxivity, R_1, of the complex. The intercept of the line in Figure 20.11 is the relaxation rate of pure water. The transverse relaxation time, T_2, shows the same qualitative behavior as T_1. Thus, a complex can be characterized by its relaxivities, R_1 and R_2, usually expressed in units of mM^{-1}sec^{-1}. Because relaxivities are

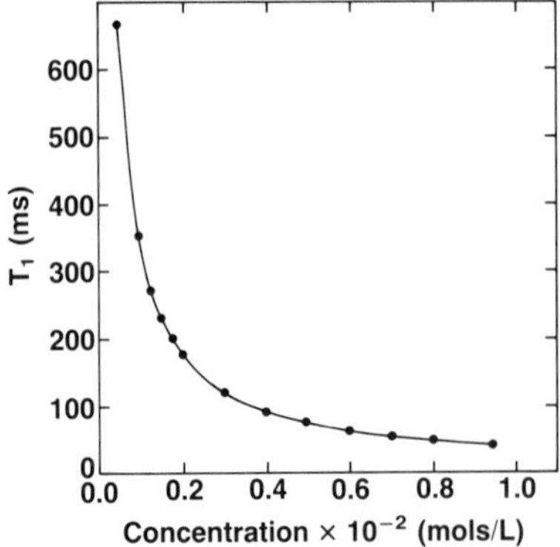

Figure 20.10 Plot of the spin-lattice relaxation time of an aqueous solution of a paramagnetic complex ($R_1 = 2.6$ (mMs)$^{-1}$) as a function of concentration of complex.

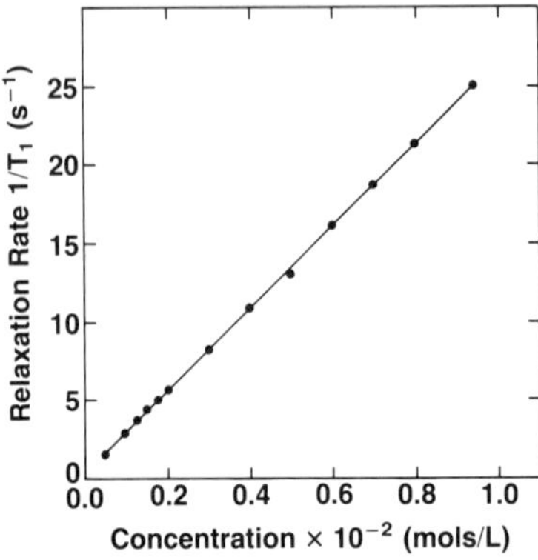

Figure 20.11 Plot of the longitudinal relaxation rate ($1/T_1$) for an aqueous solution of a paramagnetic complex ($R_1 = 2.6$ (mMs)$^{-1}$) as a function of concentration of complex.

Table 20.9 LONGITUDINAL RELAXIVITIES FOR COMPLEXES AT 20 MHz AND 37° C

COMPLEX	R_1 (mMsec)$^{-1}$	REFERENCE
$Gd(H_2O)_{8 \text{ or } 9}^{3+}$	9.1 (35° C)	a
$Gd(EDTA)(H_2O)_{2 \text{ or } 3}^{-}$	5.4	b
$Gd(DTPA)(H_2O)^{2-}$	3.7	b
$Gd(DOTA)(H_2O)^{-}$	3.4	b
$Mn(H_2O)_6^{2+}$	8.0	c
$Mn(EDTA)(H_2O)^{2-}$	2.0	b
$Mn(DTPA)^{3-}$	1.1	b
$Mn(DOTA)^{2-}$	1.1	b
$Fe(H_2O)_6^{3+}$	8.0	a
	(35° C, pH 2)	
$Fe(EDTA)(H_2O)^{-}$	1.6	b
$Fe(DTPA)^{2-}$	0.7	b
$Fe(DOTA)^{-}$	0.4	b

[a] From Dwek RA, 1973.
[b] From Koenig SH and Brown RD III, 1987a, Tweedlle MF, et al, 1988.
[c] From Chen C, et al, 1984.

dependent upon frequency and temperature, these must also be specified. Some R_1 values for metal complexes are given in Table 20.9. A more extensive list has been compiled by Lauffer (1987).

The linear relationship between relaxation rate and concentration of complex can be understood in terms of a model in which water is rapidly exchanging between the bulk solvent environment and the coordination sites of the metal complex.

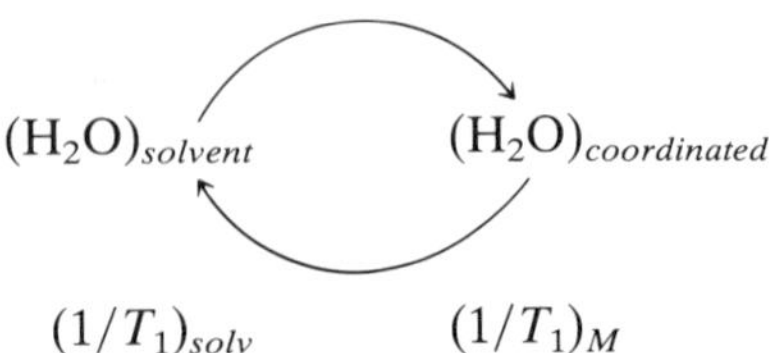

Rapid exchange

$(1/T_1)_{solv}$ is the relaxation rate of the solvent water protons and $(1/T_1)_M$ is the relaxation rate of protons in water coordinated to the metal ion M. The observed relaxation rate $(1/T_1)_{obs}$ is the sum of the mole fraction of water in each environment times the relaxation rate in that environment (Equation 13).

$$(1/T_1)_{obs} = X_{solv}(1/T_1)_{solv} + X_{coordinated}(1/T_1)_M \qquad (13)$$

The mole fraction of solvent water is well approximated by 1, and the mole fraction of coordinated water is $q[M]/55.5$, where q is the number of coordinated water molecules in the complex, $[M]$ is the molarity of the complex, and 55.5 is the molarity of water. Substituting, Equation 13 becomes

$$(1/T_1)_{obs} = (1/T_1)_{solv} + (q[M]/55.5)(1/T_1)_M \qquad (14)$$

Thus, the relaxivity, R_1, is equal to $q/55.5(1/T_1)_M$.

The relaxation rate of protons in a water molecule coordinated to a paramagnetic ion, $(1/T_1)_M$, is given by the Solomon–Bloembergen equation that expresses the rate as the sum of dipolar (through space) and scalar (through bonds) contributions (Equation 15):

$$\left(\frac{1}{T_1}\right)_M = \left(\frac{2}{15}\right)\left(\frac{\gamma_I^2 g^2 S(S+1)\beta^2}{r^6}\right)$$
$$\left\{\frac{7\tau_c}{1+\omega_s^2\tau_c^2} + \frac{3\tau_c}{1+\omega_I^2\tau_c^2}\right\}$$
$$+ \left(\frac{2}{3}\right)S(S+1)\left(\frac{A}{\hbar}\right)^2\left\{\frac{\tau_e}{1+\omega_s^2\tau_e^2}\right\} \quad (15)$$

where γ_I is the proton gyromagnetic ratio, g is the electronic g-factor, S is the total electron spin of the metal ion, β is the Bohr Magneton, r is the proton-metal ion distance, ω_s and ω_I are the electronic and proton Larmor frequencies, and $A/\hbar$ is the electron-nuclear hyperfine coupling constant. Both terms consist of the magnitude of the interaction (dipole–dipole or scalar) multiplied by a function of the correlation time, which expresses the intensity of modulation of the interaction at the Larmor frequency. The correlation times τ_c and τ_e are given by Equations 16 and 17:

$$\frac{1}{\tau_c} = \frac{1}{\tau_r} + \frac{1}{\tau_M} + \frac{1}{\tau_s} \quad (16)$$

$$\frac{1}{\tau_e} = \frac{1}{\tau_M} + \frac{1}{\tau_s} \quad (17)$$

where τ_r is the rotational correlation time (on the order of 10^{-11} sec for a moderate molecular weight complex), τ_m is the average residence time of a water molecule in the coordinated state (on the order of 10^{-6} to 10^{-9} sec for a labile metal ion), and τ_s is the electron spin relaxation time of the metal ion (see Table 20.9). It is clear that $1/\tau_c$ is dominated by the fastest of the processes, $1/\tau_r$, $1/\tau_M$, or $1/\tau_s$ to which it is related. For the metal ions most suitable for NMR contrast agents (Gd(III), Mn(II), or Fe(III)), τ_c is dominated by the rotational contribution because water exchange and electron spin relaxation are slower processes. The rotational correlation time for a molecule of radius a isotropically rotating in a medium of viscosity η can be estimated from the Stokes–Einstein equation

$$\tau_r = (4\pi\eta a^3)/(3kT) \quad (18)$$

where k and T are the Boltzmann constant and the absolute temperature. The sensitivity of the rotational correlation time to the chemical microenvironment of the complex can have a large effect on the relaxivity. Large molecules such as proteins rotate much more slowly and have τ_r on the order of 10^{-6} to 10^{-8} seconds. A paramagnetic complex bound either covalently or noncovalently to the large molecule will have τ_c between that of the free complex (10^{-11} sec) and that of the protein. This effect can cause a large increase in relaxivity, by a factor of 10 to 100, as well as dramatic changes in the frequency dependence of the relaxation rate.

In cases of metal ions with $S > 1/2$ there is an additional electron spin relaxation effect that can affect the relaxivity at low frequencies. This mechanism is due to instantaneous distortions of the complex, presumably due to collisions with solvent molecules, which modulate the zero field splitting of the metal ion. A frequency dependence in τ_s is introduced by this effect and can be reflected in a frequency dependence in τ_c for the complex. Bloembergen and Morgan (1961) developed the following equation to express the frequency dependence of τ_s:

$$\frac{1}{\tau_s} = C\left\{\frac{\tau_v}{1+\omega_s^2\tau_v^2} + \frac{4\tau_v}{1+4\omega_s^2\tau_v^2}\right\} \quad (19)$$

where C is proportional to the square of the fluctuations in the zero field splitting and τ_v is the correlation time for the fluctuations, and the other parameters are as defined above. When Equation 19 is incorporated into the definition of τ_c given in Equation 17, the resulting equation is known as the Solomon–Bloembergen–Morgan (SBM) equation. A similar series of equations can be derived for T_2 relaxation. Several excellent monographs are available that describe the treatment of relaxation mechanisms in detail and discuss the conditions under which the SBM equations apply (see Dwek A, 1973; Bertini I and Luchinat C, 1986; Koenig SH and Brown RD III, 1987b).

The most informative method for studying relaxation phenomena in metallo-aquoions, complexes, and proteins is to measure the relaxation rate as a function of frequency over a large range, most commonly from 0.01 to 50 MHz or higher. The field dependence of the relaxation rate is called relaxation dispersion; thus the curves depicting the dispersion are called nuclear magnetic relaxation dispersion profiles or NMRD profiles. These profiles will be the method of choice for evaluating the relaxation enhancement efficacy of potential contrast agents. The NMRD profiles for four aquoions are shown in Figure 20.12. Three of the ions, Fe^{3+}, Cu^{2+}, and Gd^{3+}, have one dispersion that is typical of metal ions in which the scalar contribution to the relaxation rate is negligible. Looking at Equation 15 and considering only the first (dipolar) term, it can be seen that at low frequency when both $\omega_s^2\tau_c^2$ and $\omega_I^2\tau_c^2$ are much less than 1, the relaxivity is proportional to $10\tau_c$. Since ω_s is so much greater than ω_I ($\omega_S/\omega_I = 658$ for electrons and protons),

the term proportional to $7\tau_c$ is expected to decrease as $\omega_s^2\tau_c^2$ approaches, then exceeds, 1 as the frequency is increased. Thus, the relaxivity will disperse from a low field value proportional to $10\tau_c$ to a value proportional to $3\tau_c$. At the frequency of the inflection point in the dispersion the correlation time can be estimated because $\omega_s\tau_c = 1$. Note that $\omega_s = 2\pi \times 658 \times$ frequency in Hz. An inflection point at about 10 MHz gives a correlation time on the order of 10^{-11} sec, consistent with the rotational contribution being dominant. It is also interesting to note that the $3\tau_c$ term is predicted to disperse at extremely high field, on the order of 10^6 MHz, which is presently unattainable. From Figure 20.12 it is seen that the dipolar term of Equation 15 qualitatively describes the NMRD profiles and that the dispersion inflection at about 10 MHz indicates that the correlation time is dominated by the rotational contribution (Koenig SH and Brown RD III, 1984a). The Mn^{2+} ion has an additional dispersion at low field due to the scalar term in Equation 15. The data for all the metal ions can be quantitatively fitted to a good degree of accuracy if the full SBM equations are used and a small relaxivity contribution is added due to the interaction between the metal center and solvent water molecules, which do not enter the primary coordination sphere (outer sphere contribution).

In Figure 20.13 the NMRD profiles of some small chelate complexes of Mn^{2+} and Gd^{3+} are compared (Koenig SH, et al, 1984b). All have certain features in common. The shape of the curves indicates that the dipolar mechanism describes the relaxation process. The inflection points in the vicinity of 10 MHz indicate that the rotational motion is dominant in determining the correlation time. The EDTA chelates with six coordination sites occupied by the chelate have higher relaxivity due to more exchanging water molecules than the DTPA chelates in which the ligand occupies eight coordination sites. The number of coordinated water molecules are zero and one for the Mn DTPA and EDTA complexes and approximately

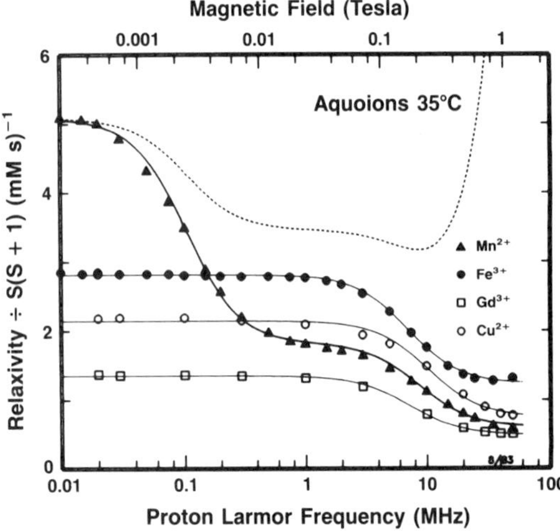

Figure 20.12 Plot of the field dependence of the relaxation rate (R_1 normalized to account for differences in the spin of the paramagnetic ions) for protons in aqueous solutions of several transition metal ions at 35° C. Plots such as this are called NMRD profiles. The dotted line is the $1/T_2$ profile for Mn^{2+} ion. The $1/T_2$ profiles of the other ions are expected to be similar to the $1/T_1$ profiles.

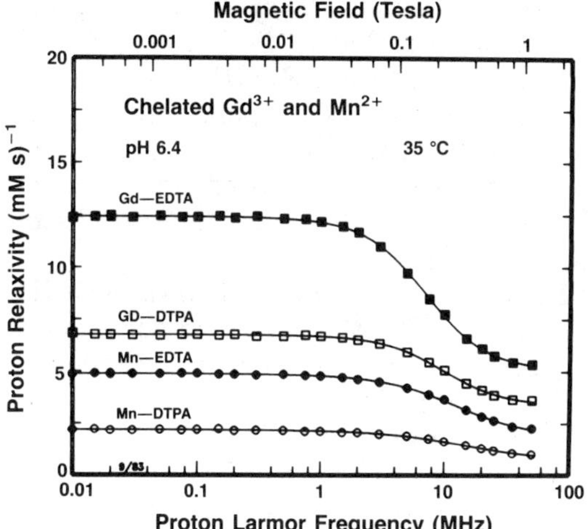

Figure 20.13 $1/T_1$ NMRD profiles for aqueous protons in solutions of Gd^{3+} and Mn^{2+} ions chelated with EDTA and DTPA.

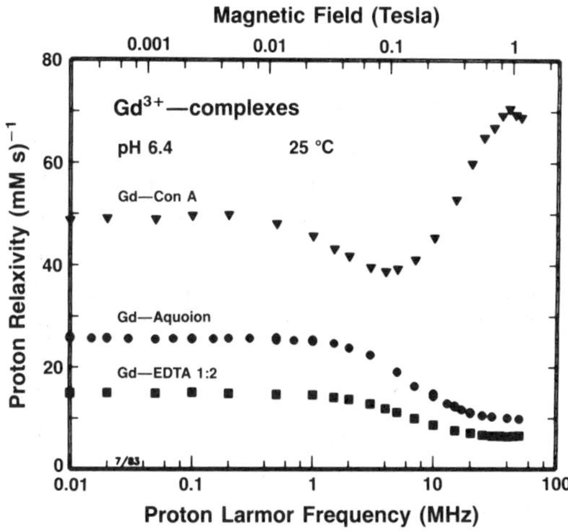

Figure 20.14 $1/T_1$ NMRD profiles for aqueous protons in solutions of Gd^{3+} ions in three chemical environments: aquoion, EDTA complex, and bound to native concanavalin A.

one and two for the Gd DTPA and EDTA complexes.

Tightly binding a metal ion to a macromolecular species such as a protein has a dramatic effect on the NMRD curve, as shown in Figure 20.14. First, due to the longer rotational correlation time, about 10^{-8} to 10^{-6} sec depending on the molecular weight, the correlation time of the molecule is dominated by the electron spin correlation time. The longer τ_c in

Equation 15 gives a much higher relaxivity per water molecule at low field. Furthermore, the strong frequency dependence of τ_s causes a dramatic increase in relaxivity in the intermediate frequency range, and the dispersion of the $\omega_s\tau_c$ term in Equation 15 is shifted to higher frequency by the longer correlation time, causing a maximum in the NMRD curve.

Studies of NMRD curves of tissue containing Gd(DTPA) indicate that the tissue environment is very similar to aqueous solution. The correlation time of the complex is not changed, presumably because the complex does not bind to tissue macromolecular structures nor does it release Gd ions. The shapes of the NMRD curves are indicative of tissue water with viscosity and other properties very similar to pure water (Koenig SH and Brown RD III, 1987b).

References

Andregg G. Komplexone XXXVI. Reactionsenthalpie und -entropie bei der Bildung der Metallkomplexe der Hohren EDTA-Homologen. *Helv Chim Acta* 1964, 47:1801–1814.

Andrew ER, Bottomley PA, Hinshaw WS, et al. NMR images by the multiple sensitive point method: Application to larger biological systems, *Phys Med Biol* 1977, 22:971–974.

Beall PT, Amter SR, Katsuri SR. *NMR Data Handbook for Biomedical Applications.* Elmsford, NY, Pergamon Press, 1984.

Bertini I, Luchinat C. *NMR of Paramagnetic Molecules in Biological Systems.* Menlo Park, CA, Benjamin/ Cummings, 1986.

Bloch F, Hansen WW, Packard M. The nuclear induction experiment. *Phys Rev* 1946, 70:474–485.

Bloembergen N. Proton relaxation times in paramagnetic solutions. *J Chem Phys* 1957, 27:572–573.

Bloembergen N, Morgan LO. Proton relaxation times in paramagnetic solutions. Effects of electron spin relaxation, *J Chem Phys* 1961, 34:842–850.

Bottomley PA. NMR in medicine, *Comput Radiol* 1984, 8:57–77.

Bottomley PA, Foster TH, Argersinger RE, Pfeifer, LM. A review of normal tissue hydrogen NMR relaxation times and relaxation mechanisms from 1–100 MHz: Dependence on tissue type, NMR frequency, temperature, species, excision and age, *Med Phys* 1984, 11:425–448.

Brasch RC, London DA, Wesbey GE, et al. Work in progress: Nuclear magnetic resonance study of a paramagnetic nitroxide contrast agent for enhancement of renal structures in experimental animals. *Radiology* 1983, 147:773–779.

Carr DH, Brown J, Bydder GM, et al. Gadolinium-DTPA as a contrast agent in MRI: Initial clinical experience in 20 patients, *Lancet* 1984, 484–486.

Chen C, Cohen JS, Myers CE, et al. Paramagnetic metalloporphyrins as potential contrast agents in NMR imaging, *FEBS Lett* 1984, 168:70–74.

Damadian R, Goldsmith M, Minkoff L. NMR in cancer: XVI. FONAR image of the live human body. *Physiol Chem Phys* 1977, 9:97–100.

Desreux JF, Merciny E, Loncin MF. Nuclear magnetic resonance and potentiometric studies of the protonation scheme of two tetraaza teraacetic macrocycles. *Inorg Chem* 1981, 20:987–991.

Dwek RA. *Nuclear Magnetic Resonance in Biochemistry: Applications to Enzyme Systems.* Oxford, Engl, Clarendon Press, 1973.

Geraldes CFGC, Sherry AD, Brown RD, Koenig, SH. Magnetic field dependence of solvent proton relaxation rates induced by Gd^{+3} and Mn^{+2} complexes of various polyaza macrocyclic ligands: Implications for NMR imaging. *Magn. Reson Med* 1986, 3:242–250.

Hanzlik RP. *Inorganic Aspects of Biological and Organic Chemistry*, New York, Academic Press, 1976, Chapter VI.

Hinshaw WS, Bottomley PA, Holland GN. Radiographic thin-section image of the human wrist by nuclear magnetic resonance, *Nature* 1977, 270:722–723.

Koenig SH, Brown RD III. Relaxation of solvent protons by paramagnetic ions and its dependence on magnetic field and chemical environment: Implications for NMR imaging, *Magn Reson Med* 1984a, 1:478–495.

Koenig SH, Baglin C, Brown RD III, Brewer CF. Magnetic field dependence of solvent proton relaxation induced by Gd^{+3} and Mn^{+2} complexes. *Magn Reson Med* 1984b 1:496–501.

Koenig SH, Brown RD III, Relaxometry of magnetic resonance imaging contrast agents, in *Magnetic Resonance Annual 1987*, Kressel HY (ed). New York, Raven, 1987a, 263–286.

Koenig SH, Brown RD III. "Relaxometry of Paramagnetic Ions in Tissue," in *Metal Ions in Biological Systems*, Sigel H (ed). Volume 21, New York, Marcel Dekker, 1987b, 229–270.

Lauffer RB, Brady TJ. Preparation and water relaxation properties of proteins labeled with paramagnetic metal chelates. *Magn Reson Imag* 1985, 3:11–16.

Lauffer RB. Paramagnetic metal complexes as water proton relaxation agents for NMR imaging: Theory and design, *Chem Rev* 1987, 87:901–927.

Lauterbur PC. Image formation by induced local interactions: Examples employing NMR, *Nature* 1973, 242:190–191.

Lauterbur PC, Mendonca-Dias MH, Rudin AM. Augmentation of tissue water proton spin-lattice relaxation rates by the in vivo addition of paramagnetic ions, in *Frontiers of Biological Energetics*, Dutton PL, et al (eds). New York, Academic Press, 1978, 364–376.

Letkeman P, Martell AE. Nuclear magnetic resonance and potentiometric protonation study of polyaminopolyacetic acids containing from two to six nitrogen atoms. *Inorg Chem* 1979, 18:1284–1289.

Magerstadt M, Gansow OA, Brechbiel MW, et al. Gd(DOTA): An alternative to Gd(DTPA) as a $T_{1,2}$ relaxation agent for NMR imaging or spectroscopy. *Magn Reson in Med* 1986, 3:808–812.

Mansfield P, Morris PG. *NMR Imaging in Biomedicine.* New York, Academic Press. 1982.

Mendonca-Dias H, Lauterbur PC. Ferromagnetic particles as contrast agents for magnetic resonance imaging of liver and spleen. *Magn Reson Med* 1986, 3:328–330.

Meyer D, Schaefer M, Bonnemain B. Gd-DOTA, A potential MRI contrast agent: Current status of physicochemical knowledge. Presented at the International Conference on Contrast Agents, 1987.

Navon G, Panigel R, Valensin G. Liposomes containing paramagnetic macromolecules as MRI contrast agents. *Magn Reson Med* 1986, 3:876–880.

Ogan MK, Brasch RC. Contrast enhancing agents in MRI imaging. Ann Repts Med Chem 1985, 20:277–286.

Partain CL, James AE, Rollo FD, et al (eds). *Magnetic Resonance Imaging.* Philadelphia, W.B. Saunders Co., 1988.

Pitt CG, Martell AE. The design of chelating agents for the treatment of iron overload, in *ACS Symposium Series No. 140*, Martell AE (ed). Washington DC, American Chemical Society, 1980, 279–312.

Ringbom A. The analyst and the inconstant constants. *J Chem Ed* 1958, 35:282–288.

Runge VM. Gd-DTPA. An i.v. contrast agent for clinical MRI, *Nucl Med Biol Int J Radiat Appl Instrum Part B* 1988, 15:37–44.

Shreve P, Alisen AM, Monoclonal antibodies labeled with polymeric paramagnetic ion chelates. *Magn Reson Med* 1986, 3:336–340.

Solomon I. Relaxation processes in a system of two spins, *Phys Rev* 1955, 99:559–565.

Tweedle MF, Brittain HG, Eckelman WC. et al. Principles of contrast enhanced MRI. In *Magnetic Resonance Imaging*, Partain CL, et al (eds). Philadelphia WB Saunders Co., 1988, pp. 793–809.

Tweedle MF, Gaughan GT, Hagan J, Wedeking PW, et al. Considerations involving paramagnetic coordination compounds as useful NMR contrast agents. *Int J Radiat Appl Instrum* 1988, Part B, 15:31–36.

Weinmann H-J, Brasch RC, Press W-R, Wesbey GE. Characteristics of gadolinium-DTPA complex: A potential NMR contrast agent. *AJR* 1984, 142:619–624.

Widder DJ, Greif WL, Widder KJ, et al. Magnetite albumin microspheres: A new MR contrast material. *AJR* 1987, 148:399–404.

Wolf GL, Popp C. *NMR: A Primer for Medical Imaging.* Thorofare, NJ, Slack, Inc., 1984.

Wolf GL, Burnett KR, Goldstein EJ, Joseph PM. Contrast agents for magnetic resonance imaging, in *Magnetic Resonance Annual 1985.* Kressel HY (ed). New York, Raven Press, 1985, 231–266.

Enhancement Agents for Magnetic Resonance Imaging: Clinical Applications

Sanjay Saini
Joseph T. Ferrucci

Even though the use of contrast media is widely recognized in diagnostic radiology, the application of contrast enhancement utilizing substances that affect paramagnetic properties is not so well known. Soon after the introduction of magnetic resonance (MR) imaging in 1973, it became apparent that a wide variety of chemical substances could be used to enhance contrast. Of these, several have been studied in laboratory settings as potential contrast agents for MR imaging, and a few are in various stages of clinical testing and development. To date, however, only a handful of the agents, called magnetopharmaceuticals (Chilton HM, et al, 1984), have shown significant clinical utility. Among the most widely studied to date is Gadolinium-DTPA (diethylene triamine pentaacetic acid, also known as gadopentetate-dimeglumine) which, in 1988, became the first MR contrast agent to be approved for clinical use in the United States. Although the discipline of MR contrast media development may be considered as still in its infancy, gadopentetate has already established a central role in neurological MR imaging. As more and more magnetopharmaceuticals are being made available, there is little doubt that contrast media will play an increasingly important role in routine MR imaging. The theoretical basis for MR image formation and contrast enhancement has been detailed in the first part of this chapter. This section deals with the clinical strategies and parameters that must be considered in the proper utilization of contrast enhancement.

Whereas x-ray imaging techniques are highly standardized and only three parameters can be manipulated to influence the effect of radiographic contrast media upon image enhancement (media dose, rate of administration, and time of imaging after drug administration), MR imaging and parameters involved in contrast enhancement are considerably more complex. The major reason for this is that there are many more operator-defined variables that can be manipulated to alter soft-tissue contrast (Wehrli FW, et al, 1984). These include: (1) choice of pulse sequences (spin echo [SE], inversion recovery [IR], gradient echo [GE]); (2) timing parameters (repetition time [TR], echo time [TE], inversion time [TI], flip angle (∞), number of excitations [NEX], etc.); and (3) imaging planes (sagittal, transverse, coronal, or oblique). For each pulse sequence, timing parameters can be infinitely varied to provide different degrees of T_1 and T_2 relaxation time-dependent soft-tissue contrast, and their selection will vary depending upon the strength of the external magnetic field and the relaxation times of tissues being imaged. Because these technical factors are not yet standardized, in routine clinical MR imaging there exist considerable machine-to-machine and site-to-site variations in their selection.

Introduction of MR contrast agents adds to this complexity. To begin with, numerous magnetopharmaceuticals, many with tissue-specific or disease-specific application, are being developed. The variety of MR contrast agents that will eventually become available is expected to exceed even the variety of radiopharmaceuticals utilized in nuclear medicine. Magnetopharmaceuticals also have a complex dose–dose dependent effect on MR images because they alter both T_1 and T_2 relaxation times, which has opposing effects on MR signal intensity (see Chapter 20). This effect is modulated by the pulse sequence and its timing parameters employed to produce the MR image. Thus appropriate use of contrast agents in MR imaging will require knowledge of the effects on tissue signal intensity of drug dose, pharmacokinetics, rate of administration, magnitude of the external magnetic field, pulse sequences, and their timing parameters. To avoid diagnostic errors, the appropriate application of MR contrast agents will require greater understanding of all relevant variables than has been necessary for conventional radiographic contrast media.

The purpose of this chapter is to describe how these technical factors can influence tissue signal intensity on contrast-enhanced MRI and to describe the appropriate imaging strategies of several prototype contrast agents.

Basis for Developing MR Contrast Agents

Soft-tissue contrast arises primarily as a result of differences in the relaxation times (T_1 and T_2) of tissues being compared (Wehrli FW, et al, 1984). Although relaxation times in pathologic tissue are generally prolonged in comparison to their normal counterparts (for example, liver cancer versus normal liver) there is large biologic variation in T_1 and T_2 times of all tissue types. Thus there is considerable overlap in relaxation times of normal and abnormal tissues and, for a given tissue pair in an individual, the differences in T_1 and T_2 relaxation times may indeed be very small. As a result, in a large population a single-screening MR pulse sequence, even when optimized for a specific organ, can not detect all pathologic processes. The evaluation of diffuse diseases is even more difficult because comparison with normal tissues is not always possible. Consequently, clinical MR imaging is performed with more than one pulse sequence. At the very least, these are selected to portray soft-tissue contrast based on differences in their T_1 and T_2 relaxation times. Still, the sensitivity of MR imaging falls well short of 100%. More specialized pulse sequences are needed to image unique physiologic phenomena such as blood flow (Wedeen VJ, et al, 1986).

In addition to the issue of disease detection, there is the objective of characterizing (tissue-typing) abnormal tissues detected. At the very least, benign processes need to be distinguished from malignant diseases. This is important because with increasing age many clinically insignificant focal and diffuse processes appear in various organs. Cavernous hemangiomas and fatty infiltration in the liver are such examples. Because benign and malignant diseases often coexist, the distinction between processes that require attention and those that may be ignored becomes imperative. In many cases, MR imaging is unable to provide this distinction.

The pharmaceutical manipulation of tissue-signal intensity has been recognized as a possible solution to overcome these deficiencies. MR contrast agents alter tissue relaxation times and can thereby influence tissue-signal intensity on MR images. The former phenomenon was first observed more than 40 years ago (Bloch, et al, 1946). The general aim of contrast-enhanced MR imaging is to augment relaxation time differences between normal and abnormal tissue that would result in greater signal intensity differences (more soft-tissue contrast) between them, allowing improved disease detection even with a standard screening pulse sequence. Alternatively MR contrast agents may be utilized to provide information on physiologic processes in vivo (for example, reticuloendothelial activity, hepatocyte function, tissue vascularity, tissue perfusion, etc.), thereby allowing tissue characterization.

Determinants of MR Signal Intensity

Tissue-relaxation times are the principal determinants of signal intensity in MR imaging (Wehrli FW et al, 1984; Moran, PR 1984). MR pulse sequence timing parameters are selected to determine the relative contribution of T_1 and T_2 relaxation time on MR signal intensity (Nelson TR et al, 1984; Hendrick RE et al, 1984). On pulse sequences in which signal intensity is based largely on the T_1 time (called T_1-weighted pulse sequences for convenience, although all pulse sequences portray signal intensity with contributions from both T_1 and T_2 relaxation times), tissues with short T_1 times (such as fat) appear hyperintense or bright, and tissues with long T_1 times (such as urine) appear hypointense or dark (Figure 21.1A). On T_2-weighted pulse sequences, this relationship is reversed. Thus tissues with short T_2 times (such as muscle) appear hypointense or dark, and tissues with long T_2 times (such as urine) appear hyperintense or bright (Figure 21.1B). Because, in general and with few exceptions, tissues with short T_1 times also possess short T_2 times, and tissues with long T_1 times have long T_2 times, hypointense structures on T_1-weighted pulse sequences will be hy-

A

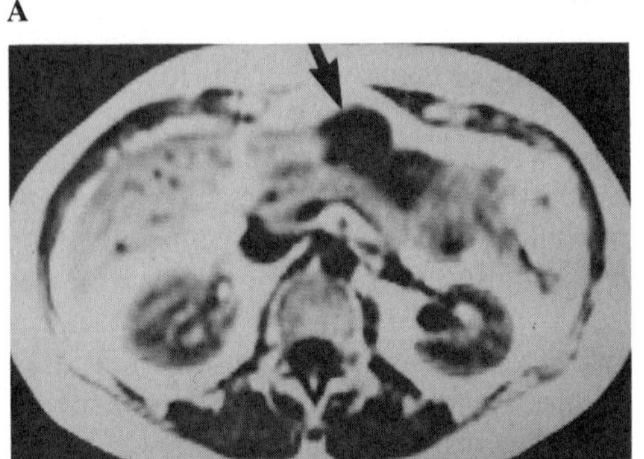

B

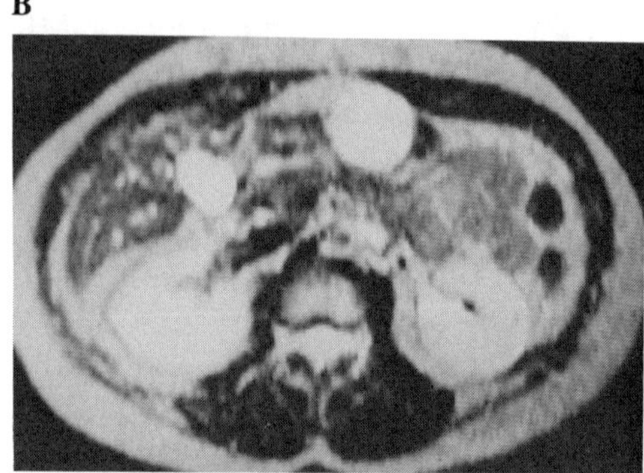

C

Figure 21.1   Manipulation of soft tissue contrast:
A. T_1-weighted image (SE 300/14); cavernous hemangioma (arrow), due to long T_1 relaxation time, is hypointense. (Similar tumor-liver soft-tissue contrast is present on an IR pulse sequence with long TI time setting (approximately 400 msec) as shown in Figure 21.14A). Note the hyperintense fatty tissues.
B. T_2-weighted image (SE 2350/180); the hemangioma is hyperintense on the T_2-weighted pulse sequence. Note the hyperintense fatty tissues.
C. $T_1 + T_2$ weighted short T1 (100 msec)-IR pulse sequence (STIR 1500/100/30). Fatty tissues are hypointense and the hemangioma is hyperintense even when soft-tissue contrast is predominantly based upon differences in the T_1 relaxation time.

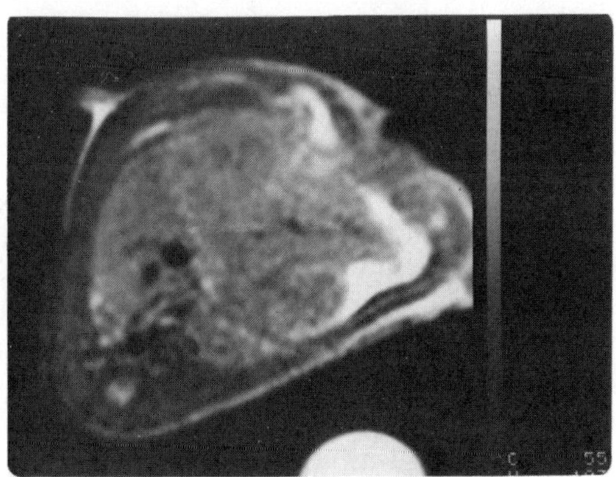

Figure 21.2 Absence of soft-tissue contrast on mixed T_1-T_2-weighted pulse sequence SE 500/30.
Transverse image of rat liver shows homogeneous signal intensity. A large tumor nodule that was visible on T_1- (see Figure 21.16A) and T_2-weighted (see Figure 21.17A) pulse sequences is obscured due to the cancellation of soft-tissue contrast when inappropriate pulse sequence timing parameters are utilized.

perintense on T_2-weighted pulse sequences, and vice versa. Thus at MR imaging, the effect of T_1 time on tissue-signal intensity is opposite the effect of T_2 time. To avoid cancellation of this divergent effect, an important aim of MR imaging is to select pulse sequences that provide as pure T_1-weighting or T_2-weighting as is practically possible. With mixed T_1-T_2 weighted pulse sequences, signal intensity from a tissue pair even with disparate relaxation times may be similar, making it impossible to distinguish them (Figure 21.2).

T_1-weighted pulse sequences can be obtained with each of the three fundamental pulse sequences, namely, spin echo (SE), inversion recovery (IR), and gradient echo (GE). For all three pulse sequences, the shortest possible TE (time of echo) must be employed. This is based on the observation that as TE values approach zero, signal loss due to T_2 relaxation (dephasing) diminishes, thereby increasing T_1 relaxation time-dependent information (Nelson TR, et al, 1984; Hendrick RE, et al, 1984). Although the TE minimum is a machine-defined variable, in the presence of contrast agents the use

of the shortest possible TE is even more important because contrast agents decrease the T_2 relaxation time and hasten the dephasing (signal loss) that necessarily occurs with TE times greater than 0 milliseconds. Reduction in the repetition time (TR), which saturates longitudinal magnetization in tissues with long T_1 times, also increases T_1 weighting, but is of much lesser importance. With GE pulse sequences, the critical factors for T_1 weighting are a large flip angle, and the shortest possible TE (Buxton RB, et al, 1987).

For T_2-weighted images, SE pulse sequences with long repetition times (approximately five times the T_1 time of tissue of interest such as to allow the longitudinal magnetization to return to equilibrium) and long echo times (greater than T_2 time of tissue of interest) must be employed (Wehrli FW, et al, 1984). Decreasing TR and TE increases T_1 information in MR images. SE pulse sequences with long TR and short TE are referred to as proton density images because on these images it is the proton density that principally determines soft-tissue contrast (Moran PR, 1984). With GE pulse sequences, the critical factors that provide T_2 weighting are a small flip angle and a long TE times (Buxton RB, et al, 1987).

Unlike SE and GE pulse sequences, IR pulse sequences are only suitable for T_1-weighted MR imaging (Wehrli FW, et al, 1984). Yet, soft-tissue contrast on the T_1-weighted IR pulse sequences may be reversed by altering the TI time (Bydder GM, et al, 1985). Thus, in the liver, for example, with long TI times, liver tumors appear hypointense. On the other hand, with short TI times, liver cancer appears hyperintense because the effect of T_1 and T_2 on soft-tissue contrast is additive (Figure 21.1C).

Whether a pulse sequence is T_1-weighted, T_2-weighted, or mixed T_1-T_2 weighted, depends both upon the pulse sequence timing parameters as well as upon the relaxation times in the tissues being imaged. For example, at 0.6T, the SE pulse sequence that provides T_1 relaxation time-dependent tissue contrast between gray and white matter typically utilizes TR times of 500 milliseconds, and TE times of 20 milliseconds (SE 500/20). However, liver relaxation times are shorter than gray and white matter, and T_1 relaxation time-dependent contrast between normal liver and liver cancer requires much shorter TE (<20 msec) and TR (<300 msec) settings (SE 300/14) (Stark DD, et al, 1985). Similarly, a T_2-weighted SE pulse sequence differentiation of structures with relatively long T_2 times, such as liver cancer and hepatic hemangiomas, requires long TR (>2000 msec) and long TE (>100 msec) times (Stark DD, et al, 1985). These factors are also influenced by the strength of the static magnetic field, because at higher field strengths, T_1 times become prolonged (Koenig SH and Brown RD, 1984).

The mathematical basis of T_1- or T_2-weighting can also be extracted from the Bloch equations that predict signal intensity in a tissue with known relaxation times and variable operator-defined pulse-sequence timing parameters (Bloembergen N, et al, 1948). For a SE pulse sequence, tissue signal intensity (SI) is proportional to

$$SI(SE) = K(1 - e^{-TR/T_1})(e^{-TE/T_2})$$

where K is a constant. When TR $\gg$ T1, the term e^{-TR/T_1} approaches 0, making signal intensity independent of T_1. If TE $\ll$ T_2, the term e^{-TE/T_2} approaches 1, making signal intensity independent of T_2. Because these equations estimate tissue signal intensity, prediction of soft-tissue contrast requires calculation of signal intensity differences between tissue being compared at a defined TR and TE. Similar formulae are available that predict signal intensity for IR pulse sequences. For GE pulse sequences, as noted previously, flip angle is an additional variable.

Pharmaceutical Manipulation of Signal Intensity

MR contrast agents shorten relaxation times and thereby alter MR signal intensity. T_1 shortening increases tissue signal intensity and T_2 shortening decreases tissue signal intensity (Figure 21.3). Each effect is best imaged with its corresponding T_1-weighted or T_2-weighted pulse sequence. Because MR contrast agents decrease both T_1 and T_2 times, one might expect one effect to cancel the other (Table 21.1). Fortunately, this does not occur because the effect of MR contrast agents on relaxation times T_1 and T_2 is not equal. For example, in its recommended doses (0.1–0.2 mmol/kg) paramagnetic Gd-DTPA produces far greater T_1 relaxation time shortening than decreases in the T_2 relaxation time. Thus the preferred pulse sequence to image the signal-enhancing effect of Gd-DTPA is a T_1-

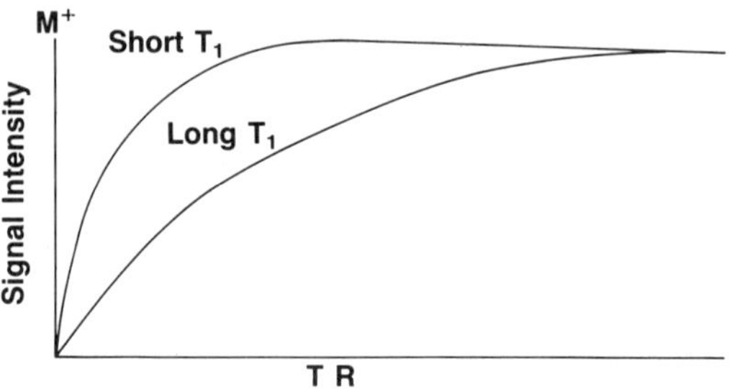

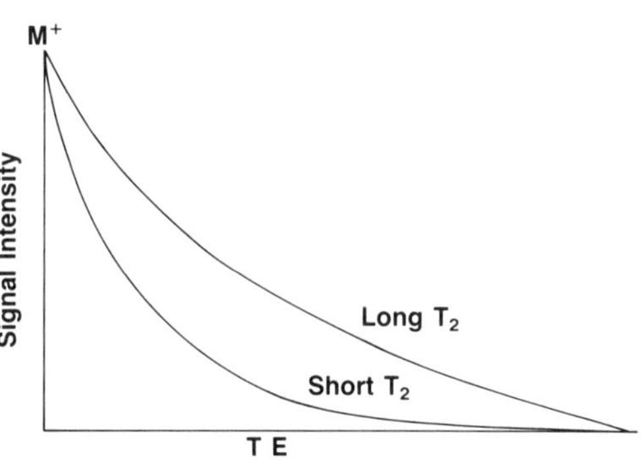

Figure 21.3 Pharmaceutical alteration of MR signal intensity. (TR: repetition time; TE: echo time).
A. Decrease in T_1 relaxation time produces increased signal intensity on a T_1-weighted pulse sequence. For a constant TE minimum, this effect diminishes as TR is prolonged, and therefore T_1 weighting is decreased.
B. Decrease in T_2 relaxation time lowers tissue signal intensity on a T_2-weighted pulse sequence. For a constant long TR, this effect decreases as T_2 weighting is reduced with smaller TE values.

Table 21.1   CLASSES OF MAGNETOPHARMACEUTICALS AND THEIR PROPERTIES

	PREDOMINANT RELAXATION TIME EFFECT	PHYSICAL STATE	NUMBER PARAMAGNETIC ATOMS/MOLECULE	EXAMPLES
Paramagnetic chelates	$\downarrow T_1$	Solute in solution	1	Gadopentetate dimeglumine (Gd-DTPA) Manganese-EDTA
Superparamagnetic particle	$\downarrow \downarrow \downarrow \downarrow T_2$	Suspensions of small particles (i. e., aggregates)	$\simeq 7{,}000$	Ferrite (Fe_3O_4) Dextran plus magnetite
Ferromagnetic	$\downarrow \downarrow \downarrow \downarrow T_2$	Suspensions of large particles (i. e., aggregates)	$\simeq 15{,}000$	

weighted pulse sequence. On the other hand, if one were interested in portraying the much smaller but real T_2 relaxation time shortening effect of Gd-DTPA, gradient echo pulse sequences that are exquisitely sensitive to magnetic susceptibility effects should be utilized. Similarly, with superparamagnetic contrast agents, the primary effect is T_2 relaxation time shortening, which is best imaged with T_2-weighted pulse sequences.

With suboptimal pulse sequences, the expected effect of MR contrast agents may be blunted or even paradoxical. Previous animal experiments with iron-EHPG showed that with a T_1-weighted pulse sequence, prolongation in TE was associated with a smaller signal-enhancing effect of the paramagnetic contrast agent (Greif WL, et al, 1985) (Figure 21.4). Furthermore, unlike radiographic contrast media, higher doses cannot compensate for inadequate T_1-weighting because at high tissue concentrations, T_2 shortening becomes significant enough to decrease tissue signal intensity. Inadequate T_2 weighting thus only makes this T_2 effect even more apparent. Superparamagnetic contrast agents, however, have a simpler dose-dependent effect on tissue signal intensity (Saini S, et al, 1987) (Figure 21.5).

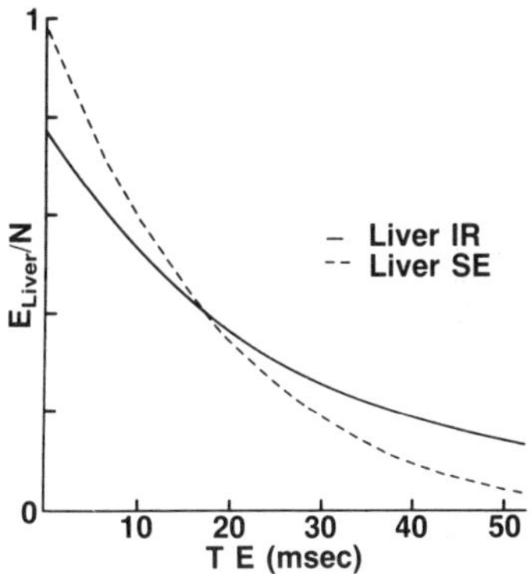

Figure 21.4 Effect of TE on tissue signal enhancement. (Reproduced with permission from Greif, et al 1985.)
Enhancement in liver (E_{liver}) signal intensity (calculated as the difference in liver signal intensity before and after administration of paramagnetic Fe-EHPG and normalized to background noise (N)), is more pronounced as TE values are reduced in both SE and IR pulse sequences. The y-axis has arbitrary units 0–1.

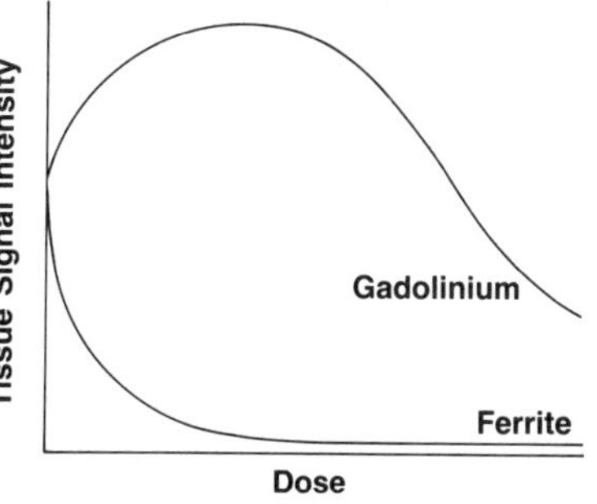

Figure 21.5 Dose-signal intensity relationship for MR contrast agents. (Reproduced with permission from Saini, et al, 1988).
At low doses, paramagnetic gadolinium has a negligible effect on T_2 relaxation time. Due to T_1 relaxation time shortening, tissue signal intensity increases. At higher doses T_2 relaxation time shortening becomes large enough to overcome T_1 effects and reduce tissue signal intensity. In comparison, superparamagnetic ferrites have a simple, monophasic relationship. They shorten T_2 relaxation time and only decrease tissue signal intensity.

The manner in which tissues process these pharmaceuticals (drug pharmacokinetics) can also influence signal intensity because at sufficiently high tissue concentrations the T_2 relaxation time shortening effect (signal depletion) of paramagnetic contrast agents on tissue signal intensity can actually mask the T_1 relaxation time shortening effects (signal enhancement). This, for example, may occur physiologically in the renal collecting system where Gd-DTPA becomes hyperconcentrated following renal excretion (Figure 21.6). This phenomenon becomes more apparent as pulse sequences with greater T_2-weighting (and therefore lesser T_1-weighting) are employed. Similarly some effects of contrast agents may be of very short duration. For example, superparamagnetic ferrite particles are removed from circulation by the reticuloendothelial cells and have blood half-life of about 15

A

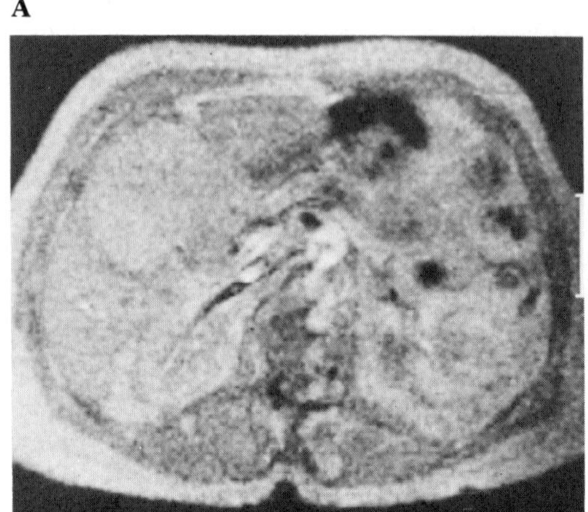

B

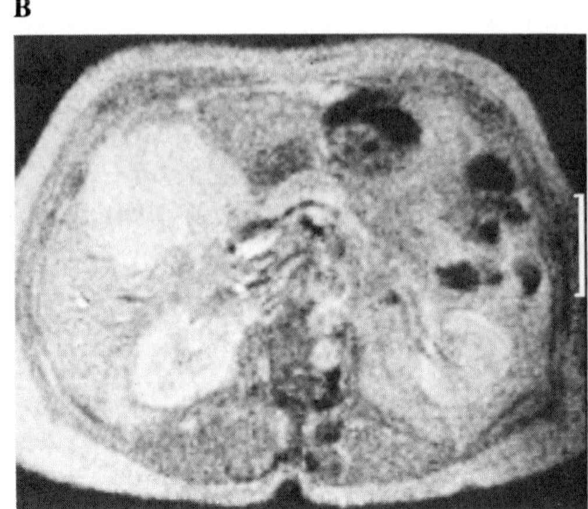

C

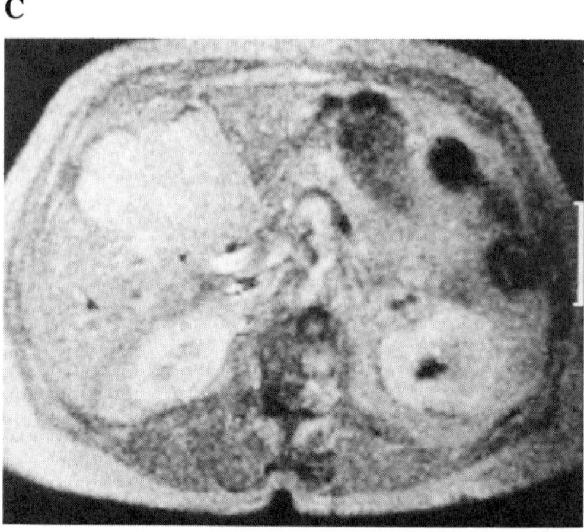

Figure 21.6 Effect of paramagnetic Gd-DTPA on tissue signal intensity. T_1-weighted GE 40/14. (Reproduced with permission from Hamm, et al, 1987.)
A. Pre-Gd-DTPA, malignant melanoma metastases and liver appear nearly isointense.
B. 1 min post 0.2 mmol/kg Gd-DTPA, the hyperperfused tumor immediately becomes hyperintense. In this setting a negative tumor-liver contrast phase does not occur. Renal parenchyma also enhances uniformly.
C. Gd-DTPA is eliminated via the kidney. Thus, 5 min post contrast infusion, Gd-DTPA is hyperconcentrated in the renal pelvis and, due to T_2 effects, decreases its signal intensity. Note the renal cortex remains hyperintense because tissue concentration remains low.

minutes (Stark DD, et al, 1988). Intravascular magnetic susceptibility effects (signal intensity depletion) can be seen in perfused tissues only briefly, while these particles are still in the intravascular compartment.

Thus far the discussion has been limited to a single tissue. Given a contrast agent of known magnetic properties, an appropriate pulse sequence can be selected to capture the expected effect on MR signal intensity (increase or decrease). However, in clinical imaging, several tissues are being evaluated simultaneously, and often two are being compared directly (for example normal liver and hepatic metastases). Thus one is really interested in maximizing signal intensity differences between tissues being compared. For example, because malignant tissues have prolonged relaxation times, in comparison to normal tissues, they are hypointense on T_1-weighted pulse sequences and hyperintense on T_2-weighted pulse sequences. On T_1-weighted pulse sequences one would seek a contrast agent that enhances signal in normal tissue (since cancer is already relatively hypointense), and on T_2-weighted pulse sequences, one would select a contrast agent that will deplete signal in normal tissue (since cancer is already hyperintense). Compounds that lack tissue specificity will enhance both the tissues that one is trying to discriminate and may reduce soft-tissue contrast (Figure 21.7). Understanding the effect of contrast agents on MR images first requires comprehension of the physical-chemical aspects of magnetic behavior.

Characteristics of MR Contrast Agents

Compounds can be used as MR contrast agents if they acquire large magnetic dipole moments (in comparison with the magnitude of the magnetic dipole moments on protons) when placed in a magnetic field. There are two physical-chemical categories of such materials (Saini S, et al, 1988).

First, paramagnetic contrast agents are ionic and have unpaired outer-shell electrons. Both manganese and iron, for example, have 5 unpaired electrons each while gadolinium has 7. These ions possess large intrinsic magnetic dipole moments because the magnetic dipole moment of an unpaired electron is approximately 1800 times that of a proton. A group of paramagnetic ions show no net magnetization due to random orientation of its constituent magnetic dipole moments. However paramagnetic ions orient parallel to an external magnetic field, and a net magnetic dipole moment then results. The magnetic dipole moments on individual paramagnetic ions interact with the nuclear magnetic dipole moments of protons and thereby alter tissue signal intensity. This dipole–dipole interaction produces T_1-shortening and, as was noted before, T_1-shortening is associated with an increase in tissue signal intensity, an effect that will be best portrayed on a T_1-weighted pulse sequence (Figure 21.5).

Second, because the electronic magnetic dipole moments on paramagnetic ions are much greater than the nuclear magnetic dipole moments on tissue protons, paramagnetic contrast agents also create inhomogeneities in a neighboring proton's local magnetic field. This enhances proton dephasing, producing T_2 shortening. At MR imaging, T_2 shortening is associated with a decrease in tissue signal intensity. This effect is best imaged with T_2-weighted GE or SE pulse sequences that are most sensitive in detecting magnetic susceptibility effects.

In recommended doses, the tissue concentration of paramagnetic contrast agents is small, and the T_1 effect predominates (Figure 21.5). Thus, members of this class of contrast agents are sometimes referred to as T_1-agents, and paramagnetic contrast-enhanced MR imaging is done with T_1-weighted pulse sequences. However, as tissue concentrations increase, T_2 shortening becomes progressively larger. Because T_2 shortening produces signal loss, with large tissue concentration of paramagnetic contrast agents, T_2 effects can mask the T_1 effects and at

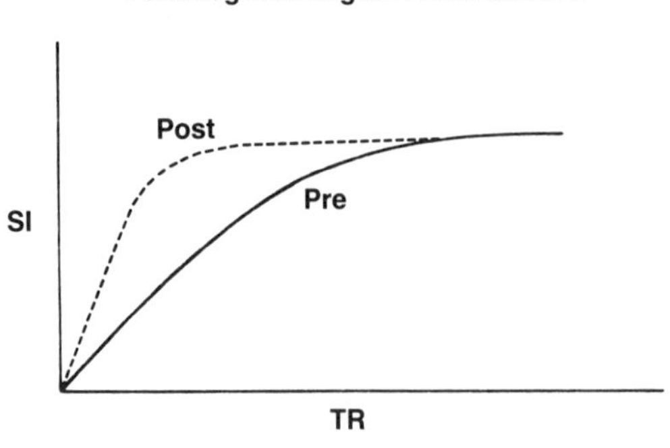

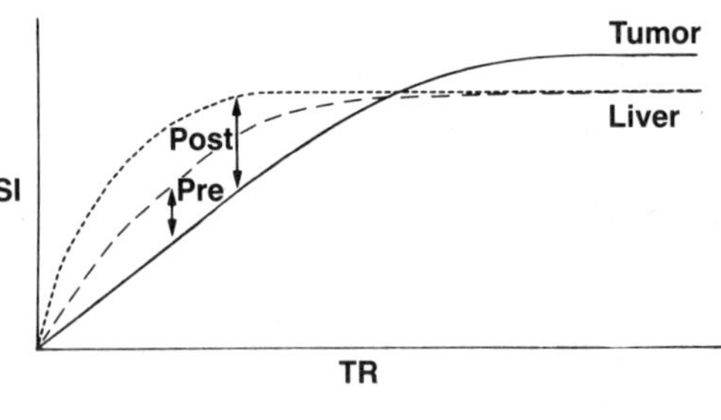

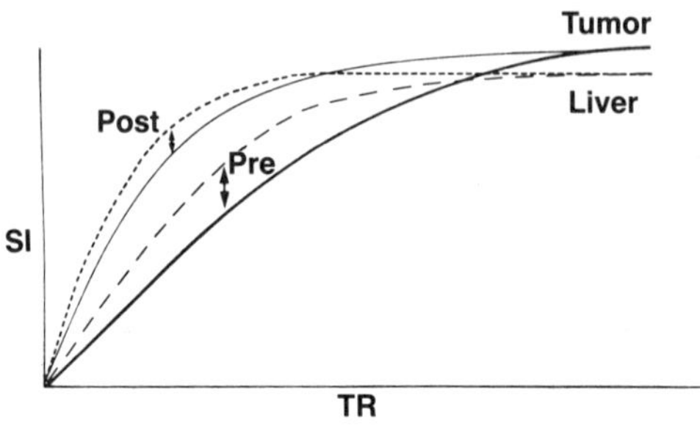

Figure 21.7 Soft-tissue contrast after selective and nonselective tissue signal enhancement. (TR: repetition time.) A. Paramagnetic contrast agents shorten T_1 relaxation time and increase tissue signal intensity. This effect is reduced as TR is increased in a SE pulse sequence which decreases T_1 weighting. B. On T_1-weighted pulse sequences (short TR times), tumors (solid line) are of lower signal intensity than normal liver (dashed line). Soft-tissue contrast before contrast agent infusion (Pre) will be augmented (Post) if the contrast media selectively increases signal in normal liver (dotted line). Hepatobiliary Fe-EHPG is such a contrast agent (see Figure 21.15). With Gd-DTPA, this occurs only in the immediate postinfusion period when the drug is in the vascular compartment and if tumors are underperfused with respect to normal liver. C. With nonselective tissue enhancement, signal intensity will increase in both liver and tumors. Thus soft-tissue contrast may be reduced after infusion of the contrast agent (Pre versus Post). With Gd-DTPA this occurs after it has equilibrated in the interstitial compartment.

MR imaging show paradoxical tissue darkening (Figures 21.5 and 21.6). Thus the relationship between tissue concentration of paramagnetic contrast agents and signal intensity is biphasic, and inadequately T_1-weighted pulse sequences cannot be compensated for with larger doses of paramagnetic contrast agents. In fact, these effects become more even evident as T_2-weighting is increased. Large tissue concentrations can result from a compact bolus injection, large doses, or physiologic hyperconcentration (Figure 21.6).

In T_2-weighted pulse sequences, especially gradient echo, paramagnetic ions such as dysprosium with large magnetic dipole moments and high magnetic field strength, will also preferentially portray the tissue-darkening effect.

Ferromagnetic, ferrimagnetic, and superparamagnetic contrast agents, on the other hand, by virtue of their even larger magnetic dipole moments, are T_2 agents, and regardless of dose decrease tissue signal intensity (Figure 21.5). This characteristic is a result of their unique physical structure. Each molecule of superparamagnetic ferrite (Fe_3O_4) for example, comprises a cluster of paramagnetic ferric iron ions bound together in a crystalline matrix. Parallel orientation of the paramagnetic dipole moments of neighboring ions is the preferred state even in the absence of an external magnetic field. Furthermore, this spontaneous magnetization is greater than the algebraic sum of the magnetic dipole moments of the constituent ions. These crystals contain regions or domains of spontaneous magnetization. In the absence of an external magnetic field, the magnetic dipole moments of domains can be oriented randomly, and these crystals may not show net magnetization. Parallel alignment however occurs quite readily, and these materials can be magnetized to saturation even in weak external magnetic fields. Single domain particles (<350 Å for ferrite) are superparamagnetic because the magnetic dipole moments on individual domains respond to the external magnetic field independent of each other (akin to paramagnetism) but with a much larger magnetization (saturation magnetization) (Bean CP and Livingston JD, 1959). When the external field is removed, domains may orient randomly and no net magnetization will be present. Permanent magnets are made of multidomain materials that retain this magnetization even when the external magnetic field is removed. Due to their large physical size (>1 μm), the net magnetic dipole moment on these molecules does not precess at a sufficiently rapid rate to produce T_1 relaxation time shortening from dipole–dipole interactions. However, because they create large perturbations in the homogeneity of the surrounding magnetic field, T_2 relaxation time shortening and signal loss results from proton dephasing. This effect is best imaged on T_2-weighted SE or GE pulse sequences that are most sensitive to T_2 or magnetic susceptibility effects. Unlike paramagnetic contrast agents, these materials show a monophasic relationship between dose and tissue signal intensity (Figure 21.7) (Saini S, et al, 1987). As tissue concentrations increase, tissue signal intensity will continue to decrease until background noise levels are reached. As T_2-weighting in pulse sequences is increased, signal intensity diminution will be even more dramatic. Thus, suboptimal pulse sequences can be partially compensated by increasing tissue concentrations.

In summary then, tissue T_1 and T_2 times are the principal determinants of tissue signal intensity. Pulse sequences display signal intensity on MR images with both T_1 and T_2 relaxation time-dependent information. To increase soft-tissue contrast, pulse sequence timing parameters are selected to maximize the information from one relaxation time and minimize the contribution from the other. MR contrast agents alter signal intensity on MR images by decreasing tissue relaxation times, The principal effect of a contrast agent is either on T_1 or on T_2 relaxation time. Thus, the pulse sequence utilized to image the effect of these pharmaceuticals should be correspondingly T_1- or T_2-weighted. Additional relevant factors are pharmaceutical dose, mode of drug administration (bolus versus drip), and the pharmacokinetic behavior of the contrast agent in tissue of interest.

Paramagnetic Contrast Agents

Numerous paramagnetic contrast agents have been investigated. These include Gadolinium-DTPA, iron-EHPG, iron-desferioxamine, manganese dipiridoxyl diphosphate, and ferric ammonium citrate. These are T_1 agents and enhance signal in tissues. MR imaging strategies employed for these contrast agents are very similar although minor differences exist due to variations in their pharmacokinetics. Following is a description for imaging with Gd-DTPA, and the general principles can be transferred to the other magnetopharmaceuticals.

Gd-DTPA (Gadolinium-diethylenetriamine-pentaacetic acid, or gadopentetate dimeglumine) was one of the earliest magnetopharmaceuticals investigated and is the first contrast agent that has been approved for clinical use (Carr DH, et al, 1984). The pharmacokinetic behavior of Gd-DTPA is entirely analogous to iodinated contrast media used in excretory urography and computed tomography (Wolf GL and Fobben ES, 1984, Wienmann H-J, et al, 1984). Gd-DTPA has rapid plasma clearance, becomes distributed in the extracellular space and is eliminated by passive filtration via the kidneys. As a dimeglumine salt, the compound is hypertonic. It has an osmolarity of 1940 mOs mol/kg water. In comparison plasma osmolarity is 285 mOs mol/kg water. Gd-DTPA is available (Magnavist Research, Berlex Laboratories) at 0.5M concentration, making a typical dose 14 cc in a 70 kg man (0.1 mMol/kg). Because the LD-50 in rats is 10 mMol/kg, it provides an extremely high safety factor (>100).

In the central nervous system, GD-DTPA enhances normal tissues that lack a blood-brain barrier (e. g., pituitary gland), extraaxial tumors (e. g., meningiomas), and regions of blood-brain-barrier breakdown (e. g., tumor margins) (Brant-Zawadski M, et al, 1986; Berry I, et al, 1986). Outside the central nervous system, Gd-DTPA rapidly equilibrates into the intersitial compartment and enhances signal in all tissues in proportion to tissue perfusion. The recommended dose for Gd-DTPA is 0.1–0.2 millimoles/kilogram body weight. In these doses, its effect on the T_2 relaxation time is quite small, and signal enhancement is the result. For best demonstration of this effect, T_1-weighted pulse sequences are utilized (Wolf GL, et al, 1986). As noted before, with less T_1-weighting and the accompanying more T_2-weighting, this effect will be blunted. Because Gd-DTPA enhances signal in interstitium of all tissues, the brain with an intact blood-brain barrier and avascular tissues such as tendons and necrotic tumors being the exceptions, it is a contrast agent that lacks tissue specificity.

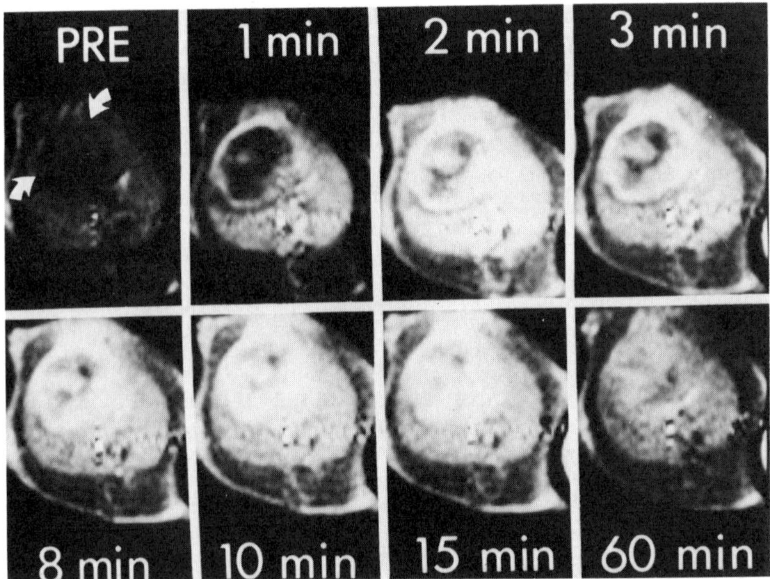

Figure 21.8 Temporal changes in tumor-liver contrast after Gd-DTPA. SE 250/15/1 (36 sec scan time). (Reproduced with permission from Saini, et al, 1986.)
Precontrast, the tumor nodule appears hypointense. In the immediate post-Gd-DTPA infusion period (0.2 mmol/kg), there is preferential enhancement of liver tissue resulting in increased tumor-liver signal differences. Later, as Gd-DTPA diffuses into tumor tissue, the tumor-liver signal differences decrease. Thus, maximal benefits of Gd-DTPA as tumor-liver contrast occur in the first 2–3 minutes after infusion. On delayed images (8–15 min) tumor appears hyperintense due to slow washout of Gd-DTPA.

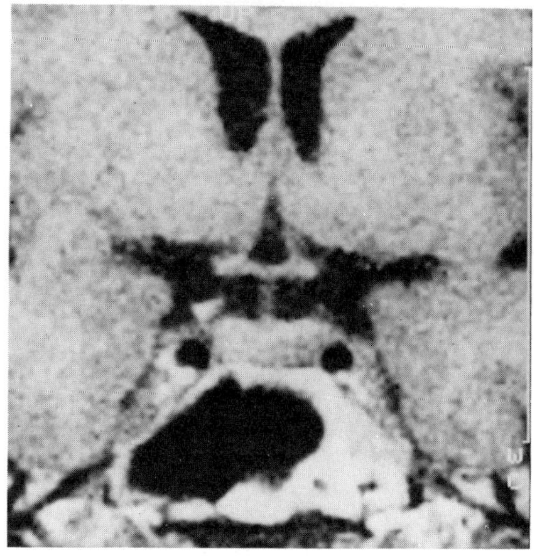

A

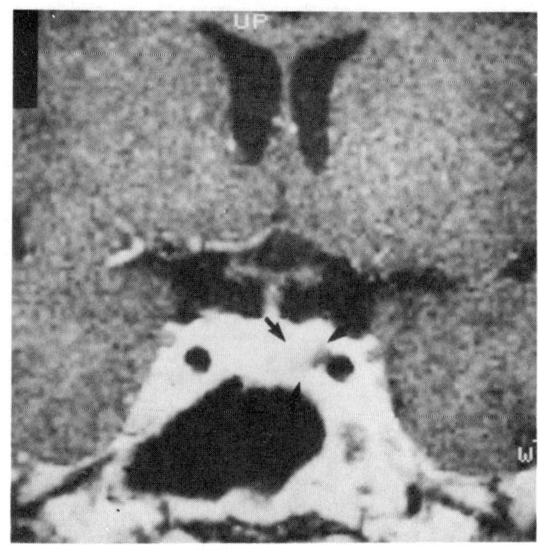

B

Figure 21.9   Increased conspicuity of pituitary microadenoma immediately after Gd-DTPA (0.1 mmol/kg). (9A versus 9B.)
The pituitary gland is an extraaxial structure and enhances after Gd-DTPA infusion. Thus microadenomas appear hypointense only in the immediate postcontrast infusion period. As Gd-DTPA passively leaks into the adenoma, it will become isointense to the pituitary on delayed scans (not shown).

Therefore, for many organs, Gd-DTPA-enhanced MR imaging requires exploitation of the perfusion differences in tissues being compared. Furthermore, because the time taken to reach equilibrium is relatively short and in the order of 2–3 minutes (where the two tissues being compared have nearly equal distribution of Gd-DTPA), pulse sequences with sufficiently short scan times must be utilized (Saini S et al, 1986) (Figures 21.8 and 21.9). Once Gd-DTPA has equilibrated into any two tissues being compared (e. g., normal liver and liver cancer, or pituitary gland and pituitary microadenoma), their signal intensity differences may actually be reduced from the precontrast infusion level (Figures 21.10 and 21.11). This may occur if delayed scanning is done or if pulse sequences with long scan times are utilized. Lesions also appear smaller because Gd-DTPA passively diffuses in from the periphery (Figure 21.12). When Gd-DTPA preferentially enhances signal in an hypointense mass (e. g., soft-tissue masses in fatty tissue such as mediastinal lymph nodes), the signal-intensity differences between these two tissues will be reduced or may be

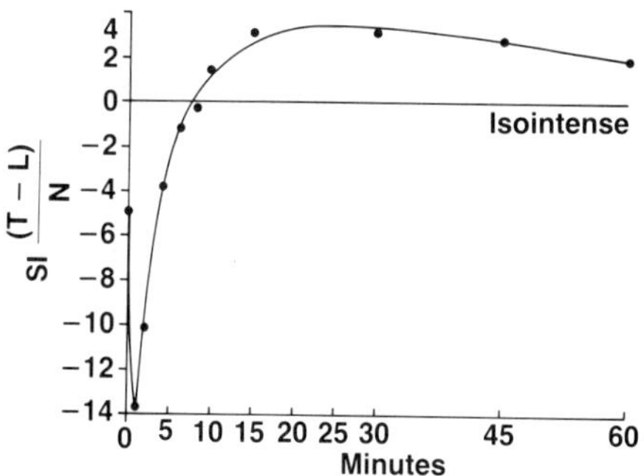

Figure 21.10   Temporal change in tumor-liver contrast after Gd-DTPA. (Reproduced with permission from Saini, et al, 1986.)
Calculation of tumor (T)-liver (L) signal intensity (SI) difference normalized to background noise (N) $[SI^{(T-L)/N}]$ 0–60 minutes after bolus infusion of Gd-DTPA (0.2 mmol/kg). In the first 2 minutes the tumor-liver contrast is increased (greater negative contrast). Then it decreases, from the case in Figure 21.8 and eventually the tumor becomes hyperintense. However this positive tumor-liver contrast is less than the negative tumor-liver contrast present prior to Gd-DTPA. Tissue will appear if MR images are acquired during the isointense period or if long pulse sequences are utilized that cancel the early negative contrast with the late hyperintense contrast.

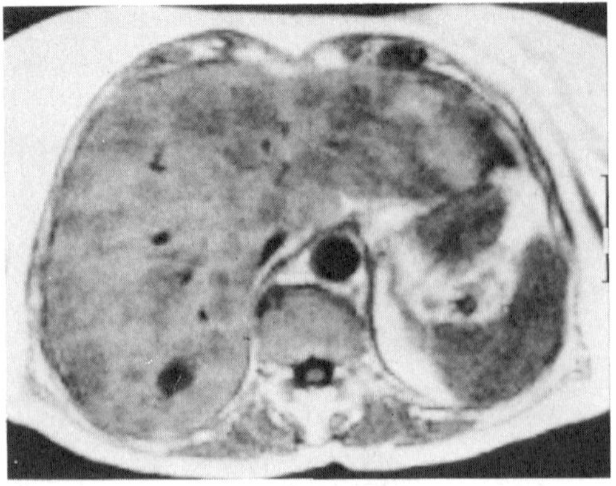

A

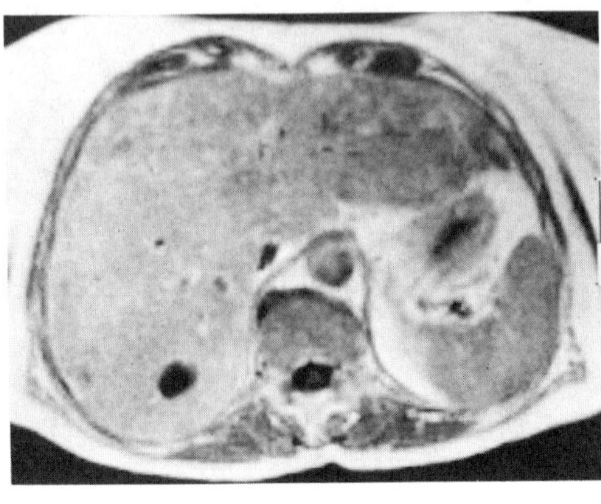

B

Figure 21.11 Obscuration of tumor-liver contrast in the equilibrium phase after Gd-DTPA; SE 200/22.
A. Pre-Gd-DTPA, the pancreatic metastases are hypointense to normal liver. There is a simple hepatic cyst as well.
B. Ten minutes after 0.1 mmol/kg Gd-DTPA, tumor-liver contrast is reduced. Because the cyst is avascular, cyst-liver contrast is higher than the pre-Gd-DTPA image.

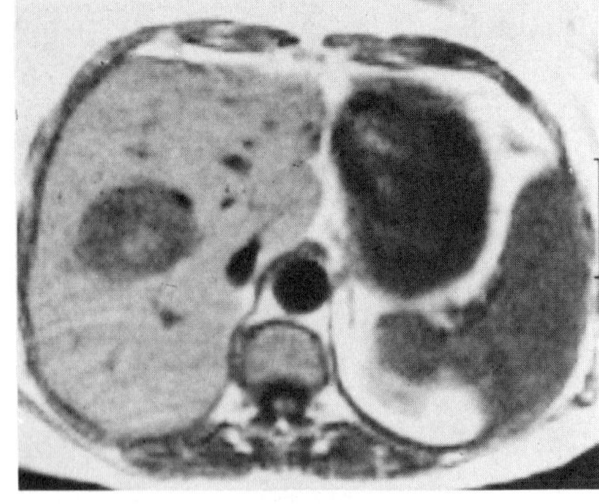

A

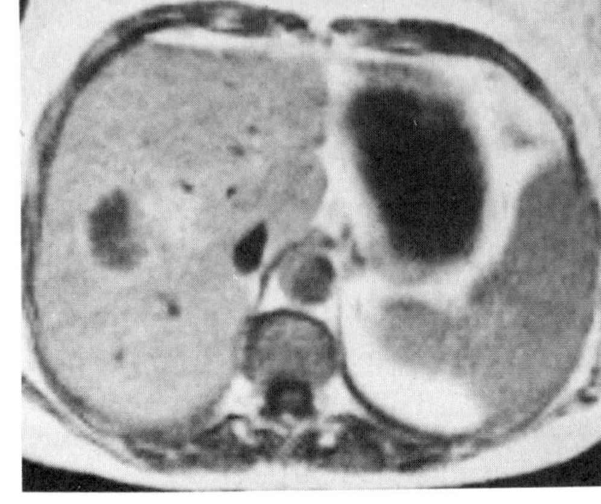

B

Figure 21.12 Decrease in tumor size after Gd-DTPA: SE 200/22. (Reproduced with permission from Hamm, et al, 1987.)
A. A 5cm liver metastasis appears hypointense on a T_1-weighted image.
B. Three minutes after Gd-DTPA (0.2 mmol/kg) there is enhancement of normal liver and only peripheral enhancement of the metastasis. This increases tumor-liver contrast and lesion conspicuity. However, due to Gd-DTPA leakage into the tumor peripherally, the metastasis appears smaller in size. It is likely that a 1–2 cm lesion might have been obscured.

paradoxically reversed (e. g., hypervascular liver metastases) even if rapid post contrast infusion imaging is done (Figure 21.6 A,B). This paradoxical contrast reversal can also occur during delayed imaging in tissues that have different rates of drug elimination. For example, cavernous hemangiomas are hypointense on T_1-weighted pulse sequences. Because Gd-DTPA will puddle in these tumors, hemangiomas become hyperintense on delayed T_1-weighted MR images (Ohtomo

K, et al, 1987). Similarly, due to slow washout of Gd-DTPA, hypovascular hepatic metastases can also become hyperintense on T_1-weighted MR images (Saini S, et al, 1986; Hamm B, et al, 1987) (Figure 21.13).

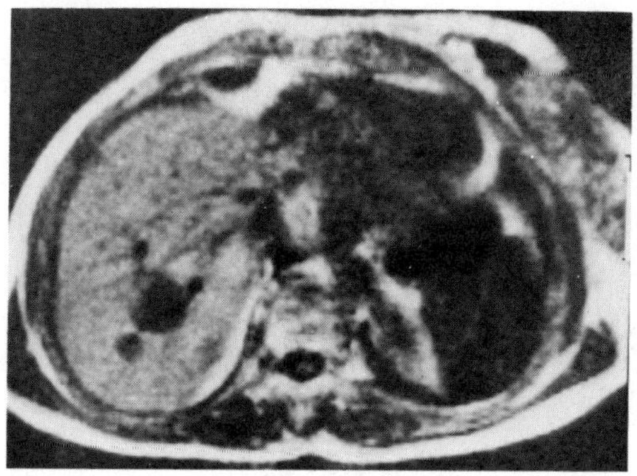

A

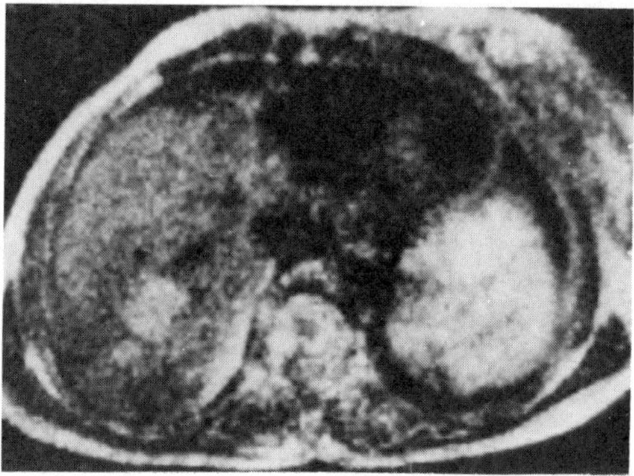

B

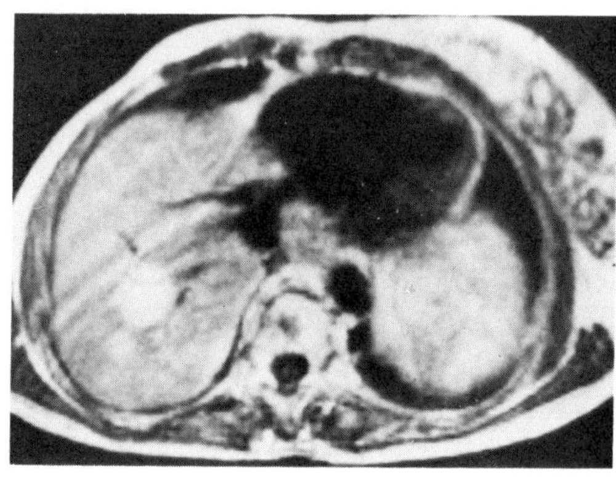

C

Figure 21.13 Reversal of tumor-liver contrast in the equilibrium phase after Gd-DTPA (0.2 mmol/kg)
A. Pre-Gd-DTPA, T_1-weighted IR 1500/400/35. Two breast metastases appear hypointense.
B. Pre-Gd-DTPA, T_2-weighted SE 1600/105. The lesions are hyperintense.
C. Ten minutes post-Gd-DTPA, T_1-weighted SE 400/30. In the equilibrium phase, there is inversion in tumor-liver contrast.

Gastrointestinal tract enhancement with Gd-DTPA requires special considerations. The major limitation is that beyond the ligament of Tritz, oral Gd-DTPA does not routinely enhance small bowel contents. This may be a result of inadequate fluid within the bowel, or hyperconcentration of the drug, or prolonged transit time. To overcome this, the addition of hypertonic mannitol (15 grams/L) administered in an oral dose of 0.01 mmol/kg Gd-DTPA has been shown to be of considerable value (Lanaido M, et al, 1988). In this regimen, Gd-DTPA enhances the entire small bowel. The effect of mannitol is to retain fluid within the bowel lumen and also to decrease gut transit time. No significant side effects from diarrhea have been reported in early clinical trials. As with intravascular Gd-DTPA, the pulse sequence that best portrays the bowel-marking effect of Gd-DTPA is a T_1-weighted pulse sequence (Figure 21.14).

Under usual circumstances, tissue concentrations of Gd-DTPA are sufficiently low so that tissue signal loss due to T_2-time shortening is not observed. There are, however, exceptions to this rule. The most common occurrence is in the kidneys where the drug is physiologically concentrated (Figure 21.6). Alternatively, if heavily T_2-weighted pulse sequences are used, and Gd-DTPA is administered as a compact bolus, transient (less than 1 minute) signal darkening has been observed in tissues with high blood flow, such as the brain and myocardium. The documentation of this phenomenon in other organs remains to be established.

Other paramagnetic contrast agents have identical imaging restrictions regarding pulse sequence timing parameters. They may differ, however, in their pharmacokinetic behavior, which may alter the imaging protocol. For example, paramagnetic contrast agents that undergo selective hepatobiliary excretion also enhance liver signal intensity. They produce a more prolonged enhancement in liver signal intensity, which eliminates the need to image with short scan times (Lauffer, et al, 1985) (Figure 21.15). In a setting

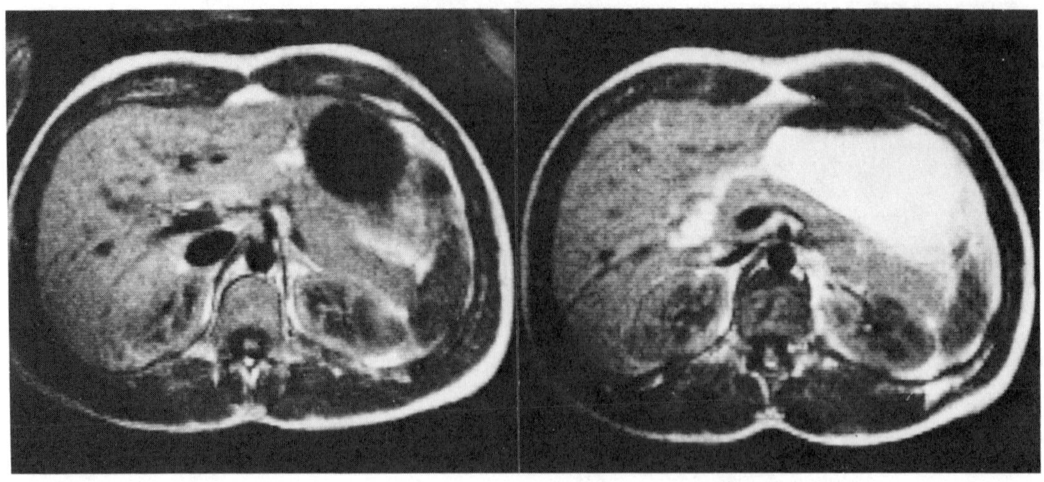

A   B

Figure 21.14 Opacification of the gastrointestinal tract after Gd-DTPA: SE 200/20. (Reproduced with permission from Lanaido, et al, 1988.)
A. The air-filled stomach is hypointense, but the gastric antrum, liver, and pancreas are inseparable (left).
B. After 0.01 mmol/kg oral Gd-DTPA, the head and body of the pancreas are easily delineated (right). The addition of mannitol (15 g/l) results in homogeneous opacification of the small bowel (not shown).

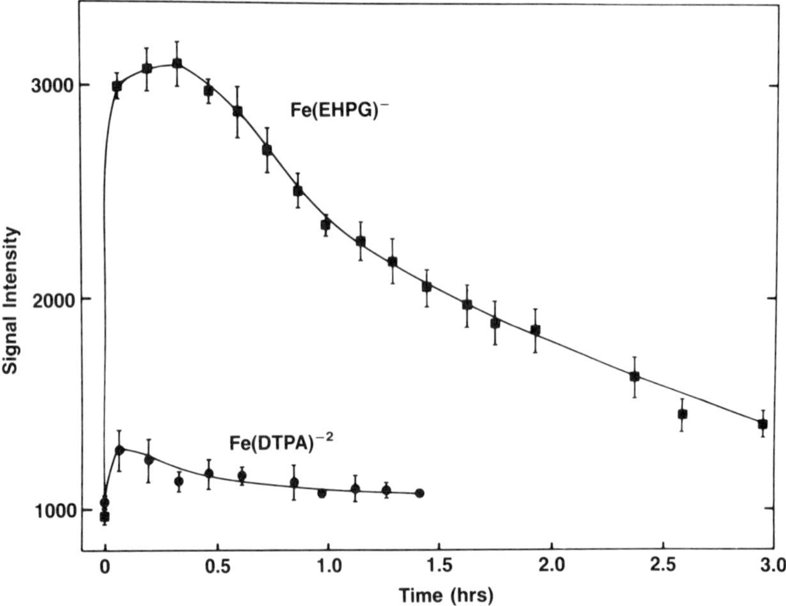

Figure 21.15 Comparison of temporal enhancement of liver signal intensity after infusion of hepatobiliary paramagnetic contrast agent Fe-EHPG and Gd-DTPA analog Fe-DTPA. (Reproduced with permission from Lauffer et al, 1985.)
Fe-DTPA is distributed in the extracellular space and, like Gd-DTPA maximal enhancement of the liver occurs early and for a brief period. In comparison, hepatic signal enhancement with Fe-EHPG is later and is prolonged. This permits much more flexibility in scan time restrictions.

of liver injury (hepatitis) or biliary obstruction, uptake by hepatocytes will be diminished, producing less enhancement in liver signal.

Superparamagnetic Contrast Agents

Recently a new class of MR contrast agents with selective and preferential T_2 relaxation time shortening has been developed (Renshaw PF, et al, 1986; Saini S, et al, 1987). Superparamagnetic materials acquire extremely large magnetic moments, even in comparison to paramagnetic compounds, which creates large perturbations in the protons' local magnetic fields (Saini S, et al, 1988). Thus, the materials show profound shortening in the T_2 relaxation time. There is a much smaller and negligible effect on the T_1 relaxation time because the relatively large molecular size prevents particle tumbling rates to match proton resonant frequency. As noted before, T_2 relaxation time shortening leads to signal loss (Figure 21.13B). This effect with ferrite particles occurs with doses that are an order of magnitude less than those employed for paramagnetic contrast agents.

Superparamagnetic ferrite is an iron ox-

ide preparation that is composed of particles that are approximately $0.3-1.0$ μm in diameter (Stark DD, et al, 1988). Since these particles are smaller than erythrocytes (5 μm), ferrite particles easily traverse the body's capillary network and are eventually removed from circulation by the reticuloendothelial system. At MR imaging ferrites reduce signal intensity in the liver, spleen, and bone-marrow (Saini S, et al, 1987). This effect can be observed within 5 minutes of intravenous administration and is maximal at 1 hour when nearly all circulating particles have been removed from circulation. During the intravascular period, signal intensity diminution can be observed in perfused tissue. To image these effects, T_2-weighted pulse sequences are required (Figure 21.16). GE pulse sequences are more sensitive to image this effect than SE pulse sequences. Ferrite degradation rates are highly variable, and the tissue signal loss may persist for up to 1 week.

Clinical and laboratory studies with superparamagnetic ferrites produce the expected effect on MR images at doses ranging from $10-20$ μmol/kg (Stark DD, et al, 1988). Dynamic scanning with pulse sequences having relatively short scan times also show intravascular signal

A   B

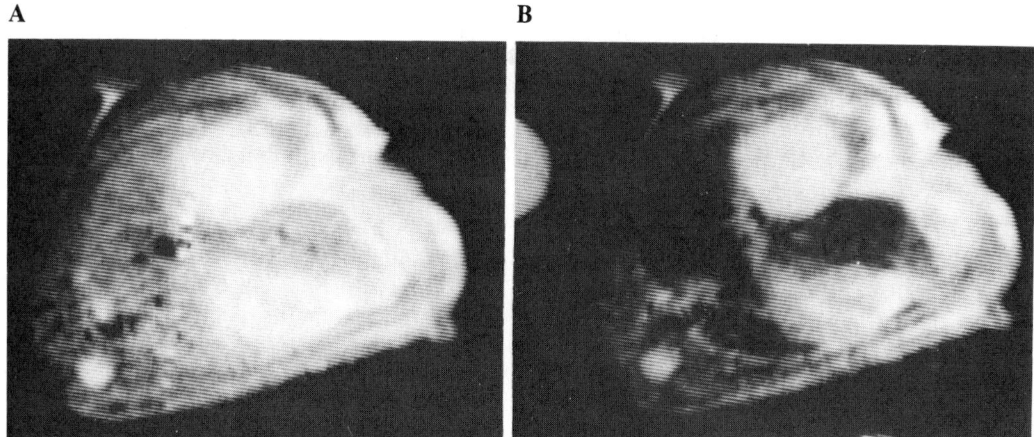

Figure 21.16 Improvement of tumor-liver contrast after ferrite; SE 1500/60.
A. Transverse image of rat liver. Preferrite, the round anteriorly located tumor nodule is slightly hyperintense on the T_2-weighted pulse sequence (left).
B. Fifteen minutes after ferrite, there is signal reduction in normal liver, which increases tumor liver contrast (right).

depletion in the first few minutes after contrast administration. The plasma half-life of these particles is approximately 15 minutes, and the drug is cleared by the reticuloendothelial cells producing signal depletion in liver, spleen, and bone marrow. The ferrite particles are eliminated from these organs within a week after administration. Thus there is considerable latitude in the time at which post ferrite administration MR imaging can be performed. There is also considerable flexibility in the selection of timing parameters. Typically, mildly T_2-weighted pulse sequences are utilized in which pre-ferrite, abnormal tissues are isointense or slightly more hyperintense than normal tissue. If T_1-weighted pulse sequences are utilized, the abnormal tissues would initially be hypointense, and decreasing signal in the relatively hyperintense normal tissue will reduce tumor-liver contrast (Figure 21.17). The only exception to this rule is with short TI-IR T_1-weighted images where liver cancer is hyperintense with respect to normal liver. In diffuse diseases, organ signal depletion is smaller than in normal tissues, and ferrite particles show some potential utility in the evaluation of diseases such as lymphoma in the spleen (Weissleder R, et al, 1987).

Investigators have also evaluated the potential of these signal-depleting magnetopharmaceuticals as a contrast agent for the gastrointestinal tract (Hahn PF, et al, 1987). The theoretical advantage for this material is that by eliminating signal from bowel lumen, both air- and fluid-filled bowel would appear hypointense. Furthermore, because no bowel lumen signal is present, peristalsis would not produce ghost artifacts. Preliminary clinical trials have shown adequate marking of the entire gastrointestinal tract. As with intravascular ferrite imaging, mildly T_2-weighted images are utilized. The relative disadvantage of T_1-weighted pulse sequences is that adjoining structures such as retroperitoneal muscle and vessels are also of low signal intensity, making soft-tissue contrast between these structures less pronounced. These effects have been

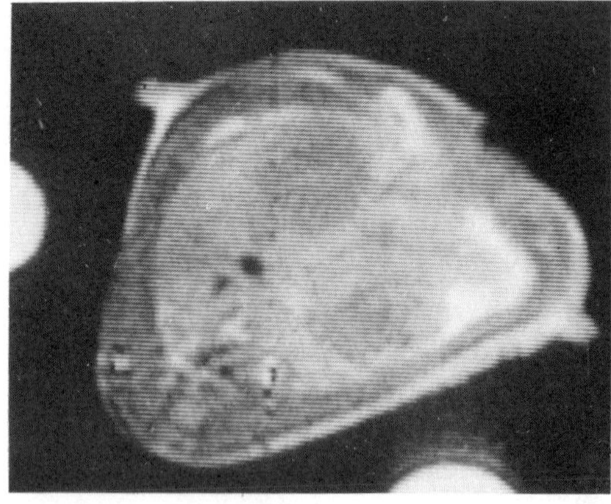

A

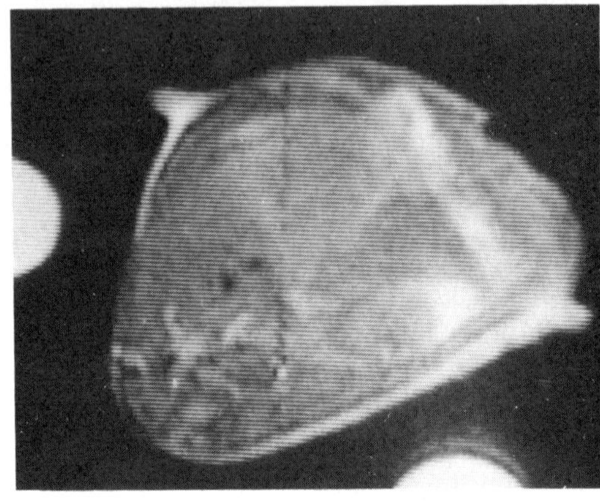

B

Figure 21.17   Decrease in tumor-liver contrast after ferrite; SE 250/15.
A. Transverse image of rat liver. Pre-ferrite, the round anteriorly located tumor nodule is slightly hypointense on the T_1-weighted pulse sequence (left).
B. Fifteen minutes after ferrite, there is signal reduction in normal liver, which reduces tumor liver contrast (right).

produced with oral doses of 0.1 mmol/kg. In excessive doses, large accumulations of ferrite can occur, especially in the gastric fundus producing metal-type artifacts (Figure 21.18).

Historical Perspective and Conclusion

The phenomenon of nuclear magnetic resonance (NMR) was first described in

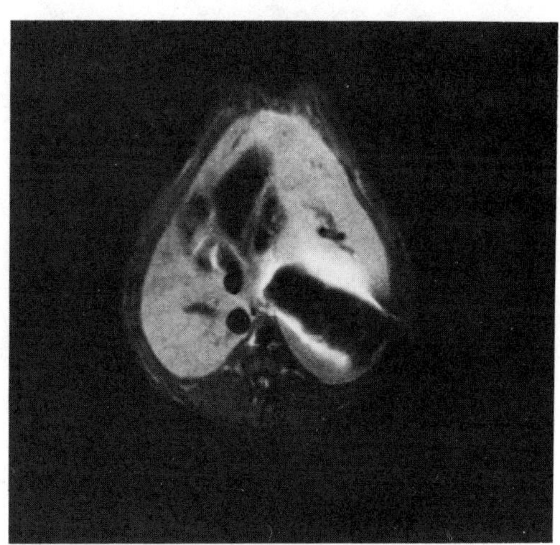

Figure 21.18 Metal-type artifact after oral ferrite administration; SE 500/32. (Reproduced with permission from Hahn, et al, 1987.) Transverse image of dog liver. Due to extremely large magnetization in ferrite particles, metal-type artifacts result from excessively large doses or inadequate suspension.

1946, for which Purcell and Block were honored with the 1952 Nobel Prize in physics. However it is only in the last 10 years that this rather simple physical phenomenon has been developed into a highly sophisticated tool for diagnostic imaging (Lauterbur PC, 1971; Damadian R, 1971; Damadian R, et al, 1973). This evolution continues to proceed at an unprecedented pace and has brought about an explosion of new ideas that has drawn together scientists from a variety of disciplines. Today high-quality magnetic resonance (MR) images are routinely able to depict clearly and with intricate detail gross human anatomy. MR images show high soft-tissue contrast (signal intensity differences) between normal tissues as well as between normal and pathologic tissues. This further improves resolution, and in many cases permits early detection of diseased tissues. Although advances in the last decade have primarily centered on machine hardware and software developments, the next major advance in MR imaging will almost certainly be with the introduction of MR contrast agents into routine clinical use. The wider application of such agents will increase still further the visualization and detection of many tumor types by enhancing the contrast between healthy tissues and those affected by diseases. With these agents it is likely that specificity will increase and imaging times may decrease. Their use is further appealing because enhancement effects can be brought about by concentrations that are safe and of low toxicity.

References

Bean CP, Livingston JD. Superparamagnetism. *J App Physics* 1959, 30: 120S–129S.

Berry I, Brant-Zawadski M, Osaki L, et al. Gd-DTPA in clinical MR of the brain. 2. Extraaxial lesions and normal structures. *AJNR* 1986, 7:789–793.

Bloch F, Hansen WW, Packard P. The nuclear induction experiment. *Physics Rev* 1946, 70:474–485.

Bloembergen N, Purcell EM, Pound RV. Relaxation effects in nuclear magnetic resonance absorption. *Phys Rev* 1948, 73:679–712.

Brant-Zawadski M, Berry I, Osaki L, et al. Gd-DTPA in clinical MR of the brain: 1. Intraaxial lesions. *AJNR* 1986, 7:781–788.

Buxton RB, Edelman RR, Rosen BR, et al. Contrast in rapid MRI: T1- and T2-weighted imaging. *JCAT* 1987, 11:7–16.

Bydder GM, Steiner E, Blumgart FLH, et al. MR imaging of the liver using short TI inversion recovery sequences. *JCAT* 1985, 9:1084–1089.

Carr DH, Brown J, Bydder GM, et al. Gd-DTPA as a contrast agent in NMI: Initial clinical experience in 20 patients. *AJR* 1984, 143:215–224.

Chilton HM, Jackels SC, Hinson WH et al. Use of a paramagnetic substance, colloidal manganese sulfide, as an NMR contrast material. *J Nucl Med* 1984, 25:604–607.

Damadian R. Tumor detection by nuclear magnetic resonance. *Science* 1971, 171: 1151–1153.

Damadian R, Zaner K, Horr D, et al. Nuclear magnetic resonance as a new tool in cancer research: Human tumors by NMR. *Ann NY Acad Sci* 1973, 222:1048–1074.

Greif WL, Buxton RB, Lauffer RB, et al. Pulse sequence optimization for MR imaging using a paramagnetic hepatobiliary contrast agent. *Radiology* 1985, 157:461–466.

Hahn PF, Stark DD, Saini S, et al. Ferrite particles for bowel contrast in MR imaging: Design issues and feasibility studies. *Radiology* 1987, 164:37–41.

Hamm B, Wolff K-J, Felix R. Conventional and rapid MR imaging of liver with Gadolinium-DTPA. *Radiology* 1987, 164:313.

Hendrick RE, Nelson TR, Hendee WR. Optimizing tissue contrast in magnetic resonance imaging. *Magn Reson Imaging* 1984, 2:193–204.

Koenig SH, Brown RD. Relaxation of solvent protons by paramagnetic ions and it's dependence on magnetic field and chemical environment: implications for NMR imaging. *Magn Reson Med* 1984, 1:478–495.

Lanaido M, Kornmesser W, Hamm B, et al. MR imaging of the gastrointestinal tract: Value of Gd-DTPA. *AJR* 1988, 150:817–821.

Lauffer RB, Grief WL, Stark DD, et al. Iron-EHPG as an hepatobiliary MR contrast agent. Initial imaging and biodistribution studies. *JCAT* 1985, 9: 431–438.

Lauterbur PC. Image formation by induced local interactions. Examples employing NMR. *Nature* 1973, 242:190–191.

Moran PR. A general approach to T_1, T_2 and spin-density discrimination sensitivities in NMR imaging sequences. *Magn Reson Imaging* 1984, 2:17–22.

Nelson TR, Hendrick RE, Hendee WR. Selection of pulse sequences producing maximum tissue contrast in magnetic resonance imaging. *Magn Reson Imaging* 1984, 2:285–294.

Ohtomo K, Itai Y, Yoshikawa K, et al. Hepatic tumors: Dynamic MR imaging. *Radiology* 1987, 163:27–31.

Renshaw PF, Owen CS, McLaughlin AC, et al. Ferromagnetic contrast agents: A new approach. *Magn Reson Med* 1986, 3:217–225.

Saini S, Frankel R, Stark DD, Ferrucci JT. Magnetism: A primer and review. *Am J Roent* 1988, 150:735–743.

Saini S, Stark DD, Brady TJ, Wittenberg J, Ferrucci JT. Dynamic spin-echo MRI of liver cancer using Gadolinium-DTPA: Animal investigation. *AJR* 1986, 147:357–362.

Saini S, Stark DD, Hahn PF, et al. Ferrite particles: Superparamagnetic contrast agents for enhanced detection of liver cancer. *Radiology* 1987, 162:217.

Saini S, Stark DD, Hahn PF, et al. Ferrite particles: A superparamagnetic MR contrast agent for the reticuloendothelial system. *Radiology* 1987, 162:211–216.

Stark DD, Felder RC, Wittenberg J, et al. MR Imaging of cavernous hemangioma of the liver: Tissue specific characterization. *Am J Roent* 1985, 145:213–220.

Stark DD, Weissleder RW, Elizondo G, et al. Superparamagnetic iron oxide: Clinical application as a contrast agent for magnetic resonance imaging of the liver. *Radiology* 1988, 168:297–302.

Stark DD, Wittenberg J, Edelman RE, et al. Detection of hepatic metastases by magnetic resonance: Analysis of pulse sequence performance. *Radiology* 1986, 159:365–370.

Wedeen VJ, Rosen BR, Buxton RB, Brady TJ. Projected MR angiography and quantitative flow volume densitometry. *Magn Reson Med* 1986, 3: 226–241.

Wehrli FW, MacFall JR, Glover GH, et al. The dependence of nuclear magnetic resonance (NMR) image contrast on intrinsic and pulse sequence timing parameters. *Magn Reson Imaging* 1984, 2:3–16.

Wienmann H-J, Brasch RC, Press WR, Wesby GE. Characterization of Gadolinium-DTPA complex: A potential NMR contrast agent. *AJR* 1984, 142: 619–624.

Weissleder R, Hahn PF, Stark DD. MRI of the spleen: Concepts of the use of contrast agents for tumor detection. *Magn Reson Imaging* 1987, 5:137–138.

Wolf GL, Fobben ES. Tissue proton T_1 and T_2 response to Gadolinium-DTPA injection in rabbits. A potential contrast agent for NMR imaging. *Invest Radio* 1984, 19:324–328.

Wolf GL, Joseph PM, Goldstein EJ. Optimal pulse sequences for MR contrast agents. *AJR* 1986, 147:367–371.

Enhancement Agents for Ultrasound: Fundamentals

Dennis P. Swanson

In ultrasound imaging, short pulses (e. g., 5 msec) of sound waves with frequencies in the megaHertz range (i. e., $3–15 \times 10^6$ cycles/sec) are generated by an ultrasound transducer and directed at an anatomical region-of-interest. Similar to x-rays, ultrasound waves pass through various tissues within this region and are attenuated by either scattering (i. e., reflection or refraction) or energy absorption. However, unlike x-ray imaging, wherein the transmitted radiation is used to produce a radiograph based on overall tissue attenuation characteristics, the production of ultrasound images is based solely on detecting the reflected portion of the attenuated sound waves. The other aspects of sound transmission and attenuation (i. e., refraction and energy absorption) play a negligible role in ultrasound image formation with the stipulation that the generated sound wave and its reflection or echo must be transmitted to a sufficient degree to permit the detection of deep-seated reflecting tissue interfaces. The transducer responsible for generating the ultrasound pulse serves as the sensing device for its echo during the interval between pulses (Christensen EE, 1978; McDicken WN, 1981).

Whether or not an ultrasound wave will be reflected at a given tissue or tissue component interface is primarily dependent on the acoustic impedance properties of the respective tissues or tissue components (Table 22.1). The greater the difference between acoustic impedance values, the greater the degree of ultrasound reflection. Sound waves behave similar to light, therefore, the percentage of an ultrasound beam that is reflected from a tissue interface is also dependent on its angle of incidence relative to the reflecting surface. As might be expected, maximum reflection occurs with a smooth interface that lies perpendicular to the path of the ultrasound wave. (Christensen EE, 1978; McDicken WN, 1981).

The acoustic impedance of a given medium is defined by the product of its density and the velocity of sound in the medium. The rate at which sound is transmitted through matter is in turn related to its density and compressibility, properties that are, in general, inversely related. Hence, sound is transmitted slowly through low density, highly compressible gases and rapidly through dense, noncompressible solids (Table 22.1).

Because, at a given temperature, the velocity of sound in a given medium is essentially constant over a wide range of frequencies, as is the medium's density, then the acoustic impedance of the medium can also be considered to be constant (Christensen EE, 1978).

The reflection of ultrasound waves at tissue or tissue component interfaces permits the ultrasonic demonstration of normal anatomical features and abnormal

Table 22.1 VELOCITY OF SOUND IN AND ACOUSTIC IMPEDANCE OF VARIOUS MATERIALS[a]

MATERIAL	VELOCITY (M/SEC)	ACOUSTIC IMPEDANCE (RAYLS: GM/CM^2 SEC $\times 10^{-5}$)
Air	331	0.0004
Fat	1450	1.38
Water (50° C)	1540	1.54
Brain	1541	1.58
Blood	1570	1.61
Kidney	1561	1.62
Liver	1549	1.65
Muscle	1585	1.70
Bone	4080	7.80

[a] Adapted from Wells PNT, 1969.

masses. As discussed, the intensity of the ultrasound signal from a tissue or tissue component interface is dependent on an acoustic impedance mismatch. Unfortunately, with the exception of air containing structures, fat and bone, the difference in acoustic impedance values between the various soft tissues are small (Table 22.1). Any such differences that do exist are primarily related to varying conformations of individual tissue components (e. g., collagen, fat, fibroelastic tissue) of heterogeneous densities.

Based on the aforementioned considerations, it is not surprising that the development of ultrasound enhancement agents, "echopharmaceuticals", has been based on an attempt to increase the acoustic impedance mismatch at tissue or tissue component interfaces. If a substance with an acoustic impedance substantially different from that of surrounding soft tissue could be made to specifically localize with sufficient concentration in a given tissue component, organ, or abnormal mass, then the ultrasound signal derived from the interface of that structure with surrounding soft tissue may be increased. Alternatively, if the inherent acoustic impedance of an organ or abnormal mass could be specifically modified (e. g., via transient thermal gradients), an augmentation of respective echo intensity may be observed (Mattrey RF, et al, 1987; Ophir J, et al, 1979).

Although the investigation of ultrasound enhancement agents has, to date, been limited, some clinical success has been achieved in the areas of gas-containing bubbles and lipid emulsions. The investigation of these agents has been obviously based on their substantial acoustic impedance differences relative to soft tissue (Table 22.1).

Microbubbles

HISTORY

The development of gas-liquid emulsions (i. e., microbubbles) as echopharmaceuticals for the enhancement of ultrasound imaging followed the initial observation that the rapid intravenous injection of indocyanine green, a diagnostic dye, produced echogenic opacification of the chambers of the right heart and of blood vessels communicating with the injection site (Gramiak R and Shah PM, 1968). Later studies revealed that a similar echogenic effect could be achieved with high-rate injections (i. e. > 20 ml/sec) of a variety of solutions (e. g., water, normal saline, 5% Dextrose in Water, U.S.P., blood, radiopaque contrast media) as a result of a cavitation phenomenon (Gramiak R, et al, 1969; Kremkau FW, et al, 1970; Ziskin MC, 1972). Pressure changes associated with the rapid alterations in fluid flow of high-rate injections can cause solubilized gases to transiently come out of solution in the form of bubbles. These intravascular gas bubbles are excellent reflectors of ultrasound waves due to their substantial difference in acoustic impedance relative to blood (Table 22.1).

CHEMISTRY

Although the high-rate hand-injection approach to the production of intravascular microbubbles is commonly utilized to enhance ultrasound studies of the right heart, it is not an optimal technique. Frequently the generation of microbubbles by this method is unsatisfactory, resulting in a low signal intensity (Goldberg SJ, et al, 1981). This problem may be related to an inadequate force of injection to induce cavitation, a situation that can be avoided if the microbubbles are present in the solution prior to its administration (Meltzer RS, et al, 1980). The rapid intravascular collapse and wide size distribution (i. e., 10–100 microns) of gas bubbles generated by the hand-injection technique may represent other factors responsible for suboptimal echogenic opacification (Feinstein SB, et al, 1984a). Furthermore, although microbubbles produced by hand injection are capable or providing ultrasound enhancement of the right heart, they are unable to survive passage through the capillary bed of the lung

(Bommer WJ, et al, 1981; Goldberg SJ, 1981). The availability of preformed microbubbles of reduced size (i.e., 4–7 microns) and increased stability may not only result in more reliable and improved echogenic enhancement of the right heart following their intravenous injection, but may also permit capillary transmission to allow noninvasive enhancement of ultrasonic studies of the left heart and/or the evaluation of tissue perfusion.

The stability of gas bubbles in a solution is dependent on several factors including bubble size, the surface tension of the solution, and the nature of the gas (Butler BD, 1986). Ultrasonic cavitation (i.e., sonification) of gas-containing aqueous solutions prior to their injection results in the formation of preformed microbubbles of a smaller and more uniform diameter than those obtained with hand agitation or rapid injection of the same solution. In general, these sonicated microbubbles are also more stable and, depending on their diameter and the surface tension of the respective solution, can survive passage through the capillary bed of the lungs following intravenous injection (Feinstein SB, et al, 1984a; Feinstein SB, 1986; Widder DJ, et al, 1986).

Reducing the surface tension of the aqueous solution that constitutes the external phase of a gas-liquid emulsion increases bubble stability. Hence, aqueous solutions of various proteinaceous, alcoholic, or carbohydrate surfactants (e.g., gelatin, albumin, glycerin, sorbitol, saccharin, dextrose, glucose) have been used to produce sonicated or hand-agitated microbubbles with increased resistance to vascular collapse (Bommer WJ, et al, 1981; Butler BD, 1986; Feinstein SB, et al, 1984b; Meltzer RS, et al, 1980). In addition to reducing the surface tension of the external phase, these surfactants also act to prevent coalescence or cohesion of the bubbles, thus maintaining a smaller and more uniform size distribution (Butler BD, 1986; Meltzer RS, et al, 1980).

Preformed microbubbles of a specific size, quantity, and composition can be manufactured using gas injection techniques (Butler BD, 1986). Compared to gas bubbles produced by the previously described cavitation approaches (i.e., hand injection or agitation, sonication), these "precision" or "calibrated" microbubbles offer advantages related to their known and controlled size range and concentration and the ability to vary their composition to increase stability (Carroll BA, et al, 1980). For example, incorporation of an insoluble gas such as nitrogen into the manufacturing process results in precision microbubbles that demonstrate a substantially longer intravascular bubble life than that observed with the use of air, carbon dioxide, oxygen, or other soluble gases (Butler BD, 1986). Such manipulation of gas or surfactant solution composition during manufacturing can result in "precision" microbubbles of virtually any desired size range or stability, thus ensuring reliable and reproducible echogenic enhancement for a variety of clinical applications.

CLINICAL CONSIDERATIONS

The forceful intravenous injection of 0.9% Sodium Chloride Injection, U.S.P. (i.e., normal saline), 5% Dextrose in Water, U.S.P, or autologous blood is frequently used to enhance echocardiographic studies of the right heart and to improve the detection of valvular abnormalities and shunts. As previously discussed, the resulting cavitation microbubbles are confined to the vascular compartment and rapidly dissipate upon entering the capillaries of the lung. Although studies have reported that small diameter (i.e., <7 microns) microbubbles produced by the sonification of various surfactant solutions or by gas injection techniques (i.e., precision microbubbles) are capable of capillary transmission (Bommer WJ, et al, 1981; Butler BD, 1986; Feinstein SB, 1984a), the use of such agents for echogenic enhancement of the left heart following intravenous administration has been extremely limited. This restricted use is most likely related to the nonavailability of appropriate surfactant solutions or precision microbubbles in a formulation indicated and approved for ultrasonic enhancement.

One approach to producing relatively stable microbubbles has involved the sonication of an intravascular radiopaque contrast medium (diatrizoate meglumine-sodium, 76% w/v) (Lang RM, et al, 1987; Feinstein SB, 1986). The resulting microbubbles have a small (i. e., approximately 4 micron diameter), fairly narrow size range and are capable of passing through capillary beds. However, unlike microbubbles derived from nonsurfactant solutions (e. g., normal saline) or solutions of carbohydrates, (e. g., dextrose, glucose) or proteins (e. g., gelatin) that demonstrate minimal physiologic effects, the pseudo-allergic and chemotoxic potential of the radiopaque contrast medium must be considered. Moreover recent experimental studies have shown that the sonication of protein solutions and intravascular contrast media to produce microbubbles results in a substantial degree of myocardial depression following coronary artery administration (Christensen CW, et al, 1988; Shapiro JR et al, 1988), an effect that may be related to bubble size (Lang RM, et al, 1987). Hence, the overall safety of such microbubble preparations must remain a consideration with their injection into the coronary arteries.

Based on their subsequent trapping in capillary beds, hand-agitated and precision microbubbles of a diameter of greater than 10 microns have been injected directly into the hepatic artery to permit the ultrasonic evaluation of normal hepatic versus hepatic tumor perfusion (Carroll BA, et al, 1982; Matsuda Y and Yabuuchi I, 1986). In these studies, viable tumor tissue frequently demonstrates echogenic enhancement relative to normal liver due to abnormalities of tumor neovascularity and/or the tumor's increased reliance on an arterial versus portal venous blood supply. Preliminary investigations (Matsuda Y and Yabuuchi I, 1986) have also shown that the pattern of ultrasonic enhancement of the tumor may correlate with its histological type (e. g., hypoechoic with rim enhancement = hepatocellular or metastatic cancer, internal spotty hyperechoic = fibrous granuloma, etc.). Again, such studies have been limited by the nonavailability of large-diameter preformed microbubbles in a formulation indicated and approved for ultrasonic enhancement.

Another approach to microbubble enhancement of ultrasound studies involves the administration of agents that react in vivo to form bubbles. For example, materials (e. g., ether, perfluorocarbon) that are liquid at room temperature but that vaporize at body temperature may represent effective intravascular ultrasonic enhancement agents provided they are nontoxic (Ziskin MC, et al, 1972). Dilute (0.2%) hydrogen peroxide solution has also been utilized clinically as an agent for echogenic opacification of the right heart (Wang X, et al, 1979; Gaffney FA, et al, 1983). This substance reacts with catalase and peroxidase enzymes of blood to form water and oxygen bubbles. Although an increase in intraluminal and right heart echogenicity has been observed following the direct administration of dilute hydrogen peroxide, a better contrast effect is achieved if it is mixed with a small amount of blood just prior to intravenous injection (Gaffney FA, et al, 1983). Prolonged incubation of dilute hydrogen peroxide with blood will, however, result in the formation of very large bubbles and should be avoided.

Lipid Emulsions

HISTORY

In addition to gases, lipid substances such as fat demonstrate acoustic impedance values that differ substantially from those of soft tissues. Hence, it is not surprising that aqueous lipid emulsions have been investigated as potential ultrasound enhancement agents. Preliminary clinical success in this area has been achieved with the intravenous injection of Fluosol-DA (Mattrey RF, et al, 1987), a yolk-phospholipid emulsion of perfluorocarbons (i. e., 14% v/v perfluorodecalin, 6% v/v perfluorotripropylamine) normally utilized in humans based on its oncotic (synthetic blood-oxygen carrier) properties.

CHEMISTRY

Perfluorocarbons are inert, dense liquids that demonstrate minimal toxicity upon intravenous administration or inhalation. Their acoustic impedance difference of approximately 30% relative to soft tissues suggests that a high degree of respective ultrasound enhancement could be achieved if these agents could be made to specifically localize with sufficient concentration in an organ or tissue of interest. Following intravenous injection of the Fluosol-DA emulsion (2.4 gm/kg), the colloidal (i. e., <0.5 micron diameter) micelle particles containing the perfluorocarbons are phagocytized by cells of the reticuloendothelial system (RES), resulting in an observed echogenic enhancement of the liver and spleen. Hepatic tumors that lack RES (i. e., Kupffer S) cells appeared as nonenhanced (hypoechoic) areas. The echogenicity of some of these hypoechoic tumors gradually increased and in many cases hyperechoic rim enhancement was observed, apparently due to the tumor localization of macrophages that also phagocytize the perfluorocarbon emulsion. Liver and spleen enhancement was optimal at 24–72 hours following Fluosol-DA injection and subsided at approximately 6 days (Mattrey RF, et al, 1987).

It may be assumed that the high density of perfluorocarbons (approximately 1.9 gm/mL) is the major factor responsible for the acoustic impedance difference that led to the demonstrated ultrasonic enhancement properties of Fluosol-DA. However, it is interesting to note that the intravenous injection (1 gm/kg) of other dense lipid emulsions (e. g., EOE-13, fat) of similar particle size failed to produce an increase in liver and spleen echogenicity in a rabbit model (Fink IJ, et al, 1985). This difference in results may be related to differences in the dosage regimens and subsequent tissue concentrations or to differences in lipid compressibility. It should also be emphasized that perfluorocarbons in the nonemulsified form vaporize at body temperature secondary to their high vapor pressure. In fact, the primary route of excretion of systemic perfluorocarbons is via the lung. Hence, the ultrasound enhancement effects of these agents may be related to lysosomal breakdown of the emulsion in the RES cells and the subsequent release of perfluorocarbon vapor in the form of microbubbles (Mattrey RF, et al, 1982). A slow rate of emulsion degradation may explain the relative lack of ultrasound enhancement of the liver and spleen at 6 hours post injection of Fluosol-DA (Mattrey RF, et al, 1987), even though rapid RES accumulation of the micellar particles would be expected.

An approach similar to the use of lipid emulsions for ultrasonic enhancement of the liver and spleen and the improved detection of hepatic lesions has involved the intravenous injection of small diameter (i. e., 2 micron) collagen particles (Ophir J, et al, 1980). In animal studies (dog model), the demonstrated enhancement of the liver and spleen exceeded the predicted results based on the acoustic impedance difference of collagen versus soft tissue. This phenomenon may be related to an increase in particle diameter associated with aggregation or surface coating by physiological proteins (Ophir J, et al, 1980; Cunningham JJ, et al, 1976).

References

Bommer WJ, Miller L, Takeda P, et al. Contrast echocardiography: Pulmonary transmission and myocardial perfusion imaging using surfactant stabilized microbubbles. *Circulation* 1981, (Suppl. IV), 64:200–203.

Butler BD. Production of microbubbles for use as echo contrast agents. *JCU* 1986, 14:408–412.

Carroll BA, Turner RJ, Tickner EG, et al. Gelatin encapsulated nitrogen microbubbles as ultrasonic contrast agents. *Invest Radiol* 1980, 15:260–266.

Carroll BA, Young SW, Rasor JS, et al. Ultrasonic contrast enhancement of tissue by encapsulated microbubbles. *Radiology* 1982, 143:747–750.

Christensen EE, Curry TS III, Dowdey JE (eds). Ultrasound. In *An Introduction to the Physics of Diagnostic Radiology*, second Edition, Philadelphia, Lea and Febiger, 1978, 361–394.

Christensen CW, Reeves WC, Holt GW. Intracoronary echo-contrast agents:

Abnormalities in myocardial function in a normal and reduced coronary perfusion model in dogs. *Ultrasound Med Biol* 1988, 14:199–211.

Cunningham JJ, Wooten W, Cunningham MA. Gray scale echography of soluble protein and protein aggregate fluid collections (in vitro study). *JCU* 1976, 4:417–419.

Feinstein SB. Myocardial perfusion imaging: Contrast echocardiography, today and tommorrow. *J Am Coll Cardiol* 1986, 8:251–253.

Feinstein SB, Shah PM, Bing RJ, et al. Microbubble dynamics visualized in the intact capillary circulation. *J Am Coll Cardiol* 1984a, 4:595–600.

Feinstein SB, TenCate FJ, Zwehl W, et al. Two-dimensional contrast echocardiography: In vitro development and quantitative analysis of echocontrast agents. *J Am Coll Cardiol* 1984b, 3:14–20.

Fink IJ, Miller DL, Shawker TH, et al. Lipid emulsions as contrast agents for hepatic sonography: An experimental study in rabbits. *Ultrason Imaging* 1985, 7:191–197.

Gaffney FA, Lin J-C, Peshock RM, et al. Hydrogen peroxide contrast echocardiography. *Am J Cardiol* 1983, 52:607–609.

Goldberg SJ, Valdez-Cruz LM, Feldman M, et al. Range-gated Doppler ultrasound detection of contrast echographic microbubbles for cardiac and great vessel blood flow patterns. *Am Heart J* 1981, 101:793–796.

Gramiak R, Shah PM. Echocardiography of the aortic root. *Invest Radiol* 1968, 3:356–366.

Gramiak R, Shah PM, Dramer DH. Ultrasound cardiography: Contrast studies in anatomy and function. *Radiology* 1969, 92:939–948.

Kremkau FW, Gramiak R, Carstensen EL, et al. Ultrasonic detection of cavitation at catheter tips. *AJR* 1970, 110:177–183.

Lang RM, Borow KM, Neumann A. Effect of intracoronary injections of sonicated microbubbles on left ventricular contractility. *Am J Cardiol* 1987, 60:166–171.

Matsuda Y, Yabuuchi I. Hepatic tumors: US contrast enhancement with CO_2 microbubbles. *Radiology* 1986, 161:701–705.

Mattrey RF, Scheible FW, Gosink BB, et al. Perfluoroctylbromide: A liver/spleen specific and tumor-imaging ultrasound contrast material. *Radiology* 1982, 145:759–762.

Mattrey RF, Strich G, Shelton RE, et al. Perfluorochemicals as US contrast agents for tumor imaging and hepatosplenography: Preliminary clinical results. *Radiology* 1987, 163:339–343.

McDicken WN, ed. Ultrasound in tissue. In *Diagnostic Ultrasonics: Principles and Use of Instruments*. Second Edition, New York, John Wiley and Sons, 1981, pp 54–70.

Meltzer RS, Tickner EG, Sahines TP, et al. The source of ultrasound contrast effect. *JCU* 1980, 8:121–127.

Ophir J, McWhirt RE, Maklad NF. Aqueous solutions as potential ultrasonic contrast agents. *Ultrason Imaging* 1979, 1:265–279.

Ophir J, Gobaty A, McWhirt RE, et al. Ultrasonic backscatter from contrast-producing collagen microspheres. *Ultrason Imaging* 1980, 2:67–77.

Shapiro JR, Xie F, Meltzer RS: Myocardial contrast two-dimensional echocardiography: dose-myocardial effect relations of intracoronary microbubbles. *J Am Coll Cardiol* 1988, 12:765–771.

Wang X, Wang J, Chen H, et al. Contrast echocardiography with hydrogen peroxide. II. Clinical application. *Chin Med J* 1979, 92:693–702.

Wells PNT, ed. *The Physical Principle of Ultrasonic Diagnosis*. New York, Academic Press, 1969, pp 1–76.

Widder DJ, Simeone JF. Microbubbles as a contrast agent for neurosonography and ultrasound-guided catheter manipulation. *AJR* 1986, 147:347–352.

Ziskin MC, Bonakdapour A, Weinstein DP, et al. Contrast agents for diagnostic ultrasound. *Invest Radiol* 1972, 67:500–505.

APPENDIX
A
▼▼▼
Units of Radioactivity

2.7 Ci	100 GBq
270 mCi	10 GBq
27 mCi	1 GBq
2.7 mCi	100 MBq
270 μCi	10 MBq
27 μCi	1 MBq
2.7 μCi	100 KBq
0.27 μCi	10 KBq
0.027 μCi	1 KBq

1 Curie (Ci) $= 3.7 \times 10^{10}$ dps $= 2.2 \times 10^{12}$ dpm

1 millicurie (mCi) $= 3.7 \times 10^{7}$ dps $= 2.2 \times 10^{9}$ dpm

1 microcurie (μCi) $= 3.7 \times 10^{4}$ dps $= 2.2 \times 10^{6}$ dpm

1 becquerel (Bq) $= 1$ dps $= 2.703 \times 10^{-11}$ Ci

1 kilobecquerel (KBq) $= 10^{3}$ dps $= 2.703 \times 10^{-8}$ Ci

1 megabecquerel (MBq) $= 10^{6}$ dps $= 2.703 \times 10^{-5}$ Ci

1 gigabecquerel (GBq) $= 10^{9}$ dps $= 2.703 \times 10^{-2}$ Ci

1 terabecquerel (TBq) $= 10^{12}$ dps $= 27.03$ Ci

1 microcurie = 37 kilobecquerels (0.037 megabecquerels)

1 millicurie = 37 megabecquerels

1 Curie = 37 gigabecquerels

Method for Prevention of Thyroid Uptake of Radioiodine

A. PHARMACEUTICALS

1. Lugol's solution (Strong Iodide Solution, U.S.P.)
    Each 100 milliliters contains:
    Iodide   5.0 grams
    Potassium iodide   10.0 grams

2. Saturated solution potassium iodide (SSKI)
    Potassium Iodide Oral Solution, U.S.P.)

    Each 100 milliliters contains:
    Potassium Iodide   100 grams

Description: Both solutions are clear, colorless, odorless.

B. PROCEDURE

SSKI, because of its higher iodide content, is usually preferred for thyroid blockade. Lugol's solution is used; however, larger amounts must be administered to ensure adequate blockade of the thyroid gland.

Dosage: Give 3–4 drops SSKI[a] 24 hours prior to radiopharmaceutical administration, then 3–5 drops SSKI b.i.d. for 1–2 weeks following radiopharmaceutical administration.

Dosing information: To protect against possible gastrointestinal injury, which has been associated with concentrated potassium salts, the oral solution should be administered in a full glass of water, fruit juice, milk, etc.

Side/adverse effects: Skin rash (hypersensitivity), salivary gland swelling or tenderness.

[a] A medicine dropper delivers approximately 20 drops/ml (U.S.P. XXI)

A P P E N D I X
C
▼▼▼

Drugs for the Mitigation of Internal Radiocontamination

Dennis P. Swanson
Terry J. Dick

The purpose of this appendix is to provide a convenient source of information on drugs that can be utilized to prevent the systemic absorption or to promote the elimination of internal radiocontaminants in the treatment of victims of radiation accidents. The material included has been condensed from less readily available government publications addressing this subject (IAEA, 1978; NCRP, 1980; Scleien, 1983) with additional precautionary statements and dosage information taken from standard drug formularies (Drug Information, 1986; Facts and Comparisons).

Immediate Actions

The first principle in treating a radiation accident victim should be an attempt to reduce or prevent the systemic absorption and distribution of the radiocontaminant(s). Obviously, external decontamination (Table C.1) should be instituted immediately to decrease external radiation exposure levels, permit safe medical access to the patient, and reduce the potential for radiocontaminant absorption through the skin. Priority attention should be given to the decontamination and treatment of open wounds. Assuming a lack of open wounds, the major routes of systemic entry of the radiocontaminants will be via the lungs and gastrointestinal tract. Although pulmonary absorption of the radiocontaminant may be difficult to prevent, several measures can be employed to reduce gastrointestinal absorption.

Table C.1 BASIC PRINCIPLES OF EXTERNAL DECONTAMINATION[a]

1. Remove contaminated clothing. Place in plastic bag(s) and label.
2. Survey body surface (including nose, mouth, ears, hair, wounds) to identify regions and associated levels of contamination.
3. Initiate external decontamination procedures:
    a. Begin with wound, followed by regions of highest contamination.
    b. Prevent the spread of contamination.
        · Restrict the use of showers to diffuse body contamination only. Cleanse from head downward.
        · Cleanse from outer regions of localized contamination inward.
        · Collect localized and, if possible, gross washings for analysis and disposal.
    c. Wounds: Irrigate with sterile normal saline, water, and/or a 3% aqueous solution of hydrogen peroxide.
    d. Intact skin: Scrub (soft brush) with soap and water or commercially available decontamination/chelating solutions (e. g., Count-Off®, Isoclean®), if available.
        · Avoid excessive scrubbing to prevent abrasion or irritation of skin.
        · Full strength or dilute (i. e., 1:5 dilution for head or whole body) liquid household bleach (aqueous hypochlorite solution) may provide additional cleansing benefits.
    e. Mucous membranes (e. g., nose, eyes, mouth, ears): Irrigate with sterile normal saline or water. Avoid swallowing of washes.
    f. Hair: Wash with shampoo and water.
        · Avoid spread of contamination to eyes, mouth, etc.
        · Clip hair if significant levels of contamination remain. (NOTE: shaving of hair presents an increased risk of laceration and internal contamination.)
    g. Continue cleansing procedures until levels of removable contamination are negligible.

---

[a] Adapted from AMA, 1984; NCRP, 1980; IAEA, 1978.

690

Mitigation of Gastrointestinal Contamination

Immediate action should include the oral administration of an appropriate aluminum or magnesium antacid or activated charcoal (Table C.2). These essentially nonabsorbable preparations strongly adsorb many chemical substances and may thereby act to reduce gastrointestinal absorption of certain of the ingested radiocontaminants. For example, a single 100 mL dose of aluminum phosphate suspension given immediately after exposure has been shown to decrease the systemic absorption of ingested radioactive strontium by 85% (NCRP, 1980).

Whether or not to initiate gastric lavage or to induce emesis is dependent on the time interval post radiation exposure. If a substantial period (i. e., > 1 hour) has elapsed, a majority of the ingested radiocontaminant(s) will be localized to the small bowel. Gastric lavage and emetics, such as ipecac syrup and apomorphine (Table C.2), primarily promote regurgitation of the contents of the stomach and upper gastrointestinal tract with negligible effect on substances in the small bowel. If employed, ipecac syrup is considered preferable to apomorphine due to its reduced potential for central nervous system and respiratory depression and the convenience of its oral administration. However, ipecac syrup must be given prior to the antacid or activated charcoal adsorbent because these latter agents will also adsorb the oral ipecac and prevent its emetic action. The subcutaneous administration of apomorphine should be reserved for those situations wherein the patient is unresponsive to ipecac syrup or the prior administration of an adsorbent has been performed.

An oral saline laxative (Table C.2) should be used to promote emptying of the small bowel and to prevent potential constipating side effects associated with the aluminum antacid or activated charcoal adsorbents. Note that the cathartic effect of a saline laxative will be additive to that of a magnesium antacid adsorbent. The saline laxatives act rapidly (i. e., within 3–6 hours) within the small bowel by exerting a hyperosmolar effect, thus resulting in the accumulation and retention

Table C.2 IMMEDIATE (NONSPECIFIC) THERAPY FOR THE MITIGATION OF INTERNAL RADIATION CONTAMINATION

GENERAL MITIGATING EFFECT	SPECIFIC DRUG THERAPY (COMMONLY AVAILABLE EXAMPLES)	SUGGESTED DOSAGE (ADULT)
I. GASTROINTESTINAL CONTAMINATION		
Adsorbent	Charcoal, activated	30–50 Gm, oral
	Aluminum hydroxide or phosphate suspension	100 mL, oral
	Magnesium hydroxide suspension	100 mL, oral
Emetic	Ipecac syrup[a]	15 mL, oral; repeat after 20 min
	Apomorphine hydrochloride	0.07–0.1 mg/kg, subcutaneous
Saline laxative (small-bowel cleansing)	Magnesium citrate solution	100–200 mL (80–140 mEq), oral
	Sodium phosphate (900 mg/5 mL)/biphosphate (2.4 Gm/5 mL) solution	30 mL (diluted to 120 mL), oral
Colonic evacuant	Sodium phosphate (60 mg/mL)/biphosphate (160 mg/mL) enema solution	120 mL, rectal
	Dulcolax suppository	10 mg, rectal
II. SYSTEMIC CONTAMINATION		
Diuretic	Furosemide	0.3–0.6 mg/kg, intravenous; 10–20 mg q 6 h, oral
	Hydrochlorothiazide	25–50 mg q 12 h, oral
Hydration	Forced fluids	3000–5000 mL/day, oral
	Dextrose 5% in Water, U.S.P	3000 mL/day, intravenous
Hydration *plus* isotopic dilution/displacement	Electrolyte replacement solutions (various)	See respective product information
Thyroid-blocking[b]	S.S.K.I. (Saturated solution of potassium iodide)	6 drops ($\cong$300 mg KI) in water/day

[a] Administer prior to adsorbent therapy.

[b] Nuclear reactor accident and/or suspected radioiodine contamination, only.

of water and a stimulation of peristaltic activity. The concomitant administration of a magnesium antacid and a magnesium saline laxative should be avoided in the presence of preexisting renal dysfunction. Caution should also be observed in administering sodium phosphate/biphosphate laxatives to edematous patients and patients on a sodium-restricted diet.

Most drugs and chemicals (e. g., radiocontaminants) are minimally or very slowly absorbed from the colon. However, rapid elimination of the colonic contents should be instituted using a saline enema or stimulant suppository (Table C.2). This step will not only reduce the potential for systemic absorption of the radiocontaminant(s), but will also result in a decrease in the radiation dose to the gastrointestinal wall and surrounding organs, including the gonads.

Nonspecific Therapy for Mitigation of Systemic Contamination

Immediately following their systemic absorption, many of the water-soluble radiocontaminants will be present in highest concentrations in the blood and the extravascular, extracellular fluid spaces. Assuming that their excretion occurs via the kidney, elimination of these radiocontaminants from the body can be promoted by the administration of a diuretic. Acute therapy may include the intravenous injection of a high-ceiling diuretic, such as furosemide, to achieve a rapid onset of action. This should be followed by daily maintenance doses of standard oral diuretics (Table C.2).

Maximum hydration of the patient should be emphasized to assist in promoting the renal elimination of water-soluble radiocontaminants and to counteract the dehydrating effects of the bowel-cleansing and diuretic regimens. Intravenous fluids (Table C.2) may be required in patients who are unable to comply with oral hydration. Consideration should be given to the intravenous infusion of multiple electro-

lyte replacement solutions, especially in those patients who suffer the gastrointestinal reactions (e. g., nausea, vomiting, diarrhea, malabsorption) of acute radiation exposure. Hydration using multiple electrolyte solutions may provide an added advantage in promoting the elimination of radiocontaminants via a dilutional or displacement mechanism (see Specific Therapy for Mitigation).

Thyroid-Blocking

If the radiation accident involves a nuclear reactor facility, the victim should receive a potassium iodide preparation (Table C.2) as soon as possible to block the thyroidal uptake of commonly associated radioiodine contaminants and to promote the systemic elimination of radioactive iodine and cesium (potassium analog) via the mechanisms of isotopic dilution and displacement (see Specific Therapy for Mitigation), respectively. Maximum benefit of this mitigation therapy is achieved if it is introduced prior to or concomitant with systemic absorption of the radioiodine.

Radiocontaminant Identification and Quantification

Urine and feces should be collected and assayed for radioactivity prior to and throughout the course of mitigation therapy. Every attempt should be made to identify and quantitate the specific radiocontaminant(s) in order to accurately assess the risks to the patient and to effectively initiate specific therapy to promote radiocontaminant elimination from the body.

Specific Therapy for the Mitigation of Systemic Contamination

Several routinely available drugs may be selectively employed to promote the systemic elimination of specific radiocontaminants. In general, these agents exert their mitigation effects via one or more of the following mechanisms (NCRP, 1980; AMA, 1984).

As the name implies, a *blocking agent* prevents or reduces organ uptake and localization of the radiocontaminant by saturating or competing for the involved transport mechanism(s) or receptor binding site(s). The unbound radiocontaminant is subsequently available for more rapid excretion. *Isotopic dilution* takes advantage of the fact that the metabolic binding of the substances in the body is in a constant state of equilibrium or flux. Thus, the administration of relatively large quantities of a stable isotope of the radiocontaminant will result in gradual dilution and elimination of the bound radioisotope. *Displacement therapy* is a form of isotopic dilution wherein stable elements with similar chemical and, hance, binding characteristics as the radiocontaminant are utilized to elicit a dilutional effect. A *mobilizing agent* increases the body's natural turnover processes and thereby also serves to enhance the rate at which a radiocontaminant would be displaced from its binding site(s) and eliminated. *Chelating agents* strongly bind heavy metals resulting in the formation of stable, water-soluble complexes that are rapidly excreted via the kidneys. If the radiocontaminant has a greater affinity for the administered chelating agent then it does for its plasma protein or organ binding site(s), it will be displaced and eliminated.

Table C.3 provides an alphabetical listing of potential radiocontaminants and the specific drugs that have been shown or suggested to enhance their systemic elimination. Note that this table includes only those drugs that are commercially and, therefore, routinely available in the United States. If more than one drug with

Table C.3 SPECIFIC DRUG THERAPY FOR THE MITIGATION OF SYSTEMIC RADIOCONTAMINATION[a]

POTENTIAL RADIOCONTAMINANT	CHEMICAL SYMBOL	NUCLEAR REACTOR BY PRODUCT (*)	MITIGATING DRUG (S)	MECHANISM (S) OF ACTION	REFERENCE(S)
Americium	Am		DTPA, Ca-, Zn-[b]	Chelation	[2,5]
			(Calcium edetate disodium)[c]	Chelation	[3]
Arsenic	As		Dimercaprol	Chelation	[2–4]
Berkelium	Bk		DTPA, Ca-Zn-[b]	Chelation	[5]
			(Calcium edetate disodium)	Chelation	[3]
Bismuth	Bi		Dimercaprol	Chelation	[3,4]
Cadmium	Cd		Calcium edetate disodium	Chelation	[2,3]
Calcium	Ca		Calcium salts	Isotopic dilution	[1,2]
			Ammonium chloride	Mobilization	—
Californium	Cf		DTPA, Ca-, Zn-[b]	Chelation	[2,5]
			(Calcium edetate disodium)	Chelation	[3]
Cerium	Ce	*	Calcium edetate disodium	Chelation	[3,4]
Cesium	Cs	*	Potassium salts	Displacement	—
Chromium	Cr		Calcium edetate disodium	Chelation	[2,3]
			(Desferoxamine)	Chelation	[1]
Curium	Cm		DTPA, Ca-, Zn-[b]	Chelation	[2,5]
			(Calcium edetate disodium)	Chelation	[3]
Europium	Eu	*	Calcium edetate disodium	Chelation	[3]
Gold	Au		Dimercaprol	Chelation	[2,4]
			(Penicillamine)	Chelation	[1–4]
Iodine	I	*	Potassium iodide	Blocking agent/Isotopic dilution	[1–4]

Table C.3 (*Continued*)

POTENTIAL RADIOCONTAMINANT	CHEMICAL SYMBOL	NUCLEAR REACTOR BY PRODUCT (*)	MITIGATING DRUG (S)	MECHANISM (S) OF ACTION	REFERENCE(S)
			Propylthiouracil	Blocking agent	[2]
			(Methimazole)	Blocking agent	[2]
Iron	Fe		Desferoxamine	Chelation	[1]
			(Penicillamine)	Chelation	[2,3]
Lanthanum	La	*	Calcium edetate disodium	Chelation	[3]
Lead	Pb		Calcium edetate disodium	Chelation	[1,2]
			(Penicillamine)	Chelation	[2–4]
			(Dimercaprol)	Chelation	[1,2]
Manganese	Mn		Calcium edetate disodium	Chelation	[1–3]
			(Desferoxamine)	Chelation	[1]
Mercury	Hg		Penicillamine	Chelation	[2–4]
			(Dimercaprol)	Chelation	[1,2,4]
Neodymium	Nd	*	Calcium edetate disodium	Chelation	[3]
Nickel	Ni		Calcium edetate disodium	Chelation	[2,3]
			(Dimercaprol)	Chelation	[2]
Niobium	Nb	*	Calcium edetate disodium	Chelation	[3]
Phosphorus	P		Phosphate salts	Isotopic dilution	[1]
Plutonium	Pu		DTPA, Ca-, Zn-[b]	Chelation	[2,4,5]
			(Calcium edetate disodium)	Chelation	[3]
			(Desferoxamine)	Chelation	[2]
Polonium	Po		Dimercaprol	Chelation	[1,2,4]
			(Penicillamine)	Chelation	[4]
Potassium	K		Potassium salts	Isotopic dilution	[1,2]
			Diuretics	Mobilization	[2]
Praseodymium	Pr	*	Calcium edetate disodium	Chelation	[3]
Promethium	Pm	*	Calcium edetate disodium	Chelation	[3]
Radium	Ra		Calcium salts	Displacement	[4]
Rare earth metals (otherwise unlisted)	Atomic nos. 64–71		Calcium edetate disodium	Chelation	[3]
Samarium	Sm	*	Calcium edetate disodium	Chelation	[3]
Scandium	Sc		Calcium edetate disodium	Chelation	[3]
Strontium	Sr	*	Ammonium chloride	Mobilization	[2,4]
			Calcium salts	Displacement	[2]
Thallium	Tl		Potassium salts	Displacement	—
Transplutonium elements (otherwise unlisted)	Atomic nos. 94–103		Calcium edetate disodium	Chelation	[3]
Tritium	^{3}H	*	Diuretics	Mobilization	[2]
			Hydration	Isotopic dilution	[1,3,4]
Uranium	U	*	Sodium bicarbonate	Mobilization	[1,3,4]
			(Calcium edetate disodium)[b]	Chelation	[3]
Yttrium	Y	*	Calcium edetate disodium	Chelation	[3]
Zinc	Zn		Calcium edetate disodium	Chelation	[3]
			Zinc salts	Isotopic dilution	[2]

[a] Adapted from [1] IAEA, 1978; [2] NCRP, 1980; [3] Scleien B, 1983; [4] Ricks RC, 1984; [5] REAC/TS, 1987.

[b] See Note in formulary section.

[c] Drugs listed in parentheses represent alternate therapy involving the same mechanism as the previously listed drug.

the same mechanism of action has been shown to be effective in promoting the excretion of a given radiocontaminant, the drug-of-choice, based on effectiveness and/or potential for adverse reactions, is listed first with the alternate agent(s) listed in parentheses. Mitigation therapy may, if indicated, employ the use of multiple drugs with differing mechanisms of action.

As a result of their limited use in special research laboratories or medical facilities, it is recognized that many of the potential radiocontaminants listed in Table C.3 would be encountered infrequently in a radiation accident. However, because information related to appropriate therapy for the systemic mitigation of these radionuclides is available, it is included. It is also recognized that the nuclear power industry represents a major area of concern and potential source of internal radiocontamination. Hence, to facilitate rapid referral, Table C.3 includes a column specifically denoting potential reactor-associated radiocontaminants.

Once an appropriate drug for systemic mitigation of a known or suspected radiocontaminant has been identified, the reader should refer to the alphabetical formulary section of this chapter for specific information on the pharmacology (i. e., mechanism of action) of the mitigation agent, cautions associated with its use, and dosage instructions. For more detailed drug information, the reader is advised to consult a standard drug formulary, reference text, or specific product information. It should be noted that the dosages suggested for mitigation therapy are, in general, consistent with the standard therapeutic dosages of these agents for electrolyte replacement or heavy metal poisoning. Because high levels of radiation exposure are commonly associated with relatively low physical quantities of the radiocontaminant, the use of such therapeutic dosages for mitigation therapy should, in general, be effective. Increasing the dose of the mitigating drug will probably have little effect on promoting more rapid excretion of the radiocontaminant but may substantially increase the potential for adverse effects.

Formulary of Mitigating Drugs (see Drug Information, 1986; Facts and Comparison [continually updated]; NCRP, 1980)

AMMONIUM CHLORIDE

PHARMACOLOGY

Ammonium chloride is normally used as a systemic acidifier in the treatment of metabolic alkalosis resulting from chloride loss due to various conditions. The systemic acidosis produced by ammonium chloride promotes the conversion of protein-bound calcium to ionic calcium, the latter form being more readily eliminated from the body by glomerular filtration. Thus, ammonium chloride is an effective mobilizing agent for the systemic mitigation of radioactive calcium or calcium analogs (e. g. strontium). Oral ammonium chloride therapy has been shown to produce a 40–75% reduction in the body burden of radiostrontium under ideal conditions (NCRP, 1980).

CAUTIONS

Side Effects. Ammonium chloride given orally is irritating to the gastrointestinal tract and may cause nausea, vomiting, or cramping. These gastrointestinal side effects can be minimized if the agent is given with food or milk. The use of enteric coated tablets should be avoided due to problems with erratic systemic absorption.

Precautions. The systemic acidosis produced by ammonium chloride may be markedly exaggerated in the presence of renal dysfunction. Should it occur, serious acidosis can be reversed with the administration of intravenous sodium bicarbonate. Adverse effects related to ammonium toxicity may be observed in the presence of severe hepatic dysfunction and the inability to metabolize ammonium to urea. Such patients should be closely monitored for signs of cardiac or central nervous system toxicity.

DOSAGE

The adult oral dosage of ammonium chloride for the mitigation of systemic radiocontamination is 12 grams daily administered in 3–4 divided doses. Children may receive up to 75 mg/kg per day in divided oral doses. Mitigation therapy with ammonium chloride may continue for up to 6 days.

CALCIUM EDETATE DISODIUM

PHARMACOLOGY

Calcium edetate disodium (Calcium-EDTA) is a chelating agent that is used primarily for the treatment of lead poisoning. It will also chelate many other divalent and trivalent heavy metal ions including cadmium, chromium, iron, manganese, nickel, zinc, and the rare earth metals (atomic numbers 57–71). Calcium edetate disodium is *not* effective for the chelation of arsenic, gold, or mercury. Administered parenterally, calcium edetate disodium can chelate and promote the renal excretion of several internal radiocontaminants (Table C.3).

NOTE: Although calcium edetate disodium is effective in chelating uranium, neptunium (Np), plutonium, and transplutonium elements (i.e., atomic numbers 94–103), it has been advised that chelating agents should *not* be utilized for the mitigation of internal uranium or neptunium radiocontaminants (IAEA, 1978; REAC/TS, 1987). In the case of uranium, increased delivery of the chelated radiocontaminant to the kidneys, combined with acidic instability and precipitation, can result in a high renal tubular radiation dose and an increased risk of severe anuric nephritis (IAEA, 1978). The administration of sodium bicarbonate is preferred for uranium contamination because the resulting uranyl bicarbonate complex

is stable, rapidly excreted, and has less nephrotoxic potential. Chelating agents form unstable complexes with neptunium and may actually contribute to its increased deposition in bone (REAC/TS, 1987).

Calcium edetate disodium should *not* be administered orally in an attempt to promote the gastrointestinal elimination of heavy metal radiocontaminants because the resulting metal-EDTA complexes may exhibit enhanced systemic absorption.

Edetate disodium is also available as a chelating agent for the systemic mitigation of divalent and trivalent metal ions. However, edetate disodium exhibits a strong affinity for the in vivo chelation and subsequent renal elimination of calcium ions resulting in serious hypocalcemic reactions including tetany, seizures, cardiac arrhythmias, and respiratory arrest. Therefore, edetate disodium is *not recommended* for the mitigation therapy of internal radiocontamination.

CAUTIONS

Side Effects. Parenterally administered calcium edetate disodium may produce pain and/or thrombophlebitis at the injection site. It is important that the drug be diluted appropriately and infused slowly to avoid these reactions. Other adverse effects may include nausea, vomiting, malaise, and hypotension.

Precautions/Contraindications. Calcium edetate disodium is potentially nephrotoxic and should be administered with extreme caution (and at reduced dosage levels) to patients with preexisting renal disease. Use of this drug is contraindicated in the presence of anuria. The nephrotoxic effects of calcium edetate disodium can usually be avoided by careful attention to the dosage regimen and the use of an intermittent therapy program. Urinalysis and BUN determinations should be performed daily throughout the course of mitigation therapy to monitor for induced renal tubular necrosis. If abnormal results (e.g., elevated BUN, proteinuria, hematuria) are observed, the therapy should be temporarily interrupted.

DOSAGE

For the treatment of heavy-metal poisoning, the intravenous dosage of calcium edetate disodium is usually 1 gm/m^2/day, administered for 3–5 days. Prior to administration, the commercially available calcium edetate disodium (200 mg/mL) must be diluted to a concentration of 2–4 mg/mL using 5% Dextrose in Water, U.S.P. or 0.9% Sodium Chloride for Injection, U.S.P. It is advisable to infuse the diluted material over a 2–8 hour interval. The daily dosage may also be given in two equally divided doses at 12-hour intervals to reduce the potential for adverse effects. If, based on continued evidence of systemic radiocontamination, a second course of therapy is required, at least 2–4 days, and preferably 2–3 weeks, should elapse prior to retreatment.

CALCIUM SALTS

PHARMACOLOGY

Calcium is essential for the maintenance of a number of physiological processes including muscular contractility, respiration, the transmission of nerve impulses, vascular and membrane permeability, and blood coagulation. Calcium salts are therefore routinely prescribed for the prevention or treatment of systemic hypocalcemia. The oral or intravenous administration of calcium salts is effective in promoting the urinary excretion of radioactive calcium by an isotopic dilution mechanism and radioactive strontium via displacement therapy.

CAUTIONS

Side Effects. Oral calcium salts, in particular the chloride salt, can be irritating to the gastrointestinal tract and may induce constipation. They should be taken with milk at approximately 1 hour after meals to reduce the gastrointestinal irritation and provide adequate systemic absorption. With the intravenous administration of calcium salts, patients may complain of tingling effects and a sensation of warmth or discomfort.

Precautions/Contraindications. The administration of calcium salts may result in hypercalcemia and associated adverse reactions (e. g., abdominal distress, dehydration, psychosis) in patients with renal dysfunction. Frequent determinations of the serum calcium concentration should be performed throughout the course of mitigation therapy. Serum calcium concentrations should be maintained at 9–10.4 mg/dL (4.5–5.2 mEq/L) and not exceed 12 mg/dL (6.0 mEq/L). In the advent of hypercalcemia, the drug should be discontinued.

Calcium salts should be administered cautiously to patients with cardiac disease. They are contraindicated in patients with ventricular fibrillation.

Drug Interactions. The myocardial contractility and electrophysiological effects of calcium salts are additive to the respective effects of the digitalis glycosides. Therefore, calcium salts should be administered with extreme caution to patients receiving cardiac glycosides.

DOSAGE

The adult oral dosage of calcium salts for the mitigation therapy of systemic radiocontamination should approach 1–1.5 Gms of elemental calcium per day administered in 3–4 divided doses. Children should receive 45–65 mg/kg of elemental calcium per day in divided oral doses. The elemental calcium content of the various commercially available calcium salts varies; therefore, the reader is advised to refer directly to the product information. For reference, 1 mEq of elemental calcium is equivalent to 20 mg.

Calcium may be administered intravenously in the form of its gluconate, gluceptate, or chloride salt. Systemic acidosis produced by the chloride salt may exert an additive mobilizing effect in promoting the elimination of the radioactive calcium or strontium contaminants; however, associated cautions should be observed (see Ammonium Chloride). Intravenous dosages of calcium salts commonly employ the slow infusion of 150–300 mg elemental calcium per day (pediatric patients: 6–7 mg elemental calcium/kg/day) at a rate not exceeding 15–30 mg (0.7–1.5 mEq)/min. Concentrated formulations of parenteral calcium salts must be diluted in large-volume, intravenous infusion fluids (e. g., 5% Dextrose in Water, U.S.P.) prior to administration. Alternately, a large-volume, calcium-containing electrolyte replacement solution may be utilized. Injection of the calcium salts too rapidly can produce systemic hypotension and negative chronotropic effects (e. g., bradycardia, ECG disturbances).

DESFEROXAMINE MESYLATE

PHARMACOLOGY

The hydroxamic ligand groups of the siderochrome, desferoxamine, readily chelate ferric ions resulting in a water-soluble complex that is readily excreted by the kidneys. Hence, desferoxamine mesylate is routinely utilized for the treatment of acute and chronic iron poisoning and can be used to promote the systemic elimination of radioactive iron contaminants. The affinity of desferoxamine for iron is greater than that of the other routinely available chelating agents. Desferoxamine chelates other metal ions to a considerably lesser degree, although it may be effective in enhancing the systemic excretion of plutonium and manganese radiocontaminants.

CAUTIONS

Side Effects. Desferoxamine produces a minimal number of minor side effects when administered intramuscularly at recommended dosage levels. Pain and induration may occur at the injection site. Rapid intravenous injection of desferoxamine can induce the release of endogenous histamine and associated flushing, erythema, abdominal distress, hypotension, and tachycardia.

Precautions/Contraindications. Because desferoxamine and its metal complexes are predominantly excreted by the kidney, caution must be observed in its administration to patients with renal failure. Its use is contraindicated in the presence of anuria.

DOSAGE

Desferoxamine mesylate should be administered intramuscularly to children and adults at a dose of 0.5–1.0 Gm per day. The intravenous route of administration should be avoided unless the patient is in shock or has severe cardiovascular disease. If the intravenous route is employed, the desferoxamine must be injected very slowly. If required, based on urine or whole-body radioassay, mitigation therapy with desferoxamine may be continued for several days.

DIMERCAPROL (BAL)

PHARMACOLOGY

The dithiol groups of dimercaprol can chelate various heavy metal ions (in particular, arsenic, gold, and mercury) and thereby prevent or reverse their systemic binding to sulfhydryl containing enzymes and proteins. The resulting dimercaprol-metal complexes are excreted rapidly by the kidney. Noncomplexed dimecaprol is metabolized by the liver, with the inactive products excreted in the urine and feces.

It has been suggested that dimercaprol may be useful in promoting the systemic elimination of arsenic, bismuth, gold, or polonium radiocontaminants. For the mitigation of radioactive mercury or lead, penicillamine and calcium edetate disodium, respectively, are more effective. Dimercaprol is ineffective for the chelation of thallium, tellurium, or vanadium. It should *not* be utilized for the treatment of iron, cadmium, selenium, or uranium contamination due to increased toxicity associated with the resultant dimercaprol-metal complexes.

The binding of radiocontaminant metal ions to dimercaprol is in equilibrium with their binding to physiological ligands. Dependent on relative binding affinities, the dimercaprol-metal complexes can readily dissociate in vivo if adequate systemic levels of dimercaprol are not maintained during mitigation therapy. The dimercaprol-metal complexes will also readily dissociate in an acidic environment. The coadministration of sodium bicarbonate (or other alkalinizing agent) should be employed to alkalinize the urine and thus minimize the nephrotoxic effects of the dimercaprol and the radioactive metal ions.

Cautions

Side Effects. The most common adverse effect of intramuscular dimercaprol is a dose-related, transient (i.e., 1–2 hours duration) elevation of systemic blood pressure accompanied by tachycardia. Other side effects typically include nausea, vomiting, headache, sweating, and a sensation of throat or chest constriction accompanied by nervous anxiety. Many of these mild adverse effects of dimercaprol can be prevented or reversed by the prophylactic or therapeutic administration of antihistamines. Seizure and coma have been reported with repeated high doses (i.e., >5 mg/kg) of dimercaprol.

Precautions/Contraindications. Dimercaprol should be administered with caution to patients with renal dysfunction or hypertension. Nonmetabolized dimercaprol is potentially nephrotoxic; therefore, the administration of this agent is contraindicated in the presence of impaired hepatic function. Dimercaprol has also been reported to cause severe hemolysis in patients with glucose-6-phosphate dehydrogenase deficiency.

Dosage

Dimercaprol is administered by deep intramuscular injection at a dose of 2.5 mg/kg. This dosage may be repeated at 4-hour intervals for the first 2 days following contamination, at 12-hour intervals on the third day, and then once daily thereafter for up to 5–10 days.

DTPA (DIETHYLENETRIAMINE-PENTAACETIC ACID), Ca-, Zn-

Pharmacology

Calcium- and Zinc- DTPA are strong chelating agents that are currently available for use under an Investigation New Drug (IND) exemption (see Note, following) for the mitigation of internal plutonium, berkelium, californium, americium, and curium radiocontaminants. Compared to the more readily available (i.e., NDA/FDA "approved") calcium edetate (EDTA) disodium chelating agent, DTPA forms more stable complexes with heavy-metal cations and is generally more effective at promoting their systemic elimination via the kidneys (NCRP, 1980).

NOTE: The IND exemptions for Ca- and Zn-DTPA are sponsored by the Radiation Emergency Assistance Center/Training Site (REAC/TS), Oak Ridge Associated Universities, Oak Ridge, Tennessee, who is also responsible for supplying these agents for use under a standard clinical protocol. Physicians desiring to maintain a supply of Ca- and Zn-DTPA on hand for the possible treatment of internal radiocontamination should directly contact the Center (REAC/TS, 1987).

Although Ca- and Zn-DTPA can effectively chelate several heavy-metal, multivalent cations including the rare earth and transuranium elements (NCRP, 1980), use of these agents under the IND exemption is limited to the treatment of plutonium, berkelium, californium, americium, and curium radiocontamination. Use of these chelators to promote the systemic elimination of other internal heavy-metal radiocontaminants requires special approval from the FDA (REAC/TS, 1987). It has been advised that DTPA-chelating agents should *not* be utilized for the mitigation of internal uranium or neptunium radiocontaminants (IAEA, 1978; REAC/TS, 1987). In the case of uranium, increased delivery of the chelated radio-contaminant to the kidneys, combined with acidic instability and precipitation, can result in a high renal tubular radiation dose and an increased risk of severe anuric nephritis (IAEA, 1978). The administration of sodium bicarbonate is preferred for uranium contamination because the resulting uranyl bicarbonate complex is stable and has less nephrotoxic potential. Chelating agents from unstable complexes with neptunium and may actually contribute to its increased deposition in bone (REAC/TS, 1987).

CAUTIONS

Side Effects. Parenterally administered Ca- and Zn-DTPA can produce nausea, vomiting, malaise, pruritis, and muscle cramps (see also respective IND materials). In general, the zinc salt produces fewer adverse effects than the calcium salt, but may be less effective in promoting the systemic elimination of radio-contaminants during the early course of therapy (NCRP, 1980).

Precautions/Contraindications. Like calcium edetate disodium, Ca- and Zn-DTPA are potentially nephrotoxic. Renal status should be evaluated prior to and throughout mitigation therapy and drug administration discontinued if an alteration in renal function is observed. The use of these agents is contraindicated in the presence of severe renal failure or clinically significant leukopenia or thrombocytopenia (NCRP, 1980).

DOSAGE

(See clinical protocol specified in respective IND exemptions). An intravenous infusion of 1 Gm of Ca- or Zn-DPTA per day diluted in 250–500 mL of 0.9% Sodium Chloride for Injection, U.S.P., or 5% Dextrose in Water, U.S.P., has been reported to be efficacious for the treatment of internal heavy-metal radiocontamination. The total dose should be administered over a 1-hour period be-cause fractionation of the dosage increases the risk for adverse reactions. It has been suggested that this dosage may be repeated for up to 5 consecutive days per week (NCRP, 1980).

METHIMAZOLE

PHARMACOLOGY

The thioimidazole derivative, methimazole, in an antithyroid agent used in the treatment of hyperthroidism. It interferes with the incorporation of thyroidal iodine into the tyrosyl residues of thyroglobulin and thereby acts to inhibit the formation and release of thyroid hormones. The administration of methimazole following radioiodine contamination will therefore reduce the organification and subsequent systemic distribution of radioiodine initially trapped in the thyroid gland. Its administration may be considered as an adjunct to the radioprotectant use of potassium iodide (NCRP, 1980).

CAUTIONS

Side Effects. Adverse reactions to methimazole occur infrequently. Minor side effects include dermatological reactions (rash, urticaria, pigmentation), nausea, vomiting, headache, edema, muscle and joint pain, and paresthesia. Methimazole-induced agranulocytosis has been reported rarely, with a dose-dependent increased likelihood in patients older than 40.

Precautions. Patients should be monitored for signs of agranulocytosis (i. e., sore throat, skin eruptions, malaise, leukopenia) throughout the course of mitigation therapy. Hypothyroidism with prolonged use of methimazole may require the supplemental administration of thyroid hormones.

DOSAGE

Methimazole is administered orally at an adult dose of 10 mg every 8 hours for 2 days following radioiodine contamination. The dosage should be subsequently reduced to 5 mg every 8 hours and continued for 6–10 days. For children, the initial dosage of methimazole is 0.4 mg/kg decreasing to 0.2 mg/kg.

PENICILLAMINE

Pharmacology

The monothiol chelating agent, penicillamine, complexes copper, iron, mercury, lead, and other heavy-metal ions and thereby promotes their systemic elimination via the kidneys. As a chelatiang agent, penicillamine is commonly used to remove copper in the treatment of Wilson's disease and less commonly for the treatment of lead and mercury poisoning. Experimental studies have shown that penicillamine will reduce systemic exposure to radioactive gold, mercury, and lead by a factor of 1.5 (NCRP, 1980).

Cautions

Side Effects. Over 30% of the patients receiving penicillamine will experience an allergic reaction usually manifesting as an acute, generalized rash or other dermatological response. Fever, arthralgia, or lymphadenopathy may also be observed. These allergic reactions to penicillamine can usually be controlled with the co-administration of an antihistamine.

Mild proteinuria is a common occurrence with penicillamine. Gastric distress and alterations in taste perception are also frequently encountered. Hematological abnormalities have been reported, including severe agranulocytosis, thrombocytopenia, and aplastic anemia.

Precautions/Contraindications. Patients should be closely monitored for symptoms of penicillamine allergy during mitigation therapy. Hematological profiles and urinalysis should be routinely performed. Clinically significant proteinuria and hematuria should be considered warning signs for the development of a nephrotoxic syndrome associated with immune complex membraneous glomerulopathy.

Extreme caution should be observed in administering penicillamine to patients with a known penicillin allergy because cross-sensitivity reactions are a definite possibility.

Drug Interactions. The gastrointestinal absorption of penicillamine is substantially reduced in the presence of iron salts, antacids, or food. It should be administered on an empty stomach at 1 hour before or 2 hours after meals.

Digoxin serum levels may be reduced by penicillamine, requiring an adjustment of dosage.

Dosage

Penicillamine is administered orally at an adult dose of 250 mg every 6 hours to promote the elimination of indicated radiocontaminants (i. e., mercury, gold, lead). It should be taken 1 hour before or 2 hours after meals. The pediatric dose is 20 mg/kg daily in divided doses.

PHOSPHATE SALTS

Pharmacology

Phosphorus is an essential intracellular anion that plays an important role in a variety of physiological processes including adenosine triphosphate (ATP) production and metabolism, acid-base equilibrium, bone deposition, and calcium metabolism. Exogenous phosphate salts are normally administered for the management of hypophosphatemia secondary to alcoholism, dietary phosphate insufficiency (e. g., altered gastrointestinal absorption, vomiting, phosphate-deficient total parenteral nutrition), and insulin therapy. The oral or intravenous administration of phosphate salts may also be used to promote the systemic elimination of radioactive phosphorus by an isotopic dilution mechanism.

Cautions

Side Effects. The oral administration of phosphate salts commonly produces diarrhea. Systemic side effects may occur as a result of the absorbed phosphate anions or the sodium or potassium cations utilized in the respective formulation. Phosphate-induced hypocalcemia can lead to paresthesia of the extremities, muscle cramping, bone and joint pain, and respiratory distress. Fluid retention and tachycardia may result from hypernatremia, whereas generalized weakness and an irregular heartbeat are associated with hyperkalemia.

Precautions/Contraindications. In general, phosphate salts should be administered with caution to patients with pre-existing renal dysfunction, cardiac disease, or hypoparathyroidism. Phosphates may accelerate deterioration of renal function. Potassium salts should be avoided in digitalized patients and in patients with, or prone to, hyperkalemia (e.g., patients on potassium-sparing diuretics, dehydrated patients). Sodium salts should be avoided in the presence of edematous conditions, hypertension, or severe liver disease.

Patients should be routinely monitored for renal functional status and serum phosphate, calcium, potassium, and sodium concentrations during mitigation therapy, especially if parenteral phosphate salts are utilized.

Drug Interactions. Magnesium or aluminum antacids can bind orally administered phosphate and prevent its systemic absorption. The concurrent administration of corticosteroids and sodium phosphate preparations may result in hypernatremia. Potassium-sparing diuretics or other potassium-containing drugs administered in conjunction with potassium phosphate preparations may result in hyperkalemia.

DOSAGE

Mitigation therapy incorporating the oral administration of phosphate salts should provide 30–90 mM (930–2790 mg) of phosphorus per day administered in 3–4 divided doses. In children under the age of 4, the oral dose is 25 mM of phosphorus daily. The oral phosphate tablets or capsules should be dissolved in water and taken with food to minimize gastric distress.

Several oral phosphate-containing preparations are commercially available. Table C.4 lists some common products and their phosphorus (and sodium and potassium) concentrations. However, the reader is advised to refer directly to the product literature to confirm the phosphorus content of the agent and the appropriate dosage regimen, and to identify the nature and respective concentrations of sodium or potassium salts.

Phosphate may be administered parenterally in the form of its sodium or potassium salt. The parenteral dose should approach 10–15 mM (310–465 mg) of phosphorus per day. Pediatric dosage is 1.5–2 mM per day. Concentrated phosphates for injection (3 mM phosphorus/mL) must be diluted in large-volume intravenous fluids and infused slowly (i.e., approximately 2 mM/hour) to prevent phosphate intoxication and/or

Table C.4 COMMERCIALLY AVAILABLE PHOSPHATE PREPARATIONS
FOR ORAL ADMINISTRATION

ORAL PHOSPHATE AGENTS®	MM PHOSPHORUS	MEQ SODIUM	MEQ POTASSIUM
Fleet Phospho-Soda	4.15/ml	4.8/ml	—
Neutra-Phos-K	8.0/cap	—	14.0/cap
Neutra-Phos	8.0/cap	7.1/cap	7.1/cap
K-Phos-Neutral	8.0/cap	13.0/tab	1.1/tab
K-Phos-Original	3.7/tab	—	3.7/tab
K-Phos M.F.	4.0/tab	2.9/tab	1.1/tab
K-Phos No. 2	8.0/tab	5.8/tab	2.3/tab
URO-KP-Neutral	5.6/tab	9.8/tab	1.3/tab

hypocalcemia. Alternately, a phosphate containing multiple electrolyte solution may be utilized.

POTASSIUM IODIDE

Pharmacology

Potassium iodide inhibits the synthesis and release of thyroid hormones. It has therefore been used as an adjunct to anti-thyroid drugs (e. g., methimazole, pro-pylthiouracil) for the treatment of hyper-thyroidism and thyrotoxicosis. Potassium iodide is frequently administered prior to thyroidectomy to induce thyroid involu-tion and a reduction in vascularity.

As a radioprotectant, the administra-tion of potassium iodide prior to radio-iodine exposure has been shown to block the thyroidal uptake of radioiodine to less than 1% of the exposure dose (Becker DV, et al, 1984). In addition to its action as a blocking agent, potassium iodide also exerts mitigational effects on radioac-tive iodine and potassium contamination via isotopic dilution and radioactive ce-sium or thallium (potassium analogs) con-tamination via displacement. Maximum benefit is obtained if potassium iodide therapy is initiated prior to radioiodine contamination. Its administration im-mediately following a reactor accident and suspected radioiodine exposure is essential. Potassium iodide will also block the organification of radioiodine pre-viously localized to the thyroid gland and prevent its systemic redistribution in the form of thyroid hormones.

Cautions

Side Effects.   Adverse reactions to potas-sium iodide are primarily associated with hypersensitivity to iodine or iodism. Side effects related to iodine hypersensitivity commonly include skin rashes, and less frequently, fever, arthralgia, eosinophilia, and lymph-node enlargement. Iodism reactions are typically associated with more prolonged dosing and are, there-fore, delayed in appearance. Common manifestations of iodism include salivary gland swelling and increased salivation, mouth and throat irritation, and head-cold symptoms. Gastrc irritation occurs frequently with the oral administration of potassium iodide and can be diminished if the preparation is given with food or milk.

Precautions/Contraindications.   Potas-sium iodide should be administered with caution to patients with preexisting hyper-kalemia or renal dysfunction. Its use is contraindicated in patients with known iodine hypersensitivity.

Drug Interactions.   Potassium iodide administered concurrently with other potassium-containing preparations or potassium-sparing diuretics may result in hyperkalemia and associated adverse effects including cardiac arrhythmias or arrest.

Dosage

As a radioprotectant, potassium iodide should be administered orally prior to or immediately following known or sus-pected exposure to radioactive iodine or potassium analogs. The adult dose is 150–300 mg of potassium iodide daily for 10–14 days following exposure. Pediatric dos-age ranges from 65 mg (<1 year) to 130 mg daily.

Potassium iodide is commercially avail-able in several formulations. The concen-tration of potassium iodide in each of these formulations is listed in Table C.5, as is the required dosage to yield 150–300 mg. Tablets should be crushed prior to administration to facilitate rapid gas-trointestinal absorption of the potassium iodide. Liquid formulations should be di-luted in water or juice prior to ingestion. All preparations should be taken with food or milk to reduce gastrointestinal irritation.

POTASSIUM SALTS

Pharmacology

Potassium is a major intracellular cat-ion essential for numerous physiological

Table C.5 COMMERCIALLY AVAILABLE POTASSIUM IODIDE PREPARATIONS

FORMULATION	POTASSIUM IODINE CONCENTRATION	DOSAGE TO YIELD 150–300 MG POTASSIUM IODIDE
Saturated Solution Potassium Iodide (SSKI)	1000 mg/mL	3–6 drops
Lugol's solution	100 mg/mL	1.5–3 mL
Potassium iodide syrup	65 mg/mL	2–5 mL
Potassium iodide tablets	130 mg/tablet	1–2 tablets

processes including the maintenance of acid–base balance and isotonicity, the activation of several enzymatic reactions, the transmission of nerve impulses, muscle contractility, renal function, and carbohydrate metabolism. The oral administration of potassium salts may be considered to promote the systemic elimination of radioactive potassium contaminants by an isotopic dilution mechanism or radioactive cesium or thallium contaminants via displacement therapy.

CAUTIONS

Side Effects. The oral administration of potassium salts commonly results in nausea, vomiting, and diarrhea. Severe reactions to potassium salts are primarily associated with hyperkalemia. Clinical signs and symptoms of potassium overdosage include paresthesia, generalized weakness, pallor, mental confusion, hypotension, cardiac arrhythmias, and heart block.

Precautions/Contraindications. Hyperkalemia is not likely with the oral administration or slow intravenous injection of potassium salts in patients with normal renal function. However, periodic assessments of ECG and plasma potassium concentration should be performed throughout mitigation therapy. In patients with renal dysfunction, routine determinations of plasma potassium concentration are a requirement. ECG changes (i. e., depression of ST segment, prolonged QT interval) are probably the best indicators of potassium toxicity.

The administration of potassium salts is contraindicated in the presence of severe renal impairment with oliguria, anuria, or azotemia. An evaluation of renal function should always be performed prior to the initiation of therapy. Potassium salts should be administered with extreme caution to patients with cardiac disease or in patients with or prone to hyperkalemia (e. g., dehydration, Addison's disease).

Drug Interactions. Potassium salts should not be administered to patients receiving potassium-sparing diuretics or other potassium-containing drugs due to the increased potential for hyperkalemia.

DOSAGE

The dosage of potassium salts is usually expressed as mEq of potassium. The suggested oral dose of potassium for mitigation therapy is 30–60 mEq per day given in 3–4 divided doses. Pediatric patients should receive 2–3 mEq/kg per day. Oral potassium salts should be administered in a liquid formulation with meals and additional liquids to minimize the potential for gastric irritation. Several formulations of potassium are commercially available for oral administration including the acetate, bicarbonate, chloride, citrate, and gluconate salts. The reader is advised to refer directly to the product information to ascertain the concentration of potassium in mEq and the appropriate dosage regimen. Note that oral potassium iodide may represent the most appropriate drug for use following a reactor accident due to its combined effects in promoting the systemic elimination of radioiodine and radiocesium contaminants.

Parenteral administration of potassium salts (acetate, chloride, phosphate) should be avoided due to the increased potential for acute hyperkalemia compared to the relatively slow intenstinal absorption of oral administration. If required, intravenous potassium salts must be administered slowly in dilute concentration. The suggested intravenous dose of potassium for mitigation therapy in adults is also 30–60 mEq daily (pediatric doses of 2–3 mEq/kg/day). In general, the concentration of the intravenous potassium solution should be less than 0.04 mEq/mL, and it should be administered at a rate not exceeding 20 mEq/hour. Routine monitoring of plasma potassium concentration and ECG is a requirement during parenteral administration. The oral administration of potassium salts should be initiated as soon as possible. Alternately, a potassium-containing multiple electrolyte solution may be considered.

PROPYLTHIOURACIL

Pharmacology

The thiourea derivative, propylthiouracil, is an antithyroid agent used in the treatment of hyperthyroidism. It interferes with the incorporation of thyroidal iodine into the tyrosyl residues of thyroglobulin and thereby acts to inhibit the formation and release of thyroid hormones. The administration of propylthiouracil following radioiodine contamination will therefore reduce the organification and subsequent systemic redistribution of radioiodine initially trapped in the thyroid gland. Its administration may be considered as an adjunct to the radioprotectant use of potassium iodide (NCRP, 1980).

Cautions

Side Effects. Adverse reactions to propylthiouracil occur infrequently. Minor side effects include dermatological reactions (rash, urticaria, pigmentation), nausea, vomiting, headache, edema, muscle and joint pain, and paresthesia. Propylthiouracil-induced agranulocytosis has been reported rarely, with an increased likelihood in patients older than 40. This serious adverse reaction to propylthiouracil does not appear to be dose related.

Precautions. Patients should be monitored for signs of agranulocytosis (i. e., sore throat, skin eruptions, malaise, leukopenia) throughout the course of mitigation therapy. Hypothyroidism with prolonged use of propylthiouracil may require the supplemental administration of thyroid hormones.

Dosage

To prevent the systemic redistribution of radioiodinated thyroid hormones following radioiodine contamination, propylthiouracil should be administered orally at an adult dose of 100 mg every 8 hours for 5–10 days. For pediatric patients, the dosage of propylthiouracil ranges from 5–10 mg/kg/day for neonates to 150 mg/m^2/day for older (age > 6) children.

SODIUM BICARBONATE

Pharmacology

The oral or parenteral administration of sodium bicarbonate results in an increase in plasma and urinary bicarbonate levels and a corresponding increase in blood and urinary pH. Sodium bicarbonate is therefore frequently used as a systemic alkalizer for the treatment of acute mild to moderate acidosis. As a urinary alkalizer, it is utilized to increase the solubility of various substances (e. g., uric acid, sulfonamides) excreted in the urine in order to prevent kidney damage associated with their renal tubular crystallization.

Sodium bicarbonate is administered concomitantly with dimercaprol mitigation therapy to increase the stability of the excreted dimercaprol-metal complexes and thereby minimize potential toxicity associated with free dimercaprol or radioactive metal ions. The administration of sodium bicarbonate should also be considered in the event of uranium radiocontamination. Uranium forms a stable, water-soluble complex in the presence of bicarbonate, thus preventing its renal tubular precipitation and associated increase in radiation exposure (IAEA, 1978; NCRP, 1980). The administration of sodium bicarbonate should be avoided in the presence of radioactive calcium or calcium analogs (e. g., strontium). The resulting systemic alkalosis will tend to reduce the mobilization and systemic elimination of these radiocontaminants (see Ammonium Chloride).

CAUTIONS

Side Effects. Excessive doses of sodium bicarbonate can result in hypokalemia-related side effects including generalized weakness, muscle cramping, and an irregular heart beat. Signs of bicarbonate-induced metabolic alkalosis include weakness, muscle pain or twitching, slow breathing, nervousness, or mood alterations.

Precautions/Contraindications. The administration of sodium bicarbonate is contraindicated in the presence of pre-existing metabolic alkolosis. Due to the potential for hypernatremia, it should be given with extreme caution to patients with renal dysfunction, edematous conditions (e. g., congestive heart failure, cirrhosis of the liver), or hypertension. Serum electrolyte (i. e., sodium, potassium) and bicarbonate levels and arterial blood pH should be routinely monitored during mitigation therapy to avoid adverse reactions associated with hypernatremia, hypokalemia, or metabolic alkalosis.

Drug Interactions. Alterations in gastrointestinal pH produced by the oral administration of sodium bicarbonate can influence the systemic absorption of many oral drugs. In general, oral medications should *not* be taken within 1–2 hours of an oral dose of sodium bicarbonate.

The concurrent administration or adrenocorticoids may increase the likelihood of hypernatremia.

DOSAGE

To produce urinary alkalization, sodium bicarbonate may be administered orally at an adult dose of 1 teaspoonful (baking soda) in a glass of water every 4 hours. Sodium bicarbonate tablets are also available, with an adult dose of 4 Gms, initially, then 1–2 Gms every 4 hours. The pediatric dosage (tablets) is 1–10 mEq/kg per day in divided doses.

The intravenous dose of sodium bicarbonate for urinary alkalinization is 2–5 mEq/kg administered over a 4–8-hour period. It is recommended that the 4.2% concentration (0.5 mEq/mL) be utilized.

These dosages should be adjusted upward or downward based on measurements of urinary and arterial pH.

ZINC SALTS

PHARMACOLOGY

Adequate dietary zinc is a requirement for normal growth, tissue repair, and enzyme function. The oral administration of zinc salts may be effective in promoting the systemic elimination of radioactive zinc contaminants via the mechanism of isotopic dilution.

CAUTIONS

Side Effects. Zinc salts administered orally are irritating to the gastrointestinal tract and should be taken with food to minimize gastric distress. Severe vomiting, dehydration, and restlessness may occur with excessive doses.

DOSAGE

The suggested oral dosage of elemental zinc for mitigation therapy is 150 mg per day in three divided doses. Zinc is available in various forms including the sulfate (0.23 mg Zn/mg), gluconate (0.12 mg Zn/mg), and chloride (0.40 mg Zn/mg) salts.

References

AMA, OP-335, *A Guide to the Hospital Management of Injuries Arising from Exposure to or Involving Ionizing Radiation*. American Medical Association, Chicago, 1984.

Becker DV, Braverman LE, Dunn JT, et al. The use of iodine as a thyroidal blocking agent in the event of a reactor accident. *JAMA* 1984, 252:659–661.

Drug Information. American Hospital Formulary Service, American Society of Hospital Pharmacists, 1986.

Facts and Comparisons, Kastrup ED, (ed). St. Louis, Facts and Comparisons, Inc.

IAEA. Safety Series No. 47, *Manual on Early Medical Treatment of Possible Radiation Injury*, Vienna, International Atomic Energy Agency, 1978.

NCRP. Report No. 65, *Management of Persons Accidentally Contaminated with Radionuclides*, National Council on Radiation Protection and Measurements, Washington, DC, 1980.

REAC/TS. Program update: DTPA chelation drugs. Radiation Emergency Assistance Center/Training Site (REAC/TS), *Newsletter* 1987, Winter/Spring: 1–2.

Ricks RC. *Hospital Emergency Department Management of Radiation Accidents*, The Federal Emergency Management Agency, Oak Ridge, TN, 1984.

Scleien B. *Preparedness and Response in Radiation Accidents*. U.S. Department of Health and Human Services HHS Publication FDA 83-8211, Rockville, MD, 1983.

INDEX

A

Abdominal and gastrointestinal imaging. *See* Gastrointestinal tract imaging; Hepatobiliary system imaging; Reticuloendothelial system imaging
Acetylcholine, 51, 58
Actinium-235, 282
Adrenal hypofunction, 367–368
Adrenocortical imaging:
  adjunctive techniques in, 364–365
  indications for, 365
    hyperaldosteronism, 366–367
    hyperandrogenism, 367
    hypercortisolism (Cushing's syndrome), 365–366
  patient preparation for, 364
Adrenocortical imaging, radiopharmaceuticals for, 360
  adrenal hypofunction and, 367–368
  adverse reactions to, 363
  chemistry of, 360–361
    NP-59, 361
  clinical considerations for, 364–367
  dosage/dosimetry for, 368
  drug interactions with, 363–364
  formulation incompatibilities, 363
  history of, 360–361
  pharmacokinetics of, 361–362
  precautions in using, 363–364
  pregnancy and breastfeeding and, 363
Adrenomedullary imaging, patient preparation for:
  catecholamine measurements, 380–381
  thyroid blockade, 381
Adrenomedullary imaging, radiopharmaceuticals for:
  adverse reactions to, 377
  chemistry of, 371–372
  clinical considerations for, 378–381
  dosage/dosimetry for, 382–386
  drug interactions with, 377–378
  history of, 368–371
  pharmacokinetics of,
    biodistribution, 372–373
    excretion and metabolism, 373–376
    mechanism of localization, 376–377
  precautions in using, 377–378
  pregnancy and breastfeeding and, 377
AEC. *See* Atomic Energy Commission
Age of patient:
  adverse reactions to contrast media and, 265
  radiation dosimetry and, 293–294
Agreement States, 296–299, 301
Allergies, contrast media and, 263, 267
Alpha decay, 281
Alpha radiation, 280
Aluminum hydroxide-containing antacids, 468
Aminophyline, 271
Ammonium chloride:
  dosage for, 696
  pharmacology of, 695
  precautions in using, 695
  side effects of, 695
Anaphylactic reactions to contrast media, 254–255
  manifestations of, 254
  treatment for, 270–272
Androgen therapy, 468
Anesthesia:
  lymphography and, 241
  reticuloendothelial imaging and, 468
Anger camera, 287

Angiographic contrast media:
   buffering agents in, 12
   chemistry of, 2–3
      buffering agents, 12
      ratio-1.5 ionic contrast media, 3–8
      ratio-3 low-osmolality contrast media,
         8–11
      sequestering agents, 11–12
   clinical considerations for, 43–61
      risk factors and, 58–61
   dosage for, 61
      concentration considerations, 62–63
      digital subtraction angiography
         considerations, 64–66
      volume considerations, 63–64
   drug interactions with, 41, 42
   history of, 2–3
   laboratory test/diagnostic procedure
         interactions with, 40, 41
   materials incompatible with, 39, 41
   pharmacokinetics of, 12
   physiological effects of, 12–13
      cardiac, 31–38
      cerebral, 27–31
      chemotoxic, 13–14
      gastrointestinal, 20–21
      pseudo-allergic reactions, 13
      pulmonary, 21–24
      renal, 24–27
   precautions in using, 39–43
   pregnancy and breastfeeding and, 41, 43
   ratio-1.5 ionic, 3–8, 10, 43, 45
   ratio-3 low-osmolality, 8–11, 45–46,
      58–61
   sequestering agents in, 11–12
Angiography, 1
   commonly used procedures for, 1
   contrast media for, 1–66
      considerations in using, 43, 45–47
   digital subtraction (DSA), 1–2
   indications for, 43, 44
   low-osmolality contrast media
         recommendations for, 58–61
   patient preparation for, 47–48
   pharmacoangiography, 48–58
Angiotensin, 52
Antigen/antibody reactions to radiographic
      contrast media, 258-259
Antigens:
   carcinoembryonic (CEA), 572
   tumor-associated (TAA), 571–572
Antihistamines:
   anaphylactic reactions to contrast media
         and, 271
   angiography and, 47–48, 58

Aortography, effects of contrast media in,
      24–27, 37–39
Artery:
   carotid, angiographic contrast media and,
      28
   coronary, angiographic contrast media
         and, 31–32
   peripheral, angiographic contrast media
         and, 38
Arthrographic contrast media:
   aspiration of, following arthrography, 226
   chemistry of, 222
   clinical considerations for, 224–226
   dosage for, 226–227
   history of, 221–222
   laboratory test/diagnostic procedure
         interactions with, 226
   pharmacokinetics of, 222–223
physiological effects of,
      hydrarthrosis, 224
         synovial irritation, 223–224
      precautions in using, 226
Arthrography, 221
   adjunctive drugs and techniques in, 226
   contraindications to, 226
   contrast aspiration and, 226
   contrast media for, 221–227
      considerations in using, 225
   double-contrast, 221
   epinephrine and, 226
   indications for, 224–225
   patient preparation for, 225–226
   pneumoarthrography, 221
   precautions in using, 226
   single-contrast, 221
Asthma, contrast media and, 263
Atomic Energy Act of 1954, 296
Atomic Energy Commission (AEC), 296,
      299, 343
Atoms:
   carrier, 283
   thallium, 287
Atropine:
   angiography and, 47
   vagal reactions to contrast media and,
      272
Attenuation of values of body structures,
      99–100

B

B$^+$ (positron) decay, 281
Barium enema, 179–181
Barium sulfate:
   biphasic examinations of upper
         gastrointestinal tract and, 172

Barium sulfate (*Cont.*)
  chemistry of, 157
    additives, 160–162
    concentration, 158
    density, 158
    viscosity, 158–160
  double-contrast evaluation of
      gastrointestinal tract and, 169–172
  drug interactions with, 163
  formulation considerations in using,
      176–177
  history of, 155
  laboratory test/diagnostic procedure
      interactions with, 163
  pharmacokinetics of, 162
  physiological effects of, 162–163
  precautions in using, 162–163
  preparations of, 112–114
  product selections for, 155–157
  single-contrast evaluation of
      gastrointestinal tract and, 166–169
  small bowel examinations and, 172–176
BATO complexes of Technetium-99m,
      438–439
BBB. *See* Blood-brain barrier
Becquerel (Bq), 282
Beta minus, 281
Beta radiation, 280
Bile concentration:
  cholangiographic contrast media and,
      207–209
  cholecystographic contrast media and,
      191–193
Biliary excretion:
  cholangiograhic contrast media and,
      207–209
  cholecystographic contrast media and,
      191–193
Bladder opacification, in computed
      tomography procedures, 114
Blocking agent, 693
Blood coagulation, 18–19
Blood flow:
  cerebral, effect of xenon on, 118
  pulmonary, angiographic contrast media
      and, 21–22
Blood pool imaging, radiopharmaceuticals
      for. *See* Radionuclide
  ventriculography
Blood pressure:
  angiographic contrast media and, 19,
      21–23, 28–29, 37–38
  pulmonary, 21–22
  systemic, 22–23, 28–29, 38

Blood transport:
  cholangiographic contrast media and, 206
  cholecystographic contrast media and, 189
Blood vessels, angiographic contrast media
      and, 19
Blood viscosity, angiographic contrast media
      and, 17
Blood volume:
  angiographic contrast media and, 14
  total. *See* Total blood volume
Blood volume measurements, 616
  indications for,
    plasma volume, 620
    red cell survival/sequestration, 620
    total blood volume, 619
  interpretation of, 621
  procedures in, 620–621
Blood volume measurements,
      radiopharmaceuticals for, 616
  chemistry of, 617–618
    Chromium-51 labeled red blood cells,
      617–618
    radioiodinated human serum albumin
      (RISA), 616–617
  clinical considerations for, 619–620
  pharmacokinetics of,
    Chromium-51 labeled red blood cells,
      618
    radioiodinated human serum albumin
      (RISA), 618
  precautions in using,
    Chromium-51 labeled red blood cells,
      619
    radioiodinated human serum albumin
      (RISA), 619
Blood-brain barrier (BBB):
  alterations in, angiographic contrast media
      and, 29–30
  deficiency in, computed tomography and,
      107–108
  radiopharmaceuticals and, 304–334
Bone marrow imaging, pharmaceuticals for
  chemistry of,
    Technetium-99m albumin colloid, 555
    Technetium-99m sulfur colloid, 555
  clinical considerations for, 557
  dosimetry for, 557
  history of, 552–555
  pharmacokinetics of, 555–556
  precautions in using, 556–557
  pregnancy and breastfeeding and, 556
  storage data for, 556–557
Bone pain, metastatic, therapeutic
      radiopharmaceuticals for:

adverse reactions to, 607
contraindications to use of, 608
dosimetry for, 609
Bradykinin, 56
Brain images:
  delayed (static), 314–315
  dynamic, 314
Brain imaging:
  indications for, 307
Brain imaging, radiopharmaceuticals for, 305
  chemistry of, 308–310
  clinical considerations in using, 312–313
  dosage/dosimetry requirements for, 313–315
  drug interactions with, 312
  history of, 305–308
  pharmacokinetics of, 310–311
  precautions in using, 312
Brain penetration, of myelographic contrast media, 138
Brain receptor-specific radiopharmaceuticals, 326–327
Brain tumor, cystic. *See* Malignant effusion
Brain, computed tomography of, 107–109, 111–112
  adrenocortical imaging and, 363
  adrenomedullary imaging and, 377
  angiographic contrast media and, 41, 43
  bone marrow imaging and, 556
  Neuron-enhanced, 116–119
Breastfeeding:
  central nervous system imaging and, 312
  glomerular filtration excretion imaging and, 509–511
  hepatobiliary system imaging and, 479
  Iodine-125 fibrinogen and, 635
  myocardial infarction imaging and, 423
  pulmonary perfusion imaging and, 398–399
  pulmonary ventilation imaging and, 409
  radioactive materials and, 294–295, 312
  radioferrokinetic studies and, 630
  radiolabeled Vitamin B_{12} and, 625–626
  renal imaging and, 519, 524
  reticuloendothelial imaging and, 468
  Schilling test and, 625–626
  skeletal imaging and, 549
  thyroid imaging and, 350–351
  treatment of polycythemia vera and, 608
  tumor imaging and, 568
  venous thrombosis detection and, 635
Bromosulphalein, 198
Bronchographic contrast media, 242

chemistry of, 244
clinical considerations for, 247
dosage requirements for, 247–248
history of, 242–244
laboratory test/diagnostic procedure interactions with, 246–247
pharmacokinetics of, 244–245
physiological effects of, 246
  foreign body reactions, 246
  pseudo-allergic reactions, 246
  pulmonary, 245–246
precautions in using, 246–247
Bronchography:
  contraindications to, 247
  contrast media for, 242–248
  indications for, 247
  patient preparation for, 247
Buffering agents, 12

C

Calcium-DTPA
    (diethylenetriamine-pentaacetic acid):
  contraindications to, 700
  dosage for, 700
  pharmacology of, 699–700
  precautions in using, 700
  side effects of, 700
Calcium edetate disodium:
  contraindications to, 696–697
  dosage for, 697
  pharmacology of, 696
  precautions in using, 696–697
  side effects of, 696
Calcium salts:
  contraindications to, 697
  dosage for, 697–698
  drug interactions with, 697
  pharmacology of, 697
  precautions in using, 697
  side effects of, 697
Camera:
  Anger, 287
  scintillation, 287
Cancer chemotherapeutic agents, 467–468
Carcinoembryonic antigens (CEA), 572
Carcinoma, thyroid. *See* Thyroid disease
Cardiac effects of angiographic contrast media, 31–39
Cardiac function studies. *See* Radionuclide ventriculography
Cardiac imaging, radiopharmaceuticals for, 419
  in myocardial infarction studies, 419–429

Cardiac imaging, radiopharmaceuticals
for (*Cont.*)
in myocardial metabolism studies, 439–442
in myocardial perfusion studies, 429–439
in ventricular function studies, 442–450
Carotid artery effects of angiography contrast
media, 28
Carrier atoms, 283
Carrier-mediated transport, 316–326
Catecholamine measure, 380–381
Captopril, 515
Cellular radiation effects, 586
Central nervous system:
angiographic contrast media and, 30–31
myelographic contrast media and, 140–142
radiopharmaceuticals for imaging of,
304–334
See also Blood-brain barrier; Brain
imaging; Cerebral function;
Cerebrospinal fluid; Receptor-specific
pharmaceuticals
Central nervous system hypothesis of
reactions to contrast media, 258–259
Cerebral effects of angiographic contrast
media, 27–31
Cerebral function, radiopharmaceuticals for
measuring, 315–316
in evaluation of cerebral perfusion,
319–323
HM-PAO
(hexamethyl-propyleneamineoxime),
323–326
transport of, 316–319
Cerebral metabolism, F-18
fluorodeoxyglucose and, 316–319
Cerebral perfusion, lipophilic
radiopharmaceuticals and, 319–323
Cerebrospinal fluid (CSF) imaging,
radiopharmaceuticals for:
clinical considerations for, 332
dosage/dosimetry for, 332–334
history of, 329–330
Indium-111 pentetate, 330–331
precautions in using, 331–443
Ytterbium-169, 330–331
Ceretec (Technetium-99m exametazime),
323
Characteristic x-rays, 281
Chelating agents, 693
Chemotoxic effects of contrast media,
253–254
angiographic, 13–20
mediating factors of, 253–254.
Cholangiographic contrast media:
chemistry of, 205–206

clinical considerations for, 213–214
differentiated from cholecystographic
contrast media, 184
dosage for, 214
drug interactions with, 211–212
history of, 184–186
laboratory test/diagnostic procedure
interactions with, 212
materials incompatible with, 211–212
pharmacokinetics of, 206
biliary excretion and bile concentration,
207–209
blood transport, 206
gallbladder concentration, 209
gallbladder excretion/enterohepatic
circulation, 209
hepatic metabolism, 207
hepatocyte uptake, 206–207
renal excretion, 209–210
physiological effects of, 210
hepatic, 211
hypotension, 210
renal, 210–211
precautions in using, 211–212
purpose of, 184
Cholangiography:
adjunctive drugs in, 213
contraindications to, 214
contrast media considerations in, 213
direct, 214
contrast media considerations in,
215–216
contrast media dosage for, 216
indications for, 213, 214–215
patient preparation for, 213
percutaneous transhepatic, 214–216
Cholangiopancreatography, endoscopic
retrograde (ERCP), 214–216
Cholecystographic contrast media:
chemistry of, 186, 187
choleretic activity of glucuronide
derivatives of, 193
clinical considerations for, 199–204
differentiated from cholangiographic
contrast media, 184
dosage for, 204–205
drug interactions with, 197–198
history of, 184–186
laboratory test/diagnostic procedure
interactions with, 198
maximum aqueous solubility of, 187
passive permeability coefficients and
benzene/water partition ratios for,
189
pharmacokinetics of, 186

biliary excretion and bile concentration, 191–193

blood transport, 189

gallbladder concentration, 193–194

gallbladder excretion and enterohepatic circulation, 194–195

hepatic metabolism, 190–191

hepatocyte uptake, 189–190

intestinal absorption, 186–189

renal excretion, 195

physicochemical properties of commercially available, 187

physiological effects of, 195–196

gastrointestinal, 196

hepatic, 197

renal, 196–197

precautions in using, 197–198

purpose of, 184

Cholecystography:

adjunctive drugs in, 202, 204

contraindications to, 204

contrast media considerations and, 199–200

indications for, 199

patient preparation for, 200–202, 203

Cholestyramine resins, 197, 213

Cholecystokinetic agents, 482–483

Chromic phosphate P-32. *See* P-32 chromic phosphate

Chromitope Sodium (Chromium-51), 617

Chromium-51:

EDTA (ethylenediamine tetraacetic acid), 503

sodium chromate, 286

labeled red blood cells:

basic steps involved in labeling, 617

chemistry of, 617–618

clinical considerations for, 619–620

dosage/dosimetry for, 620–621

pharmacokinetics of, 618

precautions in using, 619

Chromium-52 DTPA (diethylenetriamine-pentaacetic acid), 503

Chronotropic effects of angiographic contrast media, 32–35

Coagulation, angiographic contrast media and, 18–19

Cobalt, radiolabeling with isotopes of. *See* Radiolabeled Vitamin B_{12}

Cobalt-57, state authority over use of, 299

Collecting ducts, urographic contrast media and, 87–88

Collimation, 289, 290

Colon, barium studies of, 157, 179–181

Complement activation, 256–258

Computed tomography (CT):

of body, 104–107, 111

of brain, 107–109, 111–112

compared to film-based radiographic techniques, 100

contrast media for,

intracavitary, 112–116

intravascular, 100–112

reticuloendothelial, 119–122

xenon, 116–119

myelographic, 114–116, 145

renal, 109

technique of, 99–100

illustrated, 99

Contrast agents for magnetic resonance and ultrasound imaging. *See* Magnetic resonance imaging; Ultrasound imaging

Contrast media:

adverse reactions to,

age and, 265

anaphylactic, 270–272

anaphylactoid, 254–255

antigen/antibody, 258–259

central nervous system hypothesis of, 258–259

classification and terminology of, 253–255

severity of, 260

clinical manifestations and incidence of, 259–263

drugs useful in treating, 272–273

etiology of unpredictable, 255–258

factors affecting risk of, 263–266

history of previous reactions and, 263

ionic contrast media and, 260–262, 265–266

as intercurrent complications, 253

method of contrast media administration and, 265

nonionic and dimeric contrast media and, 261–262

predictable versus unpredictable, 253–254

pretesting for, 266–267

pretreatment for, 267–269

prevention of, 266–269

pseudo-allergic, 13, 232, 240, 246, 254–255

quantity of contrast medium administered and, 263–264

reporting, 273–274

route of administration and, 264

sex and, 265

Contrast Media (*Cont.*)
   therapy for, 269–274
   types of contrast media and, 260–262,
      265–266
   viscosity of contrast media and,
      266
 angiography,
   chemistry of, 2–12
   clinical considerations for, 43–61
   dosage requirements for, 61–66
   pharmacokinetics of, 12
   physiological effects of, 12–39
   precautions in using, 39–43
 arthrographic, 221
   aspiration of, following arthrography,
      226
   chemistry of, 222
   dosage for, 226–227
   history of, 221–222
   pharmacokinetics of, 222–223
   physiological effects of, 223–224
 bronchographic, 242
   chemistry of, 244
   clinical considerations for, 247
   dosage for, 247–248
   history of, 242–244
   pharmacokinetics of, 244–245
   physiological effects of, 245–246
   precautions in using, 246–247
 commercially available, chemical structures
      of, 187
 cholangiographic,
   chemistry of, 205–206
   clinical considerations for, 213–214
   differentiated from cholecystographic
      contrast media, 184
   dosage for, 214
   history of, 184–186
   pharmacokinetics of, 206–210
   physiological effects of, 210–211
   precautions in using, 211–212
   purpose of, 184–186
 cholecystographic,
   chemistry of, 186, 187
   choleretic activity of glucuronide
      derivatives of, 193
   differentiated from cholangiographic
      contrast media, 184
   dosage for, 204–205
   history of, 184–186
   maximum aqueous solubility of, 187
   passive permeability coefficients and
      benzene/water partition ratios for, 189
   pharmacokinetics of, 186–195

   physiochemical properties of
      commercially available, 187
   physiological effects of, 195–197
   precautions in using, 197–198
   purpose of, 184
 drug interactions with,
   in angiography, 41, 42
   in cholangiography, 211–212
   in cholecystography, 197–198
   in gastrointestinal studies, 163, 166
   in myelography, 130, 142–144
 gastrointestinal, 155
   barium sulfate, 155–163
   clinical considerations and dosage for,
      166–182
   iodinated, 163–166
 hysterosalpingographic, 227–228
   clinical considerations for, 232–235
   history of, 228–229
   oil-soluble, 229
   pharmacokinetics of, 230
   physiological effects of, 231–232
   precautions in using, 232–233
   water-soluble, 229–230
 intracavitary, 112–116
 intravascular, 100–112
 laboratory test/diagnostic procedure
      interactions with,
   in angiography, 41
   in arthrography, 226
   in bronchography, 246–247
   in cholangiography, 212
   in cholecystography, 198
   in gastrointestinal studies, 163
   in hysterosalpingography, 232
   in lymphography, 240
   in myelography, 130, 144
 lymphographic, 236
   chemistry of, 237–238
   clinical considerations for, 241–242
   complications associated with, 240–241
   dosage for, 242
   history of, 236–237
   pharmacokinetics of, 238–240
   physiological effects of, 239–240
   precautions in using, 240–241
 myelographic, 125
   for negative contrast myelography,
      125–126
   for positive contrast myelography,
      126–151
   iophendylate (Pantopaque), 126–130,
      145–146
   nonionic, 130–151

ratio-1.5 ionic, 3–8, 10, 43, 45
ratio-3 low-osmolality, 8–11, 45–46, 58–61
reactions to. *See* Contrast media, adverse
    reactions to
reticuloendothelial, 119–122
urographic,
    in direct urography, 95–97
    in excretory urography, 78–95
Copper-67 (Cu-67), 574
Coronary artery, angiographic contrast
    media and, 31–32
Corticosteroids:
    in angiographic procedures, 47–48, 58
    in treatment of anaphylactic reactions to
        contrast media, 271–272
Crystals, NaI, 287
CSF. *See* Cerebrospinal fluid
CT. *See* Computed tomography
Cu-67. *See* Copper-67
Curie (Ci), 282
Cushing's syndrome (hypercortisolism),
    365–366
Cystic brain tumor. *See* Malignant effusion
Cystography, radionuclide. *See* Radionuclide
    cystography

D

Dehydration, adverse reactions to contrast
    media and, 267
Delayed (static) brain images, 314–315
Department of Transportation (DOT), 301
Desferoxamine mesylate:
    contraindications to, 698
    dosage for, 698
    pharmacology of, 698
    precautions in using, 698
    side effects of, 698
Dexamethasone sodium phosphate, 271–272
Diatrizoate, 3–8
Digital subtraction angiography (DSA), 1–2,
    64–66
Dimercaprol (BAL):
    contraindications to, 699
    dosage for, 699
    pharmacology of, 698–699
    precautions in using, 699
    side effects of, 699
Dimercaptosuccinic acid (DMSA), 347
Dionosil-aqueous, 244
Dionosil-oily, 244
Dipyridamole, 57–58
Dipyridamole-adjunctive method, 435–436
Direct urography, 95–97

contraindications to, 96–97
contrast media considerations in, 96
indications for, 95–96
precautions with, 96–97
Disease, radiation dosimetry and, 294
Distal tubule, urographic contrast media
    and, 87–88
DMSA. *See* Dimercaptosuccinic acid
Dopamine, 58–59
DOT. *See* Department of Transportation
Doxycycline, 235
Drug interactions:
    with adrenocortical imaging
        radiopharmaceuticals, 363–362
    with adrenomedullary imaging
        radiopharmaceuticals, 377–378
    with angiographic contrast media, 39, 41,
        42
    with calcium salts, 697
    with cholangiographic contrast media,
        211–212
    with cholecystographic contrast media,
        197–198
    with conventional brain imaging
        radiopharmaceuticals, 312
    with ferrous (Fe-59) citrate, 630
    with gastrointestinal contrast media,
        barium sulfate, 163
        iodinated, 166
    with hepatobiliary system imaging
        radiopharmaceuticals, 479
    with myelographic contrast media, 130,
        142–144
    with penicillamine, 701
    with phosphate salts, 702
    with potassium iodide, 703
    with potassium salts, 704
    with radiolabeled Vitamin B_{12}, 624–625
    with radionuclide ventriculography
        radiopharmaceuticals, 449–450
    with radiopharmaceuticals for thyroid
        imaging, 349–350
    with reticuloendothelial system imaging
        radiopharmaceuticals, 467–468
    with sodium bicarbonate, 706
    with venous thrombosis detection
        radiopharmaceuticals, 634–635
Drugs:
    for mitigation of internal
        radiocontamination, 690–706
      ammonium chloride, 695–696
      calcium edetate disodium, 696–697
      calcium salts, 697–698
      desferoxamine mesylate, 698

Drugs (*Cont.*)
    dimercaprol (BAL), 698–699
    DTPA (diethylenetriamine-pentaacetic
      acid), 699–700
    formulary of, 695–706
    methimazole, 700–701
    penicillamine, 701
    phosphate salts, 701–703
    potassium iodide, 703
    potassium salts, 703–705
    propylthiouracil, 705
    sodium bicarbonate, 705–706
    specific, 692–695
    zinc salts, 706
  in pharmacoangiography, 48–58
  vasoactive, 48
  vasoconstrictors, 49–53
  vasodilators, 53–58
Duodenum, examination of, 179
Dynamic brain images, 314

E

Echopharmaceuticals for ultrasound imaging.
  See Ultrasound imaging
Edema, pulmonary, angiographic contrast
  media and, 23–24
Effusions. *See* Malignant effusion
Electrolyte/pH effects of angiographic
  contrast media, 14–16
Electron capture, 282
Embolization, systemic, with
  lymphography, 240
Endocrine imaging, radiopharmaceuticals
  for, 343–386. *See also*
  Adrenocortical imaging; Adrenomedullary
    imaging; Parathyroid scintigraphy;
    Thyroid imaging
Endoscopic retrograde
  cholangiopancreatography (ERCP),
  214–216
Energy Reorganization Act of 1974, 296
Energy Research and Development
  Administration, 297
Enhancement agents for magnetic resonance
  and ultrasound imaging. *See*
  Magnetic resonance imaging; Ultrasound
    imaging
Enterohepatic circulation:
  cholangiographic contrast media and, 209
  cholecystographic contrast media and,
    194–195
EOE-13, 120
Ephedrine, 47–48, 58

Epinephrine:
  in arthrography, 226
  in pharmacoangiography, 49–52
  in treatment of anaphylactic reaction to
    contrast media, 270–271, 272
Erythrocyte aggregation, angiographic
  contrast media and, 16–17
Erythromycin, 235
Esophageal reflux:
  studies of, 486–487
  therapies for, 487
Esophageal transit studies, 487–488
Esophagus, examination of, 179
Ethiodol (Lipiodol Ultrafluid):
  in hysterosalpingographic contrast
    medium, 228–230
  as lymphographic contrast medium,
    237–238
Excretory urography, 78–98

F

F-18 FDG (fluorodeoxyglucose), 439–440
  cerebral metabolism and, 316–319
  chemistry of, 317, 318, 440
  dosimetry for, 319, 441–442
  history of, 316–317
  pharmacokinetics of, 317, 318
  precautions in using, 319, 441
Fatty acids, modified, in myocardial
  metabolism imaging, 440–441
FDA. *See* Food and Drug Administration
Fe-59 ferrous citrate. See Ferrous (Fe-59)
  citrate
Ferrous (Fe-59) citrate, 629
  chemistry of, 629
  clinical considerations for,
    erythrocyte iron incorporation, 631
    organ kinetics, 631–632
    plasma iron clearance, 631
    summary of, 632
    systemic kinetics/biodistribution, 631
  dosage/dosimetry for,
    gastrointestinal absorption, 633
    systemic kinetics/biodistribution,
      632–633
  drug interactions with, 630
  pharmacokinetics of,
    gastrointestinal absorption, 629
    systemic kinetics/biodistribution,
      629–630
  precautions in using, 630
  pregnancy and breastfeeding and, 630
Fission products, 283–284

Fluorescent thyroid scanning, 358–359
Food and Drug Administration (FDA), 297,
    297, 299–301
    Investigational Review Board (IRB) of,
        300
    Radioactive Drug Research Committee
        (RDRC) of, 300
Foreign body reactions:
    with bronchography, 246
    with hysterosalpingography, 232

G

Ga-67. *See* Gallium-67
Gallbladder concentration:
    cholangiographic contrast media and, 209
    cholecystographic contrast media and,
        193–194
Gallbladder excretion:
    cholangiographic contrast media and, 209
    cholecystographic contrast media and,
        194–195
Gallbladder nonvisualization, extrabiliary
    causes of, 201
Gallium-67 (Ga-67), 347
    in inflammatory process imaging, 579–580
    in tumor imaging,
        adverse reactions to, 568
        altered biodistribution of, 567–568
        chemistry of, 565–566
        clinical considerations for 569
        dosimetry for, 569–570
        history of, 564–565
        pharmacokinetics of, 566–567
        precautions in using, 567–568
        pregnancy and breastfeeding and, 568
    state authority over use of, 299
Gamma decay (isomerism), 281–282
Gamma rays, 281
Gases, radioactive. *See* Radioactive gases
Gastric emptying:
    delayed, 489
    dosimetry for, 492
    factors affecting rate of, 491
    rapid, 489
    studies of, 488–492
    various disease states and patterns of,
        491–492
Gastric emptying curves, 489, 492
Gastrointestinal contrast media:
    adjunctive drugs for, 181–182
    barium sulfate,
        in biphasic examinations of upper
            gastrointestinal tract, 172

chemistry of, 157–162
    in double-contrast evaluation of
        gastrointestinal tract, 169–172
    drug interactions with, 163
    formulation considerations, 176–177
    history of, 155
    pharmacokinetics of, 162
    physiological effects of, 162–163
    precautions in using, 162–163
    product selections for, 155–157
    in single-contrast evaluation of
        gastrointestinal tract, 166–169
    in small bowel examinations, 172–176
iodinated, 163
    chemistry of, 164–165
    drug interactions with, 166
    gastrointestinal use of, 177–179
    laboratory test/diagnostic procedure
        interactions with, 166
    physiological effects of, 165–166
    precautions in using, 165–166
patient preparation for, 179–181
Gastrointestinal effects:
    of angiographic contrast media, 20–21
    of cholecystographic contrast media,
        196
Gastrointestinal opacification, in computed
    tomography procedures, 112–114
Gastrointestinal radiocontamination,
    mitigation of, 691–692
Gastrointestinal tract:
    biphasic examination of, 172
    double-contrast barium evaluation of,
        169–172
    imaging of,
        esophageal reflux studies, 486–487
        esophageal transit studies, 487–488
        gastric emptying studies, 488–492, 493
        Meckel's diverticulum scintigraphy,
            485–486
        rectal emptying studies, 488–492
        small bowel and colonic transit studies,
            488–492, 493
        See also Hepatobiliary system imaging;
            Reticuloendothelial system imaging
    single-contrast barium evaluation of,
        166–169
Geiger-Mueller counter, 286
Genitourinary imaging, 501–530. *See also*
    Glomerular filtration;
    Radionuclide cystography;
        Space-occupying diseases; Testicular
        imaging; Tubular secretion
GFR. *See* Glomerular filtration rate

Glomerular filtration, urographic contrast
  media and, 82–84
Glomerular filtration, radiopharmaceuticals
    excreted by:
  adverse reactions to, 511, 512
  chemistry of,
      Iodine-125 iothalamate, 506
      Technetium-99m gluceptate, 506–507
      Technetium-99m pentetate, 506
  clinical considerations for, 513
  determination of glomerular filtration rate
    and, 502–504
  dosimetry for,
      Iodine-125 iothalamate, 512
      Technetium-99m gluceptate, 513
      Technetium-99m pentetate, 512–513
  history of, 502–506
  pharmacokinetics of,
      Iodine-125 iothalamate, 507
      Technetium-99m gluceptate, 508
      Technetium-99m pentetate, 507–508
  pharmacologic intervention,
      with captopril, 515
      with Lasix (furosemide), 514–515
  precautions in using,
      Iodine-125 iothalamate, 508–509
      Technetium-99m gluceptate,
        510–511
      Technetium-99m pentetate, 509–510
  pregnancy and breastfeeding and,
      509–511
  radiolabeled complexes of soluble chelates
    and, 502–515
  renal filtration imaging and, 504–506
Gigabecqueral (GBq), 282
Glomerular filtration rate (GFR), 82–84,
    502–504
Glomerular permeability, angiographic
    contrast media and, 26
Glucagon:
  with gastrointestinal radiological studies,
    181–182
  with hystersalpingography, 235
  in pharmacoangiography, 57
Glucocorticoids, 271–272
Glucose analogues, in myocardial
    metabolism imaging, 439–440
  chemistry of, 440
  dosimetry for, 441–442
  precautions in using, 441
Gray (Gy), 290
Guide for the Preparation of Applications
    for Medical Use Programs
    (DOT, 1987), 301

H

HAM. *See* Human albumin microspheres
Heart rate, angiographic contrast media and,
    19, 22–23, 28–29, 37, 38
Hematocrit, angiographic contrast media
    and, 14
Hematological applications of
    radiopharmaceuticals. *See* Blood
    volume
  measurements; Radioferrokinetic studies;
    Schilling test; Venous thrombosis
    detection
Hepatic effects:
  of cholangiographic contrast media, 211
  of cholecystographic contrast media, 197
Hepatic metabolism:
  cholangiographic contrast media and, 207
  cholecystographic contrast media and,
    190–191
Hepatobiliary system imaging:
  adjunctive drugs in, 482–483
  patient preparation for, 479–480
  radiopharmaceuticals for,
    adverse reactions to, 479
    chemistry of, 473–475
    clinical considerations in using,
      481–483
    domimetry for, 479–481
    drug interactions with, 479
    method for, 479–481
    pharmacokinetics of, 475–478
    precautions in using, 478–479
    pregnancy and breastfeeding and, 479
    See also Reticuloendothelial imaging;
      Spleen-specific imaging
  technique used in, 480–481
Hepatocyte uptake:
  cholangiographic contrast media and,
    206–207
  cholecystographic contrast media and,
    189–190
Histamine release, radiographic contrast
    media and, 255
HM-PAD
    (hexamethyl-propyleneamineoxime),
    323–324
Hounsfield Units (HU), 99–100
Human albumin microspheres (HAM),
    395–396
  compendial requirements for, 398
  See also Technetium-99m HAM
Hydrarthrosis, with arthrography, 224
Hyperaldosteronism, 366–367
Hyperandrogenism, 367

Hypercortisolism (Cushing's syndrome), 365–366
Hyperthyroidism. *See* Thyroid disease
Hypocalcemia, angiographic contrast media and, 34
Hypotension, cholangiographic contrast media and, 210
Hysterosalpingographic contrast media, 227–228
  clinical considerations for, 233–235
  history of, 228–229
  intravasation of, 232–233
  laboratory test/diagnostic procedure interactions with, 232
  oil-soluble, 229
  pharmacokinetics of, 230
  physiological effects of,
    foreign body reactions, 232
    mucosal irritation/pain, 231–232
    pseudo-allergic reactions, 232
  precautions in using, 232–233
  water-soluble, 229–230
Hysterosalpingography, 227–228
  adjunctive drugs for, 235
  contraindications to, 232–233, 235
  contrast media for, 227–236
    considerations in using, 233–234
  indications for, 233
  pelvic inflammatory disease following, 233
  precautions with, 232–233
  pregnancy rates following, 234–235
  use of antibiotics prophylactically with, 235
Hytrast, 243

I

I-123, etc. *See* Iodine-123, etc.
ICC. *See* Interstate Commerce Commission
ICRP. *See* International Commission on Radiological Protection
Immunochemistry, 571–572
In vivo method, modified, in radionuclide ventriculography, 446–448
IND. *See* Investigational new drug
Indium-111 (In-111), 285, 574–575
  antimyosin,
    chemistry of, 426–427
    dosimetry for, 428–429
    method for, 428–429
    in myocardial infarction imaging, 426–429
    pharmacokinetics of, 427–428
    precautions in using, 428

  in bone marrow imaging, 554
  in gastric emptying studies, 490
  MAA (macroaggregated albumin), 395
  in myocardial infarction imaging, 426–429
  pentetate, 330–331
    adverse reactions to, 331–332
    in cerebrospinal fluid imaging, 331–334
    chemistry of, 331
    dosage/dosimetry for, 332–334
    in gastric emptying studies, 490
    pharmacokinetics of, 331
    precautions in using, 331–332
    pregnancy and breastfeeding and, 331
  oxine formulations, 583–584
  radiolabeled leukocytes, 580–584
  radiolabeled platelets, 637
  in tumor imaging, 580–584
  in venous thrombosis detection, 637
Inflammatory process imaging, radiopharmaceuticals for:
  Gallium-67 citrate,
    chemistry of, 579
    clinical considerations for, 580
    dosimetry for, 580
    history of, 579
    pharmacokinetics of, 570–580
  Indium-111 radiolabeled leukocytes,
    cellular radiation effects, 586
    chemistry of, 582–584
    clinical considerations for, 587–590
    dosimetry for, 590–591
    history of, 580–582
    leukocyte count and, 586
    oxine contentration and, 585–586
    pharmacokinetics of, 584–585
    precautions in using, 585–587
    quality control of, 586–587
Inotropic effects of angiographic contrast media, 35–37, 38–39
Internal radiocontamination:
  drugs for mitigation of, 690–706
    ammonium chloride, 695–696
    calcium edetate disodium, 696–697
    calcium salts, 697–698
    desferoxamine mesylate, 698
    dimercaprol (BAL), 698–699
    DTPA (diethylenetriamine-pentaacetic acid), 699–700
    formulary of, 695–706
    methimazole, 700–701
    penicillamine, 701
    phosphate salts, 701–703
    potassium iodide, 703
    potassium salts, 703–705

Internal radiocontamination (*Cont.*)
    propylthiouracil, 705
    sodium bicarbonate, 705–706
    specific, 692–695
    zinc salts, 706
  gastrointestinal, mitigation of, 691–692
  identification and quantification of
      radiocontaminant and, 692
  immediate actions for, 690
  systemic, nonspecific therapy for, 692
  thyroid blocking for, 692
International Commission on Radiological
    Protection (ICRP), 295
Interstate Commerce Commission (ICC),
    301
Intestinal absorption, cholecystographic
    contrast media and, 186–189
Intraarticular therapy. *See* Malignant effusion
Intracavitary contrast media, 112
  bladder opacification and, 114
  gastrointestinal opacification and, 112–114
  intrathecal opacification and, 114–116
Intraperitoneal effusions. *See* Malignant
    effusion
Intrapleural effusions. *See* Malignant effusion
Intrathecal opacification, in computed
    tomography procedures, 114–116
Intravasation of contrast media, in
    hysterosalpingography, 232–233
Intravascular contrast media, 100–101
  chemistry of, 101
  clinical considerations for, 104
  contraindications to, 104
  pharmacokinetics of, 101–104
  physiological effects of, 104
  precautions in using, 104
Investigational new drug (IND), 299
Investigational Review Board (IRB), 300
Iocarmate meglumine, 132
Iocetamic acid, 187
Iodamide, 78–79
Iodeikon, 185–186
Iodine-123 (I-123), 344–345, 573–574
  MIBG, 382–385
  OIHA,
    dosimetry for, 519
    in myocardial metabolism imaging,
        440–442
    pregnancy and breastfeeding and, 519
    in renal imaging, 517–520
Iodine-125 (I-125), 344, 573–574
  fibrinogen,
    clinical considerations for, 635
    dosage/dosimetry for, 635–636
    drug interactions with, 634–635

    laboratory test/diagnostic procedure
        interactions with, 634–635
    pharmacokinetics of, 634
    precautions in using, 634–635
    pregnancy and breastfeeding and, 635
    in venous thrombosis detection,
        chemistry of, 634–635
  HSA,
    in blood volume measurements, 617, 620
    chemistry of, 617
    versus Iodine-131 HSA, 620
    See also Radioiodinated human serum
        albumin (RISA)
  iothalamate,
    dosimetry for, 512
    in glomerular filtration studies, 503,
        506
    pharmacokinetics of, 507
    precautions in using, 508–509
    pregnancy and breastfeeding and, 509
Iodine-129 (I-129), 345
Iodine-130 (I-130), 345
Iodine-131 (I-131), 343–344, 573–574
  bioassay requirements for persons
      handling, 602
  commercially available formulations of,
      601
  HSA,
    in blood volume measurements, 617,
        620
    chemistry of, 617
    I-125 HSA versus, 620
  See also Radioiodinated human serum
      albumin (RISA)
  MAA (macroaggregated albumin),
      394–395
    chemistry of, 396
  MIBG (metaiodobenzylguanidine), 370
    adverse reactions to, 377
    biodistribution of, 372–373
    chemistry of, 371–372
    clinical considerations for, 378–380
    dosage/dosimetry for, 382–385
    drug interactions with, 377–378
    excretion and metabolism of, 373–376
    mechanism of localization of, 376–377
    pharmacokinetics of, 372
    pregnancy and breastfeeding and, 377
  nuclear properties of, 601
  OIHA (ortho-iodohippurate),
    compendial requirements for, 518
    dosimetry for, 519
    in genitourinary imaging, 501
    pregnancy and breastfeeding and, 519
    in renal imaging, 516–520

PIBG (para-iodobenzylguanidine),
370–374
rose bengal, in hepatobiliary system
imaging, 472–473
in treatment of thyroid disease, 600
adverse reactions to, 601–602
chemistry of, 600–601
clinical considerations for, 603
contraindications to, 603
dosimetry for, 603–605
pediatric uses of, 602–603
pharmacokinetics of, 601
precautions in using, 601–602
Iodine-132 (I-132), 345
Iodine uptake, nonthyroidal factors
influencing, 349–350, 351
Iodipamide, 205–207
Iodism, 240
Iodoaliphonic acid, 185
Iodoxamate, 205–207
Iohexol, 9–10
Ionic contrast media. *See* Contrast media *for
specific procedures*;
Ratio-1.5 ionic contrast media;
Ionic-dimeric contrast media, 10–11
iodine concentration of, 11
osmolality of, 11
viscosity of, 11
See also Contrast media *for specific
procedures*
Ions, stannous. See Stannous ions
Iopamidol, 9–10
Iopanoic acid, 186–187
Iophendylate (Pantopaque):
chemistry of, 127
contraindications to, 130
history of, 126
laboratory test/diagnostic procedure
interactions with, 130
materials incompatible with, 130
nonionic contrast media versus, 145–146
pharmacokinetics of, 127–128
physiological effects of, 128–129
precautions with, 129
Iopydol, 243
Iopydone, 243
Iothalamate, 3–8
Iotrol, 150–151
Ioversol, 66
Ioxaglate, 10–11
Ipodate, 187
IRB. *See* Investigational Review Board
Isomerism (gamma decay), 281–282
Isoproterenol, 57–58
Isotopic dilution, 693

K

Kr-81m. *See* Krypton-81m
Krypton-81m:
chemistry of, 403–404
clinical considerations for, 412
dosage/dosimetry for, 413–414
pharmacokinetics of, 406–408
precautions in using, 409
in pulmonary ventilation imaging, 403–414

L

Laboratory test/diagnostic procedure
interactions:
with angiographic contrast media, 40, 41
with arthrographic contrast media, 226
with barium sulfate, 163
with bronchographic contrast media,
246–247
with cholangiographic contrast media, 212
with cholecystographic contrast media, 198
with hysterosalpingographic contrast
media, 232
with iodinated gastrointestinal contrast
media, 166
with lymphographic contrast media, 240
with myelographic contrast media, 130
with radiopharmaceuticals for venous
thrombosis detection, 634–635
Lactation. *See* Breastfeeding
Lasix (furosemide), 514–515
Left ventriculography, angiographic contrast
media and, 37–39
Leukocyte count, in inflammatory process
imaging, 586
Leukocyte separation and collection, in
inflammatory process imaging, 583
Leukocytes, Indium-111 labeled, 580–591
Licenses, medical, for use of radioactive
materials, 298–299
Lipid emulsions, in ultrasound:
chemistry of, 686
history of, 685
Lipiodol:
as angiographic contrast medium, 2–3
as arthrographic contrast medium, 222
as bronchographic contrast medium, 242
as hysterosalpingographic contrast
medium, 228
as lymphographic contrast medium, 236
as myelographic contrast medium, 126
Lipiodol-F. *See* Ethiodol; Lipiodol Ultrafluid
Lipiodol Ultrafluid (Ethiodol):
as lymphographic contrast medium,
237–238

Lipiodol Ultrafluid (Ethiodol) (*Cont.*)
  in hysterosalpingography, 228, 229
Lipophilic radiopharmaceuticals:
  cerebral perfusion and, 319–323
  clinical considerations for, 322
  dosage/dosimetry for, 322, 323
  history of, 319–320
  HM-PAO
      (hexamethyl-propyleneamineoxime),
      323–324
  pharmacokinetics of, 321–322
  radiolabeled amines and diamines,
      320–321
  Technetium-99m PAO
      (propyleneamineoxime) derivatives,
      322–323
Liver:
  computed tomography evaluation of,
      105–107
  radiopharmaceuticals for imaging of,
      462–483.
  See also Hepatobiliary system imaging;
      Reticuloendothelial system imaging
Lung imaging, radiopharmaceuticals for:
  in regional pulmonary perfusion imaging,
      chemistry of, 395–397
    clinical considerations for, 399–402
    contraindications to, 399–402
    history of, 394–395
    pharmacokinetics of, 397
    precautions in using, 397–399
  in ventilation imaging, 402
    chemistry of, 403–406
    history of, 403
    pharmacokinetics of, 406–408
    precautions in using, 408–415
    radioaerosols and radioactive gases,
        402–415
Lymphographic contrast media, 236
  chemistry of, 237–238
  clinical considerations for, 241–242
  complications associated with, 240–241
  dosage for, 242
  history of, 236–237
  laboratory test/diagnostic procedure
      interactions with, 240
  pharmacokinetics of, 238–240
  physiological effects of,
      in lymph nodes, 239
      pulmonary, 239–240
      systemic embolization, 240
  precautions in using, 240–241
Lymphography, 236
  complications associated with, 240–241
  contraindications to, 241

  contrast media for, 236–242
  indications for, 241
  lungs and, 239–240
  lymph nodes and, 239
  lymph vessel identification in, 241
  patient preparation for, 241
  precautions with, 240–241

M

MAA. *See* Macroaggregated albumin
Macroaggregated albumin (MAA), 394–395,
      396–397
  compendial requirements for, 398
  See also Indium-113 MAA; Iodine-131
      MAA; Technetium-99m MAA
Magnetic resonance imaging (MRI):
  conventional brain imaging studies versus,
      305
  enhancement agents for,
      basis for developing, 663
      chemistry of, 650–659
      clinical applications of, 662–679
      fundamentals of, 645–648
      historical perspective on, 678–679
      history of, 648–650
      metal chelates, 650
      metal complexes, 654–655
      overview of requirements for, 650–654
      paramagnetic, 655–659, 671–677
      superparamagnetic, 677–678
  MR signal intensity in,
      determinants of, 664–665
      pharmaceutical manipulation of,
          666–671
  post-myelography computed tomography
      indications and, 115–116
Magnetopharmaceuticals. *See* Magnetic
      resonance imaging; Ultrasound
      imaging
Malignant effusion, radiopharmaceuticals for,
      609–610
  adverse reactions to, 611
  chemistry of, 610
  clinical considerations for, 611–612
  contraindications to, 611
  dosimetry for, 612–613
      in intraarticular therapy, 613
      in treatment of cystic brain tumor,
          613
      in treatment of intraperitoneal effusions,
          613
      in treatment of intrapleural effusions,
          613
  history of, 610

P-32 chromic phosphate, 610–613
  pharmacokinetics of, 610–611
  precautions in using, 611
Medical licenses for use of radioactive
    materials, 298–299
Medicine, nuclear. *See* Radiopharmaceuticals
Megabecqueral (MBq), 282
Metabolic heart agents. *See* Myocardial
    metabolism imaging
Metal chelates, in magnetic resonance
    imaging, 650
Metal complexes, in magnetic resonance
    imaging, 654–655
Metastatic bone pain. *See* Bone pain
Methiamazole:
  dosage for, 700–701
  pharmacology of, 700
  precautions in using, 700
  side effects of, 700
Methiodal sodium, 131
Methylaxanthines, 271
Metoclopramide, 182
Metrizamide, 9
Metrizoate, 3–8
Microbubbles, in ultrasound:
  chemistry of, 683–684
  clinical considerations for, 684–685
  history of, 683
Microcurie (μCl), 282
Millicurie (mCi), 282
Mo-99/Tc-99m radionuclide generator,
    284–285
Mobilizing agent, 693
MultiMediator release, radiographic contrast
    media and, 256–258
Myelographic contrast media, 125
  drug interactions with, 142–144
  formulation considerations in using, 142
  iophendylate (Pantopaque),
    chemistry of, 127
    contraindications to, 130
    history of, 126
    laboratory test/diagnostic procedure
      interactions with, 130
    nonionic contrast media versus, 145–146
    pharmacokinetics of, 127–128
    materials incompatible with, 130
    physiological effects of, 128–129
    precautions in using, 129–130
  iothalamate meglumine, 131–132
  materials incompatible with, 142
  for negative contrast myelography,
    125–126
  nonionic,
    clinical considerations in using, 144–148

development of, 130–132
    dosage for, 148–150
    iophendylate versus, 145–146
    iotrol, 150–151
    laboratory test/diagnostic procedure
      interactions with, 144
    pharmacokinetics of, 134–138
    physiological effects of, 138–142
    precautions in using, 142–144
  for positive contrast myelography, 126–151
Myelography:
  contrast media for, 125–151
  indications for, 144–145
  computed tomography and, 145
  contraindications to, 148
  negative contrast, 125–126
  patient care following, 147–148
  patient preparation for, 146–147
  positive contrast, 126–151
  procedure-induced reactions to, 139
Myocardial infarction imaging,
      radiopharmaceuticals for:
  Indium-111 antimyosin, 426
    chemistry of, 426–427
    dosimetry for, 428–429
    method for, 428–429
    pharmacokinetics of, 427–428
    precautions in using, 428
  selected and evaluated, 420
  Technetium-99m pyrophosphate, 419–420
    adverse reactions to, 422
    altered biodistribution of, 423
    chemistry of, 420–421
    clinical considerations for, 423, 425–426
    dosimetry for, 423, 424
    method for, 423, 424
    pharmacokinetics of, 421–422
    precautions in using, 422–423
    pregnancy and breastfeeding and, 423
Myocardial metabolism imaging,
      radiopharmaceuticals for, 439
  glucose analogues, 439–440
    chemistry of, 440
    dosimetry for, 441–442
    precautions in using, 441
  modified fatty acids, 440–441
  positron-emitting radionuclides, 436
  Nitrogen-13, 436
  Oxygen-15, 436–437
  Rubidium-82, 437
Myocardial perfusion imaging,
      radiopharmaceuticals for:
  Technetium-99m complexes, 437–438
    BATO (substituted oxime), 438–439
  Thallium-201 thallous chloride, 429–430

Thallium-201 thallous chloride (*Cont.*)
  chemistry of, 430
  clinical considerations for, 436
  dosimetry for, 433–436
  method for, 433–436
  pharmacokinetics of, 430–432
  precautions in using, 432–433
  pregnancy and breastfeeding and, 433
  stress testing and, 435

N

Nal crystals, 287
Narcotic analgesics, hepatobiliary system
  imaging and, 479, 483
NDA. *See* New-drug application
Nephrogram opacification, urographic
  contrast media and, 89–90
Nephrotoxicity:
  angiographic contrast media and, 24–27
  cholangiographic contrast media and,
    210–211
  cholecystographic contrast media and,
    196–197
Neurolite (Technetium-99m ECD), 326
Neurotoxicity, angiographic contrast media
  and, 30–31
Neutron activation, 283
New-drug application (NDA), 299
Nicotinic acid, hepatobiliary system imaging
  and, 479
Nitrogen-13, 436
Nitroglycerine, 57–58
Non-agreement (NRC) States, 296, 297
Nonionic contrast media, 9
  iodine concentration of, 9
  osmolality of, 10
  viscosity of, 9–10
  See also Contrast media *for specific*
    procedures
Norepinephrine, 53
NP-59, 361
  adverse reactions to, 363
NRC. See Nuclear Regulatory Commission
Nuclear magnetic resonance. *See* Magnetic
  resonance imaging
Nuclear reactors:
  fission products and, 283–284
  neutron activation and, 283
Nuclear Regulatory Commission (NRC),
  296–299, 408
  reporting misadministration of
    radiopharmaceuticals to, 300–301

O

Oxygen-15, 436–437

P

P-32 chromic phosphate:
  in diagnosing choroidal melanoma,
    dosimetry for, 609
  dosimetry for, 612–613
  in treatment of malignant effusion, 609
    adverse reactions to, 611
    chemistry of, 610
    clinical considerations for, 611–612
    contraindications to, 612
    dosimetry for, 612–613
    pharmacokinetics of, 610–611
    precautions in using, 611
  reported therapeutic applications of, 610
P-32 sodium phosphate:
  nuclear properties of, 606
  reported therapeutic applications of, 605
  in treatment of bone pain,
    adverse reactions to, 607–608
    clinical considerations for, 608
    dosimetry for, 609
  in treatment of polycythemia vera,
    adverse reactions to, 607
    chemistry of, 606
    clinical considerations for, 608
    contraindications to, 608
    dosimetry for, 609
    history of, 605–606
    pharmacokinetics of, 606
    precautions in using, 606–607
    pregnancy and breastfeeding and, 608
Pantopaque. *See* lophendylate
Papaverine, 57–58
Paramagnetic contrast agents, in magnetic
  resonance imaging, 655–659, 671–677
Parathyroid imaging, 436
Parathyroid scintigraphy,
  radiopharmaceuticals for, 359–360
Pelvic inflammatory disease, following
  hysterosalpingography, 233
Penicillamine:
  contraindications to, 701
  dosage for, 701
  drug interactions with, 701
  pharmacology of, 701
  precautions in using, 701
  side effects of, 701
Pentetate products
  commercially available, 309
  formulation information on, 309

Percutaneous transhepatic cholangiography
(PTC), 214–216
Perfluoroctylbromide, 120–122
Peripheral artery, angiographic contrast
media and, 38
Pharmacoangiography, 48–58
Phenobarbital, 483
Phentolamine:
in gastrointestinal radiology, 182
in pharmacoangiography, 55
Phosphate salts:
contraindications to, 702
dosage for, 702–703
drug interactions with, 702
pharmacology of, 701
precautions in using, 702
side effects of, 701–702
Photomultiplier tube (PMT), 287
Physical half-line, and dosimetry, 292
Physicochemical states:
dosimetry and, 292–293
mechanisms of localization for
radiopharmaceuticals and, 293
Plasma iodine concentration, factors
affecting, 80–81
Plasma kinetics, of urographic contrast
media, 79–81
Plasma volume, blood volume measurements
and, 620
Platelet aggregation, angiographic contrast
media and, 17–18
Platelets, Indium-111 labeled, 636–637
Pneumoarthrography, 221
Polycythemia vera, therapeutic
radiopharmaceuticals for:
adverse reactions to, 607
chemistry of, 606
clinical considerations for, 608
contraindications to, 608–609
dosimetry for, 609
history of, 605–606
P-32 sodium phosphate, 605–609
pharmacokinetics of, 606
precautions in using, 606–608
pregnancy and breastfeeding and, 608
Poppy-seed oil, water-insoluble iodized. *See*
Lipiodol
Positron-emitting radionuclides:
Nitrogen-13, 436
Oxygen-15, 436–437
Rubidium-82, 437
Positron-emitting tomography (PET), 436–437
Potassium iodide:
contraindications to, 703

dosage for, 703
drug interactions with, 703
pharmacology of, 703
precautions in using, 703
side effects of, 703
Potassium salts:
contraindications to, 704
dosage for, 704–705
drug interactions with, 704
pharmacology of, 703–704
precautions in using, 704
side effects of, 704
Pregnancy:
adrenocortical imaging and, 363
angiographic contrast media and, 41, 43
bone marrow imaging and, 556
central nervous system imaging and, 312
hepatobiliary system imaging and, 479
hysterosalpingographic contrast media and,
234–235
Iodine-125 fibrinogen and, 635
myocardial infarction imaging and, 423
pulmonary perfusion imaging and, 398–399
pulmonary ventilation imaging and, 409
radioactive materials and, 294–295
radioferrokinetic studies and, 630
radiopharmaceuticals excreted by
glomerular filtration and, 509–511
renal imaging and, 519, 524
reticuloendothelial imaging and, 468
skeletal imaging and, 549
thyroid imaging and, 350
treatment of polycythemia vera and, 608
tumor imaging and, 568
venous thrombosis detection and, 635
Pretesting, for reactions to contrast media,
266–267
Pretreatment, for reactions to contrast
media, 267–269
Priodax, 186
Propyliodone, as bronchographic contrast
medium, 244
Propylthiouracil:
dosage for, 705
pharmacology of, 705
precautions in using, 705
side effects of, 705
Prostaglandins, 56–57
Proton bombardment, 284
Proximal tubule, urographic contrast media
and, 84–87
Pseudo-allergic reactions to contrast media,
254–255
with angiography, 13

Pseudo-allergic reactions to
contrast media (*Cont.*)
with bronchography, 246
with hysterosalpingography, 232
with lymphography, 240
Psycho-organic syndromes, with
myelography, 141–142
Pulmonary effects:
of angiographic contrast media, 21–24
of bronchographic contrast media, 245–246
of lymphography, 239
Pulmonary perfusion imaging:
contraindications to, 401
indications for, 399–401
Pulmonary perfusion imaging,
radiopharmaceuticals for:
adverse reactions to, 398
chemistry of,
human albumin microspheres (HAM),
395–396
macroaggregated albumin (MAA),
396–397
clinical considerations for, 399–401
contraindications to, 401
dosage/dosimetry for, 401–402
history of, 394–395
pediatric uses of, 399
pharmacokinetics of, 397
precautions in using, 397–401
pregnancy and breastfeeding and, 398–399
toxicity associated with, 399
Pulmonary vasculature, 398
Pulmonary ventilation imaging:
indications for, 409–410
radiopharmaceutical considerations,
410–413
Pulmonary ventilation imaging,
radiopharmaceuticals for, 402
adverse reactions to, 409
clinical considerations for, 409–413
history of, 403
chemistry of, 403
radioaerosols, 404–406
radiogases, 403–404
dosage/dosimetry for, 413–415
pharmacokinetics of,
radioaerosols, 408
radiogases, 406–408
precautions in using, 408–409
radioaerosols and radioactives gases,
402–415
Pyelographic opacification:
factors affecting, 91
urographic contrast media and, 90–93

R

Rad (radiation absorbed dose), 290
Radiation, types of:
alpha, 280
beta, 280
characteristic x-rays, 281
dosimetry and, 291
gamma rays, 281
Radiation absorbed dose (rad), 290
Radiation detection, principles of, 286–289
Radiation dosimetry, 289–291
age and size of patient and, 293–294
amount of radioactivity administered and,
291–292
factors affecting, 291–296
physical half-life and, 292
physicochemical states and, 292–293
pregnancy and breast feeding and, 294–295
presence of disease and, 294
radiopharmaceutical elimination and, 293
types of radiation and, 291
Radiation dosimetry units:
rad (radiation absorbed dose), 290
rem (roentgen equivalent man), 290–291
roentgen, 290
Radiation Safety Committee, 298
Radioactive decay, types of:
alpha decay, 281
B+ (positron) decay, 281
beta minus, 281
electron capture, 282
gamma decay (isomerism), 281–282
Radioactive Drug Research Committee
(RDRC), 300
Radioactive gases, 402–403
adverse reactions to, 409
altered biodistribution of, 409
chemistry of, 403–404
clinical considerations for, 409–413
dosage/dosimetry for, 413–414
history of, 403
pharmacokinetics of, 406–407
physical and nuclear properties of, 403
precautions in using, 408–409
pregnancy and breastfeeding and, 409
See also Krypton; Xenon
Radioactive materials, medical licenses for
use of, 298–299
Radioactivity:
dosimetry and, 292–291
early uses of, 278–279
principles of, 279–282
production of, 282–286
units of, 282, 688

Radioaerosols, 402–403
  chemistry of, 403, 404–407
  clinical considerations for, 412–413
  dosage/dosimetry for, 414
  history of, 403
  pharmacokinetics of, 408
  physical and nuclear properties of, 403
  precautions in using, 409
  See also Technetium-99m pentetate
    (DTPA)
Radiochemistry:
  general, 572–573
  radioiodines, 573–574
  radiometals, 574–575
Radiocontamination, internal. *See* Internal
    radiocontamination
Radioferrokinetic studies,
    radiopharmaceuticals for, 629
  chemistry of, 629
  clinical considerations for,
    erythrocyte iron incorporation, 631
    organ kinetics, 631–632
    plasma iron clearance, 631
    summary of, 632
    systemic kinetics/biodistribution, 631
  dosage/dosimetry for,
    gastrointestinal absorption, 633
    systemic kinetics/biodistribution,
      632–633
  ferrous (Fe-59) citrate, 629–633
  pharmacokinetics of,
    gastrointestinal absorption, 629
    systemic kinetics/biodistribution,
      629–630
  precautions in using, 630
  pregnancy and breastfeeding and, 630
Radioiodinated human serum albumin
    (RISA):
  in blood volume measurements, 618–621
  dosage/dosimetry for, 620–621
  pharmacokinetics of, 618
  precautions in using, 619
  radiopharmaceutical considerations and,
    620
  See also Iodine-125 HSA and Iodine-131
    HSA
Radioiodinated OIHA
    (ortho-iodohippurate):
  adverse reactions to, 519
  chemistry of, 515–518
  clinical considerations for, 519–520
  compendial requirements for, 518
  dosimetry for, 519
  history of, 515

  pharmacokinetics of, 518
  precautions in using, 518–519
  pregnancy and breastfeeding and, 519
  product selection for, 517
  in renal imaging, 515–520
  stability of, 518
  storage/preparation of, 519
Radioiodines, 343–346, 573–574
  pharmacokinetics of, 348–349
  prevention of thyroid uptake of, 689
  See also Iodine
Radioisotopes:
  of iodine, 285. *See also* Iodine-123,
    Iodine-125, Iodine-131
  of Xenon, 406–407. *See also*
    Xenon-127; Xenon-133
Radiolabeled amines, 320–321
Radiolabeled antibodies, in tumor imaging,
    570
  clinical considerations for, 578
  dosimetry for, 578–579
  history of, 570–571
  immunochemistry of, 571–572
  pharmacokinetics of, 575–577
  precautions in using, 577–578
  radiochemistry of, 572–575
Radiolabeled complexes of soluble chelates,
    502–515
Radiolabeled diamines, 320–321
Radiolabeled leukocytes, 580–591
Radiolabeled platelets, 636–637
Radiolabeled red blood cells, 444–445,
    448–449
Radiolabeled Vitamin B_{12}:
  adverse reactions to, 626
  chemistry of, 622–623
  clinical considerations for, 626–628
  commercially available products
    containing, 623
  dosage/dosimetry for, 628
  drug interactions with, 624–625
  history of, 622
  laboratory test/diagnostic procedure
    interactions with, 625
  pharmacokinetics of,
    distribution, 623–624
    elimination, 624
    gastrointestinal absorption, 623
  precautions in using, 624–626
  principal emission data for, 622
  See also Schilling test
Radiometals, 574–575
Radionuclide cystography,
    radiopharmaceuticals for, 529–530

Radionuclide generators, 284
Radionuclide venography, 637–639
Radionuclide ventriculography, 442–444
  modified in vivo method of, 446–448
  removal of extracellular stannous ions in,
    445–446
  Technetium-99m radiolabeling of red
    blood cells in, 444–445
  treatment of red blood cells with
    stannous ion in, 444–445
Radionuclide ventriculography,
    pharmaceuticals for, 442–444
  chemistry of, 444–448
    Technetium-99m HSA, 444
    Technetium radiolabeled red blood cells,
      444–445
  dosimetry for, 450
  drug interactions with, 449–450
  for first-pass imaging and equilibrium
    gated blood pool imaging, 442–450
  modified in vivo method and, 446–448
  pharmacokinetics of, 448–449
    Technetium-99m HSA, 448
    Technetium radiolabeled red blood cells,
      448
  precautions in using, 449–450
    Technetium-99m HSA, 449
    Technetium radiolabeled red blood cells,
      449
Radionuclides:
  man-made, 283
  occuring in nature, 282–283
  medical use of, 282
  positron-emitting. See Positron-emitting
    radionuclides
Radiopharmaceuticals:
  for adrenocortical imaging, 360–368
  for adrenomedullary imaging, 368–386
  adverse reactions to, 295–296
    in adrenocortical imaging, 363
    in adrenomedullary imaging, 377
    in cardiac imaging, 422
    in cerebrospinal fluid imaging, 331–332
    in conventional brain imaging, 312
    in glomerular filtration studies, 511, 512
    in hepatobiliary system imaging, 479
    in cerebral function studies, 325
    in myocardial infarction imaging, 422
    in pulmonary perfusion imaging, 398
    in pulmonary ventilation imaging, 409
    in renal imaging, 519, 524–525
    in Schilling test, 624–625
    in treatent of malignant effusion, 611
    in treatment of polycythemia vera,
      607–608

    in treatment of thyroid disease, 601–603
    in tumor imaging, 567–568
  blood-brain barrier and, 304–334
  for blood volume measurements, 616
    chemistry of, 616–618
    clinical considerations for, 619–620
    dosimetry for, 620–621
    pharmacokinetics of, 618–619
  for bone marrow imaging,
    chemistry of, 555
    clinical considerations for, 557
    dosimetry for, 557
    history of, 552–555
    pharmacokinetics of, 555–556
    precautions in using, 556–557
    pregnancy and breastfeeding and use of,
      556
    storage data for, 556–557
    Technetium 99m albumin colloid, 555
    Technetium 99m sulfur colloid, 555
  for brain imaging (conventional), 305
    chemistry of, 308–310
    clinical considerations for, 312–313
    dosage/dosimetry for, 313–315
    drug interactions with, 312
    history of, 305–308
    pharmacokinetics of, 310–311
    precautions in using, 312
  brain receptor-specific, 326–327
  for cardiac imaging, 419
    in myocardial infarction studies, 419–429
    in myocardial metabolism studies,
      439–442
    in myocardial perfusion studies, 429–439
    in ventricular function studies, 442–450
  carrier-free versus no-carrier-added, 283
  for central nervous system imaging,
    304–334
  for cerebral function measurement,
    315–316
    carrier-mediated transport of, 316–319
    cerebral perfusion of, 319–323
    HM-PAO
      (hexamethyl-propyleneamineoxime),
      323–326
  for cerebrospinal fluid imaging, 329
    clinical considerations for, 332
    dosage/dosimetry for, 332–334
    history of, 329–330
    precautions in using, 331–332
    Ytterbium-169, 330–331
    Indium-111 pentetate (DTPA), 330–331
  development of, 278–279
  differentiated from traditional
    pharmaceuticals, 279

drug interactions with,
  in adrenocortical imaging, 363–362
  in adrenomedullary imaging, 377–378
  in hepatobiliary system imaging, 479
  in radioferrokinetic studies, 630
  in radionuclide ventriculography,
    449–450
  in reticuloendothelial system imaging,
    467–468
  in Schilling test, 624–625
  in thyroid imaging, 349–350
  in venous thrombosis detection, 634–635
for endocrine imaging, 343–386
for evaluating space-occupying diseases,
  521–526. *See also* Renal
  cortical imaging
excreted by glomerular filtration,
  adverse reactions to, 511, 512
  chemistry of, 506–507
  clinical considerations for, 513
  determination of glomerular filtration
    rate and, 502–504
  dosimetry for, 512–513
  history of, 502–506
  Iodine-125 iothalamate, 506, 512
  pharmacokinetics of, 507
  pharmacologic intervention and,
    514–516
  precautions in using, 509–511
  pregnancy and breastfeeding and,
    509–511
  radiolabeled complexes of soluble
    chelates, 502–515
  renal filtration imaging and, 504–506
  storage/preparation of, 511
  Technetium-99m gluceptate, 510–511,
    513
  Technetium-99m pentetate, 509–510,
    512–513
fundamentals of, 278–301
for hematological applications,
  in blood volume measurements, 616–621
  in radioferrokinetic studies, 629–633
  in Schilling test and, 621–628
  in venous thrombosis detection, 633–639
for hepatobiliary system imaging, 471–472
  adverse reactions to, 479
  chemistry of, 473–475
  clinical considerations for, 481–483
  dosimetry for, 479–481
  drug interactions with, 479
  history of, 472–473
  method for, 479–481
  pharmacokinetics of, 475–478
  precautions in using, 478–479

  pregnancy and breastfeeding and, 479
for inflammatory process imaging,
  chemistry of, 579, 582–584
  clinical considerations for, 580, 587–590
  dosimetry for, 580, 590–591
  Gallium-67 citrate, 579–580
  history of, 579, 580–582
  Indium-111 labeled leukocytes, 580–591
  pharmacokinetics of, 579–580, 584–585
  precautions in using, 585–587
laboratory test/diagnostic procedure
    interactions with,
  in Schilling test, 625
  in venous thrombosis detection, 634–635
lipophilic,
  history of, 319–320
  clinical considerations in using, 322
  dosage/dosimetry for, 322, 323
  HM-PAO
    (hexamethyl-propyleneamineoxime),
    323–324
  pharmacokinetics of, 321–322
  radiolabeled amines and diamines,
    320–321
  Technetium-99m PAO
    (propyleneamineoxime), 322–323
for lung imaging, 394
  in regional pulmonary perfusion
    imaging, 394–402
  in ventilation imaging, 402–415
for malignant effusion, treatment of,
  609–610
  adverse reactions to, 611
  chemistry of, 610
  clinical considerations for, 611–612
  contraindications to, 611–612
  history of, 610
  P-32 chromic phosphate, 610–613
  pharmacokinetics of, 610–611
  precautions in using, 611
misadministration of, 300–301
for myocardial metabolism imaging, 439
  chemistry of, 440
  dosimetry for, 441–442
  glucose analogues, 439–440
  modified fatty acids, 440–441
  precautions in using, 441
for parathyroid scintigraphy, 359–360
for polycythemia vera, treatment of,
  adverse reactions to, 607–608
  chemistry of, 606
  clinical considerations for, 608
  contradictions to, 608
  dosimetry for, 609
  history of, 605–606

Radiopharmaceuticals (*Cont.*)
  P-32 sodium phosphate, 605–609
    pharmacokinetics of, 606
    precautions in using, 606–608
    pregnancy and breastfeeding and, 608
  for radioferrokinetic studies, 629
    chemistry of, 629
    clinical considerations for, 631–632
    dosage/dosimetry for, 632–633
    pharmacokinetics of, 629–630
    precautions in using, 630
  for radionuclide cystography, 529–530
  for radionuclide ventriculography, 442–444
    chemistry of, 444–448
    dosimetry for, 50
    drug interactions with, 449–450
    for first-pass imaging and equilibrium
      gated blood pool imaging, 442–452
    pharmacokinetics of, 448–449
    precautions in using, 449–450
  receptor-specific, 326–329
  regulatory considerations involving use of,
    296–301
  for renal cortical imaging,
    adverse reactions to, 524–525
    altered distribution of, 510
    chemistry of, 521–522
    dosimetry for, 525
    history of, 521
    pediatric uses of, 524
    pharmacokinetics of, 522–524
    poor quality images with, 510
    precautions in using, 524–525
    pregnancy and breastfeeding and, 524
  for reticuloendothelial system imaging, 462
    adverse reactions to, 467
    chemistry of, 464–465
    clinical considerations for, 469–471
    drug interactions with, 467–468
    dosimetry for, 468–469
    history of, 462–464
    method for, 468–469
    pharmacokinetics of, 465–466
    precautions in using, 467–468
    toxicity associated with, 467
  for Schilling test, 621–622
    chemistry of, 622–623
    clinical considerations for, 626–628
    dosimetry for, 628
    history of, 622
    pharmacokinetics of, 623–624
    precautions in using, 624–626
  for skeletal imaging, 537
    altered biodistributions of, 549
    chemistry of, 538–546

    clinical considerations for, 549–550
    dosimetry for, 549, 550
    history of, 537–538
    pharmacokinetics of, 546–547
    precautions in using, 547–549
    pregnancy and breastfeeding and, 549
  for testicular imaging, 526–527
    method for, 527–528
    pharmaceokinetics of, 529
  for thyroid disease, treatment of,
    adverse reactions to, 601–603
    chemistry of, 600–601
    clinical considerations for, 603
    contraindications to, 603
    dosimetry for, 603–605
    history of, 600
    Iodine-125, 600, 602
    Iodine-131, 600–605
    pediatric uses of, 602–603
    pharmacokinetics of, 601
    precautions in using, 601
  for thyroid imaging, 343–359
  for tumor imaging—Gallium-67 citrate,
    adverse reactions to, 568
    altered biodistribution of, 567–568
    chemistry of, 565–566
    clinical considerations for, 569
    dosimetry for, 569–570
    history of, 564–565
    pharmacokinetics of, 566–567
    precautions in using, 567–568
    pregnancy and breastfeeding and use of,
      568
  for tumor imaging—radiolabeled
    antibodies,
    clinical considerations for, 578
    dosimetry for, 578–571
    history of, 570–571
    immunochemistry of, 571–572
    pharmacokinetics of, 575–577
    precautions in using, 577–578
    radiochemistry of, 572–573
    route of administration for, 578
  for venous thrombosis detection, 633–634
    chemistry of, 634
    clinical considerations for, 635
    dosage/dosimetry for, 635–636
    drug interactions with, 634–635
    Iodine-125 fibrinogen, 634
    Indium-111 radiolabeled platelets,
      636–637
    pharmacokinetics of, 634
    precautions in using, 634–635
    pregnancy and breastfeeding and, 635
    radionuclide venography, 637–639

therapeutic, 599–600
  for malignant effusion, 609–613
  for polycythemia vera, 605–609
  for thyroid disease, 600–605
  tubular secretion of, 515–520. *See also*
    Radioiodinated OIHA
Ratio-3 nonionic contrast media. *See* Ratio-3
  low osmolality contrast media
Ratio-1.5 ionic contrast media, 3–4
  adverse reactions to, 260–262, 265–266
  chemical structures of, 4
  considerations for, 43, 45
  iodine concentration of, 5, 10
  osmolality of, 7–8, 10
  product selection for, 43, 45
  viscosity of, 5–7, 10
  See also Contrast media *for specific*
    procedures
Ratio-3 low-osmolality contrast media, 8–9
  adverse reactions to, 261–262
  considerations for, 45–46
  iodine concentration of, 9
  osmolality of, 10
  risk factors and recommendations for,
    58–61
  viscosity of, 9–10
  See also Contrast media *for specific*
    procedures
RDRC. *See* Radioactive Drug Research
  Committee
Re-186. *See* Rhenium-186
Reactions to contrast media. *See* Contrast
  media, adverse reactions to
Reactions to radiopharmaceuticals. *See*
  Radiopharmaceuticals, adverse
  reactions to
Receptor-specific radiopharmaceuticals,
  326–329
  history of, 327
Red blood cells,
  angiographic contrast media and, 16–17
  blood volume measurements and, 619–
    621
  Chromium-51 labeled. *See* Chromium-51
    labeled red blood cells
  survival/sequestration of, 620, 621
  Technetium-99m radiolabeled. *See*
    Tc-99m radiolabeled red blood cells
  treatment of, with stannous ions, in
    radionuclide ventriculography,
    444–445
Rem (roentgen equivalent man), 290–291
Renal arteriography, effects of contrast
  media in, 24–27
Renal computed tomography, 109

Renal considerations, in angiographic
  procedures, 58–59
Renal cortical agents, for evaluation of
  space-occupying diseases. *See*
  Renal cortical imaging,
    radiopharmaceuticals for,
Renal cortical imaging, radiopharmaceuticals
  for,
  adverse reactions to, 524–525
  altered distribution of, 510
  chemistry of,
    Technetium-99m gluceptate, 521–522
    Technetium-99m succimer, 522
  clinical considerations for, 525–526
  dosimetry for,
    Technetium-99m gluceptate, 525
    Technetium-99m succimer, 525
  history of, 521
  pediatric uses of, 524
  pharmacokinetics of,
    Technetium-99m gluceptate, 522–523
    Technetium-99m succimer, 523–524
  precautions in using, 524–525
  poor quality images with, 510
  pregnancy and breastfeeding and, 524
Renal effects:
  of angiographic contrast media, 24–27,
    48
  of cholangiographic contrast media,
    210–211
  cholecystographic contrast media, 196–197
Renal excretion:
  cholangiographic contrast media and,
    209–210
  cholecystographic contrast media and, 195
Renal filtration imaging, 504–506
Renal imaging:
  altered distribution of pharmaceuticals for,
    510
  poor quality images with
    radiopharmaceuticals for, 510
  radiopharmaceuticals for, 502. *See also*
    Genitourinary imaging
Renovue, 88
Resolution, in medical imaging, 289
Respiration, angiographic contrast media
  and, 22–23, 28–29
Reticuloendothelial cells, 462
Reticuloendothelial contrast media, 119
  in computed tomography, 119–120
  EOE-13, 120
  perfluoroctylbromide, 120–122
  thoratrast, 119–120
Reticuloendothelial system imaging,
  radiopharmaceuticals for, 462

Reticuloendothelial system imaging,
    radiopharmaceuticals for (*Cont.*)
  chemistry of,
    Technetium-99m albumin colloid,
      464–465
    Techntium-99m sulfur colloid, 464
  clinical considerations for, 469–471
  drug interactions with,
    aluminum hydroxide-containing antacids
      and, 468
    androgen therapy and, 468
    anesthetic agents and, 468
    cancer chemotherapeutic agents and,
      467–468
  dosimetry for, 468–469
  history of, 462–464
  method for, 468–469
  packaging/storage data for, 468
  pharmacokinetics of, 465–467
  precautions in using, 467–468
  pregnancy and breastfeeding and, 468
  toxicity associated with, 467
  See also Hepatobiliary system imaging;
    Spleen-specific imaging
Rhenium-186, 574
RISA. *See* Radioiodinated human serum
    albumin
Roentgen (R), 290
Roentgen equivalent man (rem), 290–291
Rubidium-82, 437

S

Scanners, scintillation, 287, 289
Schilling test, 621–622
  chemistry of, 622–623
  clinical considerations for, 626–628
  contraindications to, 628
  dosage/dosimetry for, 628
  dual-isotope, advantages and
    disadvantages of, 627
  history of, 622
  indications for, 626
  limitations of, 627–62
  patient preparation for, 626
  pharmacokinetics of,
    distribution, 623–624
    elimination, 624
    gastrointestinal absorption, 623
  precautions with, 624–626
  radiopharmaceutical considerations with,
    627
  single-isotope, 627
Scintillation detector, 286–289
Scintillation scanners, 287, 289
Scintiphotos, 279, 280, 287, 289

Selenium-75 selenomethionine, 346, 359
Selenomethionine, 346
Similarity, in medical imaging, 28
Sequestering agents, 11–12
Serotonin release, radiographic contrast
    media and, 255
Sex, and adverse reactions to contrast media,
    265
Sickle cell disease, angiographic contrast
    media effects and, 17
Sievert (Sv), 290
Sinografin, in hysterosalpingography, 228
Size of patient, radiation dosimetry and,
    293–294
Skeletal imaging, radiopharmaceuticals for,
    537
  altered biodistributions of, 549
  chemistry of, 538–540
    diphosphonates, 540–541
    mechanism of localization, 542–546
    stability/storage of, 541–542
  clinical considerations for, 549–550
  dosimetry for, 549–550
  history of, 537–538
  pregnancy and breastfeeding and use of,
    549
Small bowel examinations:
  contrast media for, 172–176
  enteroclysis, 179
Society of Nuclear Medicine (SNM), 295
  Adverse Reactions Registry of, 296
Sodium bicarbonate:
  contraindications to, 706
  dosage for, 706
  drug interactions with, 706
  pharmacology of, 705–706
  precautions in using, 706
  side effects of, 706
Sodium chromate, *See* Chromium-51
Sodium phosphate P-32. *See* P-32 sodium
    phosphate
Space-occupying diseases,
    radiopharmaceuticals for evaluation
    of, 521–526. See also Renal cortical
    agents Spectrometer, 287
Spinal canal:
  computed tomography examinations of,
    114–116
  myelographic contrast media and,
    139–140
Spleen imaging. *See* Hepatobiliary system
    imaging; Reticuloendothelial
    system imaging; Spleen-specific imaging
Spleen-specific imaging,
    radiopharmaceuticals for, 483–484

clinical considerations for, 485
dosimetry for, 485
method for heat denaturation and,
484–485
Stannous ions:
removal of extracellular, in radionuclide
ventriculography, 445–446
treatment of red blood cells with, in
radionuclide ventriculography,
444–445
Static (delayed) brain images, 314–315
Stomach, examination of, 179
Stress testing, myocardial perfusion imaging
and, 435
Subarachnoid absorption of myelographic
contrast media, 134–138
Subarachnoid puncture, in myelography,
148–149
Superparamagnetic contrast agents, 677–678
Syringes, rubber, angiographic contrast
media and, 39, 41
Systemic radiocontamination, nonspecific
theraphy for, 692

R

TAA. *See* Tumor-associated antigens
Target tissues, 279
Tc-99m, *See* Technetium-99m
Technetium-99m, 574–575
albumin colloid,
in bone marrow imaging, 555–557
in reticuloendothelial system imaging,
chemistry of, 464–465
packaging/storage data for, 468
BATO complex, 438–439
complexes of, in myocardial perfusion
imaging, 438–439
DADT (diamine dithiol), 325
diphosphonates,
currently available, 543
in skeletal imaging, 540–550
DMSA (dimercaptosuccinic acid), 347
DTPA. *See* Technetium-99m pentetate
(DTPA)
ECD (ethyl cysteinate dimer), 325–326
compared to Technetium-99m
exametazime, 326
exametazime, 323–324
adverse reactions to, 325
compared to Technetium-99m ECD, 326
dosage/dosimetry for, 325
labeling of white blood cells with, 325
precautions in using, 324–325
ferpentetate, 503

gluceptate (glucoheptonate), 310
in detection of lung tumors, 526
in glomerular filtration studies, 504–513
in myocardial infarction imaging, 526
package/storage of, 310, 311
pharmacokinetics of, 311
in renal cortical imaging, 521–526
HAM (human albumin microspheres),
adverse reactions to, 398
chemistry of, 395–396
contraindications to, 401
dosage/dosimetry for, 401–402
pediatric uses of, 399
pharmacokinetics of, 397
precautions in using, 397–398
pregnancy and breastfeeding and,
398–399
toxicity associated with, 399
HSA (human serum albumin), in
radionuclide ventriculography,
chemistry of, 444
dosimetry for, 450
drug interactions with, 449–450
pharmacokinetics of, 448
precautions in using, 449
IDA (iminodiacetic acid) complexes, in
hepatobiliary system imaging,
472–473
chemistry of, 473–475
pharmacokinetics of, 475–478
precautions in using, 478
MAA (macroaggregated albumin), 395
adverse reactions to, 398
chemistry of, 396–397
contraindications to, 401
dosage/dosimetry for, 401–402
in venous thrombosis detection, 637–639
pediatric uses of, 399
pharmacokinetics of, 397
precautions in using, 397–398
pregnancy and breastfeeding and,
398–399
toxicity associated with, 399
MAG₃ (mercaptoacetyltriglycine), 520
medronate (MDP), 296
in skeletal imaging, 542, 543, 545–546,
550, 552
mertiatide, in renal imaging, 520
oxidronate, in skeletal imaging, 542, 543,
545–546, 550, 552
PAO (propyleneamineoxime), 322–323
pentetate (DPTA), 309–310
in genitourinary imaging, 501
in glomerular filtration studies,
503–513

Technetium-99m (*Cont.*)
    Nuclear Regulatory Commission rule
      permitting use of, in pulmonary
      imaging, 298
    package/storage of, 310, 311
    pharmacokinetics of, 310–311
    in pulmonary ventilation imaging,
      403–414
   pertechnetate, 346
    pharmacokinetics of, 349
    stannous pretreated red blood cells and,
      in radionuclide ventriculography, 446
   polyphosphate, in skeletal imaging, 539–540
   pyrophosphate,
    in myocardial infarction imaging, 419–426
    in pulmonary ventilation imaging, 408
    in skeletal imaging, 539–540
   radiolabeled red blood cells,
    in radionuclide ventriculography,
      444–450
    in spleen-specific imaging, 484–485
   pertechnetate,
    in Meckel's diverticulum scintigraphy,
      485–486
    in radionuclide cystography, 530
    in skeletal imaging, 539
    in testicular imaging, 527, 529
   succimer,
    in evaluation of medullary thyroid
      carcinoma, 526
    in evaluation of soft-tissue tumors and
      lung metastases of osteosarcoma, 526
    in renal cortical imaging, 524–526
   sulfur colloid,
    in bone marrow imaging, 554–557
    in esophageal reflux studies, 486–487
    in esophageal transit studies, 487–488
    in gastric emptying studies, 490–492, 493
    packaging/storage data for, 468
    in radionuclide cystography, 530
    in reticuloendothelial system imaging,
      chemistry of, 464
TechneScan MAG3, 520
Terabecquerel (TBq), 282
Testicular imaging, radiopharmaceuticals for,
    526–527
   method for, 527–528
   pharmacokinetics of, 529
Tetrabromophenophthalein, 185, 186
Tetrachlorophenophthalein, 184
Tetracycline, 235
Tetraiodophenolphthalein, 185
Thallium atoms, 287
Thallium-201 (Tl-201) thallous chloride, 347
   in myocardial perfusion imaging, 429–430

chemistry of, 430
clinical considerations for, 436
dosimetry for, 433–436
method for, 433–436
   pharmacokinetics of, 430–432
   precautions in using, 432–433
   pregnancy and breastfeeding and, 432–433
   stress testing and, 435
noncardiac applications of, 436
in parathyroid imaging, 436
state authority over use of, 299
Therapeutic radiopharmaceuticals, 599–600
   Iodine-125, 600, 602
   Iodine-131, 600–605
   P-32 chromic phosphate, 610–613
   P-32 sodium phosphate, 605–609
   selected, clinical indications for, 599
   for treatment of malignant effusion, 609–613
   for treatment of polycythemia vera, 605–609
   for treatment of thyroid disease, 600–605
Thoratrast, 119–120
Thorium-232, 282
Thrombosis, venous. *See* Venous thrombosis
Thyroid block:
   for internal radiocontamination, 692
   prior to adrenomedullary imaging, 381
Thyroid carcinoma, therapeutic
    radiopharmaceuticals for. *See* Thyroid
    disease
Thyroid disease, therapeutic
    radiopharmaceuticals for, 600
   adverse reactions to, 601–602
   chemistry of, 600–601
   clinical considerations for, 603
   contraindications, 603
   dosimetry for,
    in treatment of hyperthyroidism, 603–604
    in treatment of thyroid carcinoma, 604–605
   history of, 600
   Iodine-125, 600, 602
   Iodine-131, 600–605
   pediatric uses of, 602–603
   pharmacokinetics of, 601
   precautions in using, 601–603
Thyroid imaging:
   adjunctive techniques in, 356–357
   indications for, 351–355
   patient preparation for, 355–356
   radiopharmaceutical considerations and,
    355
Thyroid imaging, radiopharmaceuticals for,
    343
   chemistry of,
    miscellaneous agents, 346–347
    radioiodines, 343–346

Technetium-99m pertechnetate, 346
clinical considerations for, 351–357
dosage/dosimetry for, 357–358
drug interactions with, 349–350
pharmacokinetics of,
    radioiodines, 348–349
    Technetium-99m pertechnetate, 349
pregnancy and breastfeeding and, 350–351
Thyroid scanning, fluorescent, 358–359
Thyroid uptake of radioiodine, prevention
    of, 689
Tolazoline, 53–55
Total blood volume, blood volume
    measurements and, 619–620, 621
Total parenteral nutrition (TPN) therapy,
    479
Transportation, Department of (DOT), 301
Tubular secretion, radiopharmaceuticals that
    undergo:
    radioiodinated OIHA
        (ortho-iodohippurate),
        chemistry of, 515–518
        clinical considerations for, 519–520
        dosimetry for, 519
        history of, 515
        pharmacokinetics of, 518
        precautions in using, 518–519
        stability of, 518
    Technetium-99m MAG$_3$
        (mercaptoacetyltriglycine), 520
Tubule:
    distal, urographic contrast media and,
        87–88
    proximal, urographic contrast media and,
        84–87
Tumor imaging, radiopharmaceuticals for,
    564
    Gallium-67 citrate,
        adverse reactions to, 568
        altered biodistribution of, 567–568
        chemistry of, 565–566
        clinical considerations for, 569
        dosimetry for, 569–570
        history of, 564–565
        pharmacokinetics of, 566–567
        precautions in using, 567–568
        pregnancy and breastfeeding and, 568
    radiolabeled antibodies, 570
        clinical considerations for, 578
        dosimetry for, 578–579
        history of, 570–571
        immunochemistry of, 571–572
        pharmacokinetics of, 575–577
        precautions in using, 577–578
        radiochemistry of, 572–575

route of administration of, 578
T1-201. *See* Thallium-201
Tumor-associated antigens (TAA), 571–572
    representative human, 571
Tyropanoate, 187

U

Ultrasound, enhancement agents for:
    fundamentals of, 682–686
    lipid emulsions, chemistry of, 686
        history of, 685
    microbubbles,
        chemistry of, 683–684
        clinical considerations for, 684–685
        history of, 683
United States Pharmacopeial Convention,
    295–296
Units of radioactivity, 282, 688
Uranium-235, 283
Uranium-238, 282, 283
Urographic contrast media,
    in direct urography, 95
        clinical considerations for, 95–96
        contraindications to, 96–97
        dosage for, 97
        precautions with, 96–97
    in excretory urography, 78
        chemistry of, 78
        clinical considerations for, 89–94
        dosage for, 94–95
        pharmacokinetics of, 78–88
        physiological effects of, 88–89
        precautions with, 88–89
Urography,
    direct, 95
        contraindications to, 96–97
        contrast media for, 96
        indications for, 95–96
        precautions with, 96–97
    excretory, 78–95
Uterography, 228

V

V/Q imaging. *See* Pulmonary perfusion
    imaging; Pulmonary ventilation
    imaging
Vagal reactions to contrast media, 269–270,
    272
Vascular effects, of general angiography,
    14–20
Vascular endothelial permeability,
    angiographic contrast media and,
    19–20

Vasculature, pulmonary, 398
Vasoconstrictors, 49–53
  acetylcholine, 51
  angiotensin, 52
  epinephrine, 49–52
  norepinephrine, 53
  vasopressin, 52–53
Vasodilators, 53–58
  acetylcholine, 58
  bradykinin, 56
  dipyridamole, 57–58
  dopamine, 58–59
  glucagon, 57
  isoproterenol, 57–58
  nitroglycerine, 57–58
  papaverine, 57–58
  phentolamine, 55
  prostaglandins, 56–57
  tolazoline, 53–55
Vasopressin, 52–53
Vasospasm, angiographic contrast media
    and, 48
Venous thrombosis detection, 633–634
  indications for, 635
  patient preparation for, 635
  procedure for, 635–636
  radionuclide venography for, 637–639
  study interpretation in, 635–636
Venous thrombosis detection,
    radiopharmaceuticals for:
  Iodine-125 fibrinogen,
    chemistry of, 634
    clinical considerations for, 635
    dosage/dosimetry for, 635–636
    drug interactions with, 634–635
    laboratory test/diagnostic procedure
      interactions with, 634–635
    precautions in using, 634–635
    pregnancy and breastfeeding and use of,
      635
  Indium-111 radiolabeled platelets, 636–
    637
  Technetium-99m MAA (macroaggregated
    albumin), 637–639
Ventricular fibrillation, angiographic contrast
    media and, 32–35
Ventriculography:
  left, angiographic contrast media and,
    37–39
  radionuclide. See Radionuclide
    ventriculography
Viscosity of contrast media:
  adverse reactions and, 266
  reducing, in use of angiographic contrast
    media, 46–47

Vitamin B$_{12}$ absorption, measurement of.
    See Schilling Test

W
White blood cells, radiolabeling of, 325

X
X-rays, characteristic, 281
Xenon:
  blood-flow-measurements with, 414–415
  chemistry of, 116
  clinical use of, 118–119
  in computed tomography, 116–119
  contraindications to, 118–119
  dosage for, 119
  inpulmonary ventilation imaging, 403
  pharmacokinetics of, 116–117
  physiological effects of, 117–118
  precautions with radioisotopes of, 408–409
Xenon-127 (Xe-127):
  in pulmonary ventilation imaging,
    chemistry of, 403–404
    clinical considerations for, 410–412
    dosage/dosimetry for, 413
  pharmacokinetics of, 406–407
  state authority over use of, 299
Xenon-133 (Xe-133):
  chemistry of, 403–404
  clinical considerations for, 410–412
  dosage/dosimetry for, 413

Y
Y-90. See Yttrium-90
Yb-169 pentetate. See Ytterbium-169
    pentetate
Ytterbium-169 (Yb-169) pentetate, 330–331
Yttrium-90 (Y-90), 574–575

Z
Zinc salts:
  dosage for, 706
  pharmacology of, 706
  side effects of, 706
  dosage/dosimetry for, 413
Zinc-DTPA (diethylenetriamine-pentaacetic
    acid):
  contraindications to, 700
  dosage for, 700
  pharmacology of, 699–700
  precautions in using, 700
  side effects of, 700